Mosby's
RESPIRATORY
CARE
EQUIPMENT

Mosby's

RESPIRATORY
CARE
EQUIPMENT

Tenth Edition

J.M. Cairo, PhD, RRT, FAARC

Dean of the School of Allied Health Professions
Professor of Cardiopulmonary Science, Physiology, and Anesthesiology
Louisiana State University Health Sciences Center
New Orleans, Louisiana

ELSEVIER

ELSEVIER

3251 Riverport Lane
St. Louis, Missouri 63043

MOSBY'S RESPIRATORY CARE EQUIPMENT, TENTH EDITION
ISBN: 978-0-323-41636-8

Previous editions copyrighted 2014, 2010, 2004, 1999, 1995, 1992, 1989, 1986, and 1983.

International Standard Book Number: 978-0-323-41636-8

Senior Content Strategist: Yvonne Alexopoulos
Content Development Manager: Ellen Wurm-Cutter
Content Development Specialist: Charlene Ketchum
Publishing Services Manager: Julie Eddy
Project Manager: David Stein
Design Direction: Bridget Hoette

Printed in Canada

Last digit is the print number: 9 8 7 6 5 4 3 2 1

To Rhonda

CONTRIBUTORS

Arzu Ari, PhD, RRT, PT, CPFT, FAARC
Professor
Department of Respiratory Therapy
Texas State University
San Marcos, Texas

Jim Fink, RRT, NPS, PhD, FCCP, FAARC
Chief Science Officer
Aerogen Pharma Corp.
San Mateo, California

Terry L. Forrette, MHS, RRT, FAARC
Adjunct Associate Professor
Department of Cardiopulmonary Science
LSU Health
New Orleans, Louisiana

Timothy B. Op't Holt, EdD, RRT, AE-C, FAARC
Professor of Cardiorespiratory Care
University of South Alabama
Mobile, Alabama

Amanda M. Kleiman, MD
Assistant Professor
University of Virginia
Charlottesville, Virginia

Ashley Matthews Shilling, MD
Associate Professor of Anesthesiology
University of Virginia Medical Center
Charlottesville, Virginia

EVOLVE CONTRIBUTOR

Sandra T. Hinski, MS, RRT-NPS
Faculty, Respiratory Care Division
Gateway Community College
Phoenix, Arizona

Michelle L. Abreu, MHA, RCP, RRT
Director of Clinical Education/Assistant Professor
　Respiratory Care
Sinclair College
Dayton, Ohio

Valli B. Bobo, BSRT, RRT, RCP
Director of Clinical Education, Respiratory Care
Midlands Technical College
Columbia, South Carolina

Marighny Dutton, RCP, RRT, BSRC
Simulation Lab Specialist
McLennan Community College
Waco, Texas

Sanja B. Keller, MS, RCP, RRT
Program Director/Department Chair, Respiratory Care
Sinclair College
Dayton, Ohio

Jody Lester, RRT, MA
Associate Professor
Department of Respiratory Care
Boise State University
Boise, Idaho

John A. Rutkowski, MPA, MPA, RRT, FAARC, FACHE, LRCPNJ
Program Director of Respiratory Therapy
County College of Morris
Randolph, New Jersey

EVOLVE REVIEWERS

Allen Barbaro, MS, RRT
Department Chairman, Respiratory Care Education
St. Luke's College
Sioux City, Iowa

Stephen Wehrman, RRT, RPFT, AE-C
Professor
University of Hawaii
Program Director
Kapiolani Community College
Honolulu, Hawaii

PREFACE

Publication of the tenth edition of *Mosby's Respiratory Care Equipment* represents a significant milestone in the history of this text. Numerous individuals have shared their knowledge and time to help produce a textbook that has been used by respiratory therapy students and practicing respiratory therapists since 1977. Indeed, it has been an integral part of the education of generations of respiratory therapists. Steven McPherson, RRT; Charles B. Spearman, RRT; Susan P. Pilbeam, MS, RRT, FAARC; Charles, G. Durbin, MD; and many other respiratory care educators and practicing respiratory therapists have provided valuable contributions and expertise to the evolution of this textbook and are therefore part of its "DNA."

As I stated in previous editions of this text, we have witnessed significant advances in health care delivery during the past 40 years. It is reasonable to assume that these advances are the result of a better understanding of the etiology and pathophysiology of various diseases and our ability to use technology to translate this knowledge into more effective methods to diagnose and treat patients with life-threatening illnesses. This is particularly evident to critical care clinicians who treat patients afflicted with pulmonary and cardiac disorders.

Possessing a working knowledge of the various types of equipment used to treat patients with cardiopulmonary dysfunctions can be a formidable task. Assimilation of this knowledge and the wisdom required to effectively use it require a personal dedication to the idea of lifelong learning. The goal in writing this textbook has always been to provide a resource that can serve as a guide for respiratory therapy students and clinicians who choose to embark on this educational journey.

FEATURES

The hallmark of this text has been its unique comprehensive nature. The tenth edition of *Mosby's Respiratory Care Equipment* provides an up-to-date review of the devices and techniques used by respiratory therapists. As in previous editions, I have tried to ensure that the material is presented in a concise and readable fashion. You will notice throughout the text that a number of pedagogical aids have been used to assist the reader in mastering the material that is presented including:

- Full-color printing to enhance the appearance of figures, tables, and boxes throughout the text.
- Brief subject outlines.
- Measurable learning objectives.
- Lists of relevant key terms.
- Current AARC clinical practice guidelines. (See the Clinical Practice Guidelines Boxes 6.1 to 6.3 on pp. 197-199.)
- Updated reference lists to reinforce the use of evidence-based practices.
- Bulleted "Key Points" that conclude each chapter to emphasize specific concepts presented in the chapter.

- Clinical Scenarios to present practical scenarios that are encountered by respiratory therapists. You are asked several questions at the end of each scenario. Answers appear in Appendix A in the back of the book so you can assess your responses.
- Self-Assessment Questions are included at the end of each chapter, with answers in Appendix B in the back of the book, to allow readers to test their overall comprehension of the subject matter.
- Appendix C, which contains a series of boxes that provide normal reference values for commonly encountered clinical laboratory tests, as well as physiological measurements used to assess cardiovascular and pulmonary function.
- Frequently used formulae and values, which are provided in Appendix D.
- Figures, boxes, and tables, which have been updated when necessary; every effort has been made to ensure that the photographs and illustrations are descriptive and easy to follow.

ORGANIZATION

The structure of the ninth edition has been slightly altered to more closely follow a typical progression through a respiratory therapy educational program:

- Chapter 1 includes a review of the basic physical principles that the reader will encounter in later chapters.
- Chapter 2 covers important infection control topics and includes a concise review of microbiological principles and infection control procedures that apply to respiratory care equipment. The most current recommendations from the Centers for Disease Control and Prevention are addressed to educate on how to reduce the risk of infection to patients and health care providers.
- Chapters 3 and 4 provide a detailed discussion of the devices and concepts used in medical gas therapy.
- Chapter 5 presents a clinically useful approach to airway management. It includes an extensive review of the indications, application, contraindications, and complications associated with the use of various artificial airways and the related ancillary equipment. In addition, it covers advanced cardiac life support.
- Chapter 6 describes the current concepts and equipment used in the administration of humidity and aerosol therapy.
- Chapter 7 describes lung expansion and bronchial hygiene devices, including positive airway pressure devices and chest physiotherapy equipment.
- Chapters 8 and 9 provide an overview of devices and techniques routinely used to assess patients with cardiopulmonary dysfunction. Chapter 8 discusses the devices and techniques used to measure physiological function in the pulmonary diagnostic laboratory and at the bedside.

Chapter 9 provides a description of the equipment and techniques used to perform electrocardiography and hemodynamic monitoring.

- Chapter 10 includes information about invasive and non-invasive techniques and equipment used to measure and monitor arterial blood gases.
- Chapter 11 contains a conceptual approach to the diagnosis of sleep-related disorders. This approach focuses on a discussion of the physiology of sleep, pathophysiological findings associated with sleep apnea, and behavioral and electrographic criteria used to diagnose the presence of a sleep-related disorder. Many respiratory therapy educational programs now offer certificate programs in polysomnography. This chapter is not intended to be a compendium of sleep medicine but rather an overview of the equipment and procedures commonly used in sleep laboratories. Information has been included in this chapter about titration of positive airway pressure devices used in the treatment of obstructive sleep apnea.
- Chapter 12 reviews basic technical operation and physical function of ventilator components and includes coverage of such subjects as current descriptions of the types of breath delivery and current ventilator mode classification, ventilator graphics, and high-frequency ventilators. As in previous editions of this text, we have not attempted to cover management of the patient-ventilator system, which is handled in my other textbook on mechanical ventilation.*
- Chapters 13, 14, and 15 provide a systematic review of the various ventilators that are used in clinical practice:
    - Chapter 13 reviews multipurpose ventilators that are used primarily for ICU patients.
    - Chapter 14 provides an update on mechanical ventilators used in pediatric and neonatal care and also includes the neonatal and pediatric application of the general-use ICU ventilators.
    - Chapter 15 focuses on ventilators and devices that are used in patient transport, ventilation in the home setting, and noninvasive devices.

Clinicians familiar with previous editions of *Mosby's Respiratory Care Equipment* will see that the organization of the chapter on multipurpose ventilators has been maintained as a go-to guide for general information for the most widely used ventilators. Easy-to-read tables have been included throughout the chapter to provide readers the need-to-know information on basic controls, monitoring parameters, monitoring modes, alarms, and any "special features" a ventilator

may provide. Readers will find that we did not attempt to include every commercially available ventilator, but rather we have chosen to present the devices that are currently the most commonly used in clinical practice.

LEARNING AIDS

Workbook

The *Workbook for Mosby's Respiratory Care Equipment*, ninth edition, proved to be a useful learning resource for readers of this text. We have revised this edition to be new and improved. Sandra T. Hinski, MS, RRT-NPS, a seasoned educator, revised the content to reflect the changes and updates made to the text. It is an invaluable resource for students, providing the reinforcement and practice necessary for students to succeed in their study of respiratory care. The more difficult concepts from the text are broken down through a variety of exercises such as short-answer and fill-in-the-blank questions tied to each objective, critical thinking/essay questions, and NBRC-type multiple-choice questions.

Evolve Resources http://evolve.elsevier .com/Cairo/

Evolve is an interactive learning environment designed to work in coordination with this text. Instructors may use Evolve to provide an Internet-based course component that reinforces and expands the concepts presented in class. Evolve may be used to publish the class syllabus, outlines, and lecture notes; set up "virtual office hours" and e-mail communication; share important dates and information through the online class calendar; and encourage student participation through chat rooms and discussion boards. Evolve allows instructors to post exams and manage their grade books online.

For the Instructor

For the instructor, Evolve offers valuable resources to help them prepare their courses including:
- More than 1500 questions in ExamView
- PowerPoint lecture slides for each chapter
- An image collection of the figures from the book available in PowerPoint format

For Students

For students, Evolve offers valuable resources to help them succeed in their courses including:
- NBRC Correlation Guide—showing how (and where) we provide the information needed to pass the credentialing examinations

For more information, visit **http://evolve.elsevier.com/Cairo/** or contact an Elsevier sales representative.

---

*Cairo JM: *Pilbeam's mechanical ventilation—physiological and clinical applications*, ed 6, St. Louis, 2016, Elsevier.

ACKNOWLEDGMENTS

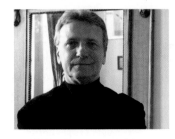

The goal of the tenth edition of *Mosby's Respiratory Care Equipment* is to continue providing a textbook that would be concise and organized in a fashion that would make it a useful reference for students, faculty, and practicing pulmonary specialists. The current edition includes contributions from a number of knowledgeable and talented colleagues. I wish to thank Amanda M. Kleiman, MD; Ashley Shilling, MD; Arzu Ari, PhD, RRT, PT, CPFT, FAARC; Jim Fink, MS, PhD, RRT, FAARC; Terry Forrette, MHS, RRT, FAARC; and Tim Op't Holt, EdD, RRT, AE-C, FAARC for their contributions. I also want to thank Kenneth Watson, MS, RRT, for his contributions in previous editions to the chapter on infant and pediatric devices, and Steven E. Sittig, RRT-NPS, C-NPT, FAARC, for his contributions to previous editions of this text on Transport, Home Care, and Noninvasive Ventilatory Devices. Stephen Wehrman, RRT, RPFT, AE-C, reviewed each question in the Test Bank for validity, structure, and format, and Allen Barbaro, MS, RRT, revised the PowerPoint lecture slides for each chapter.

I would like to acknowledge all the manufacturers and distributors who provided information about their products during the preparation of tenth edition of *Mosby's Respiratory Care Equipment*. I particularly want to thank Anthony Karle (CareFusion), Frank Caminita (Dräger Medical), Michael Champagne (Maquet), Robert Duff (GE Healthcare), and Gary S. Milne (Medtronics).

I want to express my sincere appreciation to colleagues from across the country for their insightful suggestions throughout the revision of this textbook. I especially want to thank my colleagues at LSU Health Sciences Center at New Orleans who graciously offered suggestions during this project.

The process of writing and publishing a textbook requires dedication and a significant time commitment. I have been very fortunate to work with an outstanding editorial staff at Elsevier. I want to express my sincere appreciation to Yvonne Alexopoulos, Billie Sharp, Charlene Ketchum, Julie Eddy, David Stein, and Lois Lasater for providing exceptional editorial guidance and support.

To my wife Rhonda, you are the love and joy of my life.

Jim Cairo
New Orleans, Louisiana

CONTENTS

Introduction

1

Basic Physics for the Respiratory Therapist

Physics is the most fundamental and all-inclusive of all the sciences, and has had a profound effect on all scientific development. In fact, physics is the present-day equivalent of what used to be called natural philosophy, from which most of our modern sciences arose. Students of many fields find themselves studying physics because of the basic role it plays in all phenomena.

Richard P. Feynman

Six Easy Pieces[1]

OBJECTIVES

Upon completion of this chapter, you will be able to:

1. Differentiate between kinetic and potential energy.
2. Compare the physical and chemical properties of the three primary states of matter.
3. Explain why large amounts of energy are required to accomplish the changes associated with solid-liquid and liquid-gas phase transitions.
4. Convert temperature measurements from the Kelvin, Celsius, and Fahrenheit temperature scales.
5. Define pressure and describe two devices commonly used to measure it.
6. List various pressure equivalents for 1 atmosphere (atm).
7. Calculate the density and specific gravity of liquids and gases.
8. Explain how changes in pressure, volume, temperature, and mass affect the behavior of an ideal gas.
9. Calculate the partial pressure of oxygen in a room air sample of gas obtained at 1 atm.
10. List the physical variables that influence the flow of a gas through a tube.
11. Explain how the pressure, velocity, and flow of a gas change as it moves from a part of a tube with a large radius to another part with a small radius.
12. Describe the Venturi and Coanda effects and how both can be used in the design of respiratory care equipment.
13. State Ohm's law and relate how changes in voltage and resistance affect current flow in a direct-current series circuit.
14. Describe three strategies that can be used to protect patients from electrical hazards.

OUTLINE

KEY TERMS

absolute humidity	elements	optics
acoustics	evaporation	potential energy
adhesive forces	Fahrenheit	power
ammeter	fluidic	Rankine
amorphous solids	freezing point	relative humidity
ampere	gravitational potential energy	resistors
Archimedes principle	horsepower	semiconductors
atomic theory	hydrogen bonding	sublimation
atoms	hydrometer	supercooled liquids
Avogadro's number	insulators	Système Internationale d'Unités
boiling point	joules	thermistor
Boltzmann universal gas constant	Kelvin	thermodynamics
buoyancy	kilowatt	thermometers (electrical and
Celsius	kinetic energy	nonelectrical)
cohesive forces	kinetic theory	Van der Waals forces
compounds	latent heat	vaporization
condensation	macroshock	vapor pressure
critical point	mechanics	vapors
critical pressure	melting point	volt
critical temperature	microshock	voltmeter
diffusion	mixtures	watts
dipole–dipole interactions	molecules	weight density
electricity and magnetism	ohm	Wheatstone bridge
electromotive force	Ohm's law	

Physics is the branch of science that describes the interactions of matter and energy. Classical physics comprises the fields of mechanics, optics, acoustics, electricity and magnetism, and thermodynamics. The laws of classical physics describe the behavior of matter and energy under ordinary, everyday conditions. Modern physics, which began at the end of the 19th century, seeks to explain the interactions of matter and energy under extraordinary conditions, such as in extreme temperatures or when moving near the speed of light. Modern physics also is concerned with the interactions of matter and energy on a very small scale (i.e., nuclear and elementary particle physics). It is noteworthy that, at the subatomic level, the laws of classical physics governing space, time, matter, and energy are considered no longer valid.

Knowledge of the principles of classical physics is fundamental to a clear understanding of the ways in which various types of respiratory care equipment operate. Indeed, this chapter began with a quote from Nobel laureate Richard Feynman to underscore the fact that physics is not only part of the foundation of respiratory care, it serves the same function for all of the clinical sciences.

This chapter presents a review of classical physics applicable to respiratory care equipment. It is not intended to present a compendium of physics but rather focuses on how these physical principles are commonly encountered in respiratory care equipment. Several physics textbooks are included in the references list at the end of the chapter to facilitate a more detailed study of physics.[2-4]

I. ENERGY AND MATTER

Energy and Work

The concepts of energy and work are closely related. In fact, energy usually is defined as the ability to do work, where work (W) equals the product of a force (F) acting on an object to move it a distance (d), or

$$W = F \times d$$

Note that this description of work is more specific than our everyday definition of work. In everyday life, we say that work is anything that requires the exertion of effort. In physics, work is performed only when the effort produces a change in the position of the matter (i.e., the matter moves in the direction of the force). In the Système Internationale d'Unités (SI) of measurements, energy and work are expressed in joules (J), where 1 J equals the force of 1 newton (N) acting on a 1-kilogram (kg) object to move it 1 meter (m). Power (P), which is a measure of the rate at which work is being performed (P = W/t), is expressed in watts (W) per unit of time (t = second or sec), with 1 W equivalent to 1 J/sec. Because the watt is a relatively small number, we rely more on the kilowatt (kW), which equals 1000 watts (e.g., a 2-kW motor can perform work at a rate of 2000 J/sec). Another common term used for power is horsepower (hp). Approximately, 1 hp equals 746 W of power, or 0.746 kW.

The energy required to perform work can exist in various forms, including mechanical energy, thermal energy, chemical energy, sound energy, nuclear energy, and electrical energy. According to the law of conservation of energy, energy cannot be created or destroyed but can only be transferred. For example, a fossil fuel such as coal, which is a form of chemical energy, can be converted to electrical energy, which, in turn, can provide the power to operate a fan or compressor. Therefore we can think of work as the transfer of energy by mechanical means. As such, mechanical energy usually is divided into two categories: kinetic energy and potential energy.

Kinetic and Potential Energy

Kinetic energy is the energy an object possesses when it is in motion; potential energy is stored energy, or the energy that an object possesses because of its position. The kinetic energy (KE) of an object can be quantified with the formula

$$KE = \frac{1}{2}(mv^2)$$

where m is the mass of the object and v is the velocity at which it is traveling. Intuitively, one might guess that the greater the mass, the greater the KE. It is not necessarily obvious that the KE of the substance increases to a greater extent with similar increases in the velocity at which the object is traveling. In fact, looking at the formula, one can see that KE increases exponentially when velocity increases. That is, KE is proportional to the square of the velocity at which the object is moving (e.g., a twofold increase in mass increases the KE twofold, and a twofold increase in velocity results in a fourfold increase in the KE).

Potential energy can be thought of as the energy an object has by virtue of its position. For example, an iron weight raised above your head has the potential to exert a force when it falls. The energy the weight gains as it falls is the result of gravity. (In this example, however, potential energy is more correctly referred to as gravitational potential energy.) The amount of potential energy (PE) an object has can be calculated as

$$PE = mgh$$

where m is the mass of the object, g is the force of gravity (32 feet/sec^2), and h is the height the object is raised. Potential energy also can be stored in a compressed spring or a chemical bond. With a spring, energy is required for compression. This elastic PE is then converted into KE when the spring is allowed to uncoil. Petroleum reserves of coal, oil, and gas, which represent chemical PE stores, can be converted to KE when chemical bonds are broken to provide the power required to operate lights, automobiles, and other devices we use in our daily lives.

II. STATES OF MATTER

Matter generally is defined as anything that has mass and occupies space. The atomic theory, which is the result of the work of John Dalton (1766-1844), states that all matter is composed of tiny particles, called atoms. Although it can appear in various forms, all matter is made up of approximately 100 different types of atoms, called elements.[5,6] These elements can combine in fixed proportions to form molecules, which, in turn, can form compounds and mixtures.

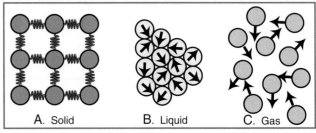

FIGURE 1.1 Simplified models illustrating the three states of matter. A, Solid. B, Liquid. C, Gas.

All matter can exist in three distinct states: solid, liquid, and gas. The physical properties of each of these states can be explained by the kinetic theory, which states that the atoms and molecules that make up matter are in constant motion. The schematic in Fig. 1.1 illustrates the three states of matter. Solids usually are characterized as either crystalline or amorphous. Notice that crystalline solids are highly organized structures in which the atoms and molecules are arranged in a lattice. Amorphous solids, such as glass or margarine, have constituent particles that are less rigidly arranged. Amorphous solids sometimes are called supercooled liquids because of this random arrangement.

Of the three states of matter, solids have the least amount of KE. Most of their internal energy is PE that is contained in the intermolecular forces holding the individual particles of solids together. In solids, these forces are strong enough to limit the motion of the atoms and molecules to what appear to be vibrations or oscillations about a fixed point. Because of these features, solids are characterized as incompressible substances that can maintain their volume and shape.

Like solids, liquids have attractive forces, but the cohesive forces in liquids are not as strong. Liquid molecules have greater freedom of movement and more KE than do molecules of solids. Illustrating exactly how liquid particles move is difficult, but one can envision that these particles are able to slide past each other, which gives liquids *fluidity*, or the ability to flow. Although the intermolecular forces holding liquids together are relatively weak compared with those in solids, these forces lend enough cohesiveness to liquid molecules to allow them to maintain their volumes. Liquids essentially are incompressible; that is, a liquid can be made to occupy a smaller volume only if an incredible amount of force is exerted upon it.

Gases have extremely weak, if any, cohesive forces between their constituent particles. Therefore gases have the greatest amount of KE of the three states of matter, and their PE is minimal compared with that of the other two states of matter. The motion of the atoms and molecules that make up gases is random. Gases do not maintain their shapes and volumes but rather expand to fill the available space. Gases are similar to liquids in that the particles composing them can move freely, thus giving gases the ability to flow. For this reason, gases and liquids are described as *fluids*.

Box 1.1 lists some of the more common substances that normally exist as gases at room temperature. Most of the gases

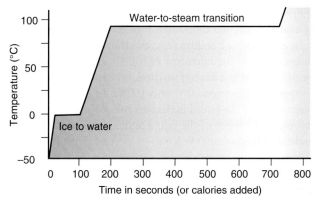

FIGURE 1.2 Energy–temperature relationship for the conversion of solid ice to liquid water to steam. Energy is added at a rate of 1 cal/sec. (Redrawn from Nave CR, Nave BC: *Physics for the health sciences,* ed 3, Philadelphia, 1985, WB Saunders.)

encountered in everyday life (e.g., nitrogen [N_2], oxygen [O_2], carbon dioxide [CO_2], and carbon monoxide [CO]) are colorless and odorless; a notable exception is nitrogen dioxide (NO_2), an atmospheric pollutant that is dark brown and has a pungent odor. The properties of individual medical gases are discussed in Chapter 3.

Change of State

It should be apparent from the discussion so far that the physical state of any substance is determined from the relation of its KE content and the PE stored in its intermolecular bonds. Changes of state involve the interconversion of solids, liquids, and gases, which can be accomplished by altering the relationship between the KE and PE of a substance, such as by changing its temperature (i.e., by adding or removing heat). Consider the example of converting the solid form of water (ice) to liquid and then to steam. Adding heat to ice increases the kinetic activity (i.e., vibration of the water molecules) in the ice, thus melting or weakening the intermolecular attractive forces and producing liquid water. (Freezing, which is the opposite of melting, can be accomplished by transferring the KE of a substance to its surroundings, such as when a substance is exposed to cold temperatures.) Adding more heat causes the liquid water molecules to move more vigorously and escape into the gaseous state, or vaporize (evaporation). The temperature at which a solid converts to a liquid is a substance's melting point. (Note that the freezing point is the same temperature as the melting point; that is, the temperature at which a liquid is changed to a solid state.) The temperature at which a liquid converts to a gaseous state is its boiling point.

Fig. 1.2 shows the phase changes associated with the conversion of 1 gram (g) of ice to steam.[7] As heat is added, ice begins to change to liquid at a temperature of 0°C. Note that although the addition of heat effects a change in state, the temperature of the water does not change immediately (i.e., there is a plateau in temperature). The temperature changes only after all of the ice is converted to liquid. The amount of heat that must be added to a substance to cause a complete change of state is called the latent heat of fusion and is expressed in calories per gram (cal/g). Therefore the amount of heat that must be added to effect the change from solid to liquid is called the *latent heat of fusion or melting.* In the case of water, approximately 80 calories (cal/g) of heat must be added to liquefy ice completely when the temperature reaches 0°C. After the ice has been completely liquefied, the temperature will increase 1°C per second if heat continues to be added

TABLE 1.1 Melting and Boiling Points and Latent Heats of Fusion and Vaporization of Some Common Substances

Substance	Melting Point (°C)	Heat of Fusion (cal/g)	Boiling Point (°C)[a]	Heat of Vaporization (cal/g)
Water	0	80	100	540
Ethyl alcohol	−114	26	78	204
Nitrogen	−210	6.2	−196	48
Oxygen	−219	3.3	−183	51
Mercury	−39	2.7	357	68

[a]At standard atmospheric pressure of 760 mm Hg.

at a rate of 1 cal/sec. This same type of phenomenon occurs at the substance's boiling point when water is converted to steam. The amount of heat that must be supplied to change liquid to steam completely (i.e., vaporize water) is the latent heat of vaporization. Obviously, a considerably greater amount of heat (540 cal/g) must be added to convert water to steam compared with the amount of heat that must be added to melt ice into water. More energy is required in the process of vaporization because intermolecular forces essentially must be removed to allow the molecules to break loose and enter into the gaseous state.[8] Table 1.1 lists the melting and boiling points for some commonly used substances, along with the latent heats of fusion and vaporization.

Sublimation

Under certain conditions, solid molecules can completely bypass the liquid state and change to gas. This process, called sublimation, occurs when the heat content of a substance increases to a point at which the molecules in the solid state gain enough energy to break loose and enter the gaseous state while remaining below its melting point. The conversion of solid carbon dioxide (i.e., dry ice) to gaseous carbon dioxide is the most common example of this process.

Evaporation and Condensation

The conversion of a liquid to the gaseous state has been discussed in terms of boiling (e.g., the transition from water to steam occurs at a temperature of 100°C). Although it may not be obvious, this phase transition (evaporation) begins at temperatures between 0°C and 100°C. Evaporation occurs when some of the liquid molecules gain enough KE to break through the surface of the liquid and convert to free gaseous molecules. The rate of evaporation increases with an increase in temperature, an increase in surface area, or a decrease in pressure.

Two forces must be overcome for evaporation to occur: the mass attraction of the molecules for each other (i.e., dipole–dipole interactions, hydrogen bonding, and Van der Waals forces) and the pressure of the gas above the liquid. We can enhance the process of evaporation either by increasing the KE of the liquid molecules or by reducing the pressure above the liquid. Raising the temperature of a liquid increases the velocity and the force of the molecules hitting each other and moves them farther apart. This increased kinetic activity increases the force that these molecules possess as they hit the surface of the liquid, thus allowing the liquid molecules to escape more easily and frequently.

Vapor pressure is a measure of the force that molecules exert as they hit the surface of a liquid and escape into the gaseous phase. The concept of vapor pressure can be used to define the boiling point of a liquid in more precise terms; that is, the boiling point is the temperature at which the vapor pressure of a liquid equals the atmospheric pressure. Reducing the pressure above the liquid lowers its boiling point, because the forces opposing the escape of molecules from the liquid are decreased. This concept explains why water boils at a lower temperature at high altitudes. It also explains the process of freeze-drying as a means of food preservation; the food is placed in a vacuum, which reduces the opposition that liquid molecules must overcome to evaporate, thereby boiling off any liquid present.

The opposite of evaporation is condensation, which is simply defined as the conversion of a substance from a gas to a liquid. In evaporation, heat energy is removed from the air surrounding a liquid and transferred to the liquid, thus cooling the air. In contrast, during condensation, heat is removed from the liquid and transferred to the surrounding air, warming it. Box 1.2 contains an example of how evaporation and condensation can affect a person's daily life.

Evaporation and condensation are essential components of respiration. Specifically, effective ventilation requires a balance between the evaporation and condensation of the moisture of respired gases so that the airway mucosa are not dried and irritated. Therapeutic procedures, such as insertion of an endotracheal tube into a patient's airway to provide mechanical ventilatory support, bypass normal physiological mechanisms that add heat and moisture to inspired air. Bypassing these mechanisms can therefore severely compromise the body's ability to maintain this balance. The potential problems associated with bypassing the body's mechanisms for humidifying inspired gases can be minimized by ensuring that all

gases delivered to the patient are adequately humidified. Devices such as humidifiers, hygroscopic condenser filters, and artificial noses can be used to ensure adequate humidification of inspired gases. These concepts are revisited in our discussion of humidity and aerosol therapy (see Chapter 6).

Critical Temperature and Critical Pressure

When a liquid is placed in a closed container, the force of the molecules trying to escape from the liquid eventually equilibrates with the force or pressure of the liquid molecules that have entered into the gaseous state, and no more liquid molecules will escape. If the temperature of the liquid is raised, however, the velocity at which its molecules are traveling will increase, whereas the mass attraction between its constituent molecules is reduced. Raising the temperature also increases the capacity of the air above the liquid to hold liquid vapor. Thus the vapor pressure also increases as the temperature rises, necessitating a higher opposing force to equilibrate the molecule's escape from the liquid state. At its boiling point the force of the molecules in the liquid equals the surrounding pressure, and the molecules may fail to escape. Therefore, in

---

BOX 1.2   Evaporation and Condensation

A fairly common example that can be used to illustrate concepts of evaporation and condensation relates to the water vapor content, or humidity, of the air surrounding us. This concept is obvious to anyone who has ever spent a hot August day somewhere in the southern part of the United States, such as New Orleans. As stated in the section on evaporation, one of the main factors influencing evaporation is temperature. Increasing the temperature increases water evaporation (in New Orleans, the water is from the lakes and bayous surrounding the city) by increasing the molecular activity of the water and increasing the capacity of the air to hold water vapor. If the actual amount of water vapor in the air is to be measured, the water vapor content must be determined. The amount or weight of water that can be contained (to capacity) in the air is called the absolute humidity and is expressed in grams of water vapor per cubic meter (g/m^3) or milligrams per liter (mg/L). The capacity of air to hold moisture increases as the temperature of the air increases. (The absolute humidity can be measured, or it can be computed with tables supplied by the U.S. Weather Bureau.[8]) Note that at a temperature of 37°C (98.6°F), a typical temperature in New Orleans during August, air that is 100% saturated will contain 43.8 mg of water per liter of air. In most cases the air is not fully saturated but typically only 90% saturated with water vapor; that is, it contains only 0.90 × 43.80 mg/L, or 39.42 mg of water in every liter of air. For this reason the National Weather Service chooses to report the relative humidity, or the ratio of actual water content to its saturated capacity, at a given temperature (in this case the relative humidity would be 90%).

One might ask how condensation can be included in this example, but consider that late in the afternoon, it is not uncommon for rain to fall in New Orleans. The rain occurs because the air cools (the sun begins to set), and the capacity of the air to hold water decreases. This decreased capacity to hold water vapor causes condensation, resulting in rain.

essence, the boiling point is the temperature at which the force exerted by the molecule of the liquid trying to escape equals the forces opposing its escape (i.e., atmospheric pressure and mass attraction). As gas molecules are heated above the boiling point, the force (pressure) required for converting them back to a liquid also increases. Ultimately, a temperature is reached above which gaseous molecules of a substance cannot be converted back to a liquid, no matter how much pressure is exerted upon them. This temperature is called the critical temperature.[7] Therefore the critical temperature can be thought of as the highest temperature at which a substance can exist in a liquid state. Critical pressure is the pressure that must be applied to the substance at its critical temperature to maintain equilibrium between the liquid and gas phases.[8] The term critical point is used to describe the critical temperature and the critical pressure of a substance. Substances that exist as liquids at ambient conditions have critical temperatures that are greater than room temperature (i.e., 20°C to 25°C). Substances that normally exist as gases at ambient conditions have critical temperatures that are usually well below room temperature.

Two commonly encountered substances can be used to demonstrate the principles of critical temperature and critical pressure. Water, for example, boils at 100°C and has a critical temperature of 374°C. At temperatures below 100°C, water exists as a liquid. As its temperature is raised above 100°C, water converts to a gas, in the form of steam. Between 100°C and 374°C, steam can be converted back into liquid by applying progressively greater amounts of pressure to it. In fact, to maintain equilibrium between the liquid and gaseous states of water at 374°C, 218 atmosphere (atm) of pressure must be applied. Furthermore, above 374°C, water can exist only as a gas—no matter how much pressure is applied. Oxygen has a boiling point of −183°C and a critical temperature of approximately −119°C. At temperatures below −183°C, oxygen can exist as a liquid. After its temperature is raised above −183°C, liquid oxygen becomes a gas. At temperatures between −183°C and −119°C, the gaseous oxygen can be converted back to a liquid by compression. As with water, greater amounts of pressure must be applied to cause this conversion until the critical temperature of −119°C is reached. At oxygen's critical temperature, a pressure of 49.7 atm must be applied to maintain equilibrium between the gaseous and liquid phases of oxygen. After the temperature is raised above the critical temperature, oxygen cannot be converted to a liquid, no matter how much pressure is applied to it.

Application of the concepts of critical temperature and critical pressure can be seen in medical gas therapy. As is discussed in Chapters 3 and 4, medical gases can be supplied in cylinders and bulk storage systems. Substances such as nitrous oxide and carbon dioxide have critical temperatures above room temperature and thus can exist as vapors (i.e., as a mixture of liquid and gas when placed in a compressed-gas cylinder [gases and vapors are discussed in the next subsection of this chapter]). Air, oxygen, and helium, on the other hand, have critical temperatures well below room temperature and exist as gases when placed under pressure in a compressed-gas

cylinder. Liquid air and oxygen, which must be kept at very low temperatures (i.e., below their boiling points), are stored in specially insulated containers. When needed, the liquid oxygen or air is allowed to exceed its critical temperature and convert to gas.[8]

Gases Versus Vapors

A gas is a state of matter that is above its critical temperature. Free molecules of the same substance below its critical temperature are a vapor. Simply stated, a vapor is the gaseous form of any substance that can exist as a liquid or a solid at ordinary pressures and temperatures. For example, under conditions of 1 atm and a room temperature of 25°C, oxygen exists in the gaseous state because it is above its critical temperature (−119°C); it therefore is classified as a true gas. Water, on the other hand, is below its critical temperature (374°C) and is considered a vapor. Water vapor can be converted back to liquid or ice if sufficient pressure is applied.

Two commonly used vapors are carbon dioxide and nitrous oxide. Both of these substances can be converted to liquid at room temperature if enough pressure is applied. In fact, both gases are supplied to hospitals in pressurized cylinders in which most of the vapor is converted to liquid. As is discussed in Chapter 3, the amount of CO_2 or N_2O remaining in cylinders containing substances below their critical temperature (liquids) must be determined by weighing the cylinders instead of reading the pressure level within the cylinder. Gases such as oxygen, nitrogen, and helium are examples of substances that usually are supplied in compressed-gas cylinders above their critical temperatures. In these cases the pressure gauge gives an accurate estimate of the amount of gas remaining in the cylinder.

III. PHYSICAL PROPERTIES OF MATTER

Temperature

As already stated, temperature is a measure of the average KE of the molecules of an object[9]; however, it is also a measure of the relative warmth or coolness of a substance. Recall that adding heat to a substance changes its physical properties. This phenomenon of changing physical properties can be used in temperature measurements and in designing temperature scales.[10]

Thermometers are devices used to measure temperature. They are made with materials that undergo physical changes as their temperature changes. Thermometers generally are classified as nonelectrical and electrical thermometers.[10] The most commonly used nonelectrical devices are mercury and alcohol thermometers. Resistance thermometers, thermistors, and thermocouples are examples of electrical thermometers.

The mercury thermometer is probably the best-known example of a nonelectrical thermometer. This device is the product of Gabriel Daniel Fahrenheit's work on temperature measurement during the early part of the 18th century. Fahrenheit (1686-1736) used mercury because he found that it expanded and contracted as its temperature changed.

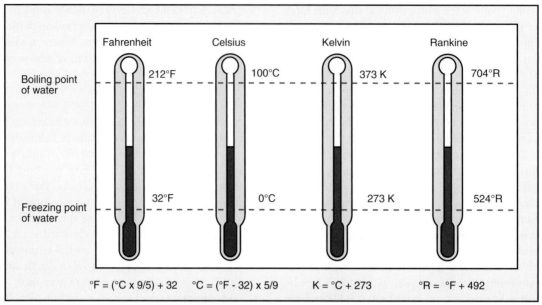

FIGURE 1.3 Temperature scales.

He constructed the first thermometer and ultimately the first mercury temperature scale (i.e., the Fahrenheit temperature scale).

Electrical thermometers operate on the principle that the electrical resistance of metal increases linearly with increases in temperature.[10] A typical resistance thermometer consists of a platinum wire resistor, a battery, and an ammeter for measuring current flow. Because the amount of current flowing through the platinum wire is directly related to the resistance of the wire, the ammeter can detect temperature changes by measuring the changes in current flow that occur when the resistor's temperature is changed.[a]

Another common example of an electrical thermometer is the thermistor. It is typically a metal oxide bead whose resistance changes according to its temperature. An ammeter connected to an electrical circuit measures temperature in a manner similar to that described for the resistance thermometer. Thermistors are incorporated into a number of medical devices, including mechanical ventilators, spirometers, capnographs, and metabolic monitors. Thermistors are also an integral part of the balloon-flotation catheters used with thermodilution cardiac output monitors. All of these devices are discussed in more detail in Chapters 8 and 9, in which monitoring of physiological function is considered.

Temperature Scales

A temperature scale is constructed by choosing two reference temperatures and dividing the difference between these points into a certain number of degrees. The size of the degree depends on the particular temperature scale being used. The most common reference temperatures are the melting point of ice and the boiling point of water, because recognizable changes take place and thus can be given a value against which other temperatures can be measured.

Three temperature scales are routinely used in science and medicine: the absolute (Kelvin) scale, the Celsius scale, and the Fahrenheit scale. A fourth temperature scale, the Rankine scale, is used in the engineering sciences.[7] Fig. 1.3 shows the scalar relationships between the Kelvin, Celsius, Fahrenheit, and Rankine scales.

The SI units for temperature are based on the Kelvin scale, with the zero point equal to 0 K, or absolute zero, and the boiling point equal to 100 K. Theoretically, absolute zero is the temperature at which all molecular motion stops. Notice that the Kelvin scale is described as a centigrade scale because there are 100 divisions between the freezing and boiling points of water.

The metric or centimeter-gram-second (cgs) system is based on the Celsius scale, which can also be characterized as a centigrade scale. In the Celsius scale the freezing point for water is designated as 0°C, whereas the boiling point for water equals 100°C. It is important to recognize that although the Celsius and Kelvin scales are both considered centigrade scales, the same temperature has a different value on each. Notice in Fig. 1.3 that a temperature of 0 K (i.e., absolute zero, or the temperature at which all the kinetic activity of a substance stops) corresponds to a temperature of −273°C, and that the zero point on the Celsius scale (0°C; i.e., the freezing point of water) therefore corresponds to a temperature of 273 K on the Kelvin scale. Similarly, the boiling point of water on the Celsius scale (100°C) corresponds to a temperature of 373 K.

The Fahrenheit scale, which is used in the English, or foot-pound-second (fps), system, sets the freezing point of water at 32°F and the boiling point of water at 212°F. The Fahrenheit scale has 180 divisions between the freezing and

---

[a]Actually, the electrical circuit consists of multiple resistors arranged in a configuration called a *Wheatstone bridge*. The principles of electronics are discussed later in this chapter. See Box 1.6 for a brief description of a Wheatstone bridge circuit.

BOX 1.3   Temperature Scales

Conversions Between the Kelvin and Celsius Scales

$$K = {}^\circ C + 273$$
$${}^\circ C = K - 273$$

Example 1

37° C equals how many Kelvin?

$$K = 37^\circ C + 273$$
$$= 310\,K$$

(Note that Kelvin is not preceded by the symbol for degrees.)

Example 2

373 K equals how many degrees Celsius?

$${}^\circ C = 373\,K - 273$$
$$= 100^\circ C$$

Conversions Between the Celsius and Fahrenheit Scales

$${}^\circ C = 5/9({}^\circ F - 32)$$
$${}^\circ F = (9/5 \times {}^\circ C) + 32$$

Example 1

98.6° F equals how many degrees Celsius?

$${}^\circ C = 5/9(98.6^\circ F - 32)$$
$$= 5/9(66.6)$$
$$= 37^\circ C$$

Example 2

25° C equals how many degrees Fahrenheit?

$${}^\circ F = (9/5 \times 25) + 32$$
$$= 45 + 32$$
$$= 77^\circ F$$

BOX 1.4   Pressure Conversions

Pressure can be measured in a variety of units, including:
- Centimeters of water (cm H_2O)
- Millimeters of mercury (mm Hg), or torr
- Pounds per square inch (lb/in^2, or psi)
- Atmospheres (atm)
- Kilopascals (kPa)

The following formulae enable conversions between these units:
- cm H_2O × 0.7355 = mm Hg (torr)
- mm Hg (torr) ÷ 0.7355 = cm H_2O
- cm H_2O × 0.098 = kPa
- kPa ÷ 0.098 = cm H_2O
- mm Hg × 0.1333 = kPa
- kPa ÷ 0.1333 = mm Hg
- mm Hg ÷ 760 = atm
- atm × 14.7 = lb/in^2 (psi)

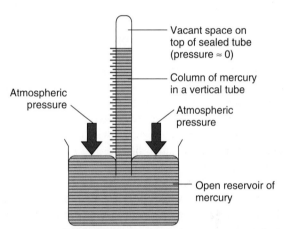

FIGURE 1.4 A mercury barometer.

---

the boiling points of water and therefore cannot be considered a centigrade scale.

Box 1.3 contains formulae for converting temperatures between the various scales. As is seen later in this chapter, the Kelvin scale is used when the gas and other physical laws are described. Also, although increased emphasis is placed on the use of the Celsius scale in the scientific literature and clinical medicine, clinicians in the United States continue to use the Fahrenheit scale for recording patient temperatures.

Pressure

When gas molecules collide with solid or liquid surfaces, they exert a pressure. Pressure (P) is usually defined as the force that a gas exerts over a given area (P = Force/Area). Pressure measurements are reported in a variety of units, including pounds per square inch (psi, or lb/in^2), millimeters of mercury (mm Hg), torr, centimeters of water (cm H_2O), and kilopascals (kPa).[11] Box 1.4 contains formulae for converting pressure units.

Atmospheric pressure is the pressure atmospheric gases exert on objects within the Earth's atmosphere. It exists because the gases that make up the atmosphere are attracted to the Earth's surface by gravity, thus forming a column of air around the Earth. Atmospheric pressure is highest near the Earth's surface; at sea level, atmospheric pressure equals 760 mm Hg. As you move away from the Earth's core, the atmospheric pressure decreases because of a reduction in the force of gravity pulling air molecules toward the Earth. For example, the atmospheric pressure in Chicago, which is located at sea level, averages approximately 760 mm Hg. The atmospheric pressure in Denver, which is located 1 mile above sea level, averages approximately 630 mm Hg.

Atmospheric pressure can be measured with a barometer similar to the one shown in Fig. 1.4. The mercury barometer, which was invented by Evangelista Torricelli (c. 1608-1647), is the most commonly used device for measuring atmospheric pressure. (Torricelli was the first person to recognize the existence of atmospheric pressure; the pressure measurement *torr* is named in his honor.) The mercury barometer uses the weight of a column of mercury to equilibrate with the force of the gas molecules hitting the surface of a mercury reservoir.

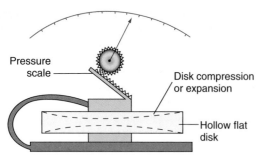

FIGURE 1.5 An aneroid barometer.

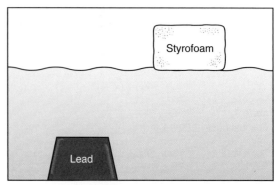

FIGURE 1.6 A Practical example of buoyancy. Notice that the block of Styrofoam floats because its weight density is less than that of water, whereas the block of lead sinks because its weight density is greater than the weight density of water.

A column is completely filled with mercury and erected with its open end below the surface of a mercury reservoir. The mercury in the column tries to return to the reservoir as a result of gravity. The force, which gas molecules exert as they hit the surface of the reservoir, counteracts the force of gravity and pushes the mercury upward in the tube. The atmospheric pressure equals the height of the mercury column.

The aneroid barometer (Fig. 1.5) measures atmospheric pressure by equilibrating the atmospheric gas pressure with a mechanical force, or the expansion force of an evacuated metal container. As atmospheric pressure increases, the pressure on the surface of the metal container tends to compress it. The change in the container's dimensions is recorded by a gearing mechanism, which changes the location of an indicator on the recording dial. Likewise, a decrease in atmospheric pressure surrounding the container allows the metal container to expand toward its normal shape.

Density

Density (d) is the measure of a substance's mass per unit volume under specific conditions of pressure and temperature, or

$$d = Mass/Volume$$

For measurements taken near the surface of the Earth, mass may be replaced by a substance's weight, so that **weight density** (d_w) equals weight divided by its volume, or

$$d_w = Weight/Volume$$

As one travels away from the surface of the Earth, the force of gravity diminishes, and thus the relationship between mass and weight changes (i.e., as the force of gravity decreases, so does weight, even though mass stays the same).

For solids and liquids, density can be expressed in grams per liter (g/L) or in grams per cubic centimeter (g/cm^3). The density of gases is also expressed in grams per liter (g/L). Because of the influence of pressure and temperature on the density of gases, density is calculated under standard temperature and pressure conditions. (*Note:* standard temperature and pressure [STPD] is defined as 0°C, 760 mm Hg, and dry.) The density of gases is covered in more detail with the discussion of Avogadro's law later in this chapter.

Buoyancy

When an object is immersed in a fluid, it appears to weigh less than it does in air. This effect, **buoyancy**, can be explained by the **Archimedes principle**.[7-9] This principle states that when an object is submerged in a fluid, it will be buoyed up by a force equal to the weight of the fluid that is displaced by the object. The weight of the displaced liquid can be calculated as the product of the volume (V) of displaced liquid and the weight density (d_w) of the liquid:

$$F_{buoyancy} = V \times d_w$$

Consider what happens when an object is submerged in water. Water has a weight density of 1 g/cm^3. If the weight density of the object being submerged is less than the weight density of water, the object will float. If the weight density of the submerged object is greater than that of water, the object will sink. Fig. 1.6 illustrates a practical example of this concept. In this case the weight density of a block of Styrofoam is considerably less than that of a block of lead. It should be apparent from this example that the Styrofoam has a weight density less than water and therefore floats, whereas the block of lead has a weight density greater than water and consequently sinks.

Measurement of the specific gravity of a liquid or gas represents another practical application of the Archimedes principle. Specific gravity is a comparison of a substance's weight density relative to a standard. For liquids, water is used as the standard, and gases are compared with air, oxygen, or hydrogen.[6] The device shown in Fig. 1.7, a **hydrometer**, is used clinically to measure the weight density or specific gravity of liquids, such as urine. The density of a liquid is measured by the level at which the hydrometer floats in the liquid. Thus if the liquid is very dense, the hydrometer floats near the surface, because only a small volume of liquid needs to be displaced to equal the weight of the hydrometer. Conversely, as the density of the liquid decreases, the hydrometer sinks toward the bottom of the beaker containing the liquid. Notice in Fig. 1.7 that the specific gravity can be read from the tube. Thus a reading of 1.025 indicates that the liquid weighs 1.025 times more than water.[8]

Viscosity

Viscosity can be defined as the force opposing deformation of a fluid. The viscosity of a fluid depends on its density and

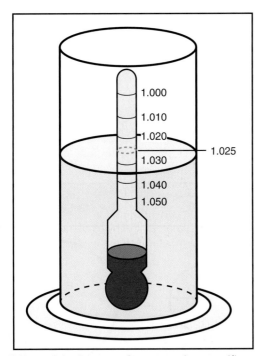

FIGURE 1.7 A hydrometer for measuring specific gravity.

BOX 1.5   Adhesive and Cohesive Forces

The properties of adhesion and cohesion can be demonstrated by placing liquid in a small-diameter glass tube, such as those shown in the figure. Notice that at the top of the column of liquid, the liquid forms a curved surface, or *meniscus*. In the tube containing water (on the left), the meniscus is concave; however, in the tube containing mercury (on the right), the meniscus is convex. In the tube with water, the meniscus is turned upward because the attractive, adhesive forces between the water and the glass cause the water to adhere to the wall of the tube. In the tube with mercury the meniscus is turned downward because the cohesive forces within the mercury are stronger than the adhesive forces between the mercury and the glass.

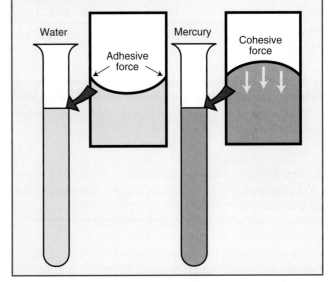

on the cohesive forces between its constituent molecules (i.e., as the cohesive forces of a fluid increase, so does its viscosity).

Viscosity is manifested differently in liquids and gases.[9] The viscosity of a liquid is primarily determined by the cohesive forces between its molecules, whereas the viscosity of a gas is determined by the number of collisions of the gas molecules. For example, raising the temperature of a liquid such as cooking oil weakens the cohesive forces between its molecules and decreases its viscosity. As the oil is heated and its temperature increases, it flows more freely than at a lower temperature (e.g., room temperature). Conversely, increasing the temperature of a gas increases its KE (i.e., the frequency of collisions of its constituent molecules). The greater number of collisions results in a higher internal friction and thus an increase in viscosity.

Viscosity is an important factor to consider when describing laminar, or streamlined, flow. The way viscosity influences fluid mechanics, specifically as it relates to Poiseuille's law, is discussed later in this chapter.

Surface Tension

Before the phenomenon of surface tension is described, the difference between adhesive and cohesive forces should be discussed. Adhesive forces are attractive forces between two different kinds of molecules. Cohesive forces, on the other hand, are attractive forces between like kinds of molecules. The difference between these two forces can be envisioned by taking two dishes and filling one with water and the other with mercury. If a paper towel is gently submerged into each liquid, the results will be different. When the towel is placed in the water dish, it absorbs the water. This is because the

attractive, adhesive forces between the molecules of the towel and the water are greater than the attractive forces of the water molecules for each other. When the towel is submerged in the mercury dish, it does not absorb the mercury, because the attractive, cohesive forces between the mercury molecules are greater than the attractive adhesive forces between the molecules of the towel and the mercury. Box 1.5 presents another application involving adhesive and cohesive forces.

Surface tension is generated by the cohesive forces between liquid molecules at a gas–liquid interface or at the interface of two immiscible (i.e., unable to mix) liquids, such as oil and water. Fig. 1.8 illustrates the molecular basis of surface tension at a gas–liquid interface. At some depth the molecules within a liquid are attracted equally from all sides, whereas the molecules near the surface experience unequal attractions.[10] Notice that near the surface of the liquid, some of the forces in the liquid act in a direction that is parallel to the surface, whereas others are drawn toward the center of the liquid mass by this net force. The forces acting parallel to the surface of the liquid cause the liquid to behave as though a film is present at the gas–liquid interface. The forces drawn toward the center of the liquid tend to reduce its exposed surface to the smallest possible area, which is usually a sphere.

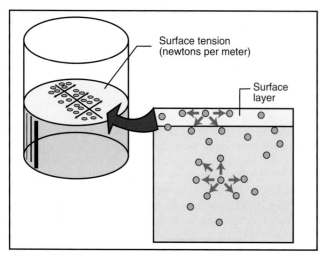

FIGURE 1.8 The molecular basis for surface tension. See text for explanation.

TABLE 1.2	**Examples of Surface Tension**	
Substance	**°C**	**Surface Tension (dyn/cm)**
Water	20	73
Water	37	70
Tissue fluid	37	50
Whole blood	37	58
Plasma	37	73

We can measure the surface tension of a liquid by determining the force that must be applied to produce a "tear" in this film.[7] As such, in the SI system of measurements, surface tension usually is expressed in dynes per centimeter (dyn/cm). Table 1.2 lists surface tensions for several liquids commonly encountered in respiratory care. Note that the surface tension of a given liquid varies inversely with its temperature. Thus surface tension decreases as the temperature of a liquid increases.

Laplace's Law

As just stated, surface tension forces cause a liquid to have a tendency to occupy the smallest possible area, which usually is a sphere. The pressure within a liquid sphere should be influenced both by the surface tension forces offered by the liquid and by the size of the sphere. Indeed, Pierre-Simon Laplace (1749-1827), a French astronomer and mathematician, found that pressure within a sphere is directly related to the surface tension of the liquid and inversely related to the radius of the sphere, or

$$P = 2(ST/r)$$

where P is the pressure within the sphere, ST is the surface tension of the liquid, and r is the radius of the sphere.

The examples in Fig. 1.9 illustrate this principle. In Fig. 1.9A, two droplets of water are shown. One droplet has a radius of 2 cm, and the other droplet has a radius of 4 cm. If we assume that the surface tension is equal in both droplets

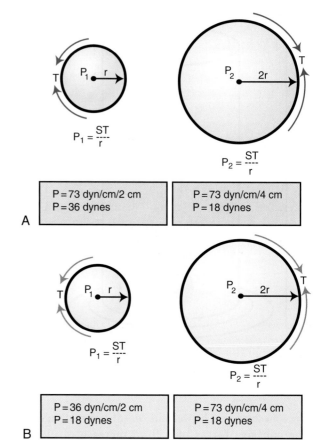

FIGURE 1.9 Laplace's law. A, Water bubble. B, Soap bubble. See text for discussion.

(i.e., the surface tension of water is 73 dyn/cm), then the pressure in the smaller droplet is twice that of the larger droplet.

Now consider what happens when the surface tension of the smaller droplet is reduced, for example, by adding a surface-active agent (e.g., soap) to the water. As shown in Fig. 1.9B, the surface tension of the larger water droplet remains at 73 dyn/cm, but the surface tension of the smaller soap bubble is reduced to half as much (36 dyn/cm). By a simple calculation, one can see that the pressures within the two spheres are now equal.

Applications of Laplace's law can be found in the discussion of aerosol therapy in Chapter 6. As will be seen, surface tension explains why liquid particles retain their spherical shape in an aerosol suspension.

IV. THE GAS LAWS

The gas laws presented in this section are important generalizations about the macroscopic behavior of gaseous substances. These laws can be seen as summaries of numerous experiments that were conducted over the course of several centuries. The importance of these laws in the development of physics and chemistry is undeniable, and their relevance to the practice of respiratory care cannot be overstated.

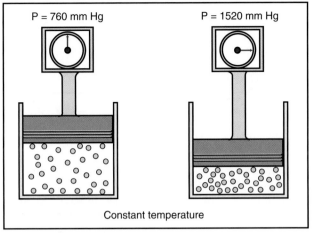

FIGURE 1.10 Boyle's law.

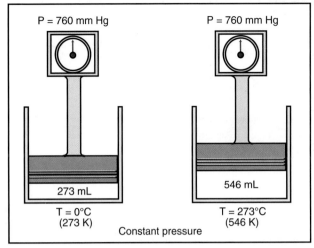

FIGURE 1.11 Charles' law.

Boyle's Law

Robert Boyle (1627-1691), a British chemist, was the first scientist to investigate the pressure–volume relationships of a gas sample systematically. Boyle found that the volume a gas occupies when it is maintained at a constant temperature is inversely proportional to the absolute pressure exerted on it, or

$$V = 1/P, \text{ or } V = k(1/P)$$

Boyle's law is illustrated in Fig. 1.10. Notice that the volume of gas in a container is reduced in half when the pressure is doubled. It is important to state that the absolute pressure of a gas equals the atmospheric pressure plus the pressure measured with a gauge. For example, the pressure of a gas compressed into a 10-L tank is measured as 29.4 psi (2 atm or 1520 mm Hg). The absolute pressure of the gas equals the atmospheric pressure (14.7 psi or 760 mm Hg) plus the gauge pressure of 29.4 psi. Thus the absolute pressure of the gas is 44.1 psi (or 3 atm).

Boyle's law can be expressed in a more useful form:

$$V_1P_1 = V_2P_2, \text{ or } V_1/V_2 = P_2/P_1$$

which allows an unknown volume or pressure to be calculated when the other variables are known. For example, one can solve for an unknown volume by rearranging the equation to read

$$V_2 = V_1P_1/P_2$$

Applications of Boyle's law can be found in a number of topics included in this text, such as the mechanics of ventilation, medical gas therapy, blood gas measurements, and pulmonary function testing, which includes spirometry and body plethysmography (see Clinical Scenario 1.1).

Charles' and Gay-Lussac's Laws

Jacques Charles (1746-1823), a French chemist, is recognized as the first scientist to demonstrate experimentally how the volume of a gas varies with changes in temperature. He showed that the volume of a given amount of gas held at a constant

CLINICAL SCENARIO 1.1

A snorkel diver is preparing to descend into a freshwater pond to a depth of 66 feet. At sea level, his lungs contain approximately 3000 mL of air. What will happen to the gas volume in his lungs as he descends to 33 feet and then to 66 feet below the surface of the pond? Remember that atmospheric pressure at sea level equals 1 atm and increases by 1 atm for every 33 feet that the diver descends below the surface. See Appendix A for the answer.

pressure increases proportionately with increases in the temperature of the gas (Fig. 1.11).[11] The relationship between volume and temperature can be explained by the fact that as the temperature of the gas increases, the KE of the gas molecules increases. This increased KE content causes the gas molecules to move more vigorously, and therefore the gas expands. Conversely, as the temperature of the gas decreases, its molecular activity diminishes, and the gas volume contracts.

William Thomson (Lord Kelvin, 1824-1907) realized the significance of these findings and suggested that there should theoretically be a temperature at which all molecular activity ceases and the associated gas volume is zero. This temperature is called *absolute zero* and has been calculated to be −273.15°C. Although the absolute zero of any substance has not been achieved in a laboratory setting, this temperature serves as a starting point for the Kelvin temperature scale. As mentioned earlier, there is a one-to-one correlation between degrees Celsius and Kelvin (i.e., 1°C corresponds to 1 K). Also, notice that temperature is expressed without degrees in the Kelvin scale (e.g., 0 K equals −273.15°C). Based on the work of Kelvin, Charles' law now is stated thusly: When the pressure of a gas is held constant, the volume of a gas varies directly with its absolute temperature expressed in Kelvin, or

$$V/T = k, \text{ or } V_1/T_1 = V_2/T_2$$

Therefore doubling the absolute temperature of a gas increases the volume of the gas twofold. Conversely, reducing

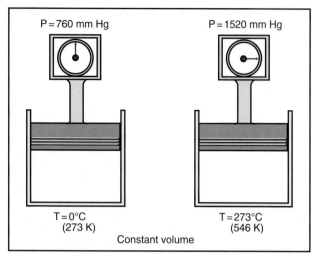

 FIGURE 1.12 Gay-Lussac's law.

 CLINICAL SCENARIO 1.2

An alarm signals that a fire has broken out in the basement of the hospital. Although the fire is confined to an area approximately 300 feet from the room where the compressed-gas cylinders are stored, you are asked to move the cylinders to a safer location. Why is it necessary to move the cylinders?
See Appendix A for the answer.

the temperature of a gas by half decreases the volume of the gas by half.

Joseph Gay-Lussac (1778-1850) extended Charles' work by showing that if the volume of a gas is held constant, the gas pressure rises as the absolute temperature of the gas increases, or

$$P/T = k, \text{ or } P_1/T_1 = P_2/T_2$$

Fig. 1.12 illustrates Gay-Lussac's law. An example of Gay-Lussac's law that might be encountered in clinical practice can be found in Clinical Scenario 1.2.

Combined Gas Law

In the discussions of the gas laws so far, it has been assumed that one or more of the variables in each law were constant. For example, Boyle's law describes the relationship between pressure and volume when temperature is constant. Charles' law specifies the relationship between temperature and volume when pressure is constant; Gay-Lussac's law describes the relationship between temperature and pressure when volume is constant.

The combined gas law describes the macroscopic behavior of gases when any or all of the variables change simultaneously. As such, the combined gas law states that the absolute pressure of a gas is inversely related to the volume it occupies and directly related to its absolute temperature, or

$$PV/T = nR$$

where *n* is the number of moles of gas (a mole is a quantity of substance with a mass equal to its molecular weight expressed in grams), and *R* is the Boltzmann universal gas constant.[3,7,8]

 CLINICAL SCENARIO 1.3

What is the new volume of a 6-L gas sample existing at 273 K and 760 mm Hg when it is heated to 37°C (310 K) and subjected to 3 atm (2280 mm Hg) of pressure?
See Appendix A for the answer.

A more practical expression of the combined gas law equation that is used throughout this text is

$$P_1 V_1 / T_1 = P_2 V_2 / T_2$$

In this form of the combined gas law, the gas constant (*R*) and the number of moles of gas (*n*) are not included, because it is assumed that they will not be affected by changes in pressure, volume, and temperature. Clinical Scenario 1.3 presents an example of a calculation using this form of the combined gas law.

Applications of the combined gas law are found throughout this text. Pressure, volume, and temperature corrections are used extensively in arterial blood gas measurements (see Chapter 10) and during cardiopulmonary function testing (see Chapters 8 and 9).

Dalton's Law of Partial Pressures

Dalton's law states that the sum of the partial pressures of a gas mixture equals the total pressure of the system. Furthermore, the partial pressure of any gas within a gas mixture is proportional to its percentage of the mixture.[7,8] The partial pressure of a gas in a mixture can be calculated by multiplying the total pressure of the mixture by the percentage of the mixture that the gas in question occupies. For example, the partial pressure of oxygen in room air when the barometric pressure equals 1 atm (760 mm Hg) can be calculated by multiplying the total barometric pressure by the percentage of oxygen in the room air. (Oxygen makes up approximately 21% of the atmosphere, or 0.21.) Therefore

$$P_{O_2} = (760)(0.21)$$
$$P_{O_2} = 159.6 \text{ mm Hg}$$

Continuing with this example, the total atmospheric pressure equals the sum of the partial pressures for oxygen (21%), nitrogen (78%), carbon dioxide (0.03%), and other trace gases (≈0.7%), or

$$P_B = P_{O_2} + P_{N_2} + P_{CO_2} + P(\text{trace gases})$$
$$P_B = (760)(0.21) + (760)(0.78) + (760)(0.0003) + (760)(0.007)$$
$$P_B = 760 \text{ mm Hg}$$

It should be noted that water vapor pressure does not follow Dalton's law, because such pressure primarily depends on temperature. Because water vapor displaces the partial pressure of other gases, the water vapor pressure (P_{H_2O}) must be subtracted from the total pressure of the gas mixture when the partial pressure of a gas saturated with water vapor is calculated.

TABLE 1.3 **Water Vapor Pressure and Content at Selected Temperatures and 760 mm Hg**	
°C	**Vapor Pressure (mm Hg)**
0	4.58
10	9.21
11	9.84
12	10.52
13	11.23
14	11.99
15	12.79
16	13.63
17	14.53
18	15.48
19	16.48
20	17.54
21	18.65
22	19.83
23	21.07
24	22.38
25	23.76
26	25.21
27	26.74
28	28.35
29	30.04
30	31.82
31	33.70
32	35.66
33	37.73
34	39.90
35	42.18
36	44.56
37	47.07
38	49.70
39	52.44
40	55.32

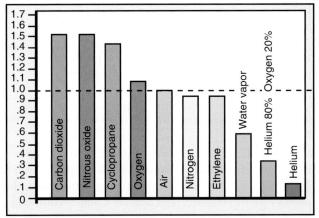

FIGURE 1.13 Specific gravity for several gases that are used in respiratory care and anesthetics. Comparisons have been made with air at 25°C and 1 atm. (Redrawn from Adriani J: *The chemistry and physics of anesthesia*, ed 3, Springfield, IL, 1979, Charles C Thomas.)

For example, to calculate the partial pressure of oxygen in a sample of gas that is saturated with water vapor at 37°C, the following formula is applied:

$$PO_2 = (P_B - P_{H_2O})(F_IO_2)$$
$$PO_2 = (760\,mm\,Hg - 47\,mm\,Hg)(0.21)$$
$$PO_2 = 149.73\,mm\,Hg$$

Notice that the vapor pressure of water at 37°C is 47 mm Hg. Table 1.3 lists the vapor pressures for water at selected temperatures.

Avogadro's Law

Avogadro's law states that equal volumes of gas at the same pressure and temperature contain the same number of molecules. It is based on the work of Amedeo Avogadro (1776-1856), who determined that 1 gram molecular weight (gmw), or mole, of any gas occupies 22.4 L at a temperature of 0°C (273 K) and a pressure of 1 atm. Subsequently, it was determined that 1 mole of gas at this volume contains 6.02×10^{23} molecules (**Avogadro's number**). For example, 1 mole of oxygen (gmw = 32 g) occupies a volume of 22.4 L and contains 6.02×10^{23} molecules when measured at 0°C (273 K) and 1 atm.

A practical application of Avogadro's law is seen in the calculation of gas densities and specific gravity. The density of a gas per unit volume can be calculated with the following formula:

$$Density(g/L) = gmw\ of\ gas/22.4\,L$$

The specific gravity of a gas is defined as the ratio of the density of a gas relative to the density of a standard gas, such as air, oxygen, or hydrogen. Fig. 1.13 shows the specific gravity of several gases used in respiratory care and anesthesia.

Laws of Diffusion

Up to this point the discussion of gases has focused on the ability of a gas to expand and to be compressed. Another property that must be discussed in any analysis of gas behavior is **diffusion**, which can be defined as the net movement of gas molecules, by virtue of their kinetic properties, from an area of high concentration to an area of low concentration. Graham's law, Henry's law, and Fick's law are used to describe diffusion and its applications in respiratory care.

Graham's Law

In 1832 Thomas Graham (1805-1869) stated that when two gases are placed under the same temperature and pressure conditions, the rates of diffusion of the two gases are inversely proportional to the square root of their masses, or

$$r_1/r_2 = \sqrt{M_2/M_1}$$

where r_1 and r_2 represent the diffusion rates of the respective gases, and M_1 and M_2 are the molar masses.

If the mass of a gas is considered directly proportional to its density at a constant temperature and pressure, then

$$r_1/r_2 = \sqrt{d_2/d_1}$$

where d_1 and d_2 are the densities of the gases in question.

Henry's Law

When a gas is confined in a space adjacent to a liquid, a certain number of gas molecules dissolve in the liquid phase. Joseph Henry (1797-1878) found that for a given temperature, the mass of a gas that dissolves (and does not combine chemically) in a specified volume of liquid is directly proportional to the product of the partial pressure of the gas and its solubility coefficient, or

$$c \alpha P \times S$$

where c is the molar concentration (in mol/L) of the dissolved gas, P is the pressure (in atm) of gas over the liquid, and S is the solubility coefficient (also known as the Bunsen coefficient) for the gas in that particular liquid (in L/atm or L/mm Hg). The solubility of a gas in a liquid is equal to the volume of gas (in liters) that will saturate 1 L of liquid at STPD (0°C and 1 atm). Henry's law is encountered in discussions of the solubility of gases, such as oxygen, in blood. In these cases the solubility of a gas is expressed in milliliters of gas dissolved in milliliters of blood. For example, it is known that 0.023 mL of oxygen dissolves in every milliliter of blood at a temperature of 38°C and 1 atm of pressure.

Fick's Law of Diffusion

Thus far we have limited our discussion to the rate of diffusion of one gas into another gas and the diffusion rate of a gas into a liquid. In respiratory physiology the diffusion of gases across semipermeable membranes (e.g., the diffusion of oxygen and carbon dioxide across the alveolar-capillary membrane) is also a concern.[12,13] A semipermeable membrane is not freely permeable to all components of a mixture. Thus the membrane may be impermeable to a substance because of its size or chemical composition (e.g., electrical charge).

Adolph Fick (1829-1901) stated that the flow of a gas across a semipermeable membrane per unit time ($\dot{V}_{gas}$) into a membrane fluid phase is directly proportional to the surface area (A) available for diffusion, the partial pressure gradient between the two compartments (ΔP), and the solubility of the gas (S). This flow is inversely proportional to the square root of the molecular weight of the gas ($\sqrt{MW}$) and the thickness of the membrane (T) (Fig. 1.14). Fick's law can be shown as

$$\dot{V}_{gas} = A \times S \times \Delta P \div \sqrt{MW} \times T$$

Considering that the diffusivity of a gas equals its solubility divided by the square root of its molecular weight, or

$$D = S \div \sqrt{MW}$$

where D is the diffusivity, S is the solubility, and MW is the molecular weight, then Fick's law can be restated as

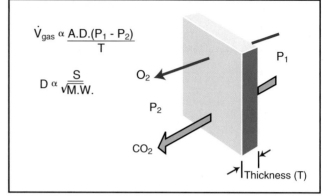

FIGURE 1.14 Fick's law of diffusion. (Modified from West JB: *Respiratory physiology: the essentials,* ed 3, Baltimore, 1985, Williams & Wilkins.)

CLINICAL SCENARIO 1.4

Using Fick's law of diffusion, describe several conditions in which the diffusion of oxygen across the alveolar-capillary membrane is reduced.

See Appendix A for the answer.

$$\dot{V}_{gas} = A \times D \times \Delta P/T$$

Test your understanding of the laws of diffusion by answering the question in Clinical Scenario 1.4.

V. FLUID MECHANICS

Fluid mechanics is the branch of physics dealing with the properties and behavior of fluids in motion. This field involves fluid dynamics, which is subdivided into hydrodynamics (the study of liquids in motion) and aerodynamics (the study of gases in motion). With diffusion, gas movement was described as being the result of the spontaneous intermingling of the individual gas molecules as a result of random thermal motion. In the subsection that follows, bulk gas flow is discussed; bulk gas flow involves the transport of whole groups of molecules (i.e., a volume of gas) from one location to another, rather than the movement of individual gas molecules.

Patterns of Flow

This text is concerned primarily with the flow of fluids through various types of tubes. Whether this flow involves the movement of liquids or gases, all fluid flow may be characterized as laminar, turbulent, or transitional in nature. Fig. 1.15 illustrates the three types of flow.

In laminar flow the fluid flows in discrete cylindrical layers, or streamlines.[8] Laminar flow normally is associated with the movement of fluids through tubes with smooth surfaces and fixed radii. With laminar flow the pressure required to produce a given flow is directly related to the viscosity of the fluid and the length of the tube and inversely related to the radius of the tube. These relationships are discussed in detail in the section on Poiseuille's law.

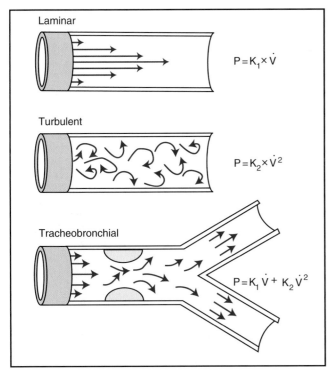

FIGURE 1.15 Three patterns of flow: laminar, turbulent, and transitional.

With turbulent flow the movement of fluid molecules becomes chaotic, and the orderly pattern of concentric layers seen with laminar flow is lost. As will be seen, Poiseuille's law cannot be used to predict the amount of pressure required for a given flow when turbulence is present. When turbulence is present, the pressure required to produce a given flow is influenced less by the viscosity of the fluid and more by its density. Additionally, the driving pressure required to achieve a given flow is proportional to the *square* of the flow. Turbulent flow occurs when the velocity at which the fluid is moving increases sharply, when the tube's radius varies, and when tubes have rough, uneven surfaces. The likelihood of turbulent flow developing can be predicted by the Reynolds number, which is discussed shortly.

Transitional flow is simply a mixture of laminar and turbulent flows. In cases when laminar flow predominates, the driving pressure varies linearly with the flow. When turbulent flow dominates, the driving pressure varies with the *square* of the flow. Transitional flow typically occurs at points where tubes divide into one or more branches. Fig. 1.15 illustrates the types of flow that can be observed as gas flows into the lungs. Gas flow in the larger airways is turbulent, but laminar flow predominates in the smaller airways. Transitional flow (or tracheobronchial flow, as it appears in Fig. 1.15) occurs at points where the airways divide (e.g., where the mainstem bronchi divide into the lobar bronchi).

Poiseuille's Law

When one considers the flow of a liquid or gas through a tube, two factors must be taken into account: the driving pressure forcing the fluid through the tube (i.e., the pressure gradient)

and the resistance the fluid must overcome as it flows through the tube. Jean L.M. Poiseuille (1797-1869), a French physiologist, described the interrelationships between pressure, flow, and resistance for a liquid flowing through an unbranched, rigid tube with the following formula:

$$\Delta P = \dot{Q} \times R$$

where ΔP is the pressure gradient from the beginning to the end of the tube ($P_1 - P_2$), $\dot{Q}$ is the flow of the liquid through the tube, and R is the resistance opposing the flow of the liquid. (Note that in discussions of the mechanics of breathing, $\dot{Q}$ is replaced with $\dot{V}$, which is used to symbolize the flow of a gas.) Poiseuille found that the factors determining resistance to flow include the viscosity of the fluid and the length and radius of the tube, or

$$R = (8\eta l)/(\pi r^4)$$

where η is the viscosity of the liquid, l is the length of the tube, and r is the radius of the tube. Incorporating these findings, Poiseuille's law can be rewritten as

$$\Delta P = \dot{Q} \times [(8\eta l)/(\pi r^4)]$$

Based on these equations, the following can be stated:
1. Poiseuille's law assumes that the fluid's flow pattern is laminar.
2. The more viscous a fluid, the greater the pressure gradient required to cause it to move through a given tube.
3. The resistance offered by a tube is directly proportional to its length; the pressure required to achieve a given flow through a tube must increase in direct proportion to the length of the tube.
4. Because the resistance to flow is inversely proportional to the fourth power of the radius, small changes in the radius of a tube cause profound decreases in the flow of the fluid through the tube. For example, decreasing the radius by one-half increases the resistance 16-fold.

Applications of Poiseuille's law are found in the discussion related to medical gas therapy, physiological pressure monitoring, and mechanical ventilation.

Reynolds Number

As was discussed earlier, fluid flow becomes turbulent when the velocity at which the liquid or gas molecules are traveling increases sharply. Several other factors also can produce turbulent flow, including changes in the density and viscosity of the gas or in the radius of the tube. These factors can be combined mathematically to determine the Reynolds number:

$$N_R = v \times d \times (2r/\eta)$$

where v is the velocity of flow, r is the radius of the tube, and d and η are the density and viscosity of the gas, respectively. The Reynolds number, which represents a ratio of momentum forces to viscous forces, provides a method to quantify the relative importance of these two types of forces for a given flow.[14] Note that the Reynolds number is dimensionless and therefore is not expressed in units of measure. Turbulent flow predominates when the Reynolds number exceeds 2000,

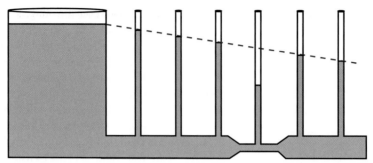

FIGURE 1.16 The Bernoulli principle. (Redrawn from Nave CR, Nave BC: *Physics for the health sciences,* ed 3, Philadelphia, 1985, WB Saunders.)

although turbulent flow may occur at lower Reynolds numbers when the surface of the tube is rough or irregular.[8]

Turbulent flow is produced by an increase in the linear velocity of the gas, the density of the gas, or the radius of the tube; it also can be produced by reductions in the viscosity of the gas. Applications of the Reynolds number are seen in the discussions of the mechanics of breathing and mechanical ventilation later in this text.

Bernoulli Principle

The Bernoulli principle is the result of work by Daniel Bernoulli (1700-1782), a Swiss mathematician who stated that as the forward velocity of a gas (or liquid) moving through a tube increases, the lateral wall pressure of the tube decreases.[7,13] This can be demonstrated using a schematic like the one shown in Fig. 1.16, which consists of a fluid flowing through a tube with a series of manometers attached to its wall. The manometers register the lateral wall pressure as the fluid flows through the tube. Notice that as the fluid flows through a tube of uniform diameter, a progressive drop in pressure occurs over the length of the tube. The gradual decrease in pressure can be determined by looking at the first three manometers in Fig. 1.16. Notice that as the fluid flows through a constriction in the tube, the pressure in the fourth manometer shows an even greater drop in pressure. If it is assumed that the total flow of liquid in the tube is the same before and after the constriction, then the velocity of flow of the liquid must accelerate as it enters the constriction (i.e., principle of continuity). Therefore it is reasonable to assume that the drop in fluid pressure is directly related to the increase in fluid speed. The Bernoulli principle is used in the design of a number of respiratory care devices (e.g., humidifiers and aerosol generators).

Venturi Principle

The Venturi principle, which is related to the work of Bernoulli, was first described by Giovanni Venturi (1746-1822) and can be illustrated with a schematic such as the one shown in Fig. 1.17. Notice that this apparatus is similar to the tube used to explain the Bernoulli principle. The Venturi principle states that the pressure that has dropped as the fluid flows through a constriction in the tube can be restored to the preconstriction pressure if a gradual dilation occurs in the tube distal to the constriction. Note that the gradual dilation of the tube must have an angle of divergence that is less than 15 degrees.[7]

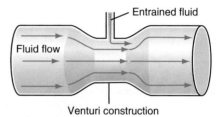

FIGURE 1.17 The Venturi principle.

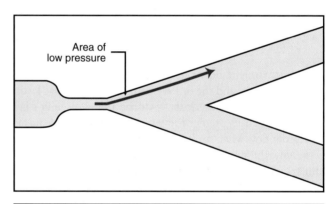

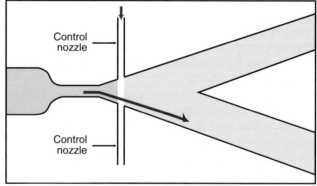

FIGURE 1.18 The Coanda effect.

Coanda Effect

The Coanda effect, which is also based on the Bernoulli principle, is illustrated in Fig. 1.18. As was previously explained, the lateral wall pressure of the tube decreases when the fluid flows through a narrowing of the tube because of the increased forward velocity of the fluid flow. If the wall does not have a side port for entraining another fluid, the low pressure adjacent to the wall draws the stream of fluid against the wall. When a specially contoured tube, such as the one in Fig. 1.18, is attached distal to the narrow part of the tube, the flow exiting the narrow part of the tube tends to adhere to the wall of the contoured tube because of two factors: (1) a negative pressure is generated past the constriction, thus drawing the fluid toward the curved extension, and (2) the ambient pressure opposite the extension pushes the fluid stream against the wall, where it remains locked until interrupted by a counter-force, such as a pulse of air.[8] Using these findings, Coanda was able to demonstrate that with careful placement of the post-constriction extensions, he could deflect a stream of air through a full 180-degree turn by extending the wall contour.[10]

The Coanda effect is the basis for fluidic devices and has been used in the design of several mechanical ventilators. Such devices use gates that are regulated by gas flow from side jets, which operate on the principle that pulses of air are used to redirect the original gas stream. The main advantage of using these fluid logic devices is that they have fewer valves and moving parts that can break (i.e., gas flow is regulated by gas jets, not typical mechanical metal or plastic valves). The primary disadvantage is that these devices consume more gas than more conventional devices because gas flow is used to power the various fluid logic gates.

VI. PRINCIPLES OF ELECTRICITY

Many respiratory care devices are powered by electricity and in many cases are also controlled by computers that use solid-state electronic circuitry. Mechanical ventilators, blood gas analyzers, physiological transducers and monitors, and strip chart and X-Y recorders are some examples. Because of the importance of these devices in respiratory therapy, a basic understanding of electronics and electrical safety is essential.

Principles of Electronics

Electricity is produced by the flow of electrons through a conductive path or circuit. Electrical current is influenced by (a) the force pushing the electrons through a conductive path (i.e., electromotive force or voltage) and (b) the resistance the electrons must overcome as they flow through the conductive path.

Electrical current, which is symbolized as I, can be measured with an ammeter. The standard unit of measurement of electrical current is the ampere (A), where 1 A is equivalent to 6.25×10^{18} electrons passing a point in 1 second. (Note that in electronics, the term *coulomb* is used as a shorthand notation for 6.25×10^{18} electrons. Thus 1 A equals 1 coulomb per second.) Amperes can be subdivided into smaller quantities, such as milliamperes (mA, or milliamp) and microamperes (μA, or microamp), using scientific notation. For example, 1 mA is $\frac{1}{1000}$ of an ampere, and 1 μA is $\frac{1}{1,000,000}$ of an ampere. Ammeters typically have scales calibrated in amperes, milliamperes, and microamperes.

As previously stated, voltage is the electrical force (more correctly termed electromotive force, or EMF) that drives electrons through the conductive path. In most physics textbooks, voltage is also described as the potential difference between two points. Voltage sources include batteries, hydro-electric generators, solar cells, and piezoelectric crystals. Voltage is measured using a voltmeter; the standard unit of measurement for voltage is the volt (V), which can be defined as the electrical potential required for 1 A of electricity to move through 1 ohm (Ω) of resistance. As with amperes, volts can be subdivided into smaller units, such as millivolts (mV) and microvolts (μV).

Resistance in electrical circuits, as with resistance in fluid circuits, is the opposition to flow. Resistance, which is measured in ohms, is a property of a conductor that is influenced by the conductor's chemical composition or specific resistance (ρ), as well as by its length and cross-sectional area. Most metals and salt solutions are good conductors (i.e., they offer low resistance to current flow). With regard to physical dimensions, the resistance of a conductor increases as its length increases or its cross-sectional area decreases. Rubber, plastic, and glass are poor conductors, because they offer high resistance to current flow. Because these materials are such poor conductors, they can be used as protective coverings on conductive wires; they therefore are often called insulators. Semiconductors are materials with conductivity characteristics that are intermediate between conductors and insulators. Semiconductors are an integral part of computer circuitry, and can also be found in thermistors and photodetectors used in diagnostic equipment.

Ohm's Law

The relationships among current, voltage, and resistance can be explained with Ohm's law:

$$V = I \times R$$

According to Ohm's law, voltage and current are directly related, which simply means that if the resistance is constant, increases in voltage cause increases in current flow. Conversely, decreases in source voltage cause a reduction in current flow (assuming resistance is constant). Now consider how changes in resistance affect current flow. If voltage is held constant, increases in resistance cause a decrease in current flow, whereas decreases in resistance cause an increase in current flow. Thus current and resistance are inversely related.

It should be apparent from this discussion that any one variable can be solved for if the other two are known. Thus, by rearranging the above equation, the current can be solved for:

$$I = V/R$$

Similarly, resistance can be solved for with the following rearrangement:

$$R = V/I$$

It is important to grasp these concepts to understand circuit analysis. These principles will now be applied in an analysis of simple electrical circuits.

Electrical Circuits

An electrical circuit consists of a voltage source, a load, and a conductive path. An applied voltage causes a current to flow through a conductive path containing one or more loads before returning to the voltage source.

Electrical circuits can be classified as series circuits and parallel circuits. Notice that in a series circuit, the current flows through one path. The current flows from the voltage source through the conductor and through a series of resistive loads, which are arranged end-to-end (i.e., through R_1, then R_2, and so on), and then back to the voltage source. In contrast, the parallel circuit may be depicted as two or more series circuits connected to a common voltage source.

One must keep in mind several principles when analyzing series and parallel circuits. These principles, which are referred to as *Kirchhoff's laws*, provide the framework for performing circuit analysis.

Kirchhoff's laws governing series circuits may be summarized as follows:

1. A series circuit can have one or more voltage sources. The total source voltage equals the sum of the individual sources if their direction of polarity is the same.
2. In a series circuit, current is the same through all components.
3. The total resistance in a series circuit can be computed by determining the sum of all resistance in the circuit. That is, $R_T = R_1 + R_2 + R_3$, and so on.
4. The sum of voltage drops across resistance in the circuit equals the applied voltage, or $V_T = IR_1 + IR_2 + IR_3$, and so on.

Parallel circuits must adhere to the following guidelines:

1. All branches of a parallel circuit have the same applied voltage.
2. Each branch of a parallel circuit may have a different current flow, depending on the resistance of the branch.
3. The total current flowing through a parallel circuit can be computed by finding the sum of the currents flowing through the various branches of the circuit. Thus, $I_T = I_1 + I_2 + I_3$, and so on.
4. The total resistance in a parallel circuit can be computed by finding the sum of the reciprocals for each resistance. That is, $R_T = 1/(1/R_1 + 1/R_2 + 1/R_3$, and so on).

Box 1.6 describes a Wheatstone bridge circuit. This type of circuitry is widely used in medical instrumentation, such as oxygen analyzers and strain gauge pressure transducers. These devices are discussed in more detail in Chapters 8 and 9.

Electrical Safety

Electrical accidents occur when current from an electrical device interacts with body tissue, impairing physiological function. It is important to recognize that electrical hazards exist only when the current path through the body is complete. That is, two connections to the body are required for an electrical shock to occur.[8,15] One connection (the "hot" wire) brings the current to the body, and the second connection (the neutral wire) completes the circuit by sending the charge to a point of lower potential or ground.

The extent of impairment depends on the amount of current flowing through the body, the duration the current is

---

BOX 1.6   Electrical Circuit Analysis: The Wheatstone Bridge

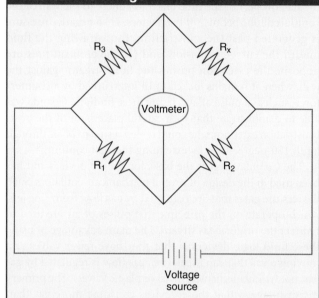

Voltage source

The Wheatstone bridge is a series-parallel circuit that consists of a direct current (DC) voltage source (e.g., a battery) and a galvanometer that connects two parallel branches containing four resistors (R_1, R_2, R_3, and R_X). The values of R_1 and R_2 are known, and R_3 is a calibrated variable resistance, for which the current value may be read from a dial on the galvanometer. The unknown resistor (R_X) is connected to the fourth side of the circuit. As the resistance of the unknown resistor changes (e.g., changes in the resistance of R_X occur when the physical dimensions of the wire are altered, such as when pressure is applied to the resistance wire), the variable resistance of R_3 is adjusted until the galvanometer reads zero.

The Wheatstone bridge circuit actually was first described by Samuel Hunter Christie in 1833. Sir Charles Wheatstone was later responsible for developing practical uses for the circuit. For example, the Wheatstone bridge is ideal for measuring small changes in resistance; it therefore can be used in devices such as the strain gauge pressure transducer, which is used to measure blood pressure in the critical care setting.

---

applied, and the path the current takes through the body.[8] Fig. 1.19 shows the approximate current ranges and the physiological effects of a 1-second exposure to various levels of 110-V, 60-Hz alternating currents applied externally to the body.[15]

Two types of electrical shock hazards usually are described: macroshock and microshock. A macroshock occurs when a relatively high current is applied to the body surface. Generally, a current of 1 mA is required to elicit a macroshock. A microshock occurs when a low current (usually less than 1 mA) is allowed to bypass the body surface and flow directly into the body.

Electrical current can damage body tissues by causing thermal burns and inadvertently stimulating excitable tissue, such as cardiac muscle. Burns are caused when electric energy dissipates in body tissues, causing the temperature of the

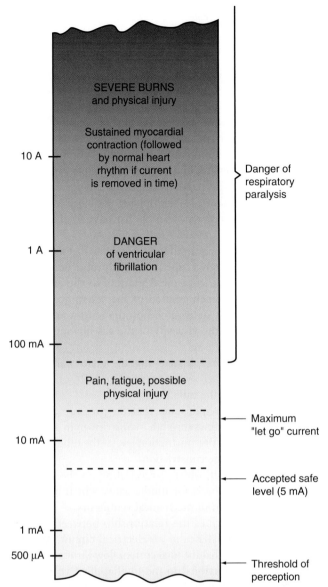

FIGURE 1.19 Physiological effects of electrical current associated with a 1-second external contact with a 110-V alternating current (AC) at 60 Hz. (Redrawn from Cromwell L, Weibell FJ, Pfeiffer EA: *Biomedical instrumentation and measurements*, ed 2, ©1980. Reprinted by permission of Pearson Education, Inc., New York, New York.)

tissues to rise. If the temperature gets high enough, it can cause severe burns. Inadvertent stimulation of excitable tissue can occur when an extraneous electrical current of sufficient magnitude causes local voltages that can trigger action potentials. Action potentials triggered in sensory nerves cause a tingling sensation that is associated with electrical shock. Action potentials generated in motor nerves and muscles result in muscle contractions, which, if the intensity of the stimulation is high enough, can cause tetanus or sustained contraction of the muscle.

It should be noted that the heart is the organ most susceptible to electrical hazards. Its susceptibility to electrical hazards

arises from the fact that when current exceeds a certain value, extra systolic contractions can occur in cardiac muscle. Further increases in current can cause the heart to fibrillate and ultimately can cause sustained myocardial contraction.

Preventing Electrical Hazards

Various strategies should be used to reduce the likelihood of electrical accidents. These include ensuring proper grounding of medical equipment, installing ground-fault circuit interrupters, and avoiding contact with transcutaneous conductors.[15]

Grounding

The principle of the grounding protection method for medical equipment is to provide a low-resistance conductive path that allows most fault current (short-circuit current) to bypass the patient and return to ground. In cord-connected electrical equipment, this ground connection is established by a third round or U-shaped contact in the plug.

It is important to recognize that grounding is effective only if a good ground connection exists. Worn or broken wires, inadvertent disconnection of ground wires from receptacles, and deliberate removal of ground contacts from plugs interfere with the protection associated with grounding. Because conventional receptacles, line cords, and plugs do not hold up to hospital use, most manufacturers provide hospital-grade receptacles and plugs that must meet UL specifications. Hospital-grade receptacles and plugs usually can be identified by a green dot.[14]

Ground-Fault Circuit Interrupters

Normally, all the power entering a device through the hot wire returns through the neutral wire. Circuit interrupters monitor the difference between the hot and neutral wires of the power line with a differential transformer and an electrical amplifier. When this difference exceeds a predetermined level (e.g., 5 mA), as occurs when the current bypasses the neutral wire and flows through the patient, the power is interrupted by a circuit breaker. Notice that this interruption occurs rapidly so that the patient does not encounter any harmful effects.

Avoiding Contact With Transcutaneous Conductors

The resistance offered by the skin represents the greatest part of the body's electrical resistance.[15] This resistance can be significantly reduced by permeating the skin with conductive fluid, by cuts and abrasions to the epithelium, or by the introduction of needles through the skin's surface. Electrically conductive catheters inserted through a vein or artery can also bypass the natural electrical resistance offered by the skin.

It should be apparent from the discussion so far that these conditions could place patients in compromised states and make them susceptible to microshock hazards. These hazardous effects can be lessened if all electrical devices used with a microshock-sensitive patient are well insulated and connected to outlets with a common low-resistance ground.[8] Additionally, devices should be inspected regularly for frayed or bare wires.

KEY POINTS

- Kinetic energy is the energy that an object possesses when it is in motion; PE is stored energy, or the energy that it possesses because of its position.
- The physical and chemical properties of all matter can be explained by the kinetic theory. The physical state of any substance is determined by the relationship between its KE content and the PE stored in its intermolecular bonds.
- Changes in state involve the interconversion of solids, liquids, and gases, which can be accomplished by altering the relationship between a substance's kinetic and potential energies.
- The amount of heat that must be added to effect the change of a solid to a liquid (latent heat of fusion) or a liquid to a gas (latent heat of vaporization) depends on the intermolecular attractive forces that must be overcome. The rate of evaporation increases with an increase in temperature, an increase in surface area, or a decrease in pressure.
- A vapor is the gaseous form of any substance that can exist as a liquid or a solid at ordinary pressures and temperatures.
- Standard temperature and pressure (STPD) is defined as 0°C, 760 mm Hg, and dry.
- Three temperature scales are routinely used in science and medicine. The SI units for temperature are based on the Kelvin scale, whereas the metric unit for temperature is the Celsius scale. The Fahrenheit scale is used in the English system of units.
- The Kelvin scale is used when describing physical laws, and the Celsius and Fahrenheit scales are used to quantify temperature measurements in the scientific literature and clinical medicine.
- Pressure is defined as the force that a gas exerts over a given area, or $P = F/A$. The pressure units most often used in respiratory care include mm Hg, cm H_2O, torr, kPa, and psi or lb/in^2.
- The density of a substance is a measure of its mass or weight per unit volume under standard conditions of temperature and pressure. The specific gravity of a liquid or gas is a comparison of its weight density relative to a standard, such as water in the case of a liquid or air in the case of gas.
- The gas laws are important generalizations about the behavior of gases. The combined gas law expresses the relationship between V, P, T, and mass for any gas. Applications of the combined gas law can be found in blood gas and pulmonary function measurements.
- According to Dalton's law, the partial pressure of a gas is the absolute pressure of that gas in a multiple gas mixture. For example, the partial pressure of oxygen in room air can be calculated by multiplying the barometric pressure by 0.21 or the percentage of oxygen that makes up room air.
- Poiseuille's law can be used to demonstrate that the laminar flow of gas through a tube is directly proportional to the pressure gradient from the beginning to the end of the tube and is inversely related to the resistance to flow. The resistance is determined by the length and radius of the tube and the viscosity of the gas flowing through the tube.
- The Bernoulli principle states that the lateral wall pressure of a tube decreases as the forward velocity of the fluid moving through the tube increases.
- The Venturi principle states that the pressure drop that occurs as a fluid flows through a constriction in a tube can be restored to the preconstriction level if the tube gradually dilates distal to the constriction.
- The Coanda effect, which is a variation on the Bernoulli principle, is the basis for fluidic gates, which have been used in the design of mechanical ventilators.
- Ohm's law describes the relationship between voltage, current, and resistance in an electrical circuit. As such, Ohm's law states that the total current flow through a circuit is directly proportional to the total applied voltage and inversely related to the total resistance of the circuit.
- The most effective methods for reducing the likelihood of electrical accidents include using proper grounding of all electrical equipment, installing ground-fault circuit interrupters, and avoiding transcutaneous conductors.

ASSESSMENT QUESTIONS

See Appendix B for the answers.

1. Convert the following temperatures:
   a. _____ °C = 102°F
   b. 25°C = _____ °F
   c. _____ K = 98.6°F
   d. 37°C = _____ K

2. Perform the following pressure conversions:
   a. _____ kPa = 30 cm H_2O
   b. _____ mm Hg = 1033 cm H_2O
   c. 20 cm H_2O = _____ mm Hg
   d. _____ lb/in^2 = 2 atm

3. Calculate the partial pressures of each of the following gases in room air when the barometric pressure is 760 mm Hg (assume that room air contains 21% oxygen, 78% nitrogen, and 0.03% carbon dioxide):
   a. PO_2 = _____ mm Hg
   b. PN_2 = _____ mm Hg
   c. PCO_2 = _____ mm Hg

4. What is the total pressure of a gas mixture if PO_2 = 90 mm Hg, PCO_2 = 40 mm Hg, PN_2 = 573 mm Hg, and PH_2O = 47 mm Hg?
   a. 573 mm Hg
   b. 713 mm Hg
   c. 750 mm Hg
   d. 760 mm Hg

5. A compressed-gas cylinder at 760 mm Hg and 25°C is moved into a room where the temperature is 38°C. What is the new pressure of the cylinder, assuming that the volume of gas within the cylinder remains constant?

6. A patient's lung capacity is measured as 6 L at an initial temperature of 25°C and an ambient pressure of 760 mm Hg. What will the new volume be if the temperature increases to 37°C and the pressure to 1520 mm Hg?

7. Calculate the densities of oxygen and carbon dioxide. The molecular weight of oxygen is 32 gmw, and the molecular weight of carbon dioxide is 44 gmw.

8. According to Poiseuille's law, the gas flow through a tube is inversely proportional to the:
   1. length of the tube
   2. driving pressure of the gas through the tube
   3. viscosity of the gas
   4. radius of the tube
      a. 1 and 3 only
      b. 2 and 4 only
      c. 1, 2, and 3 only
      d. 2, 3, and 4 only

9. Which of the following will increase the flow of a gas across a semipermeable membrane, according to Fick's law of diffusion?
   1. Increasing the surface area of the membrane
   2. Increasing the partial pressure gradient of the gas across the membrane
   3. Increasing the density of the gas
   4. Increasing the thickness of the membrane
      a. 1 and 2 only
      b. 3 and 4 only
      c. 1, 2, and 3 only
      d. 2, 3, and 4 only

10. Which of the following variables will lead to an increase in turbulent airflow?
    1. Increased density of the gas
    2. Decreased linear velocity of the gas flow

3. Increased radius of the conducting tube
4. Decreased viscosity of the gas
   a. 1 and 3 only
   b. 2 and 4 only
   c. 1, 2, and 3 only
   d. 1, 3, and 4 only

11. What is the total current flowing through an electrical circuit containing a 100-V power source and a total resistance of 50 Ω?

12. List three strategies that can be used to protect patients from electrical hazards.

13. Calculate the energy cost of operating a 1000-W air compressor for 24 hours if the electrical energy cost is 10 cents per kilowatt-hour.

14. Macroshock can occur when a person has a 1-second external contact with a 110-V alternating current (AC) at 60 Hz. What is generally considered the minimum current the person must contact to experience macroshock?
    a. 100 μA
    b. 1 mA
    c. 10 mA
    d. 1 A

15. A respiratory therapist traveling from Chicago, Illinois, to Denver, Colorado, notices that he becomes short of breath while walking to the luggage area of the airport. His wife, who is also a respiratory therapist, comments that his breathlessness is caused by the thinness of the air in Denver. He says that he knew that could explain the breathlessness, but he also remembered that the air in Denver contains 21% oxygen, just like in Chicago. Bemused by his comment, his wife asks him what is the PO_2 of the air in Denver. Note that the barometric pressure in Denver was recorded as 630 mm Hg.
    a. 147 mm Hg
    b. 132 mm Hg
    c. 122 mm Hg
    d. 90 mm Hg

REFERENCES

1. Feynman R: *Six easy pieces*, Reading, MA, 1995, Addison-Wesley.
2. Krauskoff KB, Beiser A: *The physical universe*, ed 15, New York, 2013, McGraw-Hill.
3. Asimov I: *Understanding physics*, New York, 1993, Barnes & Noble Books.
4. Bevelacqua JJ: *Basic health physics*, New York, 1999, Wiley-Interscience.
5. Brown TE, Lemay HE, Burstein BE, et al.: *Chemistry: the central science*, ed 13, New York, 2015.
6. Haynes WH, editor: *CRC handbook of chemistry and physics*, ed 97, Cleveland, 2016, CRC Press.
7. Nave CR, Nave BC: *Physics for the health sciences*, ed 3, Philadelphia, 1985, WB Saunders.
8. Kacmarek RM, Stoller JK, Heuer A, editors: *Egan's fundamentals of respiratory care*, ed 11, St. Louis, 2017, Elsevier-Mosby.
9. Wojciechowski WV: *Respiratory care sciences: an integrated approach*, ed 5, Albany, NY, 2014, Delmar.
10. Davis PD, Kenny GNC: *Basic physics and measurement in anaesthesia*, ed 5, Oxford, 2003, Butterworth-Heinemann.
11. Adriani J: *The chemistry and physics of anesthesia*, ed 3, Springfield, IL, 1979, Charles C Thomas.
12. Levitzky MG: *Pulmonary physiology*, ed 8, New York, 2013, McGraw-Hill.
13. Guyton AC, Hall JE: *Textbook of medical physiology*, ed 13, Philadelphia, 2015, Saunders.
14. Falkovich G: *Fluid mechanics*, Cambridge, UK, 2011, Cambridge University Press.
15. Cromwell L, Weibell FJ, Pfeiffer EA: *Biomedical instrumentation and measurements*, ed 2, New York, 1979, Prentice-Hall.

Principles of Infection Control

OBJECTIVES

Upon completion of this chapter, you will be able to:

1. Identify the major groups of microorganisms associated with nosocomial pneumonia.
2. List four factors that can influence the effectiveness of a germicide.
3. Define the terms *high-level disinfection, intermediate-level disinfection,* and *low-level disinfection.*
4. Describe the process of pasteurization and its application to the disinfection of respiratory care equipment.
5. Explain how quaternary ammonium compounds, alcohols, acetic acid, phenols, glutaraldehyde, hydrogen peroxide, and iodophors and other halogenated compounds are used as disinfectants.
6. Name the four physical methods commonly used to sterilize medical devices.
7. Discuss the principle of ethylene oxide sterilization.
8. Identify infection-risk devices used in respiratory care.
9. Describe three components of an effective infection surveillance program.
10. Compare standard precautions with transmission-based precautions.
11. List the most common agents associated with febrile respiratory illnesses that are potential causes of mass casualty events.

KEY TERMS

acid-fast bacillus
acid-fast stain
aerobes
airborne
airborne precautions
anaerobes
autoclave
autotrophs
bacilli
bactericide
chemical sterilant
cleaning
cocci
contact precautions
decontamination
diplobacilli
diplococci
direct contact

disinfecting
droplet precautions
endospores
eukaryotic
facultative
fomite
fungicides
germicide
Gram stain
Gram-negative
Gram-positive
health care–associated infections (HAIs)
heterotrophs
high-level disinfection
indirect contact
infection surveillance
intermediate-level disinfectants

isolation techniques
low-level disinfectants
normal flora
nosocomial
pasteurization
pathogenic
prokaryotic
spirochetes
standard precautions
staphylococci
sterilizing
streptobacilli
streptococci
transmission-based precautions
universal precautions
vegetative cells
vehicles
virucides

Preventing health care–associated infections (HAIs) is a formidable task for respiratory therapists. It is particularly challenging because devices used for respiratory care are potential reservoirs and vehicles (e.g., water, medications) for the transmission of infectious microorganisms. Additionally, many patients receiving respiratory care, especially those of extreme age (i.e., very young or very old) or who are recovering from thoracoabdominal surgery, have an increased risk for developing nosocomial pneumonia. Underlying diseases, the presence of an artificial airway, depressed sensorium, and immunosuppression can also add to the risk for acquiring a nosocomial infection.[1]

This chapter reviews the basic principles of microbiology and infection control that respiratory care practitioners must understand to prevent HAIs. Specifically, the following are described: (1) the microorganisms most often associated with nosocomial pneumonia; (2) the accepted methods for cleaning, disinfecting, and sterilizing reusable respiratory care equipment; (3) effective methods of infection surveillance; and (4) the proper use of isolation techniques to prevent person-to-person transmission of microorganisms.

I. PRINCIPLES OF CLINICAL MICROBIOLOGY

Microbiology is the study of microorganisms such as bacteria, viruses, protozoa, fungi, and algae. All of these organisms, with the possible exception of algae, are pathogenic and therefore can produce infectious diseases in susceptible hosts.[1] Clinical microbiology is primarily concerned with the isolation, identification, and control of pathogenic, or disease-producing, organisms.

The active participation of clinical microbiologists in infection control is essential for the identification and treatment of nosocomial infections, as well as for the prevention of these diseases. The process of identifying the infectious agent responsible for the nosocomial infection is fairly straightforward. Diagnosis of an infectious disease requires isolation of the suspected pathogen from the site of infection. The specimen then is inoculated onto agar or into a broth containing vital nutrients and incubated for a specified period. In many cases the organism is allowed to grow at body temperature in a specially designed incubator. It is important that those performing the collection process use aseptic techniques to prevent microbial contamination from adjacent tissue and normal flora. Normal microbial flora are microorganisms normally found in or on a particular body site. These organisms typically do not usually cause infectious disease, but they can present problems because they can overgrow the pathogen and produce erroneous results.

Identification of microorganisms is most often accomplished by direct examination of the specimen through microscopy with the aid of biological staining techniques. Metabolic and immunological tests may also help clinical microbiologists discern the nature of the invading microbe, especially with regard to its susceptibility to antibiotics.

Control of pathogenic microorganisms is based on the elimination of infections and prevention of the spread of infectious diseases through infection control techniques. Infections that overwhelm a person's immune system usually are eradicated by enhancing the host's innate immunity with antibiotics and immunizations. Decontamination of diagnostic and therapeutic medical equipment, furniture, and commonly used items and surfaces, as well as the use of barrier precautions (i.e., isolation precautions), are examples of infection control techniques.

Survey of Microorganisms

A variety of microorganisms can be isolated from the hospital environment. A brief description of the major groups of pathogenic organisms associated with hospital-acquired pneumonia follows. More detailed information about the science of microbiology can be found in the references listed at the end of the chapter.[2,3]

Bacteria

Bacteria are prokaryotic, unicellular organisms that range in size from 0.5 to 50 μm. Bacteria generally are classified according to their morphology (shape) and their staining and metabolic characteristics. Certain bacteria also can produce endospores, which are intermediate bacterial forms that develop in response to adverse condition. As discussed later in this chapter, bacterial endospores can regenerate to vegetative cells when conditions improve.

As Fig. 2.1 shows, the primary bacterial shapes are cocci (spherical), bacilli (rodlike), and spirochetes (spiral). Cocci that occur in irregular clusters are called staphylococci. Cocci and bacilli that occur in pairs are called diplococci and diplobacilli, respectively; chains of cocci and bacilli are called streptococci and streptobacilli, respectively.

The classification of bacteria according to their staining characteristics usually is accomplished with simple staining techniques, such as the Gram stain and the acid-fast stain. A Gram stain separates bacteria into two general classes: those that retain an initial gentian violet stain after an alcohol wash (Gram positive) and those that do not retain the initial violet stain (Gram negative). Gram-positive organisms appear blue or violet; Gram-negative organisms have a red appearance that results from a counterstain of the red dye safranin. Notable

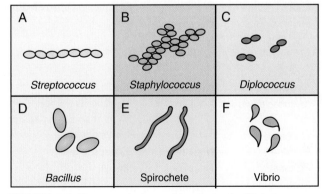

FIGURE 2.1 The morphology of bacteria. A, *Streptococcus*. B, *Staphylococcus*. C, *Diplococcus*. D, *Bacillus*. E, Spirochete. F, Vibrio.

Gram-positive pathogens are *Bacillus anthracis, Streptococcus pneumoniae, Staphylococcus aureus, Corynebacterium diphtheriae,* and *Clostridium* sp. (e.g., *C. botulinum, C. perfringens, C. tetani*). Gram-negative pathogens include *Pseudomonas aeruginosa, Acinetobacter baumannii, Escherichia coli, Klebsiella pneumoniae, Haemophilus influenzae, Serratia marcescens, Bordetella pertussis, Neisseria meningitidis,* and *Legionella pneumophila.*[2] Clinical Scenario 2.1 provides a clinical scenario that shows how Gram stains can be used in the differential diagnosis of lower respiratory tract infections.

Acid-fast stains (also called *Ziehl-Neelsen stains*) are used to identify bacteria that belong to the genus *Mycobacterium.* These microbes retain a red (carbol-fuchsin) dye after an acid wash, thus acid-fast bacillus is used synonymously with *Mycobacterium. Mycobacterium tuberculosis* organisms are responsible for pulmonary, spinal, and miliary tuberculosis. The incidence of tuberculosis has increased during the past decade, especially in patients infected with the human immunodeficiency virus (HIV; see the following discussion of viruses).

Metabolic characterization of bacteria usually involves identifying the substrate requirements for growth or the production of specific enzymes by the microbe. For example, bacteria require moisture and a source of nutrients for optimum growth. Organisms that require simple inorganic nutrients to sustain themselves are called autotrophs, whereas bacteria that require complex organic nutrients are referred to as heterotrophs. Atmospheric requirements can vary considerably among bacteria. Bacteria that require oxygen for growth are called aerobes, and those that can grow without oxygen are called anaerobes. Facultative anaerobes are bacteria that have limited oxygen tolerance. Although bacteria can be found in environments with temperatures ranging from −5°C to 80°C, pathogenic organisms typically grow at temperatures between 20°C and 40°C.[4] Metabolic characterizations may also involve the identification of various enzymes required for optimum growth of the organism. Examples of enzyme markers commonly quantified include catalase and coagulase.

As mentioned previously, certain bacteria form endospores under adverse conditions. Endospores are metabolically active life forms that can maintain their viability in the presence of dryness, heat, and poor nutrition. Their robust nature makes them especially resistant to disinfectants and a constant source of concern for infection control personnel. The most notable sources of bacterial endospores are from the aerobic *Bacillus* sp. and the anaerobic *Clostridium* sp.

Table 2.1 lists some commonly encountered bacterial genera, along with a summary of their morphological, staining, and metabolic characteristics.

Viruses

Viruses are submicroscopic parasites that consist of a nucleic acid core surrounded by a protein sheath. They range in size from 20 to 200 nm. Viruses typically are described as nonliving because they must invade a living organism to replicate. Viruses generally are classified according to their structure (i.e., icosahedral, helical, or complex) and nucleic acid content (i.e., deoxyribonucleic acid [DNA] or ribonucleic acid [RNA]).

⚖ CLINICAL SCENARIO 2-1

Laboratory examination of a sputum sample from a febrile patient with a productive cough (purulent, blood-streaked sputum) reveals the presence of Gram-positive diplococci and many segmented neutrophils. Suggest a possible diagnosis based on these findings.

See Appendix A for the answer.

TABLE 2.1 Commonly Encountered Bacteria Along With Morphological, Staining, and Metabolic Characteristics

Genus	Gram Stain	Shape/Configuration	Aerobe/Anaerobe	Species
Acinetobacter	Negative	Bacillus	Aerobe	*A. baumannii*
Bacillus	Positive	Bacillus, chains, spore forming	Aerobe	*B. anthracis*
Clostridium	Negative	Bacillus, single cell, chains, pairs, palisade, spore forming	Anaerobe	*C. tetani, C. botulinum, C. perfringens*
Diplococcus	Positive	Coccus, encapsulated pairs	Aerobe	*D. pneumoniae*
Escherichia	Negative	Bacillus	Aerobe, facultative anaerobe	*E. coli*
Haemophilus	Negative	Bacillus	Aerobe	*H. influenzae, H. haemolyticus, H. parainfluenzae*
Klebsiella	Negative	Bacillus	Aerobe	*K. pneumoniae*
Mycobacterium	Positive	Bacillus, single cell, or "cords" with two chains in a parallel arrangement	Acid-fast, aerobe	*M. tuberculosis, M. leprae*
Neisseria	Negative	Coccus, pairs	Aerobe	*N. meningitidis*
Proteus	Negative	Bacillus	Aerobe, facultative anaerobe	*P. mirabilis, P. vulgaris*
Pseudomonas	Negative	Bacillus	Aerobe, facultative anaerobe	*P. aeruginosa*
Staphylococcus	Positive	Coccus, grapelike clusters,	Aerobe, facultative anaerobe	*S. aureus*
Streptococcus	Positive	Coccus, grapelike clusters	Aerobe	Groups A, B, C, and D

Viruses also can be differentiated by the type of host they invade (i.e., animal, plant, or bacteria).

Table 2.2 lists the most commonly encountered pathogenic viruses. They include the influenza viruses, paramyxoviruses, adenoviruses, coronaviruses, rhinoviruses, enteroviruses, herpes viruses, rubella viruses, hepatitis virus, and HIV. Viruses are responsible for a number of respiratory illnesses, including the common cold, croup, tracheobronchitis, bronchiolitis, severe acute respiratory syndrome (SARS), Middle East respiratory syndrome (MERS), and pneumonia. The hepatitis

TABLE 2.2 Commonly Encountered Pathogenic Viruses

Virus	Transmission Route	Diseases
Influenza A	Respiratory tract	Tracheobronchitis Pneumonia Susceptibility to bacterial pneumonia
Paramyxoviruses Mumps	Respiratory tract	Parotitis Orchitis Pancreatitis Encephalitis
Measles (rubeola)	Respiratory tract	Rash, systemic illness Pneumonia Encephalomyelitis
Parainfluenza	Respiratory tract	Upper respiratory disease Croup, pneumonia
Respiratory syncytial virus	Respiratory tract	Bronchitis Bronchiolitis Pneumonia
Adenoviruses	Respiratory tract Conjunctivae	Tracheobronchitis Pharyngitis Conjunctivitis
Coronavirus	Respiratory tract Gastrointestinal tract	Severe acute respiratory syndrome (SARS) Middle East respiratory syndrome (MERS)
Rhinoviruses	Respiratory tract	Rhinitis Pharyngitis
Enteroviruses Coxsackie	Respiratory tract Gut	Systemic infections Meningitis Tracheobronchitis Myocarditis
Polio	Gut	Central nervous system damage (including anterior horn cells, paralysis)
Herpes Viruses Herpes simplex	Oral Genital Eye	Blisters, latent infection Keratoconjunctivitis
Varicella Herpes zoster	Respiratory tract	Vesicles—all ectodermal tissues (skin, mouth, respiratory tract)
Cytomegalovirus	Not known	Usually disseminated disease in newborns and immunodeficient individuals
Rubella	Respiratory tract	Systemic mild illness, rash, congenital anomalies in embryo
Hepatitis	Blood, body fluids	Hepatitis Systemic disease
Rabies	Bites or saliva on cut	Fatal nervous system damage
HIV	Blood, body fluids	Acquired immunodeficiency syndrome (AIDS)

HIV, Human immunodeficiency virus.

viruses and HIV are particularly important pathogens because they are spread by direct contact (i.e., through sexual contact or blood and serum). Standard isolation precautions are designed to prevent the transmission of these types of infections. Isolation precautions for blood-borne pathogens are discussed in detail later in this chapter.

Rickettsiae and *Chlamydiae* Spp.

Rickettsiae and *Chlamydiae* spp. are unusual microorganisms that are intracellular parasites. Organisms of both species are less than 1 μm in diameter. Their complex structures resemble that of bacteria, but they act like viruses because they require a living host to replicate.[4] *Rickettsiae* spp. are transmitted by insects (e.g., lice, fleas, ticks), and *Chlamydiae* spp. are transmitted by contact or the airborne route. Common rickettsial diseases include typhus, Rocky Mountain spotted fever, and Q fever. (Note that Q fever is spread by the aerosol route rather than by insect vectors.) Chlamydial infections are also associated with pneumonia, sinusitis, pharyngitis, and bronchiolitis.[4]

Protozoa

Protozoa are unicellular eukaryotes that occur singly or in colonies. Protozoan infections are common in tropical climates, especially where sanitation is poor or lacking. Common examples of protozoan infections include amebiasis, malaria, and trypanosomiasis.

Fungi

Fungi are eukaryotic organisms that include molds and yeast. Molds consist of chains of cells or filaments called *hyphae* and reproduce asexually by forming spores. Yeasts are unicellular fungi that reproduce sexually or asexually by budding. Fungal infections or mycoses can occur in otherwise normal healthy individuals. Causative organisms in these individuals include *Histoplasma capsulatum*, *Coccidioides immitis*, and *Blastomyces dermatitidis*.[3,4] Opportunistic fungal infections can occur in patients with compromised immune function (i.e., patients with HIV, transplant patients being treated with immunosuppressant drugs, and cancer patients receiving chemotherapy). Fungal infections in this latter group of patients are most often caused by *Candida albicans*, *Pneumocystis jiroveci*, and *Aspergillus fumigatus*.[3,4]

Transmission of Infectious Diseases

The public's awareness of infectious diseases has increased dramatically during the last two decades with the emergence of HIV and acquired immunodeficiency syndrome (AIDS), the Ebola and SARS viruses, H_1N_1, and the threat of bioterrorism. It is important to recognize that the transmission of infectious diseases requires three elements: (1) a source of pathogens, (2) a mode of transmission for the infectious agent, and (3) a susceptible host.

Bacteria most often cause hospital-acquired pneumonia; viruses and fungi contribute to a lesser extent. It is worth noting that although the most common source of pathogenic microorganisms is infected patients, contaminated water, food, and medications can also be sources of infectious material.

BOX 2.1   Pathogenic Organisms Commonly Associated With Ventilator-Associated Pneumonia

Gram-Negative Aerobes
Pseudomonas aeruginosa
Klebsiella pneumoniae
Escherichia spp.
Serratia marcescens
Acinetobacter calcoaceticus-baumannii
Proteus mirabilis
Haemophilus pneumoniae

Gram-Positive Aerobes
Staphylococcus aureus
Streptococcus pneumoniae

Gram-Negative Anaerobes
Bacteroides fragilis

Fungi
Candida albicans

Others
Legionella pneumophila
SARS virus
MERS virus
Influenza A virus

MERS, Middle East respiratory virus; *SARS,* severe acute respiratory syndrome.

Ventilator-associated pneumonia (VAP) represents an important subset of hospital-acquired infections affecting critically ill patients. Box 2.1 provides a list of microorganisms typically associated with VAP.[5] A discussion of the various strategies that can be used to prevent VAP is presented later in this chapter.

Infectious particles can be transmitted by four routes: contact, vehicles, airborne, and vectors (Table 2.3). Direct contact occurs when the infectious organism is physically transferred from a contaminated person to a susceptible host through touching or sexual contact. Indirect contact involves transfer of the infectious agent to a susceptible host via a fomite (e.g., clothing, surgical bandages and instruments, and equipment that have not been properly cleaned and sterilized).[2] Transfer of infectious materials by vehicles most often occurs through contaminated water and food, although intravenous fluids, blood and blood products, and medications can also occasionally harbor infectious particles.[6] Airborne or respiratory transmission involves the transfer of infectious particles through aerosol droplets or dust particles. Infectious agents are transferred by the vector route when an insect transfers the infectious particle from a host to susceptible individual.[4] Transmission of infections by vectors is rarely associated with nosocomial infections. Clinical Scenario 2.2 presents an exercise to test your understanding of infection transmission.

A variety of mechanical and immunological factors usually protect the host from becoming infected with pathogenic organisms.[6] Alterations in mechanical barriers that occur when the skin and mucous membranes are breached during surgery,

TABLE 2.3 Routes of Infectious Disease Transmission

Mode	Type	Examples
Contact	Direct	Hepatitis A Venereal disease HIV *Staphylococcus* spp. Enteric bacteria
	Indirect	*Pseudomonas* spp. Enteric bacteria Hepatitis B and C HIV
	Droplet	Measles *Streptococcus* spp.
Vehicle	Waterborne	Shigellosis Cholera
	Foodborne	Salmonellosis Hepatitis A
Airborne	Aerosols	Influenza A–H_1N_1 SARS MERS
	Droplet nuclei	Tuberculosis Diphtheria
	Dust	Histoplasmosis
Vector-borne	Ticks and mites Mosquitoes Fleas	Rickettsia, Lyme disease Malaria, Zika virus Bubonic plague

HIV, Human immunodeficiency virus; *MERS*, Middle East respiratory virus; *SARS*, severe acute respiratory syndrome.

CLINICAL SCENARIO 2-2

As previously discussed, infectious agents can be transmitted by a variety of means, including contact, droplet, airborne, and vector routes. Identify the most probable means of transmission for the following infectious particles:
- *P. aeruginosa* organisms
- Human immunodeficiency virus (HIV)
- *M. tuberculosis* organisms
- Malaria

See Appendix A for the answer.

endotracheal intubation, or placement of indwelling catheters can significantly increase an individual's risk for developing a nosocomial infection. Defects in immune function that occur because of an underlying disease or as a result of therapeutic interventions (e.g., radiation therapy, pharmacological therapies) can also increase the risk for infection. Table 2.4 lists several conditions, possible precipitating causes, and common pathogens associated with hospitalized patients at risk for developing nosocomial infections.

II. INFECTION CONTROL METHODS

The purpose of any hospital infection control program is to prevent the spread of nosocomial infections. The two most important concepts to understand about infection control

are decontamination of patient care items and isolation precautions.

Decontamination, or the removal of pathogenic microorganisms from medical equipment, is accomplished by cleaning, disinfection, and sterilization with an appropriate germicide (i.e., an agent that destroys pathogenic microorganisms). *Cleaning* is the removal of all foreign material, particularly organic matter (e.g., blood, serum, pus, fecal matter) from objects with hot water, soap, detergent, and enzymatic products. *Disinfection* is the removal of most pathogenic microorganisms except bacterial endospores. Liquid chemicals and pasteurization are the most common disinfection methods used. *Sterilization* is the elimination of all forms of microbial life. It can be accomplished with either physical or chemical processes.

Factors Influencing the Effectiveness of Germicides

As was previously stated, germicides are agents used to destroy pathogenic microorganisms. Germicides destroy these microorganisms by damaging their cell membranes, denaturing their proteins, or disrupting their cellular processes.[2] Bactericides destroy all pathogenic bacteria, virucides destroy viruses, and fungicides kill fungi. *Germicide* is a general term used to describe an agent that destroys pathogenic microorganisms on living tissue and inanimate objects; *disinfectant* is used to describe agents that destroy pathogenic microorganisms on inanimate objects only.[7] Antiseptics are germicidal agents that are applied on the skin or living tissue to destroy pathogenic microbes.

A number of factors can affect disinfection and sterilization, including the number, location, and innate resistance of the microorganisms; the concentration and potency of the germicide; the duration of exposure to the germicide; and the physical and chemical environments in which the germicide is used.[8] A brief discussion of several key points to remember when using germicides follows.

Number and Location of Microorganisms

The amount of time required to kill microorganisms is roughly proportional to the number of microorganisms present. Cleaning helps reduce the number of microbes to a manageable number. The location of the microorganisms can also influence the effectiveness of a germicide, because physical barriers can prevent contact of the germicide and the microbe. Therefore it is imperative that the germicidal agent has direct contact with any part of the device that is exposed to potential pathogens. Consequently, proper disassembly (and subsequent assembly) of equipment during the decontamination process can be a limiting factor when the effectiveness of a physical or chemical agent is assessed.

Microbial Resistance

The presence of microbial capsules can increase a microorganism's resistance to disinfection and sterilization. This resistance generally can be overcome by increasing the exposure time of the microbe to the germicide. Bacterial spores are the most resistant microbes, followed by mycobacteria, nonlipid or small

TABLE 2.4 **Medical Conditions and Common Pathogens in Hospitalized Patients With Increased Susceptibility to Nosocomial Infections**

Condition	Possible Cause	Common Pathogens
Skin and mucosal barrier disruption	Burns Foley catheter Intravenous catheter Surgical wound Endotracheal tube	*S. aureus* *P. aeruginosa* Enterobacteriaceae *Candida* spp. *P. aeruginosa, S. aureus*
Neutropenia	Oncochemotherapy Drug reactions Autoimmune process Leukemia	*P. aeruginosa* Enterobacteriaceae *S. epidermidis* *S. aureus, Aspergillus* sp.
Disruption of normal flora	Antibiotic therapy Oncochemotherapy	*C. difficile* *Candida* spp.
Altered T-cell function	Cushing syndrome Corticosteroid therapy Hodgkin disease AIDS Organ transplantation	*Mycoplasma* tuberculosis Fungal infections Herpes viruses *P. jiroveci* Toxoplasmosis
Hypogammaglobulinemia	Nephrotic syndrome Multiple myeloma	*S. pneumoniae* *H. influenzae* Enterobacteriaceae
Hypocomplementemia	Systemic lupus erythematosus Liver failure Vasculitis	*N. meningitidis* *S. pneumoniae* Enterobacteriaceae

AIDS, Acquired immunodeficiency syndrome.
From Chatburn RL: Decontamination of respiratory care equipment: what can be done, what should be done. *Respir Care* 34:98, 1989.

viruses, fungi, lipid or medium viruses, and vegetative bacteria (e.g., *Staphylococcus* and *Pseudomonas* spp.). The resistance of Gram-positive and Gram-negative microorganisms to disinfection and sterilization is similar, except for *P. aeruginosa,* which shows greater resistance to some disinfectants.[9,10]

Concentration and Potency of the Germicide

In general, a disinfectant's potency increases as its concentration increases. (Iodophors are an exception.) It is important to remember, however, that germicides are affected differently by concentration adjustments; that is, diluting a germicide influences the amount of time required for disinfection or sterilization.

Physical and Chemical Factors

The effectiveness of a germicide depends on the temperature, pH, and relative humidity of the environment in which it is used. Generally, the activity of most germicides increases as the temperature increases. Increasing the pH improves the antimicrobial activity of some disinfectants (e.g., glutaraldehyde and quaternary ammonium compounds); increasing the alkalinity of other agents reduces their effectiveness (e.g., phenols, hypochlorite, iodine). Relative humidity is an important determinant of the activity of gaseous disinfectants (e.g., ethylene oxide, formaldehyde).

Cleaning

Cleaning is the first step in the decontamination process. Fig. 2.2 is a schematic of a typical cleaning area for respiratory care equipment. Note that the space is divided into dirty and clean areas, which have separate entries and exits. The typical cleaning area includes a negative-pressure area for disinfection, a pass-through unit for drying washed equipment, and a positive-pressure area for reassembling cleaned equipment. This design helps ensure that clean equipment is not mixed with or contaminated by soiled items.

The cleaning process usually begins with disassembly of the equipment to help ensure that dirt and organic matter are removed from surfaces that are not necessarily visible when the device is assembled. Ultrasonic systems sometimes are used for cleaning equipment with crevices that are difficult to clean. These ultrasonic devices create small bubbles that can penetrate and dislodge dirt and organic material, particularly in hard-to-reach crevices.

As stated previously, cleaning usually is done with soaps, detergents, and enzymatic products. Soaps and detergents contain amphipathic molecules that help dissolve fat and grease by reducing surface tension so that water can penetrate the organic matter. The amphipathic nature of these agents relates to their ability to dissolve both polar and nonpolar molecules; that is, they can dissolve polar, or water-soluble (hydrophilic), substances and nonpolar, or water-insoluble (hydrophobic), substances. Soaps are not bactericidal but may be combined with a disinfectant. Detergents are weakly bactericidal against Gram-positive organisms, but they are not effective against tubercle bacilli and viruses.[4]

Cleaning can be done by hand with a scrub brush or with an automatic system. Automatic systems are similar to the

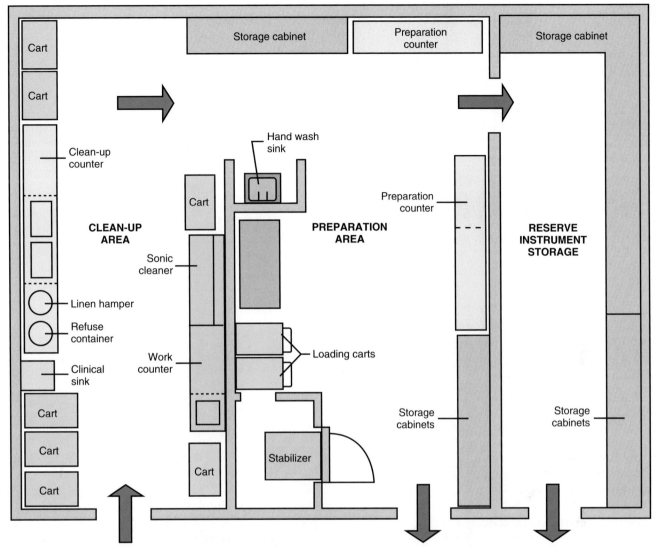

FIGURE 2.2 Schematic of a typical cleaning area for respiratory care equipment. (Redrawn from Perkins JJ: *Principles and methods of sterilization in health sciences,* Springfield, IL, 1978, Charles C Thomas.)

dishwasher found in the home. Soiled equipment goes through a series of wash and rinse cycles before automatically undergoing pasteurization or cold disinfection.

After the equipment is cleaned, it should be dried to remove residual water, because moisture can alter the effectiveness of disinfectants and sterilizing agents. For example, water can dilute the disinfectant or change its pH.[7] Residual moisture can also combine with ethylene oxide to form ethylene glycol, a toxic chemical that is difficult to remove.[4] As mentioned previously, equipment should be reassembled in a clean positive-pressure area separate from the area for processing soiled equipment to prevent recontamination. Clean equipment should never be allowed to sit on open counters for a prolonged time.

Disinfection

By definition, disinfection differs from sterilization because it lacks sporicidal properties.[8] Disinfection can be accomplished by physical and chemical methods. Pasteurization is the most common physical method of disinfection. Quaternary ammonium compounds, alcohols, acetic acid, phenols, iodophors, sodium hypochlorite, glutaraldehyde, and hydrogen peroxide are examples of chemical disinfectants. Table 2.5 lists some commonly used disinfectants and their germicidal properties.

It is important to note that certain disinfectants (e.g., hydrogen peroxide, peracetic acid, glutaraldehyde) can eliminate spores with sufficient exposure time (i.e., 3 to 12 hours). Disinfectants that can eliminate spores are called chemical sterilants. High-level disinfection occurs when chemical sterilants are used at reduced exposure times (less than 45 minutes). High-level disinfectants kill bacteria, fungi, and viruses but do not kill bacterial spores unless the spores are exposed to the disinfectant for an extended time. Intermediate-level disinfectants remove vegetative bacteria, tubercle bacteria, most viruses, and fungi but do not necessarily kill spores. Low-level disinfectants kill most vegetative bacteria, some fungi, and some viruses. Box 2.2 summarizes the properties of an ideal disinfectant.

TABLE 2.5 Germicidal Properties of Disinfectants and Sterilization Agents

Level of Germicide	Use Dilution	Level of Disinfection	INACTIVATES[a]						IMPORTANT CHARACTERISTICS								
			Bacteria	Lipophilic Viruses	Hydrophilic Viruses	*Mycobacterium tuberculosis*	Mycotic Agents	Bacterial Spores	Shelf Life >1 Week	Corrosive/ Deleterious Effects	Residue	Inactivated by Organic Matter	Skin Irritant	Eye Irritant	Respiratory Irritant	Toxic	Easily Obtainable
Isopropyl alcohol	60-95%	Int	+	+	−	+	+	+	+	±	−	+	±	+	−	+	+
Hydrogen peroxide	3-25%	CS/High	+	+	+	+	+	±	+	−	−	±	+	+	−	+	+
Formaldehyde	3-8%	High/Int	+	+	+	+	+	±	+	−	+	−	+	+	+	+	+
Quaternary ammonium compounds	0.4-1.6% aqueous	Low	+	+	−	−	±		+	−	−	+	+	+	−	+	+
Phenolic	0.4-5% aqueous	Int/Low	+	+	±	+	±		+	−	+	±	+	+	−	+	+
Chlorine	100-1000 ppm-free chlorine	High/Low	+	+	+	+	+	±	+	+	+	+	+	+	+	+	+
Iodophors	30-50 ppm-free iodine	Int	+	+	+	±	±	±	+	±	+	+	±	+	−	+	+
Glutaraldehyde	2%	CS/High	+	+	+	+	+	±	+	−	+	−	+	+	+	+	+

[a]Inactivates all indicated microorganisms with a contact time of 30 minutes or less, except bacterial spores, which require a 6- to 10-hour contact time.

Int, Intermediate; *CS*, chemical sterilant; +, yes; −, no; ±, variable results.

From Rutala WA: Disinfection, sterilization, and waste disposal. In Wenzel RP, editor: *Prevention and control of nosocomial infections*, Baltimore, 1997, Williams & Wilkins.

BOX 2.2 Properties of an Ideal Disinfectant

- *Broad spectrum:* Should have a wide antimicrobial spectrum.
- *Fast acting:* Should produce a rapid kill.
- *Not affected by environmental factors:* Should be active in the presence of organic matter (e.g., blood, sputum, feces) and compatible with soaps, detergents, and other chemicals encountered in use.
- *Nontoxic:* Should not be irritating to the user.
- *Surface compatibility:* Should not corrode instruments and metallic surfaces and should not cause the deterioration of cloth, rubber, plastics, and other materials.
- *Residual effect on treated surface:* Should leave an antimicrobial film on the treated surface.
- *Easy to use.*
- *Odorless:* Should have a pleasant odor or no odor to facilitate routine use.
- *Economical:* Should not be prohibitively expensive.
- *Solubility:* Should be soluble in water.
- *Stability:* Should be stable in concentrate and diluted.
- *Cleaner:* Should have good cleaning properties.

Modified from Rutala WA, Weber DJ, the Healthcare Infection Control Practices Advisory Committee (HICPAC): *Guidelines for disinfection and sterilization in healthcare facilities, 2008.* Atlanta, GA, Centers for Disease Control, Department of Health and Human Services.

Pasteurization

Pasteurization uses moist heat to coagulate cell proteins. The exposure time required to kill vegetative bacteria depends on the temperature. Two techniques are commonly used: the flash process and the batch process. In the flash process the material to be disinfected is exposed to moist heat at 72°C for 15 seconds. The flash process is used to pasteurize milk and other heat-labile liquids. With the batch process, equipment is immersed in a water bath heated to 63°C for 30 minutes. The batch process can kill all vegetative bacteria and some viruses, including HIV. Most respiratory care equipment can withstand the conditions of the batch process.

Quaternary Ammonium Compounds

Quaternary ammonium compounds (Quats) are organically substituted ammonium compounds that are cationic detergents containing four alkyl or heterocyclic radicals and a halide ion. The halide may be substituted by a sulfate radical. They are thought to interfere with the bacteria's energy-producing enzymes, denature its essential cell proteins, and disrupt the bacterial cell membrane.[8,11,12] Quats are bactericidal, fungicidal, and virucidal against lipophilic viruses. They are not sporicidal or tuberculocidal or virucidal against hydrophilic viruses. They are inactivated by organic material, and their effectiveness is reduced by cotton and gauze pads, which may absorb some of their active ingredients.[8] Quats are routinely used to sanitize noncritical surfaces (e.g., floors, walls, furniture) and can generally retain their activity for as long as 2 weeks if they are kept free of organic material.[7]

Alcohols

Ethyl and isopropyl alcohol are the two most common alcohols used for disinfection. Both are bactericidal, fungicidal, and virucidal, but they do not kill bacterial spores. The optimum concentrations of both alcohols range from 60% to 90%. Their ability to disinfect decreases significantly at concentrations below 50%.[8]

Alcohols are thought to kill microorganisms by denaturing proteins. This is a reasonable hypothesis considering that absolute ethyl alcohol, a dehydrating agent, is less bactericidal than an ethyl alcohol and water mixture, because proteins are denatured more quickly in the presence of water.[13] Although alcohols are effective in fairly short periods (less than 5 minutes), the Centers for Disease Control and Prevention (CDC) recommends that an exposure time of 15 minutes be required for 70% ethanol.[7]

Alcohols are used to disinfect rubber stoppers of multiple-use medication vials, oral and rectal thermometers, and stethoscopes. They also can be used to clean the surfaces of mechanical ventilators and areas used for medication preparation.[8] Alcohols are good solvents and can remove shellac from equipment surfaces. They can cause swelling and hardening of rubber and plastic tubes after prolonged and repeated use.

Acetic Acid

Acetic acid (white household vinegar) is used extensively as a means of decontaminating home care respiratory equipment. It also is used in hospitals, but on a limited basis. Because of its acidic nature (pH ≈2), its presumed mechanism of bactericidal action involves lowering a microbe's intracellular pH, thus inactivating its energy-producing enzymes.

The optimum concentration of acetic acid is 1.25%, which is the equivalent of one part 5% white household vinegar and three parts water. It has been shown to be an effective bactericidal agent (particularly against *P. aeruginosa*), but its sporicidal and virucidal activity has not been documented.[14]

Peracetic acid, or peroxyacetic acid, is acetic acid to which an oxygen atom has been added. It has been shown to be an excellent disinfectant with sterilization capabilities.[4] Peracetic acid is a strong oxidizing agent that kills microbes by denaturing proteins, disrupting cell wall permeability, and oxidizing cellular metabolites.[15] However, its strong oxidizing action is also a shortcoming because it can corrode brass, iron, copper, and steel.[8] (*Note:* Although peracetic acid mixed with hydrogen peroxide [0.23% peracetic acid and 7.35% hydrogen peroxide] has been shown to be an effective disinfectant, it is typically not used for disinfecting endoscopes because this mixture can cause physical and functional damage to the instrument.[8])

Phenols

Carbolic acid, the prototype of the six-carbon aromatic compounds known as phenols, was first used as a germicide by Lister in his pioneering work on antiseptic surgery.[8] Although carbolic acid is no longer used as a disinfectant, chemical manufacturers have synthesized numerous phenol derivatives that have been shown to be effective bactericidal, fungicidal, virucidal, and tuberculocidal agents. (Note that these derivatives are not sporicidal.) Phenol derivatives contain an alkyl, phenyl, benzyl, or halogen substituted for one of the hydrogen atoms attached to the aromatic ring. Commonly used phenols include orthophenylphenol and orthobenzylparachlorophenol.

Phenols kill microbes by denaturing proteins and injuring the cell wall. They are used primarily as surface disinfectants for floors, walls, and countertops. Phenols are readily absorbed by porous material, and residual disinfectant can cause skin irritation. They are associated with hyperbilirubinemia in neonates when used as disinfectants in nurseries.[16]

Iodophors and Other Halogenated Compounds

An iodophor is a solution that contains iodine and a solubilizing agent or carrier. This combination results in a chemical that provides a sustained release of free iodine in an aqueous solution.[8] The best known iodophor is povidone-iodine, which is used as an antiseptic and disinfectant.

Iodophors penetrate the cell wall of microorganisms, and their mode of action is thought to be disruption of protein and nucleic acid metabolism. They are bactericidal, tuberculocidal, fungicidal, and virucidal, but they are not effective against bacterial spores. Note that solutions formulated for antiseptic use are not suitable for disinfectant use because antiseptic solutions contain significantly less free iodine than those formulated as disinfectants.

Sodium hypochlorite contains free available chlorine in an aqueous solution. Three forms of chlorine are present in the sodium hypochlorite mixture: free chlorine (Cl_2), hypochlorite anion (OCl^-), and hypochlorous acid ($HOCl$). It has been suggested that these forms of chlorine kill microbes by interfering with cellular metabolism, denaturing proteins, and inactivating nucleic acids.[8,17,18] Sodium hypochlorite (household bleach) demonstrates a range of "-cidal" activities. A 1 : 100 dilution is bactericidal, tuberculocidal, and virucidal in 10 minutes and fungicidal in 1 hour. The CDC recommends that a 1 : 10 dilution be used to clean blood spills.[4,19] However, it is not sporicidal. Although sodium hypochlorite is inexpensive and relatively fast acting, it is corrosive to metals. It forms bischloromethyl ether (a carcinogen) when it comes in contact with formaldehyde and trihalomethane when hot water is hyperchlorinated. It has a limited shelf life and is inactivated by organic matter.

Glutaraldehyde

Glutaraldehyde solutions have been some of the most common disinfectants used in respiratory care departments for high-level disinfection of endoscopes, spirometry tubing, transducers, and nondisposable respiratory therapy equipment. Glutaraldehyde solutions can also be used as chemical sterilants, if exposure time is extended. They kill microbes by alkylating hydroxyl, sulfhydryl, carboxyl, and amino groups of microorganisms, which ultimately interfere with protein synthesis.[8] Alkaline and acid glutaraldehyde solutions are commercially available.

Alkaline glutaraldehyde is packaged as a mildly acidic solution (>2% glutaraldehyde) that is activated with a bicarbonate solution, yielding a solution with a pH of 7.5 to 8.5. It is bactericidal, fungicidal, tuberculocidal, and virucidal with an exposure time of 10 minutes. It is sporicidal with an exposure time of 6 to 10 hours. The average shelf life of alkaline glutaraldehyde is 14 days to 1 month. It is irritating to skin and mucous membranes (particularly the eyes). For this reason the Occupational Safety and Health Administration (OSHA) limits exposure of workers to 0.2 ppm airborne alkaline glutaraldehyde. Union Carbide, a manufacturer of glutaraldehyde, recently suggested that the threshold for exposure be lowered to 0.1 ppm. Individuals working with glutaraldehyde should wear protective eyewear, masks, gloves, and splash gowns or aprons.[20,21] Ideally, glutaraldehyde should be used under a fume hood or in a room that is under negative pressure.

Acid glutaraldehyde, which has a pH of 2.7 to 3.7, is available as a 2.4% solution that does not require activation and comes ready to use. Acid glutaraldehyde is bactericidal, tuberculocidal, and fungicidal; however, the exposure time must be extended to 20 minutes to be tuberculocidal. The activity of an acid glutaraldehyde solution can be enhanced by warming it to 60°C. At this temperature, acid glutaraldehyde is bactericidal, fungicidal, and virucidal in 5 minutes, tuberculocidal in 20 minutes, and sporicidal in 60 minutes.[4] Acid glutaraldehyde is not irritating to the skin and mucous membranes as is alkaline glutaraldehyde.

Ortho-phthalaldehyde

Ortho-phthalaldehyde (OPA) is a clear, pale blue liquid that is considered to be a high-level disinfectant. OPA contains 0.55% 1,2-benzenedicarboxaldehyde and has a pH of 7.5.[8] It has been suggested that OPA's mode of action as a disinfectant involves interaction with amino acids, proteins of microorganisms (i.e., similar to the mode of action of glutaraldehyde).[22]

OPA has been shown to be a more effective mycobactericidal agent than glutaraldehyde.[8,23] In vitro studies comparing OPA and glutaraldehyde have shown that 0.21% OPA was effective in 6 minutes compared to 32 minutes using a 1.5% glutaraldehyde solution. OPA has also been shown by in vitro analysis to be effective in destroying glutaraldehyde-resistant mycobacterial strains.[23] OPA is lipophilic, which allows its uptake by the outer layers of mycobacterial cells and Gram-negative bacteria.[8,22,23]

OPA has several advantages compared to glutaraldehyde. It does not require activation, and it has been shown to be more stable and less irritating to the nasal passages and eyes than glutaraldehyde. OPA's odor is barely perceptible and does not require activation.[8] Several points are important to mention. When using OPA to disinfect endoscopes, it is imperative to use the correct disinfection time. (*Note:* See manufacturer directions for using OPA for endoscope disinfection.) Additionally, endoscopes should be adequately rinsed following disinfection using copious amounts of sterile water because OPA can cause skin staining (i.e., OPA will stain the skin gray.). It is also important to mention that practitioners wear protective equipment (i.e., gloves, fluid-resistant gowns, goggles) when working with OPA.[8]

Hydrogen Peroxide

Commercially available 3% solutions of hydrogen peroxide are effective disinfectants of bacteria (including *Mycobacterium* sp.), fungi, and viruses, and are active within 10 minutes at room temperature. Higher concentrations (6% to 25%) and prolonged exposure are required for sterilization. Hydrogen peroxide is sporicidal in 6 hours at 20°C; it is effective against spores in 20 minutes at 50°C.[8]

Hydrogen peroxide kills microorganisms by forming hydroxyl radicals that can attack membrane lipids, nucleic acids, and other essential compounds. Note that catalase-positive aerobes and facultative anaerobic bacteria can inactivate metabolically produced hydrogen peroxide by degrading it into water and oxygen. Longer exposure times are required to kill microorganisms with high cellular catalase activity (e.g., *S. aureus, S. marcescens,* and *Proteus mirabilis*), which required 30 to 60 minutes of exposure to 0.6% hydrogen peroxide compared with organisms with lower catalase activity (e.g., *E. coli, Streptococcus* sp., and *Pseudomonas* sp.), which required only 15 minutes exposure.[8]

Sterilization

As with disinfection, sterilization techniques generally are divided into physical and chemical methods. Physical methods most often rely on heat, specifically dry heat, boiling water, steam under pressure (autoclave), and incineration. Ionizing radiation (i.e., γ-rays and x-rays) also is an effective method of sterilization; however, this method is used on a limited basis in hospitals. The most commonly used chemical for sterilization is ethylene oxide. (See Table 2.5 for a comparison of the advantages and disadvantages of various sterilization methods.)

Heat

Probably the simplest and surest means of destroying microorganisms is burning or incineration. This method is reserved for items that are disposable or are so contaminated that reuse is prohibited.[4] It should be recognized that, besides destroying the material being sterilized, incineration creates air pollution.

Dry heat is another effective method of heat sterilization. Its use is limited to items that are not heat sensitive. Temperatures must be maintained between 160°C and 180°C for 1 to 2 hours to accomplish sterilization. Dry heat is routinely used to sterilize laboratory glassware and surgical instruments, but it cannot be used for heat-sensitive items made of rubber or plastic.

Boiling water kills vegetative bacteria and most viruses in 30 minutes; however, its effectiveness against spores, especially those of thermophilic organisms, is somewhat questionable. Boiling water is commonly used to sterilize metal surgical instruments and nebulizers used in home care therapy. As with dry heat, it cannot be used for heat-sensitive equipment. Because water boils at a lower temperature at high altitudes, exposure time must be prolonged when this form of sterilization is used at high elevations.[4,6]

Steam under pressure, or autoclaving, is a highly effective and inexpensive method of sterilization. Of the aforementioned techniques, autoclaving is probably the most versatile for sterilizing laboratory glassware, surgical instruments, bacterial filters, liquids, linens, and other heat- and moisture-resistant materials. The technique of autoclaving is fairly simple. Items to be autoclaved are cleaned and wrapped in linen, gauze, or paper. They are placed in a chamber like that shown in Fig. 2.3, and the chamber is closed and secured. The chamber is evacuated of air, moisture is added (100% humidity), and the pressure inside is raised to 15 to 20 psig (pounds per square inch gauge). Air is evacuated from the chamber, because residual air prolongs the penetration time of steam, thus increasing the total autoclave cycle time. Pressure is used to raise the temperature of the steam, which is critical because the amount of time required to achieve sterilization depends on the temperature inside the autoclave. For example, at atmospheric pressure, steam has a temperature of 100°C. At 15 psig it has a temperature of 121°C, and at 20 psig it has a temperature of 132°C. At 121°C, all microbes and spores are killed within 15 minutes; at 132°C, killing occurs in 10 minutes.

Because the process of autoclaving depends on several factors, heat-sensitive and biological indicators are routinely used to ensure quality control during the process. Heat-sensitive tape used to package materials for autoclaving changes color when exposed to a given temperature for a prescribed amount of time. The most common biological indicators for autoclaving are strips of paper impregnated with *Geobacillus stearothermophilus* spores. These strips should be used weekly (at a minimum) to ensure that the autoclave is working properly.

Ethylene Oxide

Ethylene oxide (EtO) is a sterilant that has been used since the 1950s. It is a colorless gas that is flammable and explosive. It kills microorganisms by alkylating proteins, DNA, and RNA, thus interfering with cellular metabolism.[11] EtO originally was combined with chlorofluorocarbons (CFCs), which acted as a stabilizing agent. Under provisions of the Clean Air Act of 1993, CFCs were phased out in 1995 because of their detrimental effect on the ozone layer. Currently EtO is used alone or in combination with different stabilizing agents, such as carbon dioxide or hydrochlorofluorocarbons.

EtO kills all microorganisms and spores; bacterial spores are more resistant than vegetative microbes. The effectiveness of EtO depends on the gas concentration (450 to 1200 mg/L), the temperature (29°C to 65°C), the humidity (45% to 85% relative humidity), and the exposure time (2 to 5 hours).[8] Generally, increases in the EtO concentration and temperature shorten the sterilization time.

In a typical hospital or clinic setting, equipment to be sterilized with EtO is sent to central supply for processing. All equipment to be sterilized with EtO must be free of water, because water reacts with EtO to form polyethylene glycol and can interfere with the sterilization process. Additionally, equipment must be packaged in EtO-permeable materials, such as paper, muslin, or plastic bags made of polyethylene or polypropylene. The actual process of automated EtO sterilization consists of several stages: a preconditioning phase and a gas injection phase, exposure of the item to the EtO, evacuation of gas from the chamber, and an air-washing

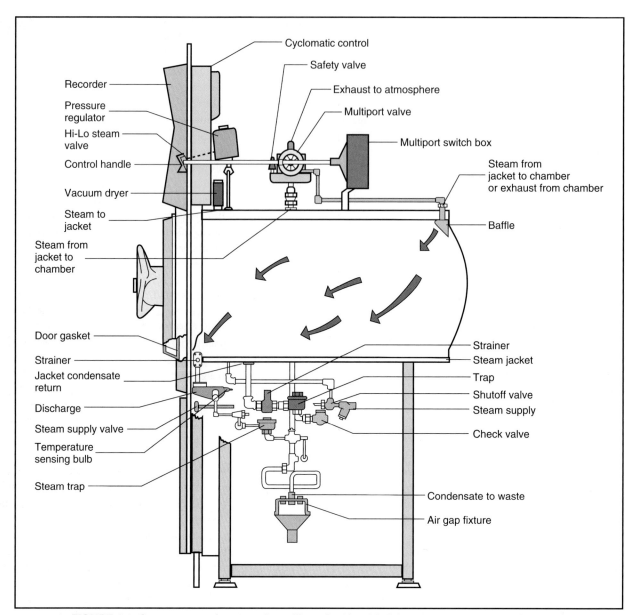

FIGURE 2.3 Components of an autoclave. (From Perkins JJ: *Principles and methods of sterilization in health sciences,* Springfield, Il, 1978, Charles C Thomas.)

period.[8] After sterilization, all equipment exposed to EtO must be aerated before use. Note that the aeration time usually is not considered part of the sterilization time and usually is accomplished by mechanical aeration for 8 to 12 hours at 50°C to 60°C. Aeration at room temperature is considered dangerous because of EtO's toxicity.

Biological indicators, similar to those used for autoclaving, must be used to monitor the effectiveness of EtO. *Bacillus subtilis* spores generally are used for this purpose. Fig. 2.4 shows a typical device for monitoring sterilization. *B. subtilis* organisms embedded in a paper strip are housed within a plastic capsule alongside a glass ampule containing a growth medium (e.g., tryptic soy broth).[8] The ampule is placed among the materials to be sterilized. After the sterilization cycle, the ampule is crushed and the paper strip is immersed in the liquid. The strip then is incubated according to the manufacturer's directions. Microbe growth is indicated by changes in the turbidity of the growth medium after incubation.[2]

Inhalation of EtO has been associated with nasal and eye irritation, dyspnea, headache, nausea, vomiting, dizziness, and convulsions.[24] Direct contact with EtO causes skin irritation and burns. OSHA and The Joint Commission (TJC) provide general guidelines for the safe use of EtO. The current OSHA standard for EtO exposure is 1 ppm in 8 hours, with a maximum short-term exposure of 5 to 10 ppm for 15 minutes.[25]

Hydrogen Peroxide Gel Plasma

This sterilization technique was patented in 1987 and introduced to the United States market in 1993 as an alternative method of sterilizing equipment that cannot tolerate high temperatures and humidity.[8] The principle of operation involves the evacuation of a chamber containing the equipment to be sterilized followed by the automated injection of hydrogen peroxide. The hydrogen peroxide is vaporized in the chamber and dispersed on the equipment surface to be sterilized. A hydrogen peroxide gas plasma is created in the chamber over

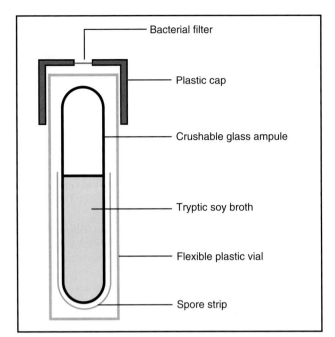

FIGURE 2.4 Biological sterilization indicators: The capsule contains a strip impregnated with bacterial spores, a pH indicator, and a culture medium (e.g., tryptic soy broth). After sterilization the ampule is crushed, releasing the culture medium onto the strip containing the spores. Incomplete sterilization is indicated if the capsule turns yellow. (Redrawn from Boyd RF, Hoerl BG: *Basic medical microbiology,* ed 3, Boston, 1986, Little, Brown.)

TABLE 2.6   Infection Risk Categories for Medical Equipment

Category	Description	Examples	Processing
Critical	Devices introduced into the bloodstream or other parts of the body	Surgical devices Intravascular catheters Implants Heart-lung and hemodialysis components	Sterilization
Semicritical	Devices in contact with intact mucous membranes	Endoscopes Trachea tubes Ventilator tubing	High-level disinfection
Noncritical	Devices that touch only intact skin or do not contact patient	Face masks Blood pressure cuffs Mechanical ventilators	Detergent washing Low- to intermediate-level disinfection

Modified from Chatburn RL: Decontamination of respiratory care equipment: what can be done, what should be done. *Respir Care* 34(2):98-109, 1989.

50 to 75 minutes. During this period radio frequency or microwave energy is used to excite H_2O_2 molecules to free radicals (i.e., hydroxyl and hydroperoxyl molecules). These highly reactive species within the plasma field are capable of interacting with cell components (e.g., nucleic acids, enzymes to disrupt microbial metabolism).[8] During the final stage of the sterilization process, excess gas is removed from the chamber, and the system is returned to atmospheric pressure by introducing high-efficiency filtered air. The by-products of the process (water vapor and oxygen) are nontoxic, and thus equipment undergoing this type of sterilization does not require aeration.[8]

Identifying Infection-Risk Devices

Not all reusable patient care items must be sterilized. Whether a medical device should be cleaned and disinfected or sterilized depends on its intended use. In 1968, E.H. Spaulding devised a classification scheme that could be used by infection control professionals in the planning of disinfection and sterilization methods for patient care items and equipment.[26,27] Spaulding's classification system placed devices into three categories based on the degree of risk for infection involved in their use. The categories are critical, semicritical, and noncritical.

Critical items must be sterilized, because they are introduced into sterile tissue or the vascular system (e.g., surgical instruments, implants, cardiac and urinary catheters, heart-lung and hemodialysis equipment, needles). Respiratory care and anesthesia equipment (e.g., ventilator tubing), endoscopes, and thermometers are examples of semicritical items. Because semicritical items come in contact with intact mucous membranes, a minimum of high-level disinfection is recommended. High-level disinfection is effective against blood-borne pathogens (i.e., HIV, hepatitis B virus) and *M. tuberculosis.* Noncritical items come in contact with intact skin but not mucous membranes. Intact skin acts as an effective barrier to most microorganisms; therefore sterility is not critical. Common examples of noncritical items are face masks, mechanical ventilators, stethoscopes, and blood pressure cuffs. Table 2.6 lists examples of medical devices and how they are classified according to Spaulding's system. Box 2.3 contains a summary of the guidelines for processing reusable respiratory care equipment.

Box 2.4 describes several strategies for preventing the spread of pathogenic organisms by in-use respiratory care equipment (e.g., nebulizers, ventilator circuits, manual resuscitators, oxygen therapy apparatuses). Of particular note is the prevention of VAP. A number of clinicians have advocated the use of various nonpharmacological and pharmacological interventions (i.e., ventilator bundles) that can be used to reduce the incidence of VAP (Box 2.5).[6] For example, several studies have focused on the incidence of VAP as a function of the time interval between ventilator circuit changes. Historically, circuits were changed daily.[28] In 1986, Craven et al.[29] found that the incidence of VAP was significantly reduced if the circuits were changed at 48-hour intervals compared with every 24 hours. Subsequent studies have suggested that the interval between ventilator circuit changes can be extended for even longer periods. Although extending the time between circuit changes clearly does not increase the incidence of VAP, the optimum interval remains unclear.[28,30,31]

BOX 2.3   Guidelines for Processing Reusable Respiratory Care Equipment

- All reusable respiratory care equipment should undergo low- or intermediate-level disinfection as part of the initial cleaning.
- All reusable breathing circuit components (including tubing and exhalation valves, medication nebulizers and their reservoirs, large-volume jet nebulizers and their reservoirs) should be considered semicritical items.
- Semicritical items should be sterilized between patient use; heat-stable items should be autoclaved, and heat-labile items should undergo EtO sterilization.
- If sterilization is not feasible, semicritical items should undergo high-level disinfection or pasteurization.
- The internal machinery of ventilators and breathing machines need not be routinely sterilized or disinfected between patients.
- Respirometers and other equipment used to monitor multiple patients should not directly touch any part of a ventilator circuit or a patient's mucous membranes. Rather, disposable extension pieces and low-resistance high-efficiency particulate air (HEPA) filters should be used to isolate the device. If the device cannot be isolated from the patient or circuit, it must be sterilized or receive high-level disinfection before use on other patients.
- After use on one patient, nondisposable resuscitation bags should be sterilized or should receive high-level disinfection before use on other patients.
- External surfaces, ports, and internal channels of bronchoscopes should be cleaned with water and a detergent before being immersed in a high-level disinfectant. All channels of the bronchoscope should be perfused for at least 20 minutes and then rinsed with sterile water, followed by an alcohol rinse, and then dried using filtered air. Forceps and specimen brushes should be sterilized separately from the bronchoscope.

Data from Chatburn RL: Decontamination of respiratory care equipment: what can be done, what should be done. *Respir Care* 34:98, 1989.

BOX 2.4   Strategies for Preventing the Spread of Pathogenic Organisms by In-Use Respiratory Care Equipment[2,6,38]

- Large-volume reusable nebulizers and humidifiers should always be filled with sterile distilled water before initial use. When fluid is replenished, any fluid remaining in these devices should be emptied and the reservoir filled completely. Prefilled, sterile disposable humidifiers should be used whenever possible.
- Large-volume room air humidifiers that create aerosols should not be used unless they can be sterilized or subjected to high-level disinfection at least daily and filled only with sterile water.
- Large-volume jet nebulizers and medication nebulizers and their reservoirs and tubing should be changed or replaced every 24 hours with equipment that has undergone high-level disinfection.
- Prefilled, sterile, disposable humidifiers that are used with oxygen-delivery devices do not need to be changed between patients in a high-use area, such as the recovery room; they can be used safely for up to 30 days. The tubing and oxygen-delivery device should be changed between patients.
- In-use ventilator circuits, including their humidifiers and nebulizers, should be changed if they malfunction or are visibly soiled. If a heat and moisture exchanger bacterial filter (i.e., artificial nose) is used instead of a water humidifier, changing the circuit between patients may be satisfactory.
- Water condensate in the ventilator and nebulizer tubing should be discarded and not drained back into the reservoir.

---

about nosocomial infections from direct smears and stains, cultures, serological tests, and antibiotic susceptibility testing. Identification of the cause of a nosocomial infection is essential for preventing and minimizing hospital epidemics.[4] Clinical Scenario 2.3 provides a test of your understanding of the principles of infection control techniques.

III. SURVEILLANCE

Ongoing surveillance is required to ensure that an infection control program is providing adequate protection for patients and health care providers. Surveillance typically consists of three components: monitoring of equipment processing procedures, routine sampling of in-use equipment, and identifying suspected pathogens microbiologically.[4] Equipment processing is monitored using the aforementioned chemical and biological indicators. In-use equipment can be routinely sampled with sterile cotton swabs, liquid broth, and aerosol impaction. Swabs can be used to obtain samples from easily accessible surfaces of respiratory care equipment. Liquid broth can be used to obtain samples when cotton swabs cannot reach many parts of the equipment (e.g., inside tubing). Aerosol impaction is used to sample the particulate output of nebulizers.

Microbiological identification requires the hospital's clinical laboratory staff to work with clinicians to identify infectious organisms. Clinical microbiologists can provide information

IV. ISOLATION PRECAUTIONS

In 2007 the CDC, in cooperation with the federal Healthcare Infection Control Practices Advisory Committee (HICPAC), revised its guideline for isolation precautions in the health care setting.[1] The revised guideline contains information on the history of isolation practices, along with recommendations for isolation precautions in a variety of health care settings. The revised recommendations are intended for acute care hospitals and for subacute and extended care facilities.

Like the 1996 recommendations, the revised recommendations establish two levels of precautions: standard precautions and transmission-based precautions. Standard precautions are to be used with all patients, regardless of their diagnosis or presumed infection status. Standard precautions represent a combination of universal precautions and body substance isolation precautions; they apply to blood, all body fluids (secretions and excretions [except sweat]), nonintact skin, and mucous membranes. Standard precautions involve the use of

BOX 2.5 Methods to Reduce the Risk for Ventilator-Associated Pneumonia

Nonpharmacological

Noninvasive ventilation

Hand washing and use of accepted infection control procedures and practices

Semirecumbent positioning of patient

Appropriate circuit changes (when grossly contaminated)

Heat-moisture exchangers when possible

Aspiration of subglottic secretions

Appropriate disinfection and sterilization techniques

Kinetic beds

Identifying a dedicated person/group for monitoring nosocomial VAP rates

Use of closed suction catheters and sterile suction technique

Avoiding large gastric volumes

Extubating and removing nasogastric tube as clinically indicated

Avoiding contamination with ventilator circuit condensate

Single-patient use of items such as monitors, O_2 analyzers, and resuscitation bags

Careful use of in-line small-volume nebulizers

Consider use of expiratory-line gas traps or filters

Oral rather than nasal intubation

Use of silver-coated endotracheal tubes to reduce biofilm formation

Pharmacological

Stress ulcer prophylaxis with sucralfate instead of histamine type 2 antagonists in high-risk patients for prevention of stress ulcers (still controversial)

Possible prophylactic intestinal decontamination (antimicrobial administration)

Avoid central nervous system depressants

Methods to improve host immunity

Maintain nutritional status

Avoid agents that impair pulmonary defenses (aminophylline, anesthetics, certain antibiotics, corticosteroids, sedative narcotics, and antineoplastic agents)

Minimize use of invasive procedures when possible

Remove or treat disease states that affect host defenses when possible (acidosis, dehydration, hypoxemia, ethanol intoxication, acid aspiration, stress, thermal injury, diabetic ketoacidosis, liver failure, kidney failure, heart failure)

VAP, Ventilator-associated pneumonia.

CLINICAL SCENARIO 2-3

The hospital infection control committee notifies your department that the incidence of nosocomial pneumonia in the recovery room increases significantly during the month of December. It has been suggested that the source of the pneumonia could be reusable, large-volume jet nebulizers. How would the respiratory therapist determine whether in-use, large-volume jet nebulizers are responsible for this outbreak of pneumonia? How could the respiratory therapist monitor the effectiveness of the sterilization of these devices?

See Appendix A for the answer.

personal protective equipment, as well as the proper handling of potentially contaminated equipment and items in the patient's environment. Standard precautions therefore are designed to reduce the risk for transmission of microorganisms from both recognized and unrecognized sources of infection in the health care setting.[1]

Transmission-based precautions are designed to interrupt transmission of known or suspected pathogens that can be transmitted by airborne or droplet routes or by direct contact with skin and contaminated surfaces. Transmission-based precautions are for the care of patients with highly transmissible or epidemiologically important pathogens that necessitate additional precautions to stop their transmission. Box 2.6 gives a synopsis of the various types of isolation precautions and a list of conditions that require each type of precaution. Table 2.7 lists clinical syndromes and conditions that warrant additional precautions to prevent the transmission of epidemiologically important pathogens upon confirmation of diagnosis.

Fundamentals of Isolation Protection

Hand washing is the most important prevention strategy for protecting health care workers from becoming infected through contact with infected patients. It also reduces the risk for health care workers transmitting infectious microorganisms from one patient to another or from a contaminated site to a clean site on the same patient.[32-35] Health care workers should wash their hands before and after caring for any patient; however, it is particularly important that they wash their hands before and after performing invasive procedures or touching wounds or patients at high risk for infection.

Routine hand washing should involve using a soap and water wash with a rubbing action to create a lather over both hands for at least 15 seconds. Hands should be rinsed thoroughly and dried with disposable or single-use towels or an air dryer.[32] The CDC updated its recommendations for hand-washing technique on October 25, 2002.[33] These updated guidelines specify that alcohol-based hand rubs should be used in conjunction with traditional soap and water to protect patients in health care settings. Alcohol-based hand rubs typically are applied to the hands after the hands have been dried after the soap and water wash. In many cases these alcohol-based hand rubs can be substituted for the traditional hand washing with soap and water. As effective as these agents can be as an adjunct to infection control, it is important to recognize that frequent use of alcohol-based formulations for hand antisepsis can cause drying of the skin unless skin conditioning agents are added to the formulations. In addition, alcohol-based hand rubs are flammable and have flash points in the range of 21°C to 24°C, depending on the type and concentration of alcohol. Therefore alcohol-based hand rubs should be stored away from high temperatures and flames, in accordance with the recommendations of the National Fire Protection Association.[33]

Gloves are worn for several reasons: (1) to protect the health care worker from contact with blood and body fluids (i.e., blood-borne pathogens); (2) to provide a barrier so that resident and transient microorganisms on the hands of health

---

BOX 2.6   Infection Control Precautions and Patients Who Require Them

Standard Precautions
Use standard precautions for the care of all patients.

Airborne Precautions
In addition to standard precautions, use airborne precautions for patients known to have or suspected of having serious illnesses transmitted by airborne droplet nuclei. Examples of such illnesses include:
- Measles
- Varicella (including disseminated zoster)[a]
- Tuberculosis[b]

Droplet Precautions
In addition to standard precautions, use droplet precautions for patients known to have or suspected of having serious illnesses transmitted by large-particle droplets. Examples of such illnesses include:
- Invasive *H. influenzae* type b disease (meningitis, pneumonia, epiglottitis, and sepsis)
- Invasive *N. meningitidis* disease (meningitis, pneumonia, and sepsis)
- Other serious bacterial respiratory infections spread by droplet transmission, including:
  - Diphtheria (pharyngeal)
  - *Mycoplasma* pneumonia
  - Pertussis
  - Pneumonic plague
  - Streptococcal pharyngitis, pneumonia, or scarlet fever in infants and young children
- Serious viral infections spread by droplet transmission, including:
  - Adenovirus[a]
  - Influenza

- Mumps
- Parvovirus B19
- Rubella

Contact Precautions
In addition to standard precautions, use contact precautions for patients known to have or suspected of having serious illnesses easily transmitted by direct patient contact or by contact with items in the patient's environment. Examples of such illnesses include:
- Gastrointestinal, respiratory, skin, or wound infections or colonization with multidrug-resistant bacteria (judged by the infection control program to be of special clinical and epidemiological significance based on current state, regional, or national recommendations).
- Enteric infections with a low infectious dose or prolonged environmental survival, including *C. difficile* organisms.
- For diapered or incontinent patients: Enterohemorrhagic *E. coli*, *Shigella* sp., hepatitis A, or rotavirus.
- Respiratory syncytial virus, parainfluenza virus, or enteroviral infections in infants and young children.
- Skin infections that are highly contagious or that may occur on dry skin, including:
  - Diphtheria (cutaneous)
  - Herpes simplex virus (neonatal or mucocutaneous)
  - Impetigo
  - Noncontained abscesses, cellulitis, or decubiti
  - Pediculosis
  - Scabies
  - Staphylococcal furunculosis in infants and young children
  - Zoster (disseminated or in an immunocompromised host)[a]
- Viral/hemorrhagic conjunctivitis
- Viral hemorrhagic infections (Ebola, Lassa, or Marburg)

[a]Certain infections require more than one type of precaution.
[b]See the CDC guidelines for environmental infection control in health care facilities.[40]
CDC, Centers for Disease Control and Prevention.
Modified from Garner JS: Guideline for isolation precautions in hospitals, *Infect Control Hosp Epidemiol* 17:53, 1996.

---

care workers are not transferred to patients during patient care or medical or surgical procedures; and (3) to prevent health care workers from indirectly transmitting pathogens from an infected patient to another patient.[32,36] It is important to remember that hand washing is essential after removing gloves after each patient contact, because hands can be contaminated during glove removal. Defects or tears in gloves also can allow contamination of the hands.[37,38]

Gowns and other protective apparel (e.g., shoe covers) are worn to prevent contamination of clothing and to protect the skin from blood and body fluid exposure.[31] This protective apparel should be impermeable to liquids and worn only once, then discarded. OSHA's final rule on blood-borne pathogens requires gowns and protective apparel to be worn.[39]

Face shields or masks with protective eyewear should be worn whenever splashing or spraying of blood or body fluid is possible (e.g., when obtaining arterial blood gas samples and inserting intravascular catheters). They may also be mandated in special circumstances stated in OSHA's final rule on blood-borne pathogens.[39] Face masks are used to prevent the

spread of large-particle droplets transmitted by close contact (e.g., when working with patients who are coughing or sneezing). Note that the efficacy of wearing a mask to prevent the transmission of *M. tuberculosis* organisms is questionable. The most recent guidelines established by the National Institute for Occupational Safety and Health (NIOSH) require that health care workers use respiratory protective devices, such as the N95 respirator, to prevent the inhalation of airborne droplet nuclei, particularly when caring for patients with SARS, MERS, tuberculosis (TB), or smallpox.[1] A wide range of respirators that meet NIOSH standards are available to prevent the inhalation of droplet nuclei. (Historical Note 2.1 presents a brief discussion of the several types of protective respirators currently available.)

Patient care equipment and articles that may serve as fomites for the transmission of infectious particles (e.g., needles, scalpels, and other sharp objects) should be disposed of in specially designated containers. Disposable medical gas therapy devices, such as nebulizers and tubing, should be discarded in a sturdy bag or container. Reusable items should be

TABLE 2.7 Clinical Syndromes and Conditions Warranting Additional Empirical Precautions to Prevent the Transmission of Infectious Disease[a]

Clinical Syndrome or Condition[b]	Clinical Syndrome or Condition[c]	Empirical Precautions
Diarrhea		
Acute diarrhea with a likely infectious cause in an incontinent or diapered patient	Enteric pathogens[d]	Contact
Diarrhea in an adult with a history of recent antibiotic use	C. difficile	Contact
Meningitis	N. meningitidis	Droplet
Rash or exanthems, generalized, etiology unknown	N. meningitidis	Droplet
Petechia/ecchymosis with fever	Varicella	Airborne, contact
Vesicular Condition		
Maculopapular with coryza fever	Rubeola (measles)	Airborne
Respiratory Infections		
Cough/fever/upper lobe pulmonary infiltrate in an HIV-negative patient or a patient at low risk for HIV infection	M. tuberculosis	Airborne
Cough/fever/pulmonary infiltrate in an HIV-negative patient or a patient at high risk for HIV infection	M. tuberculosis	Airborne
Paroxysmal or severe, persistent cough during periods of pertussis activity	B. pertussis	Droplet
Respiratory infections, particularly bronchiolitis and croup, in infants and young children	Respiratory syncytial or parainfluenza virus	Contact
Risk for multidrug-resistant microorganisms	Resistant bacteria[e]	Contact
History of infection or colonization with multidrug-resistant organisms		
Skin, wound, or urinary tract infection in a patient with a recent hospital or nursing home stay in a facility where multidrug-resistant organisms are prevalent	Resistant bacteria[e]	Contact
Skin or wound infection	S. aureus	Contact
Abscess or draining wound that cannot be covered	Group A Streptococcus	

[a]Infection control professionals are encouraged to modify or adapt this table according to local conditions. To ensure that appropriate empirical precautions are always implemented, hospitals must have systems in place for evaluating patients routinely according to these criteria as part of their preadmission and admission care.

[b]Patients with the syndromes or conditions listed may present with atypical signs or symptoms (e.g., pertussis in neonates and adults may not cause a paroxysmal or severe cough). The clinician's index of suspicion should be guided by the prevalence of specific conditions in the community and by clinical judgment.

[c]The organisms listed are not intended to represent the complete, or even the most likely, diagnosis but rather are possible etiological agents that require additional precautions until they can be ruled out.

[d]These pathogens include enterohemorrhagic E. coli, Shigella sp., hepatitis A, and rotavirus.

[e]Resistant bacteria as judged by the infection control program to be of special clinical or epidemiological significance, based on current state, regional, or national recommendations.

HIV, Human immunodeficiency virus.

Modified from Garner JS: Guideline for isolation precautions in hospitals. Infect Control Hosp Epidemiol 17:52, 1996.

HISTORICAL NOTE 2.1

Personal protective respirators that are used in hospital infection control programs must be certified by the NIOSH and the U.S. Food and Drug Administration (FDA). Each type of mask typically is identified with a letter and a number code. The letter specifies whether the mask is not resistant (N), somewhat resistant (R), or strongly resistant (P) to oil degradation; the number following the letter refers to its particulate filtering efficiency. For example, an N95 mask is not oil resistant, and it filters out 95% of the particles that attempt to flow through it. More information about personal protective respirators can be found at the NIOSH Personal Protective Technology Laboratory website: http://www.cdc.gov/niosh/npptl/default.html.

NIOSH, National Institute for Occupational Safety and Health.

sterilized or disinfected by standard procedures to prevent the transmission of infectious microorganisms from patient to patient. Disposable items should be disposed of according to hospital and applicable government regulations. Care must be taken not to contaminate the outside of the bag when it is handled and transported.

Fluids and medications used to treat patients should be sterile; therefore only sterile water should be used to fill nebulizers and humidifiers. Unused portions of large bottles of sterile water should be discarded within 24 hours. Single-dose ampules of sterile water and normal saline are ideal for small-volume nebulizers. Multidose vials should be stored according to manufacturers' specifications (e.g., refrigerated after opening). Single-dose and multidose vials should not be used beyond the expiration date on the label.[2]

Standard Precautions

As was stated previously, standard precautions are a synthesis of previous CDC guidelines for universal precautions and body substance isolation techniques. Hands should be washed between patients and between tasks and procedures on the same patient to prevent cross-contamination of different body sites.[1,28] Gloves, masks, protective eyewear, and splash-proof gowns should be worn when there is a chance of splashing blood, body fluids, secretions, and excretions, or contact with contaminated items. Needles and other sharp objects should be handled with care to prevent injuries. Needles should not be recapped; when recapping a syringe is necessary, both hands should never be used, instead, the one-hand "scoop" technique or a mechanical device to recap syringe needles safely should be used.[32]

Three new elements have been added to standard precautions to reinforce existing infection control recommendations: respiratory hygiene/cough etiquette, safe injection practices, and the use of masks by clinicians performing catheter insertion or injection of materials into spinal or epidural spaces via lumbar puncture procedures. Note that these recommendations focus on protection of the patient, whereas the other recommendations evolved from the original universal precautions, which were designed to protect health care personnel.

Respiratory hygiene/cough etiquette has five components: (1) education of health care staff, patients, and visitors; (2) signage that provides instructions about isolation procedures for family members and visitors accompanying the patient; (3) source control measures, such as using a surgical mask on a coughing patient when tolerated; (4) hand hygiene after contact with respiratory secretions; and (5) spatial separation of patients with respiratory infections in common waiting areas.[1]

Safe injection practices focus on reinforcing the importance of using proper aseptic techniques. Specifically, safe injection practices involve the use of a sterile, single-use, disposable needle and syringe for each injection. Additionally, single-dose medication vials should be used whenever possible to avoid contamination of injection equipment and medication.

Finally, recent evidence suggests that the use of face masks by health care providers participating in procedures involving lumbar puncture, spinal and epidural anesthesia, and the insertion of central venous lines can significantly limit the dispersal of oropharyngeal droplets and thus protect the patient from droplet-borne infectious materials.[41]

Airborne Precautions

Airborne precautions have two major components: (1) placement of the infected patient in an area with appropriate air handling and ventilation and (2) use of respiratory protective equipment by health care workers and visitors entering the patient's room.[28,32] When an infected patient must be transported, the patient should wear a surgical mask to minimize dispersal of droplet nuclei. Current standards require that infected patients be placed in a private, negative-pressure isolation room. Negative air pressures in the room should be monitored relative to other areas of the hospital. SARS, H_1N_1, measles, chickenpox (primary varicella zoster), and tuberculosis are illnesses that require airborne precautions. Because varicella zoster organisms can also be transmitted by direct contact, infected patients may also require contact isolation.

Droplet Precautions

Droplet precautions are designed to prevent the transmission of microorganisms contained in droplets generated by sneezing, coughing, or talking, or during procedures such as bronchoscopy and suctioning.[28] Precautions include donning gloves, masks, and protective eyewear. Special air handling and ventilation are not required. *H. influenzae* type b organisms and *N. meningitidis* organisms are transmitted by this route. Other serious infections are adenovirus, influenza, parvovirus B19, pertussis, streptococcal pharyngitis, pneumonia, and scarlet fever.[32] As with airborne precautions, infected patients should wear a surgical mask to minimize transmission of droplet nuclei.

Contact Precautions

Contact precautions are recommended for patients infected with pathogenic organisms that can be spread by direct patient contact or through contact with items in the patient's environment.[28] Contact precautions require the patient to be isolated in a private room with a bath. Health care workers should wear masks, gloves, and gowns when caring for these patients. Illnesses that require contact isolation include gastrointestinal, respiratory, and skin infections. Some organisms responsible for these illnesses are *Clostridium difficile*, *Shigella* sp., hepatitis A, respiratory syncytial virus, and the parainfluenza virus. Patients colonized with multidrug-resistant organisms of special clinical and epidemiological significance (e.g., methicillin-resistant *Staphylococcus aureus* [MRSA]) also require contact isolation. Table 2.8 summarizes the HICPAC infection control guidelines for standard and transmission-based precautions. Clinical Scenario 2.4 provides a problem-solving exercise on isolation precautions typically required in the clinical setting.

V. INFECTION CONTROL ISSUES IN MASS CASUALTY SITUATIONS

Considerable time and effort have been devoted to the development of an effective rapid response plan for a mass casualty event, such as a severe influenza pandemic. Federal, state, and local governments, as well as many health-related

 CLINICAL SCENARIO 2-4

A respiratory therapist is on call in the emergency department when one adult and two children are admitted after a house fire. The children incurred only minor cuts and bruises, but the adult sustained third-degree burns over 60% of his body. What precautions should the respiratory therapist take when treating a burn patient?

See Appendix A for the answer.

TABLE 2.8 HICPAC Guidelines for Standard and Transmission-Based Precautions

Precautions	Scenario	Hand Hygiene	Gowns/Gloves	Mask and Eye Protection	Environmental Controls
Standard	Use for all patients, regardless of confirmed or suspected presence of an infectious agent.	Should be performed before patient contact, after touching blood, body fluids, and contaminated items, immediately after removing gloves, and between patient contacts.	Gowns should be worn when contact of clothing or exposed skin with blood or body fluids is anticipated. Gloves should be worn for touching blood, body fluids, contaminated items, mucous membranes, or nonintact skin.	A surgical mask and eye protection should be worn during procedures and patient care activities likely to generate splashes or sprays of blood or body fluids, especially suctioning and endotracheal intubation.	Routine care, cleaning, and disinfection of environmental surfaces.
Contact[a]	Use for infectious agents spread by direct or indirect contact with patients or their environment (e.g., vancomycin-resistant *Enterococcus, C. difficile*, respiratory syncytial virus).	As above.	Gowns and gloves should be worn for all interactions that involve contact with the patient or contaminated areas of the patient's environment. Gown and gloves should be donned on room entry for pathogens known to be transmitted through environmental contamination.	As above.	Single-patient room is preferred. When a single-patient room is not available, consultation with infection control practitioners is recommended to assess other options, such as cohorting.
Droplet[a]	Use for infectious agents that are spread through close respiratory or mucous membrane contact with respiratory secretions (e.g., *B. pertussis,* influenza, *N. meningitidis*).	As above.	Per standard precautions.	A mask should be donned on room entry. Eye protection should be used per standard precautions.	As above. Curtains should be drawn between beds in shared patient rooms, and the patient should wear a mask when transported out of the hospital room.
Airborne[a]	Use for infectious agents that remain infectious over long distances when suspended in air (e.g., *M. tuberculosis* and varicella and rubeola viruses).	As above.	Per standard precautions.	A fit-tested N95 respirator or a powered air-purifying respirator should be worn whenever the patient's room is entered.	Patients should be placed in a monitored, airborne infection isolation room, maintained with 6 to 12 air exchanges per hour and negative pressure relative to surrounding areas.

[a]Transmission-based precautions (always used in addition to standard precautions).

HICPAC, Healthcare Infection Control Practices Advisory Committee.

From Daugherty EL: Health care worker protection in mass casualty respiratory failure: infection control, decontamination, and personal protective equipment. *Respir Care* 53(2):201-214, 2008. Adapted from Siegel JD, Rhinehart E, Jackson M, et al.: The healthcare infection control practices advisory committee. 2007 Guideline for isolation precautions: preventing transmission of infectious agents in healthcare settings. June, 2007. http://www.cdc.gov/ncidod/dhqp/pdf/guidelines/isolation2007.pdf.

organizations and professional societies, have presented documents to guide clinicians on the epidemiology and treatment of community-acquired severe respiratory ilnesses.[42,43]

Febrile respiratory illness (FRI) caused by community-acquired pneumonia is a common reason for admission to the intensive care unit. Although bacterial and viral organisms are most often cited in the etiology of FRI, a relatively small group of agents have the potential to cause widespread epidemics that can severely affect our health care system.[44] Box 2.7 provides a list of naturally occurring or intentional causes of FRIs that can lead to a sustained mass casualty event. Although it is beyond the scope of this text to discuss every aspect of infection control in an FRI mass casualty event, it should be apparent that early detection and isolation of infected patients are the cornerstones of an effective disaster infection control plan. It is imperative that all potentially involved health care workers be knowledgeable about the plan and receive education in the proper use of personal protective equipment.

Table 2.9 provides a summary of isolation precautions for five specific infectious biological agents associated with mass casualty respiratory failure. More detailed information about emergency preparedness can be found on the Evolve Resources site that accompanies this text.

BOX 2.7 Naturally Occurring or Intentional Causes of Febrile Respiratory Illness That Can Lead to a Mass Casualty Event

Influenza[a]
Viral hemorrhagic fevers[a] SARS coronavirus[a] Smallpox[a] Plague[a] Tularemia
Anthrax

[a]Contagious condition (e.g., H_1N_1 virus).
From Sandrock CE: Severe febrile respiratory illnesses as a cause of mass critical care. *Respir Care* 53:40, 2008.

TABLE 2.9 Recommended Precautions for Biological Agents Associated With Mass Casualty Respiratory Failure

Agent	Mode of Transmission	Patient Placement	Type and Duration of Precautions
Smallpox	Inhalation of droplets or aerosols	Patients should be placed in airborne isolation whenever possible. In a mass exposure situation, cohorting may be appropriate.	Standard, contact, and airborne precautions should be used until all scabs have separated (3-4 weeks). Only immune health care workers should care for infected patients. Nonimmune individuals who are exposed should receive postexposure vaccination within 4 days.
Anthrax	Person-to-person transmission does not occur with respiratory or gastrointestinal tract anthrax. Person-to-person transmission of cutaneous anthrax is extremely rare.	No restrictions.	Standard precautions. If presence of aerosolized powder or environmental exposure is suspected, airborne precautions should be used, and exposed persons should be decontaminated.
Pneumonic plague	Inhalation of respiratory droplets. Risk of transmission is low during the first 20 to 24 hours of illness.	Patients should be placed in private rooms whenever possible, and cohorted if private rooms are unavailable.	Use standard precautions. Droplet precautions should be used until the patient has received at least 48 hours of appropriate therapy.
SARS, MERS	Droplet and contact transmission. Opportunistic airborne transmission is possible.	Airborne infection isolation.	Standard, droplet, and airborne precautions with eye protection should be continued for the duration of potential infectivity.
Pandemic influenza	Presumed transmission is primarily via large respiratory droplets, but opportunistic airborne transmission also is possible.	Airborne infection isolation.	Standard, droplet, and airborne precautions with eye protection should be continued for 14 days after the onset of symptoms or until an alternative diagnosis is made.

MERS, Middle East respiratory virus; *SARS,* severe acute respiratory syndrome.
From Daugherty EL: Health care worker protection in mass casualty respiratory failure: infection control, decontamination, and personal protective equipment. *Respir Care* 53(2):201-214, 2008. Adapted from Siegel JD, Rhinehart E, Jackson M et al.: The healthcare infection control practices advisory committee. 2007 Guideline for isolation precautions: preventing transmission of infectious agents in healthcare settings. June, 2007. http://www.cdc.gov/ncidod/dhqp/pdf/guidelines/isolation2007.pdf; and Centers for Disease Control and Prevention: Public health guidance for community-level preparedness and response to severe acute respiratory syndrome (SARS), version 2; supplement I: Infection control in healthcare, home, and community settings; III: infection control in healthcare facilities. January 8, 2004. http://www.cdc.gov/ncidod/sars/guidance/i/pdf/healthcare.pdf.

KEY POINTS

- Three elements are required for spread of an infectious disease: a source of pathogens, a mode of transmission of the infectious agent, and a susceptible host.
- Hospital-acquired pneumonia is most often caused by bacteria, but viruses, protozoa, and fungi contribute to a lesser extent. Most nosocomial bacterial pneumonias are described as polymicrobial, and Gram-negative bacilli are the predominant microbes identified.
- The four routes of transmission of HAIs are the contact route, vehicle route, airborne route, and vector route.
- A number of factors can affect disinfection and sterilization, including the number, location, and innate resistance of the microorganism. The effectiveness of a germicide depends on its concentration and potency, the duration of exposure to the germicide, and the physical and chemical environment in which the germicide is used.
- Three levels of disinfection are possible: high-level disinfection kills bacteria, fungi, and viruses. Spores can also be destroyed with high-level disinfection, but an extended exposure time is required. Intermediate-level disinfection removes vegetative bacteria, tubercle bacteria, some viruses, and fungi but does not kill spores. Low-level disinfection kills most vegetative bacteria, some fungi, and some viruses.
- Quats, alcohols, acetic acid, phenols, glutaraldehyde, hydrogen peroxide, and halogenated compounds are highly effective chemicals used to disinfect floors, countertops, and the outer surface of respiratory care equipment.
- Individuals working with glutaraldehyde should wear protective eyewear, masks, gloves, and splash gowns or aprons. Ideally, glutaraldehyde should be used under a fume hood or in a room that is under negative pressure.
- The activity of an acid glutaraldehyde solution can be enhanced by warming it to 60°C. At this temperature, acid glutaraldehyde is bactericidal, fungicidal, and virucidal in 5 minutes, tuberculocidal in 20 minutes, and sporicidal in 60 minutes.
- Acetic acid is commonly used as a disinfectant in the home care environment. The optimum concentration of acetic acid is 1.25%, which is the equivalent of one part 5% white household vinegar and three parts water.
- Five methods are commonly used to sterilize medical devices: (1) dry heat, (2) boiling water and steam under pressure (autoclave), (3) ionizing radiation, (4) EtO, and (5) hydrogen peroxide gel plasma.
- Reusable medical equipment can be categorized as critical, semicritical, or noncritical, depending on the degree of risk for infection involved in their use.
- The effectiveness of an infection control program should be monitored routinely with mechanical, chemical, and biological indicators.
- Standard precautions are used for all patients, regardless of confirmed or suspected presence of an infectious agent. Transmission-based precautions involve specific requirements for dealing with possible contaminants that can be spread by airborne, droplet, and contact routes.

ASSESSMENT QUESTIONS

See Appendix B for the answers.

1. Which of the following organisms is a Gram-negative bacterium often associated with VAP?
   a. *Pseudomonas aeruginosa*
   b. *Diplococcus pneumoniae*
   c. *Clostridium botulinum*
   d. *Mycobacterium tuberculosis*

2. *Mycobacterium tuberculosis* organisms are:
   a. Gram-negative bacilli
   b. An anaerobic infection
   c. Acid-fast bacteria
   d. Spore-producing bacteria

3. All of the following are transmitted through the respiratory route *except*:
   a. H_1N_1 virus
   b. Adenoviruses
   c. Varicella
   d. HIV

4. Briefly describe the most recent CDC guidelines for proper hand hygiene.

5. Which of the following disinfectants can be used as a chemical sterilant?
   a. Povidone-iodine
   b. Acetic acid
   c. Glutaraldehyde
   d. Isopropyl alcohol

6. Indicate whether each of the following presents a critical, semicritical, or noncritical risk for infection.
   a. Ventilator tubing
   b. Swan-Ganz catheter
   c. Blood pressure cuff
   d. Endoscope (bronchoscope)
   e. Endotracheal tubes

7. Which of these clinical conditions warrants additional precautions to prevent the spread of epidemiologically significant pathogens?
   a. Meningitis
   b. Pertussis
   c. Measles
   d. Diarrhea in an adult with a history of recent antibiotic use

8. The best method of decontaminating a flexible bronchoscope is:
   a. Intermediate-level disinfection with 70% isopropyl alcohol
   b. High-level disinfection with 1.5% glutaraldehyde
   c. Low-level disinfection with 5% acetic acid
   d. High-level disinfection with ortho-phthalaldehyde

9. Which of the following methods should *not* be used to disinfect plastic oxygen masks?
   a. Ethylene oxide
   b. Steam autoclave
   c. 1.25% acetic acid
   d. 2% alkaline glutaraldehyde

10. Which of the following conditions requires the application of contact precautions?
    a. Legionellosis
    b. Diphtheria
    c. Hepatitis
    d. Rubella

11. Which of the following are potential causes of skin and mucosal barrier disruption?
    1. Foley catheters
    2. Intravenous catheters
    3. Endotracheal tubes
    4. Burns
       a. 1 and 2 only
       b. 2 and 3 only
       c. 1, 2, and 4 only
       d. 1, 2, 3, and 4

12. *Bacillus anthracis* is a(n):
    a. Gram-negative bacterium
    b. Anaerobic infection
    c. Acid-fast bacterium
    d. Spore-producing bacterium

13. Name three elements that must be present for the spread of infectious materials.

14. Describe various techniques that are routinely used to determine the effectiveness of sterilization.

15. Which of the following precautions should be taken with a patient under respiratory isolation?
    1. The patient should have a private room.
    2. Gowns should be worn by all those entering the room.
    3. Articles contaminated with secretions must be disinfected or discarded.
    4. Masks must be worn by all individuals who will be in close contact with the patient.
       a. 2 and 3 only
       b. 3 and 4 only
       c. 1, 2, and 3 only
       d. 1, 3, and 4 only

16. Define standard precautions.

17. Match the following:
    1. _____ HIV
    2. _____ Respiratory syncytial virus
    3. _____ Parainfluenza
    4. _____ Influenza
    5. _____ Histoplasmosis
       a. Bronchitis, bronchiolitis
       b. Fungal infection virus
       c. Croup, pneumonia
       d. Tracheobronchitis
       e. AIDS

18. Give an example of a disease that is transmitted by each of the following routes of transmission:
    a. Contact (direct)
    b. Vehicle (foodborne)
    c. Airborne (droplet nuclei)
    d. Vector-borne (fleas)

REFERENCES

1. Siegel JD, Rhinehart E, Jackson M, et al.: *Guideline for isolation precautions: preventing transmission of infectious agents in healthcare settings*, Atlanta, 2007, Centers for Disease Control and Prevention.
2. Kacmarek RM, Stoller JK, Heuer AH: *Egan's fundamentals of respiratory care*, ed 11, St. Louis, 2017, Elsevier.
3. Niederman MS, Sarosi GA, Glassroth J: *Respiratory infections: a scientific basis for management*, Philadelphia, 2001, WB Saunders.
4. Kacmarek RM, Mack CW, Dimas S, editors: *The essentials of respiratory care*, ed 4, St. Louis, 2005, Elsevier-Mosby.
5. Chastre J, Fagon J-V: Ventilator-associated pneumonia. *Am J Respir Crit Care Med* 165:872, 2002.
6. Cairo JM: *Pilbeam's mechanical ventilation: physiological and clinical applications*, ed 6, St. Louis, Elsevier, 2016.
7. Chatburn RL: Decontamination of respiratory care equipment: what can be done, what should be done. *Respir Care* 34:8, 1989.
8. Rutala WA, Weber DJ, the Healthcare Infection Control Practices Advisory Committee (HICPAC): *Guidelines for disinfection and sterilization in healthcare facilities*, Atlanta, GA, 2008, Centers for Disease Control, Department of Health and Human Services.
9. Favero MS, et al.: Gram-negative water bacteria in hemodialysis systems. *Health Lab Sci* 12:321, 1987.
10. Rutala WA, Cole EC: Ineffectiveness of hospital disinfectants against bacteria: a collaborative study. *Infect Control* 8:501, 1987.
11. Sykes G: *Disinfection and sterilization*, ed 2, London, 1965, E & FN Spon.
12. Petrocci AN: Surface active agents: quaternary ammonium compounds. In Block SS, editor: *Disinfection, sterilization, and preservation*, ed 3, Philadelphia, 1983, Lea & Febiger.
13. Morton HE: Alcohols. In Block SS, editor: *Disinfection, sterilization, and preservation*, ed 3, Philadelphia, 1983, Lea & Febiger.
14. Chatburn RE, Kallstrom TJ, Bajaksouzian MS: A comparison of acetic acid with a quaternary ammonium compound for the disinfection of hand-held nebulizers. *Respir Care* 33:179, 1988.
15. Block SS: Peroxygen compounds. In Block SS, editor: *Disinfection, sterilization, and preservation*, ed 3, Philadelphia, 1983, Lea & Febiger.
16. Rutala WA: APIC guideline for selection and use of disinfectants. *Am J Infect Control* 18:99, 1990.
17. Bloomfield SF, Uso EE: The antibacterial properties of sodium hypochlorite and sodium dichloroisocyanurate as hospital disinfectants. *J Hosp Infect* 6:20, 1985.

18. Favero MS, Bond WW: Chemical disinfection of medical and surgical materials. In Block SS, editor: *Disinfection, sterilization, and preservation*, ed 3, Philadelphia, 1983, Lea & Febiger.

19. U.S. Department of Labor: *Bloodborne pathogens and acute care facilities*, OSHA 3128, 1992, Washington, DC.

20. Gorman SP, Scott EM, Russell AD: A review: antimicrobial activity, uses, and mechanisms of action of glutaraldehyde. *J Appl Bacteriol* 48:161, 1980.

21. Association for the Advancement of Medical Instrumentation: *American National Standard—safe use and handling of glutaraldehyde-based products in health care settings*, ANSI/AAMI ST58, 1996, Arlington, VA.

22. Walsh SE, Maillard JY, Russell AD: Ortho-phthalaldehyde: a possible alternative to glutaraldehyde for high level disinfection. *J Appl Microbiol* 86:1039-1046, 1999.

23. Fraud S, Maillard JY, Russell AD: Comparison of the mycobacterial activity of ortho-phthalaldehyde, glutaraldehyde, and other dialdehydes by a quantitative suspension test. *J Hosp Infect* 48:214-221, 2001

24. Gross JA, Haas MI, Swift TR: Ethylene oxide neurotoxicity: report of four cases and review of the literature. *Neurology* 29:978, 1979.

25. Occupational Safety and Health Administration: Occupational exposure to ethylene oxide—OSHA, final standard. *Fed Regist* 49:25734, 1984.

26. Garner JS: Guideline for isolation precautions in hospitals. *Infect Control Hosp Epidemiol* 17:53, 1996.

27. Spaulding EH: Chemical disinfection of medical and surgical materials. In Lawrence CA, Block SS, editors: *Disinfection, sterilization, and preservation*, ed 3, Philadelphia, 1968, Lea & Febiger.

28. Branson RD: The ventilator circuit and ventilatory-associated pneumonia. *Respir Care* 50:774, 2005.

29. Craven DE, Connolly MG, Lichtenbery DA, et al.: Risk factors for pneumonia and fatality in patients receiving continuous mechanical ventilation. *Am Rev Respir Dis* 133:792, 1986.

30. Fink JB, Krause SA, Barrett L, et al.: Extending ventilator circuit change interval beyond 2 days reduces the likelihood of ventilator-associated pneumonia. *Chest* 113:405, 1998.

31. Hess DR, Kallstrom TJ, Mottram CD, et al.: American Association for Respiratory Care: care of the ventilator circuit and its relation to ventilator associated pneumonia. *Respir Care* 48:869, 2003.

32. Larson E: APIC guideline for handwashing and hand antisepsis in health care settings. *Am J Infect Control* 23:251, 1995.

33. Boyce JM, Pittet D; Healthcare Infection Control Practices Advisory Committee; HICPAC/SHEA/APIC/IDSA Hand Hygiene Task Force: Guideline for hand hygiene in health-care settings. *MMWR Recomm Rep* 51(RR16):1, 2002.

34. Damani N: *Handbook of infection prevention and control*, ed 3, New York, 2012, Oxford University Press.

35. Garner JS, Favero MS: Guideline for handwashing and hospital environmental control. *Infect Control* 7:231, 1986.

36. Olsen R, et al.: Examination gloves as barriers to hand contamination and clinical practice. *JAMA* 270:350, 1993.

37. Doebbeling B, et al.: Removal of nosocomial pathogens from the contaminated glove: implications for glove reuse and handwashing. *Ann Intern Med* 109:394, 1988.

38. Cadwallader HL, Bradley CR, Ayliffe GA: Bacterial contamination and frequency of changing ventilator circuits. *J Hosp Infect* 5:65, 1990.

39. U.S. Department of Labor, Occupational Safety and Health Administration: Occupational exposure to bloodborne pathogens: final rule. *Fed Regist* 56:64175, 1991.

40. Sehulster L, Chinn RY; CDC; HICPAC: Guidelines for environmental infection control in health-care facilities. *MMWR Recomm Rep* 52(RR-10):1, 2003.

41. O'Grady NP, Alexander M, Dellinger EP, et al.: Guidelines for the prevention of intravascular catheter-related infections. *MMWR Recomm Rep* 51(RR10):1, 2002.

42. Branson RD, Rubinson L: Mechanical ventilation in mass casualty scenarios. I. *Respir Care* 53:41, 2008.

43. Branson RD, Rubinson L: Mechanical ventilation in mass casualty scenarios. II. *Respir Care* 53:130, 2008.

44. Sandrock CE: Severe febrile respiratory illnesses as a cause of mass critical care. *Respir Care* 53:40, 2008.

Medical Gases

Manufacture, Storage, and Transport of Medical Gases

OBJECTIVES

Upon completion of this chapter, you will be able to:

1. Describe the chemical and physical properties of the medical gases most often encountered in respiratory care.
2. Identify various types of medical gas cylinders (e.g., types 3, 3A, 3AA, and 3AL).
3. Identify the following cylinder markings: Department of Transportation (DOT) specifications, service pressure, hydrostatic testing dates, manufacturer's identification, ownership mark, serial number, and cylinder size.
4. List the color codes used to identify medical gas cylinders.
5. Discuss United States Pharmacopeia and The National Formulary (USP–NF) purity standards for medical gases.
6. Compare the operation of direct-acting cylinder valves with that of diaphragm-type cylinder valves.
7. Explain the American Standards Safety System (ASSS), the Pin Index Safety System (PISS), and the Diameter Index Safety System (DISS).
8. Identify and correct a problem with cylinder valve assembly.
9. Calculate the gas volume remaining in a compressed-gas cylinder and estimate the duration of gas flow based on the cylinder's gauge pressure.
10. Describe the components of a bulk liquid oxygen system and discuss the recommendations of the National Fire Protection Association (NFPA) for the storage and use of liquid oxygen in bulk systems.
11. Discuss the operation of a portable liquid oxygen system and describe NFPA recommendations for these systems.
12. Calculate the duration of a portable liquid oxygen supply.
13. Identify three types of medical air compressors and describe the operational theory of each.
14. Summarize NFPA recommendations for medical air supply safety.
15. Compare continuous and alternating central supply systems.
16. Identify a DISS station outlet and a quick-connect station outlet.
17. Compare the operational theory of a membrane oxygenator with that of a molecular sieve oxygenator.

OUTLINE

KEY TERMS

alternating supply systems
American Standards Safety System (ASSS)
check valves
continuous supply system
cryogenic
Diameter Index Safety System (DISS)
diaphragm compressors
diaphragm valves
direct-acting valves

fractional distillation
fusible plugs
Joule-Kelvin (Joule-Thompson) effect
liquefaction
molecular sieves
oxygen concentrators
physical separation
Pin Index Safety System (PISS)
piston compressors

pressure swing adsorption (PSA) method
quick-connect adapters
rotary compressors
rupture disks
semipermeable membranes
spring-loaded devices
Thorpe tube flowmeter
volume–pressure constants
Wood's metal

Compressed gases are routinely used in the diagnosis and treatment of patients with cardiopulmonary dysfunction. The appropriate quality, purity, and potency of these medical gases are subject to government regulations. These regulations, along with recommendations proposed by the Compressed Gas Association (CGA) and other private agencies, provide guidelines for the manufacture, storage, and transport of compressed gases. As such, the primary purpose of these guidelines is to protect public safety. Respiratory therapists should be familiar with these regulations, as well as the indications, contraindications, and adverse effects associated with breathing medical gases.

I. PROPERTIES OF MEDICAL GASES

Air

At normal atmospheric conditions, air is a colorless, odorless gas mixture that contains varying amounts of water vapor. For practical purposes, we can assume that atmospheric air contains approximately 78% nitrogen and 21% oxygen by volume. Trace gases, including argon, carbon dioxide, neon, helium, methane, krypton, nitrous oxide, and xenon, make up the remaining 1% of atmospheric air. Table 3.1 shows a typical analysis of dry air at sea level.

Air is a nonflammable gas, but it supports combustion. It has a density of 1.29 kg/m^3 at 21.1°C (70°F) and 760 mm Hg.[1] Because air is used as a standard for measuring the specific gravity of other gases, it is assigned a value of 1 at 21.1°C and 1 atmosphere (atm).[1] At its freezing point, −195.6°C (−320°F), air is a transparent liquid with a pale bluish cast.

Compressed air is prepared synthetically from nitrogen and oxygen and shipped as a gas in cylinders at high pressure. Liquid air can be obtained through a process called liquefaction and shipped in bulk in specially designed cryogenic containers. For many medical applications, air is filtered and compressed at the point of use. The theory of operation of portable air compressors is described later in this chapter.

Oxygen (O₂)

Oxygen is an elemental gas that is colorless, odorless, and tasteless at normal temperatures and pressures. It makes up 20.9% of the Earth's atmosphere by volume and 23.2% by weight. It constitutes approximately 50% of the Earth's crust by weight. Oxygen is slightly heavier than air, having a density of 1.326 kg/m^3 at 21.1°C and 760 mm Hg (specific gravity = 1.105).[1] At temperatures less than −183°C (−297.3°F), oxygen exists as a pale bluish liquid that is slightly heavier than water.

Oxygen is classified as a nonflammable gas, but it readily supports combustion (i.e., the burning of flammable materials is accelerated in the presence of oxygen). Some combustibles, such as oil and grease, burn with nearly explosive violence if ignited in the presence of oxygen.[1] All elements except the inert gases combine with oxygen to form oxides; oxygen therefore is characterized as an oxidizer.

The two methods most commonly used to prepare oxygen are the fractional distillation of liquid air and the physical separation of atmospheric air. The fractional distillation of liquid air, which relies on the Joule-Kelvin (or Joule-Thompson) effect, was introduced by Karl von Linde in 1907.[2] Box 3.1 describes the fractional distillation process; Fig. 3.1 illustrates the components of a typical fractional distillation system. The fractional distillation process is used commercially to produce bulk oxygen, which can be stored as a liquid in cryogenic storage tanks or converted into a gas and shipped in metal cylinders.

The physical separation of atmospheric air is accomplished with devices that use molecular sieves and semipermeable membranes to filter room air. These devices, called oxygen concentrators, are used primarily to provide enriched oxygen mixtures for oxygen therapy in the home care setting. The operation of oxygen concentrators is discussed in more detail later in this chapter.

TABLE 3.1 Composition of Room Air		
Component	% by Volume	% by Weight
Nitrogen	78.084	75.5
Oxygen	20.946	23.2
Argon	0.934	1.33
Carbon dioxide	0.0335	0.045
Neon	0.001818	—
Helium	0.000524	—
Methane	0.0002	—
Krypton	0.000114	—
Nitrous oxide	0.00005	—
Xenon	0.0000087	—

From the Compressed Gas Association: *Handbook of compressed gases,* ed 3, New York, 1990, Van Nostrand Reinhold.

BOX 3.1   Fractional Distillation of Liquid Air

1. Room air is drawn through scrubbers to remove dust and other impurities.
2. Air is cooled to near the freezing point of water (0°C) to remove water vapor.
3. Air is compressed to 200 atm, causing the temperature of the gas mixture to increase.
4. Compressed air is cooled to room temperature by passing nitrogen through coils surrounding the gas mixture.
5. As the temperature drops, the gas mixture expands. The temperature achieved is less than the critical temperature of nearly all gases in air, and a liquid gas mixture is produced.
6. The liquid air is transferred to a distilling column, where it is warmed to room temperature. As the air warms, various gases boil off as their individual boiling points are reached.
7. Liquid oxygen is obtained by maintaining the temperature of the gas mixture just below the boiling point of oxygen (−183°C [−297.3°F] at 1 atm).
8. The process is repeated until the liquid oxygen mixture is 99% pure with no toxic impurities.
9. The liquid oxygen is transferred to cold converters for storage and later transported either in bulk as a liquid or in compressed-gas cylinders as a gas.

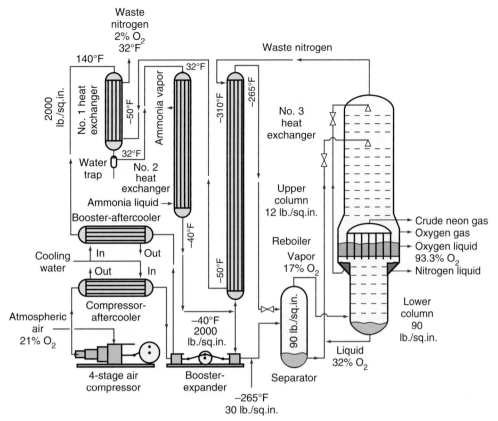

FIGURE 3.1 Fractional distillation apparatus for producing liquid oxygen. (Copyright © 2013 Medtronic Minimally Invasive Therapies. All rights reserved. Reprinted with permission of Medtronic Minimally Invasive Therapies.)

Carbon Dioxide (CO₂)

Carbon dioxide is a colorless, odorless gas at normal atmospheric temperatures and pressures. It has a density of 1.833 kg/m^3 at 21.1°C and 1 atm; it therefore is approximately 1.5 times heavier than air (specific gravity = 1.522).[1] Carbon dioxide is nonflammable and does not support combustion or life.

Carbon dioxide can exist as a solid, liquid, and gas at a temperature of −56.6°C (−69.9°F) and a pressure of 60.4 psig (pounds per square inch gauge), carbon dioxide's triple point.[1] (The triple point is a specific combination of temperature and pressure in which a substance can exist in all three states of matter in a dynamic equilibrium.) At temperatures and pressures below its triple point, carbon dioxide exists as a solid ("dry ice") or a gas, depending on the temperature. At temperatures and pressures above its triple point but below its critical temperature (31.1°C [87.9°F]), carbon dioxide can exist as a liquid or as a gas. Therefore, when carbon dioxide is stored at these temperatures in a pressurized container, such as a metal cylinder, the liquid and gaseous forms of carbon dioxide exist in equilibrium. Above 31.1°C, carbon dioxide cannot exist as a liquid, regardless of the pressure.[1]

Unrefined carbon dioxide can be obtained from the combustion of coal, natural gas, or other carbonaceous fuels.[1] Carbon dioxide can also be obtained as a by-product in the production of ammonia, lime, and kilns, among other products. Purified carbon dioxide is prepared through the liquefaction and fractional distillation processes.

Solid carbon dioxide is used to refrigerate perishable materials while in transport (e.g., food and laboratory specimens). Liquid carbon dioxide can be used as an expendable refrigerant[1] and is used extensively as a fire-extinguishing agent in portable and stationary fire-extinguishing systems. Gaseous carbon dioxide is used in food processing (e.g., carbonation of beverages) and water treatment, and as a growth stimulant for plants.[1]

Utilization of carbon dioxide for medical purposes is a relatively small percentage compared to its use for industrial (manufacturing) purposes. It has been used for the treatment of singultus (hiccups) and as a stimulant/depressant of the central nervous system. Because carbon dioxide cannot support life, it must be combined with oxygen before it can be administered to patients. Carbon dioxide–oxygen mixtures (carbogen mixtures) are prepared by combining 5% to 10% carbon dioxide with 90% to 95% oxygen. The US Food and Drug Administration (FDA) purity standard requires that carbon dioxide used for medical purposes is 99% pure.[3] It is important to recognize that breathing carbon dioxide–oxygen mixtures can have adverse effects on other medications that a patient may be taking (e.g., blood pressure medications, muscle relaxants, chemotherapy drugs, and antibiotics). As discussed in Chapters 8 and 10, carbon dioxide is also used in pulmonary diagnostic testing as a standard calibration gas for blood gas analyzers, transcutaneous partial pressure of carbon dioxide (PCO₂) electrodes, and capnographs.

Helium (He)

Helium is the second lightest element, having a density of 0.165 kg/m^3 at 21.1°C and 1 atm (specific gravity = 0.138).[1] It is an inert gas that has no color, odor, or taste. Helium is only slightly soluble in water and is a good conductor of heat, sound, and electricity.[4]

Helium occurs naturally in the atmosphere in very small quantities (see Table 3.1). It can be prepared commercially from natural gas, which contains as much as 2% helium.[1] Helium can also be obtained by heating uranium ore. Purity standards for the preparation of helium require that commercially available helium be 95% pure. Helium is chemically and physiologically inert and is classified as a nonflammable gas that will not support combustion or life. Indeed, breathing 100% helium can lead to severe hypoxemia. Because of its low density, helium is combined with oxygen (e.g., heliox is a mixture of 80% helium and 20% oxygen; however, heliox mixtures containing 70% helium and 30% oxygen, and 60% helium and 40% oxygen, are also available) to deliver oxygen therapy to patients with severe airway obstruction (i.e., it decreases the work of breathing by decreasing turbulent airflow).[3] It also is used in pulmonary function testing to measure residual volume and diffusing capacity.

Nitric Oxide (NO)

Nitric oxide is a diatomic molecule that exists as colorless gas with a slight metallic odor at room temperature. It is nonflammable and will support combustion. It has a density of 1.245 kg/m^3 and a specific gravity of 1.04 (at 21.1°C, 760 mm Hg).[1] Nitric oxide is highly unstable in the atmosphere and can exist in three biologically active forms in tissues: as nitrosonium (NO^+), as nitroxyl anions (NO^-), and as a free radical ($NO^{\cdot}$).

In the presence of air, nitric oxide combines with oxygen to form brown fumes of nitrogen dioxide (NO_2), a strong oxidizing agent. It is not corrosive, and most structural materials are unaffected; in the presence of moisture, however, it can form nitrous and nitric acids, both of which can cause corrosion. Nitric oxide and nitrogen dioxide combined form a potent irritant that can cause chemical pneumonitis and pulmonary edema.[4]

Nitric oxide can be prepared by oxidizing ammonia at high temperatures (500°C [932°F]) in the presence of a platinum catalyst or by reducing acid solutions of nitrates.[1] Chemiluminescent analysis is used to determine the final concentration of nitric oxide and nitrogen dioxide, with a stated accuracy of 62% (see Chapter 8 for a discussion of chemiluminescent analysis of nitric oxides). Nitric oxide is supplied with nitrogen in compressed-gas aluminum alloy cylinders. Before 1997 nitric oxide was supplied in cylinders with a volume capacity of 152 cu ft with 660 Compressed Gas Association (CGA) valve outlets. It now is supplied in smaller cylinders (82 cu ft) with 626 CGA valve outlets. Inhaled nitric oxide (iNO) can be delivered via a dedicated nitric oxide delivery system using a flow-based oxygen delivery system (e.g., nasal cannula, O_2 mask) or entrained during mechanical ventilation using a specially designed delivery system (see Chapter 4).[5]

Although nitric oxide is toxic in high concentrations, experimental results indicate that low doses are a powerful pulmonary vasodilator.[5] Very low concentrations (2 to 80 parts per million [ppm]) combined with oxygen have been used successfully to treat persistent pulmonary hypertension of the newborn[6] and hypoxic respiratory failure in term and near-term newborns in whom conventional ventilator therapy has failed.[7,8] Although many investigators have suggested that inhalation of low-dose nitric oxide is relatively safe, special precautions apply. Specifically, the levels of nitrogen dioxide and nitrogen trioxide, as well as the patient's methemoglobin levels, should be monitored throughout the procedure. Additional details on the administration of iNO are provided in Chapter 4.

Nitrous Oxide (N₂O)

Nitrous oxide is a colorless gas at normal temperatures and atmospheric pressures. It is odorless, tasteless, and nonflammable but will support combustion and is slightly soluble in water, alcohol, and oils. Nitrous oxide is noncorrosive and therefore may be stored in commercially available cylinders. Because it is an oxidizing agent, it will react with oils, grease, and other combustible materials.

Nitrous oxide is prepared commercially by the thermal decomposition of ammonium nitrate and as a by-product of the adipic acid manufacturing processes.[1] At elevated temperatures (>649°C [1200°F]), it decomposes into nitrogen and oxygen.

Nitrous oxide is used primarily as a central nervous system depressant (i.e., an anesthetic). It is a potent anesthetic when administered in high concentrations; in low concentrations, other depressant drugs must be used concomitantly to achieve effective anesthesia. (Nitrous oxide often is called "laughing gas," a term coined in 1840.[9]) Note that inhalation of nitrous oxide without provision of a sufficient oxygen supply may cause brain damage or be fatal.

Long-term exposure of health care workers to nitrous oxide has been associated with adverse side effects, including neuropathy and fetotoxic effects (spontaneous abortion).[1] The National Institute of Occupational Safety and Health has recommended limits on exposure to nitrous oxide for health care providers working in surgical suites and dental offices. Systems that trap exhaled nitrous oxide are used to capture any unused gas, preventing inadvertent exposure of health care workers.

Table 3.2 provides a summary of the properties of commonly used medical gases. Clinical Scenario 3.1 provides an exercise to help you test your understanding of the medical gases just discussed.

II. STORAGE AND TRANSPORT OF MEDICAL GASES

Medical gases can be classified as nonliquefied and liquefied. Nonliquefied gases are stored and transported under high pressure in metal cylinders. Liquefied gases are stored and transported in specially designed bulk liquid storage units. The design of compressed-gas cylinders, bulk storage containers, and their valve outlets, as well as their transportation,

TABLE 3.2   Properties of Commonly Used Medical Gases

Medical Gas	Chemical Symbol	Molecular Weight	PHYSICAL CHARACTERISTICS			Boiling Point (°C)	Critical Temperature (°C)	Physical State	Combustion Characteristics
			Color	Odor	Taste				
Air	Air	28.97	Colorless	Odorless	Tasteless	−194.3	−140.6	Gas/liquid	NF/SC
Oxygen	O_2	31.99	Colorless	Odorless	Tasteless	−182.9	−118.4	Gas/liquid	NF/SC
Carbon dioxide	CO_2	44.01	Colorless	Odorless	Slightly acidic	−29.0	+31.0	Liquid/gas	NF
Carbon monoxide	CO	28.01	Colorless	Odorless	Tasteless	−191.5	−140.2	Gas	F
Nitrous oxide	N_2O	44.01	Colorless	Odorless	Tasteless	−88.5	+36.4	Liquid/gas	NF
Nitric oxide	NO	30.01	Colorless	Slightly metallic	Tasteless	−151.8	−92.9	Gas	NF
Helium	He	4.00	Colorless	Odorless	Tasteless	−268.9	−267.0	Gas	NF

F, Flammable; *NF,* nonflammable; *SC,* supports combustion.

CLINICAL SCENARIO 3.1

Based on the discussion of compressed gases, name the appropriate gas for each of the following situations:
1. Use as a refrigerant.
2. For reducing the work of breathing in a patient with airway obstruction.
3. To treat hypoxemia in a patient with chronic obstructive pulmonary disease.
4. For reducing pulmonary vasoconstriction, such as occurs in persistent pulmonary hypertension of the newborn.

See Appendix A for the answer.

---

testing, and periodic examination, are subject to national standards and regulations. Box 3.2 lists the agencies that provide recommendations and regulations for the manufacture, storage, transport, and use of medical gases.

Cylinders

Metal cylinders have been used for storing compressed gases since 1888.[10] Federal regulations issued by the Department of Transportation (DOT) require that all cylinders used to store and transport compressed gases conform to well-defined specifications. These specifications, along with recommendations from the National Fire Protection Association (NFPA) and the CGA, provide industry standards for cylinder design and maintenance and the safe use of compressed gases. Box 3.3 contains a summary of NFPA and CGA recommendations for compressed-gas cylinders.

Construction and Maintenance of Compressed-Gas Cylinders

Compressed-gas cylinders are constructed of seamless, high-quality steel, chrome-molybdenum, or aluminum that is either stamped into shape using a punch press die or spun into shape by wrapping heated steel bands around specially designed molds. The bottom of the cylinder is welded closed, and the top of the cylinder is threaded and fitted with a valve stem (Fig. 3.2).

Type 3AA cylinders are produced from heat-treated, high-strength steel; type 3A cylinders are made of carbon-steel (non–heat treated). Type 3AL cylinders are constructed of specially prescribed seamless aluminum alloys. Type 3 cylinders, which are made of low-carbon steel, are no longer produced. Note that the steel used in the construction of cylinders must meet the chemical and physical standards set by the DOT. (In Canada the specifications for the construction of cylinders are set by Transport Canada.[8])

Compressed-gas cylinders should be capable of holding up to 10% more than the maximum service pressure as marked.[11,12] This added capacity is required because of variations in cylinder pressure that occur with changes in ambient temperature. The Bureau of Alcohol, Tobacco, Firearms, and Explosives, an agency of the US Department of the Justice, requires that all cylinders contain a pressure-relief mechanism to prevent explosion.[12]

Types 3AA and 3A cylinders must be hydrostatically tested every 10 years to determine their expansion characteristics. (An asterisk following the reexamination date on the cylinder markings [see Fig. 3.4] indicates that the cylinder must be retested every 10 years.[11]) Type 3AL cylinders must be reexamined every 5 years to test their expansion characteristics. Hydrostatic examination involves measuring a cylinder's expansion characteristics when it is filled to a pressure of five-thirds its working pressure. This examination consists of placing a cylinder filled with water in a vessel that is also filled with water. When pressure is applied to the interior of the cylinder, the cylinder expands, displacing water from the jacket surrounding the cylinder. The volume of water displaced when pressure is applied equals the total expansion of the cylinder. The permanent expansion of the cylinder equals the volume of water displaced when the pressure is released. This information is used to calculate the elastic expansion of the cylinder, which is directly related to the thickness of the cylinder. Increases in the elastic expansion of a cylinder indicate a reduction in the wall thickness. Reductions in wall thickness can occur when the cylinder is physically damaged or is subject to corrosion.[1]

Regulating Agencies

- Center for Devices and Radiological Health (CDRH)
  An agency of the FDA that provides standards for medical devices.
- Department of Health and Human Services (DHHS)
  Department of the federal government that oversees health care delivery in the United States. Formerly known as the Department of Health, Education, and Welfare (DHEW).
- Department of Transportation (DOT)
  Provides regulations for the manufacture, storage, and transport of compressed gases.
- Environmental Protection Agency (EPA)
  Government agency that establishes standards and administers regulations concerning potential and actual environmental hazards.
- Food and Drug Administration (FDA)
  An agency of the DHHS that sets purity standards for medical gases.
- Occupational Safety and Health Administration (OSHA)
  An agency of the Department of Labor (DOL) that oversees safety issues related to the work environment.
- Transport Canada (TC)
  Canadian government agency that administers regulations concerning the manufacture and testing of compressed-gas cylinders and their distribution.

Recommending Agencies

- American National Standards Institute (ANSI)
  Private, nonprofit organization that coordinates the voluntary development of national standards in the United States. Represents US interests in international standards.
- American Society of Mechanical Engineers (ASME)
  Issues information on the design, manufacture, and structural standards for components of central piping systems.
- Compressed Gas Association (CGA)
  Comprises companies involved in the manufacture, storage, and transport of all compressed gases. Provides standards and safety systems for compressed-gas systems.
- International Organization for Standardization (ISO)
  International agency that provides standards for technology.
- National Fire Protection Association (NFPA)
  Independent agency that provides information on fire protection and safety.
- United States Pharmacopeia/The National Formulary (USP–NF)
  A not-for-profit private organization founded to develop officially recognized quality standards for drugs, including medical gases.
- Z-79 Committee
  ANSI committee for establishing standards for anesthetic and ventilatory devices, including anesthetic machines, reservoir bags, tracheal tubes, humidifiers, nebulizers, and other oxygen-related equipment.

Filling of Medical Cylinders

As you might expect, filling and refilling a medical gas cylinder is a potentially dangerous process. The DOT, the FDA, and the United States Pharmacopeia and The National Formulary (USP–NF) have established a series of guidelines (i.e., good manufacturing practices) that set strict controls over large commercial cylinder-filling operations, as well as small home medical equipment dealers refilling relatively small numbers of cylinders.[9] Companies performing cylinder filling and refilling procedures must register with the FDA, which monitors compliance through biannual on-site inspections.

Good manufacturing practices are designed to ensure that only properly trained individuals are involved in the refilling process and that the procedure is performed using certified equipment. These guidelines also specify that only safe and clean cylinders can be refilled. Gases used in this process must meet USP–NF standards for purity, and each cylinder must have a current, intact label that is readable and meets FDA and DOT regulations. Additionally, each batch of cylinders must be identified with an assigned lot number that is traceable if recall is necessary.

The process of filling and refilling gas cylinders involves four steps: (a) cylinder prefill inspection, (b) cylinder filling, (c) postfill procedures, and (d) appropriate documentation.[8] Cylinder prefill inspection focuses on removal of any residual gas before refilling, visual inspection of each cylinder for any signs of damage, verification that the last hydrostatic testing date does not exceed DOT retest criteria, and ensuring that the cylinder is properly labeled. As mentioned, cylinder refilling must be done with certified equipment. Cylinders are attached to a specially designed manifold (Fig. 3.3) that allows for cylinder evacuation before filling of the cylinder from a gas supply source. Gas from the supply source is introduced into the cylinders at a controlled flow that permits a filling rate of no more than 200 psig/min until the permitted full pressure is attained. (Note that the full pressure is corrected for temperature so that the accurate volume is present at standard temperature and pressure [STP] conditions.[8]) Once the cylinders are filled, the valves of the cylinders are closed and removed from the manifold. A postfill procedure is then performed on each cylinder to ensure that the cylinder valve does not leak and that the cylinder's contents meet the minimum purity standards set by the USP–NF. Documentation of each of the previous steps and the signature of the individual who filled the cylinders must be recorded in a transfilling log. Company records should also include daily calibration of the oxygen analyzers used to test the purity of the cylinders' contents, along with evidence that the manifold and gauges are inspected according to an established schedule.

Cylinder Sizes and Capacities

Table 3.3 summarizes the weights and volume capacities of various cylinders and gases used in respiratory care. The most commonly used cylinders for medical gas therapy are the E and H types. D cylinders are used for the storage of nitric oxide.

BOX 3.3   National Fire Protection Association and CompressedN Gas Association Recommendations for Compressed-Gas Cylinders

Storage

1. Storage rooms must be dry, cool, and well ventilated. Cylinders should not be stored in an area where the temperature exceeds 51.67°C (125°F).
2. No flames should have the potential of coming in contact with the cylinders.
3. The storage facility should be fire resistant where practical.
4. Cylinders must not be stored near flammable or combustible substances.
5. Gases that support combustion must be stored in a separate location from those that are combustible.
6. The storage area must be permanently posted.
7. Cylinders must be grouped by content.
8. Full and empty cylinders must be segregated in the storage areas.
9. Below-ground storage should be avoided.
10. Cylinders should never be stored in the operating room.
11. Large cylinders must be stored upright.
12. Cylinders must be protected from being cut or abraded.
13. Cylinders must be protected from extreme weather to prevent rusting, excessive temperatures, and accumulations of snow and ice.
14. Cylinders should not be exposed to continuous dampness or corrosive substances that could promote rusting of the cylinder and its valve.
15. Cylinders should be protected from tampering.
16. Valves on empty cylinders should be kept closed at all times.
17. Cylinders must be stored with protective caps in place.
18. Cylinders must not be stored in a confined space, such as a closet or the trunk of a car.

Transportation

1. If protective valve caps are supplied, they should be used whenever cylinders are in transport and until they are ready for use.
2. Cylinders must not be dropped, dragged, slid, or allowed to strike each other violently.
3. Cylinders must be transported on an appropriate cart secured by a chain or strap.

Use

1. Before connecting equipment to a cylinder, make sure that connections are free of foreign materials.
2. Turn valve outlet away from personnel and crack cylinder valve to remove any dust or debris from outlet.
3. Cylinder valve outlet connections must be American Standard or CGA pin indexed, and low-pressure connections must be CGA diameter indexed.
4. Cylinders must be secured at the administration site and not to any movable objects or heat radiators.
5. Outlets and connections must be tightened only with appropriate wrenches and must never be forced on.
6. Equipment designed to use one gas should not be used with another.
7. Never use medical cylinder gases when contamination by backflow of other gases may occur.
8. Regulators should be off when the cylinder is turned on, and the cylinder valve should be opened slowly.
9. Before equipment is disconnected from a cylinder, the cylinder valve should be closed and the pressure released from the device.
10. Cylinder valves should be closed at all times except when in use.
11. Do not transfill cylinders, because this is hazardous.
12. Cylinders may be refilled only if permission is secured from the owner.
13. Cylinders must not be lifted by the cap.
14. Equipment connected to cylinders containing gaseous oxygen should be labeled: OXYGEN—USE NO OIL.
15. Enclosures intended to contain patients must have the minimum text regarding NO SMOKING, and the labels must be located (a) in a position to be read by the patients and (b) on two or more opposing sides visible from the exterior. It should be noted that oxygen hoods fall under the classification of oxygen enclosures and require these labels as well. In addition, another label is required that instructs visitors to obtain approval from hospital personnel before placing toys in an oxygen enclosure.
16. High-pressure oxygen equipment must not be sterilized with flammable agents (e.g., alcohol and ethylene oxide), and the agents used must be oil-free and nondamaging.
17. Polyethylene bags must not be used to wrap sterilized, high-pressure oxygen equipment because when flexed, polyethylene releases pure hydrocarbons that are highly flammable.
18. Oxygen equipment exposed to pressures of less than 60 pounds per square inch (psi) may be sterilized with either a nonflammable mixture of ethylene oxide and carbon dioxide or with fluorocarbons.
19. Cylinders must not be handled with oily or greasy hands, gloves, or clothing.
20. Never lubricate valve outlets or connecting equipment. (Oxygen and oil under pressure cause an explosive oxidation reaction.)
21. Do not flame test for leaks. (Usually a soap solution is used.)
22. When a cylinder is in use, open the valve fully and then turn it back a quarter- to a half-turn.
23. Replace the cap on an empty cylinder.
24. Position the cylinder so that the label is clearly visible. The label must not be defaced, altered, or removed.
25. Check the label before use; it should always match the color code.
26. No sources of open flames should be permitted in the area of administration. A NO SMOKING sign must be posted at the administration site. It must be legible from a distance of 5 feet and displayed in a conspicuous location.
27. Inform all area occupants of the hazards of smoking and of the regulations.
28. Equipment designated for use with a specific gas must be clearly and permanently labeled accordingly. The name of the manufacturer should be clearly marked on the device. If calibration or accuracy depends on gas density, the device must be labeled with the proper supply pressure.
29. Cylinder carts must be of a self-supporting design with appropriate casters and wheels, and those intended for use in surgery where flammable anesthetics are used must be grounded.

Continued

BOX 3.3   National Fire Protection Association and CompressedN Gas Association Recommendations for Compressed-Gas Cylinders—cont'd

30. Cold cylinders must be handled with care to avoid hand injury resulting from tissue freezing caused by rapid gas expansion.
31. Safety-relief mechanisms, noninterchangeable connections, and other safety features must not be removed or altered.
32. Control valves on equipment must be closed both before connection and when not in use.

Repair and Maintenance

1. Use only the service manuals, operator manuals, instructions, procedures, and repair parts that are provided or recommended by the manufacturer.

2. Allow only qualified personnel to maintain the equipment.
3. Designate and set aside an area clean and free of oil and grease for the maintenance of oxygen equipment. Do not use this area for the repair and maintenance of other types of equipment.
4. Follow a scheduled preventive maintenance program.

CGA, Compressed Gas Association.

Reproduced with permission from NFPA99-2012: Health Care Facilities, Copyright © 2011, National Fire Protection Association. This reprinted material is not the complete and official position of the NFPA on the referenced subject, which is represented only by the standard in its entirety.

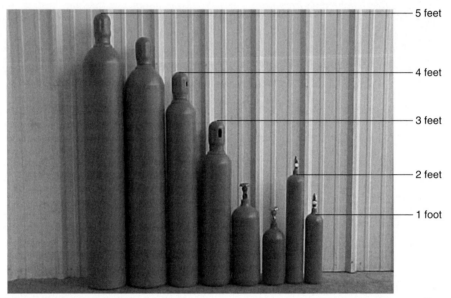

FIGURE 3.2 Various types of high-pressure cylinders used in medical gas therapy. (Courtesy nexAir, LLC, Memphis, TN.)

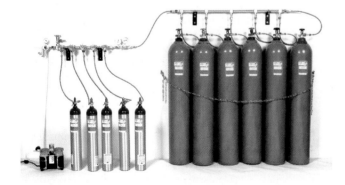

FIGURE 3.3 Example of a transfilling manifold.

E cylinders frequently are used as a source of oxygen in emergency situations (e.g., cardiopulmonary resuscitation carts ["crash carts"]) and for transporting patients requiring oxygen therapy. These smaller cylinders also store gases used in anesthetics, as well as calibration gases for portable diagnostic equipment (e.g., capnographs and pulse oximeters).

H cylinders are used as the primary source of oxygen and other medical gases in smaller hospitals that do not have bulk liquid systems (see the following subsection). Hospitals and other facilities with bulk liquid oxygen systems use these larger cylinders as a secondary or reserve source of medical gases in case of electrical power failure. Large cylinders are often used for home care patients who need long-term oxygen therapy. H cylinders can also serve as a backup oxygen source in the event of electrical power failure in the home care setting. These larger cylinders are also routinely used to store the calibration

TABLE 3.3 Physical Characteristics of Common-Size Aluminum and Steel Cylinders

| | ALUMINUM | | | | | | | STEEL | | | | |
	B or M6	ML6	C or M9	D	E	N or M60	M or MM	D	E	M	H	T
Service pressure (psig)	2216	2015	2015	2015	2015	2216	2216	2015	2015	2015	2015	2400
Height without valve (inches)	11.6	7.7	10.9	16.5	25.6	23	35.75	16.75	25.75	43	51	55
Diameter (inches)	3.2	4.4	4.4	4.4	4.4	7.25	8	4.2	4.2	7	9	9.25
Weight without valve (pounds)	2.2	2.9	3.7	5.3	7.9	21.7	38.6	7.9	11.3	58	117	139
Capacity at Listed Pressure at STPD												
Oxygen (cubic feet)	6	6	9	15	24	61.4	122	15	24	110	244	300
Oxygen (liters)	170	170	255	425	680	1738	3455	425	680	3113	7075	8490

STPD, Standard temperature and pressure, dry.
From Hess D, MacIntyre N, Mishoe S, et al: *Respiratory care: principles and practice,* ed 2, Sudbury, MA, 2012, Jones & Bartlett Learning.

gases required in blood gas and pulmonary function laboratories.

Cylinder Identification

Cylinders are engraved with information that is designed primarily to identify where the cylinder was manufactured, the type of material used in its construction (i.e., 3AA, 3A, or 3AL), the service pressure of the cylinder, the date of its original hydrostatic test, and its reexamination dates.[1] Additionally, the manufacturer's name, the owner's identification number, and the size of the cylinder are usually engraved on the cylinder. Fig. 3.4 shows the standard markings that appear on compressed-gas cylinders. Note that a "+" following the stamped hydrostatic examination date indicates that the cylinder complied with requirement of the examination. A "+" does not follow the reexamination date on aluminum cylinders.

Medical gas cylinders are color coded for easy identification. Table 3.4 shows the color codes prescribed by the NF.[3] Generally, these colors conform to an international cylinder color-coding system. Two major exceptions in the international system are oxygen cylinders, which are painted white, and compressed-air cylinders, which are painted yellow or black and white. In the United States the color code for oxygen is green, and compressed air cylinders are painted yellow. Cylinders containing gas mixtures (e.g., helium–oxygen and carbon dioxide–oxygen) are divided into two categories of color coding, each based on the percentage of gases contained. For example, cylinders of carbon dioxide–oxygen mixtures that contain more than 7% carbon dioxide are predominantly gray with the shoulder of the tank painted green. Cylinders

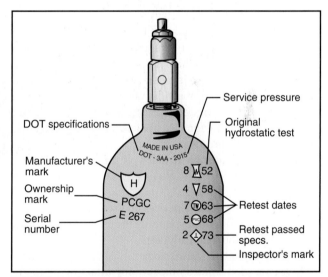

FIGURE 3.4 Standard markings for compressed-gas cylinders. *DOT,* Department of Transportation. (Copyright © 2013 Medtronic Minimally Invasive Therapies. All rights reserved. Reprinted with permission of Medtronic Minimally Invasive Therapies.)

containing carbon dioxide–oxygen mixtures with less than 7% carbon dioxide are predominantly green with a gray shoulder. Helium–oxygen cylinders containing more than 80% helium are painted brown with a green shoulder. Cylinders of helium–oxygen mixtures containing less than 80% helium (balanced with oxygen) are predominantly green with a brown shoulder.

TABLE 3.4 Color Codes for Medical Gases

Gas	Chemical Symbol	Purity[a] (%)	Color Code
Air	—	99.0	Yellow or black and white[b]
Carbon dioxide	CO_2	99.0	Gray
Carbon dioxide/oxygen	CO_2/O_2	99.0	Gray and green[c]
Cyclopropane	C_3H_6	99.0	Orange
Ethylene	C_2H_4	99.0	Red
Helium	He	99.0	Brown
Helium/oxygen	He/O_2	99.0	Brown and green[c] or brown and white
Nitrogen	N_2	99.0	Black
Nitrous oxide	N_2O	97.0	Light blue
Nitric oxide	NO	99.0	Teal and black
Oxygen	O_2	99.0	Green or white[b]

[a]National Formulary Standards.
[b]International color code for oxygen is white; in the United States the color code for oxygen cylinders is green.
[c]Always check labels to determine the percentages of each gas.

Color codes are only a guide; printed labels are still the primary means of identifying the contents of a gas cylinder. Fig. 3.5 is a standard label for an oxygen cylinder. The CGA and the American Standards Safety System (ASSS) specify that all labels should include the name and chemical symbol of the gas in the cylinder. The label should also show the volume of the cylinder (in liters) at a temperature of 21.1°C (70°F).[1] Generally, labels also include any specific hazards related to use of the gas and precautionary measures and instructions in case of accidental exposure or contact with the contents.

The FDA requires that compressed gases used for medical purposes meet certain minimum requirements for purity, and the purity of the gas must be indicated on the label identifying the contents of the cylinder. These standards are listed in the USP–NF (see Table 3.4 for a list of these purity requirements). The FDA also requires that the names of the manufacturer, packer, and distributor be included on the label.

Cylinder Valves

Cylinder valves are control devices that seal the contents of a compressed cylinder until it is ready for use. A cylinder valve is composed of the following parts:
1. A chrome-plated, brass body
2. A threaded inlet connector for attachment to the cylinder
3. A stem that opens and closes the cylinder when turned by a hand wheel or handle
4. An outlet connection that allows for attachment of regulators and pressure-reducing valves
5. A pressure-relief valve

Fig. 3.6 shows the two types of cylinder valves affixed to compressed medical gas cylinders: direct-acting valves and diaphragm valves. A direct-acting valve (see Fig. 3.6A) contains two fiber washers and a Teflon packing to prevent gas leakage around the threads. The term *direct-acting* is derived from the arrangement of movements in the valve wheel. These movements are directly reflected in the valve seat because it

is one piece moved by threads. Direct-acting valves can withstand high pressures (i.e., more than 1500 pounds per square inch [psi]).

Diaphragm valves (see Fig. 3.6B) use a threaded stem in place of the packing found on the direct-acting valves. The stem is separated from the valve seat and spring by two diaphragms, one made of steel and one made of copper. When the stem is turned counterclockwise and raised because of the threading, the diaphragm is pushed upward with the stem by the valve seat and spring, causing the valve to open. Turning the stem clockwise resets the diaphragm and closes the valve.

Diaphragm valves have several advantages: (1) the valve seat does not turn and therefore is resistant to scoring, which could cause leakage; (2) no stem leakage can occur because of the diaphragm; and (3) the stem can be opened with a partial rotation rather than with two turns of the wheel, as in direct-acting valves. Diaphragm valves generally are preferable when pressures are relatively low (i.e., less than 1500 psi). They also are ideal for situations in which no gas leaks can be allowed, such as with flammable anesthetics.

Pressure-Relief Valves

Fig. 3.7 illustrates three types of pressure-relief mechanisms: rupture disks, fusible plugs, and spring-loaded devices.[1] A rupture disk (also called a *frangible disk*) is a thin, metal disk that ruptures or buckles when the pressure inside the cylinder exceeds a certain predetermined limit. A fusible plug is made of a metal alloy that melts when the temperature of the gas in the tank exceeds a predetermined temperature. Fusible plugs operate on the principle that as the pressure in a tank increases, the temperature of the gas increases, causing the plug to melt. After the plug melts, excess pressure is released. (A commonly used metal alloy is called Wood's metal; fusible plugs made of this alloy generally have melting temperatures of 98°C to 104°C [208°F to 220°F].) Spring-loaded devices are designed to release excessive cylinder pressure and reseal,

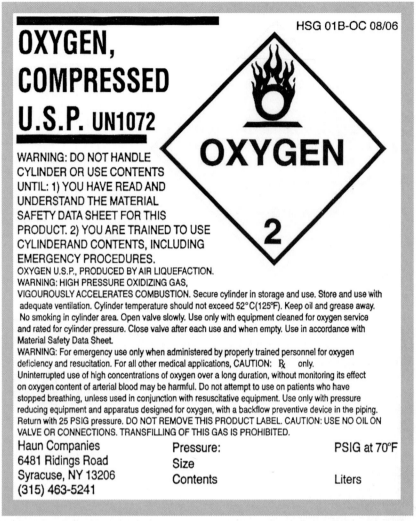

FIGURE 3.5 Example of compressed-gas cylinder labeling. (From dailymed.nlm.nih.gov; US National Library of Medicine, Bethesda, MD.)

preventing further release of gas from the cylinder after the cause of the excessive pressure is removed.[1] With these devices a metal seal is held in place by an adjustable spring. The amount of pressure required to force the seal open depends on the tension of the spring holding the metal seal in place. Spring-loaded devices usually are more susceptible to leakage around the metal seal than are rupture disks and fusible plugs.[1] Note that spring-loaded devices may also be affected by changes in environmental conditions (i.e., freezing conditions can cause these devices to stick). Rupture disks and fusible plugs are often incorporated into smaller cylinders, whereas spring-loaded devices are found on larger cylinders.[8]

Safety Systems

Outlet connections of cylinder valves are indexed according to standards designed by the CGA and adopted by the American National Standard Institute and the Canadian Standards Association. (***Note:*** This indexing system is referred to as the American Standard Safety System or ASSS.) ASSS connections are noninterchangeable to prevent the interchange of regulating equipment between gases that are not compatible.

The ASSS includes separate systems for large and small cylinders. Large cylinder valve outlets and connections (e.g., for sizes H and K) are indexed by thread type, thread size, right- or left-handed threading, external or internal threading, and nipple-seat design.[12] Fig. 3.8 illustrates the ASSS connections for medical gases that are commonly used in respiratory care. Look at the oxygen connection shown in this figure. The diameter of the cylinder's outlet is listed in thousandths of inches (e.g., the oxygen connection is 0.903 inch). (***Note***: Diameter Indexing Safety System (DISS) is a term used to describe the ASSS safety system used for large cylinders.) The letters following these numbers indicate the type of threading used (i.e., right-handed [RH] versus left-handed [LH]). The abbreviations *Ext* and *Int* specify whether the threads are external or internal. Note that the connections for oxygen and other life support gases are right-handed and external. The remaining information indicates whether the outlet requires a nipple attachment. Oxygen valves require a rounded nipple.

Small cylinders (e.g., sizes AA to E) with post-type valves use a different ASSS indexing called the Pin Index Safety

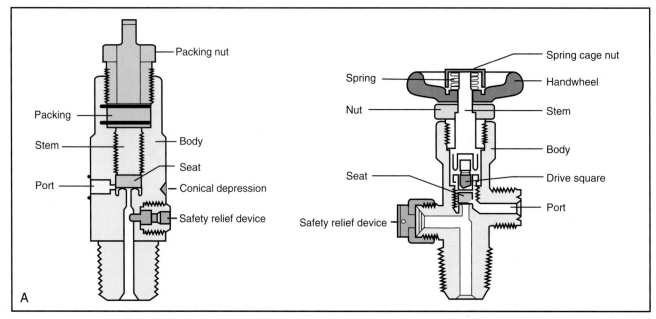

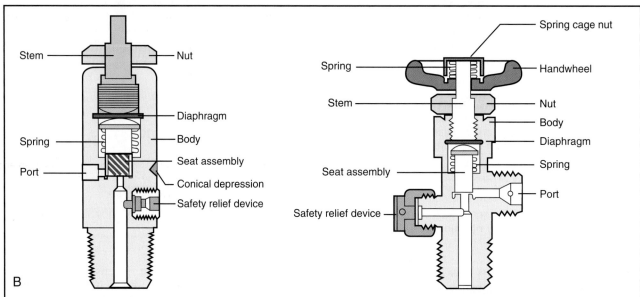

FIGURE 3.6 Cylinder valves. A, Direct-acting valve. B, Diaphragm valve. (Copyright © 2013 Medtronic Minimally Invasive Therapies. All rights reserved. Reprinted with permission of Medtronic Minimally Invasive Therapies.)

System (PISS). In this system, indexing is accomplished by the exact placement of two pins into holes in the post valve. Note that the hole positions are numbered from 1 to 6; each medical gas uses a specified pin sequence. Fig. 3.9 shows the different combinations used to differentiate the most common medical gases. For example, the pins for an oxygen regulator must be placed in the 2 and 5 positions for it to attach to the oxygen cylinder's post valve. Cylinder regulators are discussed in Chapter 4.

Setting Up and Troubleshooting Compressed-Gas Cylinders

Box 3.4 presents the steps that should be followed in setting up a compressed-gas cylinder.[13] The following is a list of simple

suggestions that should be kept in mind in the handling of compressed-gas cylinders:

1. The cylinder's contents should be clearly labeled. If the contents of a cylinder are questionable, do not use it.
2. Full and empty cylinders should be appropriately labeled and kept separate.
3. Cylinder valves should be fully opened when in use and always closed when the gas contained in the cylinder is not being used. Cylinder valves should be closed if the cylinder is empty.
4. Large cylinders have a protective cap that fits over the valve stem. This cap should be kept on the cylinders when they are moved or stored. Small cylinders with PISS valve stems do not have protective caps but have

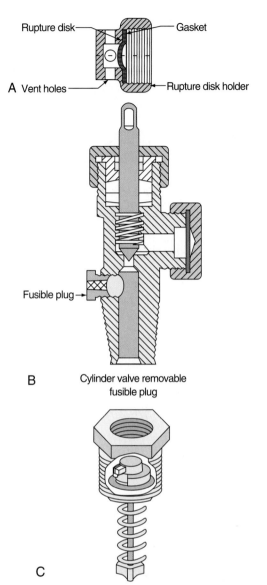

FIGURE 3.7 Pressure-relief valves. A, Rupture (frangible) disks. B, Fusible plug. C, Spring-loaded device. (Redrawn from the Compressed Gas Association: *Handbook of compressed gases*, ed 3, New York, 1990, Van Nostrand Reinhold.)

an outlet seal that must be removed before the appropriate regulator is attached.

5. Regulators and other appliances intended for use with a specific gas should not be used with other gases.
6. Cylinders should be properly secured at all times, either in a stand, chained to a wall, or in a cart, to prevent them from tipping over.

Most problems encountered with cylinders and regulators involve (1) gas leakage at the valve stem or in the regulator and (2) failure to achieve adequate gas flow at the cylinder regulator outlet. Leaks typically occur from large cylinders because of loose connections between the regulator and the cylinder valve. Gas leaks from small cylinders most often are associated with damage to the plastic washer that fits between the valve stem and the regulator. Gas leaks at the regulator outlet can be caused by a loose connection between the regulator and attached equipment (Clinical Scenario 3.2). Failure

CLINICAL SCENARIO 3.2

A respiratory therapist "cracks" an H cylinder of oxygen and then attaches an oxygen regulator to the cylinder outlet. She slowly opens the valve stem and hears a sudden, loud hissing sound coming from the connection between the cylinder outlet and the regulator. What should she do?
See Appendix A for the answer.

to achieve a desired gas flow from a cylinder regulator can result from inadequate pressure (e.g., low gauge pressure) or from an obstruction at the regulator outlet.

Determining the Volume of Gas Remaining in a Cylinder and the Duration of Cylinder Gas Flow

Calculation of the gas volume remaining in a cylinder requires knowledge of either the pressure or the weight of the cylinder (see Table 3.3 for a list of values for commonly used medical gas cylinders). For nonliquefied-gas cylinders (e.g., compressed air, oxygen, helium), the gas volume contained in a cylinder is directly related to the regulator's gauge pressure. Table 3.5 shows these volume–pressure constants, or "tank factors," for the more commonly used medical gas cylinders. The volume of gas remaining in a cylinder can then be calculated by multiplying the cylinder's volume-pressure constant by the gauge pressure. Box 3.5 presents an example of this calculation. The resultant volume can then be divided by the flow rate of gas being used to determine the duration of gas flow remaining in minutes.

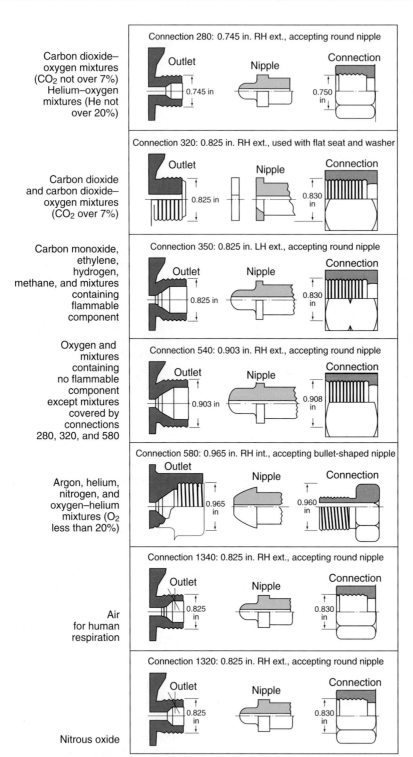

FIGURE 3.8 American Standard Safety System indexing system for large cylinders. (Courtesy Datex-Ohmeda, Madison, WI.)

TABLE 3.5	Volume–Pressure Conversion Factors	
Cylinder Size	**Conversion Factor**
E	622.0 L/2200 psi = 0.28
G	5264.0 L/2200 psi = 2.39
H or K	6900.0 L/2200 psi = 3.14

Determining the gas volume remaining in a liquefied-gas cylinder (e.g., carbon dioxide and nitrous oxide) is more of a challenge. The gas volume remaining in a liquefied-gas cylinder cannot be determined by the method just described because the liquid remains in equilibrium with the gas above it until the liquid is depleted. The volume of liquefied gas remaining is best determined by weighing the cylinder before and after it is filled. Thus the volume of liquid gas remaining in the cylinder

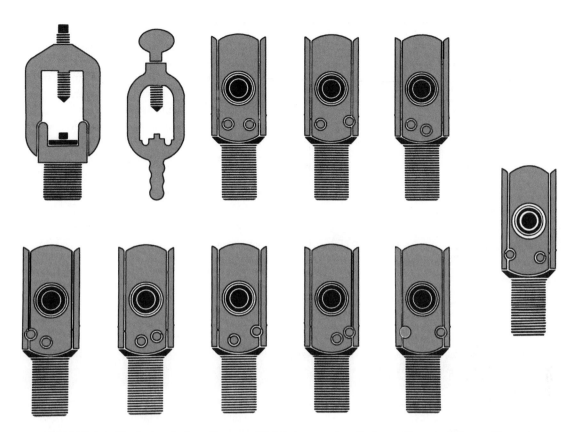

FIGURE 3.9 Pin Index Safety System (PISS) for small cylinders. (Courtesy Datex-Ohmeda, Madison, WI.)

BOX 3.5 Estimating the Duration of a Medical Gas Cylinder Supply

The amount of time it will take a cylinder filled with compressed gas to provide a set flow rate of gas can be calculated with the following formula[a]:

$$\frac{\text{Cylinder Pressure (psi)} \times \text{Cylinder factor}^a}{\text{Flow rate of gas (L/min)}} = \frac{\text{Duration of flow}}{\text{in minutes}}$$

Example
You are asked to transport a patient who is receiving oxygen from a nasal cannula at 4 L/min. The pressure gauge on the cylinder reads 1800 psi. How long will the cylinder provide the appropriate oxygen flow?

1800 psi × (0.28) ÷ 4 L/min = 126 minutes, or about 2 hours

---

[a]The cylinder factor represents the relationship between the cylinder volume and the gauge pressure. For example, an E cylinder can hold 622 L of gas at a filling pressure of 2200 psi. The volume–pressure cylinder factor for E cylinders equals 622 L/2200 psi, or 0.28 L/psi. Table 3.5 shows the cylinder factors for the several commonly used cylinders.

is directly related to the weight of the cylinder. After the volume is determined, the duration of gas flow can be calculated by dividing that volume by the flow rate of gas being used.

Liquid Oxygen Systems

Hospitals and larger health care facilities typically rely on bulk liquid supply systems for medical air and oxygen needs. The increased use of bulk liquid supply systems is the result of a couple of factors: (1) gases shipped in bulk are less expensive than gases shipped in cylinders, and (2) liquefied oxygen occupies a fraction of the space required to store gaseous oxygen. Note that gaseous oxygen occupies a volume 860 times that of liquid oxygen.

The construction of bulk reservoir systems is regulated by the NFPA and the American Society of Mechanical Engineers (ASME). The NFPA requirements also address installation, inspection, testing, maintenance, performance of safe practices for facilities, material, equipment, and appliances.[12]

Bulk Liquid Oxygen Systems

The NFPA defines a bulk oxygen system as more than 20,000 cu ft of oxygen (at atmospheric temperature and pressure), including unconnected reserves, that are on hand at a site.[12] Fig. 3.10 shows the major components of a bulk oxygen system. It consists of an insulated reservoir, a vaporizer with associated tubing attached to the reservoir, a pressure-reducing valve, and an appropriate pressure-release valve. The reservoir stores a mixture of liquid and gaseous oxygen. The vaporizer acts as a heat exchanger, where heat is absorbed from the environment and used to warm the liquid oxygen to room temperature, thus forming gaseous oxygen. The pressure-reducing valve serves to reduce the working pressure of the gas to a desired level (usually 50 psi for hospitals and other health care facilities) before it enters the hospital's compressed-gas piping system (see Fig. 3.19 for a description of piping systems). The pressure-release valve allows some of the gas

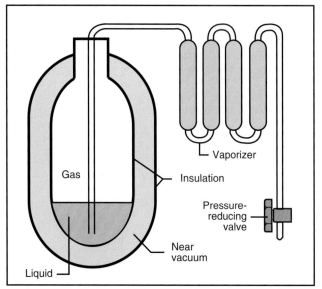

FIGURE 3.10 Components of a bulk oxygen supply system.

on top of the liquid to escape if the contents are warmed too much. This release of gas allows the gas within the container to expand, thus lowering the temperature (see Gay-Lussac's law in Chapter 1). This keeps the gas under pressure between its boiling point and its critical temperature, so that most of the reservoir's contents are maintained in the liquid state.

As previously stated, bulk reservoir systems must meet specifications established by the NFPA.[12] Box 3.6 contains a summary of the NFPA recommendations and regulations for bulk oxygen systems. Proper installment of these systems is critical to maintain public safety. Fig. 3.11 shows the minimum distances between bulk oxygen storage facilities and other structures.

Portable Liquid Oxygen Systems

Smaller versions of the bulk oxygen system are available for the home care setting. A typical home liquid oxygen system consists of two components: a stationary base reservoir and a portable unit. The main unit contains a liquid reservoir, a

---

BOX 3.6   National Fire Protection Association Recommendations and Regulations for Bulk Oxygen Systems

1. Containers that are permanently installed should be mounted on noncombustible supports and foundations.
2. Liquid oxygen containers should be constructed from materials that meet the impact test requirements of paragraph UG-48 of the ASME Boiler and Pressure Vessel Codes, Section VII, and must be in accordance with DOT specifications and regulations for 4-L liquid oxygen containers. Containers operating above 15 psi must be designed and tested in accordance with the ASME Boiler and Pressure Vessel Code, Section VII, and the insulation of the liquid oxygen container must be of noncombustible material.
3. All high-pressure gaseous oxygen containers must comply with the construction and test requirements of ASME Boiler and Pressure Vessel Code, Section VIII.
4. Bulk oxygen storage containers must be equipped with safety-release devices as required by ASME Code IV and the provisions of ASME S-1.3 or DOT specifications for both the container and safety releases.
5. Isolation casings on liquid oxygen containers shall be equipped with suitable safety-release devices. These devices must be designed or located so that moisture cannot either freeze the unit or interfere in any manner with its proper operation.
6. The vaporizing columns and connecting pipes shall be anchored or sufficiently flexible to provide for expansion and contraction as a result of temperature changes. The column must also have a safety-release device to properly protect it.
7. Any heat supplied to oxygen vaporizers must be done in an indirect fashion, such as with steam, air, water, or water solutions that do not react with oxygen. If liquid heaters are used to provide the primary source of heat, the vaporizers must be electrically grounded.
8. All equipment composing the bulk system must be cleaned to remove oxidizable material before the system is placed into service.

9. All joints and connections in the tubing should be made by welding or using flanged, threaded slip, or compressed fittings, and any gaskets or thread seals must be of suitable substance for oxygen service. Any valves, gauges, or regulators placed into the system must be designed for oxygen service. The piping must conform to ANSI B 31.3; piping that operates below −28.8°C (−20°F) must be composed of materials meeting ASME Code, Section VIII.
10. Storage containers, piping valves, and regulating equipment must be protected from physical damage and tampering.
11. Any enclosure containing oxygen control or operating equipment must be adequately ventilated.
12. The location shall be permanently posted to indicate OXYGEN—NO SMOKING—NO OPEN FLAMES or an equivalent warning.
13. All bulk systems must be regularly inspected by qualified representatives of the oxygen supplier.
14. Weeds and tall grass must be kept a minimum of 15 feet from any bulk oxygen container. The bulk oxygen system must be located so that its distance provides maximum safety for other areas surrounding it. The minimum distances for location of a bulk oxygen system near the following structures (see Fig. 3.11) are as follows:
    a. 25 feet from any combustible structure.
    b. 25 feet from any structure that consists of fire-resistant exterior walls or buildings of other construction that have sprinklers.
    c. 10 feet from any opening in the adjacent walls of fire-resistant structures.
    d. 25 feet from flammable liquid storage above ground that is less than 1000 gallons in capacity, or 50 feet from these storage areas if the quantity is in excess of 1000 gallons.
    e. 15 feet from an underground flammable liquid storage that is less than 1000 gallons, or 30 feet from one in excess of 1000 gallons capacity. The distance from the

BOX 3.6   National Fire Protection Association Recommendations and Regulations for Bulk Oxygen Systems—cont'd

oxygen storage containers to connections used for filling and venting of flammable liquid must be at least 25 feet.

f. 25 feet from combustible gas storage above ground that is less than 1000 gallons capacity, or 50 feet from the storage of over 1000 gallons capacity.

g. 15 feet from combustible liquid storage underground and 25 feet from the vent or filling connections.

h. 50 feet from flammable gas storage less than 5000 cu ft; 90 feet from flammable gas in excess of 5000 cu ft NTP (normal temperature and pressure).

i. 25 feet from solid materials that burn slowly (e.g., coal and heavy timber).

j. 75 feet away in one direction and 35 feet away at an approximately 90-degree angle from confining walls unless they are made from a fire-resistant material and are less than 20 feet high. (This is to provide adequate ventilation in the area in case venting occurs.)

k. 50 feet from places of public assembly.

l. 50 feet from nonambulatory patients.

m. 10 feet from public sidewalks.

n. 5 feet from any adjoining property line.

o. Must be accessible by a mobile transport unit that fills the supply system.

15. The permanent installation of a liquid oxygen system must be supervised by personnel familiar with the proper installation and construction as outlined in the NFPA 50.

16. The oxygen supply must have an inlet for the connection of a temporary supply in emergency and maintenance situations. The inlet must be physically protected to prevent tampering or unauthorized use and must be labeled EMERGENCY LOW-PRESSURE GASEOUS OXYGEN INLET. The inlet is to be installed downstream from the main supply line shutoff valve and must have the necessary valves to provide the emergency supply of oxygen as well as isolate the pipeline to the normal source of supply. There must be a check valve in the main line between the inlet connection and the main shutoff valve and another check valve between the inlet connection and the emergency supply shutoff valve. The inlet connection must have a pressure-relief valve of adequate size to protect the downstream piping from pressures in excess of 50% above normal pipeline operating pressure.

17. The bulk oxygen system must be mounted on noncombustible supports and foundations.

18. A surface of noncombustible material must extend at least 3 feet beyond the reach of liquid oxygen leaks during system operation or filling. Asphalt or bitumastic paving is prohibited. The slope of the area must be considered in the sizing of the surface.

19. The same type of surface must extend at least the full width of the vehicle that fills the bulk unit and at least 8 feet in the transverse direction.

20. No part of the bulk system should be underneath electrical power lines or within reach of a downed power line.

21. No part of the system can be exposed to flammable gases or to piping containing any class of flammable or combustible liquids.

22. The system must be located so as to be readily accessible to mobile supply equipment at ground level, as well as to authorized personnel.

23. Warning and alarm systems are required to monitor the operation and condition of the supply system. Alarms and gauges are to be located for the best possible surveillance, and each alarm and gauge must be appropriately labeled.

24. The master alarm system must monitor the source of supply, the reserve (if any), and the mainline pressure of the gas system. The power source for warning systems must meet the essentials of NFPA 76 A.

25. All alarm conditions must be evaluated and necessary measures taken to establish or ensure the proper function of the supply system.

26. Two master alarm panels, with alarms that cannot be canceled, are to be located in separate locations to ensure continuous observation. One signal must alert the user to a changeover from one operating supply to another, and an additional signal must provide notification that the reserve is supplying the system.

27. If check valves are not installed in the cylinder leads and headers, another alarm signal should be initiated when the reserve reaches a 1-day supply.

28. All piping systems must have both audible and visible signals that cannot be canceled to indicate when the mainline pressure increases or decreases 20% from the normal supply pressure. A pressure gauge must be installed and appropriately labeled adjacent to the switch that generates the pressure alarm conditions.

29. All warning systems must be tested before being placed in service or being added to existing service. Periodic retesting and appropriate recordkeeping are required.

ANSI, American National Standards Institute; *ASME,* American Society of Mechanical Engineers; *DOT,* Department of Transportation; *NFPA,* National Fire Protection Association.
Reproduced with permission from NFPA99-2012: Health Care Facilities, Copyright © 2011, National Fire Protection Association. This reprinted material is not the complete and official position of the NFPA on the referenced subject, which is represented only by the standard in its entirety.

vaporizer coil, and a pressure-relief valve. Fig. 3.12 shows various sizes of stationary liquid oxygen reservoirs that are available for the home care setting. The portable device is filled from the main unit.

Stationary reservoirs have capacities of 12 to 60 L of liquid oxygen, whereas portable units have capacities of 0.5 to 1.2 L.[9] Stationary reservoir systems can provide an economical source

of oxygen for home care patients who require long-term oxygen therapy. These systems generally can provide a reliable source of oxygen for 4 to 6 weeks, depending on the demand. Portable units can provide an 8- to 10-hour supply of oxygen for patients during times of greater mobility. Newer portable devices, such as the Helios unit shown in Fig. 3.13, weigh less than 4 lb when filled and can provide continuous oxygen for

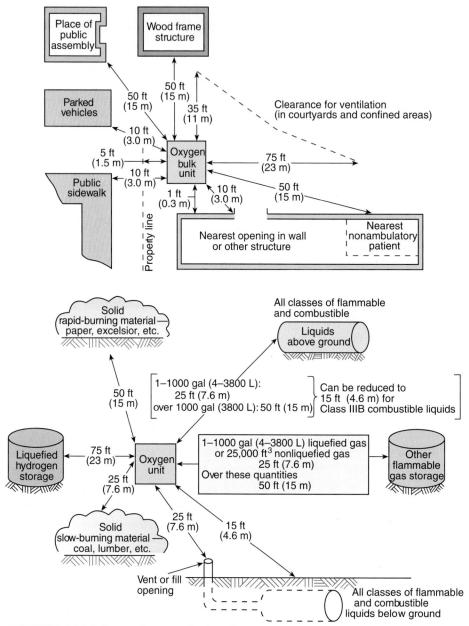

FIGURE 3.11 Minimum distances for locating structures around a bulk oxygen supply.

6 to 10 hours, depending on the flow rate used. As is discussed in Chapter 4, oxygen-conserving devices can increase the amount of time these smaller systems can provide oxygen. Box 3.7 explains how to calculate the duration of a liquid oxygen supply. Remember that the amount of time a supply will last depends on the weight of the liquid remaining in the reservoir—not the pressure, as for cylinders. Because 1 L of liquid oxygen weighs 2.5 lb, the number of liters of liquid oxygen present can be calculated by dividing the weight of the liquid oxygen by 2.5. Considering that oxygen expands to 860 times its liquid volume at 25°C (77°F) and 1 atm, the total volume of gaseous oxygen available can be calculated by multiplying the number of liters of liquid oxygen by 860. The amount of time in minutes that the supply will last can be determined by dividing this volume by the flow rate of the gas being delivered.

Most portable systems are designed to provide working pressures of approximately 20 psi. It is important to know the operating pressure of the device before flowmeters or restrictors are attached to control gas flow out of the system. Failure to recognize the actual delivery pressure of these devices can result in injury to the patient or damage to the attached equipment. The actual flow delivered can be determined with a calibrated Thorpe tube flowmeter (see Chapter 4 for a discussion of flowmeters). Box 3.8 lists the NFPA safety recommendations for portable liquid oxygen systems.

Medical Air Supply
Portable Air Compressors

Compressed air is used to power many respiratory care devices. In many cases, air can be compressed at the point of administration by portable air compressors. Larger portable systems

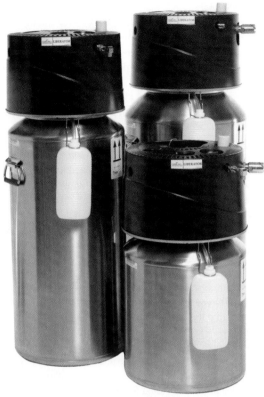

FIGURE 3.12 Stationary liquid oxygen reservoirs. (Copyright © 2013 Medtronic Minimally Invasive Therapies. All rights reserved. Reprinted with permission of Medtronic Minimally Invasive Therapies.)

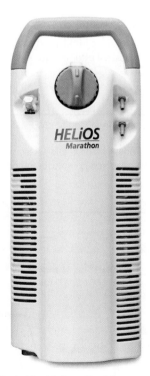

FIGURE 3.13 Portable Helios liquid oxygen system. This system uses an oxygen-conserving mechanism that relies on a demand valve, which delivers oxygen on inhalation and stops during exhalation. (Courtesy CAIRE Medical, Chart Industries, Ball Ground, GA.)

BOX 3.7 Calculating the Duration of a Liquid Oxygen Supply

1. A liter of liquid oxygen weighs 2.5 lb, therefore:
   Liquid weight ÷ 2.5 = Number of liters of liquid oxygen
2. Gaseous oxygen occupies a volume that is 860 times the volume of liquid oxygen, therefore:
   Liters of liquid × 860 = Liters of gas
3. Duration of supply (minutes) = Gas supply remaining (in liters) ÷ Flow (L/min).

Example

How long would a liquid oxygen supply weighing 10 lb last if a patient were receiving oxygen through a nasal cannula at 2 L/min?

Amount of gas (liters) = (10 lb ÷ 2.5 lb/L) × 860

Amount of gas = 3440 L

Duration of supply (minutes) = Amount of gas ÷ Flow (in liters)

Duration of supply = 3440 L ÷ (2 L/min)

Duration of supply = 1720 minutes or approximately 28 hours and 40 minutes

---

can produce compressed air with a standard working pressure of 50 psi; these units can therefore be used to power devices such as pneumatically powered ventilators. Smaller portable compressors, which are unable to achieve these high working pressures, are used for bedside applications (e.g., powering small-volume nebulizers).

Three types of compressors are currently available: piston, diaphragm, and rotary units. **Piston compressors** use the action of a motor-driven piston to compress atmospheric air. The piston is seated within a cylinder casing and is sealed to it with a carbon or Teflon ring. Fig. 3.14 shows the operational principle of a typical piston air compressor used to power a mechanical ventilator. As the piston retracts, atmospheric air is drawn in through a one-way intake valve. When the piston protracts, the intake valve closes, and the gas is compressed before it leaves through a one-way outflow valve. A small gas reservoir is placed in a coiled tube to allow the hot, compressed gas to cool to room temperature before it is delivered to the output valve. The reservoir also removes some of the humidity from the intake gas. Usually a water drain is located near the compressor's output, and a water trap should be placed between the output and the device to be attached to the compressor to prevent problems with moisture accumulation. Examples of portable piston compressors include the Bennett MC-1 and MC-2 compressors, the Ohio High Performance Compressor, and the Timeter PCS-1 units.

Diaphragm compressors (Fig. 3.15) use a flexible diaphragm attached to a piston to compress gas. As the piston moves down, the diaphragm is bent outward, and gas is drawn through a one-way valve into the cylinder. Upward movement of the piston forces the gas out of the cylinder through a separate one-way outflow valve. Examples of diaphragm compressors are the Air-Shields Dia-Pump and the DeVilbiss small nebulizer compressor.

BOX 3.8   National Fire Protection Association Safety Recommendations and Regulations for Portable Liquid Oxygen Systems

1. Liquid oxygen units will vent gas when not in use, creating an oxygen-enriched environment. This can be particularly hazardous in the following situations:
   a. When the unit is stored in a closed space.
   b. When the unit is tipped over.
   c. When the oxygen is transferred to another container.
2. Liquid oxygen units should not be located adjacent to heat sources, which can accelerate the venting of oxygen.
3. The unit surface should not be contaminated with oil or grease.
4. Verify the contents of liquid containers when setting up the equipment, changing the containers, or refilling the containers at the home.
5. Connections for containers are to be made with the manufacturer's operating instructions.
6. The patient and family must be familiar with the proper operation of the liquid devices, along with all precautions, safeguards, and troubleshooting methods.
7. Transfill one unit from another in compliance with CGA pamphlet p-26, "transfilling of low pressure liquid oxygen to be used for respiration," and in accordance with the manufacturer's operating instructions.
8. All connections for filling must conform to CGA v-1, and the hose assembly must have a pressure release set no higher than the container's rated pressure.
9. Liquid containers must have a pressure release to limit the container pressure to the rated level, and a device must also be incorporated to limit the amount of oxygen introduced into a container to the manufacturer's specified capacity.
10. Delivery vehicles should be well-vented to prevent the buildup of high oxygen levels, and transfilling should take place with the delivery vehicle doors wide open.
11. "No Smoking" signs must be posted, and there can be no sources of ignition within 5 feet.
12. The transfiller must affix the labels required by DOT and FDA regulations, and records must be kept stating the content and purity. Instructions must be on the container, and the color coding and labeling must meet CGA and NFPA standards.
13. All devices used with liquid oxygen containers must be moisture free, and pressure releases must be positioned correctly to prevent freezing and the buildup of high pressures.
14. When liquid oxygen is spilled, both the liquid and gas that escape are very cold and will cause frostbite or eye injury. When filling liquid oxygen containers, wear safety goggles with side shields as well as loose-fitting, properly insulated gloves. High-top boots with cuffless pants worn outside of the boots are recommended.
15. Items exposed to liquid oxygen should not be touched, because they can not only cause frostbite, they can stick to the skin. Materials that are pliable at room temperature become brittle at the extreme temperatures of liquid oxygen.
16. If a liquid oxygen spill occurs, the cold liquid and resulting gas condense the moisture in the air, creating a fog. Normally the fog will extend over an area larger than the area of contact danger, except in extremely dry climates.
17. In the event of a spill, measures should be taken to prevent anyone from walking on the surface or wheeling equipment across the area for at least 15 minutes. All sources of ignition must be kept away from the area.
18. Liquid oxygen spilled onto asphalt or oil-soaked concrete constitutes an extreme hazard because an explosive reaction can occur.
19. If liquid oxygen or gas comes in contact with the skin, remove any clothing that may constrict blood flow to the frozen area. Warm the affected area with water at about body temperature until medical personnel arrive. Seek immediate medical attention for eye contact or blistering of the skin.
20. Immediately remove contaminated clothing and air it away from sources of ignition for at least one hour.

CGA, Compressed Gas Association; *DOT,* Department of Transportation; *FDA,* US Food and Drug Administration; *NFPA,* National Fire Protection Association.

Reproduced with permission from NFPA99-2012: Health Care Facilities, Copyright © 2011, National Fire Protection Association. This reprinted material is not the complete and official position of the NFPA on the referenced subject, which is represented only by the standard in its entirety.

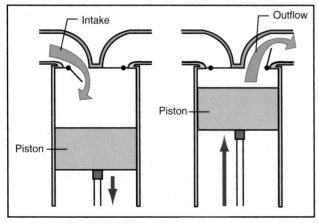

FIGURE 3.14 Piston air compressor.

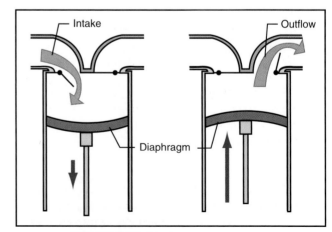

FIGURE 3.15 Diaphragm compressor.

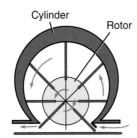

FIGURE 3.16 Rotary compressor.

Rotary compressors use a rotating vane to compress air from an intake valve. As the rotating vane turns, gas is drawn into the cylinder through a one-way valve (Fig. 3.16). As the rotor turns, the gas is compressed as the oval-shaped cylinder becomes smaller. The compressed gas is then forced out of the compressor through another one-way outflow valve. Low-pressure, rotary compressors are used in ventilators such as the CareFusion AVEA.

Bulk Air Supply Systems

Most bulk air systems use two compressors that can operate together or independently, depending on the demand for compressed air. Each compressor should also be able to deliver 100% of the average peak demand if the other compressor is turned off for maintenance or fails to operate. Box 3.9 summarizes the NFPA recommendations for safely operating medical air supply systems.

Air compressors used in bulk supply systems are usually piston or rotary compressors. Large piston compressors typically can provide a high-flow output and working pressures of at least 50 psi. A reservoir is incorporated into the design of the compressor unit to accommodate varying peak flow needs. The reservoir receives the compressed air and stores it at a higher pressure than in the piping system. A dryer attached to the outflow of the reservoir removes humidity (from refrigeration) from the air entering the piping system. A reducing valve on the reservoir outflow line reduces the pressure to 50 psi or the desired working pressure. In most cases a pneumatic sensing unit turns off the compressor when the reservoir pressure reaches a preset high level. This sensing unit also turns the compressor back on when the reservoir pressure falls below 50 psi.

High-pressure rotary units require a liquid sealant to produce high pressures efficiently. These systems typically include a reservoir for storing gas under high pressure, a dryer to remove humidity, and a pressure-relief valve to control the output pressure of the compressed gas. A pneumatic sensing unit, such as those used in piston compressors, is also used to maintain a constant working pressure of 50 psi and to prevent unnecessary high pressures.

Central Supply Systems

Hospitals and other health care facilities, such as freestanding clinics, rehabilitation centers, and diagnostic laboratories, typically rely on central supply systems to provide medical gases to multiple sites in the institution.

BOX 3.9   National Fire Protection Association Recommendations for Medical Air Supply

1. The source of medical air must be from the outside atmosphere and should not contain contaminants such as particulate matter, odor, or other gases.
2. The air intake port must be located outdoors, above roof level, at a minimum distance above the ground and 10 feet from any door, window, or other intake opening in the building. Intake ports must be turned downward and screened.
3. Air taken into the system must contain no contamination from engine exhaust, fuel storage vents, vacuum system discharges, or other particulate matter, because odor of any type can be drawn into the system.
4. A minimum of two oil-free compressors must be duplexed together, with provisions for operating alternately or simultaneously, depending on the demand. Each compressor or duplex must be capable of maintaining the air supply to the system at peak demand.
5. Backflow through compressors that are cycled off must be prevented automatically.
6. Each duplex system should be provided with disconnection switches, motor-starting devices with overload protection, and a means of automatically alternating the compressor or compressors. Use of the compressors should be divided evenly, and automatic means of activating an additional compressor or compressors should be provided in case the supply source unit becomes incapable of maintaining adequate pressure.
7. Air storage tanks or receivers must have a safety valve, an automatic drain, a pressure gauge, and the capacity to ensure practical on-off operation.
8. The type of medical air compressor and the local atmospheric conditions govern the need for intake filters/mufflers, after-coolers for air dryers, and additional downstream regulators.
9. Anti-vibration mountings are to be installed (in accordance with the manufacturer's recommendations) under the components and flexible couplings that connect the air compressors, receivers, and intake and supply lines.
10. A maintenance program must be established following the manufacturer's recommendations.

Large hospitals usually rely on continuous supply systems. A **continuous supply system** contains two sources of gas supply, one of which serves as a reserve source for use only in an emergency.[12] The primary source is usually a large liquid oxygen or air reservoir, whereas the reserve supply is a smaller liquid reservoir or a bank of compressed-gas cylinders. The primary source must be refilled at regular intervals. NFPA regulations require that the reserve supply contain an average day's supply of oxygen. The NFPA also requires that these systems include a pressure regulator, **check valves**, and a pressure-relief valve between each gas supply and main piping system.

Alternating supply systems usually consist of two banks of cylinders, one designated as the primary source and the other as the secondary source. Each bank of cylinders must contain a minimum of two cylinders or at least an average day's supply of oxygen or air. After the primary source is depleted or unable to meet system demands, the secondary system automatically becomes the primary source of oxygen or air. The empty bank is simply refilled or replaced. As a safety feature, an actuating switch must be connected to the master control panel to indicate when the change to the secondary bank is about to occur.[12] Check valves are installed between each cylinder and the manifold to prevent loss of gas from the manifold cylinders in the event the pressure-relief devices on an individual cylinder function or a cylinder lead fails.

Fig. 3.17 shows an alternating system that contains liquid oxygen cylinders as the primary and secondary oxygen sources, along with a reserve oxygen supply of compressed-gas cylinders. The reserve supply is used only when the primary and secondary sources are unable to supply system demands.[12] Note that the system must contain check valves and pressure-relief devices between the gas source and the main supply line. As with the previously described alternating system, an actuating switch signals when the changeover from the primary to the secondary source occurs.

Piping Systems

Gases stored in central supply units are distributed to various sites or zones in a hospital or health care facility via a piping system such as the one shown in Fig. 3.18. NFPA regulations govern the construction, installation, and testing of these systems.[12] Pipes used to transport gases must be seamless type K or L (ASTM B-8) copper tubing or standard weight brass pipe. The size of the pipes must be sufficient to maintain proper delivery volumes and to conform to good engineering practices. The gas contents of the pipeline must be labeled at least every 20 feet and at least once in each room or story through which the pipeline travels.

Pressure-regulating devices located between the bulk and the main supply lines must be capable of maintaining a minimum delivery pressure of 50 psi to all station outlets at the maximum delivery line flow. Pressure-relief valves should be installed downstream from the mainline pressure regulator. A pressure-relief valve should also be installed upstream of any zone valve to prevent excessive pressure in a zone where the shutoff valve is closed. All pressure-relief valves are set 50% higher than the system working pressure (e.g., 75 psi for a 50-psi system pressure).

As previously stated, piping systems in hospitals are organized into zones, which allow for quick isolation of all independent areas if maintenance is required. In case of fire, affected zones can be isolated, preventing the problem from spreading to other areas of the hospital (Clinical Scenario 3.3). Shutoff valves are located at the point where the main line enters the hospital, at each riser, and between each zone and

the main supply line. Zone shutoff valves for oxygen must be located outside of each critical care unit. Shutoff valves for every oxygen or nitrous oxide line must also be located outside of each surgical suite.

Shutoff valves generally are located in a large box with removable windows large enough to permit manual operation of the valve. They should be installed at a height where they can be operated from the standing position in an emergency. All valves must be labeled as shown in Fig. 3.19.

Piping systems must be tested for leaks and to ensure that gas supply lines have not become crossed. Visual inspection of the system can identify obvious problems, such as worn or loose connections; damaged pipes; pipes soiled with oil, grease, or other oxidizable materials; and crossing of gas supplies (e.g., crossing of compressed air and oxygen supply lines). Crossing of supply lines can be checked by reducing the system pressure to atmospheric and then purging each supply line separately with oil-free dry air or nitrogen. Whether the gas lines are crossed can also be determined by analyzing gas samples from the appropriate station outlets. Gases used to purge the supply lines should be passed through a white filter at a flow of 100 L/min to determine whether the purge gas is clean and odor-free. The content of gas lines should be tested for purity with the appropriate gas analysis.

All medical gas supply lines should have alarm systems that alert hospital personnel of system malfunctions (e.g., loss of system pressure, change from the primary system supply source to the secondary and reserve supplies, reduction in reserve supply below an average day's amount). Alarm panels should include visual and audible alerting signals and should be placed in locations that allow continuous surveillance (e.g., in the engineering department of the hospital). Alarm systems should also be located in critical care areas where life support systems (e.g., mechanical ventilators) are used. The Joint Commission mandates a written policy for responding to alarms and requires that personnel working in areas where alarms are located be instructed in how to respond.[14] Failure to respond appropriately can result in disaster. Response plans should include ensuring that all patient equipment is working properly and that appropriate personnel (i.e., respiratory care services and engineering) are notified immediately.

Station Outlets

Station outlets provide connections for gas delivery devices, such as flowmeters and mechanical ventilators. These outlets consist of a body mounted to the supply line, an outlet faceplate, and primary and secondary check valves, which are safety valves that open when the delivery device's adapter is inserted into the station outlet and close automatically when

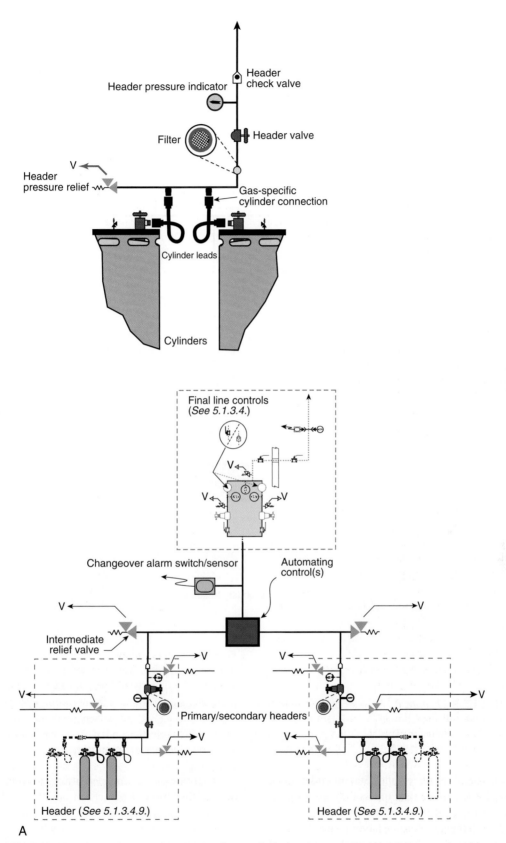

FIGURE 3.17 Alternating supply systems for medical air or oxygen. A, Alternating supply without reserve supply. *Continued*

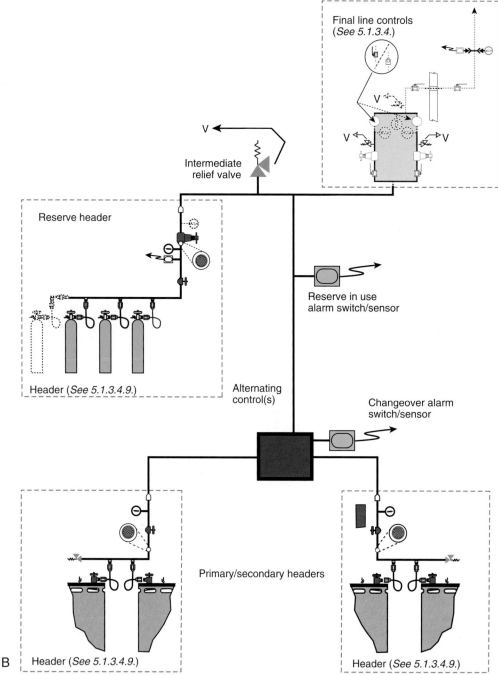

Final line controls
(*See 5.1.3.4.*)

V

Intermediate
relief valve

Reserve header

Reserve in use
alarm switch/sensor

Header (*See 5.1.3.4.9.*)

Alternating
control(s)

Changeover alarm
switch/sensor

Primary/secondary headers

Header (*See 5.1.3.4.9.*)

Header (*See 5.1.3.4.9.*)

B

FIGURE 3.17, cont'd. B, Alternating supply with primary and secondary cylinders. (Reproduced with permission from NFPA99-2015: Health Care Facilities, Copyright© 2014, National Fire Protection Association. This reprinted material is not the complete and official position of the NFPA on the referenced subject, which is represented only by the standard in its entirety.)

the adapter is disengaged from the outlet. Station outlets must not be supplied directly from a riser unless they are supplied through the manual shutoff valve located in the same story as the outlet. Outlet faceplates must be labeled with the name or symbol of the delivered gas. They may also be color coded for easy identification.

Station outlets are designed with safety systems that prevent the connection of incompatible devices. Two safety systems are currently available: **Diameter Index Safety System (DISS)** and **quick-connect adapters**. Fig. 3.20 shows an outlet that uses DISS. This system, which was designed by the CGA, uses

noninterchangeable, threaded fittings to connect gas-powered devices to station outlets. Each outlet must be fitted with a cap on a chain or installed in a recessed box that is equipped with a door to protect the outlet when not in use. Outlets typically are located approximately 5 feet above the floor or are recessed to prevent physical damage to the valve or control equipment. Delivery lines that serve anesthetic devices must have a backflow of gas into the system, and the check valves must be able to hold a minimum of 2400 psi.[1,12]

Fig. 3.21 shows a schematic of a quick-connect connection, and Fig. 3.22 shows examples of quick-connect adapters. These

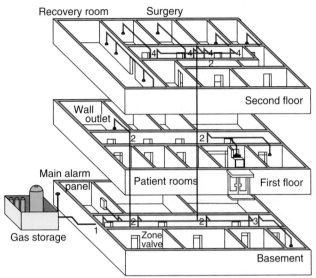

FIGURE 3.18 Hospital piping system. Zone valves must be placed (1) at the entrance to the hospital, (2) at each riser, (3) at each branch supplying an area, and (4) at each operating room. (Courtesy Nellcor Puritan Bennett, Pleasanton, CA.)

connections use a plunger that is held forward by a spring to prevent gas from leaving the outlet. Insertion of the appropriate adapter pushes the plunger backward, allowing gas to flow into the striker and into the equipment attached to the adapter. When the adapter is removed, the spring resets the plunger and closes the outlet.

Oxygen Concentrators

Oxygen concentrators are devices that produce enriched oxygen from atmospheric air. They provide an alternative to compressed-gas cylinders, particularly in the delivery of respiratory therapy to home care patients. Two types of concentrators are currently available: those using semipermeable plastic membranes and those using molecular sieves.

Concentrators using semipermeable membranes to separate oxygen from room air are composed of plastic membranes containing pores that are 1 mm in diameter (1 mm = 1/25,000 in). Atmospheric gases diffuse through the membrane at different rates. The rate at which a gas diffuses depends on its diffusion constant and solubility for the plastic membrane and the pressure gradient for the gas across the membrane. A diaphragm compressor is used to provide a constant vacuum across the membrane.

Oxygen and water vapor diffuse through these membranes faster than nitrogen. Generally, a constant flow of humidified 40% oxygen can be provided at a flow of 1 to 10 L/min.[13] Fig. 3.23 is a functional diagram of an oxygen concentrator that uses a semipermeable membrane.

Fig. 3.24 shows a typical oxygen concentrator that relies on molecular sieves to produce an enriched oxygen mixture. Such systems use a compressor to pump room air at pressures of 15 to 25 psig to one of two sets of sieves. Nitrogen is removed by passing room air through sodium-aluminum silicate (zeolite) pellets, producing an enriched oxygen mixture. It is important to mention that nitrogen and other gases absorbed by the

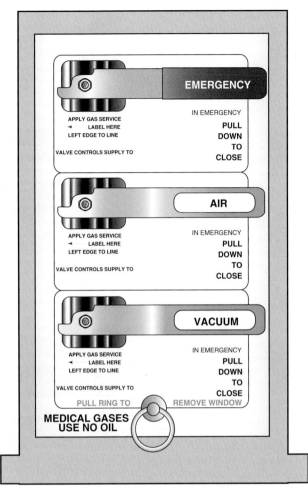

FIGURE 3.19 Zone shutoff valves for a bulk oxygen supply.

zeolite pellets must be purged to ensure that the unit functions properly. In the pressure swing adsorption (PSA) method, intermittent pressurization of one of the sieve beds occurs while the other bed is purged to remove any absorbed gases and moisture.

The concentration of oxygen leaving the system depends on the flow rate set. For example, at flows less than 6 L/min, the gas contains approximately ±93% oxygen.[8] Note that flowmeters calibrated for low inlet pressures must be used to ensure accurate delivery of oxygen to the patient, because the outlet pressure from these concentrators is approximately 5 to 10 psig. Examples of molecular sieve concentrators include the AirSep NewLife, LifeStyle, and FreeStyle, and VisionAire oxygen concentrators, and the DeVilbiss 303 DS/DZ and 515 DS/DZ oxygen concentrators.

Fig. 3.25 shows several examples of compact oxygen concentrators used for home care treatment of patients requiring long-term oxygen therapy. The larger devices shown are equipped with alarms that signal power failure, high and low pressure, and low oxygen concentration. These devices weigh approximately 30 lbs and provide nearly silent operation (i.e., approximately 40 decibels) and are therefore ideal for in-home oxygen therapy. The smaller devices shown in Fig. 3.25 are portable oxygen concentrators that permit

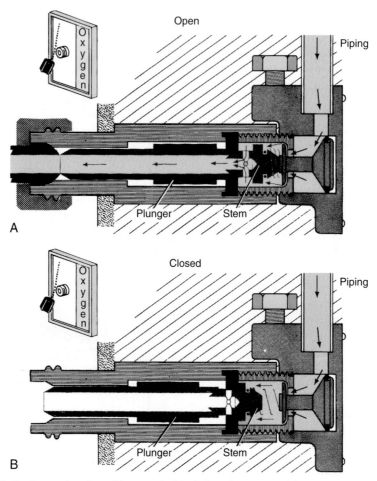

Open

Piping

Plunger   Stem

A

Closed

Piping

Plunger   Stem

B

FIGURE 3.20 Station outlets for a Diameter Index Safety System (DISS). (Courtesy Nellcor Puritan Bennett, Pleasanton, CA.)

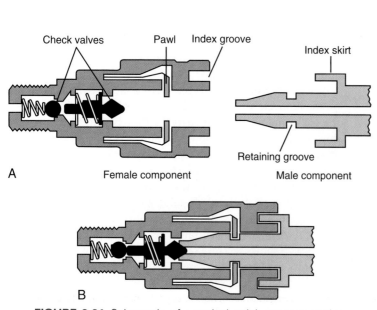

Check valves   Pawl   Index groove

Index skirt

Female component   Male component

Retaining groove

A

B

FIGURE 3.21 Schematic of a typical quick-connect station outlet.

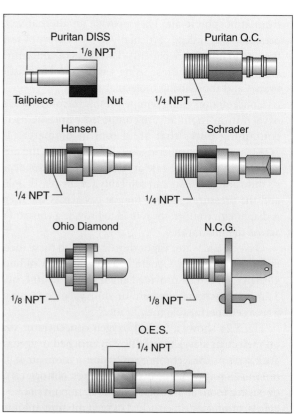

Puritan DISS

1/8 NPT

Tailpiece   Nut

Puritan Q.C.

1/4 NPT

Hansen

1/4 NPT

Schrader

1/4 NPT

Ohio Diamond

1/8 NPT

N.C.G.

1/8 NPT

O.E.S.

1/4 NPT

FIGURE 3.22 Examples of various quick-connect adapters from different manufacturers and suppliers.

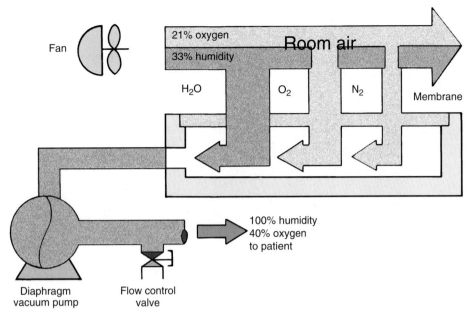

FIGURE 3.23 Oxygen concentrator that uses a semipermeable membrane. (Courtesy Oxygen Enrichment, Schenectady, NY.)

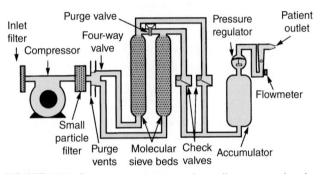

FIGURE 3.24 Oxygen concentrator that relies on a molecular sieve.

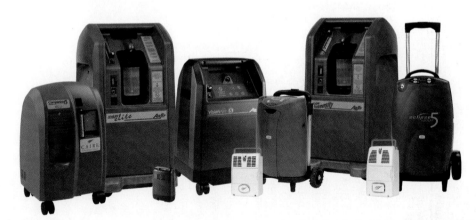

FIGURE 3.25 Stationary and portable oxygen concentrators. (Courtesy AirSep, Buffalo, NY.)

greater mobility for patients requiring long-term oxygen therapy. The smaller portable devices can be powered by an internal battery, an alternating current (AC) power supply, a direct current (DC) power supply, or an optional rechargeable battery belt that can be used in combination with the unit's internal battery. The battery belt pack, when used with a fully charged internal battery, can supply power to the unit for up to 10 hours between charges. Table 3.6 provides a comparison of several commercially available portable oxygen concentrators.

TABLE 3.6   Portable Oxygen Concentrators

Portable Oxygen Concentrators	Features	Dimensions	Weight	O₂ Flow Settings	Battery Run Time	Battery Recharge Time	Additional Optional External Battery	Power Supply	FAA-Approved Altitude Operating Range
AirSep Focus	Small size	6.4" H × 4.8" W × 2.5" D	Under 2 lb	2 LPM pulse only	Up to 3 hours	4 hours	Yes	AC 100-240 VAC DC Vehicle	Up to 10,000 feet above sea level
LifeChoice ActivOx	Small size Long battery life Active/sleep mode	9.05" W × 7.875" H × 4.38" D	3.9 lb	1-3 LPM pulse only	Up to 5.5 hours	4 hours	Yes	AC 100-240 VAC DC Vehicle	Up to 10,000 feet above sea level
AirSep Freestyle 5	On demand up to 5 LPM Small size	6.6" W × 10.7" H × 4.4" D	6.2 lb	1-5 LPM pulse only	Up to 3 hours	3 hours	Yes	AC 100-240 VAC DC Vehicle	Up to 12,000 feet above sea level
SeQual Eclipse 5	Continuous and pulse flow High oxygen settings Use with CPAP and BiPAP	12.3" W × 19" H × 7.1" D	18.4 lb	1-9 LPM pulse settings Up to 3 LPM continuous settings	Up to 5 hours Pulse 2 hours continuous	Up to 5 hours	Yes	AC 100-240 VAC DC Vehicle	Up to 13,000 feet above sea level
SeQual eQuinox	High oxygen settings Use with CPAP and BiPAP	10.6" W × 13.6" H × 7.5" D	14-16 lb	1-9 LPM pulse settings Up to 3 LPM continuous settings	Up to 3.5 hours	Up to 3.5 hours	Yes	AC 100-240 VAC DC Vehicle	Up to 13,130 feet above sea level
Invacare Solo 2	Continuous and pulse use 24/7	16.5" W × 20.2" H × 8" D	19.9 lb	1-5 LPM pulse settings Up to 3 LPM continuous settings	Up to 9 hours	Up to 5 hours	Yes	AC 100-240 VAC DC Vehicle	Up to 10,000 feet above sea level
Respironics SimplyGo	Home and portable unit Use 24/7 Use with CPAP and BiPAP	10" W × 11.5" H × 6" D	9.5 lb	1-6 LPM pulse settings 2 LPM continuous setting	3.5 hours @ 2 LPM pulse 1 hour @ 2 LPM continuous	Up to 3 hours	Yes	AC 100-240 VAC DC Vehicle	Up to 10,000 feet above sea level

AC, Alternating current; *BiPAP,* bilevel positive airway pressure; *CPAP,* continuous positive airway pressure; *D,* depth; *DC,* direct current; *FAA,* Federal Aviation Administration; *H,* height; *LPM,* liters per minute; *VAC,* volts alternating current; *W,* width.
Modified from Portable Oxygen Concentrator Comparison Review, Courtesy of Portable Oxygen Solutions, Charlotte, NC (www.portableoxygensolutions.com).

KEY POINTS

- An understanding of the properties of the commonly used medical gases is essential for safe and effective use of these agents in the clinical setting.
- Medical gases typically are classified as nonliquefied and liquefied. Nonliquefied gases are stored and transported under pressure in metal cylinders; liquefied gases are stored and transported in specially designed bulk storage units.
- Compressed-gas cylinders are available in a variety of sizes. Smaller cylinders typically are used as a portable source of oxygen in emergency situations and for transporting patients requiring O_2 therapy. Larger cylinders are used as a primary source of medical gases in medical facilities that do not have bulk storage units.
- The contents of compressed-gas cylinders must be easily identifiable. Standard labels should include the name and chemical symbol of the gas in the cylinder, along with information about hazards associated with use of the gas. The label should also include information about precautionary measures that should be taken when exposure to the contents leads to an adverse reaction.
- American Standard Safety System connections are noninterchangeable to prevent the interchange of regulating equipment between gases that are not compatible.
- Color codes are only a guide; printed labels are still the primary means of identifying the contents of a gas cylinder.
- Types 3AA and 3A cylinders must be hydrostatically retested every 10 years to determine their expansion characteristics. Type 3AL cylinders must be reexamined every 5 years to test their expansion characteristics.
- The volume of gas remaining in a cylinder and the duration of cylinder gas flow can easily be determined if one knows the cylinder gauge pressure and the cylinder's volume-pressure factor. To determine the volume of gas in a cylinder containing liquefied gas (e.g., carbon dioxide or nitrous oxide cylinders), one must weigh the cylinder, because a liquid remains in equilibrium with gas above it until the liquid is depleted.
- Bulk liquid storage systems for medical gases are cost-effective and require considerably less space than compressed-gas cylinders. Lightweight portable units are particularly advantageous for patients who require long-term oxygen therapy. Note that gaseous oxygen occupies a volume 860 times that of liquid oxygen.
- Compressed air is used to power many respiratory care devices, ranging from small handheld nebulizers to pneumatically powered ventilators. Bulk systems for hospitals and other health care facilities use multiple compressors that operate together or independently, depending on the demand for compressed air. In many cases, such as the home care setting, air can be compressed at the point of care by portable air compressors.
- Hospitals and other health care facilities typically rely on central supply systems to provide medical gases to multiple sites in the institution. Gases are stored in central supply units and distributed to the various sites through standardized piping systems. Alarm panels and shutoff valves throughout the facility allow continuous surveillance and control of the system. Standardized station outlets provide connections for gas delivery devices, such as flowmeters and mechanical ventilators.
- Pressure-reducing valves serve to reduce the working pressure of the gas to a desired level (usually 50 psi for hospitals and other health care facilities) before it enters the hospital's compressed-gas piping system.
- NFPA regulations require that hospitals maintain a reserve supply of oxygen. The available reserve should be an average day's supply of oxygen.
- Oxygen concentrators are an effective alternative to compressed-gas cylinders for home care patients.

ASSESSMENT QUESTIONS

See Appendix B for the answers.

1. Which of the following is classified as a nonflammable gas that does not support combustion?
   a. Oxygen
   b. Carbon dioxide
   c. Nitrous oxide
   d. Nitric oxide
2. Medical gas cylinders are color coded for easy identification. E cylinders of carbon dioxide are painted:
   a. Yellow
   b. Green
   c. Black
   d. Gray
3. A respiratory therapist is having trouble attaching a regulator to an E cylinder. One possible cause might be:
   a. The outlet threads of the cylinder do not match the threads of the regulator.
   b. The regulator diaphragm is jammed.
   c. The pin positions of the regulator are not the same as those on the cylinder.
   d. The cylinder has not been cracked.
4. Bulk liquid oxygen supplies should not be closer than _____ to public sidewalks.
   a. 2 feet
   b. 4 feet
   c. 7 feet
   d. 10 feet
5. Calculate the duration of the liquid oxygen supply if the liquid supply weighs 30 lb and the oxygen demand is 4 L/min.
   a. 10 hours
   b. 23 hours
   c. 35 hours
   d. 43 hours

6. What is the duration of oxygen flow from an H cylinder containing 1200 psi of oxygen when the flow to a nasal cannula is 4 L/min?
   a. 9 hours, 42 minutes
   b. 12 hours, 15 minutes
   c. 15 hours, 42 minutes
   d. 16 hours, 10 minutes

7. Large piston air compressors used in bulk supply systems typically can provide working pressures of:
   a. 50 psi
   b. 75 psi
   c. 100 psi
   d. 120 psi

8. Alternating supply systems for medical gases that are used in hospitals should include a reserve supply for oxygen in case the primary system fails. How much reserve oxygen should be available?
   a. An average 8-hour supply
   b. An average day's supply
   c. An average 3-day supply
   d. An average week's supply

9. Oxygen concentrators that use semipermeable membranes usually can provide what percentage of oxygen at flows of 1 to 10 L/min?
   a. 24%
   b. 40%
   c. 60%
   d. 100%

10. The percentage of oxygen delivery provided by molecular sieve O_2 concentrators depends on which of the following factors?
    1. The size of the concentrator
    2. The rate of gas flow
    3. The temperature of the refrigeration unit
    4. The age of the sieve beds
       a. 2 only
       b. 2 and 4 only
       c. 1, 2, and 3 only
       d. 1, 2, and 4 only

11. The pressure inside a cylinder increases dramatically when the cylinder is exposed to extremely high temperatures.

What prevents cylinders with frangible disks from exploding when exposed to extremely high temperatures?
   a. The frangible disk ruptures from the increased pressure, allowing gas to escape from the cylinder.
   b. The cylinder stem blows off when the temperature reaches 93.3°C (200°F).
   c. The stem diaphragm ruptures, allowing gas to escape.
   d. The frangible disk melts when the temperature reaches 37.8°C (100°F).

12. A respiratory therapist is checking cylinder markings to determine whether any of the cylinders need to be tested. The labeling reads as follows:
   9   83+
   6   94+
   This information indicates:
   a. The cylinder is due for retesting.
   b. The time between the test dates shown exceeds recommendations.
   c. The cylinder is made of aluminum.
   d. The owner of the cylinder.

13. Before using an H cylinder of oxygen, a respiratory therapist opens it, and gas at high pressure comes out of the cylinder outlet. Which of the following statements is true?
   a. This was an accident and should not be repeated.
   b. Allowing gas to escape from the cylinder lets the therapist smell the gas to ensure that it is oxygen.
   c. This action clears debris from the connector.
   d. This action should be performed after a regulator is attached to the cylinder outlet.

14. A respiratory therapist is helping design a new hospital wing. Which of the following agencies should be contacted so that the piping system of oxygen and air is correctly installed?
   a. NFPA
   b. FDA
   c. HHS
   d. DOT

15. A hospital uses a large air compressor system to supply air through its piped gas lines. This gas will be free of pollutants found in the local environment. True or false? Why?

REFERENCES

1. Compressed Gas Association: *Handbook of compressed gases,* ed 4, New York, 1999, Van Nostrand Reinhold.
2. Dorsch JA, Dorsch SE: *Understanding anesthesia equipment: construction, care, and complications,* ed 5, Baltimore, 2008, Williams & Wilkins.
3. Kacmarek RM, Dimas S, Mack CW: *The essentials of respiratory care,* ed 4, St. Louis, 2005, Elsevier-Mosby.
4. Wilkins RL, Stoller JK, Scanlon C: *Egan's fundamentals of respiratory care,* ed 8, St. Louis, 2003, Mosby.
5. Katz I: Inhaled nitric oxide: therapeutic uses and potential hazards. *PCCSU,* vol. 25, lesson 22, 2012.
6. Kinsella JP, Neish SR, Dunbar I, et al.: Clinical response to prolonged treatment of persistent pulmonary hypertension of the newborn with low doses of inhaled nitric oxide. *J Pediatr* 123:103, 1993.
7. Van Meurs KP, Wright LL, Ehrenkranz RA: Preemie inhaled nitric oxide study for premature infants with severe respiratory failure. *N Engl J Med* 353(1):13-22, 2005.
8. US food and Drug Administration: INOmax (nitric oxide) for inhalation: highlights of prescribing information. http://www.accessdata.fda.gov/drugsatfda_docs/label/2010/020845s011lbl.pdf, accessed March 4, 2012.

9. Hess D, MacIntyre N, Mishoe S, et al.: *Respiratory care: principles and practice*, ed 2 Sudbury, MA, 2012, Jones & Bartlett Learning.

10. McPherson S: *Respiratory care equipment*, ed 5, St. Louis, 1995, Mosby.

11. *Code of Federal Regulations*: Title 49, Parts 1-199, Washington, DC, 1974, US Government Printing Office.

12. National Fire Protection Association: *Standard for health care facilities,* (ANSI/NFPA 99), New York, 2002, Author.

13. Kacmarek RM: Delivery systems for long-term oxygen therapy. *Respir Care* 45:84, 2000.

14. Klein BR, editor: *Health care facilities handbook*, ed 4, Quincy, MA, 1993, National Fire Protection Association.

Administering Medical Gases:
Regulators, Flowmeters, and Controlling Devices

OBJECTIVES

Upon completion of this chapter, you will be able to:

1. Compare the design and operation of single-stage and multistage regulators.
2. Identify the components of preset and adjustable regulators.
3. Explain the operational theory of a Thorpe tube flowmeter, a Bourdon flowmeter, and a flow restrictor.
4. Demonstrate a method for determining whether a flowmeter is pressure compensated.
5. Compare low-flow and high-flow oxygen delivery systems.
6. Name several commonly used low-flow oxygen delivery systems.
7. Describe the components of a high-flow nasal cannula system and the benefits of using these systems in the treatment of hypoxemia.
8. Discuss the advantages and disadvantages of using oxygen-conserving devices in the treatment of patients requiring long-term oxygen therapy.
9. Explain the operational theory of air entrainment devices.
10. Compare the operation of oxygen blenders with that of oxygen mixers and adders.
11. Describe the physiological effects of hyperbaric oxygen therapy.
12. List the indications and contraindications of inhaled nitric oxide therapy.
13. Describe the appropriate use of mixed gas (e.g., heliox, carbogen) therapy.

OUTLINE

KEY TERMS

adjustable, multiple-orifice flow restrictors
adjustable regulators
Boothby-Lovelace-Bulbulian (BLB) mask
Bourdon flowmeters
carbogen
driving pressure
fixed-orifice flow restrictors
flow restrictors

French
heliox
high-flow (fixed-performance) oxygen delivery system
low-flow (variable-performance) oxygen delivery system
monoplace hyperbaric chamber
multiplace hyperbaric chamber
multistage regulators
mustache cannula

non–pressure compensated
oxygen adder
oxygen blender
pendant cannula
preset regulators
pressure compensated
pulse-demand oxygen delivery systems
single-stage regulator
Thorpe tube flowmeters

Administering medical gases is one of the primary responsibilities of respiratory therapists. This responsibility stems from work that began in several 18th-century physiology laboratories and came to fruition in the clinical settings of the mid-20th century. Scheele, Priestly, Lavoisier, Barcroft, Davies and Gilchrist, Barach, Petty, and others made significant contributions to the theory and practice of oxygen therapy by designing apparatuses to deliver oxygen to dyspneic patients.[1,2] Cogent studies performed by these and other scientists demonstrated the value of oxygen therapy and laid the foundation for the respiratory care profession.

As the responsibilities of respiratory therapists continue to grow, all practitioners must understand the principles of oxygen therapy, as well as other forms of medical gas therapy,

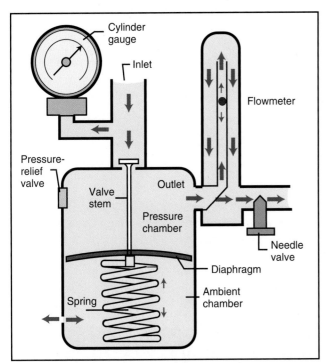

FIGURE 4.1 Components of a single-stage regulator.

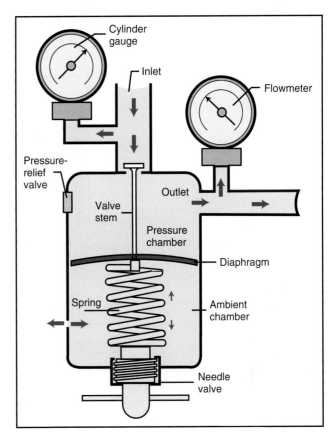

FIGURE 4.2 Components of an adjustable single-stage regulator.

including nitric oxide (NO) and hyperbaric oxygen therapy. Therefore this chapter reviews the operational principles of devices commonly used to administer medical gases.

I. REGULATORS AND FLOWMETERS

Regulators (or reducing valves) are devices that reduce high-pressure gases from cylinders or bulk storage units to lower working pressures, usually to 50 pounds per square inch (psi). Flowmeters are devices that control and indicate the gas flow delivered to patients.

Regulators

Regulators generally are classified as single-stage or multistage. They can be further divided into preset and adjustable regulators. Preset regulators deliver a specific outlet pressure; adjustable regulators can deliver a range of outlet pressures.

Single-Stage Regulators

Fig. 4.1 shows the components of a typical preset single-stage regulator, which consists of a body that is divided in half by a flexible metal diaphragm. The area above the diaphragm is a high-pressure chamber. The lower chamber has a spring attached to the lower surface of the diaphragm and is exposed to ambient pressure. A valve stem attached to the upper half of the diaphragm sits on the high-pressure inlet to the upper chamber. Note that excess pressures in the upper chamber can be released through a pressure-relief valve, which opens if the regulator malfunctions and the pressure inside the high-pressure chamber rises to 200 pounds per square inch gauge (psig).

The gas flow into the high-pressure side of the regulator depends on the effects of two opposing forces: gas pressure

above the diaphragm and spring tension below the diaphragm. When the force offered by the high-pressure gas above the diaphragm equals the force offered by spring tension, the diaphragm is straight and the inlet valve is closed. If the force offered by the spring exceeds the force offered by the gas pressure, the spring expands the diaphragm and opens the inlet valve.

For a preset single-stage regulator, the spring tension is calibrated to deliver gas at a preset pressure (usually 50 psig). Adjustable regulators, such as the one shown in Fig. 4.2, allow the operator to adjust the spring tension (and thus control the outlet pressure) by using a threaded hand control attached to the spring-diaphragm apparatus. Most adjustable regulators can be set to deliver pressures between 0 and 100 psig.

Multistage Regulators

Multistage regulators are simply two or more single-stage regulators in a series. Fig. 4.3 is a schematic of a two-stage regulator. Notice that the tension of the spring in the first stage of the regulator is usually preset by the manufacturer, but the spring tension in the second stage typically is adjustable. Each stage of the regulator contains a pressure-relief valve to release excess pressure if a malfunction occurs in either stage. (The number of stages of a regulator can be determined by counting the number of pressure-relief valves on the regulator.)

Multistage regulators operate on the principle that gas pressure is gradually reduced as gas flows from a high-pressure

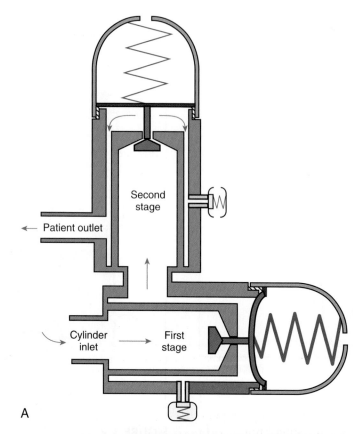

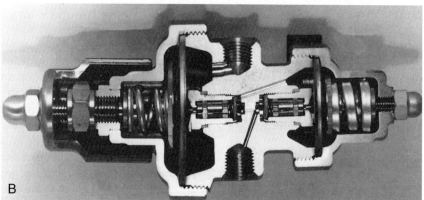

FIGURE 4.3 A, Multistage reducing valve. A double-stage valve is functionally two single-stage reducing valves in tandem. Gas enters the first stage (first reducing valve), and its pressure is lowered. Gas then enters the second stage (second reducing valve), and the pressure is lowered to the desired working pressure (usually 50 psig). A three-stage reducing valve has one more reducing valve in the series. B, National double-stage reducing valve. (Courtesy National Welding Equipment Co., Richmond, CA.)

source through a series of stages to the outlet. For example, gas from a compressed cylinder (e.g., 2200 psig) enters the first stage of a two-stage regulator, and the gas pressure is reduced to an intermediate pressure (e.g., 700 psig). This lower-pressure gas then enters the second stage of the regulator, where the gas pressure is further reduced to the desired working pressure (e.g., 50 psig) before the gas reaches the outlet.

Multistage regulators can control gas pressures with more precision than single-stage regulators because the pressure is reduced gradually. Additionally, multistage regulators produce

gas flow that is much smoother than that from single-stage regulators. Multistage regulators are more expensive and larger than single-stage regulators; therefore they usually are reserved for tasks requiring precise gas flow (e.g., research purposes).

Flowmeters

As mentioned previously, flowmeters are devices that control and indicate flow. Three types usually are described: **Thorpe tube flowmeters**, **Bourdon flowmeters**, and **flow restrictors**.

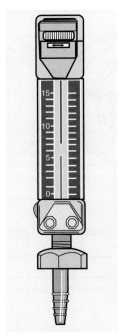

FIGURE 4.4 Thorpe tube flowmeter.

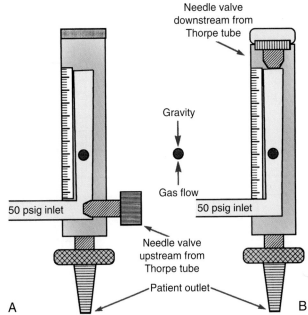

FIGURE 4.5 A, Non–pressure-compensated Thorpe flowmeter. B, Pressure-compensated Thorpe flowmeter. The two opposing forces are (1) gravity pulling the float downward and (2) the driving pressure of the gas flow pushing the float upward. When these two forces reach a balance (equilibrium), the float remains stationary, "floating" in the gas column. Because the gas column consists of a tapered tube, as the gas flow increases and the float is displaced upward, greater volumes of gas pass by the float and enter the patient outlet. Needle valve placement determines whether the device is back pressure–compensated.

Thorpe Tube Flowmeters

Thorpe tubes are the most common flowmeters used in respiratory care. As Figs. 4.4 to 4.6 show, the Thorpe tube consists of a tapered, hollow tube engraved with a calibrated scale (usually in L/min), a float, and a needle valve for controlling the flow rate of gas. (Flowmeters used in neonatal and pediatric care may be calibrated in mL/min.) The flow rate of gas delivered is read by locating the float on the calibrated scale. It is important to use the center of the float as the reference point when reading flow rates on the calibrated scale. This is particularly evident when trying to adjust flows of 1 to 3 L/min.

The operational principle for these devices can be explained as follows: As gas flows through the unit, it pushes the ball float higher. As the ball float moves higher in the Thorpe tube, more gas is allowed to travel around it as a result of the gradually increasing diameter of the indicator tube. The height that the ball float is raised depends on the force of gravity pulling down on it and the force of the molecules trying to push it up. The ball float rises until enough molecules can go around it to restore the equilibrium between gravity and the number of molecules hitting the bottom of the ball float.

Back pressure compensation. Thorpe tube flowmeters usually are described as pressure compensated or non–pressure compensated. On pressure-compensated flowmeters (see Fig. 4.5), the needle valve controlling gas flow out of the flowmeter is located downstream of the Thorpe tube. This arrangement allows the pressure in the indicator tube to be maintained at the source gas pressure (e.g., 50 psig). Pressure-compensated flowmeters provide accurate estimates of flow, regardless of the downstream pressure. (Note that pressure-compensated flowmeters indicate actual flow unless the source gas pressure varies, the flowmeter is set to deliver a higher flow than is

actually available from its source gas supply, or the float in the tube is not set in a vertical position.[1]) The following example may help illustrate how these devices operate: When a restriction or high-resistance device is attached to a pressure-compensated flowmeter, the pressure gradient between the source gas pressure and the outlet pressure is decreased. The float within the Thorpe tube registers the true gas flow out of the flowmeter, because back pressure created by downstream resistance increases only the pressure distal to the needle valve. It should be apparent, however, that if the back pressure exceeds the source gas pressure (e.g., 50 psig), gas flow stops.

With non–pressure-compensated flowmeters (see Fig. 4.6), the needle valve is located before the indicator tube. Restriction or high-resistance devices attached to the outlet of a non–pressure-compensated Thorpe tube flowmeter create back pressure, which is transmitted back to the needle valve. Because the needle valve is located proximal to the Thorpe tube, the back pressure causes the float to fall to a level that indicates a flow lower than the actual flow.

Pressure-compensated flowmeters usually are labeled as such on the back of the flowmeter. A flowmeter can also be determined to be pressure compensated if the following test is performed: With the needle valve closed, the flowmeter is plugged into a high-pressure gas source (i.e., bulk storage wall outlet). If the float in the indicator tube jumps and then falls

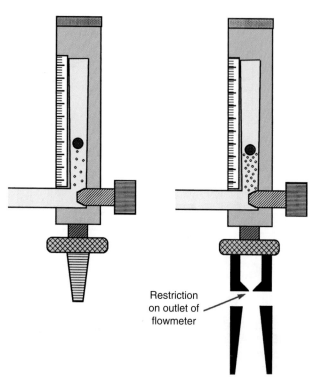

FIGURE 4.6 Non–pressure-compensated Thorpe tube flowmeter. Attaching a restriction or high-resistance devices to the outlet of a non–pressure-compensated Thorpe tube flowmeter creates back pressure, which causes the float to fall to a level that indicates a flow lower than actual flow.

to zero, the flowmeter is pressure compensated. This float movement occurs because the source gas must pass through the indicator tube before it reaches the needle valve.[1]

The most common problem associated with Thorpe tube flowmeters is gas leakage resulting from faulty valve seats. This problem usually is detected when the flowmeter is turned off completely but gas can be heard continuing to flow from the flowmeter outlet; these flowmeters should be replaced.

Bourdon Flowmeters

As Fig. 4.7 shows, the Bourdon flowmeter is actually a reducing valve that controls the pressure gradient across an outlet with a fixed orifice. The operational principle of this device is simple: as the driving pressure is increased, the flow from the flowmeter outlet increases.

The flow rate of gas can be measured because the Bourdon flowmeter gauge is calibrated in liters per minute. As long as the pressure distal to (i.e., downstream from) the orifice remains atmospheric, the indicated flow is accurate. As resistance to flow increases, the indicated flow reading becomes inaccurate (i.e., these devices are not back pressure–compensated and will therefore show a higher than actual flow in the presence of increased downstream resistance). Fig. 4.8 shows how increasing resistance at the gas outlet affects the flow reading. Note that although the outlet becomes totally occluded, the flow reading remains constant. Fig. 4.9 shows a commonly used Bourdon flowmeter.

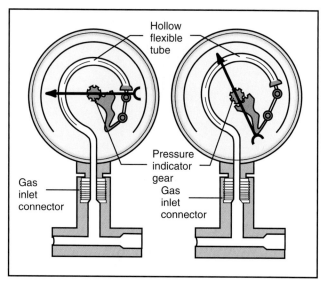

FIGURE 4.7 Schematic of a Bourdon flowmeter.

Flow Restrictors

Flow restrictors operate on the same principle as Bourdon flowmeters (i.e., the gas flow through these devices can be increased by raising the driving pressure across a fixed resistance). Like Bourdon flowmeters, flow rate readings are inaccurate when resistance increases downstream from the gas outlet. The two types of flow restrictors are fixed-orifice and adjustable, multiple-orifice models (although fixed-orifice devices are no longer manufactured). The adjustable, multiple-orifice flow restrictor uses a series of calibrated openings in a disk that can be adjusted to deliver different flows. As with the fixed-orifice flow restrictor, the operating pressure is crucial to the accuracy of the device. Fig. 4.10 is a schematic illustrating the principle of operation for a variable-orifice flow restrictor.

For these devices to function properly, it is essential to use the appropriate operating pressure. Some of the devices are designed for use with hospital gas sources (i.e., 50-psi gas sources), and others are designed to work on portable liquid oxygen equipment used in the home care setting (i.e., 20-psi gas source).

II. DEVICES FOR ADMINISTERING MEDICAL GASES

Oxygen Therapy

The goal of oxygen therapy is to treat or prevent hypoxemia. Many different devices can be used to achieve this goal in spontaneously breathing patients. It is important that respiratory therapists understand how to select and assemble these devices and ensure that they are working properly. The American Association for Respiratory Care has developed clinical practice guidelines for oxygen administration in acute care facilities, alternative site health care (e.g., extended care) facilities, and the home setting.[3-5] These guidelines inform practitioners of indications, contraindications, precautions, and possible complications of oxygen therapy. Each guideline lists

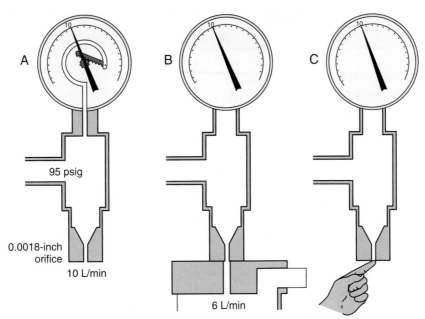

A 95 psig

0.0018-inch
orifice

10 L/min

6 L/min

FIGURE 4.8 A, Bourdon gauge operating under normal conditions. The actual flow delivered equals the flow registered on the flowmeter. B, The effect when resistance is added downstream of the flowmeter at the outlet. Notice that the flow registered on the flowmeter is higher than the actual flow. C, Complete occlusion of the outlet has a similar effect; that is, the flow registered on the flowmeter is erroneously high. (Copyright © 2013 Medtronic Minimally Invasive Therapies. All rights reserved. Reprinted with permission of Medtronic Minimally Invasive Therapies.)

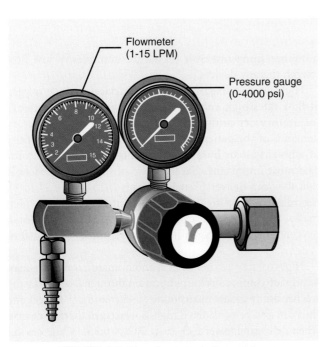

Flowmeter
(1-15 LPM)

Pressure gauge
(0-4000 psi)

FIGURE 4.9 Bourdon gauge flowmeter.

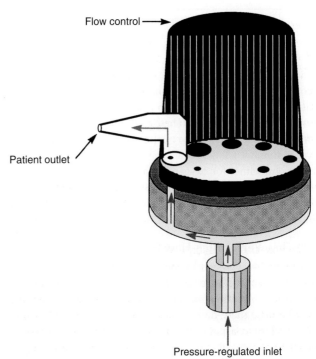

Flow control

Patient outlet

Pressure-regulated inlet

FIGURE 4.10 Schematic of a variable-orifice flow restrictor. These devices use a series of calibrated ports to deliver a set flow at a designated pressure. Per the requirements of the National Fire Protection Association (NFPA), the delivery pressure is included on the restrictor label.

CLINICAL PRACTICE GUIDELINE 4.1   Oxygen Therapy for Adults in the Acute Care Facility—2002 Revision and Update

Definition/Description

Oxygen therapy is the administration of oxygen at concentrations greater than ambient air with the intent of treating or preventing the symptoms and manifestations of hypoxia. The procedure addressed is the administration of oxygen therapy in the acute care facility other than with mechanical ventilators and hyperbaric chambers.

Indications

- Documented hypoxemia. Defined as a decreased PaO_2 (partial pressure of arterial oxygen) in the blood below normal range (i.e., PaO_2 <60 mm Hg or SaO_2 [arterial oxygen saturation]) <90% in patients breathing room air, or with a PaO_2 or SaO_2 below desirable range for the specific clinical situation.
- An acute situation in which hypoxemia is suspected; substantiation of hypoxemia is required within an appropriate period after initiation of therapy.
- Severe trauma.
- Acute myocardial infarction.
- Short-term therapy (postanesthesia) or surgical intervention.

Precautions and/or Complications

- With a PaO_2 ≥60 mm Hg, ventilatory depression may occur in spontaneously breathing patients with a chronically elevated $PaCO_2$.
- With a fraction of inspired oxygen (F_IO_2) ≥0.50, absorption atelectasis, oxygen toxicity, and/or depression of ciliary and/or leukocyte function may occur.

- Bacterial contamination associated with certain nebulization and humidification systems is a possible hazard.
- Oxygen should be administered with caution to patients suffering from paraquat poisoning and those receiving bleomycin.
- During laser bronchoscopy, minimal levels of supplemental oxygen should be used to avoid intratracheal ignition.

Limitations

- Oxygen therapy has only limited benefit for the treatment of hypoxia resulting from anemia and may be of limited benefit with circulatory disturbances.
- Oxygen therapy should not be used in lieu of, but in addition to, mechanical ventilation when ventilatory support is indicated.

Monitoring

- Patient monitoring should include clinical assessment along with oxygen tension or saturation measurements. This should be done at the following times: when therapy is initiated; within 12 hours of initiation of therapy for F_IO_2 levels <0.40; within 8 hours for F_IO_2 levels ≥0.40; within 72 hours of an acute myocardial infarction; within 2 hours for patients diagnosed with chronic obstructive pulmonary disease (COPD).
- All oxygen delivery systems should be checked at least once per day. More frequent checks with calibrated analyzers are indicated for systems susceptible to variations in the F_IO_2.

Modified from the American Association for Respiratory Care: Clinical practice guideline: oxygen therapy for adults in the acute care facility—2002 revision and update. *Respir Care* 47:717, 2002.

the devices that can be used to administer oxygen to spontaneously breathing patients, along with a brief description of criteria that should be used to assess the need for and the outcome of oxygen therapy. These guidelines should be reviewed and used as a resource in the treatment of patients who require oxygen therapy. Clinical Practice Guidelines 4.1 and 4.2 summarize guidelines for oxygen therapy for adults in acute care and alternative site health care facilities. Clinical Practice Guideline 4.3 summarizes the guidelines for oxygen therapy for neonatal and pediatric patients.

Low-Flow Versus High-Flow Devices

Oxygen delivery systems generally are classified as low-flow (variable performance) and high-flow (fixed performance) devices.[4,5] The terms *low flow* and *variable performance* are used because these devices supply oxygen at flow rates that are lower than a patient's inspiratory demands; therefore varying amounts of room air must be added to provide part of the inspired volume. Low-flow devices deliver fractional inspired oxygen (F_IO_2) levels that can vary from 0.22 to approximately 0.8, depending on the patient's inspiratory flow and tidal volume and the oxygen flow used. Nasal cannulas and catheters (Historical Note 4.1), transtracheal catheters, simple oxygen masks, partial rebreathing reservoir masks, and

nonrebreathing reservoir masks are examples of low-flow oxygen therapy devices.

High-flow, or fixed-performance, devices provide oxygen at flow rates high enough to completely satisfy a patient's inspiratory demands. Such devices supply the inspiratory demands of the patient either by entraining fixed quantities of ambient air or by using high flow rates and reservoirs. The most important characteristic of high-flow devices is that they can deliver fixed F_IO_2 levels (i.e., from 0.24 to 1), regardless of the patient's breathing pattern. Air entrainment masks, high-flow nasal cannulas, isolettes (i.e., incubators), oxygen tents, and oxygen hoods are examples of high-flow systems.

High-volume aerosol devices and humidifiers that are used to provide continuous humidification through face masks and tracheostomy collars incorporate air entrainment devices and thus can also be considered high-flow oxygen therapy devices when delivering lower F_IO_2 (e.g., F_IO_2 ≈ 0.35). These devices may not meet all of the patient's needs at high F_IO_2s. A common misconception is that low-flow systems can deliver only a low F_IO_2 and high-flow systems can deliver only a high F_IO_2. As will be seen, both low- and high-flow systems can deliver a wide range of F_IO_2 levels. Do not confuse the terms *low-flow* and *high-flow* with the terms *low F_IO_2* and *high F_IO_2*.

CLINICAL PRACTICE GUIDELINE 4.2   Oxygen Therapy in the Home or Alternative Site Health Care Facility—2007 Revision and Update

Setting

This guideline is confined to oxygen administration in the home or in an alternative site health care facility (i.e., skilled nursing facility, extended care facility).

Indications: Documented Hypoxemia

- In adults, children, and infants older than 28 days: As evidenced by a PaO_2 (partial pressure of arterial oxygen) ≤55 mm Hg or an SaO_2 (arterial oxygen saturation) ≤88% in patients breathing room air, or a PaO_2 of 56 to 59 mm Hg or an SaO_2 or SpO_2 (oxygen saturation as measured using pulse oximetry) ≤89% in association with specific clinical conditions (e.g., cor pulmonale, congestive heart failure, or erythrocythemia with a hematocrit >56%).
- Some patients may not demonstrate a need for oxygen therapy at rest but become hypoxemic during ambulation, sleep, or exercise. Oxygen therapy is indicated during these specific activities when the SaO_2 is shown to fall to ≤88%.

Precautions and Complications

Precautions and complications are the same as those cited for oxygen therapy in the acute care setting.

Resources

- Low-flow oxygen devices, such as nasal cannulas, transtracheal oxygen catheters, pulse-dose oxygen delivery devices, demand oxygen delivery systems, oxygen reservoir cannulas.
- High-flow oxygen devices, such as tracheostomy collars and T-tube adapters that are associated with high-flow supplemental oxygen systems.

- Oxygen supply systems, including oxygen concentrators, liquid oxygen systems, and compressed-gas cylinders.

Monitoring

- Initial and ongoing clinical assessment of the patient should be performed by a licensed and/or credentialed respiratory therapist or other professional functioning within the scope of practice required by the state standards under which the professional is licensed.
- Baseline oxygen tension and/or saturation levels must be measured before oxygen therapy is started; these measurements should be repeated when clinically indicated or to follow the course of the disease as determined by the attending physician.
- SpO_2 should be measured to determine the appropriate oxygen flow and pulse-dose or demand oxygen delivery settings for sleep, exercise, or ambulation.
- Oxygen therapy should be administered in accordance with the physician's prescription.

Infection Control

Normally, low-flow oxygen systems without humidifiers do not present a clinically important risk for infection and need not be routinely replaced. High-flow systems that use heated humidifiers or aerosol generators, especially when applied to patients with artificial airways, should be cleaned and disinfected regularly.

Modified from the American Association for Respiratory Care: Clinical practice guideline: oxygen therapy in the home or alternative site health care facility—2007 revision and update. *Respir Care* 52:1063, 2007.

Low-Flow Devices

Low-flow nasal cannulas. Nasal cannulas (Fig. 4.11) are used extensively to treat spontaneously breathing, hypoxemic patients in emergency departments, in general and critical care units, during exercise in cardiopulmonary rehabilitation, and for long-term oxygen therapy in the home care setting.[2,6] The standard nasal cannula is a blind-ended, soft plastic tube with two prongs that fit into the patient's external nares. The prongs are approximately $\frac{1}{2}$-inch long and can be straight or curved. The cannula is held in place either with an elastic band that fits over the ears and around the head or with two small-diameter pieces of tubing that fit over the ears and can be tightened with a bolo tie–type device that fits under the chin. Cannulas are available in infant, child, and adult sizes.

The most common problems with nasal cannulas are related to (1) nasopharyngeal-mucosal irritation, (2) twisting of the connective tubing between the patient and the oxygen flowmeter, and (3) skin irritation at pressure points where the tubing holding the cannula in place touches the patient's face and ears. Irritation of the nasal mucosa and the paranasal sinuses occurs most often when high flow rates of oxygen are used. The problem appears to be greater with nasal cannulas

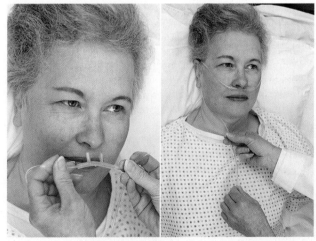

FIGURE 4.11 Nasal cannula.

that use straight rather than curved prongs. With straight prongs, oxygen flow is directed toward the superior aspects of the nasal cavity, which promotes turbulent flow; with curved prongs, oxygen entering the nose is directed across the nasal turbinate, thus enhancing laminar flow as the gas flows through

CLINICAL PRACTICE GUIDELINE 4.3   **Selection of an Oxygen Delivery Device for Neonatal and Pediatric Patients—2002 Revision and Update**

Definition/Description

The administration of supplemental oxygen to neonatal and pediatric patients requires the selection of an oxygen delivery system that suits the patient's size and needs and the therapeutic goals.

Indications

- Documented hypoxemia.
- An acute situation in which hypoxemia is suspected or in which suspected regional hypoxia may respond to an increase in PaO_2 (partial pressure of arterial oxygen). Verification of the PaO_2 level is required within an appropriate period after initiation of therapy.

Contraindications

- No specific contraindications exist to the delivery of oxygen when indications are judged to be present.
- Nasal cannulas and nasopharyngeal catheters are contraindicated in patients with nasal obstruction (e.g., nasal polyps, choanal atresia).
- Nasopharyngeal catheters are contraindicated in patients with maxillofacial trauma and in those with or suspected of having a basal skull fracture or coagulation problems.
- It is the expert opinion of the Clinical Practice Guideline Steering Committee (2002) that nasopharyngeal catheters are not appropriate for oxygen administration in the neonatal population.

Hazards/Precautions/Possible Complications

- The etiology of retinopathy of prematurity, especially the role of oxygen, is controversial. Care should be taken when supplemental oxygen is provided to preterm infants (<37 weeks' gestation). It is suggested that oxygen supplementation should not result in a PaO_2 >80 mm Hg.
- Administration of supplemental oxygen to patients with certain congenital heart lesions (e.g., hypoplastic left heart, single ventricle) may cause an increase in alveolar oxygen tension and compromise the balance between pulmonary and systemic blood flow.
- Administration of supplemental oxygen to patients suffering from paraquat poisoning or to patients receiving certain chemotherapeutic agents (e.g., bleomycin) may result in pulmonary complications (e.g., oxygen toxicity and pulmonary fibrosis).
- Stimulation of the superior laryngeal nerves in an infant may cause alterations in the respiratory pattern if the gas flow from the oxygen source is cool and is directed at the infant's face.
- Inappropriate selection of the fractional delivered oxygen concentration (F_DO_2) or oxygen flow may result in hypoxemia or hyperoxemia.
- Skin irritation can result from material used to secure the cannula or from local allergic reaction to polyvinyl chloride. Improper sizing can lead to nasal obstruction or irritation.
- Displacement can lead to loss of oxygen delivery.
- Inadvertent continuous positive airway pressure (CPAP) may be administered, depending on the size of the nasal cannula, the gas flow, and the infant's anatomy.

- Irritation can result if flows are excessive; improper insertion can cause gagging and nasal or pharyngeal trauma; improper sizing can lead to nasal obstruction or irritation.
- Excessive secretions and/or mucosal inflammation can result.
- Excessive flow may cause gastric distention.
- Transtracheal catheters may be associated with an increased risk for infection compared with nasal cannulas and catheters.
- Aspiration of vomitus may be more likely with oxygen masks. Rebreathing of carbon dioxide (CO_2) may occur if the total oxygen (O_2) flow to the mask is inadequate.
- It is the expert opinion of the Clinical Practice Guideline Steering Committee (2002) that partial rebreathers or nonrebreathers are not appropriate for the neonatal population.

Limitations

- *Nasal cannulas:* Changes in minute ventilation and inspiratory flow affect air entrainment and result in fluctuations in F_IO_2 (fraction of inspired oxygen). Prongs are difficult to keep in position, particularly with small infants. The effect of mouth versus nose breathing on the F_IO_2 remains controversial. Use may be limited by the presence of excessive mucus drainage, mucosal edema, or a deviated septum. Maximum flow should be limited to 2 L/min in infants and newborns. Care should be taken to keep the cannula tubing and straps away from the neck to prevent airway obstruction in infants. Discrepancies between the set and the delivered flow can occur in the same flowmeter at different settings and among different flowmeters. Discrepancies in flow and oxygen concentration between set and delivered values can occur in low-flow blenders at flows below the recommended range of the blender.
- *Transtracheal catheters:* This method is less commonly used because of the complexity of care. Frequent medical monitoring is required, and replacement catheters are costly. Increased time is needed for candidate evaluation and teaching.
- *Masks:* Masks provide a variable F_IO_2, depending on the inspiratory flow and the construction of the mask's reservoir. Masks are not recommended when precise concentrations are required. Also, they are confining and may not be well tolerated; they interfere with feeding; they may not be available in sizes appropriate for all patients; and they require a minimum flow, per the manufacturer's instructions, to prevent possible rebreathing of CO_2. The maximum F_IO_2 attainable with a simple nonrebreathing or partial rebreathing mask in neonates, infants, and children has not been well documented. The performance of air entrainment masks may be altered by resistance to flow distal to the restricted orifice (resulting in a higher F_DO_2 and a lower total flow delivered). The total flow from air entrainment masks at settings greater than 0.40 may not equal or may exceed the patient's inspiratory flow. Performance is altered if the entrainment ports are blocked.
- *Hoods:* O_2 concentrations may vary within the hood. O_2 concentrations should be measured as near the nose and mouth as possible. Opening of any enclosure reduces the O_2 concentration. For infants and children confined to hoods, nasal O_2 may need to be supplied during feeding and nursing care. Flows greater than 7 L/min are required to wash out

---

CLINICAL PRACTICE GUIDELINE 4.3   Selection of an Oxygen Delivery Device for Neonatal and Pediatric Patients—2002 Revision and Update—cont'd

CO_2. Devices can be confining and isolating. Concentration in a hood can be varied from 0.21 to 1.0. The temperature of the gases in the hood should be maintained to provide a neutral thermal environment. High gas flows may produce harmful noise levels.

Assessment of Need

Need is determined by measurement of inadequate oxygen tensions and saturations by invasive or noninvasive methods and/or the presence of clinical indicators as previously described. Supplemental oxygen flow should be titrated to maintain adequate oxygen saturation as indicated by pulse oximetry SpO_2 or appropriate arterial or venous blood gas values.

Monitoring

- Clinical assessment should include but should not be limited to cardiac, pulmonary, and neurological status and apparent

work of breathing; noninvasive or invasive measurement of oxygen tensions or saturation should be performed within 1 hour of initiation of therapy in any neonate treated with oxygen.

- All oxygen delivery systems should be checked at least once each day. More frequent checks by calibrated analyzer are necessary in systems susceptible to variation in oxygen concentration or that are applied to patients with artificial airways. Continuous analysis is recommended in hoods. Oxygen should be analyzed as close as possible to the infant's face.
- All heated delivery systems should be monitored continuously for temperature.

Modified from the American Association for Respiratory Care: Clinical practice guideline: selection of an oxygen delivery device for neonatal and pediatric patients—2002 revision and update. *Respir Care* 47:707, 2002.

HISTORICAL NOTE 4.1

Nasal Catheters

Nasal catheters were introduced by Lane in 1907.[1,6] It is important to recognize that although these devices are still available, they are used infrequently. Nasal catheters consist of a hollow, soft plastic tube that contains a blind distal tip with a series of holes. They are available in 8 to 10 French (Fr) for children and 12 to 14 Fr for adults.

Note that the term **French** is a method of sizing catheters according to the outside diameter (OD). Each unit in the French scale is approximately 0.33 mm; a 10-Fr tube therefore has an outside diameter of 3.3 mm.

The catheter can be placed with relative ease and minimal patient discomfort if done properly. First, it should be coated with a water-soluble lubricant, and its patency should be checked (by observing whether oxygen flows through it unobstructed). Once the patency has been confirmed, the catheter is inserted into an external naris and advanced along the floor of the nasal cavity until it can be seen at the back of the patient's oropharynx. It should then be positioned just behind the uvula. For blind insertion the distance the catheter must be inserted can be estimated by measuring the distance from the tip of the patient's nose to the earlobe; this length can then be marked on the catheter with a small piece of surgical tape. The catheter can be held in place by taping it to the nose.

Nasal catheters can deliver an F_IO_2 of approximately 0.24 to 0.35 when the oxygen flow is set at 2 to 5 L/min. A higher F_IO_2 can be obtained by increasing the oxygen flow to the patient. Notice that the actual F_IO_2 varies considerably, depending on the patient's tidal volume and respiratory rate and whether respiration occurs primarily through the nose or the mouth.

F_IO_2, Fractional inspired oxygen.

the nasal cavity. Twisting of connective tubing is an insidious problem that is difficult to prevent. Avoiding excessive lengths of connective tubing and periodically checking for patency appear to be the most reliable means of dealing with this problem. The problems of skin irritation and pressure point soreness can be minimized by placing cotton gauze padding between the tubing and the patient's face and ears.

For adult and pediatric patients, nasal cannulas theoretically can produce F_IO_2 levels of 0.24 to 0.44 at oxygen flow rates of 1 to 6 L/min. Oxygen flows higher than 6 L/min delivered with a traditional nasal cannula system do not produce a significantly higher F_IO_2 and are poorly tolerated by patients because they may cause nasal bleeding and drying of the nasal mucosa. For neonates, clinicians typically use oxygen flows of 0.25 to 2 L/min.[5,6] Keep in mind that the actual F_IO_2 delivered is influenced by the patient's tidal volume and respiratory rate, total respiratory time, inspiratory time, inspiratory flow and pattern, and whether breathing is occurring predominantly through the nose or the mouth.

Table 4.1 lists the approximate F_IO_2 levels delivered by flow rates of 1 to 6 L/min to an adult patient. It should be emphasized that this is simply an estimate and that the actual delivered F_IO_2 for any given oxygen flow rate may be significantly different.[2] In a clinical setting, adjusting the flow rate of oxygen delivered to the patient is generally an empirical process (i.e., it is adjusted according to the patient's oxygen needs). This empirical approach should be based on observations of the patient's breathing pattern and level of comfort, as well as pulse oximetry or arterial blood gas data, if available. A problem-solving exercise for calculating the approximate F_IO_2 when using a variable-performance device such as a nasal cannula is provided in Clinical Scenario 4.1.

Oxygen-conserving devices. Transtracheal oxygen (TTO) catheters, reservoir cannulas, and pulse-demand oxygen delivery systems are recent developments that have significantly

TABLE 4.1 **Guidelines for Estimating F_IO_2 With Low-Flow Oxygen Delivery Systems**

100% Oxygen Flow Rate (L/min)	F_IO_2
Nasal Cannula or Catheter	
1	0.24
2	0.28
3	0.32
4	0.36
5	0.40
6	0.44
Simple or Partial Rebreathing Oxygen Mask[a]	
5-6	0.40
6-7	0.50
7-8	0.60
10	0.70
Nonrebreathing Mask With Reservoir Bag	
6	0.60
7	0.70
8	0.80
9	0.80+
10	0.80+

[a]A partial rebreathing mask is capable of delivering an F_IO_2 of 0.7 at flows of 10 L/min

F_IO_2, Fractional inspired oxygen.

📌 **CLINICAL SCENARIO 4.1   A Simple Method for Estimating the Theoretical F_IO_2**

A 150-lb, spontaneously breathing patient is receiving oxygen at the rate of 6 L/min through a nasal cannula. The patient's tidal volume is 500 mL, and the respiratory rate is 20 breaths per minute (inspiratory time = 1 second; expiratory time = 2 seconds). Estimate the theoretical F_IO_2.
   See Appendix A for the answer.

F_IO_2, Fractional inspired oxygen.

---

improved the delivery of oxygen therapy, especially with regard to conserving oxygen supplies during long-term oxygen therapy.

Transtracheal catheters. The concept of TTO therapy was first described by Heimlich[7] in 1982. The guiding principle for such oxygen therapy is that oxygen delivered directly into the trachea should provide the patient with adequate oxygen while reducing the amount of oxygen used; that is, direct delivery of oxygen into the trachea reduces dilution with room air on inspiration because the upper airways (the anatomical reservoir) are filled with oxygen. Consequently, lower oxygen flows from the source gas (e.g., 0.25 to 2 L/min) are required to achieve a desired level of oxygenation. Indeed, TTO catheters can produce overall oxygen savings of 54% to 59%.[1]

Catheter placement requires minor surgery. A small, plastic stent is inserted into the patient's trachea between the second and third tracheal rings.[1,8] The stent remains in place for approximately a week to ensure that a permanent tract is

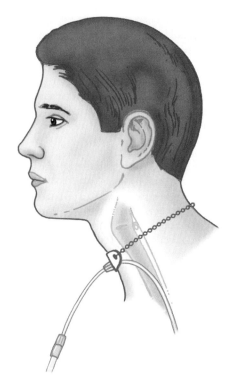

FIGURE 4.12 Transtracheal catheter. (From Kacmarek RM, Stoller JK, Heuer AJ: *Egan's fundamentals of respiratory care,* ed 10, St. Louis, 2013, Mosby-Elsevier.)

formed between the trachea and the outer skin. Removal of the stent is accomplished over a guide wire. After the stent is removed, a 9-Fr Teflon catheter is inserted into the tract over the guide wire. The catheter is held in place with a neck chain to prevent inadvertent dislodgment or removal (Fig. 4.12). It is recommended that catheters are replaced at 90 days or sooner, before they become cracked, kinked, or occluded by pus or mucus.[1,9,10] Patients must be taught the proper care of these devices to prevent complications. Routine care should include cleaning, lavage, and use of a cleaning rod to remove mucus that can occlude the lumen of the catheter.[8,11]

As previously stated, transtracheal catheters reduce oxygen costs by requiring lower oxygen flows to prevent hypoxemia. Therefore patients can purchase smaller, lighter cylinders or reservoirs for greater convenience. The use of special low-flow regulators or flow restrictors may also lead to greater cost savings.[1,11] Other important advantages of transtracheal catheters include improved patient compliance with oxygen therapy because of cosmetic appearance (these devices are relatively inconspicuous), increased patient mobility, and the avoidance of nasal irritation associated with the use of nasal cannulas. Finally, it should be mentioned that TTO devices use standard oxygen therapy equipment; this is important because if a problem arises with the catheter, emergency equipment (e.g., a conventional nasal cannula) can easily be set up and used by the patient.

The primary disadvantage of transtracheal catheters is complications associated with minor surgery (i.e., hemoptysis, infection, and subcutaneous emphysema).[8,11] Mucous obstruction and occlusion of the distal end of the tube can also cause

📌 CLINICAL SCENARIO 4.2

A home-care patient who requires continuous oxygen therapy is instructed to use a nasal cannula at a flow of 2 L/min. After a short period the patient is admitted to the hospital with signs of hypoxemia. When asked if he had been using the prescribed oxygen, the patient explains that he used it only intermittently because it was uncomfortable, and furthermore he felt self-conscious about wearing the equipment in public. What would you suggest to help this patient overcome the problems he described?

See Appendix A for the answer.

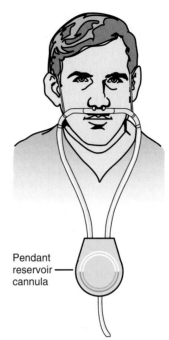

FIGURE 4.14 Pendant reservoir cannula.

Pendant reservoir cannula

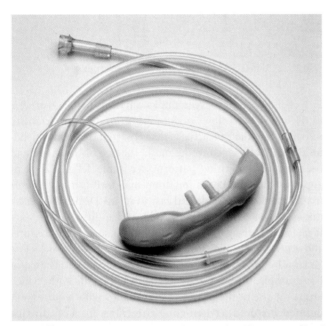

FIGURE 4.13 Mustache reservoir cannula. (Courtesy Chad Therapeutics, Chatsworth, CA.)

complications; however, these can be minimized with proper care, including saline instillation and periodic clearing of the catheter lumen with a guide wire or cleaning rod. Clinical Scenario 4.2 presents a common example of how TTO can increase patient compliance with oxygen therapy.

Reservoir cannulas. Two commercially available reservoir cannulas are the mustache cannula (Fig. 4.13) and the pendant cannula (Fig. 4.14). The mustache cannula can hold approximately 20 mL of gas. During the early part of exhalation, gas derived from the patient's dead space inflates the reservoir. As exhalation continues, oxygen from the source gas (e.g., 100% oxygen from a 50-psi source) flows into the lateral aspects of the cannula, forcing the dead space gas medial and out of the nasal prongs and filling the reservoir with 100% oxygen. On inspiration the initial part of the inhaled gas entering the patient's airway is drawn from this reservoir. As the reservoir collapses, the device functions like a conventional nasal cannula. Thus the reservoir adds 20 mL of 100% oxygen as a bolus in addition to the continuous oxygen flow from the supply source. The added bolus of gas reduces the amount of oxygen that must be derived from the continuous-flow source to achieve a desired F_IO_2.

Pendant cannulas operate in a similar manner, except that the reservoir is attached with connective tubing that serves as a conduit to a pendant that hangs below the chin. The added tubing between the reservoir and the pendant increases the amount of gas that can be stored; therefore these types of devices can hold nearly 40 mL of 100% oxygen. As with mustache cannulas, the main advantage of these devices is their ability to conserve gas flow.

Mustache and pendant cannulas can significantly reduce oxygen supply use compared with continuous-flow nasal cannulas. Studies indicate that mustache and pendant systems may reduce oxygen supply use by 50%,[12] although the cost of reservoir cannulas is higher than that of standard nasal cannulas. Also, many patients feel that mustache cannulas are heavier, larger, and more obvious than conventional nasal cannulas. Pendant cannulas, however, can be concealed by the patient's clothing.

Pulse-demand oxygen delivery systems. As the name implies, pulse-demand oxygen delivery systems deliver oxygen to the patient on demand; that is, they provide oxygen only during inspiration. Electronic, fluidic, and combined electronic-fluidic sensors are used to control gas delivery to the patient. Demand systems can operate with nasal catheters, nasal cannulas, and transtracheal catheters.[9,12] Fig. 4.15 is a schematic of a demand system for a conventional nasal cannula.[1] With this type of system, oxygen is delivered to the patient only after a sufficient inspiratory effort is made (i.e., <−1 cm H_2O). After it is activated, the demand valve opens, delivering oxygen at a preset flow rate; it closes during exhalation to conserve oxygen. Because the demand valve connects directly to the oxygen source (50 psig), it replaces the flowmeter used with continuous-flow cannulas. Note that demand systems can function as pulsed- or continuous-flow sources of oxygen. Settings allow the operator to select the equivalent of 1 to 5 L/

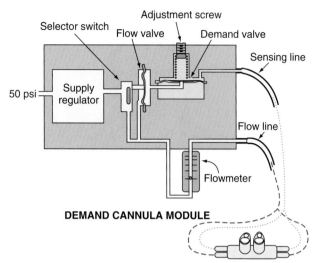

FIGURE 4.15 Pulse-demand oxygen delivery system for nasal cannula.

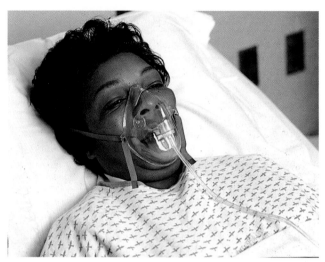

FIGURE 4.16 Simple oxygen mask.

min of oxygen flow from a conventional flowmeter. Shigeoka and Bonnekat[9] calculated that a patient receives approximately 17 mL of oxygen at the 1 L/min setting, 35 mL at the 2 L/min setting, 51 mL at the 3 L/min setting, and so on. It should be pointed out that oxygen delivered from these devices is not humidified, because the system is delivering small pulses of oxygen. Humidification is not necessary because drying of the mucous membranes, as might occur with continuous-flow delivery systems, does not occur with these devices.

A common problem with demand devices is improper placement of the sensor; this can result in interference with detection of an inspiratory effort, malfunction of the demand (solenoid) valve, and inadequate inspiratory flows. Improper placement of the sensor and malfunction of the demand valve usually can be detected by careful observation of the patient during the initial setup. Determining the adequacy of inspiratory flow requires feedback from the patient, either through verbal comments or oximetric analysis.

Simple oxygen mask. Although modern oxygen masks are made of different materials from those used in earlier masks, their overall design has hardly changed since their introduction in the late 18th century.[6] Modern oxygen masks, such as the one shown in Fig. 4.16, are cone-shaped devices that fit over the patient's nose and mouth and are held in place with an elastic band that fits around the patient's head. During inspiration the patient draws gases both from oxygen flowing into the mask through small-bore tubing connected to the base of the mask and from room air via ports on the sides of the mask. These ports also serve as exhalation ports. A typical adult oxygen mask has a volume of approximately 100 to 200 mL and may be thought of as an extension of the anatomical reservoir, because the patient inhales its contents during the early part of inspiration. As such, simple oxygen masks can deliver higher F_IO_2 levels than nasal cannulas because of a "reservoir effect." Note that the oxygen flow into the mask must be sufficient to wash out exhaled carbon dioxide, which can accumulate in this potential reservoir.

Generally, simple oxygen masks can deliver an F_IO_2 of 40% to 60% at oxygen flows of 5 to 8 L/min. It is important to recognize that the F_IO_2 actually delivered to the patient depends on the flow of oxygen to the mask, the size of the mask, and the patient's breathing pattern (see Table 4.1 for a list of approximate F_IO_2 levels for flows of 5 to 8 L/min). Simple oxygen masks are reliable and easy to set up. Disposable plastic masks are available in infant, child, and adult sizes. They are ideal for delivering oxygen during minor surgical procedures and emergency situations.

However, the use of oxygen masks has several disadvantages. For example, the delivered F_IO_2 can vary significantly, which limits the use of these devices for patients who require well-defined inspired oxygen concentrations. Carbon dioxide rebreathing can occur if the oxygen flow to the mask is not sufficient to wash out the patient's exhaled gases. For this reason, it generally is recommended that the minimum flow set on an oxygen mask should be 5 L/min. Oxygen masks are confining and may not be well tolerated by some patients. Furthermore, they must be removed during eating, drinking, and facial and airway care. Patients often complain that oxygen masks cause skin irritation, especially when they are tightly fitted. Finally, aspiration of vomitus may be more likely when the mask is in place.

Partial rebreathing masks. The partial rebreathing mask is derived from the Boothby-Lovelace-Bulbulian (BLB) mask, which was introduced by Boothby et al. in 1938.[10] As Fig. 4.17 shows, the partial rebreathing mask consists of a facepiece, which is similar to the simple oxygen mask described previously, and a reservoir bag that is attached to the base of the mask. In a typical adult partial rebreathing mask, the reservoir bag has a volume capacity of approximately 300 to 500 mL. Gas flow from the oxygen source is directed into the mask and the reservoir via small-bore tubing that connects at the junction of the mask and bag.

The operational theory of these devices is fairly straightforward. When the patient inhales, gas is drawn from the bag, the source gas flowing into the mask, and potentially from the room air through the exhalation ports. As the patient

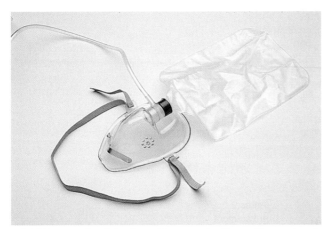

FIGURE 4.17 Partial rebreathing mask. (From Sorrentino S: *Mosby's textbook for long-term care nursing assistants*, ed 6, St. Louis, 2011, Mosby-Elsevier.)

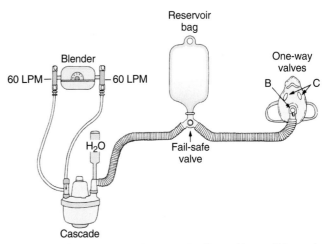

FIGURE 4.18 Nonrebreathing mask. (From Foust GN, et al: Shortcomings of using two jet nebulizers in tandem with an aerosol face mask for optimal oxygen therapy. *Chest* 99:1346, 1991.)

exhales, the first third of the exhaled gas fills the reservoir bag, and the last two-thirds of the exhaled gas are vented through the exhalation ports. Notice that the volume that fills the reservoir bag is roughly equivalent to the volume of the patient's anatomical dead space volume. Because the volume that fills the reservoir bag represents gas that has not participated in gas exchange, it has a high partial pressure of oxygen (PO_2) and a low partial pressure of carbon dioxide (PCO_2). The patient inhales this gas mixture during the next breath.

Partial rebreathing masks can deliver an F_IO_2 of 0.4 to 0.7 for an oxygen flow of 10 L/min. The actual percentage of oxygen delivered is also influenced by the patient's ventilatory pattern. Note that the minimum flow of oxygen should be sufficient to ensure that the bag does not completely deflate when the patient inhales (i.e., a minimum flow of 10 L/min should be sufficient to maintain the reservoir bag at least one-third to one-half full on inspiration).[4,13] Partial rebreathing masks are available in child and adult sizes.

Nonrebreathing masks. Nonrebreathing masks look very similar to partial rebreathing masks except that they have two types of valves attached to the mask, as Fig. 4.18 illustrates. The first set of valves is a one-way valve (B) located between the reservoir bag and the base of the mask. This valve allows gas flow to enter the mask from the reservoir bag when the patient inhales and prevents gas flow from the mask back into the reservoir bag during the patient's exhalation, as occurs with the partial rebreathing mask. The second set of valves is at the exhalation ports (C). These one-way valves prevent room air from entering the mask during inhalation and allow the patient's exhaled gases to exit the mask on exhalation. As with the partial rebreathing mask, the flow of oxygen to the mask should be sufficient to maintain the reservoir bag at least one-third to one-half full on inspiration.

Nonrebreathing masks theoretically can deliver 100% oxygen, assuming that the mask fits snugly on the patient's face and the only source of gas being inhaled is derived from the oxygen flowing into the mask-reservoir system. In actual practice, disposable nonrebreathing masks can deliver an F_IO_2 of 0.6 to 0.8.[13] The discrepancy between disposable nonrebreathing masks and the original BLB masks is primarily related to the fact that manufacturers usually supply disposable masks with one of the exhalation valves removed. The valve is removed as a precaution in case the oxygen flow to the mask is interrupted or inadequate for the patient's needs (i.e., according to safety regulations, the patient must still be able to entrain room air if source gas flow is interrupted). Original BLB masks contain a spring-disk safety valve that opens if oxygen flow to the mask is interrupted.

Nonrebreathing masks are effective for administering a high F_IO_2 to spontaneously breathing patients for short periods. Prolonged use of these masks can be associated with valve malfunctions (i.e., sticking as a result of moisture accumulation or deformity from wear).

High-Flow Oxygen Systems

Air entrainment masks. Air entrainment masks are the result of the pioneering work of Barach and associates[14,15] and Campbell.[16] Fig. 4.19 is a schematic of a typical air entrainment mask. It consists of a plastic mask connected to a jet nozzle, which is encased within a plastic housing that contains air entrainment ports. Oxygen flowing through the nozzle "drags" in room air through the entrainment ports as a result of viscous, shearing forces between the gas exiting the jet nozzle outlet and the surrounding ambient air.[17] The concentration of oxygen delivered to the patient therefore depends on the flow of oxygen exiting the jet nozzle, the size of the jet nozzle outlet, and the size of the entrainment port.

For most commercially available masks the oxygen concentration is varied by changing the size of the nozzle outlet or the entrainment ports. The flow of oxygen to the nozzle is constant and set to a minimum value, usually 2 to 10 L/min. Note that partial obstruction of oxygen flow downstream of the jet orifice or partial obstruction of the entrainment ports reduces the amount of room air entrained, thus raising the F_IO_2 of the delivered gas.[18-20]

Fig. 4.20 presents a simple method for calculating the air-to-oxygen entrainment ratio and the total gas flow delivered

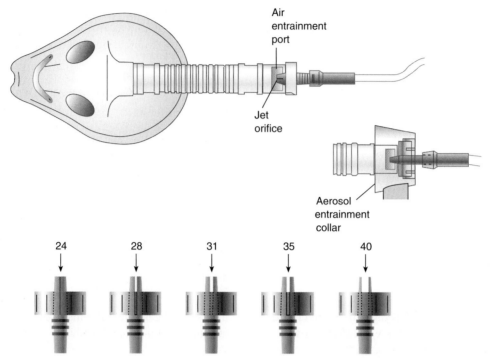

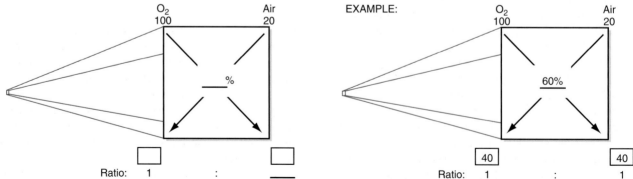

FIGURE 4.19 Schematic of the components of an air entrainment mask. The aerosol collar allows high humidity or aerosol entrainment from an air source. (From Kacmarek RM, Stoller JK, Heuer AJ: *Egan's fundamentals of respiratory care,* ed 10, St. Louis, 2013, Mosby-Elsevier.)

$$O_2 \text{ flow} = \frac{\text{Total flow} \times (FIO_2 - 0.2)}{0.8}$$

EXAMPLE:
Known: Total flow = 10 L/min
        $FIO_2 = 0.4$

$$O_2 \text{ flow} = \frac{10 \times (0.4 - 0.2)}{0.8}$$

$$O_2 \text{ flow} = \frac{10 \times 0.2}{0.8}$$

$$O_2 \text{ flow} = \frac{2}{0.8}$$

O_2 flow = 2.5 L/min

(Air flow = Total flow − O_2 flow)

$$FIO_2 \text{ flow} = \frac{O_2 \text{ flow} + (0.2 \times \text{Air flow})}{\text{Total flow}}$$

EXAMPLE:
Known: O_2 flow = 2.5 L/min
        Air flow = 7.5 L/min
        Total flow = 10 L/min

$$FIO_2 = \frac{2.5 + (0.2 \times 7.5)}{10}$$

$$FIO_2 = \frac{2.5 + 1.5}{10}$$

$$FIO_2 = \frac{4}{10}$$

$FIO_2 = 0.4$

$$\text{Total flow} = \frac{O_2 \text{ flow} \times 0.8}{FIO_2 - 0.2}$$

EXAMPLE:
Known: O_2 flow = 2.5 L/min
        $FIO_2 = 0.4$

$$\text{Total flow} = \frac{2.5 \times 0.8}{0.4 - 0.2}$$

$$\text{Total flow} = \frac{2}{0.2}$$

Total flow = 10 L/min

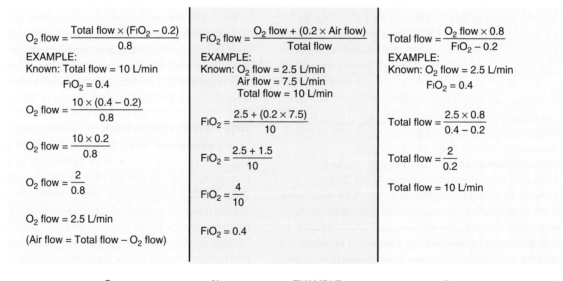

FIGURE 4.20 Method of calculating air-to-oxygen entrainment ratios.

TABLE 4.2 Approximate Entrainment Ratios for Commonly Used Oxygen Concentrations[a]

Oxygen Percentage	Air:Oxygen Ratio	Total Parts[b]
100	0:1	1
70	0.6:1	1.6
60	1:1	2
50	1.7:1	2.7
40	3:1	4
35	5:1	6
30	8:1	9
28	10:1	11
24	25:1	26

[a]Assuming the F_IO_2 of room air is 20.9%.
[b]Total parts × Oxygen flow = Total flow estimate.
F_IO_2, Fractional inspired oxygen.

for a given F_IO_2.[19] Table 4.2 presents a list of the air-to-oxygen entrainment ratios required to achieve a given F_IO_2, showing that the total flow of gas delivered is greater for a low F_IO_2 than for a high F_IO_2. Air entrainment masks function much better as fixed-performance devices at a low F_IO_2 (less than 0.4) than at a higher F_IO_2 (greater than 0.4).[18,20,21] The discrepancy between the set F_IO_2 and the actual delivered F_IO_2 is exaggerated by abrupt increases in inspiratory flow. Campbell and Minty[22] suggest that many commercially available masks produce a variable F_IO_2 when patients generate high inspiratory flows because of insufficient mask volume.

Air entrainment masks are excellent for providing oxygen therapy to hypoxemic patients with chronic obstructive pulmonary disease (COPD); these patients typically require a fixed F_IO_2 that is between 0.24 and 0.35.[16] The total flow of gas delivered by such masks (oxygen plus air) for lower F_IO_2 levels usually is sufficient to meet the peak inspiratory flow requirements of these patients. Supplemental humidification of the delivered gas usually is not required when the oxygen flow is low (i.e., less than 4 L/min) because the oxygen flow is a small percentage of the total flow. Increased moisture can be delivered by attaching a compressed, air-driven aerosol to the air entrainment port via an open plastic collar (such collars work best with masks that have large air entrainment ports). Alternatively, high humidity can be delivered with a fixed F_IO_2 with large-volume aerosol nebulizers and humidifier units that use air entrainment devices, which can provide increased levels of moisture at several fixed oxygen percentage settings (e.g., 0.4, 0.6, and 1). A number of appliances, including aerosol masks, face tents, T-tubes, and tracheostomy collars, can be used to deliver these moisture-rich gases. Care should be taken to not allow moisture to accumulate in the tubing downstream from the air entrainment device. Accumulated moisture acts as an obstruction, which can reduce the amount of room air entrained and raise the F_IO_2 delivered to the patient. Notice that the total flow of gas provided by this type of apparatus may not be sufficient to meet patients' high ventilatory demands. Thus the F_IO_2 may vary considerably in these

situations, because the patient is forced to entrain room air to meet increased ventilatory needs.[23,24] Large-volume nebulizers and humidifiers are discussed in more detail in Chapter 6.

High-flow nasal cannulas. Another approach for delivering a high F_IO_2 (>0.6) via nasal cannula to patients with moderate hypoxemic respiratory failure involves using *high-flow nasal cannula* (HFNC) systems. HFNC can achieve these high F_IO_2 levels by washing out CO_2 from the nasopharyngeal dead space and generating gas flows that exceed the inspiratory flow needs of most patients. These higher flows reduce the patient's need to entrain room air, resulting in a more reliable delivery of high F_IO_2 levels.[25,26] Additionally, it has been suggested that these devices enhance patient comfort by providing warmed and humidified gas that preserves the rheology and volume of secretions, thus facilitating mucociliary clearance.[25]

HFNC systems include a patient interface, a gas delivery device to control oxygen flow, and a humidifier.[27] Monitoring the efficacy of these devices relies on physical findings related to breathing frequency and pulse oximetry. Commercial systems are available from Salter Labs, Vapotherm, Teleflex, and Fisher and Paykel.[27]

The Salter Labs 1600HF high-flow system uses a standard nasal cannula tubing that is connected to a humidifying system that resembles an unheated bubble humidifier. The diffuser for the humidifiers has a lower resistance than standard bubble humidifiers. The 1600HF system can provide nonheated, humidified oxygen at flows up to 15 L/min (F_IO_2 >0.6), and a relative humidity of 72% to 78%.

The Vapotherm 2000i system can deliver heated and humidified oxygen (relative humidity of 99%) at flows of 5 to 40 L/min and an F_IO_2 greater than 0.9 through a specially designed nasal cannula. The device requires the addition of a high-flow air/O_2 blender and flowmeter. The core of the system uses a *vapor transfer cartridge,* which is composed of a continuous-feed high-efficiency heated humidifier system.[27] The Vapotherm 2000i system allows water vapor to be added to the oxygen flow via a semipermeable membrane. The manufacturer reports that the pores of the membrane are less than 0.1 μm in diameter and thus are small enough to prevent the transfer of bacteria into the gas stream. The Vapotherm Precision Flow high-flow humidification system was released in 2008. The Vapotherm Precision Flow system (Fig. 4.21) uses a cartridge humidifier similar to Vapotherm 2000i, but it differs from the latter device because it includes an air/O_2 blender and oxygen analyzer incorporated into the humidifier module.[11]

The Teleflex Comfort Flo system can deliver flows of 1 to 40 L/min of heated, humidified oxygen through a nasal cannula interface. The Comfort Flo system is equipped with a sterile ConchaTherm Neptune heated humidifier, which contains sterile water, thus minimizing the risks associated with cross-contamination and bacteria growth. Teleflex Comfort Flo Nasal Cannulas are available in adult, pediatric, infant, and premature sizes.

The Fisher and Paykel Optiflow system uses specially-designed oval-shaped nasal prong orifices that connect via large-bore corrugated tubing to a Fisher and Paykel 850 heated

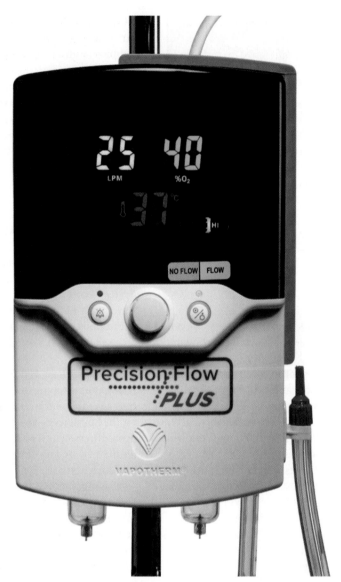

FIGURE 4.21 Vapotherm Precision Flow high-flow humidification system. (Courtesy Vapotherm, Annapolis, MD.)

humidifier. The humidifier is connected to a separate air/O_2 blender or a Maxtec MaxVenturi combination air/O_2 entrainment device and flowmeter. An external oxygen analyzer is required. The system also includes a single-limb heated-wire circuit to minimize condensation within the tubing, which can obstruct oxygen flow to the cannula.[27]

Oxygen hoods. Oxygen hoods were introduced in the 1970s as a means of maintaining a relatively constant F_IO_2 to infants requiring supplemental oxygen. Fig. 4.22 shows a typical hood used to deliver oxygen therapy to pediatric patients. It is a clear plastic enclosure that is placed around the patient's head. Fixed oxygen concentrations (from an air entrainment device or an oxygen–air blender [see the section on oxygen blenders later in this chapter]) can be connected to the hood via an inlet port at the rear of the hood. The flow rate of gas entering the hood is set to ensure that the exhaled carbon dioxide is

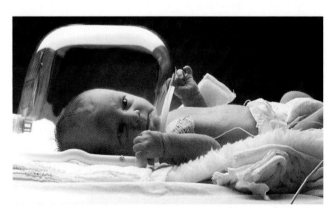

FIGURE 4.22 Oxygen hood. (Courtesy Utah Medical Products, Midvale, UT.)

flushed out (i.e., the flow rate should be approximately 5 to 10 L/min).

The F_IO_2 must be measured intermittently or monitored continuously with an oxygen analyzer. Several studies have shown that in hoods, the oxygen seems to be layered, with the highest concentration near the bottom of the hood. The partial pressure of oxygen in the arteries (PaO_2) should also be measured by arterial blood gas analysis at regular intervals. The noise levels inside an oxygen hood can present problems, and every effort should be made to minimize this effect.[28]

Isolettes (incubators). Isolettes (i.e., incubators), along with oxygen tents, can be classified as environmental delivery systems because they provide large volumes of oxygen-enriched gas to the atmosphere immediately surrounding the patient. The first incubator was designed by Denuce in 1857.[19] Several years later (c.1880), Tarnier designed an enclosed incubator to provide a warm environment for premature infants.[19]

The Dräger Isolette 8000 incubator (Dräger Medical AG & Co.) (Fig. 4.23) is an example of an incubator used in the care of newborn infants. The Dräger Isolette 8000 includes a micro air intake filter with 99.9% efficiency. The temperature and humidity of the gas in the incubator are regulated by a servo-controlled mechanism. It allows for variable control of the environmental temperature (20.0°C to 37.0°C [68°F to 98.6°F]), humidity (30% to 95% relative humidity), and F_IO_2 (21% to 65%).

It is important to remember that the actual concentration of oxygen delivered to the patient can vary considerably when the enclosure is opened for nursing care procedures. Because of the variability in oxygen concentrations that can occur when oxygen is provided through the incubator's oxygen inlet, supplemental oxygen may need to be delivered directly to the infant via a standard nasal cannula, high-flow nasal cannula, nasal prongs, or an oxygen hood placed directly over the infant's head inside the incubator.[8] Regardless of the method used to deliver oxygen to the infant, the actual F_IO_2 in the incubator should be measured intermittently or continuously monitored. Additionally, arterial oxygenation (e.g., pulse oximetry, arterial blood gas levels) should be monitored at regular intervals to ensure that the infant is receiving the appropriate oxygen therapy. The PaO_2 should be monitored in infants receiving oxygen therapy. High PaO_2 values in these patients are associated with a high incidence of retinopathy and loss of sight.

Clinical studies have demonstrated that noise levels in incubators can be quite high.[28] Although noise may be a difficult problem to control, every effort must be made to minimize it inside these devices.

Oxygen tents. Sir Leonard Hill is credited with being the first clinician to use the oxygen tent,[3] but Alvin Barach improved the operation of these devices by conditioning the air inside the tent.[4] (Barach accomplished this early form of air conditioning by adding a fan to circulate the air over a cooling tower containing ice.) During the early 1900s, oxygen tents were often used to provide oxygen to hypoxemic adults and children. Currently, oxygen tents are used primarily for pediatric patients who require enriched oxygen and high humidity levels. Today's oxygen tents can provide environmental control of (1) oxygen concentration, (2) humidity, and (3) temperature (Fig. 4.24). The F_IO_2 and the humidity content delivered to the patient are controlled by a high-flow aerosol unit, which is incorporated into the tent. Ultrasonic nebulizers (see Chapter 6) can also be used to increase the humidity inside the tent. The temperature is controlled with refrigeration coils containing Freon. These systems typically can reduce the temperature inside the tent from 5.5°C to 6.7°C (10°F to 12°F) below room temperature.

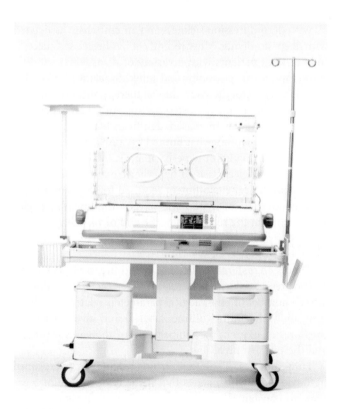

FIGURE 4.23 Infant incubator. (Courtesy Dräger Medical AG & Co., Lübeck, Germany.)

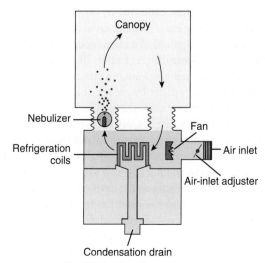

FIGURE 4.24 Oxygen tent.

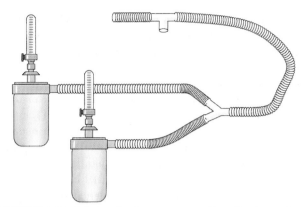

FIGURE 4.25 Schematic of an oxygen adder. (Redrawn from Kacmarek RM, Stoller JK, Heuer AJ: *Egan's fundamentals of respiratory care,* ed 10, St. Louis, 2013, Mosby-Elsevier.)

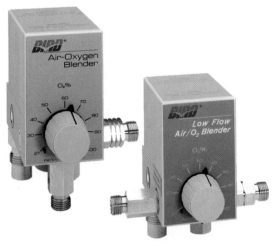

FIGURE 4.26 Oxygen blenders. (Courtesy CareFusion, San Diego, CA.)

Oxygen Proportioners

Oxygen adders. The simplest example of an oxygen proportioner is an oxygen adder, such as the one shown in Fig. 4.25. Although these devices are not commonly used clinically, the principle of operation can be used to describe how oxygen proportioners work. The typical oxygen adder system consists of two flowmeters: one attached to an oxygen supply and the other attached to an air supply. The outputs of the two flowmeters are directed to humidifiers and then to the patient via any of the delivery systems previously described. The F_IO_2 of the gas delivered to the patient depends on the ratio of air-to-oxygen flow. The concentration can be calculated using the same principle as that for calculating air-to-oxygen entrainment ratios for air entrainment masks. For example, if the air and oxygen flowmeters are each set to deliver 15 L/min, the ratio is 1:1, which corresponds to an F_IO_2 of 0.6. However, if the air flowmeter is set to 15 L/min and the oxygen flowmeter is set to 5 L/min, the air-to-oxygen entrainment ratio is 3:1, corresponding to an F_IO_2 of 0.4 (see Table 4.2).

Oxygen blenders and mixers. A more sophisticated device for accomplishing air-oxygen mixing is the oxygen blender (or oxygen mixer). Fig. 4.26 shows typical oxygen blenders and their components. Compressed air and oxygen from a high-pressure source enter a chamber, where the pressures of the two gases are equalized. An alarm system is incorporated into the design of these devices to alert the practitioner if the pressures of the source gases are not comparable (i.e., the air and oxygen pressures differ by greater than 10 psi). Unequal source gas pressures can cause the blender to malfunction and deliver unreliable F_IO_2 levels. Unequal pressures are remedied by reducing the higher-pressure gas to match the lower-pressure gas, which is usually 50 psig. The gases then are routed to a precise metering device that controls the amount of each gas reaching the outlet. This metering device can be adjusted with a rotary mixing control knob on the faceplate. Turning the knob counterclockwise reduces the amount of oxygen reaching the outlet, thereby reducing the delivered F_IO_2. Conversely, turning the knob clockwise reduces the amount of air reaching the outlet, increasing the F_IO_2.

Oxygen blenders are a reliable means of providing a variety of F_IO_2 levels. Flowmeters can be connected to the blender's outlet, as can ventilators or any other devices that use 50-psig source gas. Because moisture and particulate matter introduced into the blender by the source gases can cause the blender to malfunction, it is important to filter the gas before it enters the blender housing.

Hyperbaric Oxygen Therapy

Hyperbaric oxygen therapy exposes patients to a pressure greater than atmospheric pressure while they breathe 100% oxygen, either continuously or intermittently. Historically, hyperbaric therapy has been used most often to treat individuals with decompression sickness and air embolism associated with deep-sea diving. More recently, it has been used successfully to treat patients with a variety of disorders, including carbon monoxide poisoning and smoke inhalation, anaerobic infections refractory to conventional therapy, thermal injuries, skin grafts, and refractory osteomyelitis. Although hyperbaric oxygen therapy has increased significantly during the past decade, its use is somewhat limited because it is expensive to purchase and maintain hyperbaric units. A brief discussion of the physiological basis of hyperbaric oxygen therapy and a description of the equipment required follows. For a more detailed analysis of hyperbaric oxygen therapy, the reader should consult the references at the end of this chapter.[29-35]

Physiological Principles

Effects on respiratory function. Exposure to elevated barometric pressures during hyperbaric oxygen therapy can directly affect a number of physiological parameters related to respiration, including lung volume, arterial and alveolar partial pressures of oxygen, the temperature of the gases breathed, and the work of breathing.

Lung volumes. The effects on lung volume can be explained by Boyle's law, which states that if the temperature of a gas remains constant, the volume of a gas is inversely related to its pressure. That is, as pressure exerted on the container increases, the gas volume decreases. Therefore, when a person

Depth in feet	Pressure in ATM	Relative volume	Relative diameter
0	1	100%	100%
33	2	50%	79.3%
66	3	33.3%	69.3%
99	4	25%	63%
132	5	20%	58.5%
165	6	16.6%	55%

FIGURE 4.27 Pressure–volume relationships during hyperbaric oxygen therapy. *ATM,* Atmosphere(s). (Redrawn from Davis JC, Hunt TK: *Hyperbaric oxygen therapy,* Kensington, MD, 1977, Undersea Medical Society.)

is exposed to elevated pressures, the gas volume contained in any body cavity tends to be compressed. For example, as the ambient pressure is doubled (1520 mm Hg, or 2 atmospheres [atm]), the air volume in the lung is reduced to one-half of what it would occupy at a normal ambient pressure (760 mm Hg, or 1 atm). Fig. 4.27 shows the pressure–volume relationships typically encountered during hyperbaric oxygen therapy.

Alveolar and arterial partial pressures of oxygen. The effect of increased ambient pressure on the partial pressure of alveolar oxygen (P_AO_2) can be explained by Dalton's law, which states that the total pressure of a gas mixture, such as air, equals the sum of the partial pressures of each of the constituent gases in the mixture. Considering that air is 21% oxygen and 79% nitrogen, then ambient air (assuming that the barometric pressure is 760 mm Hg) has a PO_2 of approximately 160 mm Hg (0.21×760 mm Hg) and a partial nitrogen pressure of approximately 600 mm Hg (0.79×760 mm Hg). This same logic can be applied to the alveolar air equation for calculating the P_AO_2:

$$P_AO_2 = [(P_{bar} - PH_2O) F_IO_2 - P_aCO_2]/0.8$$

Therefore, if the barometric pressure (P_{bar}) equals 760 mm Hg, the PH_2O equals 47 mm Hg, the $PaCO_2$ equals 40 mm Hg, and the F_IO_2 equals 0.21, the P_AO_2 would be approximately 100 mm Hg. Consider the case if the barometric pressure is doubled to 1520 mm Hg, or 2 atm. If all other variables in the equation remain constant, the P_AO_2 would equal 259 mm Hg.

Henry's law is used to explain the changes in the P_aO_2 that occur with exposure to elevated ambient pressures. Henry's law states that the degree to which a gas enters into physical solution in body fluids is directly proportional to the partial pressure of gas to which the fluid is exposed. Remember that

Henry's law states that the relative quantities of gas entering a fluid are related to the pressure of gas exerted on the fluid and the solubility of the gas in the fluid in question. Oxygen's solubility in plasma is approximately 0.003 volume percent (vol%) (milliliters of oxygen/100 mL of whole blood) for every 1 mm Hg of PaO_2. If it is assumed that the ventilation–perfusion relationship for a patient's lungs is normal, the P_aO_2 would be slightly less than 100 mm Hg when the patient is breathing room air at 1 atm. Furthermore, the P_aO_2 would be approximately 259 mm Hg for breathing room air when the ambient pressure is increased to 2 atm. Then it can be calculated that as the P_aO_2 increases from approximately 100 mm Hg (at 1 atm) to approximately 259 mm Hg (at 2 atm), the amount of dissolved oxygen increases from 0.3 vol% (100 mm Hg × 0.003 vol%/mm Hg) to 0.78 vol% (259 mm Hg × 0.003 vol%/mm Hg). As can be seen, the oxygen-carrying capacity of plasma increases considerably under hyperbaric conditions. Therefore it is reasonable to assume that this form of therapy is beneficial in the treatment of patients with abnormally functioning hemoglobin and consequently a reduced ability to carry oxygen attached to hemoglobin, such as occurs with carbon monoxide poisoning.

Gas temperatures. According to Gay-Lussac's law, if the volume of a gas remains constant, a direct relationship exists between the absolute pressure of a gas and its temperature. It is reasonable to suggest that if the volume of a hyperbaric chamber remains constant, increasing the pressure would raise the temperature inside the chamber. (Indeed, this problem should limit the usefulness of this form of therapy.) In practice, gas temperature changes encountered during hyperbaric therapy are easily controlled by regulating the rates at which pressures are increased and decreased, the temperature of the air used for compression and decompression, and the flow rate of ventilation used to dissipate heat.[30,31]

Work of breathing. As the barometric pressure increases, the density of the gas being breathed also increases. The increase in gas density results in an increased work of breathing, which is not noticeable and can easily be accommodated in normal patients. In patients with reduced lung reserves, however, this increased work may present problems and require ventilatory support. It also is important to recognize that many ventilators malfunction when placed in a hyperbaric chamber.[32]

Vascular function. Several studies have demonstrated that hyperbaric oxygen therapy increases the synthetic ability of tissues by increasing collagen deposition, thus enhancing the growth of new blood vessels in damaged tissues and the revascularization of these tissues.[29] This effect has been used to successfully treat patients with skin grafts.

Immunological function. It is well established that leukocyte function is enhanced during hyperbaric oxygen therapy. This improved function is thought to be related to an increase in the oxygen available for microbicidal metabolism (i.e., H_2O_2, OH^-). Coupled with this enhanced microbicidal activity of leukocytes, oxygen appears to directly inhibit the growth of certain bacteria, particularly those involved in anaerobic infections, such as *Clostridia* spp., which are responsible for gas gangrene.

Equipment

Hyperbaric chambers generally are classified as either monoplace or multiplace units (Fig. 4.28). Monoplace hyperbaric chambers are categorized by the National Fire Protection Association (NFPA) as class B chambers and are rated for single occupancy.[30] Several models of monoplace units are available commercially. Although they differ considerably in appearance, they all use the same principle of operation, generally relying on a single gas source for compression and respiration. Some newer systems provide connections for a separate gas source for respiration.

A typical chamber generally is approximately 8 to 10 feet long and 3 feet in diameter. The outer shell of the unit is constructed of steel and clear, double-layered acrylic. Some newer units contain a separate chamber compartment to accommodate attendants working with the patient. Most units are mounted on wheels for portability, but they usually are treated as stationary systems and are placed in a room designated for the purposes of hyperbaric therapy.

Multiplace hyperbaric chambers are walk-in units that provide enough space to allow two or more patients to be treated simultaneously. They vary in size (2 to 13 occupants) but usually contain a main chamber for treating patients and a smaller chamber that allows attendants to enter and leave without altering the pressure in the main chamber. Multiplace chambers provide two gas sources, one for compression and one for respiration. Hyperbaric oxygenation is achieved by having the patient breathe oxygen by mask or through a specially designed hood while exposed to elevated barometric pressures in the compressed air chamber. Treatment schedules (i.e., the amount of time the patient breathes 100% oxygen vs. air) are tailored to the specific needs of the patient. Generally, patients are placed on schedules in which intermittent air breathing periods of 5 minutes or longer are programmed approximately every 20 minutes. This intermittent air breathing is used to prevent oxygen toxicity.

Monitoring devices. All hyperbaric facilities should have the capability to monitor the oxygenation status of patients undergoing hyperbaric oxygen therapy. Transcutaneous monitoring has proven to be valuable in assessing the overall oxygenation status of a patient undergoing this treatment. Selective placement of the probe also can provide information

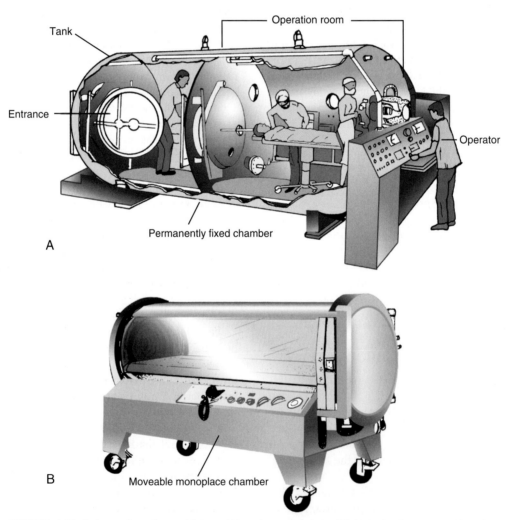

FIGURE 4.28 Schematics of a multiplace (A) and a monoplace (B) hyperbaric oxygen chamber. (From Kacmarek RM, Stoller JK, Heuer AJ: *Egan's fundamentals of respiratory care*, ed 10, St. Louis, 2013, Mosby-Elsevier.)

on the localized effects of hyperbaric oxygen therapy on ischemic tissue.

Arterial blood gas monitoring can provide information on the oxygenation status of patients receiving hyperbaric therapy and is also an indication of their ventilatory status. Arterial blood samples can be drawn from patients and removed from the chamber for analysis. Care must be taken to ensure that the sample remains tightly sealed until it is analyzed. Transcutaneous monitoring and arterial blood gas analysis are discussed further in Chapter 10.

Indications and Contraindications for Hyperbaric Oxygen Therapy

As stated previously, hyperbaric oxygen therapy is most often associated with the treatment of individuals who have experienced decompression sickness and other maladies associated with deep-sea diving. Box 4.1 lists several other conditions that have been successfully treated with this type of oxygen therapy.[33-35] Although the effectiveness of hyperbaric oxygen therapy may vary among patients, those with any of these conditions should respond to it.

Box 4.2 lists some of the known contraindications to hyperbaric oxygen therapy. The only absolute contraindication is pneumothorax. If pneumothorax occurs during hyperbaric treatment, chest tubes should be inserted immediately; failure to treat pneumothorax can have dire consequences. The other conditions listed are relative contraindications. Note that

---

BOX 4.1   Indications for Hyperbaric Oxygen Therapy

- Air or gas embolism
- Carbon monoxide poisoning
- Acute thermal burns injuries
- Acute traumatic and ischemic syndromes
- Decompression sickness
- Clostridial myositis and myonecrosis (gas gangrene)
- Necrotizing soft tissue infections
- Refractory osteomyelitis
- Compromised skin grafts
- Wound healing

BOX 4.2   Contraindications for Hyperbaric Oxygen Therapy

- Congenital spherocytosis
- High fevers
- Hypercapnia (>60 mm Hg)
- Obstructive airway disease
- Optic neuritis
- Pneumothorax
- Seizure disorders
- Sinusitis
- Upper respiratory infections
- Viral infections

From Kindall EP: Clinical hyperbaric oxygen therapy. In Bennett P, Elliot D, editors: *Physiology and medicine of diving*, ed 4, Philadelphia, 1993, WB Saunders.

---

serious problems can arise when patients with obstructive bronchial disease caused by asthma, bronchitis, or emphysema are treated with hyperbaric therapy. Gas trapping can result in barotrauma. Similarly, patients who have upper respiratory infections and nasal congestion usually are unable to clear their ears during compression and decompression and thus are prone to eardrum rupture during treatment.

Inhaled Nitric Oxide Therapy

As was discussed in Chapter 3, inhaled nitric oxide (iNO) has been shown to be a potent pulmonary vasodilator. It has been used to treat persistent pulmonary hypertension of the newborn, hypoxic respiratory failure in term and near-term newborns in whom conventional ventilator therapy has failed, as an adjunct to the treatment of congenital cardiac defects, and possibly to reverse the bronchoconstriction induced by histamine and methacholine.[36-40]

Nitric oxide is supplied as a compressed-gas mixture of nitric oxide and nitrogen (minimum purity 99%) in cylinders constructed of aluminum alloy.[41] It is supplied this way because it is a highly reactive molecule that is rapidly oxidized to nitrogen dioxide in the presence of oxygen and to nitric acid in the presence of water. Nitrogen dioxide and nitric acid are toxic if inhaled. In low concentrations, they can cause a chemical pneumonitis; higher concentrations can cause lung injury, such as pulmonary edema, which ultimately can lead to death.[33,42]

The initial therapeutic dose of iNO is 5 to 80 ppm.[36] Three US Food and Drug Administration (FDA)–approved commercially available delivery devices are available for the administration of iNO, including the INOmax DS_{IR} Plus (Ikaria), the INOvent (GE Healthcare), and the AeroNOx (International Biomedical).

The INOmax DS_{IR} Plus (Fig. 4.29) delivers NO for inhalation into the inspiratory limb of the patient breathing circuit in a way that provides a constant concentration of NO, as set by the user, throughout the inspired breath.[41] The INOmax DS_{IR} system can be used to deliver NO with conventional mechanical ventilators, high-frequency ventilators, and anesthesia machines. It can also be used with spontaneously breathing patients via low-flow and high-flow nasal cannula systems and nasal continuous positive airway pressure (CPAP) devices.[37] (*Note:* Ventilator operation manuals should always be reviewed before using NO to ensure proper set up and patient safety.)

The INOmax nitric oxide drug is stored in an aluminum cylinder as a gas mixture of NO/N_2 at a concentration of 800 ppm. The aluminum cylinder is attached to a high-pressure regulator that is attached to the INOmax DS_{IR} using one of two NO/N_2 quick-connect inlets located on the back of the device.[41]

Using a dual-channel design, the first channel uses a delivery central processing unit (CPU), flow controller, and an injector module to ensure the accurate delivery of NO (Fig. 4.30). The specially designed injector module enables tracking of the ventilator flow waveforms and the delivery of a synchronized and proportional dose of NO. The second channel is the monitoring system, which uses a separate monitor CPU, electrochemical gas sensors, and a graphically enhanced user

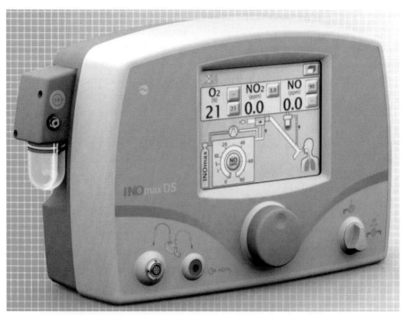

FIGURE 4.29 INOmax DS. (Courtesy Ikaria, Clinton, NJ).

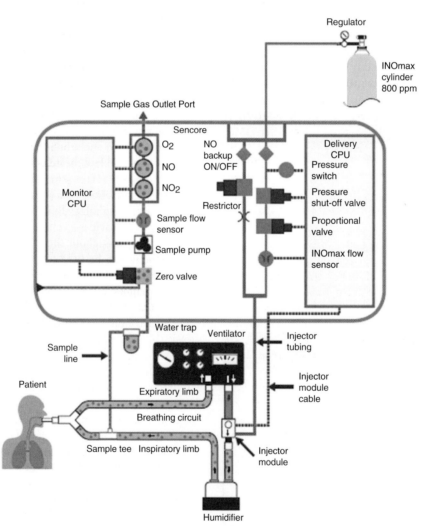

FIGURE 4.30 Schematic illustrating the principle of operation of the INOmax DS. (See text for description.) (Courtesy Ikaria, Clinton, NJ).

interface. The dual-channel design for delivery and monitoring allows the INOmax monitoring system to shut down INOmax delivery if it detects a fault in the delivery system (e.g., delivered NO concentration >100 ppm).[41]

The INOmax gas monitoring system allow for continuous monitoring of inspired oxygen (O_2), nitrogen dioxide (NO_2), and NO. Several alarm systems are available to alert staff members when problems arise, including alarms for high and low NO, high NO_2, and high and low O_2. Other alarms can be set to notify the user when source gas pressure is lost, the electrochemical cells fail, and calibration is required.[42]

Helium–Oxygen (Heliox) Therapy

Helium–oxygen (heliox) mixtures have been used on a limited basis to treat patients with airway obstruction.[43-45] Specifically, heliox has been used to manage asthmatic patients with acute respiratory failure, to treat postextubation stridor in pediatric trauma patients, as an adjunct to the treatment of pediatric patients with refractory croup, to administer anesthetic gases to patients with small-diameter endotracheal tubes, and to provide ventilatory support for patients with severe airway obstruction caused by chronic bronchitis and emphysema.[46-49]

Heliox mixtures are supplied in compressed-gas cylinders. Three concentrations are generally available: an 80%-to-20% (helium-to-oxygen) mixture, a 70%-to-30% mixture, a 65%-to-35% mixture, and a 60%-to-40% mixture. As was stated in Chapter 3, the benefit of breathing heliox is related to its lower density compared with pure oxygen or air. Remember that the density of an 80%-to-20% (helium-to-oxygen) mixture is 0.43 g/L, and that 100% oxygen has a density of 1.43 g/L. Therefore an 80%-to-20% mixture is 1.8 times less dense than 100% oxygen. A 70%-to-30% mixture of heliox has a density of 0.55 g/L and is therefore 1.6 times less dense than 100% oxygen, and a 60%-to-40% mixture has a density of 0.58 g/L and is 1.4 times less dense than 100% oxygen. (The density of a helium–oxygen mixture can be calculated using the following relationships: The density of 100% helium is 0.179 g/L, and the density of 100% oxygen is 1.43 g/L. Therefore the density of an 80%-to-20% heliox mixture equals [0.8 × 0.179 g/L] + [0.2 × 1.43 g/L], or 0.43 g/L.) The lower density promotes laminar flow and reduces the amount of turbulent flow. This relationship is important to remember when administering heliox because the actual flow rate of gas delivered is greater than the set flow. Table 4.3 presents a list of correction factors that can be applied to calculate the actual flow when a typical oxygen flowmeter is used to deliver a heliox mixture; Clinical Scenario 4.3 presents an example of this concept.[50]

TABLE 4.3 Heliox Correction Factors for Oxygen Flowmeters	
Helium:Oxygen Ratio	**Correction Factor**
80:20	1.8 × liter flow
70:30	1.6 × liter flow
60:40	1.4 × liter flow

Modified from Myers TR: Use of heliox in children. *Respir Care* 51:619, 2006.

Heliox usually is administered to intubated patients with an intermittent positive-pressure device. For nonintubated patients, a well-fitted, nonrebreathing mask attached to a reservoir bag should be used. The flow rate of gas should be high enough to prevent the reservoir bag from collapsing during inspiration. Nasal cannulas are ineffective for delivering heliox because of leakage. Large-volume enclosures, such as hoods, also are unsatisfactory because helium tends to concentrate at the top of these devices.

It is important to monitor the fractional concentration of oxygen delivered to the patient when a heliox mixture is administered. In some cases, commercial cylinders containing helium and oxygen may be "unmixed" (i.e., because of the difference in densities between helium and oxygen, a layering effect can occur). If a sufficient amount of oxygen is not mixed with the helium inspired by the patient, hypoxemia can result.[51] (Clinical Scenario 4.4 presents a problem-solving exercise involving heliox therapy.)

Carbon Dioxide–Oxygen (Carbogen) Therapy

Carbon dioxide–oxygen mixtures (carbogen) have used to treat hiccoughs and carbon monoxide poisoning, as a stimulant/depressant of ventilation, and to prevent the complete washout of carbon dioxide during cardiopulmonary bypass. The frequency of this procedure is limited because of the adverse effects associated with breathing elevated concentrations of carbon dioxide. Box 4.3 lists the clinical manifestations of carbon dioxide toxicity.

Carbogen is supplied in compressed-gas cylinders as either 5%-to-95% (carbon dioxide-to-oxygen) or 7%-to-93% (carbon dioxide-to-oxygen). It can be administered to patients with a nonrebreathing mask connected to a reservoir bag. The mask should fit snugly on the patient's face, and the flow rate of gas should be high enough to prevent the bag from collapsing when the patient inhales.

CLINICAL SCENARIO 4.3

You are asked to set up a large-volume nebulizer for the treatment of a patient with an acute asthma exacerbation. The attending physician asks you to use an 80%-to-20% heliox gas mixture as the driving gas for nebulizing the β_2-bronchodilator. What is the actual flow of gas being administered to the patient if the set flow on the oxygen flowmeter used is 10 L/min?

See Appendix A for the answer.

CLINICAL SCENARIO 4.4

You are the therapist on call when an asthmatic patient is admitted to the emergency department of the hospital. The attending physician requests that you administer heliox containing 30% oxygen to the patient. While you are administering the gas from a cylinder labeled 70%-to-30% (helium-to-oxygen), the patient becomes progressively more dyspneic and cyanotic. What should you do?

See Appendix A for the answer.

BOX 4.3 Clinical Manifestations of Carbon Dioxide Toxicity[a]

- Extrasystole (premature ventricular contractions)
- Flushed skin
- Full and bounding pulse
- Hypertension
- Muscle twitching

[a]Note that hypercapnia cannot be reliably diagnosed on clinical examination only. Arterial blood gas levels (measurement of the partial pressure of arterial carbon dioxide) should be determined in case of doubt.

To prevent adverse reactions when this type of therapy is administered, it is essential to monitor the patient's pulse, blood pressure, and respiration, as well as mental status. Pulse, arterial blood pressure, and minute volume normally increase as the patient breathes carbogen, but the rapidity and level of these changes depend on the concentration of the mixture. Changes occur faster and the effects are greater if the patient breathes a 7%-to-93% (carbon dioxide-to-oxygen) mixture than with a 5%-to-95% mixture. The treatment should be stopped immediately if any of the monitored parameters increase or decrease abruptly or significantly.

KEY POINTS

- Multistage regulators can control gas pressures with more precision than single-stage regulators because the pressure is reduced gradually. Additionally, multistage regulators produce a much smoother gas flow than do single-stage regulators.
- Flowmeters are devices that control and indicate flow. Pressure-compensated Thorpe tube flowmeters, the most commonly used flowmeters in respiratory care, provide accurate estimates of flow, regardless of the downstream pressure. Bourdon flowmeters and adjustable, multiple-orifice flow resistors are actually reducing valves that control the pressure gradient across an outlet with a fixed orifice.
- Oxygen therapy systems generally are classified as *low-flow (variable performance)* and *high-flow (fixed performance)* devices.
- Low-flow devices are also called *variable-performance devices* because they supply oxygen at flow rates that are lower than a patient's inspiratory demands.
- High-flow (fixed-performance) devices provide oxygen at flow rates high enough to satisfy the patient's inspiratory demands.
- Examples of low-flow devices include nasal cannulas, simple oxygen masks, and partial rebreathing masks. The most common example of a high-flow device is the air entrainment mask.

- Hyperbaric oxygen therapy exposes patients to a pressure greater than atmospheric pressure while they breathe 100% oxygen either continuously or intermittently.
- Hyperbaric oxygen therapy is indicated for air embolism, carbon monoxide poisoning, and decompression sickness and as an adjunct to the treatment of gas gangrene, refractory osteomyelitis, and wound healing.
- NO delivery systems are designed for use with most conventional critical care ventilators and can be adapted for use with both adult and pediatric ventilators.
- NO therapy has been shown to be effective in the treatment of persistent pulmonary hypertension of the newborn and as an adjunct to the treatment of congenital cardiac defects.
- Heliox has been successfully used in the management of airflow obstructive diseases. It has been used successfully to improve oxygen delivery and as an adjunct to aerosol therapy in spontaneously breathing patients with acute asthmatic exacerbations and refractory croup.
- Helium–oxygen mixtures have been used to administer anesthetic gases to patients with small-diameter endotracheal tubes and to provide ventilatory support for patients with severe lower airway obstruction.

ASSESSMENT QUESTIONS

See Appendix B for the answers.

1. Describe an easy method of determining the number of stages in a multistage regulator.
2. Which of the following devices is/are considered fixed-performance oxygen delivery system(s)?
   1. Simple oxygen mask
   2. Nasal catheter
   3. Air entrainment mask
   4. Partial rebreathing mask
      a. 1 and 2 only
      b. 1, 2, and 3 only
      c. 3 only
      d. 1, 2, 3, and 4
3. Which of the following statements is true regarding back pressure–compensated flowmeters?

   a. The needle valve is positioned before the indicator tube.
   b. High-resistance devices attached to these flowmeters cause erroneously high flow readings.
   c. Faulty valve seats do not affect flow readings.
   d. Gas flow from these flowmeters stops if resistance creates a back pressure that exceeds the source gas pressure.
4. Which of the following are advantages of using transtracheal oxygen (TTO) therapy catheters?
   1. They do not require periodic replacement.
   2. The incidence of infection is considerably lower than with other low-flow oxygen devices.
   3. They require lower oxygen flows to achieve a given F_IO_2 than do standard nasal cannulas.

4. They are less obtrusive (i.e., more cosmetically pleasing) than nasal cannulas.
   a. 1 and 3 only
   b. 2 and 3 only
   c. 3 and 4 only
   d. 2, 3, and 4 only

5. What is the air-to-oxygen entrainment ratio for delivering 40% oxygen through an air entrainment mask?
   a. 2:1
   b. 1:2
   c. 1:3
   d. 3:1

6. Studies have shown that mustache and pendant cannulas can reduce the cost of oxygen therapy by as much as:
   a. 10%
   b. 30%
   c. 50%
   d. 80%

7. What is the approximate partial pressure of inspired oxygen of room air if the barometric pressure is raised to 2 atm?
   a. 150 mm Hg
   b. 300 mm Hg
   c. 200 mm Hg
   d. 1520 mm Hg

8. Hyperbaric oxygen therapy is indicated for:
   1. Air embolism
   2. Hypercapnia (>60 mm Hg)
   3. Carbon monoxide poisoning
   4. Sinusitis
      a. 1 and 3 only
      b. 2 and 4 only
      c. 1, 2, and 3 only
      d. 2, 3, and 4 only

9. Administration of heliox can be an effective form of therapy in which of the following situations?
   1. Managing postextubation stridor in pediatric trauma patients
   2. Providing ventilatory support for patients with severe airway obstruction resulting from chronic bronchitis and emphysema
   3. Administering anesthetic gases to patients with small-diameter endotracheal tubes
   4. Delivering oxygen therapy to asthmatic children
      a. 1 and 2 only
      b. 1 and 3 only
      c. 1, 2, and 3 only
      d. 1, 2, 3, and 4

10. You are asked to administer a helium–oxygen mixture to an asthmatic patient who is admitted to the emergency department with acute respiratory distress. Which of the following devices is the most appropriate method of delivering this form of medical gas therapy?
    a. Air entrainment mask
    b. Partial rebreathing mask
    c. Nasal cannula
    d. Nonrebreathing mask

11. Which of the following is an indication for NO therapy?
    1. It has been used successfully to treat persistent pulmonary hypertension of the newborn.
    2. It can be used as an adjunct to the treatment of congenital cardiac defects.
    3. It can be used to reverse vasoconstriction associated with systemic hypertension.
    4. It can be used to treat refractory croup.
       a. 1 and 3 only
       b. 2 and 4 only
       c. 1 and 2 only
       d. 1, 2, 3, and 4

12. The gas flow delivered to a patient receiving a 70%-to-30% (helium-to-oxygen) mixture is indicated on the standard oxygen flowmeter as 10 L/min. What is the actual gas flow delivered to the patient?
    a. 5.6 L/min
    b. 6.25 L/min
    c. 16 L/min
    d. 18 L/min

13. When carbogen is administered, which of the following vital signs should be monitored?
    1. Pulse
    2. Blood pressure
    3. Respirations
    4. Mental status
       a. 1 and 2 only
       b. 1 and 3 only
       c. 1, 3, and 4 only
       d. 1, 2, 3, and 4

14. Which of the following statements are true regarding NO therapy?
    1. NO is a potent vasoconstrictor.
    2. NO is supplied in compressed-gas cylinders constructed of steel.
    3. Nitrogen dioxide and NO are toxic if inhaled.
    4. The therapeutic dose of NO is 5 to 80 parts per million (ppm).
       a. 1 and 2 only
       b. 2 and 3 only
       c. 3 and 4 only
       d. 1, 3, and 4 only

15. Which of the following would be considered clinical manifestations of carbon dioxide toxicity?
    1. Hypertension
    2. Bounding pulse
    3. P_aCO_2 >70 mm Hg
    4. Multiple premature ventricular contractions
       a. 1 and 2 only
       b. 2 and 3 only
       c. 1, 2, and 3 only
       d. 1, 2, 3, and 4

REFERENCES

1. Heffner JE: The story of oxygen. *Respir Care* 58(1):18, 2013.
2. Petty TL: Historical highlights of long-term oxygen therapy. *Respir Care* 45:29, 2000.
3. American Association for Respiratory Care: Clinical practice guideline: oxygen therapy in the home or alternative site health care facility—2007 revision and update. *Respir Care* 52:1063, 2007.
4. American Association for Respiratory Care: Clinical practice guideline: oxygen therapy for adults in the acute care facility—2002 revision and update. *Respir Care* 47:717, 2002.
5. American Association for Respiratory Care: Clinical practice guideline: selection of an oxygen delivery device for neonatal and pediatric patients—2002 revision and update. *Respir Care* 47:707, 2002.
6. Vain NE, Prudent LM, Stevens DP, et al.: Regulation of oxygen concentrations delivered to infants by nasal cannulas. *Am J Dis Child* 143:1458, 1989.
7. Heimlich HJ: Respiratory rehabilitation with a transtracheal oxygen system. *Ann Otol Rhinol Laryngol* 91:643, 1982.
8. Saponsnick AB, Hess D: Oxygen therapy: administration and management. In Hess D, MacIntyre N, Adams A, et al., editors: *Respiratory care: principles and practice*, Philadelphia, 2002, WB Saunders.
9. Shigeoka JW, Bonnekat HW: The current status of oxygen-conserving devices. *Respir Care* 30:833, 1985.
10. Boothby VM, Lovelace WR, Bulbulian AH: I. Oxygen administration: the value of high concentration of oxygen for therapy. II. Oxygen for therapy and aviation: an apparatus for the administration of oxygen or oxygen and helium by inhalation. III. Design and construction of the masks for oxygen inhalation apparatus. *Mayo Clin Proc* 13:641-656, 1938.
11. Johnson JT, Dauber JH, Hoffman LA, et al.: Transtracheal delivery of oxygen: efficacy and safety for long-term continuous therapy. *Ann Otol Rhinol Laryngol* 100:108, 1991.
12. Tieb BL, Lewis MI: Oxygen conservation and oxygen conserving devices. *Chest* 92:263, 1987.
13. Kacmarek RM: Methods of oxygen delivery in the hospital. *Probl Respir Care* 3:563, 1990.
14. Barach AL, Eckman BS: A physiologically controlled oxygen mask apparatus. *Anesthesiology* 2:421, 1941.
15. Barach AL: Symposium: inhalation therapy historical background. *Anesthesiology* 23:407, 1962.
16. Campbell EJM: A method of controlling oxygen administration which reduces the risk of carbon dioxide retention. *Lancet* 2:12, 1960.
17. Scacci R: Air entrainment masks: jet mixing is how they work; the Bernoulli and Venturi principles are how they don't. *Respir Care* 24:928, 1979.
18. Cohen JL, Demers RR, Sakland M: Air entrainment masks: a performance evaluation. *Respir Care* 22:279, 1977.
19. McPherson S: *Respiratory care equipment*, ed 5, St. Louis, 1995, Elsevier-Mosby.
20. Wilkins RL, Stoller JK, Scanlan CL: *Egan's fundamentals of respiratory care*, ed 8, St. Louis, 2003, Elsevier-Mosby.
21. Cox D, Gilbe C: Fixed performance oxygen masks. *Anesthesiology* 36:958, 1981.
22. Campbell EJM, Minty KB: Controlled oxygen at 60% concentration. *Lancet* 2:1199, 1976.
23. Fourst GN, Potter MA, Wilons MD, et al.: Shortcomings of using two jet nebulizers in tandem with an aerosol face mask. *Chest* 99:1346, 1991.
24. Kuo CD, Lin SE, Wang JH: Aerosol, humidity, and oxygen levels. *Chest* 99:1325, 1991.
25. Spoletini G, Alotaibi M, Blasi F, et al.: Heated humidified high-flow nasal oxygen in adults: mechanisms of action and clinical implications. *Chest* 148(1):253-261, 2015.
26. Jones PG, Kamona S, Doran O, et al.: Randomized controlled trial of humidified high-flow nasal oxygen for acute respiratory distress in the emergency department: The HOT-ER Study. *Respir Care* 61(3):291-299, 2016.
27. Ward JJ: High-flow oxygen administration by nasal cannula for adult and perinatal patients. *Respir Care* 58(1):98-122, 2013.
28. Mishoe SC, Brooks CW, Dennison FH, et al.: Octave waveband analysis to determine sound frequencies and intensities produced by nebulizers and humidifier used with hoods. *Respir Care* 40:1120, 1995.
29. Harch PG, McCullough V: *The oxygen revolution*, New York, 2007, Hatherleigh.
30. Kindall EP: Clinical hyperbaric oxygen therapy. In Bennett P, Elliott D, editors: *The physiology and medicine of diving*, ed 4, Philadelphia, 1993, WB Saunders.
31. Tibbles PM, Eldelsberg JS: Hyperbaric-oxygen therapy. *N Engl J Med* 334:1642-1647, 1996.
32. Gallagher TJ, Smith RA, Bell GC: Evaluation of mechanical ventilators in a hyperbaric environment. *Aviat Space Environ Med* 49:375, 1978.
33. Lustbader D, Fein A: Other modalities of oxygen therapy: hyperbaric oxygen, nitric oxide, and ECMO. *Respir Care Clin N Am* 6:659, 2000.
34. Moon RE: Hyperbaric oxygen treatment for air or gas embolism. *Undersea Hyperb Med* 41:159-166, 2014.
35. Myers RAM, Snyder SK, Lindberg S, et al.: Value of hyperbaric oxygen in suspected carbon monoxide poisoning. *JAMA* 246:2478, 1981.
36. DiBlasi RM, Myers TR, Hess DR: Evidence-based clinical practice guideline: inhaled nitric oxide for neonates with acute hypoxic respiratory failure. *Respir Care* 55(12):1717-1745, 2010.
37. Sosenko IR, Bancalari E: NO for preterm infants at risk for bronchopulmonary dysplasia. *Lancet* 376: 308-310, 2010.
38. Bone RC: A new therapy for the adult respiratory distress syndrome. *N Engl J Med* 328:431, 1993.
39. Bigatello LM, Hurford WE, Kacmarek RM, et al.: Prolonged inhalation of low concentrations of nitric oxide in patients with severe adult respiratory distress syndrome: effects on pulmonary hemodynamics and oxygenation. *Anesthesiology* 80:761, 1994.
40. Brown RH, Zerhouni EA, Hirshman C: Reversal of bronchoconstriction by inhaled nitric oxide: histamine versus methacholine. *Am J Respir Crit Care Med* 150:233, 1994.
41. *INOmax DS_{IR} Plus Operation Manual*, Hampton, NJ, 2014, INO Therapeutics LLC.
42. Hess DH, Bigatello LM, Hurford WE: Toxicity and complications of inhaled nitric oxide. *Respir Care Clin N Am* 3:487, 1997.
43. Barach AL: The therapeutic use of helium. *JAMA* 107:1273, 1935.
44. Hess SE, Fink JB, Venkastaraman ST, et al.: The history and physics of heliox. *Respir Care* 51:608, 2006.

45. Kim K, Saville AL, Sikes KL, et al.: Heliox-driven albuterol nebulization for asthma exacerbations: an overview. *Respir Care* 51:613, 2006.

46. Stillwell PC, Quick JD, Munro PR, et al.: Effectiveness of open-circuit and Oxy-Hood delivery of helium–oxygen. *Chest* 95:1222, 1989.

47. Skrinskas GJ, Hyland RH, Hutcheon MA: Using helium–oxygen mixtures in the management of acute upper airway obstruction. *Can Med Assoc J* 128:555, 1983.

48. Kemper KJ, Ritz RH, Benson MS, et al.: Helium–oxygen mixtures in the treatment of postextubation stridor in pediatric patients. *Crit Care Med* 19:356, 1991.

49. Nelson DS, McClellan L: Helium–oxygen mixtures as adjunctive support for refractory viral croup. *Ohio State Med J* 78:729, 1982.

50. Myers TR: Use of heliox in children. *Respir Care* 51:619, 2006.

51. Emergency Care Research Institute: Cylinders with unmixed helium–oxygen. *Health Devices* 19:146, 1990.

SECTION III

Airway Management

Airway Management Devices and Advanced Cardiac Life Support

Amanda M. Kleiman, Ashley Matthews Shilling

OBJECTIVES

Upon completion of this chapter, you will be able to:

1. Recognize normal airway anatomy.
2. Describe a complete airway examination.
3. Describe ways to displace the tongue to improve gas exchange in unconscious patients
4. List patient characteristics that may contribute to difficult mask ventilation or intubation.
5. List several complications associated with improper placement of oral and nasopharyngeal airways
6. Identify various types of manual resuscitators and discuss the common hazards associated with use of these devices.
7. Explain how to place the laryngeal mask airway and the Combitube in an unconscious patient.
8. Describe the appropriate sequence of steps for inserting an endotracheal tube using laryngoscopy to provide a secure airway.
9. Identify at least three ways to confirm proper placement of an endotracheal tube.
10. Name three airway devices that can facilitate the placement of an endotracheal tube in the event of difficult laryngoscopy.
11. Understand the use of ultrasonography in point-of-care airway management.
12. Discuss the most common problems facing intubated patients and identify strategies to avoid any equipment used to treat these complications.
13. Identify the equipment necessary to perform invasive ventilation (transtracheal or surgical airway) and describe a procedure for airway entry.
14. Understand changes in basic advanced cardiac life support regarding the prioritization of airway management and chest compressions.

OUTLINE

The loss of the ability to breathe spontaneously can be one of the more dramatic emergencies seen in the medical field and can be associated with significant morbidity and mortality. Loss of spontaneous ventilation can be caused by upper airway obstruction, as with foreign body aspiration; lower airway obstruction, as with severe bronchospasm or a tension pneumothorax; or altered respiratory drive, as with depressant drugs or secondary to a neurological insult. Failure to restore adequate respiratory gas exchange can result in hypoxic brain injury or death within 3 minutes. In these scenarios, sustaining life depends on the important task of airway management and restoring the ability to oxygenate and ventilate patients who are unable to do so themselves. Because of the importance of effective and rapid airway management, significant resources, including websites, task forces, and teaching seminars that focus solely on airway management, have been developed and are easily accessible and available to clinicians.

This chapter reviews normal airway anatomy, techniques used to establish and maintain a patent upper airway and respiratory gas exchange, and primary and ancillary devices used for controlled or supported ventilation. The discussion includes minimally invasive techniques, such as bag-mask-valve ventilation (or face mask ventilation [FMV]) and supraglottic airway devices, as well as infraglottic devices such as the endotracheal tube (ETT) and tracheostomy tube (TT). Table 5.1 briefly describes some of these devices and techniques and separates them into supraglottic and infraglottic airways. Additional equipment used for patients with artificial airways, and some of the risks and problems encountered in their use, are also described in this chapter. Further, the chapter reviews changes to current advanced cardiac life support (ACLS) algorithms, techniques, and the use of airway management in the acutely unstable patient.

With improvements in knowledge as well as technology, many airway devices and tools for airway management have been developed over the years as alternatives or adjuncts to direct laryngoscopy. Although scientific evidence substantiates the use and safety of many of these devices, others are novel and have yet to prove their practicality. With the ever-evolving alternatives to laryngoscopy and the traditional ETT, we have improved our ability to manage the difficult airway on multiple levels and in many different settings (including prehospital environments), thereby reducing the need for emergency surgical airway intervention. Because it would be impractical to cover all the new and changing artificial airways and their adjuncts, this chapter focuses on selected equipment that is commonly used and that can serve as models for other equipment.

I. AIRWAY ANATOMY

To understand airway management, one must have an appreciation of normal airway anatomy. Fig. 5.1 shows the normal upper airway and tracheal anatomy in an adult. The airway has two natural access routes—the nasopharynx and the oropharynx—both of which lead to the pharynx, the larynx, and ultimately the trachea. The larynx consists of three large cartilaginous structures: the thyroid and cricoid cartilages and the epiglottis. Although it is essential to identify the true vocal cords and the glottic opening, one also should understand the spatial relationships of the surrounding structures, including the vestibular folds (the false cords), the arytenoid cartilages, and the vallecula, as well as the relationship of the epiglottis to these structures.

The glottic opening, formed by the thyroarytenoid ligaments, or vocal cords, is the narrowest portion of the adult airway and usually the limiting factor determining the size of the tube that can safely be placed into the trachea. The cricoid cartilage, which is the only complete tracheal ring, is usually found at the sixth cervical vertebra level (C6) in the adult and at the C4 level in the infant and young child. Unlike in the adult, the cricoid cartilage is the narrowest portion in the pediatric airway until approximately age 6. This is an important distinction and is the reason that adults are typically intubated with a cuffed ETT, whereas infants and young children may be intubated with an uncuffed ETT without a significant leak. Additionally, the cricoid cartilage is an important landmark for cricothyroidotomy (discussed later in the chapter). In the adult the trachea divides at the carina into the mainstem bronchi, typically at the level of the fifth thoracic vertebral body (T5).

TABLE 5.1   Devices and Techniques Used to Establish and Maintain a Patent Upper Airway and Respiratory Gas Exchange

Device or Maneuver	Description	Concerns and Contraindications
Supraglottic Airway Maneuver or Device		
Extreme extension (sniffing position)	Extension of the occiput with the head extended	Unstable cervical spine
Jaw thrust or chin lift	Anterior displacement of the mandible with or without dislocation of the temporomandibular joints	Temporomandibular joint disease, fractured mandible, or unstable cervical spine
Anesthesia face mask	Assisted or controlled ventilation using a rubber or plastic mask contoured to fit the patient's face	Trauma to the face, presence of a beard, or abnormal anatomy, with resultant poor mask fit
Oropharyngeal airways	Rigid, curved device with an air passage that is placed through the mouth with the end resting distal to the tongue above the glottic opening	Gagging or vomiting, improper size, incorrect placement
Nasopharyngeal airways	Soft or semirigid hollow tube placed through the nares, the tip lying distal to the tongue above the glottic opening	Gagging or vomiting (usually better tolerated in patients who are not comatose); posterior pharyngeal wall dissection; severe bleeding
Laryngeal mask airways	Custom-formed, soft mask with a hollow tube fitting into the pyriform sinuses directly above the larynx	Placement may be difficult, mask may fold, epiglottis may obstruct laryngeal opening, trachea is not protected from aspiration, positive-pressure ventilation is more difficult to generate
Combitube	Double-lumen device inserted blindly, with one lumen providing ventilation and the other commonly in the esophagus	Not considered a secure airway device; should not be used in patients with intact gag reflex or esophageal disease; may cause injury to the esophagus, trachea, or surrounding soft tissue
Infraglottic Airway Device		
Endotracheal tubes (ETTs)	Semirigid hollow tube placed into the trachea with or without an inflatable cuff	Usually requires special devices (e.g., laryngoscopy) and technical skill for consistent correct placement; tracheal placement must be objectively confirmed and esophageal placement and ETT displacement avoided
Intubating laryngeal mask airways (LMAs)	Laryngeal mask airway designed to align the glottis with the LMA and allow blind endotracheal intubation through the hollow channel of the LMA	Requires training and practice; placement may be difficult
Lightwand	Rigid, light stylet that relies on transillumination of the trachea to confirm ETT placement	Ambient lights must be turned off during placement; difficult to use in patients with thick, short neck; blunt trauma
Indirect laryngoscope	Uses mirrors, lenses, or fiberoptic technology to view the glottis and allow insertion of the ETT under direct visualization	Often expensive and more cumbersome
Flexible fiberoptic bronchoscopy	Flexible fiberoptic bronchoscope that allows visualization of the airway with minimal neck extension; procedure can be done with the patient awake or asleep; also can be done with an oral or nasal intubation; considered the gold standard for an unstable cervical spine	Expensive and requires practice to master technique; fragile equipment that is prone to damage; blood and secretions can easily obscure view
Transtracheal invasive airway	Emergent, direct entry into the trachea below the larynx with a large-bore needle, or surgical incision with insertion of an ETT	Hypoxia, bleeding, nerve or esophageal injury; failure to establish an airway; gas dissection or pneumothorax
Tracheostomy tubes	Hollow tube, with or without a cuff, that is electively inserted directly into the trachea through a surgical incision or with a wire-guided progressive dilation technique	Hypoxia, bleeding, nerve or esophageal injury; failure to establish the airway as a result of nontracheal placement; displacement

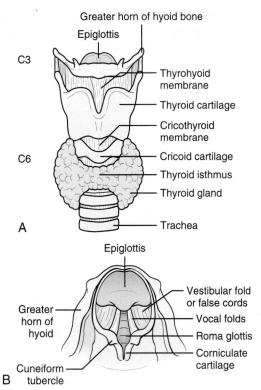

FIGURE 5.1 A, Anterior view of the adult larynx. B, View from above the vocal cords as would be seen during laryngoscopy.

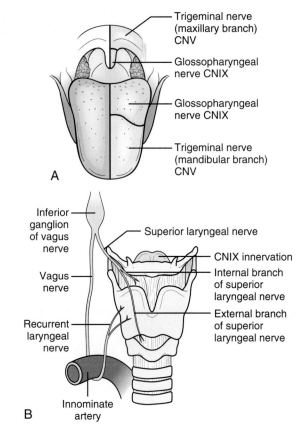

FIGURE 5.2 Sensory innervation of the airway and trachea. *CNV*, Cranial nerve V; *CNIX*, cranial nerve IX.

Fig. 5.2 shows the sensory innervation of the oropharynx and the trachea. The anterior part of the tongue is innervated by the fifth cranial nerve (CN V), the trigeminal nerve. The posterior third of the tongue, extending to the superior surface of the epiglottis, is supplied by the ninth cranial nerve (CN IX), the glossopharyngeal nerve. Understanding this innervation pattern is important because it is responsible for an active gag reflex. The inferior surfaces of the epiglottis and the vocal cords are innervated by a branch of the vagus nerve (CN X), the internal branch of the *superior laryngeal nerve*. The region of the trachea below the vocal cords is supplied by another branch of the vagus nerve, the *recurrent laryngeal nerve*. All the muscles of the larynx are innervated by the recurrent laryngeal nerve except for the cricothyroid muscles, which are controlled by the external branch of the superior laryngeal nerves. Understanding the innervation of the airway is crucial when performing an awake intubation because it allows the practitioner to block the sensory nerves. During an awake intubation, thorough anesthesia of the airway is needed to prevent coughing and gagging, provide patient comfort, decrease risk for aspiration, and allow for successful intubation.

II. AIRWAY EXAMINATION

The risks of airway management in the critically ill are greater than for patients undergoing elective procedures.[1] A number of different predictors of difficult laryngoscopy have been

developed; however, no specific test is useful in predicting difficulty in laryngoscopy in all patients. The incidences of both difficult airway management and inadvertent esophageal intubation are significantly higher in emergent scenarios than with airway management in the controlled environment of the operating room.[2] During elective surgery the incidence of failed intubation is quite low (0.05% to 0.35%), and the incidence of failed intubation and inability to provide mask ventilation is even lower (0.01% to 0.03%).[3-7] Because difficulties with airway management occur even under ideal conditions, reliable methods of predicting these problems are critical to decreasing associated morbidity. Specialized equipment and advance planning can improve success and prevent a catastrophe with an unanticipated difficult airway.

It is imperative to obtain any available airway history from the patient or review past medical records before attempting to establish an artificial airway. Important points that may predict a more difficult airway include (1) a known history of difficult intubation; (2) the presence of obstructive sleep apnea (OSA); (3) temporomandibular joint disease; (4) previous airway surgery or radiation to the airway; (5) anatomical abnormalities of the head, neck, or airway, including significant micrognathia; (6) a small mouth opening—patients may have been told this by their dentist; or (7) significant overbite of the teeth. Although a complete airway examination might be impossible in an emergency or on a comatose or uncooperative patient, a cursory examination of the airway for various

TABLE 5.2 Suggested Components of the Preoperative Airway Physical Examination

Airway Examination Component	Concerning Findings
1. Length of upper incisors	Relatively long
2. Relation of maxillary and mandibular incisors during normal jaw closure	Prominent "overbite" (maxillary incisors extend anterior to mandibular incisors)
3. Relation of maxillary and mandibular incisors during voluntary protrusion	Mandibular incisors unable to be placed anterior to (mandible in front of) maxillary incisors
4. Interincisor distance	Less than 3 cm with maximum voluntary mouth opening
5. Visibility of uvula	Not visible when tongue is protruded with patient in sitting position (e.g., Mallampati class higher than II)
6. Shape of palate	Highly arched or very narrow
7. Compliance of mandibular space	Stiff, indurated, occupied by mass, or nonresilient
8. Thyromental distance	Less than three ordinary finger breadths
9. Neck length	Short
10. Neck bulk	Thick
11. Range of motion of head and neck	Patient cannot touch tip of chin to chest or cannot extend head on neck

TABLE 5.3 Mallampati Classification With Samsoon and Young Modifications to Airway Classes

Class	View With Patient Sitting, Without Phonation
I	Faucial pillars, soft palate, and uvula visible
II	Uvula masked by base of tongue
III	Only base of uvula and soft palate visible
IV	No visualization of uvula or soft palate; only hard palate visible

Data from Mallampati SR, Gatt SP, Gugino LD, et al.: A clinical sign to predict difficult tracheal intubation: a prospective study. *Can Anaesth Soc J* 32:429, 1985; and Samsoon GL, Young JR: Difficult tracheal intubation: a retrospective study. *Anaesthesia* 42:487, 1987.

At times, intubation may be difficult or impossible, and predicting the patients at high risk can help the practitioner assemble back-up devices and prepare to use advanced techniques. Predictors of difficult intubation include (1) a Mallampati airway class III or IV, (2) a thyromental distance of less than 6 cm, (3) mouth opening of less than 4 cm, (4) reduced atlanto-occipital neck extension, (5) increased body mass index (BMI), and (6) a large neck circumference.[10-12]

In addition to other airway parameters noted earlier, ultrasonography of airway structures may be useful in assessing different components of the airway before induction of anesthesia if difficulty in direct laryngoscopy is suspected. Point-of-care ultrasonography of the airway could provide a real-time, noninvasive assessment of airway structures to more adequately predict potential difficulty. Specifics of airway ultrasonography are found later.

When difficult intubation is anticipated, additional personnel should be available, supplies gathered, and plans for either advanced airway techniques and/or surgical airway should be established beforehand. The American Society of Anesthesiologists (ASA) has proposed a difficult airway algorithm (Fig. 5.3) to help direct airway management and improve patient outcome in the event of a difficult airway.[8] If difficult mask ventilation or intubation is encountered, it is essential to document the reason to provide valuable information for future caregivers. For example, a patient who has a bloodied airway secondary to trauma may not present with the same challenges during a future intubation, whereas a patient with a small mouth opening and anterior larynx is unlikely to show improvements in the ease of future intubations. *It is essential to document the characteristics that make an airway challenging, as well as the technique that was ultimately responsible for securing the airway.* This is critical to avoiding similar issues in future intubation attempts and to ensure that a patient is not extubated without appropriate resources and personnel available should extubation fail. Making patients aware that they experienced a difficult intubation is essential, and patients should be told to inform future caregivers of their history of a difficult airway, just as they would tell a physician of a known drug allergy. Ideally, the patient should be given a letter describing the reasons for the difficulty and the means in which the

characteristics and gross abnormalities can be beneficial in many instances. Table 5.2 lists important points of the airway examination and findings that are cause for concern.[8]

Patient mouth opening, a dental examination, cervical range of motion, and the thyromental distance are all common components of the airway examination. Several classification systems have been developed to help predict the ease or difficulty of providing face mask ventilation (FMV) or intubating patients. One of the most commonly used systems was described by Mallampati et al.[9] and later modified by Samsoon and Young.[4] This system (Table 5.3) attempts to predict the difficulty of visualizing the glottic structures during laryngoscopy. The examination should be performed with the patient sitting upright, and the individual should not be asked to phonate because this may elevate the palate and improve the view while the airway is examined. Despite the use of this classification system and other components of the airway examination, a difficult intubation is often unanticipated even by experienced providers. A number of prospective and retrospective studies have attempted to correlate the airway examination and patient characteristics with the ease of FMV and intubation.

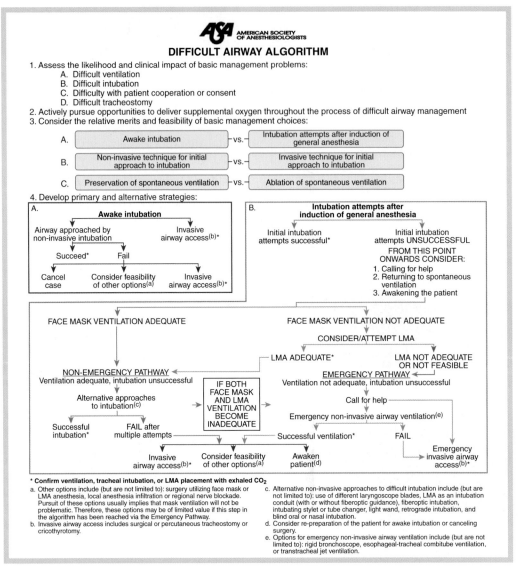

FIGURE 5.3 Difficult airway algorithm established by the American Society of Anesthesiologists. *LMA,* Laryngeal mask airway. (From the American Society of Anesthesiologists Task Force: Practice guidelines for management of the difficult airway. *Anesthesiology* 98:1269, 2003.)

airway was finally established. In addition, wearing a medical alert bracelet may be advisable, especially in a patient with a significantly high likelihood of needing invasive airway management in the future.

III. ESTABLISHING A PATENT AIRWAY AND MASK VENTILATION

Displacing the Tongue

Often, simple maneuvers can restore breathing in patients with upper airway obstruction. When in the supine position, if the pharyngeal and tongue muscles lose tone, the tongue falls backward and may occlude the pharynx. Elevating the head and extending the neck advance the jaw and move the tongue forward, helping to open an obstructed or closed airway. This so-called sniffing position (Fig. 5.4) opens the upper airway and places the long axes of the mouth, pharynx,

and larynx in alignment. This head position also provides for a tighter fit for a bag-mask-valve manual resuscitator and is also optimal for endotracheal intubation under direct vision. Forcing the jaw anteriorly with a jaw thrust or a chin lift maneuver moves the tongue farther from the hard and soft palates, and a patent upper airway that allows air exchange may be achieved. Figs. 5.5 and 5.6 demonstrate these techniques.

Mask Ventilation

The anesthesia face mask is a noninvasive means of ventilating and oxygenating an apneic patient. Traditionally made of black rubber, most modern masks are latex-free, disposable, and usually made of silicone or plastic. Clear face masks have the advantage of allowing visualization of the patient's face for condensation (indicating successful FMV) or cyanosis, as well as the presence of vomit or blood in the mask. In addition,

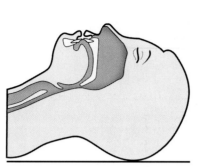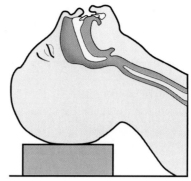

FIGURE 5.4 Sniffing position, the optimum position for opening the upper airway, can be achieved by supporting the occiput on a solid surface and extending the head. This is also the optimum position for oral intubation with a curved laryngoscope blade.

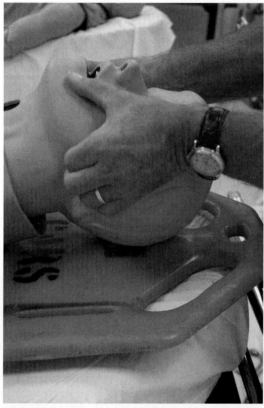

FIGURE 5.5 The index fingers of both hands are used to perform a jaw thrust maneuver, which displaces the temporo-mandibular joints anteriorly, achieving a patent airway without neck extension. This is particularly useful for patients with cervical spine injuries.

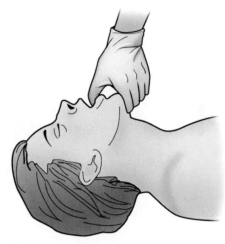

FIGURE 5.6 The chin lift is another maneuver for opening the upper airway by moving the tongue anteriorly, and it can be performed successfully without extending the cervical spine.

awake and responsive patients find the clear plastic less claustrophobic than the opaque rubber. Most face masks have an inflatable cushion to optimize the mask seal, which allows a better fit to the patient's unique facial configuration and contour (Fig. 5.7). Most adult masks come with a device for attaching a mask strap to improve the success of mask ventilation, reduce air leakage around the mask, and also reduce the work of providing FMV. Additionally, masks typically have a standard 15-mm attachment for the ventilator tubing or a manual resuscitator. Most mask manufacturers provide six to eight numbered sizes to fit patients ranging from the neonate to the adult. Sizes 3, 4, and 5 typically are used for adults.

To provide FMV, the E and C configuration is used; the fingers of the left hand rest on and elevate the mandible to prevent bruising of the soft tissue and obstruction of the oropharynx with submandibular soft-tissue pressure (Fig. 5.8). The mask should fit over the bridge of the nose and form a tight seal. The mask should not be pushed onto the face as this may obstruct the airway; rather, the patient's mandible should be pulled up into the mask. Two-handed bag-mask-valve techniques may be needed for obese or bearded patients or patients with a difficult mask fit.

Ventilatory pressures less than 20 cm H_2O should be used to prevent the forcing of gas into the patient's stomach. Jaw thrust, maximized sniffing positioning, two-handed mask technique, and oral or nasal airways, as discussed later, help facilitate successful FMV at lower ventilatory pressures. Signs of effective mask ventilation include the presence of carbon dioxide (CO_2) on capnography, condensation in the mask, a taut and refilling (non–self-inflating or anesthesia) bag, adequate bilateral breath sounds, and symmetrical chest rise.

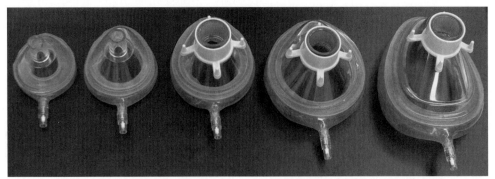

FIGURE 5.7 The anesthesia face mask is made of plastic and contains an inflatable rim to form a tight seal with the face.

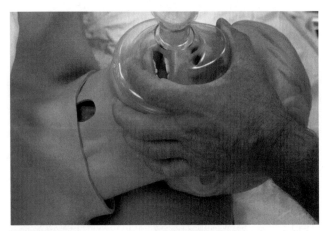

FIGURE 5.8 Note the **E** and **C** formation of the hand during mask ventilation.

The skills needed to provide adequate ventilation by a bag-mask-valve device are of paramount importance and must be acquired by all who want to manage an airway successfully. Practitioners must always remember that even if a patient cannot be intubated, providing FMV allows for adequate oxygenation and CO_2 removal. Simple, effective mask ventilation can be sufficient until a definitive airway can be established.

Although manual resuscitation ventilation with a bag-mask-valve device is one of the mainstays of airway management, it is not without complications. Common problems include injury to the surrounding soft tissues and nerves, such as the mandibular branch of the facial nerve and the mental nerves. Attention must be taken to avoid placing pressure on the eyes because corneal abrasions or other eye injury may occur. Using the minimal ventilatory pressures needed to adequately ventilate the patient helps to avoid insufflation of the stomach leading to gastric distention and regurgitation. An inability to ventilate the patient adequately is the most serious complication associated with mask ventilation, and unfortunately inadequate ventilation may go unrecognized by the provider.

Difficulty in providing mask ventilation is indicated by a poor mask seal despite proper technique, excessive gas leakage, and difficulty initiating ingress or failure of egress of respiratory gases. The incidence of difficult mask ventilation ranges from 1% to 5%, with impossible mask ventilation ranging from 0.1% to 0.2%.[12,13] Patient characteristics shown to reduce the success of mask ventilation include obesity (BMI greater than 30), Mallampati airway class III or IV, age greater than 55 years, poor mandible protrusion, lack of teeth, and history of snoring.[12,13] Presence of a beard is the only acutely modifiable risk factor. Troubleshooting for failed manual ventilation in a patient with a beard includes placing an occlusive adhesive dressing over the beard to improve the mask seal or using a water-soluble lubricant on the beard to smooth down the facial hair and form a better seal. In addition, the mask may be removed and the patient can be ventilated by placing the end of the airway circuitry in the patient's mouth and occluding the patient's nose. In extreme situations the beard can be shaved before induction, especially in those with a history of difficult mask ventilation or difficult airway. Additionally, patients with poor lung or chest wall compliance are more difficult to mask ventilate and may require higher pressures to achieve adequate ventilation.

IV. MANUAL RESUSCITATORS

Manual resuscitators (or resuscitator bags) are portable, hand-held devices that provide a means of delivering positive-pressure ventilation to a patient's airway. These devices incorporate a self-inflating bag, an air intake valve, a nonrebreathing valve mechanism, an oxygen inlet nipple, and an oxygen reservoir, which may be an attached tube or bag.[14,15] Manual resuscitators can deliver room air, oxygen, or air–oxygen mixtures via a mask or through an adapter that attaches directly to a patient's ETT.

As their name implies, manual resuscitators originally were designed to ventilate patients during cardiopulmonary resuscitation (CPR), but they have become an indispensable part of the management of mechanically ventilated patients. They can be used to hyperinflate patients with enriched oxygen mixtures before and after suctioning procedures, to generate airway pressures and large tidal volumes to expand atelectatic lung segments, and to ventilate bradypneic or apneic (ventilator-dependent) patients as they are transported from one area of the hospital to another. Resuscitators differ in the type of valve used (see the following subsections), the stroke and tidal volume potential, the amount of dead space, and the type of oxygen reservoir.

All types of manual resuscitators have various features that allow for adaptation to specific situations. These include syringe ports for administration of medication, metered-dose inhaler (MDI) connections, and specialized coverings to allow use in toxic environments. In addition, resuscitators allow for the addition of positive end-expiratory pressure (PEEP) valves, which have resistance characteristics that allow the addition of 1 to 20 mm Hg of PEEP.

Types of Manual Resuscitators (Bag-Valve Units)

Manual resuscitators can be classified by the type of nonrebreathing valve used.[16] Therefore two classes of resuscitators usually are described: those that use a spring-loaded mechanism and those that rely on pressure to affect diaphragm valves. Diaphragm valves can be subdivided into two types: a duckbill valve and a leaf valve.

Spring-Loaded Valves

Spring-loaded devices use a nonrebreathing valve that consists of a disk or ball supported or attached to a spring. When the operator compresses the self-inflating bag, the spring-loaded disk or ball is pushed against the exhalation port, occluding it, and gas is directed to the patient's airway. After the flow from the bag stops, the spring returns the disk or ball to the open position, and gas exhaled by the patient is vented to the atmosphere. Simultaneously, as gas enters the self-inflating bag through the one-way air inlet valve (which is attached to a reservoir), the bag inflates. The air inlet valve can be attached directly to the nonrebreathing valve or located separately at the bottom of the bag.

The most common examples of this type of manual resuscitator are the early Ambu (air-mask-bag unit) system, the Ohio Hope II bag, the Air Viva, and the Vital Signs Stat Blue Resuscitator. Early versions of the Ambu system used a spring-loaded, disk-type nonrebreathing valve that is no longer produced. The Hope II (Fig. 5.9) and the Vital Signs Stat Blue (Fig. 5.10) resuscitators both rely on the spring-disk–type

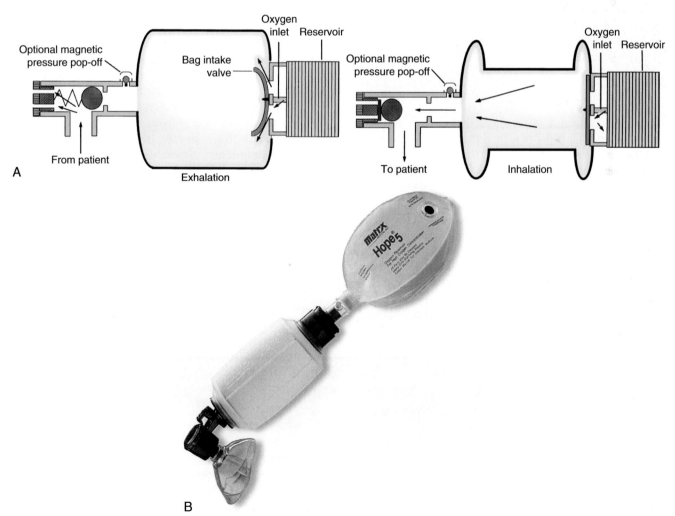

FIGURE 5.9 A, Valves for the Ohio Hope II resuscitator. B, The adult model of the Hope II with an oxygen reservoir. (B courtesy MDS Matrix, Orchard Park, NY.)

nonrebreathing valve. Notice that the reservoir of the Hope II resuscitator, which allows for oxygen accumulation and potential delivery of 100% oxygen, is located on the bottom of the self-inflating bag. This reservoir is designed so that the angle of the oxygen inlet valve allows oxygen flows in excess of 30 L/min to be used without interrupting normal function. The Vital Signs Stat Blue Resuscitator differs from the Ohio

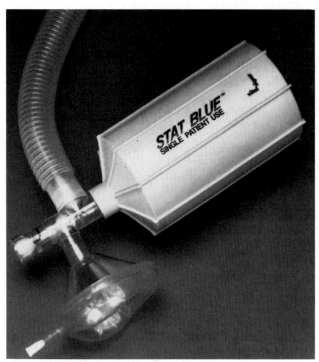

FIGURE 5.10 Vital Signs Stat Blue Resuscitator. (Courtesy Vital Signs, Totowa, NJ.)

Hope II bag because oxygen is drawn in through the neck, where a reservoir is attached.

Diaphragm Valves

Duckbill valves. A duckbill valve incorporates a diaphragm-type nonrebreathing valve in place of spring-loaded mechanisms. The Laerdal Silicone Resuscitator, the Laerdal adult resuscitator, the Laerdal infant and child resuscitators (Fig. 5.11), and the Hudson Lifesaver II resuscitator are examples of devices that use the duckbill-type diaphragm valve.

The operating principle of these devices is comparable with that of spring-loaded resuscitators. Compression of the bag pushes a diaphragm against the exhalation ports. At the same time, the duckbill valve opens, and gas flows to the patient. After the flow from the bag ceases, the duckbill valve closes, and the diaphragm is pushed away from the exhalation port. Exhaled gas exits through the exhalation ports. During reexpansion of the bag, the bag inlet valve allows air or oxygen from the reservoir to enter the self-inflating bag. Notice that the inlet valve is a simple one-way leaf valve that closes when the bag is compressed to prevent gas leakage. The one-way valve opens when the bag reexpands as a result of subatmospheric pressure inside the bag.

Leaf valves. Resuscitators that use a leaf valve operate similarly to duckbill resuscitators. As shown in Fig. 5.12, when the bag is compressed, a diaphragm swells and occludes the exhalation ports. The leaf valve in the middle of the diaphragm is pushed open, and gas is directed to the patient. During exhalation the bag reexpands, creating a negative pressure that causes the diaphragm to move away from the exhalation ports. The leaf then closes and prevents exhaled gas from leaking into the bag. The bag inlet valve is opened, and the bag reinflates. The Respironics disposable resuscitator, the Hudson

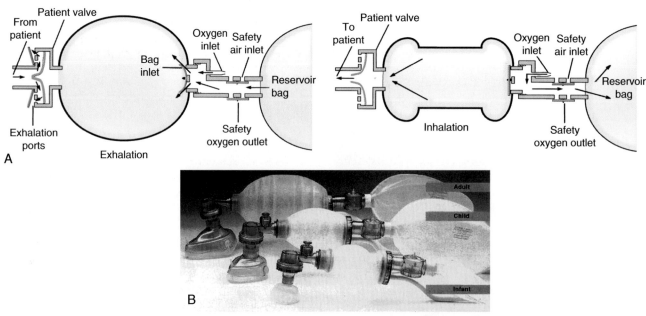

FIGURE 5.11 A, Valves for the adult and child with an oxygen reservoir system for adults. B, The Laerdal adult and infant resuscitators with oxygen reservoir systems. (B courtesy Laerdal Medical, Wappingers Falls, NY.)

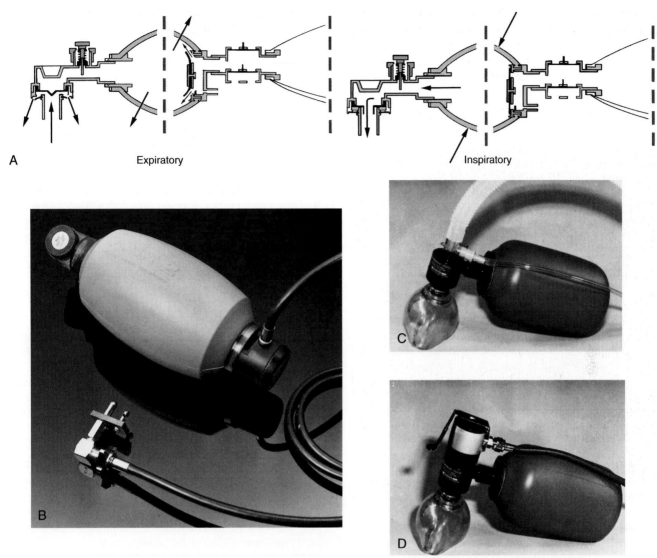

A   Expiratory   Inspiratory

FIGURE 5.12 A, Operation of the leaf diaphragm valve for a Hudson manual resuscitator (as well as for a Robertshaw bag resuscitator). B, Hudson RCI Lifesaver manual resuscitator with a manufacturer-supplied reservoir system attached. C, A modified reservoir system with 22-mm T-connection used for attaching the oxygen inlet at a right angle to the bag-inlet valve. D, Robertshaw demand valve attached to the bag inlet for providing 100% oxygen or other source gas to the bag. (A courtesy Hudson Oxygen Therapy Sales, Temecula, CA.)

Lifesaver, and Robertshaw resuscitators are examples of devices that use leaf valves.

Standards for Manual Resuscitators

Standards for the design, construction, and use of manual resuscitators are published by ASTM International (formerly the American Society for Testing and Materials) and the International Organization for Standardization (ISO).[17,18] The ECRI Institute (formerly the Emergency Cardiac Care Committee) and the American Heart Association (AHA) also provide standards for the use and evaluation of manual resuscitators, specifically relating to the level and timing of ventilation during CPR.[19] (Box 5.1 summarizes these standards.)

Table 5.4 compares the performance patterns required by the ASTM International, ISO, and AHA standards; however, delivery of a tidal volume of 800 mL (as specified by the AHA) may not be possible unless a patient is intubated. Fig. 5.13 shows the results of several studies in which investigators measured the average tidal volumes delivered by one-handed compression of the bag.[20-25] It has been suggested that the lower tidal volumes could have resulted either from an inability to maintain an adequate mask seal while ensuring a patent airway or from gastric expansion. Another consideration is that the operator may be unable to deliver an appropriate tidal volume unless the bag is compressed with both hands.

BOX 5.1   Standards for the Design and Construction of Manual Resuscitators

1. ASTM International and the ISO recommend that manual resuscitators be capable of delivering a fractional inspired oxygen (F_IO_2) of 0.85 with an oxygen flow of 15 L/min. Recognize that these are minimum requirements and may not be optimal for treating patients during cardiopulmonary resuscitation. It therefore is prudent to choose a device that can deliver an $F_IO_2 \geq 0.95$.
2. Manual resuscitators must be able to operate at extreme temperatures (–180°C to 600°C [–292°F to 1112°F]) and at a relative humidity of 40% to 96%.
3. Adult resuscitators should deliver a tidal volume of at least 600 mL into a test lung set at a compliance of 0.02 L/cm H_2O and a resistance of 20 cm H_2O/L/s.
4. The resuscitator's nonrebreathing valve must be designed so that the valve will not jam at oxygen flow rates up to 30 L/min.
5. If the resuscitator valve malfunctions because of a foreign obstruction (e.g., vomitus), the valve must be restored to proper function within 20 s.
6. Patient connectors of the resuscitator valve must have a 15:22-mm (internal diameter–to–outside diameter [ID:OD]) fitting.
7. Resuscitators used for adults should not have a pressure-limiting system. Bag-valve devices used for children must incorporate a pressure-release valve that limits peak inspiratory pressure to 40 ± 10 cm H_2O; devices used for infants may incorporate a pressure-release valve that limits peak inspiratory pressure to 40 ± 5 cm H_2O.
8. When a pressure-limiting system is incorporated into a resuscitator, an override capability must exist that is readily apparent to the operator (i.e., it should be easily visible that the valve is on or off), and an audible signal should indicate that the gas is being vented. The override mechanism should be provided for times when lung impedance is high and the patient has an endotracheal tube in place.
9. The resuscitator must be able to operate after being dropped from a height of 1 m onto a concrete floor.

BOX 5.2   Features of an Ideal Manual Resuscitator

1. The resuscitator should be lightweight and easily held in one hand.
2. It should have standard 15:22-mm (internal diameter–to–outside diameter [ID:OD]) patient adapters.
3. The bag-valve device should be easy to disassemble, clean, and reassemble.
4. It should be constructed of durable materials (e.g., rubber, silicone, polyvinyl chloride).
5. The nonrebreathing valve should prevent back-leaking of patient-exhaled gases into the bag. It should have a low resistance to inspiratory and expiratory airflow and a small dead space volume (<30 mL for adult models). The non-rebreathing valve should be transparent to allow detection of vomitus or any other obstruction.
6. A manual resuscitator should be able to deliver oxygen concentrations of 0.4 when oxygen is available.
7. The bag construction should allow rapid refill so that faster respiratory rates can be achieved as necessary.
8. The volume of the self-inflating bag should be at least twice the volume to be delivered, because not all of the bag volume is delivered when the bag is compressed. For example, adult resuscitators should have a volume of 1600 mL or more to be able to deliver a tidal volume of 800 mL. Resuscitation bags used for children should have a volume of at least 500 mL, and infant bags should hold at least 240 mL.
9. The bag-valve device should allow a positive end-expiratory pressure valve or spirometer attachments to measure exhaled volumes. It should be equipped with a tap for monitoring airway pressure with an aneroid manometer.
10. Every manual resuscitator should be supplied with a face mask that attaches to the standard patient connector of the resuscitator. The mask should provide an effective seal when applied to the patient's face.

Although manual resuscitators may differ in design, it is generally agreed that the ideal manual resuscitator should have certain characteristics.[26-28] Box 5.2 lists the characteristics of the ideal manual resuscitator.

Oxygen-Powered Resuscitators

Oxygen-powered resuscitators are pressure-limited devices that work similarly to reducing valves. A typical oxygen-powered resuscitator consists of a demand valve that can be manually operated or patient triggered. Oxygen-powered resuscitators can deliver 100% oxygen at flows of less than 40 L/min. Inspiratory pressures generally are limited to 60 cm H_2O, but the pressure-relief valve may be set to 80 cm H_2O if necessary.

Fig. 5.14 shows an example of an oxygen-powered resuscitator. When the manual control actuator is depressed, oxygen enters the device from a 50-psig gas source and flows to the patient through a standard 15:22-mm (internal diameter–to–outside diameter [ID:OD]) connector. The connector can be coupled to a mask, an ETT, a TT, or an esophageal obturator airway.

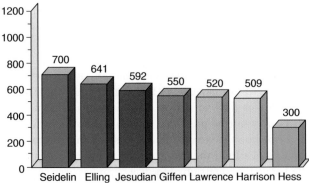

FIGURE 5.13 Tidal volumes produced by bag-valve-mask devices. (From Barnes TA: *Core textbook of respiratory care practice,* ed 2, St. Louis, 1994, Mosby.)

TABLE 5.4 Ventilation Patterns Specified by Standards for Fractional Delivered Oxygen and Ventilation for Bag-Valve Devices

Specification	VENTILATION PATTERN (mL × cycles/min) ASTM[4]	ISO[5]	AHA[6]	O₂ Flow (L/min)	Compliance L/cm H₂O	Resistance cm H₂O/L/sec
Fractional Delivered Oxygen (F$_D$O$_2$)						
Adult	600 × 12	600 × 12	800 × 12	15	0.020	20
Child	300 × 20	15/kg × 20	N/A	15	0.010	200
Infant	20 × 60	20 × 60	6-8 kg × 40	15	0.001	400
Ventilation						
Adult	600 × 20	600 × 20	800 × 12		0.020	20
Child 1	300 × 20	15/kg × 20	N/A		0.010	20
Child 2	70 × 30	150 × 25	N/A		0.010	20
Infant 1	70 × 30	20 × 60	6 to 8/kg × 40		0.010	20
Infant 2	20 × 60	N/A	N/A		0.010	400

AHA, American Heart Association; *ASTM*, American Society for Testing and Materials; *ISO*, International Organization for Standardization; *N/A*, not available.
From Barnes TA: *Core textbook of respiratory care practice*, ed 2, St. Louis, 1994, Mosby.

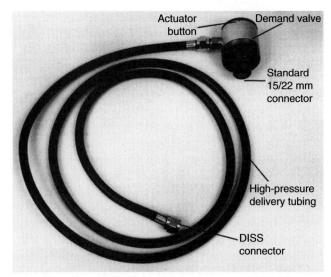

FIGURE 5.14 Oxygen-powered resuscitator. *DISS*, Diameter Index Safety System. (From Scanlan CL, Wilkins RL, Stoller JK: *Egan's fundamentals of respiratory care*, ed 7, St. Louis, 1998, Mosby.)

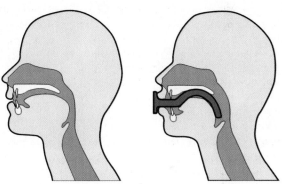

FIGURE 5.15 Anatomical insertion of an oral airway.

Hazards Associated With Manual Resuscitators

The most common hazards encountered with manual resuscitators are delivery of excessively high airway pressures, a defective or malfunctioning nonrebreathing valve, and faulty pressure-relief valves.[29] Excessively high airway pressures are more likely in patients who are intubated than in patients ventilated with a bag-mask-valve device. A nonrebreathing valve that is stuck in the inspiratory position because of improper assembly, inadvertent squeezing of the bag while the patient exhales, or obstruction of the exhalation port (e.g., by a mucous plug) can all produce dramatic increases in airway pressure. Defective nonrebreathing valves may cause an inspiratory leak, resulting in part of the tidal volume escaping through the exhalation port and decreased volumes being delivered to the patient. Low tidal volumes also can occur with the use of an inappropriately sized mask or failure to maintain an adequate seal between the mask and the patient's face. Additionally, improper setting of the pressure-relief valve can cause gas delivery at excessively high pressures and increase the risk for barotrauma.

V. OROPHARYNGEAL AIRWAYS

In some patients, providing FMV can be difficult, and simple manual maneuvers are ineffective at opening an air passage past an obstructing tongue. A number of devices have been developed to displace or bypass the tongue and create a passage for air during FMV. The most common device for this purpose is the oropharyngeal airway (Fig. 5.15).

A Guedel airway (Fig. 5.16) consists of a hollow, central channel for air passage, a buccal flange, a bite block portion, and a curved part that follows the contour of the hard palate. Most are single-use, plastic devices with color-coded inserts based on size. Size is determined by the size of the oropharynx, and the airway must extend past the posterior part of the

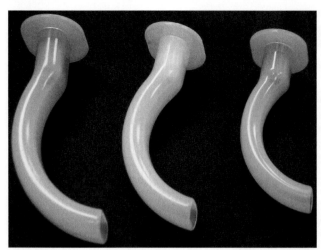

FIGURE 5.16 The Guedel oral airway is available in multiple sizes to fit patients ranging from neonates to adults.

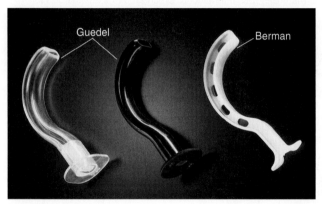

FIGURE 5.17 The Guedel and Berman airways are upper airway devices used to provide air passage distal to an obstructing tongue. (Courtesy Cardinal Health Respiratory Care Products and Services, McGaw Park, IL.)

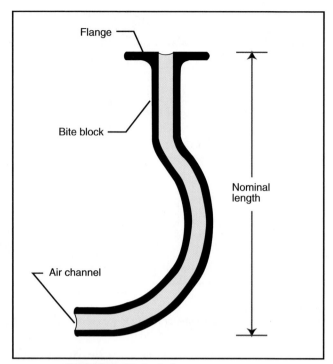

FIGURE 5.18 Oral airway components.

tongue to allow air to pass. Variants of these airways are available, such as the Cath-Guide, which includes three internal channels, the middle channel being a dedicated suction port. Oral airways are available in six sizes and cost roughly $1 each. The Berman airway (Fig. 5.17) is similar in shape to the Guedel airway but has a different cross-sectional profile, and it does not have a protected central channel.

Oral airways are available in a variety of lengths. The standard for oral airways established by the American National Standards Institute (ANSI) is that the size is the "nominal" length in millimeters. Fig. 5.18 shows this measurement convention. Because jaw sizes differ markedly among individuals, the correct-size oropharyngeal airway can be estimated to be the one that reaches from the angle of the jaw or the meatus of the ear to the lips. Choosing an airway that is too large is safer than choosing one that is even slightly too small because the tongue will not be bypassed by an airway that is too short, and therefore the obstruction will not be relieved. If the airway is too long, the excess length protrudes from the mouth, but the airway may be adequate.

An oropharyngeal airway may be inserted into an unconscious person in several ways. Using a tongue blade or gloved fingers, the practitioner can open the mouth and then insert the airway, following the curve of the hard palate and seated with the tip past the back of the tongue. Getting the tip past the flaccid tongue is sometimes difficult, but it is essential for success. To reduce the likelihood of the airway tip getting hung up on the back of the tongue, the practitioner can insert the airway upside down. The airway can then be advanced with the tip riding along the hard palate until it is past the tongue and then rotated 180 degrees to the correct position. A modification of this technique that may be less traumatic to the palate is to insert the airway rotated 90 degrees from the side of the mouth, using the airway as a tongue blade to displace the tongue forward, and then rotate it back 90 degrees to seat the device. Fig. 5.19 illustrates these three insertion techniques.

The correct size of airway and proper seating are essential for creating an open air passage with an oropharyngeal airway. An important sign that the distal airway tip may not have passed the back of the tongue is protrusion of the flange from the patient's mouth. If attempts to advance the airway farther result in resistance or the airway bouncing outward, it is likely catching on the back of the tongue and should be removed and replaced immediately using one of the previously described methods of insertion. An alternative technique for seating an airway that has failed to pass the tongue is to perform a jaw thrust and use the thumbs to push the airway in past the anteriorly displaced tongue (Fig. 5.20).

Care must be taken when placing an oropharyngeal airway in alert patients. Oropharyngeal airways are contraindicated in patients who retain protective airway reflexes because

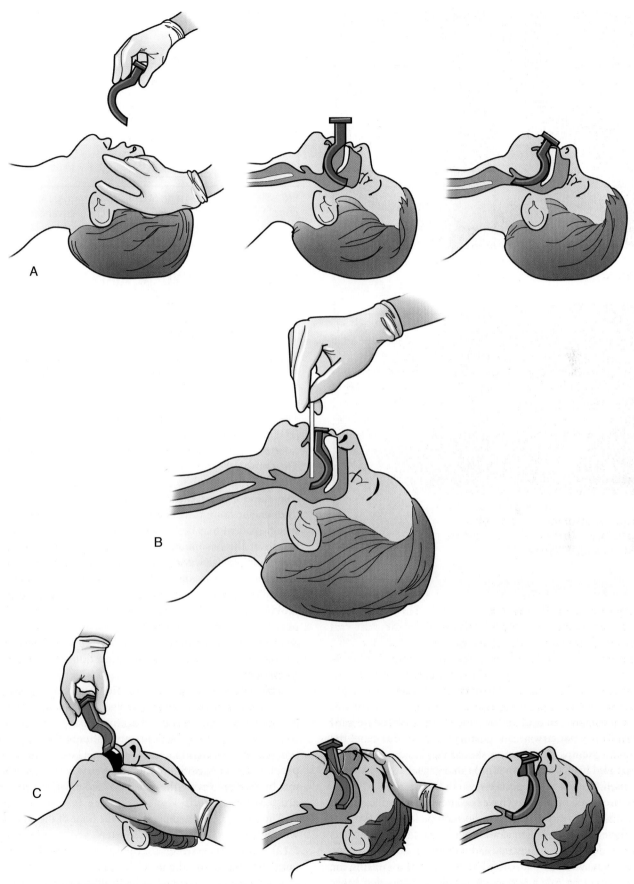

FIGURE 5.19 A, Antianatomical insertion of an oral airway. B, Anatomical insertion of an oral airway with a tongue blade. C, Insertion of an oral airway from the side of the mouth. The airway itself can be used as a tongue blade to displace the tongue while the airway is inserted.

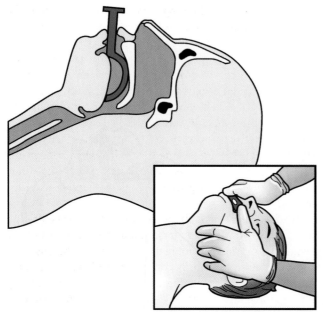

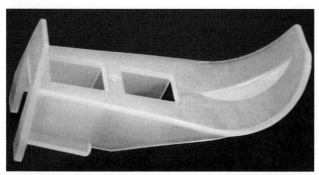

FIGURE 5.20 A jaw thrust is performed to seat the oropharyngeal airway, which has become blocked by the tongue. If the correct-size oropharyngeal airway fails to seat properly and protrudes from the mouth, performing a jaw thrust and using the thumbs to insert the airway provides proper placement.

FIGURE 5.21 Intubating airways can be used to support and direct a fiberoptic bronchoscope and endotracheal tube into the trachea with direct vision. The incomplete channel allows separation of the scope from the airway after tracheal intubation.

gagging, vomiting, or laryngospasm may result. Additionally, dental damage can occur if the patient forcibly bites the hard plastic or metal airway. If the patient struggles to expel the airway, attempts at insertion should be abandoned and an improved head position or a nasopharyngeal airway should be used to open the upper airway.

Specialized oral airways have been developed to allow blind and fiberoptic-directed endotracheal intubation. The simplest of these is an Ovassapian airway, a hollow bite block that acts as a guide for a bronchoscope and also protects the endoscope from damage if the patient reflexively bites down during the procedure (Fig. 5.21). Airways that facilitate intubation either have open channels or are split devices that can be removed, leaving the ETT in place.

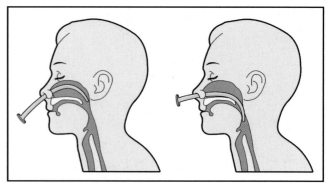

FIGURE 5.22 Placement of a nasopharyngeal airway. For correct insertion of the device, the tip is advanced directly posteriorly—not upward—because the nasopharynx lies directly behind the external nares.

VI. NASOPHARYNGEAL AIRWAYS

Nasopharyngeal airways, which are also called *nasal trumpets* or *nasal airways,* are better tolerated than are oral airways by alert patients who retain some protective airway reflexes.

Nasopharyngeal airways resemble shortened, uncuffed ETTs. Most are made for single use and are composed of soft latex or polyethylene. The end is flanged to prevent the tube from falling back into the airway and being lost in the patient. The ANSI sizing system requires that the internal diameter (ID) be given in millimeters, although French sizes (i.e., the external circumference in millimeters) are also frequently used. The critical size for these airways is the airway length, which must be long enough to pass beyond the tongue base but not enter the esophagus. Each manufacturer uses a different length-to-diameter ratio; thus, determining the proper airway for a specific patient may be a matter of trial and error. The correct length of the nasopharyngeal airway can be estimated by positioning the airway along the side of the head. For proper function, the tip should extend past the angle of the jaw. An airway that is too long may enter the esophagus and not provide an air passage. Unlike oropharyngeal airways, nasopharyngeal airways that are too short will not make a bad airway worse, they just will not improve the problem.

Nasal bleeding can complicate insertion of the nasopharyngeal airway. Caution should be used with patients who are coagulopathic. The correct insertion technique, generous lubrication, and vasoconstrictive agents can reduce the frequency of nasal bleeding. A mixture of a local anesthetic solution (i.e., 4% lidocaine) and phenylephrine (Neo-Synephrine) or oxymetazoline (Afrin) can be effective for this purpose. In emergency situations the airway should only be well lubricated to avoid the delay involved in waiting for these drugs to take effect.

The airway is inserted parallel to the floor of the nasopharynx and slightly medially with constant, gentle pressure (Fig. 5.22). Clinicians often make the mistake of attempting to insert the airway "up the nose" (i.e., parallel to the long axis of the nose), which increases the likelihood of bleeding and fails to secure placement. If undue resistance is met on one side of the nose, insertion should be attempted on the other

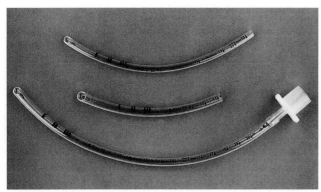

FIGURE 5.23 Uncuffed endotracheal tubes can be used as nasopharyngeal airways.

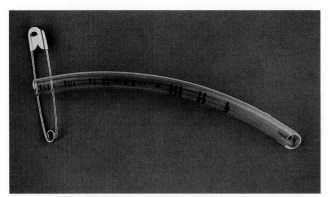

FIGURE 5.24 Inserting a safety pin just through the tube wall helps secure a custom-cut endotracheal tube used as a nasopharyngeal airway.

side, or a smaller-diameter airway may be needed. Softer airways are less likely to cause bleeding and conform to a distorted passageway as they pass through a narrow nasal channel. However, they also are more likely to obstruct and prevent passage of a suction catheter. If only a small airway can be passed through the external nasal passage, it may not function because of its concomitant short length.

Uncuffed ETTs can be used as nasopharyngeal airways (Fig. 5.23). The tube length can be customized to fit the individual patient's anatomy. A long, thin tube can be created by trimming the tube to the proper length. The tube connector can be used to prevent the tube from disappearing into the nose; however, the friction fit may be inadequate to prevent accidental separation. Also, the connector's ID is smaller than that of the tube and may prevent passage of a suction catheter and limit gas flow during ventilation. Leaving extra length so that the tube can be taped at the correct distance is another solution, but it may reduce the efficiency of ventilation. Accidental movement can be prevented by placing a safety pin through the side of the tube, avoiding compromise of the center lumen of the tube with tape (Fig. 5.24).

As mentioned previously, nasal bleeding is a concern; thus nasopharyngeal airways should be used with caution in coagulopathic patients, those on blood thinners, and parturients. If bleeding occurs, topical vasoconstrictors can be applied, and the bleeding source can be directly tamponaded by leaving

the device in place or holding direct pressure just below the bridge of the nose for at least 5 minutes. Significant hemorrhage does occasionally occur and may necessitate a transfusion. A relative contraindication for use of a nasopharyngeal airway is a Le Fort II or III facial fracture or a basilar skull fracture. Entry into the maxillary antrum, orbit, or base of the skull or penetration of the brain by the airway is possible, although unlikely. The risk must be weighed against the urgency of the need for the airway and the failure of other techniques. Many clinicians avoid placing nasal airways in parturients due to engorgement of nasal tissues and possible bleeding. Sinus infection is a long-term risk of nasopharyngeal tube placement.

As with oral airways, fiberoptic or blind tracheal entry can be facilitated with a nasopharyngeal airway. Removal of the device after intubation is more difficult, however, because split devices are not commercially available. Nasopharyngeal airways are also useful for protecting the nose from trauma during blind nasotracheal suctioning. Once securely in place, they are usually well tolerated, even by awake individuals.

VII. SUPRAGLOTTIC AIRWAYS

Laryngeal Mask Airway

The laryngeal mask airway (LMA) was invented by Dr. Archie Brain in the 1980s and was approved by the US Food and Drug Administration (FDA) in 1991 as a substitute for the face mask. The LMA has become part of the difficult airway algorithm, as seen previously, as well as a staple airway device for elective surgeries performed in the operating room. It is also a mainstay found in the toolboxes of many emergency medical technicians (EMTs) and respiratory therapists.

The LMA consists of a plastic tube attached to a silicone laryngeal mask (Fig. 5.25). It is designed to form a low-pressure seal in the laryngeal inlet by means of an inflated cuff. Note that the cuff pressures should not exceed 60 cm H_2O. The LMA is placed blindly, with the tip resting against the upper esophageal sphincter (cricopharyngeus muscle) and the cuff seated laterally in the pyriform fossa. It is equipped with a standard 15-mm slip fitting. A properly seated LMA allows for positive-pressure ventilation to be delivered if necessary. Ventilating with pressures exceeding 20 cm H_2O may result in volume loss, gas leakage, and ventilation around the cuff and potentially into the stomach. This device does not replace endotracheal intubation, because the lung is not protected from aspiration. Put simply, the LMA essentially acts as a modified FMV technique and should not be used in patients at risk for aspiration except as a temporary bridge to a more definitive airway as seen in the difficult airway algorithm.

The LMA is a useful emergency airway device for several reasons: (1) insertion is simple, can be done blindly, and is easy to teach and learn; (2) it provides a patent airway that usually is superior to that obtained with an oral or nasopharyngeal device; (3) it does not require airway manipulation or extreme head positioning and minimizes flexion and extension of the cervical spine; (4) it eliminates the need to place a foreign body in the patient's trachea and causes less

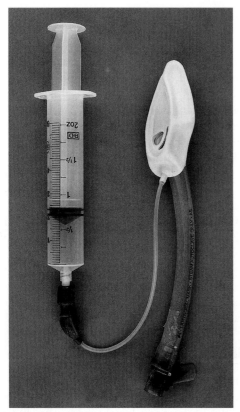

FIGURE 5.25 For correct insertion of a laryngeal mask airway, the cuff should be deflated completely with the mask forming an upward, open-bowl configuration. This minimizes the risk for oral damage and helps prevent the mask from folding over during insertion.

BOX 5.3   Contraindications to Use of a Laryngeal Mask Airway

Contraindications to Elective Use of a Laryngeal Mask Airway
- Full stomach or inability to confirm fasting status
- Retained gastric contents
- Severe gastroesophageal reflux
- Decreased pulmonary compliance that necessitates high ventilation pressures

Contraindications to Emergent Use of a Laryngeal Mask Airway
- Patient conscious and/or resisting placement of the LMA

LMA, Laryngeal mask airway.

TABLE 5.5   Sizing of Laryngeal Mask Airways

Mask Size	Age Group	Patient Weight (kg)
1	Neonates/infants	Up to 5
1½	Infants	5-10
2	Infants/children	10-20
2½	Children	20-30
3	Children	30-50
4	Adults	50-70
5	Adults	70-100
6	Large adults	>100

bronchospasm and coughing in patients with asthma and irritable airways; and (5) once the LMA is in place, the user's hands are free for other tasks. A major drawback of the LMA is aspiration from gastroesophageal reflux disease (GERD) or a full stomach because the LMA does not reliably seal the tracheal inlet and ensure that the patient's airway is protected.

Contraindications to elective use of the LMA include a nonfasted patient or a patient in whom fasting cannot be confirmed, retained gastric contents, and decreased pulmonary compliance. Box 5.3 lists the major contraindications to use of an LMA. Sizes are based on weight and range from 1 (neonates) to 6 (adults who weigh more than 100 kg) (Table 5.5). Normal adult women usually tolerate a size 4, and adult men tolerate a size 5. Use of a larger size with less air in the cuff often improves the ability to ventilate and may reduce the risk for mucosal damage and a sore throat. Cuff pressures of the LMA may be tested using manometry to ensure there is less risk for mucosal damage.

Before the LMA is inserted, the cuff is inflated and examined for ability to maintain inflation; it can be placed with or without air depending on practitioner preference. A water-soluble lubricant is used on the back side of the cuff to help it slide past the hard and soft palates. Fig. 5.26 shows the insertion technique. A black line along the length of the tube marks the center of the device and is used to prevent and detect rotation during and after placement. The head may be extended and a finger used to guide the deflated cuff past the tongue and pharynx. The tube is held in place with the other hand while the guiding fingers are withdrawn. The tube then is advanced until it is fully seated and resistance to further insertion is felt. With the tube free in the mouth, the cuff is inflated. If it is seated correctly in the pyriform sinuses, the tube will move approximately 1 to 2 cm out of the mouth. This should be done "hands free" and without any ventilation equipment attached to the tube. If the mask is too small, it may pass down the esophagus, and no backward movement will occur on cuff inflation. Adding a small amount of air to the LMA before insertion may be useful in preventing the cuff from folding over on itself and failing to seat.

The final test of correct placement is the presence of adequate breath sounds over both lung fields and not over the stomach with manual ventilation. End-tidal CO_2 ($ETCO_2$) should also be present. If ventilation fails, the head position may be extended or altered, or the LMA can be repositioned by inserting further or removing and reinserting. If the patient has a significant air leak and peak inspiratory pressures less than 20 cm H_2O, a larger LMA may be needed.

After the device has been properly placed and a patent airway obtained, the tube is secured with tape. Either spontaneous or positive-pressure ventilation can be used. Tidal

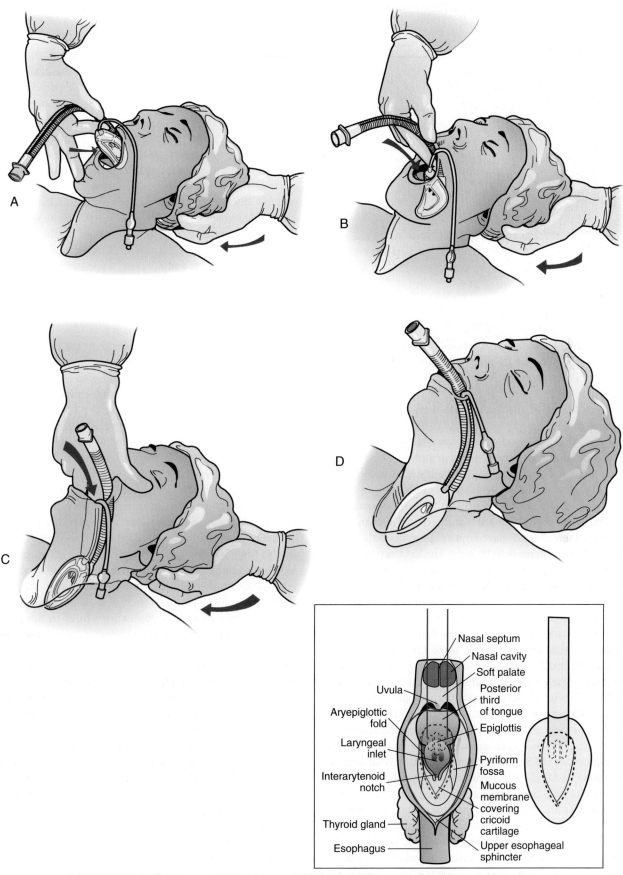

Nasal septum
Nasal cavity
Soft palate
Uvula
Posterior third of tongue
Aryepiglottic fold
Epiglottis
Laryngeal inlet
Pyriform fossa
Interarytenoid notch
Mucous membrane covering cricoid cartilage
Thyroid gland
Esophagus
Upper esophageal sphincter

FIGURE 5.26 A, The laryngeal mask airway (LMA) is held like a pencil and inserted into the open mouth with only the slightest neck extension. B, The LMA is directed posteriorly and down to the oropharynx. C, The LMA is advanced with the opposite hand and guided into the posterior pharynx. D, The final location of the LMA after correct placement.

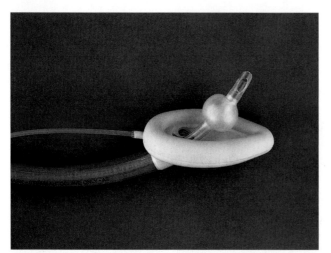

FIGURE 5.27 The laryngeal air mask can be used as a conduit for intubation.

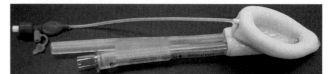

FIGURE 5.28 The LMA ProSeal contains a port for gastric suction and venting of the stomach.

volumes less than 8 mL/kg are recommended for manual ventilation. Close attention still must be paid to the airway when it is secured with the LMA because loss of airway patency can occur, often caused by dislodgment or twisting of the device, foreign body aspiration, obstruction of the LMA, or laryngospasm.

Blind or fiberoptic intubation with a cuffed ETT can be performed through an LMA to establish a definitive or secure airway (Fig. 5.27). (A modification specifically designed for this purpose, the intubating LMA, is described later.) Occasionally the epiglottis is trapped in the LMA (it usually lies on top of the mask cuff), but this seems to have little effect on its function. The LMA is particularly beneficial in patients known or expected to have a difficult airway. Pregnant and obese patients predictably have improved ventilation with an LMA compared with mask techniques. The LMA is potentially lifesaving when intubation and other ventilation devices have failed. It is an excellent bridge, allowing for acquisition of more resources and, ultimately, a more definitive airway.

Use of LMAs is becoming widespread outside the operating room because mastering the necessary skills for LMA placement is easier than mastering those needed for effective mask ventilation or endotracheal intubation. Emergency personnel anecdotally report excellent results in field use. Increased use of these devices in infants and pediatric patients is especially encouraging, because the skills necessary for other airway techniques in these patients are difficult to learn and maintain. The AHA recommends instruction in the use of the LMA in basic life support (BLS) training as an alternative to bag-mask ventilation. In ACLS, use of the LMA is considered a IIa (acceptable to use) recommendation.

Most LMAs are made in a disposable, single-use form in a multitude of sizes, and reusable LMAs are becoming rare. In the case of reusable LMAs, they should be mechanically washed with a mild soap solution and autoclaved at a temperature of 124°C (255°F) or less. The cuff must be evacuated completely, or it will rupture during the sterilization process. Glutaraldehyde should not be used, because it is absorbed

into the silicone and is quite toxic to the laryngeal mucosa. LMAs may be resterilized 100 to 200 times. Marked discoloration and failure of the pilot tube and cuff to hold pressure are indications that the tube should be discarded. Although reusable silicone rubber LMAs can cost as much as $200, the disposable models cost around $10. It is important to emphasize that these disposable devices *should not* be reused. In addition to the LMA Classic (multiuse) and LMA Unique (single use), there are a number of "second-generation" LMAs that offer specific benefits over the first-generation models. The LMA Flexible has a wire-reinforced tubing that allows greater flexion and greater adaptability for attaching the LMA to an airway circuit or during surgery. The LMA ProSeal has an additional lateral tube that ends at the tip of the LMA and allows venting of the stomach (Fig. 5.28). A gastric tube can be placed through this additional channel and may reduce gastric distention and the risk for pulmonary aspiration.[30] It is worth mentioning that the ProSeal is touted as capable of generating 50% higher seal pressures. In addition to the aforementioned supraglottic airway devices, the LMA has been modified to act as a conduit for intubation (see later discussion).

LMA North America manufactured the first supraglottic airway device. Since then a multitude of supraglottic and extraglottic airway devices have arrived on the market, including the Cobra (Engineered Medical Systems); King Laryngeal Tubes (King Systems), which have a gastric access port; the Aura laryngeal mask (Ambu, Inc.); the Portex Soft-Seal Laryngeal Mask (Smiths Medical), and i-gel (Intersurgical). Each device has unique features, including single use to reduce cross-contamination, clear tubes with built-in bite blocks, reinforced tips to prevent folding during insertion, and various characteristics relating to the angle and composition of the tube portion to prevent malposition or twisting (Figs. 5.29 and 5.30). A recent version of the supraglottic airway device is the air-Q (Mercury Medical), which is designed with a wider, shorter lumen; an easily removable connector; a narrow inflated cuff; and a large keyhole-shaped ventilating distal port. It is designed with the specific purpose of acting as a conduit for performing fiberoptic or blind intubation through the lumen with a conventional ETT once the device is in place. This device can help the clinician in the instance of difficult mask ventilation and facilitate intubation.

Fastrach Laryngeal Mask Airway

As mentioned previously, a modification of the LMA has been developed to facilitate blind intubation in patients who need a secure airway. This modified version takes advantage of the fact that the LMA is simple to place and rests directly above

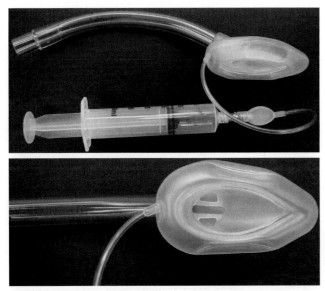

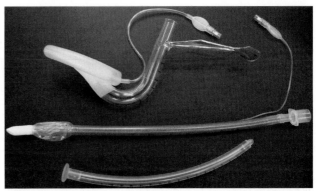

FIGURE 5.31 The Fastrach laryngeal mask airway (LMA) allows intubation through the LMA. The intubating LMA is shown with its special silastic endotracheal tube and tube pusher, which is used to help remove the LMA and leave the endotracheal tube in place.

FIGURE 5.29 The LMA Unique is disposable to reduce the risk for cross-contamination.

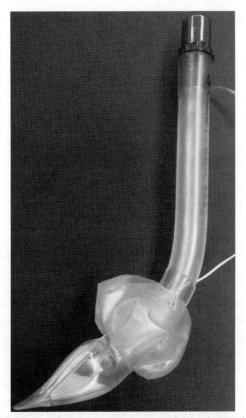

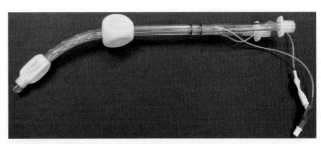

FIGURE 5.32 The Combitube is a supraglottic airway device that is useful for saving patients from failed intubations.

FIGURE 5.30 The Cobra is another supraglottic airway device.

the larynx. Fig. 5.31 shows the prototype of this intubating LMA, the Fastrach (LMA North America). It consists of an LMA cuff mounted on a curved, hollow metal shaft, preformed to fit into an average-size airway. Originally the Fastrach was a nondisposable, metal tube device with an attached silicone cuff. It was packaged with a wire-reinforced ETT and an ETT stabilizer, allowing for removal of the device while maintaining intubation. Newer, disposable versions made of polyvinyl

chloride are now available. The Fastrach has a flexible epiglottic elevating flap and a handle that allows control and manipulation of the mask orientation, which improves the chances of successful blind intubation. After intubation the Fastrach is removed using the ETT stabilizer or stylet to prevent the ETT from becoming dislodged during removal of the LMA portion.

One benefit of the Fastrach includes the fact that it can be used with minimal mouth opening (3 cm). More importantly, the Fastrach allows for ventilation of the patient during the various steps of placement of the LMA and, finally, the ETT. Placement is blind. Thus this is a useful technique for a bloodied airway in which fiberoptic visualization would prove to be difficult. In addition, minimal cervical neck motion is involved compared with direct laryngoscopy. Major disadvantages of the Fastrach are its cost ($500 for the reusable model and $90 for the disposable device) and the fact that it is available only in adult sizes. Despite these drawbacks, the Fastrach has become an important part of emergency and difficult airway equipment carts.

Combitube

The esophageal tracheal Combitube is a double-lumen device designed to provide a patent upper airway when inserted blindly in comatose patients with airway difficulty or after failed intubation. The two cuffs, proximal and distal, are designed to seal the esophagus and the pharynx (Fig. 5.32). The tube can be placed blindly or during a failed laryngoscopy

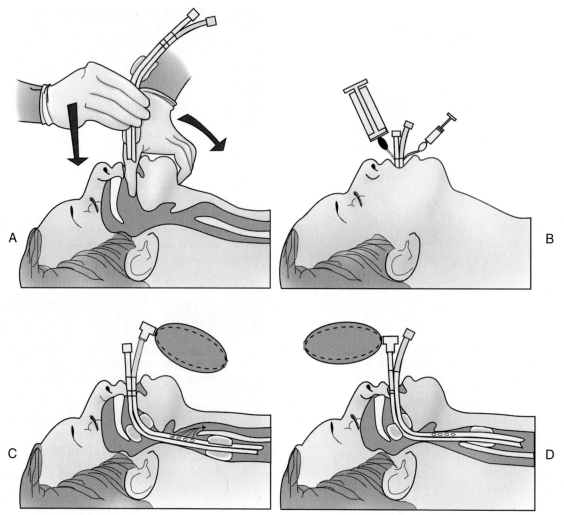

FIGURE 5.33 The Combitube is inserted with the head in the neutral position (A) and both cuffs inflated (B). The two possible locations of the distal lumen are the usual esophageal location (C) and, in rare cases, the trachea (D).

procedure. With blind insertion the tube should be lubricated and inserted through the mouth, following the contour to the pharynx. Insertion continues until the depth mark reaches the lips or significant resistance is encountered. The distal cuff should be inflated with 12 to 15 mL of air, and the chest and abdomen should be auscultated for breath sounds or gurgling in the epigastrium. The small distal lumen usually advances into the esophagus, but in the case of a tracheal entry of the distal lumen, the Combitube can be used as a conventional ETT (Fig. 5.33). If the distal tip enters the esophagus, both cuffs need to be inflated (the proximal cuff with 85 to 100 mL of air and the distal with 15 mL of air) to prevent air from escaping through the esophagus. Ventilation is then provided through the proximal lumen, which opens in a series of holes into the hypopharynx.

The benefits of the Combitube are that it is a blind technique, it is easy to learn, and it allows the patient's head to remain in the neutral position. The esophageal cuff affords some protection from regurgitation, but as with the LMA, the Combitube is not considered a secure, protective airway device. A nasogastric tube can be inserted through the esophageal lumen into the stomach for decompression with reduction in the risk for pulmonary aspiration. The Combitube is made in two sizes, 37 and 41 French (Fr). The 41-Fr size is recommended for patients over 60 in in height. As of now, the Combitube is not suitable for pediatric use. The device is contraindicated for patients with a vigorous gag, in the presence of esophageal disease, or after ingestion of a caustic substance. Complications from the Combitube include dysphagia, a sore throat, and injury to the pyriform sinus and esophageal wall. Injury to the pyriform sinus or esophageal wall can result in subcutaneous emphysema, pneumomediastinum, pneumoperitoneum, or esophageal rupture.

VIII. SUBGLOTTIC AIRWAY DEVICES

Endotracheal Tubes

The ETT was first described in the 1800s and has since become the gold standard of airway management. ETTs allow ventilation with high levels of positive pressure, provide direct access to the lower airway for secretion removal and drug delivery, prevent aspiration of foreign material into the lung, and permit

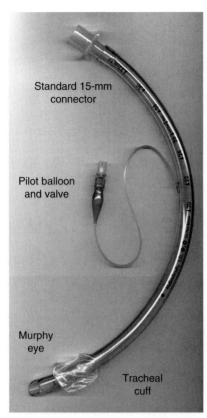

FIGURE 5.34 The components of a cuffed endotracheal tube.

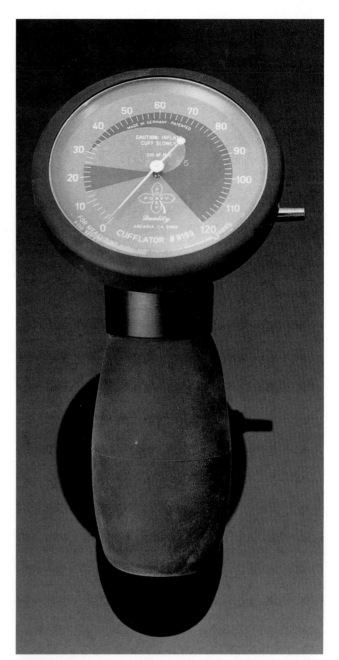

FIGURE 5.35 A manometer is a device used for measuring endotracheal tube cuff pressure.

bronchoscopic examination of the peripheral airways. Placement of an ETT requires a high degree of skill and specialized equipment (e.g., laryngoscopes). Risks during placement attempts include hypoxia, hypercarbia, and cardiovascular changes. Ideally, before an ETT is placed, adequate gas exchange should be established with mask ventilation or another device such as an LMA. Intubation may be an urgent procedure, but it should rarely be performed in a patient without a previously established patent airway and some evidence of reasonable gas exchange. Exceptions include patients who are full-stomach who require a rapid-sequence intubation without ventilation to reduce the risk for aspiration.

As shown in Fig. 5.34, the conventional, or Murphy-type, ETT consists of a round, plastic tube with a beveled tip, a side hole (Murphy eye) opposite the bevel, a cuff attached to a pilot balloon with a spring-loaded valve, and a 15-mm standard connector. The tube has distance markers and a radiopaque marker embedded along its length. The Murphy eye allows gas flow if the bevel tip becomes occluded. ETTs that lack a Murphy eye are called Magill-type tubes. ETTs are sized by ID (in millimeters), although occasionally French sizes are reported. After the ETT is in place in the trachea, the cuff can be used to form a seal with the tracheal wall. Usually air is inflated through the one-way valve in the pilot balloon until a seal forms or high pressure develops. Most ETT cuffs are large-volume, low-pressure devices meant to contact a large portion of the tracheal wall with a low pressure. Because of tracheal mucosal blood pressure flow characteristics, the cuff pressure should be below 25 mm Hg to prevent tracheal

ischemic damage. Fig. 5.35 shows a manometer for determining and regulating cuff pressure. If a manometer is not available, a "just seal" or "minimal leak" technique can be used to minimize the lateral tracheal wall pressure from the inflated cuff. For some patients who require high airway pressure for mechanical ventilation, the cuff pressure cannot be kept below 25 mm Hg without significant volume loss. The amount of pressure used should be enough to guarantee adequate ventilation and protection from aspiration. An alternative to an inflatable cuff is a self-inflating cuff that is filled with foam. Before insertion, this type of cuff must be actively deflated and clamped; the clamp then is removed, and the cuff is allowed to expand to form a seal. The pilot port of foam-filled cuffs does not have a valve.

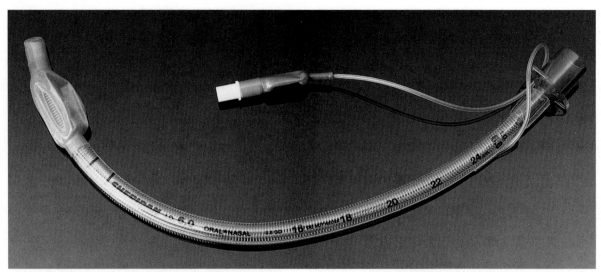

FIGURE 5.36 Spiral wire–reinforced endotracheal tube.

Uncuffed tubes generally are used for children because the smaller lumen necessary to accommodate a cuff would further compromise an airway that is already small in diameter. Additionally, the narrowest part of an infant or child's airway is below the larynx at the cricoid ring, and a snug fit at this level permits positive-pressure ventilation. The correct size of tube for an infant or a child can be determined only during actual intubation; a tube that will not pass easily down the trachea should be exchanged for a smaller-diameter tube. To prevent postintubation croup or subglottic stenosis, an air leak at approximately 20 cm H_2O should be obtained in children intubated with an uncuffed ETT. ETTs with a significant leak at less than 20 cm H_2O may need to be exchanged for a larger size. Additionally, manometers can be used to test ETT cuff pressure in cuffed ETTs to prevent mucosal ischemia or injury.

Many variants of the basic ETT design have been developed to solve clinical problems related to patient anatomy as well as surgical positioning and manipulation. The plastic tube tends to collapse and obstruct when bent at an acute angle, which frequently occurs in the posterior pharynx with a nasally placed ETT. A spiral wire-embedded tube (Fig. 5.36) helps prevent this problem, but these tubes are flimsy and do not hold a preformed arch shape, which makes them difficult to place in the trachea. Another solution to the bending and kinking problem is the Ring-Adair-Elwyn (RAE) tube, which has a preformed bend for oral or nasal intubation.

IX. TOOLS AND AIDS TO ENDOTRACHEAL INTUBATION

Laryngoscopes

The ETT is placed through the mouth or nose into the trachea, and the cuff forms a seal against the tracheal wall. Placement of the ETT is usually performed using a laryngoscope, which allows direct visualization of the larynx and control of the supraglottic structures. The first glottiscope was invented in the 1800s (Historical Note 5.1).[31-33] The modern laryngoscope was not invented until the 1940s and consisted of a handle

---

HISTORICAL NOTE 5.1 **History of the Laryngoscope**

Benjamin Guy Babington, a medical student, created a glottiscope in 1829 that used sunlight to illuminate the glottis. The device consisted of one arm that depressed the tongue and another that was placed along the palate to reflect the sunlight for illumination and allow visualization of the glottis.

In 1854, Manuel Garcia, a singing professor at the Royal Academy of Music in London, used a dental mirror and a handheld mirror to reflect sunlight and visualize his larynx and trachea during vocalization. Part of his success in visualizing his glottis was a result of his absent gag reflex and vocal control. This discovery was called autolaryngoscopy. At the age of 100 years, Garcia was honored with the title "Father of Laryngology."

---

containing a battery and a detachable blade with a light bulb. Fig. 5.37 shows the two basic types of laryngoscope blades: a straight blade (Miller blade) and a curved blade (Macintosh blade). Note that direct laryngoscopy is performed slightly differently with the two types of blades. With either blade attached, the handle is held like a hammer in the left, usually nondominant, hand (although "left-handed" models have been made, which are made to be held in the right hand) with the blade below the hand and the long axis directed forward (Fig. 5.38). The mouth is opened, and the blade is inserted along the right side of the tongue. After the blade is inserted past the base of the tongue, it is brought back to the midline of the oral cavity, moving the tongue completely to the left. With the straight blade the epiglottis is identified and lifted with the tip of the blade, and the jaw and epiglottis are lifted forward and upward (not rocked backward, which could cause trauma to the upper teeth). Using good technique, the light should illuminate the larynx, the vocal cords, and the glottis aperture leading to the trachea. With a curved blade the epiglottis is identified and the tip inserted above it into the vallecula, the space between the tongue base and the epiglottis.

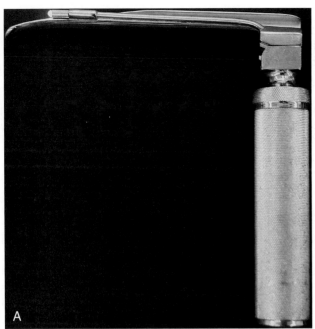

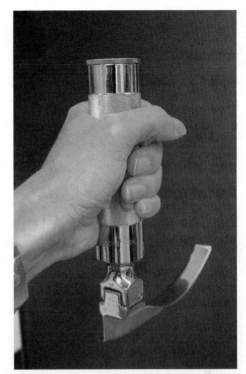

FIGURE 5.38 The laryngoscope is held like a hammer in the left hand.

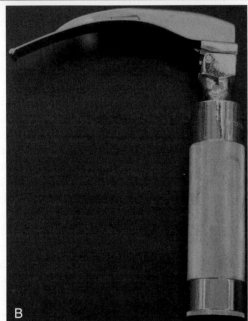

FIGURE 5.37 A, The Miller blade is a common version of the straight blade. B, The Macintosh blade is a type of curved blade.

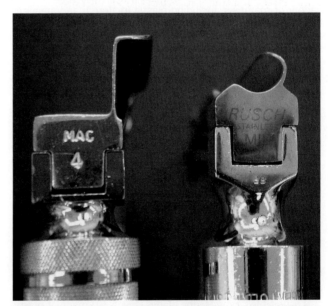

FIGURE 5.39 Cross-section of straight and curved blades. The broad flange of the curved blade gives better tongue control and working room during intubation.

Using the same forward and upward lift, the larynx is illuminated, and the ETT can be passed through the vocal cords into the trachea. The light is located farther down toward the blade tip on straight blades and brightly illuminates the larynx, whereas the light on curved blades is approximately midway down the blade and illuminates the pharynx and supraglottic area. The broad flange of the curved blade (Fig. 5.39) gives better tongue control and more working room for tube insertion than does the straight blade. In children the epiglottis is less rigid and longer than in adults, and often a straight-blade technique (i.e., lifting the epiglottis) is necessary, even if a

curved blade is used. Table 5.6 shows the standard Cormack-Lehane classification of the glottic view with laryngoscopy.[34]

The basic laryngoscope blades have been modified over the years to deal with an anterior larynx, small mouth opening, cervical spine immobility, and a small sternal space. The size and shape of the flange and the location of the light on the curved blade are common features for innovation. Ports for suction or oxygen insufflation have been added. Straight blades

TABLE 5.6 Cormack-Lehane Grades of Glottic Exposure During Direct Laryngoscopy

Grade	Description
I	Full vocal cords exposure
II	Only posterior commissure of glottis visible
III	Only epiglottis visible
IV	No exposure of glottis or epiglottis

From Cormack RS, Lehane J: Difficult tracheal intubation in obstetrics. *Anaesthesia* 39:1105, 1984.

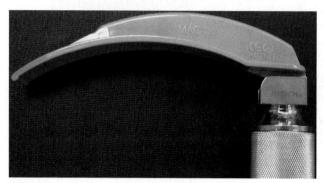

FIGURE 5.40 Disposable laryngoscope blades come in a variety of materials, including plastic (pictured) and stainless steel.

have been modified in their cross-sectional shape to give better tongue control or working room during insertion of an ETT. No standardized size equivalency is represented in blade numbers, but a #0 or #1 blade generally is correct for infants, and a #3 or #4 blade is usually appropriate for average adults. The angle at which the blade leaves the handle is another area of modification. An acute angle may improve visualization, and an obtuse or offset angle may allow insertion of the blade when pendulous breasts or an orthopedic apparatus is in the way. An angled blade tip, a mirror, or a prism may allow the clinician to see "around the corner" into the larynx. In addition, short handles have been made to help with blade insertion in patients with a small sternal space. These specialized devices are often expensive and require considerable practice to master.

Disposable laryngoscope blades (Fig. 5.40) made of plastic or aluminum have gained popularity because of convenience, less need for maintenance, and the reduced risk for cross-contamination. Both the straight and curved blades come in sterile packaging and in the traditional sizes of the reusable blades. Another benefit of disposables is the elimination of sterilization because some evidence indicates that blades still contain protein matter even after sterilization.[35] In some cases the disposable plastic blades have been reported to bend or break. Other studies have shown that disposable blades lead to increased intubation times, greater peak force generated during intubation, and increased failed intubations during rapid-sequence intubations.[36] The quality of disposable

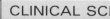
laryngoscope blades and handles continues to improve with more acceptance by large medical centers.

Although the ability to see the laryngeal structures is useful, a good view does not guarantee easy ETT insertion. Manipulation of the ETT into the trachea can be facilitated in several ways. The first consideration is proper head position. The sniffing position is ideal for opening the upper airway and aligning the trachea for intubation. The next consideration is the position of the intubator's head. The intubator's head should be far enough away from the patient's mouth to allow binocular vision (Fig. 5.41). If the laryngoscopist is too close to the airway (see Fig. 5.41B), depth perception is compromised. In general, if the arm holding the laryngoscope is 90 degrees or more at the elbow, the eye distance is correct. In difficult intubations the larynx is often described as "anterior." This means that the laryngeal opening is above the field of vision with the laryngoscope inserted. A malleable stylet can be inserted into the ETT to provide stiffness and can be bent to give the tube an upward hook at its end. This "hockey stick curve" is very useful if the problem is an anterior location of the larynx. Intubation often can be accomplished with this curved tip, even if a direct laryngeal view is not possible. The stylet should be lubricated before it is placed into the ETT so that it can be easily withdrawn. Another solution to controlling the ETT tip is the Endotrol Tracheal Tube (Medtronic Minimally Invasive Therapies). With this device an implanted string with a pull-ring directs the tip anterior when pulled (Fig. 5.42). This device is particularly well suited for blind nasotracheal intubation.

Endotracheal Tube Guide/Intubating Stylet

Even when the larynx cannot be seen during laryngoscopy, it may be possible to pass a rigid stylet blindly into the trachea. Called the *Eschmann stylet, gum elastic bougie, or intubating introducer catheter,* this device is useful with an anterior larynx or when the epiglottis can be seen but little or no glottic opening can be visualized. Ranging from 35 cm (pediatric) to 100 cm and averaging 5 mm in diameter, the ETT guide has a 35-degree angle several centimeters from the tip (Fig. 5.43). A washboard feeling or tracheal clicks are often felt when the device is advancing down the trachea over the tracheal rings, which may reassure the clinician that the bougie is in the trachea as opposed to the esophagus. An ETT can then be threaded over the stylet to achieve intubation. Variations include hollow centers that allow oxygenation and ventilation and a channel for a fiberoptic scope to allow visual guidance through the glottic opening (Clinical Scenario 5.1).

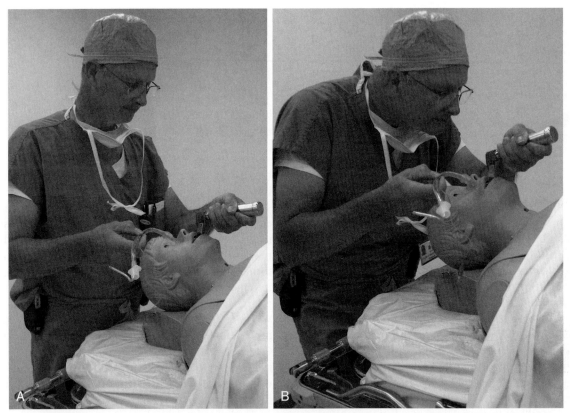

FIGURE 5.41 A, The correct head to trachea distance during intubation allows depth perception to be maintained. B, If the intubator is too close to the airway, the proper distance for depth perception is not present, and intubation becomes more difficult.

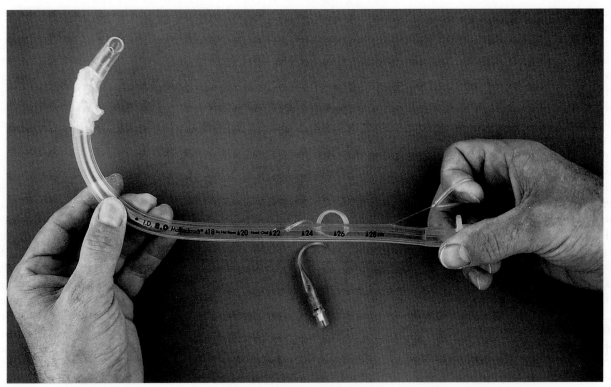

FIGURE 5.42 The Endotrol Tracheal Tube has a string that when pulled directs the tip of the endotracheal tube anteriorly during intubation attempts.

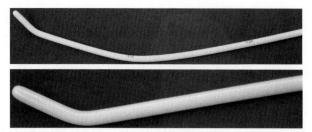

FIGURE 5.43 An intubating stylet or gum elastic bougie can be useful when a patient has an anterior larynx.

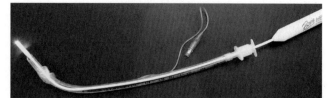

FIGURE 5.44 The lightwand can be useful in patients with cervical immobility or instability.

Blind Intubation

Another approach to tracheal intubation is through the nasal passage. Blind nasotracheal intubation is typically performed in spontaneously breathing, semiconscious individuals. As with a nasopharyngeal airway, a well-lubricated ETT is inserted posteriorly, directly through the nares into the nasopharynx. Topical local anesthetics and vasoconstrictors should reduce patient discomfort and bleeding. Instead of the sniffing position, a neutral or slightly flexed head position is optimal for blind nasal intubation. Breath sounds or moisture in the tube is used to identify the tip location and the timing of tube advancement. Breath sounds or moisture disappears when the tube enters the esophagus. The ETT is placed just above the larynx and rapidly advanced 1 to 2 cm during inspiration when the cords are maximally abducted. If tracheal topical anesthesia is not used, a vigorous cough follows successful tracheal intubation. If initially unsuccessful, turning the head to one side or the other, flexing the neck further, or pushing the thyroid cartilage posteriorly may lead to success. Use of a fiberoptic bronchoscope may be necessary to guide nasotracheal intubation in some difficult circumstances. A nasally inserted ETT can be directed anteriorly into the trachea using a laryngoscope in the mouth and Magill forceps in an anesthetized patient, although care must be taken not to rip the cuff with the sharp teeth of the Magill forceps.

Blind oral ETT insertion techniques have been described. Proper placement can be achieved by using two fingers to retract the epiglottis and direct the tube tip anteriorly. The Berman intubating airway (Berman II) is an oropharyngeal airway with a hooked end and an open channel for an ETT. The ETT is placed through the channel while the tip is used to lift the vallecula. The tube can be passed into the trachea blindly and then separated from the open channel of the airway. The effectiveness of these blind techniques depends on patient anatomy and the experience and skill of the individual because they are unlikely to be successful in the hands of a novice.

X. ADJUNCTS TO ENDOTRACHEAL INTUBATION

Lighted Stylets or Lightwand

Lighted stylets or the lightwand can be used to blindly place ETTs (Fig. 5.44). This technique relies on pharyngeal and tracheal transillumination to identify the correct location of the stylet in the trachea. The stylet should be lubricated before it is inserted into the ETT to allow for easier placement. The stylet can be molded into roughly a 90-degree bend to achieve entry into the anterior trachea. The patient's neck should be in the neutral position, although a jaw thrust can help with movement of the stylet and tube. The room lights should be turned off or dimmed, and the stylet should be placed blindly into the patient's oropharynx or nasopharynx. A dim, diffuse glow is characteristic of esophageal entry, whereas a bright, V-shaped light can be seen with tracheal entry. A lateral transillumination often indicates entry into the pyriform fossae. Once the characteristic pattern of light is seen on the neck, the ETT should be advanced off the stylet and the stylet withdrawn. As with any form of intubation, the position of the tube in the trachea must be confirmed.

The lighted stylet technique is most commonly used when direct laryngoscopy is not possible because of cervical neck injury with the neck stabilized to prevent extension. A mouth opening of only 6 to 8 mm is required, and this can be useful in patients with an anterior larynx or a bloody airway. One drawback of this intubating technique is the need to turn the ambient lights off to perform transillumination through the neck tissues. Furthermore, this procedure can prove challenging, if not impossible, in a patient with a short or excessively large, thick neck or darkly pigmented skin. It can prove equally difficult in a patient with a thin neck because esophageal entry can look bright on transillumination and can be misleading. Although generally safe, this technique may cause blunt trauma to the airway and, less frequently, heat damage from the light source.

Indirect Laryngoscopy

Another procedure that has gained popularity among clinicians is indirect laryngoscopy. Indirect laryngoscopy devices rely on lenses, mirrors, or fiberoptic technology to obtain a clear view of the glottic opening and cords. Many of these devices have an optional attached video camera, which can be a useful aid for teaching airway anatomy and intubation skills. One of the first indirect, rigid fiberoptic laryngoscopes was the Bullard scope, an anatomically shaped device with a curved blade on the end and a fiberoptic bundle that allows visualization of the glottis without alignment of the oropharynx with the larynx (Fig. 5.45). The Bullard scope has a built-in adjustable focusing system, suction port, and an introducing stylet. The fiberoptic bundle allows visualization of the cords and placement of the ETT under direct visualization. This device has proven useful for patients with temporomandibular

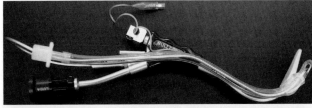

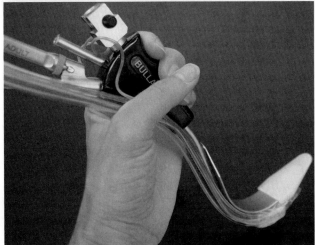

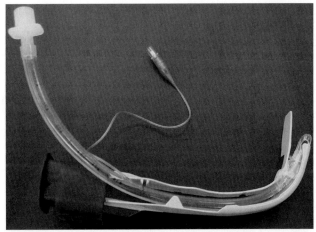

FIGURE 5.47 The Airtraq is a battery-operated, disposable device for indirect laryngoscopy.

FIGURE 5.45 The Bullard scope is used for indirect laryngoscopy.

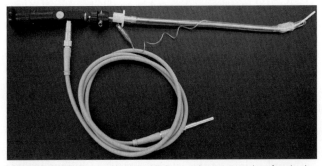

FIGURE 5.46 The optical stylet is another example of a device used for indirect laryngoscopy.

immobility, micrognathia, and an anterior larynx. Because it requires less neck movement than direct laryngoscopy, it also has been helpful in patients with cervical spine instability.[37] Other rigid fiberoptic laryngoscopes include the WuScope and Upsherscope, which are variations of the Bullard scope.

A simpler, rigid fiberoptic stylet, often called the *optical stylet* or Bonfils, consists of an anatomically shaped tube with a light on the distal end and an adjustable eyepiece proximally (Fig. 5.46). An ETT can be mounted on the tube and advanced into the airway under fiberoptic guidance once the stylet is advanced into the airway. Like the Bullard scope, the optical stylet allows visualization of the larynx without requiring alignment of the various axes of the airway.

A myriad of optical indirect laryngoscopes allow visualization of the airway but do not rely on fiberoptics for visibility. The Airtraq (Prodol Meditec) (Fig. 5.47) is an example of a battery-operated, disposable device that provides an angular, mirrored, magnified view during the laryngoscopic procedure. It consists of one optical channel and a guiding channel for ETT placement. As with the Bullard scope, this device is beneficial in patients with minimal mouth opening (18 mm is necessary), an unstable cervical spine, and an anterior larynx.

Video Laryngoscopes

Video laryngoscopes, which combine indirect laryngoscopy with a mounted video camera, are becoming increasingly popular for use in the anticipated difficult airway, and multiple studies demonstrate that they afford superior views of the glottis compared to direct laryngoscopy.[38-39] Additional benefits include decreased movement of the cervical spine, which can offer advantages, especially in emergent airway management of the patient with unknown cervical stability.[40-41] There are a number of different video laryngoscopes on the market, and they differ in their various features, including portability, reusability, USB port access, channel for ETT placement, and antifog features.

The GlideScope (Verathon Medical) is an example of a video laryngoscope that comes in either a reusable or single-use form. The operator places a rigid, curved blade resembling a Macintosh blade into the mouth of the patient, and the ETT can be placed under direct visualization by a digital video camera near the end of the blade.

Maintaining a clear view with all these devices is mandatory, and blood and excessive secretions reduce their success rates. Experience is a primary determinant of success, and the devices with cameras may offer better opportunities in learning environments where both the anesthesiologist and resident can view the image at the same time.

The King Vision (Ambu) is a lightweight, battery-powered, portable video laryngoscope that can be easily carried in an emergency airway bag or by EMT personnel. The video display is mounted at the base of the laryngoscope handle for easy visualization during manipulation. The King Vision offers two different blade choices: a standard blade that requires the use of a stylet and a channeled blade that allows for guidance of the ETT from the end of the blade. The blade covers are

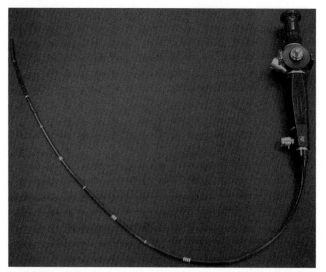

FIGURE 5.48 A flexible fiberoptic bronchoscope is useful for intubation in an awake patient known to have a difficult airway.

disposable and low cost, making it a practical and portable option for clinicians.

The C-MAC system (Karl Storz) is another USB video laryngoscope. The C-MAC combines the optics of Karl Storz bronchoscopes (discussed in the next section) and a video laryngoscope into a portable, single unit. The user can switch between a video laryngoscope with disposable blade and a bronchoscope quickly and easily if necessary. Both the blades and the bronchoscopes come in a variety of sizes, including pediatric sizes.

Flexible Fiberoptic Bronchoscopy

Flexible fiberoptic bronchoscopy generally is considered the gold standard for intubation of a patient known to have a difficult airway or an unstable cervical spine. Laryngoscopy with a flexible fiberoptic bronchoscope allows ETT insertion under laryngeal visualization using the scope as a guide for the ETT (Fig. 5.48). The ETT is threaded over the scope before endoscopy and need only be advanced off the scope once the bronchoscope enters the airway. After airway entry with the scope is confirmed visually, the tube can be advanced over the scope and into the trachea. Because the scope is smaller than the ETT, the tube may need to be rotated gently to allow passage between the vocal cords and into the trachea. The fiberoptic technique can be used for either oral or nasal intubations. Indications include a history or suspicion of difficult intubation, cervical spine instability or inability to move the cervical spine, anatomical abnormalities, and also ETT placement conformation and assessment. Contraindications to the use of this device include lack of skill or training in its use, inability to maintain oxygenation in the patient during the procedure, and significant bleeding or upper airway debris that blocks visualization. In addition, the fiberoptic bronchoscope is expensive and prone to damage without careful handling. Skill and practice in fiberoptic examination of patients is a prerequisite for use of this technique (Clinical Scenario 5.2). Fiberoptic intubation can be performed in awake,

anesthetized, or comatose patients. During intubation of an alert patient, complete topical anesthesia is needed to prevent hemodynamic consequences, including coughing, bronchospasm, and laryngospasm. Forms of topical anesthesia include nebulized lidocaine, spraying or gargling local anesthetics, and various nerve blocks that anesthetize the tongue, pharynx, and trachea.

Retrograde Wire Intubation

The retrograde wire intubation technique is another method of placing an ETT with the added benefit of not requiring manipulation of the cervical spine. Because this technique takes several minutes or longer, it should not be performed on a patient who is acutely hypoxic. The retrograde wire technique requires a thin-walled needle or an intravenous (IV) catheter-over-a-needle device, a guidewire, and forceps. The IV catheter (or needle) should be placed through the cricothyroid membrane directed in a cephalad direction and the needle withdrawn, leaving the catheter in the trachea. The guidewire is then advanced through the catheter in a cephalad direction until it can be retrieved through the nose or mouth. The wire should be pulled taut, and the ETT should be passed over the guidewire either orally or nasally and advanced into the trachea. Once the ETT is in the trachea, the guidewire should be removed, and ETT placement should be confirmed using one or more of the techniques described earlier (Fig. 5.49).

Complications of the retrograde wire technique include failure to establish an airway, bleeding or hematoma at the needle puncture site, subcutaneous emphysema at the needle puncture site, laryngospasm, pneumothorax, and cord damage. Although this is a viable technique in a controlled situation, it takes more time than other techniques and requires practice to perform quickly and successfully. A kit with all the required components is available commercially and includes a wire stiffener to help advance the ETT.

Airway Ultrasonography

Ultrasonography of the airway is emerging as a means by which one can evaluate an airway as well as a tool in assisting with intubation and predicting difficult intubation as described earlier. Although the tongue, oropharynx, epiglottis, larynx, true and false vocal cords, cricoid cartilage, cricothyroid membrane, and anterior trachea may be easily visualized, the posterior pharynx, posterior commissure, and posterior wall of the trachea are difficult to see due to artifacts from intratracheal air.[42] Indeed, ultrasonography has been shown to be comparable to computed tomography (CT) in visualization of airway

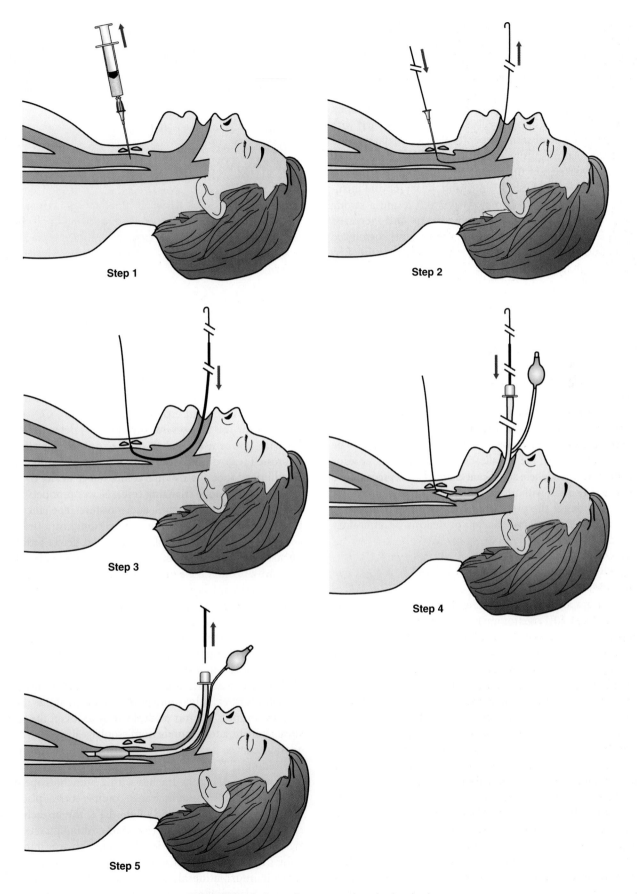

Step 1

Step 2

Step 3

Step 4

Step 5

FIGURE 5.49 Steps in retrograde wire intubation.

structures as well as in quantification of nearly all airway structure dimensions, including suprahyoid and infrahyoid measurements.[43] Pinto et al. found a statistically significant correlation between difficult laryngoscopy and an increase in the distance between the skin and the epiglottis at the level of the thyrohyoid membrane measured using ultrasonography. This correlation was improved when it was combined with modified Mallampati examination.[44] Likewise, Adkikari et al.[45] showed a relationship between difficult laryngoscopy and increased thickness of the soft tissue at both the level of the hyoid bone (16.9 mm vs. 13.7 mm) and the thyrohyoid membrane (34.7 mm vs. 23.7 mm). Wu el al.[46] found a strong correlation between difficult laryngoscopy and increased anterior soft tissue measurements at the hyoid bone, thyrohyoid membrane, and at the level of the anterior commissure. Ezri et al. looked specifically at the use of ultrasonography to evaluate the airway in obese patients. They found that an increased anterior soft tissue measurement at both the vocal cords (28 mm vs. 17.5 mm) as well as at the suprasternal notch (33 mm vs. 27.4 mm) was associated with difficult laryngoscopy in obese patients.[47] In addition to measurements of soft tissue, Hui and Tsui examined the use of sublingual ultrasonography to predict difficult airways. The inability to view the hyoid bone with sublingual ultrasonography was associated with more difficult laryngoscopic view. They found that sublingual ultrasonography had a 75% sensitivity and 97% specificity for predicting difficult airways.[48] Ultrasonography can also be particularly useful in the visualization of neck masses for signs of airway invasion where significant changes from preoperative CT scan may occur with tumor growth. Ultrasonography may be used to detect the presence of subglottic hemangiomas, pharyngeal pouches, laryngeal cysts or stenosis, or respiratory papillomatosis.[49]

Determining Correct Endotracheal Tube or Tracheostomy Size

Ultrasonography of the upper airway can be useful in estimating the proper ETT size for a particular patient. Ultrasonography of the subglottic area in children and young adults correlates well with magnetic resonance imaging measurements used to determine the appropriate size for endotracheal or tracheostomy tubes.[50-51] In the case of lung surgery, ultrasonography of the outer diameter of the trachea above the sternoclavicular joint can be used to estimate the diameter of the left mainstem bronchus and correlates with CT and chest x-ray examination measurements.[52] The diameter of the left mainstem bronchus helps guide clinicians in choosing the correct size of double-lumen ETT to place.

XI. CONFIRMATION OF TRACHEAL INTUBATION

Objective confirmation of tracheal placement, rather than esophageal intubation, is imperative. This is especially true after intubation using a blind technique. In addition to auscultation of the chest and confirmatory chest x-ray examination, the most sensitive way to immediately confirm correct

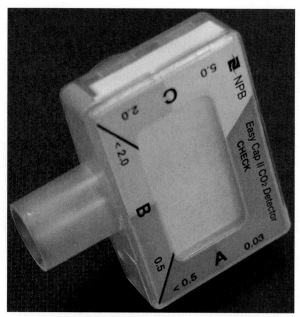

FIGURE 5.50 Calorimetric capnometer.

placement is to detect expired CO_2 with a capnograph or a color-change capnometry device like the one shown in Fig. 5.50. Even during an esophageal intubation, CO_2 may be detected for the first several breaths. CO_2 detection devices also are not as useful when cardiac output is profoundly depressed (e.g., during chest compressions for cardiac arrest). In addition, once a traditional color-change device or capnogram is wet, it stops changing color. Newer products include 24-hour capnogram devices and moisture-repellant devices that maintain function despite 100% humidity.

A syringe or bulb can also be used to detect esophageal versus tracheal intubation. With this technique, because of negative pressure, the syringe or rubber bulb expands if the ETT is in the trachea, but it remains collapsed if the ETT is in the esophagus (Fig. 5.51). The primary advantage of this technique is that it does not depend on cardiac function or CO_2 delivery to the lungs to confirm correct tube placement. False-positive and false-negative results have been reported with this device in obese and pregnant patients. Auscultation should be performed in at least three areas after intubation. Auscultatory examination should reveal bilateral thoracic breath sounds but no audible sounds over the gastric area. Unfortunately, sounds from esophageal and gastric ventilation can be heard transmitted to the chest and may be misleading.

Directly viewing the trachea with a bronchoscope passed through the ETT is another way to confirm correct placement. After exiting the distal end of the ETT, the bronchoscope should be above the carina (Fig. 5.52). Although chest radiography (anteroposterior view) is useful for determining the tube depth in the chest relative to the carina, it does not provide information about the appropriate location in the trachea. A lateral film can identify tracheal rather than esophageal placement, but the other techniques described give more rapid feedback on incorrect placement in enough time to

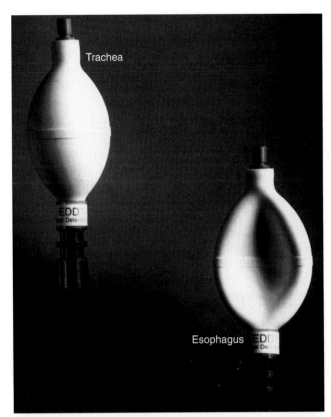

FIGURE 5.51 An esophageal detection device is another means of detecting tracheal or esophageal intubation. (Courtesy ARC Medical, Tucker, GA.)

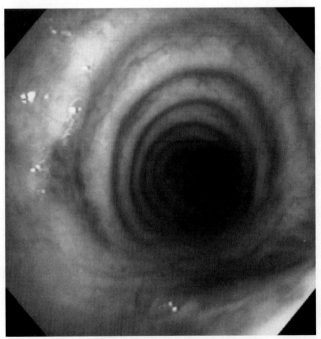

FIGURE 5.52 Bronchoscopic view of the trachea.

prevent disaster (Clinical Scenario 5.3). Other indications that the ETT is in the trachea include seeing the chest rise and condensation in the tube with each breath. The ETT cuff can also be palpated in the trachea in thinner patients during rapid inflation.

In addition to its utility in the evaluation of difficult airways, ultrasonography can also be useful to confirm ETT placement if capnography is unavailable or thought to be inadequate, as with circulatory arrest. Placing the ultrasound probe at the level of the cricoid cartilage and directing the probe cranially 45 degrees or transversely superior to the suprasternal notch, passage of the ETT into the trachea can be visualized as a "flutter" deep to the thyroid cartilage. Esophageal intubation using the same ultrasonographic methods appears as a hyperechoic line deep to the trachea.[53,54] Esophageal intubation may also be confirmed by visualizing ventilation with lung ultrasonography of the third and fourth intercostal spaces. Lung sliding should be seen bilaterally if the tube is located in the trachea.[55] Endobronchial intubation should be suspected if lung sliding is seen on one side and absent on the other side.[56] The absence of lung sliding on both sides is consistent with esophageal intubation. The ability to diagnose an esophageal intubation quickly is important to avoid additional harm. Pfeiffer et al. found the use of ultrasonography in experienced providers to confirm endotracheal intubation was as fast as auscultation alone and faster than combined ausculatation and capnography, suggesting it may be superior to these methods in quickly diagnosing inadvertent esophageal intubation.[54] Transverse ultrasonography of the neck may additionally be used to determine the correct position of an LMA cuff. Ultrasonography correlates with fiberoptic visualization of LMA position. Ultrasonography can be useful in ill-seated LMAs to diagnose the cause of a potential leak and poor ventilation when an LMA is in place.[57,58]

If ETTs are inserted or migrate too far into the trachea, the cuff may obstruct a bronchus, or only one lung may be ventilated inadvertently. Right mainstem intubation is most common because the angle of takeoff of the right main bronchus is less than that of the left. This is especially common in children because the distance between the glottis and the carina is small.

XII. SPECIALIZED ENDOTRACHEAL TUBES

Sometimes the need arises to provide selective ventilation to a single lung or a different kind of ventilatory support to each lung. Specialized ETTs that allow independent lung ventilation are available. These tubes were developed for bronchoalveolar lavage (to treat alveolar proteinosis) and for performing differential lung function tests before a pneumonectomy. They have been refined and frequently are used to improve surgical exposure and reduce risks during anesthesia for lung surgery or resection. Sometimes a double-lumen endotracheal tube

(DLT) is used outside the operating room to protect the "good," or healthy, lung from blood contamination, as in patients with massive hemoptysis or infection from an empyema (Fig. 5.53). They may also be useful in patients with a bronchopleural fistula. Probably the most common use of these devices outside the operating room is after single-lung transplantation, when the compliance of the native lung and that of the transplanted lung are very different. Two ventilator systems can be used to titrate the appropriate support for each lung independently. More detail about DLTs is available on the Evolve website.

Other specialized ETTs have additional distal airway channels. One is the Hi-Lo Jet ETT, in which the additional lumen can be used for distal airway pressure monitoring during jet ventilation (Fig. 5.54). Another specialized ETT has a lumen designed for tracheal drug delivery (Fig. 5.55). Recognition that aspiration of small amounts of infective oral secretions into the lung around the ETT cuff plays a role in the development of ventilator-associated pneumonia (VAP) has led to the production of a specialized ETT with a large suction port opening above the cuff (Fig. 5.56). Using this ETT, removal

of subglottic secretions with continuous or intermittent aspiration through the suction lumen reduces the risk for VAP. Use of this specialized ETT is recommended to help reduce nosocomial pneumonia in patients requiring prolonged translaryngeal intubation.

XIII. SURGICAL AIRWAY DEVICES

On rare occasions, establishment of a patent airway with the previously described techniques (i.e., head position, oral and nasal airways, LMA, and Combitube) is unsuccessful. If the patient cannot be ventilated at all with a mask and an airway cannot be secured, invasive airway access should be established quickly to prevent hypoxia, cardiovascular compromise or collapse, and anoxic brain or organ injury. (Historical Note 5.2 presents a description of the first surgical airways.) The

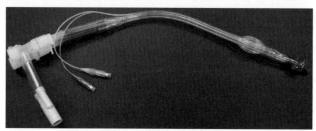

FIGURE 5.53 Double-lumen endotracheal tube (DLT) used for lung isolation.

> **HISTORICAL NOTE 5.2** **History of Tracheostomy**[59]
>
> - As early as 2000 BC, the Rgveda described a healed tracheostomy incision.
> - Around 400 BC, Hippocrates condemned tracheostomy because of the risk to the carotid arteries.
> - In 1546, Brasavola became the first person known to perform a tracheostomy for tonsillar obstruction.
> - In the 17th century, tracheostomy became lifesaving and honored as a procedure to be performed in patients with severe diphtheria.
> - Lorenz Heister coined the term *tracheotomy* in 1718 as a substitute for laryngotomy or bronchotomy.

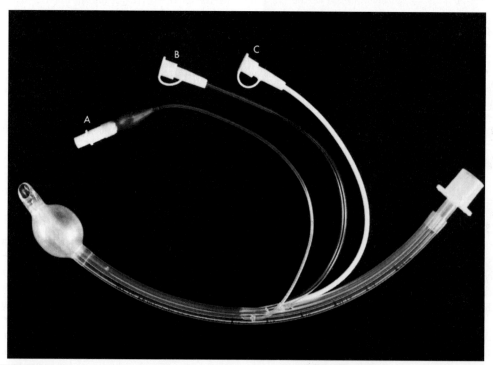

FIGURE 5.54 An endotracheal tube (ETT) with multiple lumens for jet ventilation and airway pressure measurement. (Courtesy Cardinal Health Respiratory Care Products and Services, Dublin, OH.)

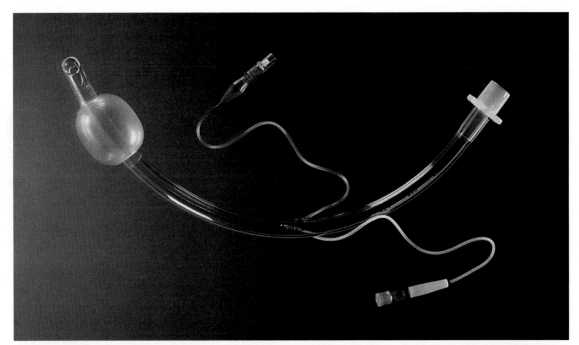

FIGURE 5.55 An endotracheal tube (ETT) with an additional port to be used for the instillation of medications. (Courtesy Cardinal Health Respiratory Care Products and Services, Dublin, OH.)

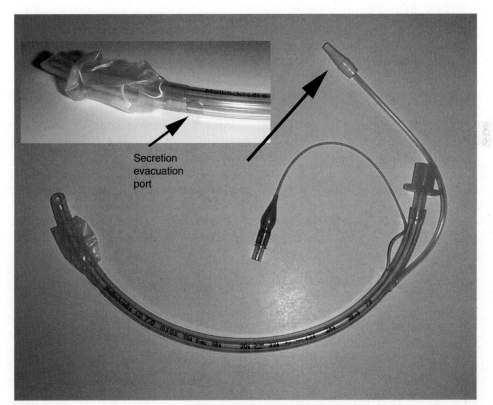

Secretion
evacuation
port

FIGURE 5.56 The Hi-Lo Evac tube has a portal for suctioning subglottic secretions and is used as part of a program to reduce the incidence of ventilator-associated pneumonia in intubated patients.

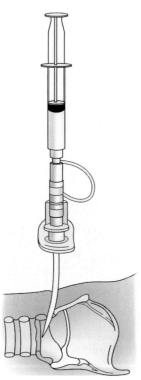

FIGURE 5.57 Transtracheal jet ventilation can be performed through a large-bore intravenous catheter or a special tracheal entry device placed through the cricothyroid membrane or trachea.

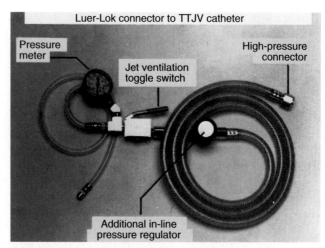

FIGURE 5.58 High-pressure jet ventilator system. *TTJV,* Transtracheal jet ventilation. (From Benumof JL: *Airway management: principles and practice,* St. Louis, 1996, Mosby.)

simplest invasive airway device is a large-bore IV catheter inserted percutaneously through the cricothyroid membrane (a procedure known as a needle cricothyroidotomy). The cricothyroid membrane is an easily identified space between the thyroid cartilage and the cricoid ring. A 14-gauge or larger catheter over a needle IV device is attached to a syringe and inserted through the cricothyroid membrane at a slightly caudad direction. Continuous aspiration is applied to the syringe until air or bubbles are aspirated, a sign that the needle has entered the trachea. The catheter then is advanced off the needle into the trachea in a caudad direction. Fig. 5.57 shows the position of the catheter. To provide adequate gas delivery through a tracheal needle, a high-pressure gas source (50 pounds per square inch [psi]) must be used. A pressure interrupter or Saunders valve (Fig. 5.58) is attached to the catheter with a Luer-Lok system to prevent disconnection from the catheter during ventilation. Expiration is passive and occurs through the upper airway. With brief jets of gas and intermittent pauses to allow for passive exhalation, ventilation and oxygenation can be maintained with this technique. It must be kept in mind, however, that the patient will become hypercarbic with time, and a needle cricothyroidotomy is merely a temporizing measure. With complete apnea, CO_2 rises approximately 2 to 3 mm Hg every minute.

It is important to use caution with the bursts of high-pressure gas to minimize the risk for barotrauma. The amount of pressure delivered should be enough to cause the chest to rise and to maintain oxygenation. If a high-pressure system is unavailable, the catheter can be connected to a plungerless

3-mL syringe, which can then be adapted to fit with the tube connector of a size 7 ETT. This can be used in an emergency, and the patient can be ventilated by hand for a short time while an alternative ventilation method is established. For successful emergency use the appropriate equipment must be assembled and ready for use ahead of time. Complications of catheter–jet ventilation include formation of a false passage into subcutaneous tissue, development of subcutaneous emphysema, pneumothorax, bleeding, failure to ventilate, and damage to neck structures.

A cricothyroidotomy is a surgical incision into the trachea that passes through the cricothyroid membrane. A conventional ETT or TT can be placed through the incision. Routine airway equipment can then be used to provide ventilation and oxygenation with the tube in place. A single, horizontal slash incision through the skin all the way to the trachea is placed. In an adult a small, uncuffed ETT or TT (5 mm) may be placed through the wound into the trachea to allow for the smallest surgical incision to minimize bleeding and to prevent potential damage to the trachea from scarring or stenosis. If there is a significant gas leak around the tube through the cricothyroid incision, it can be reduced by packing the wound with sterile Vaseline gauze. Bleeding usually is minimal because no large vascular structures lie in the area of the incision. Complications of cricothyroidotomy include false placement and failure to provide adequate gas exchange, bleeding, infection, and damage to other neck structures. Subglottic or laryngeal stenosis may be a long-term problem after cricothyroidotomy. Most authorities suggest elective conversion of an emergency cricothyroidotomy to a formal tracheostomy within 24 hours to reduce the likelihood of these severe problems. Cricothyroidotomy is not recommended for infants or small children because of a higher frequency of more severe complications.

To improve the ease, speed, and safety of performing an emergency cricothyroidotomy, several self-contained percutaneous devices have been developed. In general, these consist of a needle to enter the trachea through the cricothyroid membrane, a wire to guide the stoma creation, and a dilator or cutting device to open the stoma combined with a small TT.[60] Although use of these devices in an airway emergency is intuitively attractive, the device must be immediately available, and the user must have been previously trained if successful placement and patient survival are to be achieved. Practice on models before clinical use is essential to build confidence in the provider and to achieve success in practice because expert manual airway management using simple devices and needle cricothyroidotomy is more likely to save a life than a complex, specialized device used under duress for the first time in a human.

Although not considered an emergency airway technique, percutaneous dilatory tracheostomy (PDT) has become a common means of providing direct tracheal access for long-term airway management. Because of its effectiveness, simplicity, and relatively low incidence of complications, this technique for placement of a TT is often performed in the intensive care unit. Recently PDT has become accepted as an alternative means of securing an emergency airway.

PDT can be performed by several different methods. The most common is the Ciaglia method, in which a guidewire is placed between the first and second or second and third tracheal rings, and a series of stiff, plastic, tapered dilators is pushed through and compresses the soft tissues and the tracheal wall over the wire until an opening of sufficient size to accommodate the desired TT is created. PDT is typically performed on an anesthetized or a comatose patient and can be done in the intensive care unit or the operating room. It is worth mentioning that PDT requires some neck extension (a concern with the trauma patient) and is a sterile procedure.

Although some clinicians continue to perform PDT with blind entry into the trachea, most have adopted a technique of observing and directing needle and wire placement using fiberoptic bronchoscopy.[61] This may help prevent inadvertent injury of the membranous tracheal (posterior) wall or placing the tracheostomy too laterally.[62] A respiratory therapist often is requested to assist with the bronchoscopy and sometimes to administer sedative medications (in jurisdictions where the scope of practice laws and demonstrated competence allow). To allow visualization of the upper rings of the trachea with the bronchoscope, the ETT must be withdrawn until the tip rests in the larynx. This creates a significant gas leak during ventilation, because the ETT cuff is no longer in the trachea. Patients experiencing severe hypoxic respiratory failure may deteriorate during this time and may benefit from conversion to open surgical tracheostomy rather than persistence with attempting PDT.

In patients who require a tracheostomy only for airway access or protection, an LMA often can replace the ETT to provide the route for bronchoscopic visualization. The view of the larynx is unhampered when bronchoscopy is performed using an LMA, allowing for accurate identification of the tracheal anatomy. The bronchoscopic view of wire placement shown in Fig. 5.59 was obtained this way.

Griggs et al.[63] developed an alternative to the sequential dilator technique. Their technique uses a tracheal spreader

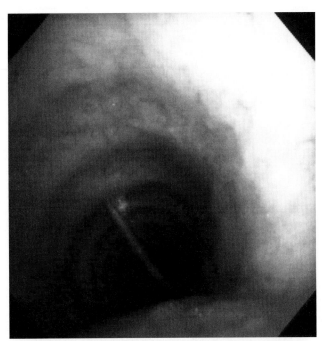

FIGURE 5.59 Wire is placed in the trachea in preparation for percutaneous dilatory tracheostomy.

modified to thread over the wire and a cutting forceps to create the skin path and tracheal stoma. As with the Ciaglia technique, the trachea is entered between the appropriate tracheal rings with an IV catheter. Aspiration of air confirms tracheal entry. Bronchoscopy can also be used to assist with correct placement. Note that the risk for tracheal injury is higher with this technique than with the other PDT techniques, especially if the procedure is performed without bronchoscopy.

The Blue Rhino dilator is a single, tapered dilator that is used instead of the sequential dilators of the Ciaglia method (Fig. 5.60).[64] It has a lubricated coating that makes insertion very easy. It is softer and therefore may be less likely to damage the membranous tracheal wall. Because only a single dilator must be passed, insertion of the tracheal tube is accomplished more quickly.[65] Unfortunately, a significant amount of downward force is required to advance the stomal dilators and TT. This pressure often collapses the trachea and occasionally fractures a tracheal ring. The long-term significance of ring fracture is not known, but it has sometimes caused airway obstruction after decannulation.

As stated, PDT has been used as a technique for establishing an emergency airway. Divatia et al.[66] reported a patient who self-extubated but could not be intubated or ventilated. They used a needle cricothyroidotomy to maintain oxygenation initially. After tracheal entry with a needle and high-pressure oxygen insufflation, a second needle was placed, followed by the guidewire, stomal dilator, and TT. With appropriate experience, PDT is likely to be more rapidly successful than a surgical tracheostomy in patients requiring emergency surgical airways.[67]

Ultrasonography has emerged as an adjunct to the surgical airway because anatomical identification of the cricothyroid and thyroid membranes can be particularly challenging in the

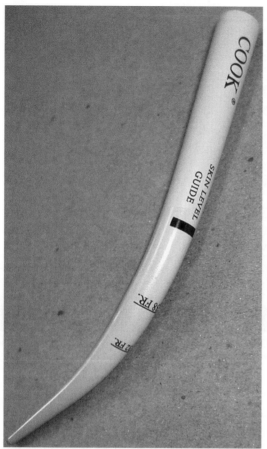

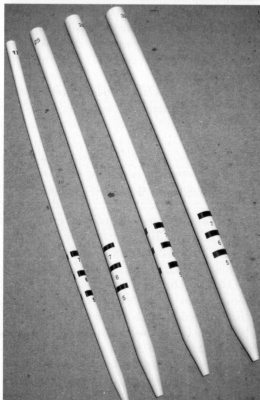

FIGURE 5.60 The Blue Rhino dilator is a single tapered dilator used for percutaneous dilation *(top figure)* in place of the sequential dilator described by Ciaglia *(bottom figure)*.

obese or in patients with pathology leading to abnormal anatomy or tracheal deviation (masses, prior radiation, prior surgery).[68] Even in patients with normal anatomy, palpation and landmark techniques may correctly identify the cricothyroid membrane in only approximately 30% of patients by anesthesiologists.[69] Airway ultrasonography can be particularly useful to quickly and reliably identify both the cricothyroid and thyroid cartilage when abnormal anatomy is encountered either electively in the case of a difficult airway or especially in an emergent situation. The cricothyroid membrane can be visualized by placing an ultrasound probe transversely and scanning until the cricothyroid membrane is visualized as an echogenic structure with surrounding cricothyroid muscle.[70] Once the cricothyroid membrane is located, percutaneous cricothyroidotomy may be achieved using a standard kit. Ultrasonography can also be used for correct placement of percutaneous dilatational tracheostomies via localization of the anterior wall of the trachea, intercartilaginous space, and surrounding structures.[71] The use of ultrasonography is associated with a decrease in cannula misplacement compared with landmark-based techniques.[72] Ultrasonography may also be useful in determining the correct size of the puncture cannula as well as length of the tracheostomy cannula.[73]

XIV. TRACHEOSTOMY TUBES

Similar to an ETT, a TT consists of a round, plastic tube—with or without a cuff, pilot balloon, and valve—with a standard 15-mm connector. Metal TTs (Jackson tubes) are sometimes used to maintain a patent stoma and to allow for suctioning and for the size of the stoma to be gradually reduced. These tubes are rarely equipped with a cuff and need adapters to be mated with standard airway equipment. TTs are bent at approximately a 90-degree angle to fit flat against the skin and lie parallel to the axis of the trachea. As with ETTs, TT sizes are assigned as the ID in millimeters, although the use of French sizes is still popular. TTs generally are more rigid than ETTs, although some are flexible. TTs are now available that are less likely to kink and must be carefully selected to fit the patient correctly. TTs typically have a collar that is used to secure the tube. There is no universal standard for manufacturing TTs, and individual tube geometry varies by manufacturer. The distance from the collar to the bend, the length of the tube distal to the bend (Fig. 5.61), and the size and shape of the cuff vary by manufacturer and may be quite different. Some tubes have movable collars that accommodate different skin-to-trachea distances. The standard adapter may be part of a removable connector or inner cannula.

TTs usually are supplied with the lumen occluded with a blunt, solid obturator that makes passage through the tissues less traumatic. The obturator is removed after the tube is in place but should remain with the patient and should be conveniently available for reinsertion in the TT if it is accidentally dislodged. Some surgeons place strong tagging sutures at the corners of the tracheal incision that can be grasped and pulled forward to expose the tract and facilitate reinsertion of a displaced TT. If ventilation is found to be difficult after urgent

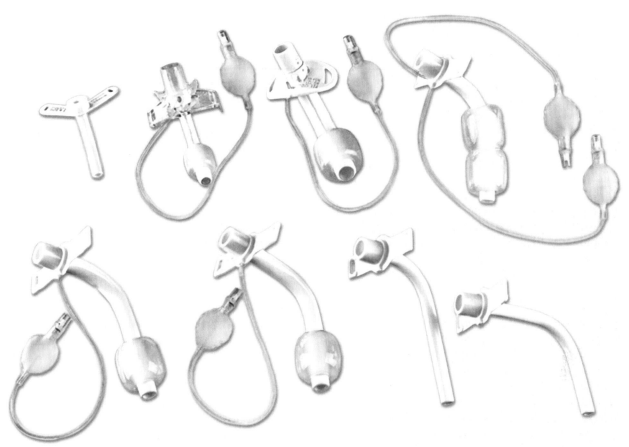

FIGURE 5.61 Tracheostomy tubes (TTs) come in preformed shapes with lengths that are not standardized. TTs are bent at approximately a 90-degree angle to fit flat against the skin and lie parallel to the axis of the trachea. A solid obturator is usually supplied for occluding the lumen to make passage through the tissues less traumatic. (Courtesy Medtronic Minimally Invasive Therapies, Boulder, CO.)

replacement of a dislodged TT, the problem may be that the TT is not in the trachea and is instead in a false passage. **If this occurs, manual ventilation through the upper airway should be initiated without delay.** TT cuffs come in various sizes and, as with ETT cuffs, can cause mucosal ischemia if overpressurized (i.e., cuff pressure should not exceed 25 cm H_2O). Cuff pressure monitoring and low-pressure cuff design are methods of reducing complications associated with the maintenance of TTs.

Another device used to maintain a tracheostomy stoma is the tracheal button (Fig. 5.62). It protrudes slightly into the airway but usually is less obstructive than a small TT. It usually is kept capped or plugged unless airway access is needed. Of note, it cannot be effectively used to provide positive-pressure ventilation, but it can be exchanged for a cuffed TT if necessary.

XV. POSITIONING ADJUVANTS

As discussed earlier, the importance of good patient positioning before attempted intubation or airway manipulation cannot be stressed enough. Because successful airway management is often dependent on maximizing patient position, several positioning products are available. One of the most commonly

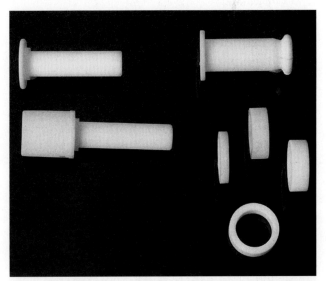

FIGURE 5.62 Olympic tracheostomy button.

used is the Troop Elevation Pillow (Mercury Medical). The Troop pillow provides patients and providers with the head elevated laryngoscopy position (HELP). It is most helpful in morbidly obese patients and establishes a position that maximizes alignment of the oropharyngeal axis. In addition, it is helpful in the obese, awake patient because it allows the patient to breathe more comfortably and helps to unload the weight of a large chest from the lungs.

XVI. EQUIPMENT USED TO MANAGE ARTIFICIAL AIRWAYS

Airflow to patients who have been intubated or those with TTs bypasses the nasopharynx and oropharynx during respirations. Humidifying and warming of inspired gases are primary functions of the upper airway. Active or passive humidification systems should be used in patients with ETTs or TTs for a prolonged period. Fig. 5.63 shows a passive humidification system. (Chapter 6 presents a more detailed description of humidification systems available for patients with artificial airways.) Even with these devices, airway secretions may be increased because of tracheal irritation and thickened as a result of inadequate humidification or infection. In addition to the lack of humidification, the ability to cough is severely compromised because the glottis cannot be closed when the patient is intubated. Secretions must be aspirated from the lung in most intubated patients. Suction catheters are illustrated in Fig. 5.64A. Suction catheters are available in a variety of sizes and designs; however, the general recommendation is that the catheter diameter should be no more than half the ID of the artificial airway. It is important to recognize that suction catheters are sized according to the tube's circumference (i.e., French size). The tube's inner diameter can be converted to the catheter's circumference, or French size, by multiplying the ID by 3 (actually 3.14, or *pi*). The appropriate catheter size for the tube can then be determined by dividing the product by 2. For example, a size 8 (ID) TT requires a 12-Fr catheter.

$$(8 \times 3) \div 2 = 12\,Fr$$

Preoxygenation, sterile preparation, and standard infection precautions should be used during endotracheal suctioning. In-line closed-system suction devices (see Fig. 5.64B) may reduce the caregiver's and patient's risk for exposure to infectious disease, lower costs, and compromise ventilation less during suctioning. Sterile sputum samples can be obtained using a Lukens sputum trap (Fig. 5.65). Care must be taken during suctioning to prevent mucosal trauma and injury.

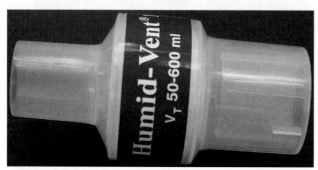

FIGURE 5.63 The Humid-Vent is a passive humidification system. (Courtesy Hudson RCI/Teleflex, Research Triangle Park, NC.)

Many devices have been developed to help secure ETTs and TTs. Effective methods of securing these tubes are especially important in children. In addition to tube holders and securing devices, judicious use of sedation and physical restraints is important for the comfort and safety of the intubated patient and to prevent inadvertent extubation.

Changing an ETT may pose significant risk to critically ill patients. A tube exchanger designed specifically for this purpose is shown in Fig. 5.66. The tube exchanger is inserted through the ETT, and the tube is withdrawn and removed. Oxygen can be insufflated through the tube exchanger during the procedure. A new ETT can be slipped over the tube exchanger and threaded down into the trachea. Sometimes the new tube may catch on the vocal cords or larynx and may need to be gently rotated into position. ETT exchange using a tube exchange device is not always successful, and equipment for primary reintubation must be on hand.

A common indication of the need to change a tube is failure of the cuff to hold pressure. If the pilot balloon does not hold pressure at all, the cuff is likely compromised. If the pilot balloon remains inflated and the tube transiently seals when more air is added but quickly develops a leak again, the cuff probably has herniated through the vocal cords. This can be remedied by deflating the cuff completely, advancing the ETT 2 to 3 cm, and reinflating the cuff. If the pilot balloon holds pressure while the syringe is attached but deflates when it is disconnected, the pilot tube valve probably is defective. This can be overcome by inserting a stopcock into the valve, inflating the cuff, and turning the stopcock off toward the cuff. The pilot balloon and valve can be replaced with a blunt needle, and the stopcock inserted into the pilot tube after the balloon has been cut off (Fig. 5.67). These methods of valve and pilot balloon repair may save patients the risk and trauma of reintubation.

XVII. COMPLICATIONS OF AIRWAY MANAGEMENT

Intubating patients is not a benign procedure, and the incidence of complications during intubation has been reported to be as high as 30%.[1] Complications from intubation can be conveniently grouped into traumatic and cardiorespiratory complications. Traumatic problems include damage to the teeth and soft tissues of the lips and mouth, vocal cord injury, laryngeal cartilage dislocation, and perforation or rupture of the pharynx, larynx, trachea, or esophagus. In addition, corneal abrasions or injuries to the face, eyes, or cervical spine may occur during attempted laryngoscopy. Cardiorespiratory complications include the hemodynamic consequences of intubation or placement of a foreign body in the trachea, such as hypertension, tachycardia, vagal reactions (bradycardia and fainting), and ventricular arrhythmias. Respiratory complications include hypoxia, hypercarbia, aspiration, laryngospasm, and bronchospasm. Increased intracranial and intraocular pressure may also occur during intubation.

Although modern materials are less toxic than the hard rubber from which ETTs and TTs originally were made, these

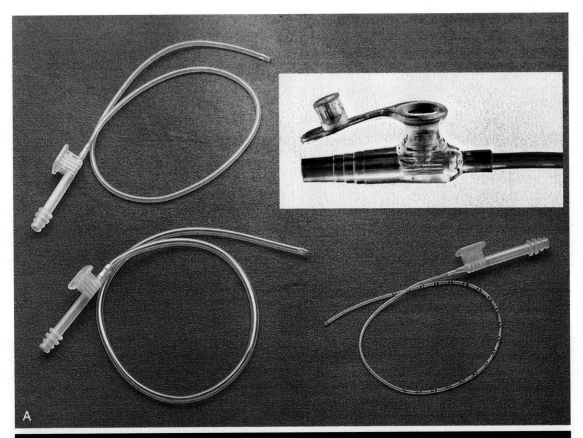

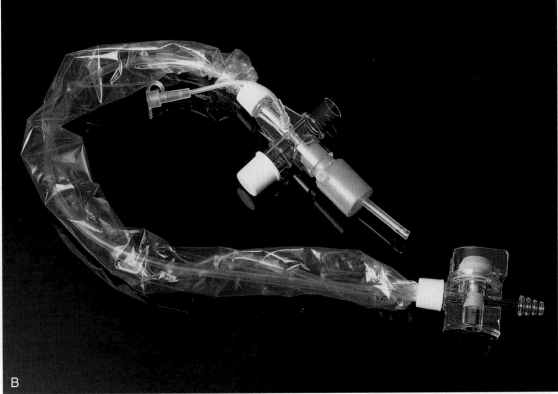

FIGURE 5.64 A, Types of suction catheters. B, Closed-system suction catheter. (A courtesy Cardinal Health Respiratory Care Products and Services, Dublin, OH.)

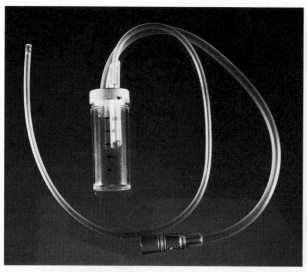

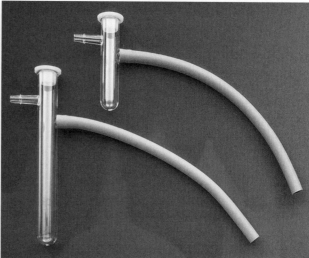

FIGURE 5.65 Uncontaminated sputum samples can be collected with a Lukens sputum trap. (Courtesy Cardinal Health Respiratory Care Products and Services, McGaw Park, IL.)

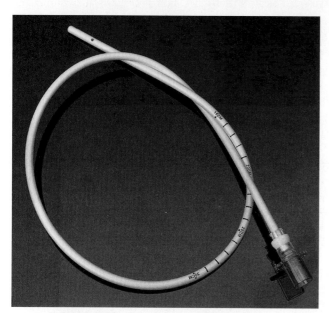

FIGURE 5.66 An endotracheal tube changer.

artificial airways can damage the structures through which they pass. TTs and ETTs can damage the larynx, as well as the trachea, from cuff pressure and tip trauma. TTs can cause damage at cuff and tip locations and at the tracheal stoma. Severe vocal cord damage and laryngeal stenosis are dreaded complications of translaryngeal intubation. These complications typically are difficult to treat and may permanently disable the patient. They increase with the duration of intubation and the larger diameter of the tube.

Long-term endotracheal intubation can lead to granuloma formation, mucosal ulceration or necrosis from high ETT cuff pressures, and vocal cord paralysis. Subglottic stenosis is another potential consequence of long-term intubation. If the need for tracheal intubation is predicted to exceed 1 to 2 weeks (in adults), a tracheostomy is often performed to reduce laryngeal complications. Trauma to the trachea from the tube cuff or

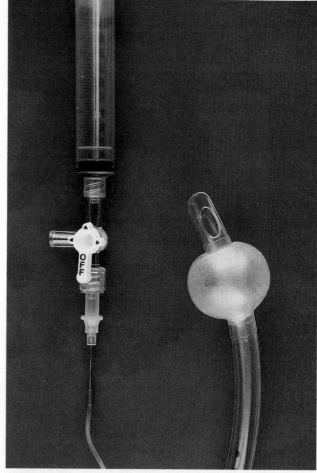

FIGURE 5.67 If the pilot balloon or pilot balloon valve fails to hold air, the entire assembly may be temporarily replaced by inserting a cut-off 19-gauge needle with a stopcock into the pilot tubing.

tip can result in ulcers, cartilage loss, tracheomalacia, or rupture, which are complications of both TTs and ETTs. Granulation tissue may form at the TT stoma; also, after removal of the TT, stenosis at the stomal site may occur in up to 10% of patients. Treatment of these complications is difficult and often requires resection of tracheal segments or placement of a stent.

XVIII. BASIC LIFE SUPPORT AND ADVANCED CARDIAC LIFE SUPPORT

Adult Basic Life Support

Periodically the AHA releases guidelines for both Basic Life Support and Advanced Cardiac Life Support to help to guide practitioners as well as lay rescuers in supportive care in the event of a cardiac arrest. In 2010 the AHA reoriented the traditional "A-B-C" sequence of resuscitation to "C-A-B," prioritizing circulation and chest compressions during basic life support (Box 5.4). In fact, the 2015 guidelines recommend untrained providers provide chest compression-only CPR for adults with suspected out-of-hospital circulatory arrest. Trained providers should provide 30 chest compressions followed by

---

> **BOX 5.4 Basic Life Support and Advanced Cardiac Life Support Techniques Updates**
>
> - Despite the importance of airway management in critically ill patients, in the event of a cardiac arrest, there have been changes to the long-standing "A-B-Cs" of resuscitation. The 2010 guidelines of the American Heart Association (AHA) now no longer recommend mouth-to-mouth ventilation during bystander cardiopulmonary resuscitation (CPR).
> - The emphasis is on restoration of circulation as the primary goal for CPR by providing chest compressions at a rate of 100 compressions per minute in a person who is found unresponsive and/or pulseless. In the hospital setting, mask ventilation or intubation can occur concomitantly, but CPR should NOT be stopped for airway management. The reasons for this are multifactorial. In the outpatient setting, it has been shown that bystanders can perform chest compressions more easily than mouth-to-mouth resuscitation and the intervention time is quicker if chest compressions are performed first. There is a significant delay in chest compressions if first responders attempt to provide two breaths. Second, patients with sudden collapse who have just been breathing typically have oxygen reserves that can be circulated with CPR alone. There are important distinctions in specific patient populations, and health care providers should certainly tailor their response and interventions to the likely cause of unresponsiveness. An example is a postoperative patient who is thought to have just suffered an apneic episode from a narcotic overdose. Establishing an airway and ventilating the patient are clearly the first priorities.

From Berg RA, Hemphill R, Abella BS, et al.: Part 5: Adult basic life support: 2010 American Heart Association guidelines for cardiopulmonary resuscitation and emergency cardiovascular care. *Circulation* 122(18 Suppl 3):S685-S705, 2010.

---

2 breaths until an advanced airway is in place, at which time CPR should not be interrupted, and instead 1 breath should be delivered every 6 seconds.[74-75]

In the most recent recommendations, the AHA again reemphasized high-quality chest compressions. Providers should perform chest compressions at a rate of 100 to 120/min at a depth of at least 2 in (5 cm) but not greater than 2.4 in. Components of high-quality CPR include adequate rate, adequate depth, allowing full recoil between chest compressions, minimizing interruptions, and avoiding excessive ventilation. If at all possible, there should be simultaneous chest compressions, airway management, rescue breathing, rhythm detection, medication administration, and shock delivery if warranted.[74-75]

Adult Advanced Cardiac Life Support

No high-quality evidence exists to support improved survival or neurological outcome with the use of an ETT when compared to bag-mask ventilation or supraglottic airway. In fact, several retrospective studies show worse outcomes with endotracheal intubation. Likewise, the use of a supraglottic airway has also not been shown to be superior to bag-mask ventilation. The 2015 ACLS guidelines recommend advanced airway placement only if the provider has the necessary training, skills, and experience to insert the airway and confirm position with minimal interruptions in CPR. The use of continuous wave capnography to confirm placement following endotracheal intubation remains a class I recommendation. Additionally, capnography can be used to evaluate resuscitative efforts because a low end-tidal carbon dioxide in intubated patients after 20 minutes of CPR was noted to be associated with inadequate resuscitation. Maximal inspired oxygen should be used during CPR because blood flow is the major limiting factor to oxygen delivery.[76]

Pediatric Life Support

Pediatric cardiac arrest is different in that the cause is much more likely to be hypoxic than a primary cardiac issue, as is seen in adults. Although no studies have examined the use of the C-A-B resuscitation versus the classic A-B-C, current recommendations from 2015 support the use of C-A-B to provide consistency and increase the effectiveness of bystander CPR. Chest compressions should be at least one-third of the anteroposterior depth of the chest (approximately 1.5 in or 4 cm) at a rate of 100 to 120/min. Once puberty has been reached, adult compression depth should be used. One breath should be delivered every 3 to 5 seconds. Unlike adults, in whom chest compression–only CPR may be adequate, many pediatric arrests are respiratory in nature. In children, compression-only CPR is associated with worse 30-day outcomes.[77,78]

Neonatal Resuscitation

Positive-pressure ventilation is the recommended treatment for preterm or term neonates with apnea. Positive-pressure ventilation can be delivered by a flow-inflating or self-inflating resuscitation bag or T-piece resuscitator. Laryngeal mask airways or endotracheal intubation may be considered when bag-mask ventilation is ineffective or prolonged. Of note, unlike adult and pediatric life support, neonatal resuscitation should be initiated with a low oxygen concentration (21% to 30%) unless cardiac arrest requiring chest compressions occurs to limit the potential negative effects of high oxygen concentrations in the neonate. Whenever possible, high oxygen concentrations should be titrated to minimize harm in neonates. Chest compressions should be delivered on the lower part of the sternum with a depth of approximately one-third of the anteroposterior diameter of the sternum. Compressions may be delivered with two thumbs with the fingers encircling the chest and supporting the back (the two-thumb technique) or with two fingers with a second hand supporting the back (the two-finger technique). The two-thumb technique is preferred by most clinicians because it can be delivered from the head of the bed. One breath should be delivered for every three compressions to maximize ventilation.[79]

KEY POINTS

- Inadequate gas exchange is an acute emergency. Failure to restore adequate respiratory gas exchange can result in hypoxic brain injury or death within minutes.
- An understanding of the normal airway anatomy is essential for effective airway maintenance.
- The incidence of difficult airway management and inadvertent esophageal intubation is significantly higher in the critical care setting than when intubation is performed in the operating room.
- Various devices, such as oral and nasopharyngeal airways, LMAs, and other supraglottic airway devices, can be used in emergency situations to improve the patency of the upper airway and permit manual ventilation.
- ETTs and TTs are definitive devices for airway management, allowing for ventilation with high levels of positive pressure as well as directing access to the lower airways for secretion removal and drug delivery.
- Correct sizing, proper placement, and securing of ETTs and TTs are essential for creating and maintaining an open airway.
- Objective confirmation of tracheal tube placement rather than esophageal intubation is imperative.

- Complications from endotracheal intubation typically are divided into traumatic and cardiorespiratory complications. Traumatic problems include damage to the teeth and soft tissues. Cardiorespiratory complications included hemodynamic compromise and hypoxia, hypercapnia, and aspiration.
- An adjunct to endotracheal intubation, such as lighted stylets, indirect laryngoscopy, and rigid fiberoptic stylets, can significantly improve the probability of successful ETT placement.
- Providing adequate, routine bronchial hygiene should be a primary concern of respiratory therapists caring for patients with ETTs or TTs.
- Manual resuscitators can be classified according to the type of nonrebreathing valve used. Two types of devices typically are described: those that rely on a spring-loaded mechanism and those that rely on pressure to affect diaphragm valves.
- The most common hazards encountered with manual resuscitators include delivery of excessively high airway pressures, a defective or malfunctioning nonrebreathing valve, and faulty pressure-relief valves.

ASSESSMENT QUESTIONS

See Appendix B for the answers.

1. The most important concern in an unconscious person is:
   a. Establishing a patent airway
   b. Calling for help
   c. Administering oxygen by mask
   d. Beginning chest compressions
2. A finding on the physical examination that may indicate a difficult intubation is:
   a. A large mouth opening
   b. A thyromental distance of 8 cm
   c. Prominent incisors
   d. A long neck
3. The laryngeal mask airway (LMA):
   a. Is a definitive, secure airway
   b. Can be easily inserted in a conscious patient
   c. Bypasses upper airway obstructions
   d. Can be used to provide positive-pressure ventilation in patients with reduced pulmonary compliance

4. Benefits of the LMA include all of the following *except*:
   a. Requires less cervical range of motion during placement than direct laryngoscopy
   b. Requires less training to insert than an endotracheal tube
   c. Can be a conduit to fiberoptic intubation
   d. Prevents pressure injuries and damage to pharyngeal tissues
5. Endotracheal tube (ETT) placement can be confirmed by all of the following *except*:
   a. Capnogram color change
   b. Breath sounds over the epigastrium
   c. Fiberoptic bronchoscopy through the ETT to visualize the carina
   d. Easy expansion of the syringe of an esophageal detection device
6. Which of the following is the preferred artificial airway for a patient with liver failure who is vomiting blood?
   a. Nasotracheal intubation with a cuffed tube
   b. Oral intubation with a cuffed tube

c. Laryngeal mask airway

d. Cricothyroidotomy with a cuffed tube

7. A Combitube is placed in an unconscious patient. If breath sounds are clearly heard when ventilating through the pharyngeal lumen with both cuffs inflated, which of the following is true?

   a. A gastric tube should not be passed through the esophageal lumen.

   b. The lung is not protected from aspiration.

   c. Oxygen should be added to the esophageal lumen.

   d. More air should be placed in the pharyngeal cuff.

8. During placement of an appropriately sized oropharyngeal airway, the flange protrudes from the mouth. Attempts to insert it result in the device popping back out. This could be caused by:

   a. The airway catching on the back of the tongue

   b. The use of an airway that is too small

   c. A foreign body in the pharynx

   d. False teeth

9. Which of the following is a complication of performing a cricothyroidotomy?

   a. Gas embolism syndrome

   b. Cervical spinal cord injury

   c. Stroke

   d. Subcutaneous emphysema

10. The most important concern with blind nasal intubation is:

    a. Failure to recognize esophageal intubation

    b. Nasal hemorrhage

    c. Sinusitis

    d. Loss of the ability to speak

11. After oral intubation, no CO_2 is detected during exhalation. This could be caused by:

    a. Esophageal intubation

    b. Cardiac arrest

    c. Low cardiac output

    d. All of the above

12. A patient has a size 7 (internal diameter [ID]) tracheostomy tube (TT) in the trachea. What size suction tube should be used?

    a. 10 French (Fr)

    b. 12 Fr

    c. 14 Fr

    d. 16 Fr

13. List three important points in an airway examination.

14. Which size of laryngoscope blade should be used to attempt intubation of an average adult?

    a. #0

    b. #1

    c. #3

    d. #6

15. Which of the following are complications associated with TT placement?

    1. Hypoxia

    2. Hemorrhage

    3. Nerve injury

    4. Gas dissection of the tissues surrounding the tracheotomy site

    a. 1 and 2 only

    b. 2 and 3 only

    c. 1, 2, and 4 only

    d. 1, 2, 3, and 4

16. Trauma from overinflation of an ETT cuff can result in:

    1. Tracheal ulcers

    2. Tracheal cartilage loss

    3. Tracheal malacia

    4. Tracheal rupture

    a. 1 only

    b. 1 and 2 only

    c. 2, 3, and 4 only

    d. 1, 2, 3, and 4

17. The proper ETT size for a premature infant is:

    a. 2-mm ID

    b. 3-mm ID

    c. 4-mm ID

    d. 4.5-mm ID

18. A large adult male patient has a 7-mm (ID) ETT in place and is being mechanically ventilated. Cuff pressures of 35 cm H_2O are required to maintain an adequate cuff seal. Which of the following strategies would you suggest to correct this problem?

    a. Lower cuff pressures to no more than 25 cm H_2O

    b. Change the ETT to an 8.5-mm (ID) tube

    c. Request placement of a TT

    d. Periodically deflate and inflate the cuff

19. A patient who has undergone a single-lung transplant is to be ventilated with two ventilators connected in tandem. What is the most appropriate type of airway to use?

    a. Magill-type ETT

    b. Murphy-type ETT

    c. Double-lumen endotracheal tube (DLT)

    d. Combination of TT and oral ETT

20. What is the minimum fraction of inspired oxygen (F_IO_2) that a manual resuscitator with a reservoir should deliver according to ASTM International and International Organization for Standardization (ISO) recommendations?

    a. 0.4 with an oxygen flow of 8 L/min

    b. 0.7 with an oxygen flow of 10 L/min

    c. 0.85 with an oxygen flow of 15 L/min

    d. 1 with an oxygen flow of 6 L/min

21. Which of the following are standards recommended for the design and construction of manual resuscitators?

    1. Manual resuscitators must be able to operate at a relative humidity of 40% to 96%.

    2. Adult resuscitators must deliver a tidal volume of at least 600 mL into a test lung set at a compliance of 0.02 L/cm H_2O.

    3. The resuscitator's nonrebreathing valve must be designed so that the valve will not jam at oxygen flows up to 40 L/min.

    4. Resuscitators that are used for adults should have a pressure-limiting system.

    a. 1 only

    b. 1 and 2 only

    c. 1, 2, and 3 only

    d. 1, 2, 3, and 4

REFERENCES

1. Jaber S, Amraoui J, Lefrant JY, et al.: Clinical practice and risk factors for immediate complications of endotracheal intubation in the intensive care unit: a prospective, multiple-center study. *Crit Care Med* 34:2355-2361, 2006.
2. Walz J, Zayaruzny M, Heard S: Airway management in critical illness. *Chest* 131:608-620, 2007.
3. Hawthorne L, Wilson R, Lyons G, et al.: Failed intubation revisited: 17-year experience in a teaching maternity unit. *Br J Anaesth* 76:680-684, 1996.
4. Samsoon GL, Young JR: Difficult tracheal intubation: a retrospective study. *Anaesthesia* 42:487-490, 1987.
5. Rocke DA, Murry WB, Route CC, et al.: Relative risk analysis factors associated with difficult intubation in obstetric anesthesia. *Anesthesiology* 77:67-73, 1992.
6. Lyons G: Failed intubation. *Anaesthesia* 40:759-762, 1985.
7. Adnet F, Racine SX, Borron SW, et al.: A survey of tracheal intubation difficulty in the operating room: a prospective observational study. *Acta Anaesthesiol Scand* 45:327-332, 2001.
8. American Society of Anesthesiologists Task Force: Practice guidelines for management of the difficult airway. *Anesthesiology* 98:1269-1277, 2003.
9. Mallampati SR, Gatt SP, Gugino LD, et al.: A clinical sign to predict difficult tracheal intubation: a prospective study. *Can Anaesth Soc J* 32:429-434, 1985.
10. Iohom G, Ronayne M, Cunningham AJ: Prediction of difficult tracheal intubation. *Eur J Anaesthesiol* 20:31-36, 2003.
11. el-Ganzouri AR, McCarthy RJ, Tuman KJ, et al.: Preoperative airway assessment: predictive value of a multivariate risk index. *Anesth Analg* 91:1197-1204, 1996.
12. Kherterpal S, Han R, Tremper K, et al.: Incidence and predictors of difficult and impossible mask ventilation. *Anesthesiology* 105:885-891, 2006.
13. Langeron O, Huraux C, Guggiari M, et al.: Prediction of difficult mask ventilation. *Anesthesiology* 92:1229-1236, 2000.
14. Fink JB: Volume expansion therapy. In Burton GC, Hodgkin JE, Ward JJ, editors: *Respiratory care: a guide to clinical practice*, ed 4, Philadelphia, 1997, JB Lippincott.
15. McPherson SP: *Respiratory care equipment*, ed 5, St. Louis, 1995, Mosby.
16. Barnes TA, Watson ME: Cardiopulmonary resuscitation and emergency cardiac care. In Barnes TA, editor: *Core textbook of respiratory care practice*, ed 2, St. Louis, 1994, Mosby.
17. American Society for Testing and Materials: *Standard specification for performance and safety requirements for resuscitators intended for use with humans*, Designation F-920-985, Philadelphia, 1988, The Society.
18. ISO Technical Committee ISO/TC 121: *Anesthetic and respiratory equipment: International Standard ISO 8382: resuscitators intended for use with humans*, Geneva, Switzerland, 1988, The Organization.
19. Emergency Cardiac Care Committee, American Heart Association: *Textbook on advanced cardiac care*, ed 4, Dallas, 1996, The Association.
20. Eiling R, Plitis J: An evaluation of emergency medical technicians' ability to use manual ventilation devices. *Ann Emerg Med* 12:765-768, 1983.
21. Giffen PR, Hope CE: Preliminary evaluation of a prototype tube-valve-mask ventilator for emergency artificial ventilation. *Ann Emerg Med* 20:262-266, 1991.
22. Harrison RR, et al.: Mouth-to-mask ventilation: a superior method of rescue breathing. *Ann Emerg Med* 11:74-76, 1982.
23. Hess D, Baran C: Ventilatory volumes using mouth-to-mouth, mouth-to-mask, and bag-valve-mask techniques at various resistances and compliances. *Respir Care* 32:1025, 1987.
24. Jesudian MC, et al.: Bag-valve-mask ventilation: two rescuers are better than one—preliminary report. *Crit Care Med* 13:122-123, 1985.
25. Seidelin PH, Stolarek IH, Littlewood DG: Comparison of six methods of emergency ventilation. *Lancet* 2:1274-1275, 1986.
26. Hess D, Goff G, Johnson K: The effects of hand size, resuscitator brand, and the use of two hands on volume delivered during adult bag-valve ventilation. *Respir Care* 34:805-810, 1989.
27. Barnes TA: Emergency ventilation techniques and related equipment. *Respir Care* 37:673-690, 1992.
28. Melker RJ, Banner MJ: Ventilation during CPR: two rescuer standards reappraised. *Ann Emerg Med* 14:397-402, 1985.
29. Dorsch JA, Dorsch SE: *Understanding anesthesia equipment*, ed 4, Philadelphia, 1998, Lippincott, Williams & Wilkins.
30. Brain AL, Verghese C, Strube PJ: The LMA "ProSeal": a laryngeal mask with an oesophageal vent. *Br J Anaesth* 84:650-654, 2000.
31. Bailey B: Laryngoscopy and laryngoscopes: who's the first?—The forefathers/four fathers of laryngology. *Laryngoscope* 106:939-943, 1996.
32. Bailey BJ: What's all the fuss about? The laryngoscope pages cause an international incident. *Laryngoscope* 106:925-927, 1996.
33. Cooper R: Laryngoscope: its past and future. *Can J Anaesth* 51:R6, 2004.
34. Cormarck RS, Lehane J: Difficult tracheal intubation obstetrics. *Anaesthesia* 39:1105-1111, 1984.
35. Miller DM, Youkhana I, Karunaratne WU, et al.: Presence of protein deposits on "cleaned" re-usable anaesthetic equipment. *Anaesthesia* 56:1069-1072, 2001.
36. Evans A, Vaughan RS, Hall JE, et al.: A comparison of the forces exerted during laryngoscopy using disposable and non-disposable laryngoscope blades. *Anaesthesia* 58:869-873, 2003.
37. Hastings RH, Vigin AC, Yand BY, et al.: Cervical spine movement during laryngoscopy with the Bullard, Macintosh, and Miller laryngoscopes. *Anesthesiology* 82:859-869, 1995.
38. De Jong A, Molinari N, Conseil M, et al.: Video laryngoscopy versus direct laryngoscopy for orotracheal intubation in the intensive care unit: a systematic review and meta-analysis. *Intensive Care Med* 40:629-639, 2014.
39. Brown CA, Bair AE, Pallin DJ, et al.: Improved glottic exposure with the Video Macintosh Laryngoscope in adult emergency department tracheal intubations. *Ann Emerg Med* 56:83-88, 2010.
40. Kill C, Risse J, Wallot P, et al.: Videolaryngoscopy with glidescope reduces cervical spine movement in patients with unsecured cervical spine. *J Emerg Med* 44:750-756, 2013.
41. Robitaille A, Williams SR, Tremblay MH, et al.: Cervical spine motion during tracheal intubation with manual in-line stabilization: direct laryngoscopy versus GlideScope videolaryngoscopy. *Anesth Analg* 106:935-941, 2008.
42. Kristensen MS: Ultrasonography in the management of the airway. *Acta Anaesthesiol Scand* 55(10):1155-1173, 2011.
43. Prasad A, Yu E, Wong DT, et al.: Comparison of sonography and computed tomography as imaging tools for assessment of airway structures. *J Ultrasound Med* 30(7):965-972, 2011.

44. Pinto J, Cordeiro L, Pereira C, et al.: Predicting difficult laryngoscopy using ultrasound measurement of distance from skin to epiglottis. *J Crit Care* 33:26-31, 2016.

45. Adhikari S, Zeger W, Schmier C, et al.: Pilot study to determine the utility of point-of-care ultrasound in the assessment of difficult laryngoscopy. *Acad Emerg Med* 18(7): 754-758, 2011.

46. Wu J, Dong J, Ding Y, et al.: Role of anterior neck soft tissue quantifications by ultrasound in predicting difficult laryngoscopy. *Med Sci Monit* 20:2343-2350, 2014.

47. Ezri T, Gewürtz G, Sessler DI, et al.: Prediction of difficult laryngoscopy in obese patients by ultrasound quantification of anterior neck soft tissue. *Anaesthesia* 58(11):1111-1114, 2003.

48. Hui CM, Tsui BC: Sublingual ultrasound as an assessment method for predicting difficult intubation: a pilot study. *Anaesthesia* 69(4):314-319, 2014.

49. Kristensen MS, Teoh WH, Graumann O, et al.: Ultrasonography for clinical decision-making and intervention in airway management: from the mouth to the lungs and pleurae. *Insights Imaging* 5(2):253-279, 2014.

50. Milling TJ, Jones M, Khan T, et al.: Transtracheal 2-D ultrasound for identification of esophageal intubation. *J Emerg Med* 32:409-414, 2007.

51. Muslu B, Sert H, Kaya A, et al.: Use of sonography for rapid identification of esophageal and tracheal intubations in adult patients. *J Ultrasound Med* 30:671-676, 2011.

52. Weaver B, Lyon M, Blaivas M: Confirmation of endotracheal tube placement after intubation using the ultrasound sliding lung sign. *Acad Emerg Med* 13:239-244, 2006.

53. Blaivas M, Tsung JW: Point-of-care sonographic detection of left endobronchial main stem intubation and obstruction versus endotracheal intubation. *J Ultrasound Med* 27:785-789, 2008.

54. Pfeiffer P, Rudolph SS, Børglum J, et al.: Temporal comparison of ultrasound vs. auscultation and capnography in verification of endotracheal tube placement. *Acta Anaesthesiol Scand* 55:1190-1195, 2011.

55. Gupta D, Srirajakalidindi A, Habli N, et al.: Ultrasound confirmation of laryngeal mask airway placement correlates with fiberoptic laryngoscope findings. *Middle East J Anesthesiol* 21:283-287, 2011.

56. Shibasaki M, Nakajima Y, Ishii S, et al.: Prediction of pediatric endotracheal tube size by ultrasonography. *Anesthesiology* 113:819-824, 2010.

57. Lakhal K, Delplace X, Cottier JP, et al.: The feasibility of ultrasound to assess subglottic diameter. *Anesth Analg* 104:611-614, 2007.

58. Sustić A, Miletić D, Protić A, et al.: Can ultrasound be useful for predicting the size of a left double-lumen bronchial tube? Tracheal width as measured by ultrasonography versus computed tomography. *J Clin Anesth* 20:247-252, 2008.

59. Lindman JP, Morgan CE, Dixon S: Tracheostomy, http://emedicine.medscape.com/article/865068-overview.

60. Metterlein T, Frommer M, Ginzkey C, et al.: A randomized trial comparing two cuffed emergency cricothyrotomy devices using a wire-guided and a catheter-over-needle technique. *J Emerg Med* 41(3):326-332, 2011.

61. Oberwalder M, Weis H, Nehoda H, et al.: Videobronchoscopic guidance makes percutaneous dilational tracheostomy safer. *Surg Endosc* 18:839-842, 2004.

62. Fernandez L, Norwood S, Roettger R, et al.: Bedside percutaneous tracheostomy with bronchoscopic guidance in critically ill patients. *Arch Surg* 131:129-132, 1996.

63. Griggs W, Worthley L, Gilligan J, et al.: A simple percutaneous technique. *Surg Gynecol Obstet* 170:543-545, 1990.

64. Bewsher M, Adams A, Clarke C, et al.: Evaluation of a new percutaneous dilational tracheostomy set apparatus. *Anaesthesia* 56:859-864, 2001.

65. Byhahn C, Wilke H, Habig S, et al.: Percutaneous tracheostomy: Ciaglia Blue Rhino versus the basic Ciaglia technique of percutaneous dilational tracheostomy. *Anesth Analg* 91:882-886, 2000.

66. Divatia J, et al.: Failed intubation managed with subcricoid transtracheal jet ventilation followed by percutaneous tracheostomy. *Anesthesiology* 96:1519-1520, 2002.

67. Dult M, Ault B, Ng P: Percutaneous dilational tracheostomy for emergent airway access. *J Intensive Care Med* 18:222-226, 2003.

68. Munir N, Hughes D, Sadera G, et al.: Ultrasound guided localisation of trachea for surgical tracheostomy. *Eur Arch Otorhinolaryngol* 267:477-479, 2010.

69. Elliott DS, Baker PA, Scott MR, et al.: Accuracy of surface landmark identification for cannula cricothyroidotomy. *Anaesthesia* 65:889-894, 2010.

70. Nicholls SE, Sweeney TW, Ferre RM, et al.: Bedside sonography by emergency physicians for the rapid identification of landmarks relevant to cricothyrotomy. *Am J Emerg Med* 26:852-856, 2008.

71. Hatfield A, Bodenha A: Portable ultrasonic scanning of the anterior neck before percutaneous dilatational tracheostomy. *Anaesthesia* 54:660-663, 1999.

72. Sustić A, Kovac D, Zgaljardić Z, et al.: Ultrasound-guided percutaneous dilatational tracheostomy: a safe method to avoid cranial misplacement of the tracheostomy tube. *Intensive Care Med* 26:1379-1381, 2000.

73. Muhammad JK, Patton DW, Evans RM, et al.: Percutaneous dilatational tracheostomy under ultrasound guidance. *Br J Oral Maxillofac Surg* 37:309-311, 1999.

74. Neumar RW, Shuster M, Callaway CW, et al.: Part 1: Executive Summary: 2015 American Heart Association Guidelines Update for Cardiopulmonary Resuscitation and Emergency Cardiovascular Care. *Circulation* 132(suppl 2):S315-S367, 2015.

75. Kleinman ME, Brennan EE, Goldberger ZD, et al.: Part 5: Adult Basic Life Support and Cardiopulmonary Resuscitation Quality: American Heart Association Guidelines Update for Cardiopulmonary Resuscitation and Emergency Cardiovascular Care. *Circulation* 132:S414-S435, 2015.

76. Link MS, Berkow LC, Kudenchuck PJ, et al.: Part 7: Adult Advanced Cardiac Life Support: American Heart Association Guidelines Update for Cardiopulmonary Resuscitation and Emergency Cardiovascular Care. *Circulation* 132:S444-S464, 2015.

77. Atkins DL, Berger S, Duff JP, et al.: Part 11: Pediatric Basic Life Support and Cardiopulmonary Resuscitation Quality: American Heart Association Guidelines Update for Cardiopulmonary Resuscitation and Emergency Cardiovascular Care. *Circulation* 132:S519-S525, 2015.

78. de Caen AR, Berg MD, Chameides L, et al.: Part 12: Pediatric Advanced Life Support: American Heart Association Guidelines Update for Cardiopulmonary Resuscitation and Emergency Cardiovascular Care. *Circulation*. 132:S526-S542, 2015.

79. Wyckoff MH, Aziz K, Escobedo MB, et al.: Part 13: Neonatal Resuscitation: American Heart Association Guidelines Update for Cardiopulmonary Resuscitation and Emergency Cardiovascular Care. *Circulation* 132:S543-S560, 2015.

Humidity and Aerosol Therapy

Arzu Ari, Jim Fink

OBJECTIVES

Upon completion of this chapter, you will be able to:

1. Differentiate humidity from aerosol.
2. Differentiate the roles of humidity and aerosol in respiratory care.
3. Describe the mechanisms of humidification.
4. Describe the natural physiological humidification process throughout the respiratory tract.
5. Identify the indications, contraindications, and hazards associated with humidity therapy.
6. Describe how various types of humidifiers work.
7. Compare and contrast low-flow and high-flow humidifiers.
8. Explain the importance of monitoring and maintaining humidity therapy.
9. Describe the physical characteristics of an aerosol.
10. Discuss factors that influence aerosol deposition.
11. Describe the therapeutic indications for aerosol therapy.
12. Identify special considerations for administering aerosol therapy.
13. Determine the optimum technique for administering aerosol—small-volume nebulizer, large-volume nebulizer, pressurized metered-dose inhaler, or dry powder inhaler.
14. Explain how pneumatic, ultrasonic, and vibrating mesh aerosol generators work.
15. Discuss criteria for device selection.
16. Describe how each type of device should be set up, used, and maintained.

OUTLINE

KEY TERMS

absolute humidity
adiabatic
aerosol
aerosol output
aging
atomizer
baffle
body temperature and pressure saturated (BTPS)
breath-actuated nebulizers (BANs)
breath-enhanced nebulizers (BENs)
Brownian motion
bubble humidifiers
chlorofluorocarbons (CFCs)

condensation
deposition
diffusion
dry powder inhalers (DPIs)
emitted dose
evaporation
fine-particle fraction (FPF)
geometric standard deviation (GSD)
heat and moisture exchangers (HMEs)
heated wires
heterodisperse
humidifier
humidity

humidity deficit
hydrofluoroalkane
hydrophobic
hygrometer
hygroscopic
inertial impaction
inhaled mass
inhaler
inspissated
International Organization for Standardization (ISO)
isothermic saturation boundary (ISB)
large-volume jet nebulizer

large-volume nebulizer (LVN)

mass median aerodynamic diameter (MMAD)

monodisperse

nebulizer

passover humidifier

piezoelectric ceramic transducer

pressurized metered-dose inhaler (pMDI)

relative humidity (RH)

residual drug volume

respirable mass

sedimentation

servo-controlled systems

small-volume nebulizer (SVN)

spacer

therapeutic index

ultrasonic nebulizer (USN)

volume median diameter (VMD)

wick humidifier

Vapors and mists have been used for thousands of years to treat patients with respiratory diseases. Respiratory therapists use these treatments routinely at the bedside in the form of water vapor (humidity), bland water aerosols, and active medicated aerosols. This chapter reviews the principles, methods, and devices typically used to deliver humidity and aerosol therapy.

Humidity is water that exists in the form of individual molecules in the vaporous or gaseous state. Molecules of water (0.001 μm) are much smaller than medical aerosols, which can range from 0.2 to 50 μm. A vapor consists of individual free molecules of a substance that exist below its critical temperature; humidity therefore often is described as water vapor. An aerosol is a suspension of solid or liquid particles in a gas. Aerosols occur in nature as pollens, spores, dust, smoke, smog, fog, and mist.[1] Medical aerosols, which are generated with an atomizer, a nebulizer, or an inhaler, can be used to deliver bland water solutions to the respiratory tract or to administer drugs to the lungs, throat, or nose for both local and systemic effects.

Water vapor exerts a pressure (P_{H2O}) that results from the continuous random movement of water molecules (i.e., kinetic activity). As the temperature of a gas increases, water vapor pressure also increases because gas molecules move faster, resulting in a greater number of molecular collisions. As molecular collisions increase, kinetic activity increases, and water molecules leave the liquid state and evaporate (i.e., enter into a vaporous, or molecular, state).

As discussed in Chapter 1, the energy required to vaporize a liquid is called the *latent heat of vaporization*. As water is heated to its boiling point and molecules leave the liquid state, water vapor is produced. The boiling point of water is influenced by the pressure above the water's surface. If this pressure increases, the boiling point increases (this is the principle by which pressure cookers and steam autoclaves work). Similarly, if the pressure decreases, the boiling point decreases (this is the reason water boils faster at a lower temperature in the mountains). Evaporation occurs when liquid molecules near the surface contain enough kinetic energy to break free and enter a vaporous state, reducing the volume and energy contained in the liquid.

Humidity usually is described in terms of *absolute humidity* or *relative humidity*. Absolute humidity is the actual content or weight of water present in a given volume of gas (expressed in grams per cubic meter [g/m³] or milligrams per liter [mg/L]). Relative humidity (RH) is the ratio of the actual content or weight of the water present in a gas sample relative to the

sample's capacity to hold water at that temperature. The RH is calculated by dividing the amount of water in the gas (content) by the amount of water the gas can hold at that temperature (capacity). This ratio is expressed as a percentage and can be calculated using humidity measurements of weight (mg/L) or partial pressure (P_{H2O}). Box 6.1 shows an example of how to calculate the RH.

Humidity can be measured with a hygrometer. Hygrometers can work on a variety of principles. For example, a psychrometer uses two thermometers (one with a wet wick surrounding the bulb and one with a dry bulb). The device is rotated rapidly through the air producing evaporation and cooling of the wet wick, and the difference between the temperatures of the two thermometers is used to calculate the RH. Electronic hygrometers use a transducing element with electrical properties that change with water content. Some electronic hygrometers have sensors small enough to be used to monitor humidity and temperature in a ventilator circuit. However, some problems exist with this technology, and once saturated, these

---

BOX 6.1   Calculating the Relative Humidity

The actual water content (absolute humidity) of a sample of room air is measured with a hygrometer and is found to be 12 mg/L. If the room air temperature is 20°C (68°F), what is the relative humidity (RH)?

Step 1
Refer to Table 6.1 and locate 20°C and note the water content, which is the maximum amount of water a gas sample at this temperature can hold.

Step 2
The RH is the ratio of the actual amount of water in the gas sample (content) to the amount the gas sample can hold when saturated with water vapor (capacity). To calculate the relative humidity, divide the content by the capacity:

$$\frac{\text{Measured humidity (content)}}{\text{Water capacity}} \times 100 = \text{Relative humidity}$$

$$\frac{12\,\text{mg/L}}{17\,\text{mg/L}} = 71\%$$

Step 3
Interpret the answer. In this case the room air is holding 71% of what it is capable of holding at 20°C.

What would the RH be at body temperature?

TABLE 6.1 Absolute Humidity and Water Vapor Pressure at Various Temperatures When the Gas Is Saturated With Water

Temperature (°C)	Absolute Humidity (mg/L)	Water Vapor Pressure (mm Hg)
19	16.3	16.5
20	17.3	17.5
21	18.4	18.6
22	19.4	19.8
23	20.6	21.0
24	21.8	22.3
25	23.0	23.7
26	24.4	25.1
27	25.8	26.7
28	27.2	28.3
29	28.8	29.9
30	30.4	31.7
31	32.0	33.6
32	33.8	35.5
33	35.6	37.6
34	37.6	39.8
35	39.6	42.0
36	41.7	44.4
37	43.9	46.9
38	46.2	49.5
39	48.6	52.3
40	51.1	55.1
41	53.7	58.1

hygrometers are not reliable for reporting changes in humidity over time. At best, they should be used only for spot checks.

When the amount of water a gas contains is equal to the capacity of the gas to hold water, the RH is 100% and the gas is saturated. Table 6.1 shows the relationship between absolute humidity and water vapor pressure at various temperatures when the gas is saturated with water. Note that at sea level a gas at body temperature and pressure saturated (BTPS) has a water vapor pressure of 47 mm Hg and contains 43.9 mg of water per liter of gas. As is discussed later in this chapter, these are the conditions found in the lung under normal circumstances.

It is important to understand that when the absolute humidity is held constant, increasing the temperature of the gas decreases the RH, because the higher temperatures increase the gas's capacity to hold water. In contrast, a decrease in the temperature of the gas decreases the capacity of the gas to hold water. Water molecules in excess of the amount of water vapor the saturated gas can hold combine to condense into liquid droplets. In nature, this is described as *fog formation*. The liquid particles suspended in gas (aerosols) continue to collect water molecules, growing larger and heavier. As the particles collide and coalesce (on each other and on surfaces), they condense, fall out of suspension, and form larger bodies of liquid.

In many respiratory care devices, this condensation can accumulate in the lowest point of delivery tubing, and it must be removed to eliminate the possibility of the water obstructing the gas delivery tube, disrupting gas and humidity delivery to the patient.

I. HUMIDITY THERAPY

Humidity therapy involves adding water vapor to inspired gas. An understanding of the respiratory system's control of heat and moisture exchange is essential for determining the need for and the appropriate level of humidity therapy.

Physiological Control of Heat and Moisture Exchange

Heat and moisture exchange is one of the primary functions of the respiratory tract.[1] The upper airways add heat and humidity to inspired gases during inhalation and cool and reclaim water during exhalation. The nasal mucosa is kept moist by secretions from mucous glands, goblet cells, transudation of fluid through cell walls, and condensation of exhaled humidity. The vascular mucosa lining the sinuses, trachea, and bronchi promote effective heat transfer by serving as an active energy source for heating and humidifying inspired gases. The tortuous path of gas through the turbinates increases contact between the inspired air and the mucosa. As the inspired air enters the nose, it is warmed by convection and picks up water vapor from the moist mucosal lining by evaporation, thus cooling the mucosal surface.

During exhalation the expired gas transfers heat back to the cooler tracheal and nasal mucosa by convection. As the saturated gas cools, the water vapor in the exhaled gas condenses because it holds less water vapor, and water is reabsorbed by mucus (rehydration). In cold environments the formation of condensate may exceed the ability of mucus to reabsorb water (resulting in a "runny nose"). The mouth is less efficient than the nose because of the relatively low ratio of gas volume to moist surface area of the less vascular squamous epithelium lining the oropharynx and hypopharynx. When a person inhales through the mouth at normal room temperature, temperatures at the hypopharynx are approximately 3°C lower and the RH is approximately 20% less than when a person inhales through the nose. During exhalation the mouth is much less efficient than the nose at reclaiming heat and water.[2]

As Fig. 6.1 shows, the isothermic saturation boundary (ISB) is the point at which inhaled gas reaches saturation (100% RH at a body temperature of 37°C [98.6°F]); this point typically is 5 cm below the carina.[3] Below the ISB, temperature and RH remain constant (BTPS). Temperature and humidity decrease with inspiration and increase with exhalation. The ISB shifts deeper into the lungs when a person inhales through the mouth; breathes cold, dry air through an artificial tracheal airway; or simply increases the minute ventilation. Prolonged and severe shifts of the ISB can damage the airways and compromise the body's normal heat and moisture exchange mechanisms.

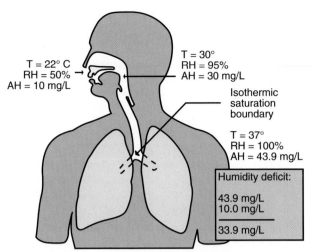

FIGURE 6.1 When a person breathes typical ambient air, the upper airway adds 20 mg/L of water vapor and the lower airway adds 13.9 mg/L. If all that humidity were exhaled, this would represent a 33.9 mg/L humidity deficit. *AH*, Absolute humidity; *RH*, relative humidity; *T*, temperature.

BOX 6.2   Clinical Signs and Symptoms of Inadequate Airway Humidification

- Atelectasis
- Dry, nonproductive cough
- Increased airway resistance
- Increased incidence of infection
- Increased work of breathing
- Substernal pain
- Thick, dehydrated secretions

Indications for Humidification and Warming of Inspired Gases

The primary goal of humidification is to maintain normal physiological conditions in the airways. Proper levels of heat and humidity help ensure normal functioning of the mucociliary transport system. When the airways are exposed to relatively cold, dry air, ciliary motility is reduced and the airways become more irritable. The production of mucus increases, and pulmonary secretions become thick and **inspissated** (i.e., *dried, heavy,* or *intense*). The hazards of breathing dry gas are even greater when the upper airway is bypassed, as occurs with endotracheal intubation[4]; prolonged breathing of improperly conditioned gases through a tracheal airway can lead to serious consequences. Box 6.2 summarizes the signs and symptoms associated with breathing cold, dry gases.

When the RH of inspired gas is greater than 60% of BTPS conditions, no injury is believed to occur in normal lungs.[5,6] As Fig. 6.1 shows, the targeted level of heat and humidity depends on the site of gas delivery (e.g., nose/mouth, hypopharynx, or trachea). Box 6.3 summarizes the recommended humidity levels for administering medical gases based on current standards.[7,8]

In addition to maintaining normal humidity levels in the airway, warm, humidified gases are used to raise the core temperature of hypothermic patients, to prevent intraoperative

---

BOX 6.3   Humidity Requirements for Gas Delivery at Various Sites in the Upper and Lower Airway

Gas Delivered to the Nose or Mouth
50% relative humidity with an absolute humidity level of 10 mg/L at 22°C (71.6°F)

Gas Delivered to the Hypopharynx
95% relative humidity with an absolute humidity level of 28 to 34 mg/L at 29°C to 32°C (84.2°F to 89.6°F)

Gas Delivered to the Midtrachea
100% relative humidity with an absolute humidity level of 36 to 40 mg/L at 31°C to 35°C (87.8°F to 95°F)

BOX 6.4   Physical Principles Governing Humidifier Function

- *Temperature:* The higher the temperature of a gas, the more water vapor it can hold (increased capacity). The colder the gas, the less water vapor it can hold.
- *Surface area:* The greater the surface area of contact between water and gas, the more opportunity for evaporation to occur.
- *Contact time:* The longer a gas remains in contact with water, the greater the opportunity for evaporation to occur. For example, the slower the gas flow through a heated body of water or chamber, the more heat and water vapor are transferred to the gas. In contrast, a humidifier that fully heats and humidifies gas at low to moderate flows may fail to maintain that level of humidity with high peak flows.
- *Thermal mass:* The greater the mass of water or the core element of a humidifier, the greater its capacity to hold and transfer heat. As heat is transferred from the thermal mass, the differential between the core and the gas is reduced, and the speed of heat transfer is reduced.

hypothermia, and to alleviate bronchospasm in patients with reactive airways when they breathe cold air.[9-12] Cool, humidified gas often is used with bland aerosol delivery to treat upper airway inflammation caused by croup, epiglottitis, and postextubation edema.

Contraindications and Hazards of Humidity Therapy

Although providing heat and humidity to inspired gas is generally not contraindicated during spontaneous breathing or invasive or noninvasive mechanical ventilation, humidity devices may be contraindicated in specific clinical conditions. Table 6.2 lists indications, contraindications, and hazards of each device used for humidification therapy.

Types of Humidifiers

A **humidifier** is a device that adds molecular water to gas. This occurs by means of evaporation of water from a surface, such as a reservoir, a wick, or a sphere of water in suspension (i.e., aerosol). Box 6.4 summarizes the various factors that can

TABLE 6.2   Indications, Contraindications, and Hazards of Devices Used for Humidity Therapy

Device	Indications	Contraindications	Hazards
Bubble humidifiers	To humidify the inspired gas given by a nasal cannula or face mask to spontaneously breathing patients	• Patients with artificial airways such as tracheostomy tubes or ETTs • Patients with thick and tenacious secretions • Not recommended for use at flow rates greater than 10 L/min	• Obstruction in the small bore tubing due to excessive condensate, when heated • Dysfunctional pressure-relief valve with prolonged use
Passover humidifiers	To provide heat and humidity to inspired gas during invasive and noninvasive ventilator support	None	• Risk for electrical shock • Hypothermia or hyperthermia due to inadequate adjustment of the temperature • Risk for contamination, patient-ventilator asynchrony due to accumulation of condensate
Heated humidifiers	To provide high level of heat and humidity to inspired gas during mechanical ventilation	None	• Risk for electrical shock • Hypothermia, hyperthermia, thermal injury, and burns with inadequate adjustment of temperature • Tubing meltdown due to incompatible circuits and heated humidifiers • Patient-ventilator asynchrony and nosocomial infection due to accumulated and contaminated condensate
Large-volume nebulizers	• Presence of upper airway edema, postextubation edema, and subglottic edema • Laryngotracheobronchitis • To mobilize secretions • To obtain a sputum specimen	• Patients with upper airway hyperresponsiveness • Patients who are at risk for bronchoconstriction	Inadequate production of mist with the misalignment of the jet orifices, obstruction in the siphon tube, or inadequate flow
Heat and moisture exchangers (HMEs)	To provide heat and humidity during patient transport, anesthesia, and short-term mechanical ventilation (<72 h)	• Thick, copious secretions • Body temperature less than 89.6°F (32°C) • High minute ventilation • In ventilator-dependent patients receiving in-line aerosol drug administration • During noninvasive ventilation with large mask leaks • In patients with minute ventilation greater than 10 L/min • Patients with an expired V$_T$<70% of the delivered V$_T$ (e.g., large bronchopleurocutaneous fistula, incompetent or absent ETT cuffs)	• Increased volume of secretions • Thick, dehydrated secretions • Hypothermia • Large V$_T$ (>700 mL) • Small V$_T$ with large-rebreathed-volume HME (i.e., HME volume > −30% of V$_T$) • Uncuffed ETTs • Large leak around an ETT, such as might occur with a large bronchopleurocutaneous fistula or leaking ETT cuff • Exhaled V$_T$ < 70% of inhaled V$_T$ • Cannot be placed between nebulizer and airway during aerosol therapy • Cannot be used with heated humidification • Hypothermia in using HMEs with low humidity outputs (<25 mg/L) • An increase in airway resistance and work of breathing due to water accumulation in the HME • An increase in the dead space during mechanical ventilation • Underhydration and impaction of mucous secretions • Ineffective low-pressure alarm during disconnection because of resistance through HME

ETT, Endotracheal tube; *V$_T$,* tidal volume.

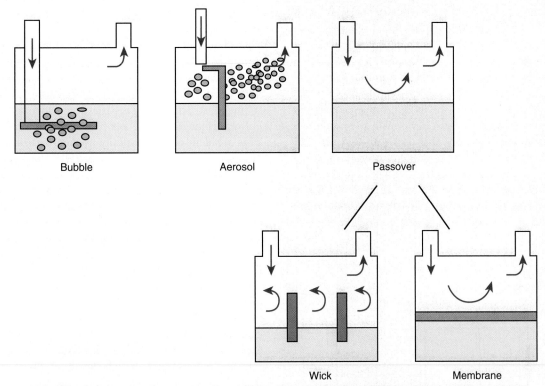

Bubble   Aerosol   Passover

Wick   Membrane

FIGURE 6.2 Primary types of active humidifiers. Gas passes through the water (bubble) or around drops of water (bland aerosol), or gas passes over the surface of water (passover), a saturated material (wick), or a semipermeable membrane (membrane).

affect the quality of a humidifier's performance. These factors include (1) temperature, (2) surface area, (3) time of contact, and (4) thermal mass.

Humidifiers generally are classified as active and passive devices. Fig. 6.2 shows the three primary types of active humidifiers: (1) bubble, (2) aerosol, and (3) passover, which includes wick and membrane devices. The most common examples of a passive humidifier are heat and moisture exchangers (HMEs). Design and performance requirements for all medical humidifiers are established by ASTM International (formerly the American Society for Testing and Materials).[13]

Bubble Humidifiers

Bubble humidifiers direct gas through a tube or channel into the bottom of a water reservoir, where the gas stream produces bubbles that rise through the water and pass through the device outlet to the patient (Fig. 6.3). The gas within the bubbles is humidified as the bubbles rise to the water's surface. Increasing the height of the water column above the gas outlet increases the humidity content of the bubbles by allowing a longer contact time.

Standard low-flow bubble humidifiers incorporate pressure-relief gravity or spring-loaded valves that release high pressures (>2 pounds per square inch [psi]) to prevent bursting of the humidifier bottle and warn of flow path obstruction. Humidifier pop-off valves typically provide both audible and visible alarms, which automatically resume normal operation once the excess pressure has been vented.[13] If the system is obstructed at or near the patient interface and the pop-off sounds, the

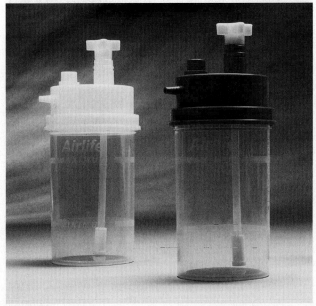

FIGURE 6.3 Bubble humidifier. (Courtesy Cardinal Health, Dublin, OH.)

system is leak-free. Failure of the pop-off valve to produce an alerting sound may indicate a leak (or a faulty pop-off valve).

Unheated bubble humidifiers are commonly used with low-flow oral-nasal oxygen delivery systems when the goal is to raise the water vapor content of the gas to ambient levels. An unheated bubble humidifier can provide an absolute humidity level of 10 to 20 mg/L.[14-16] An absolute humidity of 10 mg/L in a gas corresponds to a 50% RH at standard room temperatures, but only a 20% RH at BTPS. Notice that as gas flow increases, the reservoir cools by as much as 10°C, thus limiting the effectiveness of providing humidity at flow rates higher than 10 L/min.

Bubble size is governed by the design of the gas outlet at the bottom of the capillary tube. A device with an open lumen makes larger bubbles than one that uses a diffuser made of plastic foam, porous metal, or a plastic or metal mesh (Fig. 6.4). Diffuser humidifiers are designed to create a large number of small bubbles, allowing a greater surface area for gas and water interaction.[8] It is important to recognize that although larger bubbles have greater surface area, the greater internal volume of these bubbles produces a lower surface-to-volume ratio than smaller bubbles.

Adding heat to a bubble humidifier increases the absolute humidity in the gas. However, in bubble humidifiers designed for low-flow oxygen applications, condensation can occur with heating, and liquid droplets can form in the narrow tubing, obstructing the gas pathway. Condensate therefore is an important issue with any heated humidification system. This problem can be partially averted by using large-bore (10- to 22-mm internal diameter [ID]) corrugated tubing, which results in a less immediate risk for obstruction, and by placing a water trap at the lowest point of the tubing circuit to collect condensate. Heated wires also can be added to the circuit to minimize the formation of condensate.

High-flow bubble humidifiers are available for use during mechanical ventilation. They were designed to accommodate flow rates of gas delivered up to 100 L/min. It is worth mentioning that absolute humidity decreases during periods of peak flow with these devices. Consequently, the absolute humidity of gas passing through a heated humidifier can change during the course of an individual breath. Manufacturers have attempted to address this issue by using 22-mm ID inlet and outlets ports on high-flow humidifiers. In addition, these devices typically have shallower reservoirs than low-flow humidifiers, and they use bubble diffusers, which allow for a greater air–liquid interface. Note that the system compensates for the reduced water contact time by heating the reservoir (up to 50°C [122°F]). Fig. 6.5 shows how the exiting gas cools as it passes through a 6-ft corrugated aerosol tube to the patient and yet still is 37°C at the patient's airway. Because the gas in the standard corrugated aerosol tubing is hotter than the ambient air surrounding it, the gas cools as it travels through the 5- to 6-ft inspiratory limb of the ventilator circuit. Water content drops from 84 mg/L to 44 mg/L as vapor, the

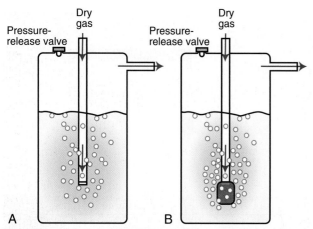

FIGURE 6.4 Bubble humidifiers pass gas under the surface of the water using an open lumen (A) or a diffuser (B). Diffusers tend to make smaller bubbles with a higher surface-to-volume ratio for humidification.

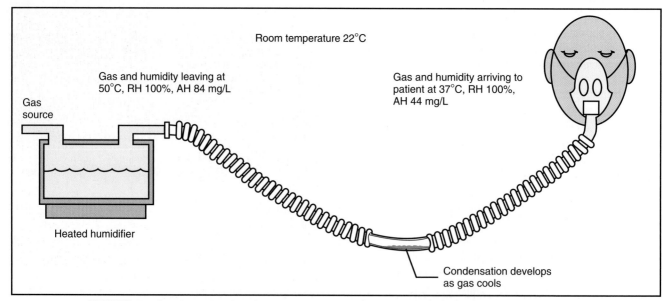

FIGURE 6.5 Condensation forms in a gas delivery tube as heated humidity is cooled by ambient conditions surrounding the tube. As the temperature of the gas cools (up to 1°C [1.8°F] per foot of 22-mm corrugated tubing), excess water leaves the gas and accumulates in the gravity-dependent loops of the delivery tubing. *AH*, Absolute humidity; *RH*, relative humidity.

difference forming condensate in the circuit tubing. High-flow humidifiers do not typically have internal pop-off valves.

Aerosol Generators

Humidity is simply water in the gas phase; a bland aerosol, however, consists of liquid particles suspended in a gas providing both humidity and additional liquid applied locally to the airway. Bland aerosol therapy involves the delivery of sterile water or hypotonic, isotonic, or hypertonic saline aerosols. The American Association for Respiratory Care (AARC) has published a Clinical Practice Guideline on Bland Aerosol Administration.[17] Devices used to generate bland aerosols include large-volume jet nebulizers and ultrasonic nebulizers. Aerosol delivery systems can include a variety of direct airway appliances, such as aerosol face masks, tracheostomy masks, face tents, and enclosures such as mist tents.

Large-volume jet nebulizers. A large-volume jet nebulizer is the device most commonly used to generate bland aerosols. Liquid particle aerosols are generated by passing gas at a high velocity through a small "jet" orifice (Fig. 6.6). The resulting low pressure generated at the jet draws fluid from the reservoir up to the top of a siphon tube, where it is sheared off and shattered into liquid particles (i.e., the Bernoulli principle). The larger, unstable particles fall out of suspension and strike the internal surfaces of the device and the fluid surface, a process called *baffling*. The smaller particles remaining in

suspension leave the nebulizer through the outlet port and are carried in the gas stream.

Jet nebulizers typically operate at a flow of 6 to 15 L/min; however, higher flows may be required to meet a patient's inspiratory needs. Devices with air entrainment ports can be used to increase inspiratory flows by allowing for air mixing (Fig. 6.7). Also, various levels of fractional inspired oxygen (F_IO_2) can be achieved with these devices. Closed dilution nebulizers use a primary gas to drive the jet nebulizer, and a second gas inlet port can be used to add gas to the nebulizer at a rate greater than 40 L/min (Fig. 6.8). Depending on the design, input flow, and air entrainment setting, the total water output of an unheated, large-volume jet nebulizer can vary from 26 to 35 mg/L. If the device is heated, the output increases to 33 to 55 mg/L, mainly because of increased vapor

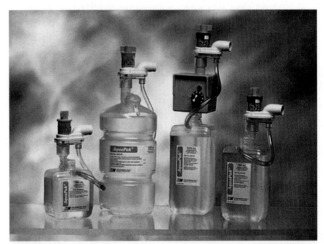

FIGURE 6.7 Hudson RCI Prefilled Precision Nebulizer. (Courtesy Hudson Respiratory Care, Temecula, CA.)

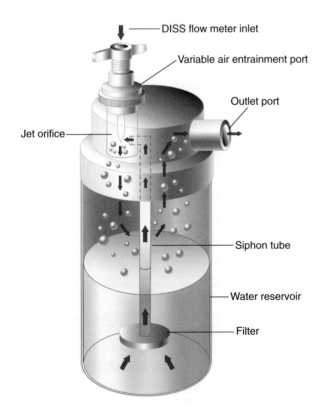

FIGURE 6.6 Diagram of a large-volume jet nebulizer with a variable entrainment port. *DISS*, Diameter Index Safety System. (From Kacmarek RM, Stoller JK, Heuer AJ: *Egan's fundamentals of respiratory care*, ed 10, St. Louis, 2013, Mosby-Elsevier.)

Labels in Figure 6.6:
- DISS flow meter inlet
- Variable air entrainment port
- Outlet port
- Jet orifice
- Siphon tube
- Water reservoir
- Filter

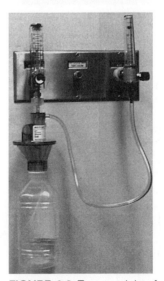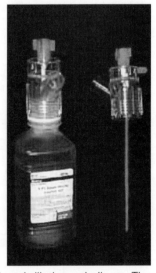

FIGURE 6.8 Two models of closed dilution nebulizers. The primary gas is delivered to the jet, which delivers limited flows up to 40 L/min; the secondary gas port allows additional flow up to 80 L/min. The ratio of oxygen to airflow determines the oxygen concentration and total flow to the patient. (Courtesy Vital Signs, a GE Healthcare company, Totowa, NJ.)

capacity.[18,19] Heating options include a hot plate, wraparound, yoke (collar), or immersion element (Fig. 6.9). Unfortunately, many of these devices do not have servo-controlled systems to regulate the delivery temperature and therefore do not shut down when the reservoir empties. In addition, failure of the heating element can cause a loss of heating, without any warning to the clinician.

Babington nebulizer. In this type of nebulizer, fluid is spread over the surface of a glass sphere and struck by compressed gas passing from the inside of the sphere through one or more orifices on its surface. The liquid is sheared from the thin layer and directed against a baffle (Fig. 6.10). The Hydrosphere and the Solosphere, two models of large-volume Babington nebulizers, are no longer manufactured. These devices generated aerosol with a relatively small particle size (<2 μm) and had a relatively high aerosol output.

Spinning disk devices. Sometimes referred to as a *centrifugal nebulizer*, the spinning disk nebulizer is a mechanical aerosol generator. It operates on the principle that a spinning disk with a hollow shaft draws liquid from the reservoir (Fig. 6.11). As the liquid leaves the shaft, it is spread across the top of the disk and contacts a system of baffles attached to the disk, producing an aerosol. This mechanism is used in many commercially available, large-volume room humidifiers intended for home use.

Larger versions of spinning disk nebulizers (2- to 3-L reservoirs) are used to deliver bland aerosols into mist tents. These enclosure systems can generate flow rates greater than 20 L/min, with water outputs as high as 5 mL/min (300 mL/h). Because heat buildup is a problem in enclosures, these systems are always unheated.

Ultrasonic nebulizers. An ultrasonic nebulizer (USN) is an electrically powered device that uses a piezoelectric ceramic transducer that vibrates at 1.3 to 2.3 MHz (Fig. 6.12). These

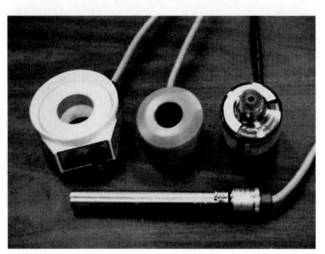

FIGURE 6.9 Heaters used with large-volume nebulizers. (From Scanlan CL, Wilkins RL, Stoller JK: *Egan's fundamentals of respiratory care*, ed 7, St. Louis, 1999, Mosby.)

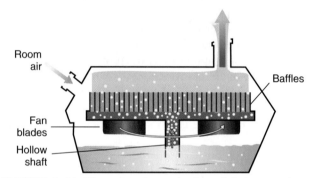

FIGURE 6.11 Diagram of a spinning disk large-volume nebulizer.

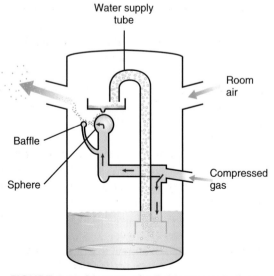

FIGURE 6.10 Diagram of a Babington nebulizer.

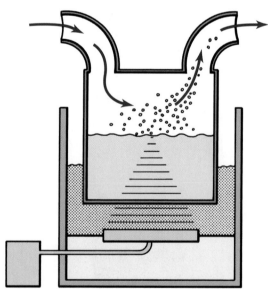

FIGURE 6.12 Ultrasonic nebulizer. High-frequency sound waves from a transducer are transmitted through a tap water couplant to the medication cup, where the fluid forms standing waves, producing aerosol. A gas source (e.g., a fan or compressed gas) is used to move the aerosol from the unit to the patient. (From Barnes TA: *Core textbook for respiratory care practice*, ed 2, St. Louis, 1994, Mosby.)

vibrations are transmitted through a liquid to create a cavitation in the liquid, forming a standing wave or "geyser" that sheds aerosol droplets. The vibrational energy is transmitted through a water-filled couplant reservoir or directly to a drug solution chamber. Although gas is not required to generate the aerosol, gas flow is required to convey the aerosol particles from the nebulizer to the patient. Some large-volume USNs use a built-in fan to direct room air through the nebulizer chamber. The airflow can be adjusted by changing the fan speed or by using a simple damper valve. As an alternative, compressed anhydrous gases can be delivered to the chamber inlet through a flowmeter. If necessary, the clinician can precisely control the delivered oxygen concentration by attaching a flowmeter with an oxygen blender or air entrainment system to the chamber inlet. Fig. 6.13 shows a commercially available USN manufactured by Nouvag AG.

The size of the particles produced by a USN is inversely proportional to the transducer's signal frequency, which is set by the manufacturer. The rate of aerosol production is directly related to the signal's amplitude. In some large-volume USNs, the signal amplitude can be adjusted by the clinician. The flow and amplitude settings interact to determine the density of the aerosol (mg/L) and the total water output (mL/min). At a given amplitude setting, the greater the flow through the chamber, the less dense the aerosol. Conversely, low flows result in higher density aerosols. The total aerosol output (mL/min) is greatest when both flow and amplitude are set at the maximum level. Using these settings, some units can achieve a total water output as high as 7 mL/min. High density and high aerosol output make the large-volume USN a valuable clinical tool for inducing sputum specimens for diagnostic analysis. USNs yield a higher quantity and quality of sputum for analysis than other nebulizers, but at some cost in increased airway reactivity.[20]

It is important to recognize that the particle size, aerosol density, and output of USNs are also affected by the RH of the carrier gas. Because of the considerable energy required to generate aerosols with a USN, the temperature of the solution increases by as much as 20°C during use of the device.

USNs marketed as "cool mist" devices are sold as room humidifiers for home use. The wet, large-volume reservoirs of these devices can easily become contaminated, resulting in airborne transmission of pathogens. Care should be taken to ensure that these units are cleaned according to the manufacturer's recommendations and that water is discarded from the reservoir periodically between cleanings. In the absence of a manufacturer's recommendation, these units should undergo appropriate disinfection at least every 6 days. As is discussed later in this chapter, passover and wick humidifiers present less risk for cross-contamination than does a USN used as a room humidifier.

Patient interface appliances. Airway appliances used to deliver bland aerosol therapy include the aerosol mask, face tent, T-tube, and tracheostomy mask. In all cases, large-bore tubing (22-mm ID) is used to minimize flow resistance and prevent occlusion by condensate. The aerosol mask and face tent are used with patients who have intact upper airways. T-tubes and tracheostomy masks are used for patients who have been intubated with an endotracheal tube or who have a tracheostomy tube in place. Tracheostomy masks can be used only for patients with tracheostomies.

For short-term therapy in patients with intact upper airways, the aerosol mask is the device of choice. However, some patients cannot tolerate masks and may do better with a face tent. No data are available to support preferential use of an open aerosol mask versus a face tent.

Although the T-tube is the most common application for tracheostomy patients, unless moderate to high F_IO_2 levels are needed, a tracheostomy mask may be a better choice. Unlike T-tubes, tracheostomy masks exert no traction on the airway, and they allow secretions and condensate to escape from the airway, reducing airway resistance.

A limitation of standard aerosol masks is the large venting holes that allow room air to be inhaled, which dilutes the gas and aerosol delivered. As mentioned previously, standard

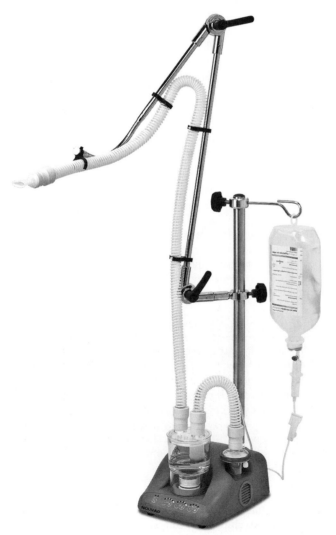

FIGURE 6.13 The Ultrasonic 2000, a large-volume ultrasonic nebulizer, which has controls for adjusting the fan flow and the nebulizer output rate. (Courtesy Nouvag AG, Goldach, Switzerland.)

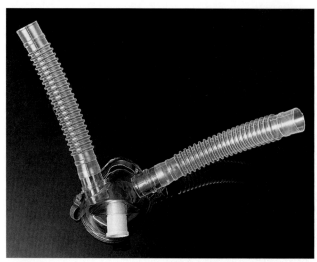

FIGURE 6.14 Aerosol mask modified with two 6-in sections of 22-mm internal diameter (ID) aerosol tubing. Each 6-in section has a 50-mL internal volume.

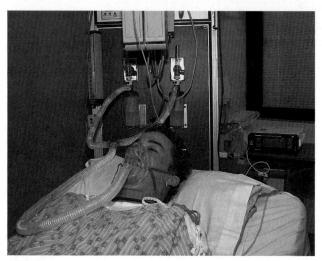

FIGURE 6.15 Two entrainment large-volume nebulizers are combined to create a high-flow system.

large-volume nebulizers do not have sufficient output to match the peak inspiratory flow of many patients. Aerosol masks can be modified by adding 6-in sections of the 22-mm ID aerosol tubing to the ports, which provides a small reservoir when peak inspiratory flow exceeds gas flow delivered to the mask (Fig. 6.14). An alternate strategy is to increase the aerosol output to the patient by setting up two aerosol devices in tandem and connecting them by a T-piece to the aerosol mask (Fig. 6.15).

Box 6.5 provides a step-by-step approach to setting up a large-volume jet nebulizer (also see Clinical Scenario 6.1).

Mist tents and hoods. Infants and small children may not easily tolerate direct airway appliances such as masks; therefore enclosures such as mist tents and aerosol hoods are used to deliver bland aerosol therapy to these patients. Recent studies have shown that in infants, aerosol hoods can provide aerosol delivery with efficiency similar to that of a properly fitted aerosol mask, with less discomfort for the patient.

BOX 6.5 **Setting Up a Cool or Heated Air Entrainment Large-Volume Jet Nebulizer**

1. Obtain the appropriate equipment:
   Oxygen flowmeter
   Nebulizer
   Large-bore corrugated tubing
   Drain bag
   Appropriate patient interface (i.e., aerosol mask, face tent, tracheostomy collar, or T-piece)
   Oxygen analyzer
   Thermometer (heated aerosol)
   Heating device (heated aerosol)
2. Attach flowmeter to 50-psi outlet.
3. Assemble the nebulizer. Aseptically fill the device with sterile water for inhalation if it was not prefilled.
4. Attach the nebulizer to the flowmeter.
5. Attach the large-bore corrugated tubing to the nebulizer.
6. Position the tubing so the drain bag is in the lowest position.
7. Attach the patient interface.
8. Turn on the gas flow to the nebulizer, and adjust the entrainment collar to the appropriate fractional delivered oxygen (F_DO_2). Verify the F_DO_2 with the oxygen analyzer, and adjust the entrainment collar as necessary to obtain the F_DO_2.
9. Make sure that the device is producing an adequate gas flow, and then apply the interface to the patient. Confirm adequacy of the gas flow by observing the aerosol escaping from the patient interface; the aerosol should not completely disappear during inspiration. If total flow remains inadequate (as demonstrated by complete disappearance of the aerosol during inspiration), increase the oxygen flow to the nebulizer. If the total flow continues to be inadequate and the oxygen flow is at maximum level, change the device to an injection nebulizer or a high-flow heated humidifier.
10. If a heated aerosol is clinically indicated, add the appropriate heating device to the nebulizer. Place a thermometer close to the patient interface, and verify that the aerosol has been warmed to a safe operating temperature.

CLINICAL SCENARIO 6.1

After abdominal surgery, a 50-year-old man is brought to the recovery room and started on an aerosol mask at a fractional inspired oxygen (F_IO_2) of 0.5. While performing your initial assessment of this patient, you notice that his respiratory rate is 20 breaths per minute and he shows signs of respiratory distress. You also note that during inspiration, the aerosol stops flowing from the mask. How would you remedy this situation to ensure that the patient is receiving 50% oxygen? See Appendix A for the answer.

Because mist tents were used for more than 40 years mainly to treat croup, clinicians often still refer to these devices as "croup tents." The use of this device to treat croup patients is based on the theory that a cool mist promotes vasoconstriction, reduces edema, and diminishes upper airway obstruction.

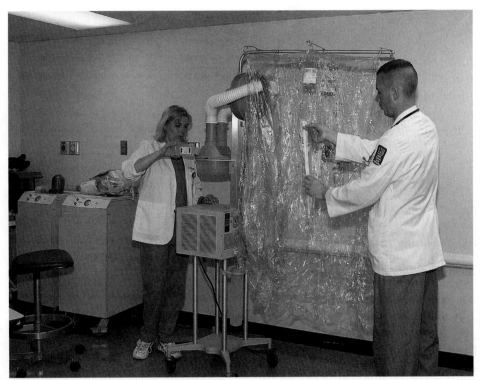

FIGURE 6.16 For this large aerosol tent, a large-volume reservoir and jet nebulizer have been integrated with a compressor-driven cooling unit to dissipate heat buildup in the tent.

Mist tents and hood enclosures present two major problems for many patients: carbon dioxide (CO_2) buildup and heat retention. The buildup of CO_2 can be reduced by providing sufficiently high gas flow rates. High flows of fresh gas circulate continually through the enclosure and "wash out" CO_2 while helping maintain the desired oxygen concentrations. Heat retention is handled differently by each manufacturer. Some devices (e.g., the Maxicool) use high flows of fresh gas to prevent heat buildup. Others incorporate a separate cooling device. Some tent devices (e.g., the Air Shields Croupette) use a simple ice compartment to cool the aerosol.

The Ohmeda Ohio Pediatric Aerosol Tent (Fig. 6.16) and the Mistogen CAM-2M Tent use electrically powered refrigeration units to cool the circulating air. The cooling from these refrigeration units produces a great deal of condensation, which must be drained into a collection bottle outside the tent. The problem was resolved in the Mistogen CAM-3M Tent through the use of a thermoelectric cooling system, in which an electric current passing through a semiconductor augments heat absorption and release. As warm air is taken from the tent, heat is transferred and released in the room while cool air is returned to the tent.

Problem solving and troubleshooting for bland aerosol systems. The most common problems with bland aerosol delivery systems involve infection control, environmental safety, inadequate mist production, overhydration, bronchospasm, and noise.

Infection control can be aided by rigorous adherence to infection control guidelines, especially those covering equipment processing. For example, water should be changed regularly, and the couplant compartments and nebulizer chambers of USNs should be disinfected or replaced regularly. Careful compliance with these measures helps minimize the risks involved in the use of aerosol systems.

Environmental safety concerns regarding secondhand and exhaled aerosol arise mainly when aerosol therapy is prescribed for immunosuppressed patients or patients who have been diagnosed with active tuberculosis. Respiratory therapists may be at increased risk for developing asthmalike symptoms, attributed in part to secondhand exposure to aerosols such as ribavirin. To minimize the risk, all clinicians should strictly follow the standards and airborne precautions established by the Centers for Disease Control and Prevention (CDC).

Inadequate mist production is a common problem with all nebulizer systems. With pneumatically powered jet nebulizers, poor mist production can be caused by inadequate input flow of driving gas, loose connections that cause a leak between the source gas and the nebulizer input, siphon tube obstruction, or jet orifice misalignment. Except for inadequate driving gas flow and loose connections, these problems require repair or replacement of the unit. For USNs that are not functioning properly, the electrical power supply (cord, plug, and fuse or circuit breakers) should be checked first. The clinician then should confirm that (1) carrier gas is actually flowing through the device and (2) the amplitude, or output, control is set above minimum. If the unit still has no visible mist output, the clinician should inspect the couplant chamber to confirm that the device has been filled to the proper level and that the nebulizer cup or crystal is free of any visible dirt, debris, or corrosion. Finally, the clinician must make sure that the solution in the couplant chamber meets the manufacturer's specifications (some units do not function properly with distilled water).

Overhydration is a potentially serious problem for patients treated with heated jet nebulizers and USNs. Because large-volume USNs are capable of high water outputs, they should never be used for continuous therapy. The risk for overhydration is greatest for infants, small children, and those with preexisting fluid or electrolyte imbalances. Even if used only to meet BTPS conditions, bland aerosol therapy effectively eliminates insensible water loss through the lungs and thus should be equated to a daily water gain (approximately 200 mL/day for the average adult). Another complication associated with overhydration is the potential for inspissated pulmonary secretions to swell after high-density aerosol therapy, which ultimately can lead to worsening airway obstruction. Careful patient selection and monitoring can prevent most potential problems with overhydration.

Bland water aerosols can cause bronchospasm in some patients. In fact, ultrasonic nebulization of distilled water is used in some pulmonary function laboratories to provoke bronchospasm and to assess bronchial hyperactivity.[21] To avoid this complication at the bedside, the clinician should always review the patient's history and diagnosis before administering any bland aerosol, especially a hypotonic water solution. As indicated in the AARC Clinical Practice Guideline, patients receiving continuous bland aerosol therapy initially should be monitored closely (including breath sounds and subjective response) and reevaluated every 8 hours or with any change in the patient's clinical condition.[17] If bronchospasm occurs during therapy, treatment must be stopped immediately, oxygen must be provided, and appropriate bronchodilator therapy should be initiated as soon as possible. If the physician still requests bland aerosol therapy for such a patient, pretreatment with a bronchodilator may be required. Also, these patients may better tolerate isotonic solutions (0.9% saline) than water.

A problem unique to large-volume air entrainment jet nebulizers is the noise they generate, especially at high flows. The American Academy of Pediatrics recommends that sound levels be kept below 58 dB to prevent hearing loss in infants cared for in incubators and oxygen hoods. Because a number of commercially available nebulizers exceed this noise level when in operation, careful selection of equipment is necessary.

Passover Humidifiers

A passover humidifier directs gas over a liquid or a liquid-saturated surface. The three common types of passover humidifiers are (1) simple reservoir models, (2) wick units, and (3) membrane devices.

The simple reservoir model directs gas over the surface of a volume of water or fluid. The surface for gas–fluid interface is limited. These systems typically are used to provide heated humidified gases during mechanical ventilation. Fig. 6.17 shows the Fisher & Paykel MR850. Passover humidifiers are also used for noninvasive nasal continuous positive airway pressure or bilevel ventilation.

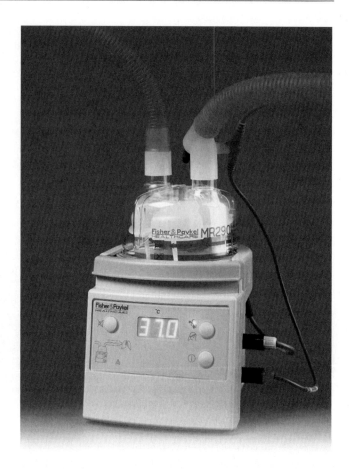

FIGURE 6.17 Fisher & Paykel MR850 heated humidifier. (Courtesy Fisher & Paykel Healthcare, Irvine, CA.)

In a wick humidifier, gas passes over or through water-saturated material. Fig. 6.18 shows a cross-section of a wick humidifier designed for placement in a ventilator circuit. The wick (a cylinder of absorbent material) is placed upright with the gravity-dependent end in a water reservoir and surrounded by a heating element. Capillary action continually draws up water from the reservoir and keeps the wick saturated. As dry gas enters the chamber, it flows around the wick, quickly picking up heat and moisture, leaving the chamber fully saturated with water vapor. No bubbling occurs; therefore no aerosol is produced. The Hudson RCI ConchaTherm IV (Hudson Respiratory Care) is an example of this type of humidifier (Fig. 6.19).

In a membrane humidifier the water is separated from the gas stream by a hydrophobic membrane. Water vapor molecules can pass through the membrane, but liquid water (and pathogens) cannot. As with wick humidifiers, bubbling and aerosol generation do not occur. Moreover, if a membrane humidifier were to be inspected while in use, no liquid water would be seen in the humidifier chamber.

The Vapotherm 2000i (Vapotherm) is a membrane cartridge system (see Fig. 4.12) that can heat and humidify oxygen at flows up to 40 L/min. This system has been used to provide high-flow oxygen via nasal cannula to a range of patients from infants to adults. The manufacturer maintains that this

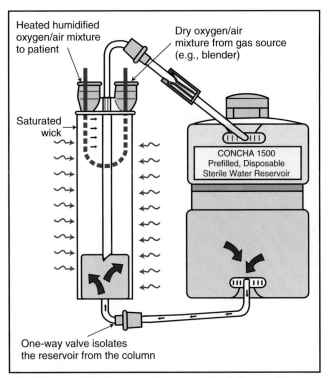

FIGURE 6.18 The low-compliance ConchaColumn with water reservoir assembly. Water enters the bottom of a metal column and saturates an absorbent wick lining the column. The column is inserted into a wraparound heating element. (Redrawn from Hudson Respiratory Care, Temecula, CA.)

technology allows molecular water vapor to pass into the gas stream but prevents direct contact between the water source and breathing gas, thereby creating a bacterial filter. The Hummax II (Metran Co., Ltd.) consists of a heated wire and polyethylene microporous hollow fiber placed in the tubing of the inspiratory circuit so that water vapor is delivered throughout the circuit.

Humidifier Heating Systems

Six types of heating elements and strategies are currently available:

- A hot-plate element at the base of the humidifier (e.g., the Fisher & Paykel MR850).
- A wraparound element that surrounds the humidifier chamber (e.g., the ConchaTherm IV and the Vapotherm).
- A yoke (or collar) element that sits between the water reservoir and the gas outlet.
- An immersion heater, with the element actually placed in the water reservoir (e.g., Cascade humidifier [Medtronic Minimally Invasive Therapies Puritan Bennett, Nellcor Puritan Bennett]).
- A heated wire in the inspiratory limb that warms a saturated wick or hollow fiber (e.g., Anamed [Vital Signs, Inc., a GE Healthcare Company] and Hummax II).
- A thin-film, high-surface-area boiler (e.g., Hydrate [PARI Respiratory Equipment]).

The Hydrate device (Fig. 6.20) represents a relatively new technology that uses C-force technology based on capillary

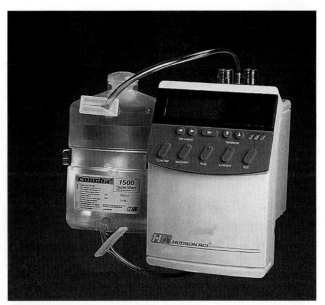

FIGURE 6.19 Hudson RCI ConchaTherm IV Heater Humidifier. (Courtesy Hudson Respiratory Care, Temecula, CA.)

force vaporization (CFV) (Vapore, LLC). The capillary force vaporizer is a thin-film, high-surface-area boiler that combines capillary force and phase transition to impart pressure onto an expanding gas (water vapor) and ejects it. The CFV is driven by software that controls a heater element and water flow. The disk, which is 19 mm in diameter, can deliver up to 2.2 mg/min of water vapor at 37°C. The single-patient-use C-force device, which includes the CFV disk mounted in a plastic housing, can be used for mechanical ventilation or high-flow gas. The unit includes a PC board, temperature probe, water and gas flow connecters, and a cable to the controller (Hydrate). Data from prototypes suggest that the temperature can be regulated from 33°C to 41°C (91.4°F to 105.8°F) for flows from 2 to 40 L/min.[22,23]

Humidifier heating systems generally have a controller that regulates the power to the heating element. In the simplest systems the controller monitors the heating element, varying the delivered current to match either a preset or an adjustable temperature. These systems might use a thermistor placed at the outlet of the humidifier, with the heater set to control output temperature. Servo-controlled heating systems monitor the temperature at the humidifier's outlet and at the patient's airway using a thermistor probe. The controller then adjusts heater power to achieve the desired airway temperature. Both types of controller units usually incorporate alarms and an alarm-activated heater shutdown function.

Reservoir and Feed Systems

Manual systems. Simple large reservoir systems may be manually refilled with sterile or distilled water. It is important to recognize that manually refilling the reservoir can change the reservoir temperature. Opening the reservoir for refilling can also interrupt mechanical ventilation and increase the risk for cross-contamination. Changing water levels alter the gas compression factor and thus the delivered volume during

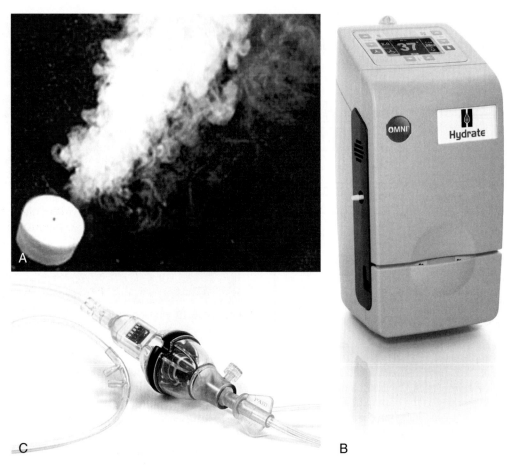

FIGURE 6.20 Hydrate humidification system for high-flow oxygen. (From Kacmarek RM, Stoller JK, Heuer AJ: *Egan's fundamentals of respiratory care,* ed 10, St. Louis, 2013, Mosby-Elsevier.)

mechanical ventilation, a critical factor during mechanical ventilation of the neonate.

Gravity feed system. A small inlet port in the wall of the humidifier chamber attached to a gravity-fed water bag allows refilling without interruption of ventilation. Such systems still require constant checking and manual replenishment by opening the line valve or clamp. If not checked regularly, the reservoir in these systems can go dry, placing the patient at risk.

Automatic feed systems avoid the need for constant checking and manual refilling of humidifiers. The simplest type of automatic feed system is the level-compensated reservoir (see Fig. 6.18). In these systems an external reservoir is aligned horizontally with the humidifier, maintaining relatively consistent water levels between the reservoir and the humidifier chamber. The addition of a siphon tube allows the low-compliance ConchaColumn to maintain the same water level independent of the water level in the reservoir.

Flotation valve controls can be used to maintain the fluid volume of the humidifier. In flotation systems a float rises and falls with the water level. If the water level falls below a preset value, the float opens the feed valve; as the water rises back to the set fill level, the float closes the feed valve (Fisher & Paykel MR290 chamber). Membrane humidifiers typically do

not require a sophisticated flow control system. Because the liquid water chamber underlying the membrane cannot overfill, membrane humidifiers require only an open gravity-feed system to ensure proper function.

Condensation. In standard heated humidifier systems, saturated gas cools as it leaves the point of humidification en route to the patient. As the gas cools, its water vapor capacity decreases, resulting in condensation, or "rainout." Factors that influence the amount of condensation include (1) the temperature difference across the system (humidifier to airway); (2) the ambient temperature; (3) the gas flow; (4) the set airway temperature; and (5) the length, diameter, and thermal mass of the breathing circuit.

Consider the following example, which illustrates how condensation forms in a ventilator circuit. Gas flowing from the ventilator to the patient is cooled as it flows through the circuit. To compensate for this cooling, the humidifier temperature must be set to a higher level (50°C) than that desired at the airway. At 50°C the humidifier fully saturates the gas to an absolute humidity of 84 mg/L of water. The capacity of the gas to hold water vapor decreases as cooling occurs along the tubing path. By the time the gas reaches the patient, its temperature has dropped to 37°C, and it is capable of holding only 44 mg/L of water vapor. Although BTPS conditions have

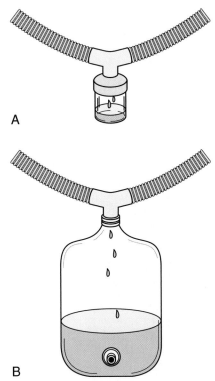

FIGURE 6.21 When condensate forms, the ribs in the 22-mm internal diameter (ID) corrugated tubing catch and hold it, and overflow tends to pool in the tubing. Placement of a trap (A) or drain bag at the low point of the circuit prevents condensate from obstructing the tubing.

been achieved, 40 mg/L, half the total output of the humidifier (84 − 44 mg/L = 40 mg/L), has condensed in the inspiratory limb of the circuit.

Condensation can disrupt or occlude gas flow through the circuit, potentially altering the F_1O_2 or ventilator function (or both), and it may even be aspirated by the patient. Typically, patients contaminate ventilator circuits within hours, and condensate is colonized with bacteria that can pose an infection risk.[24] To avoid problems in this area, health care personnel should treat all breathing circuit condensate as infectious waste.

To reduce the negative impact of condensate, circuits must be positioned to drain condensate away from the patient, and excess condensate must be drained from the circuit on a regular basis (Fig. 6.21). Water traps placed at low points in the circuit (both the inspiratory and expiratory limbs of ventilator circuits) allow emptying without disruption of ventilation. Several approaches can be used to collect condensate. Large-bore, corrugated tubing and small-volume taps can help minimize early pooling, which can obstruct the tubing. Small-volume traps can also help minimize pooling of condensate and do not cause large changes in ventilator circuit compliance. Some have spring-loaded valves that maintain a closed circuit during emptying. Drain system bags can collect large volumes of condensate over time, and the bag can be drained without breaking the ventilator circuit; however, the compressible volume may change a great deal.

It is worth mentioning that nebulizers with medication reservoirs below the aerosol generator that are placed in the ventilator circuit can act as a water trap, collecting contaminated condensate. This presents considerable risk that contaminated aerosols can be generated and pathogens delivered to the deep lung. To minimize this risk, nebulizers should be placed in a superior position so that any condensate travels downstream from the nebulizer. In addition, these nebulizers should be removed from the ventilator circuit between treatments. These devices should be rinsed with sterile water and air-dried or disposed of and replaced, if necessary.

Some other techniques that can be used to deal with the potential problems associated with condensation include adding insulation or increasing the thermal mass of the circuit and using coaxial circuits. With the insulation technique, condensation is reduced because the circuit is kept at a constant temperature. In a coaxial circuit, the inspiratory limb of the ventilator circuit is within the expiratory limb, which insulates the inspiratory limb with the ambient air (i.e., the warm exhaled gas surrounds the inspiratory limb, reducing the temperature gradient). These circuits have been more popular for use with anesthesia ventilators, but they are gaining some acceptance for use in the intensive care unit.

Heated-wire circuits, which are quite common in the intensive care unit, offer another approach to addressing the problems associated with condensation. Placing wire-heating elements in the ventilator circuit allows the gas delivered to the patient to remain at a constant temperature. Most heated-wire circuits use a dual-control mechanism with two temperature sensors, one that monitors the temperature of the gas leaving the humidifier and the other placed at or near the patient's airway (Fig. 6.22). The controller regulates the temperature difference between the humidifier output and the patient's airway. When heated-wire circuits are used, the humidifier heats gas to a lower temperature (32°C to 40°C [89.6°F to 104°F]) than it does with conventional circuits (45°C to 50°C [113°F to 122°F]). Management of this temperature gradient is critical to proper humidification.[24a-24d] When the humidifier is warmer than the circuit, rainout occurs. When the circuit is warmer than the humidifier output, the inspired gas will not be fully saturated, and a humidity deficit can be created. Notice that heated-wire circuits can produce unwanted levels of condensate. Fine tuning with the temperature differential is important. An additional strategy is to provide absorptive material in the inspiratory limb of the ventilator circuit, which acts as a wick warmed by the heated-wire system (e.g., Fisher & Paykel Healthcare, and Vital Signs, a GE Healthcare Company).

The use of heated-wire circuits in the treatment of neonates is complicated by the use of incubators and radiant warmers. Incubators provide a warm environment surrounding the child, and radiant warmers use radiant energy to warm objects that intercept radiant light. In both cases a temperature probe placed in the heated environment will affect the humidifier's performance, resulting in reduced humidity received by the patient. Therefore temperature probes should always be placed outside of the radiant field or incubator (Fig. 6.23).

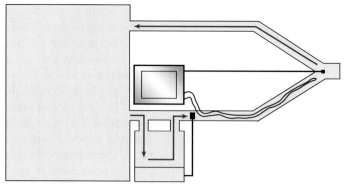

FIGURE 6.22 A heated-wire circuit in the inspiratory limb of the gas delivery tube. (From Kacmarek RM, Stoller JK, Heuer AJ: *Egan's fundamentals of respiratory care,* ed 10, St. Louis, 2013, Mosby-Elsevier.)

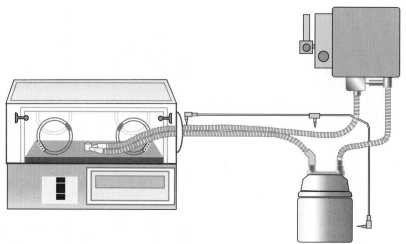

FIGURE 6.23 Neonatal breathing circuit configuration with incubator. The temperature probe is placed outside of the warming environment, and an unheated portion of the inspiratory circuit passes into the incubator and attaches to the Y-piece. (From Kacmarek RM, Stoller JK, Heuer AJ: *Egan's fundamentals of respiratory care,* ed 10, St. Louis, 2013, Mosby-Elsevier.)

Heat and Moisture Exchangers

The HME, or artificial nose, is classified as a passive humidifier. Like the nose, an HME captures and returns up to 70% of exhaled heat and humidity to the patient to heat and humidify the next inspiration (Fig. 6.24). Unlike the nose, with its rich vasculature and endothelium, most HMEs do not actively add heat or water to the system.

HMEs have been used successfully to meet the short-term humidification needs of spontaneously breathing and mechanically ventilated patients with endotracheal and tracheostomy tubes.[25] Earlier methods of classifying HMEs included (1) simple condenser humidifiers, (2) hygroscopic condenser humidifiers, and (3) hydrophobic condenser humidifiers.

Simple HMEs contain a condenser element with high thermal conductivity, usually consisting of metallic gauze, corrugated metal, or parallel metal tubes with or without an additional fibrous element. On inspiration, inspired air cools the condenser element. On exhalation, expired water vapor condenses directly on the element's surface and warms it. On the next inspiration, cool, dry air is warmed and humidified

as its passes over the condenser element. Simple condenser humidifiers are only able to recapture less than 50% of a patient's exhaled moisture (50% efficiency). Fibrous material aids in moisture retention and reduces pooling of condensate. Moisture output ranges from 10 to 14 mg H_2O per liter. The addition of filtering capability to the HME has increased its efficiency. These heat and moisture exchanging filters (HMEFs) have an increased internal surface area of the medium and can provide a moisture output in the range of 18 to 28 mg H_2O per liter.

Hygroscopic heat and moisture exchangers (HHMEs) provide higher efficiency by (1) using a condensing element of low thermal conductivity (e.g., paper, wool, or foam) and (2) impregnating this material with a hygroscopic salt (calcium or lithium chloride). During exhalation, some water vapor condenses on the cool condenser element, whereas other water molecules bind directly to the hygroscopic salt. During inspiration the lower water vapor pressure in the inspired gas liberates water molecules directly from the hygroscopic salt, without cooling. These devices typically achieve approximately

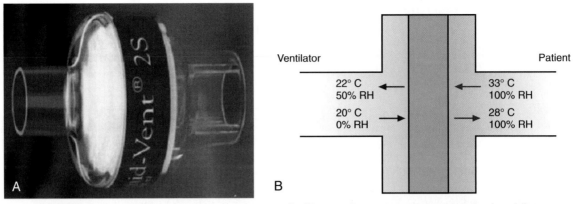

FIGURE 6.24 A, Heat and moisture exchanger. B, Changes in temperature and relative humidity (RH) as gas passes from the patient to the ventilator circuit during exhalation and from the vent to the patient during inhalation. (Courtesy Telefax Medical, Research Triangle Park, NC.)

70% efficiency. Moisture output ranges from 22 to 34 mg H_2O per liter.

Hygroscopic heat and moisture exchangers with filter (HHMEF) combine the HHME with a water-repellent and often electrostatically charged medium with a large surface area with filtration capabilities and low thermal conductivity. The filter medium often is placed between the HHME and the ventilator circuit. In efficiency, these devices are comparable with hygroscopic condenser humidifiers; they offer a small increase in moisture output but with increased airway resistance. Fig. 6.25 shows examples of several different types of HMEs.

Design and performance standards for HMEs are set by the International Organization for Standardization (ISO).[26] Ideally, an HME should operate at 70% efficiency or better (providing at least 30 mg/L of water vapor). HMEs use standard connections, have a low compliance, and add minimal weight, dead space, and flow resistance to a breathing circuit.[27] HMEs come in a broad range of shapes and sizes. Their performance varies from brand to brand and may differ from manufacturers' specifications (Lemmens & Brock-Utne, 2004).[27a] The moisture output of HMEs tends to fall at high volumes and high rates of breathing. In addition, high inspiratory flows and high F_1O_2 levels can reduce the HME's efficiency.[27] When an HME is dry, resistance across most devices is minimal. However, because of water absorption, HME flow resistance increases after several hours' use.[28,29] In some patients the increased resistance imposed by the HME may not be well tolerated, particularly if underlying lung disease already causes increased work of breathing.

Because HMEs eliminate the problem of breathing circuit condensation, many consider these devices (especially HMEs with hydrophobic filters) to be helpful in preventing nosocomial infections. Although HMEs show less bacterial colonization of ventilator circuits than active humidification systems, circuit colonization plays a minor role in the development of nosocomial infections, provided the usual maintenance precautions are applied.[30] Because HMEs delivering at least 30 mg H_2O or more per liter are associated with a lower incidence

of endotracheal tube (ETT) occlusion, they are recommended for use.[24c,27a]

The position of the HME relative to the patient's airway can affect the device's ability to both heat and humidify inhaled gas. Intuitively, placing the HME directly at the patient airway would seem to be best; however, secretions can occlude an HME attached directly to the airway. The use of equipment such as closed-suction catheters and airway monitor ports requires placement of the HME closer to the ventilator circuit's Y-piece. Inui et al. tested the performance of HMEs placed in two different positions: directly at the airway (10 cm from an endotracheal tube) and proximal to the ventilator circuit.[29] Both HMEs tested performed best at the airway, although one model did not perform adequately at either site. The other HME model exceeded recommended performance standards (≥30 mg/L absolute humidity and 30°C [86°F]) at both sites. Clinicians should select the HME that performs adequately when placed at the intended site.

Although use of HMEs has been associated with thickened secretions in some patients, the incidence of ETT occlusion is lower with HMEs than when heated humidifiers are used.[31] HMEs are not recommended for use with infants for several reasons. HMEs add 30 to 90 mL of mechanical dead space, often exceeding the tidal volume of a 5-kg infant (25 mL). Uncuffed ETTs in small infants allow a portion of exhaled gas to leak around the tube, bypassing the HME and reducing its ability to capture exhaled heat and humidity. The provision of heated humidity at temperatures less than 35°C (95°F) has been associated with narrowing and obstruction of ETTs in infants. A simple set of questions can help determine when use of an HME is appropriate.

HMEs have been developed for use by patients with a tracheostomy who no longer require mechanical ventilation but only room air or low-flow oxygen. Devices to fit on an ETT vary by design, but they typically allow an inlet port for low-flow oxygen and in some cases have silicon suction ports that act as one-way valves.

Patients who no longer need an artificial airway and can breathe through an open stoma may benefit from HMEs like

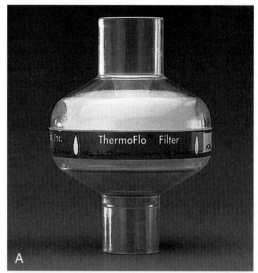

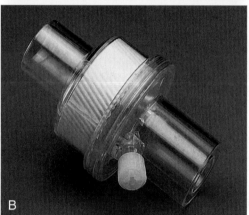

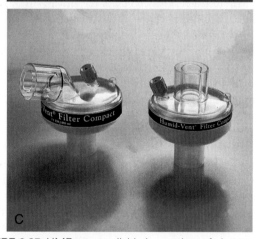

FIGURE 6.25 HMEs are available in a variety of shapes, sizes, and types. A, ThermoFlo HME (ARC Medical, Inc). B, Hygrolife HME Heat and Moisture Exchanger Hygroscopic (Medtronic Minimally Invasive Therapies). C, Humid-Vent Filter with gas sampling port (Teleflex).

the one shown in Fig. 6.26. This combines the benefit of heat and humidity with the filtration of gross particulates from inhaled gas.

Active Heat and Moisture Exchangers

Active HMEs add humidity or heat (or both) to inspired gas by chemical or electrical means. These devices have been

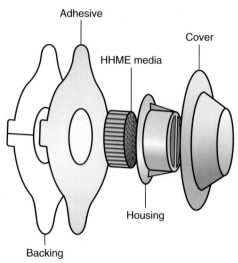

FIGURE 6.26 Components of a hygroscopic heat and moisture exchanger (HHME) for use with a tracheal stoma.

shown to be equivalent to mainstream active humidifiers in both in vitro and in vivo use. Active HMEs add weight and complexity at the patient airway.

The Humid-Heat (Louis Gibeck AB) consists of a supply unit with a microprocessor, water pump, and a humidification device, which is placed between the Y-piece and the ETT. The humidification device is based on an HHME, which absorbs expired heat and moisture and releases it into the inspired gas. External heat and water are then added to the patient side of the HME so that the inspired gas should reach 100% humidity at 37°C (44 mg H_2O per liter of air). The external water is delivered to the humidification device via a pump onto a wick and then evaporated into the inspired air by an electrical heater. The microprocessor controls the water pump and the heater by an algorithm using the minute ventilation (which is fed into the microprocessor) and the airway temperature measured by a sensor mounted in the flex-tube on the patient side of the humidification device.

The HME-Booster (King Systems), which was designed for use as an adjunct to a passive HME, consists of a T-piece containing an electrically heated element (Fig. 6.27). The heating element heats water so that water vapor passes into the airway between the artificial airway and the ETT, through a Gore-Tex membrane and aluminum. Water is fed to the heater from a gravity feed bag via a flow regulator that limits flow to 10 mL/h. The heater operates at 110°C (230°F) and adds 3 to 5.5 mg/L of humidity and 3°C to 4°C of inhaled gas compared with an HME alone. It is designed for patients with minute volumes of 4 to 20 L, and it is not appropriate for use with pediatric patients or infants. Box 6.6 presents information about the clinical findings for use of a heat and moisture exchanger.

Setting Humidification Levels

The American National Standards Institute (ANSI) recommends that the minimum level of humidity for intubated patients exceed 30 mg/L; however, the ANSI has not recommended an optimum level of humidification for nonintubated

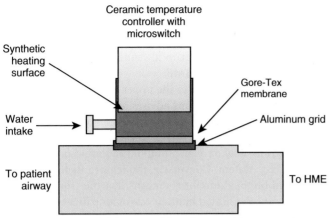

FIGURE 6.27 HME-Booster (King Systems) is a membrane humidifier that is placed between the patient's airway and the heat and moisture exchanger. *HME,* Heat and moisture exchanger.

> ### BOX 6.6 Clinical Findings for Use of a Heat and Moisture Exchanger
>
> - Are there bloody secretions or thick sputum? Is the core temperature less than 32°C (89.6°F)?
> - If not, a hygroscopic condenser humidifier (HCH) can be used. Evaluate the quality and quantity of secretions.
> - If yes, heated humidification at 32°C to 34°C (89.6°F to 93.2°F) and 100% relative humidity at proximal airway is recommended.
> - If more than four HCHs are used within a 24-h period, then heated humidification as described above is recommended.

---

patients. One suggestion is to deliver the temperature and level of humidity for normal conditions at the point where the gas enters the airway. For example, air entering the carina typically has a humidity level of 35 to 40 mg/L. Studies have suggested that operating a humidifier at a temperature less than 32°C for adults and less than 35°C for infants can lead to increased airway plugging. Furthermore, active heated humidifiers may perform differently under the same conditions. Nishida[32] compared the performance of five active humidifiers (MR290 with MR730, MR310 with MR730 [Fisher & Paykel], ConchaTherm IV, and Hummax II), which were set to maintain the temperature of the airway opening at 32°C and 37°C under a variety of ventilator parameters. The greater the minute ventilation, the lower the humidity delivered with all the devices except the Hummax II. When the devices' airway temperature control was set at 32°C, the ConchaTherm IV, the MR310, and the MR730 did not deliver 30 mg/L of vapor, the minimum level recommended by the ANSI. These results point to the need to set humidifiers to maintain airway temperatures in the range of 35°C to 37°C.

The appropriate temperature and humidity of inspired gas delivered to mechanically ventilated patients with artificial airways are the subject of controversy. The current AARC Clinical Practice Guideline recommends a temperature of 33°C ± 2°C and a minimum humidity level of 30 mg/L.

Williams[33] suggests that inspired gas be delivered at 37°C with 100% RH and a water vapor level of 44 mg/L to prevent complications. Theoretically, optimum humidity improves mucociliary clearance. To guide practitioners in the use of humidity therapy for patients receiving ventilatory support, AARC has published its *Clinical Practice Guideline: Humidification During Mechanical Ventilation.*[7]

Problem Solving and Troubleshooting for Humidification Systems

Common problems with humidification systems include dealing with condensation, preventing cross-contamination, and ensuring proper conditioning of the inspired gas.

Cross-Contamination

Aerosol and condensate from ventilator circuits are known sources of bacterial colonization.[24] However, advances in both circuit and humidifier technology have reduced the risk for nosocomial infection with the use of these systems. Wick or membrane passover humidifiers prevent the formation of bacteria-carrying aerosols. Heated-wire circuits reduce the production and pooling of condensate within the circuit. In addition, the high reservoir temperatures in humidifiers are bacteriocidal.[22] In fact, in ventilator circuits using wick humidifiers with heated-wire systems, circuit contamination usually occurs from the patient to the circuit rather than vice versa.

For decades the traditional way to minimize the risk for circuit-related nosocomial infection in critically ill patients receiving ventilatory support was to change the ventilator tubing and its attached components every 24 hours. It is now known that frequent ventilator circuit changes actually increase the risk for nosocomial pneumonia.[23] Current research indicates that minimal risk for ventilator-associated pneumonia exists with weekly circuit changes and that circuits may not need to be changed unless they are visibly soiled.[23,34] In addition, substantial cost savings can accrue with fewer frequent circuit changes.

Monitoring Proper Conditioning of the Inspired Gas

All respiratory therapists are trained to monitor patients' F_IO_2 levels regularly and, in ventilatory care, to monitor selected pressures, volumes, and flows. However, few clinicians take the steps needed to ensure proper conditioning of the inspired gas received by their patients. The most accurate and reliable way to ensure that patients receive gas at the expected temperature and humidity level is to measure these parameters. Portable, battery-operated digital hygrometer-thermometer systems are available for less than $300 and are invaluable for ensuring proper conditioning of the inspired gas.

Many heated-wire humidification systems have a humidity control. However, this control does not reflect either the absolute humidity or the RH, but only the temperature differential between the humidifier and the airway sensor. If the heated wires are set warmer than the humidifier, less RH is delivered to the patient. To ensure that the inspired gas is properly conditioned, clinicians should always adjust the temperature differential to the point where a few drops of condensation form near the patient's Y-adapter. Lacking direct measurement of humidity, observation of this minimal condensate is the most reliable indicator that the gas is fully saturated at the specified temperature. If condensate cannot be seen, there is no way of knowing the level of RH without direct measurement; it could be anything from 99% to 0%! HME performance can be evaluated in a similar manner.[35]

Selecting the Appropriate Humidity and Bland Aerosol Therapy

Fig. 6.28 presents a basic algorithm for selecting or recommending the appropriate therapy to condition a patient's inspired gas. Key considerations include (1) the gas flow, (2) the presence or absence of an artificial tracheal airway, (3) the character of the pulmonary secretions, (4) the need for and expected duration of mechanical ventilation, and (5) contraindications to use of an HME.

For delivering oxygen to the upper airway, the American College of Chest Physicians advises against using a bubble humidifier at flow rates of 4 L/min or less.[36] For the occasional patient who complains of nasal dryness or irritation when receiving low-flow oxygen, a humidifier should be added to the delivery system. Conversely, the relative inefficiency of unheated bubble humidifiers means that the clinician may need to consider heated humidification for patients receiving

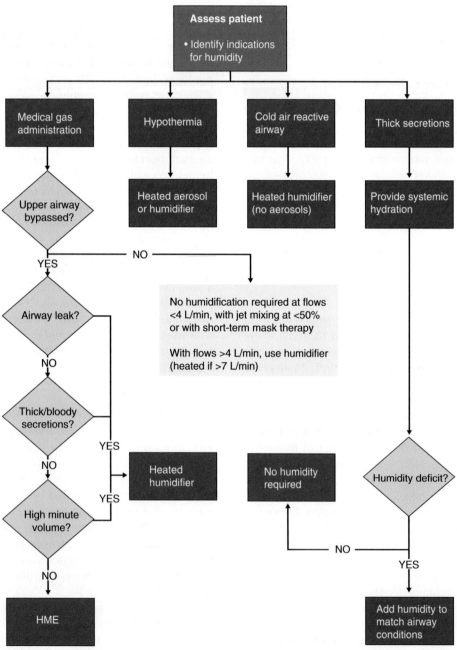

FIGURE 6.28 Algorithm for selecting the correct humidity and bland aerosol therapy. *HME*, Heat and moisture exchanger. (From Kacmarek RM, Stoller JK, Heuer AJ: *Egan's fundamentals of respiratory care*, ed 10, St. Louis, 2013, Mosby-Elsevier.)

long-term oxygen at high flow rates (>10 L/min without air entrainment).

HMEs provide an inexpensive alternative to heated humidifiers when used for ventilation of patients who do not have complex humidification needs. However, passive HMEs may not provide sufficient heat or humidification for long-term management of certain patients. When an HME is used, its selection should be based on the individual patient's ventilatory pattern, as well as the unit's performance, efficiency, and size. Moreover, all patients using HMEs should be reevaluated regularly so that the appropriateness of continued use can be confirmed.[37]

Clinical Scenario 6.2 presents an exercise to test your ability to select the appropriate device for patients requiring humidity therapy.

II. AEROSOL THERAPY

The goal of medical aerosol therapy is to deliver a therapeutic dose of a selected agent (i.e., drug) to the desired site of action.[38] The indications for delivering a particular agent depend on the condition being treated. For patients with pulmonary disorders, the administration of drugs by aerosol offers the advantage of achieving higher local drug concentrations in the lung with lower systemic levels compared with other forms of administration. Improved therapeutic action with fewer systemic side effects provides a higher therapeutic index.

Characteristics of Therapeutic Aerosols

Effective use of medical aerosols requires an understanding of the characteristics of aerosols and their effect on drug delivery to the desired site of action. Key concepts include aerosol output, particle size, and deposition.

Aerosol Output

Aerosol output is the mass of fluid or drug produced or emitted by a nebulizer. The emitted dose is the mass of drug leaving the mouthpiece of a nebulizer or inhaler as aerosol. Output is expressed as either the total mass emitted or as a percentage of the dose placed in the nebulizer. The output rate is the mass emitted per unit of time.

Aerosol output is measured by collecting the emitted aerosol on filters and measuring either the weight (gravimetric analysis) or the amount of drug (assay). Gravimetric measurements of drugs in aerosols are less reliable than drug assay techniques because weight changes caused by water evaporation cannot be differentiated from changes in drug mass.

Particle Size

Aerosol particle size depends on the method used to generate the aerosol, the substance nebulized, and the environmental conditions surrounding the particle. The unaided human eye cannot see particles smaller than 50 μm in diameter (the size of a small grain of sand). The most common laboratory methods used to measure aerosol particle size are liquid impingers, cascade impactors, and laser diffraction. Liquid impingers capture particles of different sizes on fluid placed in serial reservoirs. Cascade impactors collect aerosol particles of different size ranges on a series of stages or plates. For both methods the mass of aerosol deposited is quantified by drug assay, and a distribution of particle sizes is calculated. With laser diffraction a computer is used to estimate the range and frequency of droplet volumes crossing the laser beam.

Because medical aerosols contain particles of many different sizes (i.e., they are heterodisperse), the average particle size is expressed with a measure of central tendency, such as mass median aerodynamic diameter (MMAD) for cascade impaction or volume median diameter (VMD) for laser diffraction. These measurement methods may report different sizes for the same aerosol.

In an aerosol distribution with a specific MMAD or VMD, 50% of the particles are smaller and have less mass, and 50% are larger and have greater mass. The variability of particle sizes in an aerosol distribution set at 1 standard deviation (SD) above or below the median (15.8% and 84.13%, respectively) is the geometric standard deviation (GSD). The greater the GSD, the wider the range of particle sizes and the more heterodisperse the aerosol. Monodisperse aerosols consisting of particles of similar size have a GSD less than or equal to 1.4. Nebulizers that produce monodisperse aerosols are used mainly in laboratory research and nonmedical industries.

Deposition

The inhaled mass is the amount of drug inhaled. It represents only a portion of the emitted dose. The fine-particle fraction (FPF) is the percentage of the aerosol small enough to have a good chance of depositing in lung (1 to 5 μm). The product of the inhaled mass multiplied by the FPF is the respirable mass.

In inertial impaction a particle of sufficient (relatively large) mass, which is moving in a gas stream that changes direction, tends to remain on its initial path and collide with the airway surface. This is the primary mechanism of deposition for particles larger than 5 μm. Inertia involves both mass and velocity. Turbulent flow patterns, obstructed or tortuous pathways, and inspiratory flow rates greater than 30 L/min are associated with increased inertial impaction.

Sedimentation occurs when aerosol particles settle out of suspension as a result of gravity. The greater the mass of a

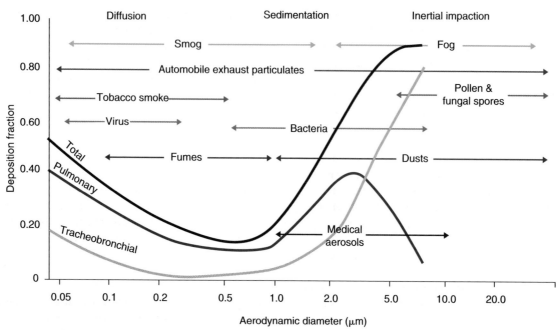

FIGURE 6.29 Range of particle size for common aerosols in the environment and the influence of particle size on diffusion, sedimentation, and inertial impaction. (Modified from Yu CP, Nicolaides P, Soong TT: Effect of random airway sizes on aerosol deposition. *Am Ind Hyg Assoc J* 40(11):999-1005, 1979.)

particle, the faster it settles. During normal breathing, sedimentation is the primary mechanism of deposition for particles 1 to 5 μm. Sedimentation occurs mostly in the central airways and increases with time.

Diffusion, or Brownian motion, is the primary mechanism of deposition for small particles (<3 μm), mainly in the respiratory region, where bulk gas flow ceases and most aerosol particles reach the alveoli by diffusion. These aerosol particles have very low mass and are easily bounced around by collisions with carrier gas molecules. These random molecular collisions cause some particles to contact and become deposited on surrounding surfaces. Particles between 0.5 and 1 μm are so stable that most remain in suspension and are cleared with the exhaled gas, whereas particles smaller than 0.5 μm have a greater retention rate in the lungs. Fortunately, these small particles do not have much mass; therefore they represent only a small percentage of the total drug dose that is lost on exhalation (typically 1% to 5% of an inhaled drug).

Aging is the process by which aerosol particles grow, shrink, coalesce, and fall out of suspension over time. The way an aerosol ages depends on the composition of the aerosol, the initial size of its particles, the time in suspension, and the ambient conditions to which it is exposed. Aerosol particle size can decrease or increase as a result of evaporation or hygroscopic water absorption, respectively. The relative rate of particle size change is inversely proportional to the size of a particle; therefore small particles grow or shrink faster than larger particles.

Aerosol deposition is affected by the inspiratory flow rate and pattern, respiratory rate, inhaled volume, ratio of inspiratory time to expiratory time (I:E ratio), and breath-holding.

Airway obstruction is one of the most important factors influencing aerosol deposition. Kim[39] demonstrated that total pulmonary deposition is greater in smokers and patients with obstructive airway disease than in healthy individuals. Similarly, when inspiratory flow rates are constant, the deposition fraction of monodisperse aerosols increases with increased tidal volume, length of respiratory (inspiratory) period, and particle size.

Relatively simple in vitro models simulating a range of tidal volumes, inspiratory flow rates, I:E ratios, and respiratory rates have been useful in predicting the inhaled mass of drug and the relative performance of nebulizers.[40] Fig. 6.29 summarizes the relationships between particle size and aerosol deposition in the respiratory tract. Notice that the depth of penetration and deposition of a particle in the respiratory tract can vary with particle size and tidal volume.[41]

Hazards of Aerosol Therapy

In addition to an adverse reaction to the medication administered, the hazards of aerosol therapy include infection, airway reactivity, systemic effects of bland aerosols, and drug concentration changes during nebulization.

Infection

Aerosol generators can contribute to nosocomial infections by allowing the airborne spread of bacteria. Common sources of bacteria include contaminated solutions (i.e., multiple-dose drug vials), caregivers' hands, and the patient's own secretions. The organisms most often associated with these types of nosocomial infections are Gram-negative bacilli, particularly *Pseudomonas aeruginosa* and *Legionella pneumophila*.[42]

According to CDC guidelines, nebulizers should be either sterilized between patients or replaced every 24 hours. In the home care setting, the generally accepted practice is to rinse the nebulizer with sterile water (not tap water) and air-dry it after each treatment. Weekly disinfection of these devices with a diluted acetic acid (white vinegar) solution can also help to reduce the infection risk in the home care environment.

Airway Reactivity

Cold and high-density aerosols can cause reactive bronchospasm and increased airway resistance.[43] Medications such as acetylcysteine, antibiotics, steroids, cromolyn sodium, ribavirin, and distilled water are associated with increased airway resistance and wheezing during aerosol therapy. Administration of bronchodilators before or with administration of these agents may reduce the risk or duration of increased airway resistance.

The risk for inducing bronchospasm always should be considered when aerosols are administered. Monitoring for reactive bronchospasm should include peak flow measurements or measurement of the percentage of the forced expiratory volume in 1 second (% FEV_1) before and after therapy; auscultation for adventitious breath sounds; observation of the patient's breathing pattern and overall appearance; and, the most essential part, communicating with the patient during therapy to determine the perceived work of breathing.[44]

Pulmonary and Systemic Effects

Aerosols have the potential to cause both local and systemic effects (i.e., effects at the site of delivery or effects caused by absorption into the systemic circulation). These effects largely depend on the drug concentration delivered, but they also may be associated with the size, temperature, and volumes of aerosols delivered.

As has already been mentioned, aerosols can have a local irritating effect, resulting in bronchospasm. Animal data indicate that long-term, continuous administration of bland aerosols can cause localized inflammation and tissue damage, atelectasis, and pulmonary edema. Continuous high-output aerosol administration also can increase the risks for overhydration and electrolyte disturbances, such as hypernatremia (the latter risks are especially important in pediatric patients).

Preliminary assessment therefore should balance the need versus the risk of aerosol therapy, especially among patients at high risk, such as infants, those prone to fluid and electrolyte imbalances, and patients with atelectasis or pulmonary edema. Care must be taken to ensure that patients are capable of clearing secretions once the secretions are mobilized by aerosol therapy. Appropriate airway clearance techniques should accompany any aerosol therapy designed to help mobilize secretions.

Drug Concentration Changes

During the evaporation, heating, baffling, and recycling of drug solutions undergoing jet or ultrasonic nebulization, the solute concentration may increase significantly.[45] This process may expose the patient to increasingly higher concentrations of the drug over the course of a therapeutic session. An increase in concentration therefore is time dependent, with the greatest effect occurring when medications are nebulized over extended periods. Although the clinical implications of this change in drug concentration have not been well documented, the clinician should keep this factor in mind during continuous aerosol drug delivery.

Eye Irritation

Eye irritation may be an issue during aerosol drug delivery via a face mask with nebulizers or open-mouth technique with pressurized metered-dose inhalers as a result of inadvertent drug deposition in the eyes. Some mask designs have been shown to reduce drug deposition in the eyes. Clinicians should exercise caution when a face mask is used during aerosol therapy.

Exposure to Secondhand Aerosol Drugs

Exposure to secondhand aerosol drugs may be a problem for health care providers and bystanders because it was shown that repeated secondhand exposure to bronchodilators is associated with increased risk for occupational asthma. According to Ari et al.,[46] up to 40% of aerosols delivered during mechanical ventilation are exhausted to the environment if there is no filter placed in the expiratory limb. Therefore, developing and implementing an occupational health and safety policy are important to minimize the risk for secondhand aerosol exposure.[47-49]

Aerosol Drug-Delivery Systems

Aerosol generators in clinical use include pressurized metered-dose inhalers (pMDIs), dry powder inhalers (DPIs), jet nebulizers (small and large volume), USNs, hand-bulb atomizers (including nasal spray pumps), vibrating mesh nebulizers, and a number of emerging technological devices. Device selection and proper operation can make the difference between successful and unsuccessful therapy; consequently, clinicians must have in-depth knowledge of the operating principles and performance characteristics of the various systems and how best to select and apply them.

Metered-Dose Inhalers

The pressurized metered-dose inhaler (pMDI) is the most commonly prescribed method of aerosol delivery. pMDIs are compact, portable, relatively easy to use, and offer multidose convenience. Unlike most nebulizers, the pMDI was developed as a drug-device combination, with the actuator boot and canister designed for the specific drug formulation and dose volume to be delivered. pMDIs can be used to administer short- and long-acting bronchodilators, anticholinergics, and steroids. Indeed, more formulations of these drugs are available for use by pMDI than for any other type of nebulizer.

Although pMDIs appear to be rather simple and relatively easy to use, they represent sophisticated technology and engineering and are often misused by patients. When properly used, pMDIs are at least as effective as other nebulizers for drug delivery. For this reason, pMDIs often are the preferred method for delivering bronchodilators to spontaneously breathing patients, as well as to those who are intubated and undergoing mechanical ventilation.[50]

Equipment design. A typical pMDI consists of a pressurized canister that contains a drug (a micronized powder or aqueous solution) in a volatile propellant combined with surfactants, dispersing agents, preservatives, and flavoring agents (Fig. 6.30). The active drug represents 1% or less of the mixture emitted from the pMDI. Chlorofluorocarbons (CFCs), such as Freon, were the propellants used in pMDIs since their introduction in 1956. However, because of Freon's contribution to the effects of global warming, other pMDI propellants have been developed, such as hydrofluoroalkane (HFA-134a). The most common dispersal agents are surfactants (e.g., soy lecithin, sorbitan trioleate, and oleic acid), which help keep the drug suspended in the propellant and lubricate the valve mechanism. Solvents used to dissolve the drug and surfactant include ethanol, glycerol, and propylene glycol.

A pMDI is designed to deliver smaller doses than a nebulizer and DPI. Metering valve volumes of 25 to 100 μL limit dose per actuation to typically 50 μg to 5 mg, depending on the drug formulation. When the canister is inverted (nozzle down) and placed in its actuator, or "boot," the volatile suspension fills a metering chamber that controls the amount of drug delivered. Pressing down on the canister aligns a hole in the metering valve with the metering chamber. The high-propellant

vapor pressure quickly forces the metered dose out through this hole and through the actuator nozzle.

Aerosol production takes approximately 20 milliseconds (msec). As the liquid suspension is forced out of the pMDI, it forms a plume, within which the propellants vaporize, or "flash." Once the pMDI is actuated, the initial velocity of this plume is high (>30 m/sec), and the particles are large (35 μm). Within 0.1 second, the plume velocity decreases more than 50%, and propellant particle size reduces (to 3 to 5 μm) as the plume extends 10 cm from the actuator nozzle.[51]

Nozzle size may be different with each type of pMDI and actuator, and debris or moisture on the nozzle/actuator reduces aerosol drug delivery. Therefore the pMDI nozzle actuator should be cleaned based on manufacturer's recommendations, and the pMDI canister should never be placed under water.

Before initial use and after prolonged storage, every pMDI should be primed by actuating the device one to four times (see the label for the specific pMDI). Without priming, the initial dose actuated from a new pMDI canister contains less active substance than subsequent actuations.[52] A reduction in the emitted dose with the first actuation commonly occurs with a pMDI after storage, particularly when the pMDI is stored with the valve pointed in the downward position. This "loss of dose" from a pMDI occurs when drug particles rise to the top of the canister over time, like cream rising to the top of milk. This development is related to valve design and occurs when propellant leaks from the metering chamber during periods of nonuse (in as little as 4 hours).[52]

Improved metering valve designs have been developed for use with HFA propellants in an attempt to reduce these losses. Unlike CFC pMDIs that have not been used for 8 to 12 hours, pMDIs containing HFA propellants may not require wasting of dose for periods ranging from 2 days to 2 weeks. Because each pMDI is different, the clinician and the patient need to be aware of the priming requirements for the specific formulation being used.

A cold ambient temperature (<10°C [50°F]) dramatically reduces the output of CFC pMDIs. This is an issue during cold weather, when people with asthma tend to keep their pMDIs in an outer coat pocket for easy access. Patients should be instructed to keep the pMDI closer to the body and to warm the pMDI to body temperature before inhalation by rubbing the canister with their hands. Reduction of dose at lower temperatures is less of an issue with the pMDIs that use HFA and other, newer propellants.[13]

Aerosol delivery characteristics. Pulmonary deposition ranges from 10% to 20% with a standard CFC pMDI.[53] Although many of the new HFA pMDIs were designed to match this low level of dose efficiency, some pMDIs containing HFA propellants (e.g., QVAR, 3M, St. Paul, MN) can deposit as much as 50% of the emitted dose. As aerosol is emitted from the pMDI, particles are as large as 30 μm. Although pMDIs can produce particles in the respired range (MMAD of 3 to 6 μm), this transition occurs at approximately 10 cm from the nozzle.[52] Consequently, when pMDIs are used as directed, the initial velocity and larger particles that are generated when the device is placed between the lips result in

Metered-Dose Inhaler

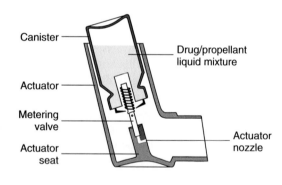

Metered-Valve Function

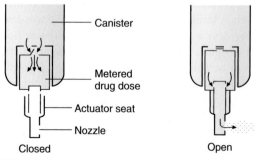

FIGURE 6.30 Key components of a pressurized metered-dose inhaler. (From Gardenhire DS: *Rau's respiratory care pharmacology*, ed 8, St. Louis, 2012, Mosby-Elsevier.)

approximately 80% of the dose being deposited in the oropharynx.

New pressurized metered dose inhaler technology. The Aerospan (Meda Pharmaceuticals) was developed to deliver flunisolide hemihydrate using a built-in valveless spacer to eliminate the hand-breath coordination. It does not need to be cleaned on a regular basis to maintain proper orientation. The disadvantage of the Aerospan is that it does not have a built-in dose counter.

Techniques of administration, cleaning, and maintenance. Administration of aerosol drugs by pMDI is technique dependent. It has been estimated that as many as two-thirds of patients and of health professionals who teach patients how to use a pMDI do not perform the procedure properly.[54] Preliminary patient instruction can last 10 to 30 minutes and should include demonstration, practice, and confirmation of patient performance (demonstration pMDIs with a placebo should be available from manufacturers for this purpose). Repeated instruction usually improves performance and can be performed on follow-up clinic or home visits. Repeat demonstrations may be required several times to ensure that the patient is using the device properly. When the pMDI is new or has not been used for 24 hours or more, it needs to be primed by shaking the device and releasing two or more sprays into the air. Through priming, the drug inside the canister is mixed with the propellant, and an adequate dose is given to the patient during therapy. Also, it must be noted that manufacturers recommend 30 seconds to 1 minute between actuations. However, Fink et al.[55] found that pMDI output is similar at 15-second intervals for up to eight actuations. In contrast, more rapid multiple actuations decreased the drug inhaled per puff.

Box 6.7 outlines the recommended steps for self-administering a bronchodilator using a simple pMDI. The pMDI should be actuated at the beginning of a slow, deep inspiration. Hand-breath coordination problems include actuating the pMDI before or after the breath. Infants, young children, the elderly, and patients in acute distress may not be able to coordinate actuation of the pMDI with inspiration. The "cold Freon effect" occurs when the cold aerosol plume reaches the back of the mouth and the patient stops inhaling. All of these problems reduce aerosol delivery to the lung.

Most pMDI labels instruct patients to place the mouthpiece between the lips. Positioning the outlet of the pMDI approximately 4 cm (two fingers' width) in front of an open mouth with a low inspiratory flow rate can increase the dose delivered to the lower respiratory tract of an adult from approximately 7% to 10% to 14% to 20%, as well as reduce oropharyngeal impaction.[56] However, this technique is more difficult for patients to perform reliably than is the closed-mouth technique. Concerns have been raised about use of the open-mouth technique with ipratropium bromide, because poor coordination can result in the drug being sprayed into the eyes.

Proper cleaning and maintenance of pMDIs is important. Medication and debris may build up on the nozzle or actuator orifice over time and reduce the emitted dose.[56a] According to manufacturer's recommendations, the pMDI actuator should

---

BOX 6.7 Optimum Technique for Using a Simple Pressurized Metered-Dose Inhaler

1. Remove the cap from the actuator mouthpiece.
2. Inspect the mouthpiece, and clear it of any debris.
3. Shake the inhaler well, and prime it by releasing one to four test sprays into the air, away from your face. (The inhaler should be primed before it is used for the first time and when it has not been used for longer than 1 day.)
4. Breathe out fully through your mouth.
5. Insert the mouthpiece fully into your mouth with the canister above the mouthpiece, and close your lips around the mouthpiece. Alternatively, place the mouthpiece 4 cm from your mouth. (*Note:* Do not use the latter technique with anticholinergic drugs.)
6. Depress the top of the metal canister at the beginning of a breath while breathing in deeply and slowly.
7. Hold your breath for up to 10 s.
8. Repeat at 30- to 60-s intervals.
9. Replace the cap on the mouthpiece.
10. Clean the actuator mouthpiece at least once a week. Rinse it under running water, shake off the excess water, and allow the mouthpiece to air-dry.
11. Discard the canister after you have taken the labeled number of doses. Never immerse the canister in water to determine how full it is.

---

be rinsed with warm running tap water from each end of the actuator for 30 seconds once a week, and the final rinse should be with sterile water for infection control.

Breath-Actuated Pressurized Metered-Dose Inhalers

Breath-actuated pMDIs trigger during inhalation, reducing the need for the patient or caregiver to coordinate actuation with inhalation.[57] The Tempo Inhaler (Fig. 6.31) (MAP Pharmaceuticals), a new-generation pMDI, is a breath-actuated pMDI that uses impinging flow to lower the force of the plume exiting the mouthpiece, reducing oropharyngeal deposition and increasing lung dose. After approval from the U.S. Food and Drug Administration, the Tempo Inhaler will be used for the treatment of migraines.

Techniques of Administration

A lever mechanism on the top of the unit is cocked, setting in motion a downward spring force. As the patient inhales through the mouthpiece using the closed-mouth technique, exceeding an inspiratory flow threshold (such as 20 to 30 L/min), a vane releases the spring, forcing the canister down and actuating the pMDI. Some models can only be breath-actuated, so small children and patients experiencing an acute exacerbation of bronchospasm may not be able to generate sufficient flows to trigger the breath-actuated inhaler. This theoretical concern has not been widely observed in clinical studies of patients with severe exacerbation of asthma who were receiving treatment in emergency departments. Nevertheless, caution may be appropriate in ordering breath-triggered

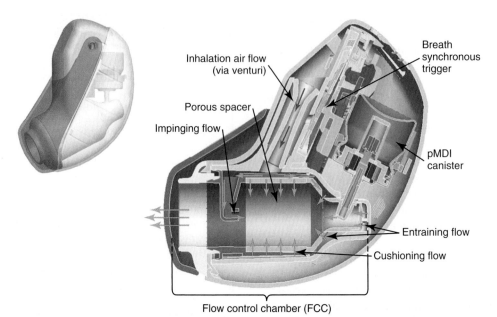

FIGURE 6.31 Tempo is breath actuated with mechanism to "cushion" flow exiting the canister, reducing the force of the aerosol plume, thereby reducing impaction in the oropharynx. *pMDI,* Pressurized metered-dose inhaler. (Courtesy MAP Pharmaceutical. The TEMPO inhaler is a registered trademark of MAP Pharmaceuticals, Inc., Mountain View, CA.)

pMDIs for small children and patients prone to severe levels of airway obstruction.

Pressurized Metered-Dose Inhaler Accessory Devices

A variety of pMDI accessory devices have been developed to overcome problems such as hand-breath coordination, dose counting, and high oropharyngeal deposition.

Dose counters. Dose counters indicate the number of doses remaining in the pMDI canister. Historically, pMDIs have had no mechanism that tells the patient how many doses remain in the canister. Depending on the drug and the manufacturer, a pMDI may contain 60 to 240 doses. After the number of labeled doses has been administered, the pMDI may appear and sound as though it can emit as many as 20 to 60 additional doses. The term *tail-off effect* refers to the variability of drug dispensed at the end of the canister's "label" life, with swings from normal to almost no dose emitted from one breath to the next. With no dose counter, patients frequently use a pMDI long after any active medication is emitted from the canister. The only reliable way to track the remaining doses is to count the number of actuations.

In the past, some manufacturers' labels recommended floating the pMDI canister in water to estimate the percentage of medication remaining in the device; however, this does not provide an accurate estimate of the amount of drug remaining, and water in the nozzle of the pMDI impairs its performance and output. The U.S. Food and Drug Administration now requires all new pMDIs to include an accurate method of tracking the pMDI actuations used. An integrated light-emitting diode dose counter lets the patient know when to reorder and replace the pMDI (Fig. 6.32).

Tracking the number of actuations remaining in the pMDI can be done with either of the following two techniques:

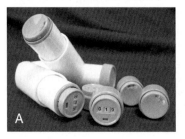
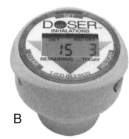

FIGURE 6.32 Dose counters mounted on top of a pMDI canister. A, AeroCount. B, Doser. *pMDI,* Pressurized metered-dose inhaler. (A Courtesy Trudell Medical International, London, Ontario, Canada. B Courtesy Meditrack, Hudson, MA.)

- *With Dose Counters:* The user should[49]:
  1. Determine the number of puffs available in the pMDI when it is full.
  2. Learn how to read the counter display because each dose counter has a different way of displaying doses left in the pMDI.
  3. Properly dispose of the pMDI after the last dose is dispensed and replace it with a new pMDI.
- *Without Dose Counters:* The user should[49]:
  1. Read the label to determine the number of puffs of drug available in the pMDI.
  2. Calculate how long the pMDI will last by dividing the total number of puffs in the pMDI by the total puffs used per day.
  3. Determine the date that all the puffs will be used and mark it on the canister or on a calendar.
  4. Track the number of puffs of drug administered on a daily log sheet and subtract them from the remaining puffs.

5. Keep the daily log sheet in a convenient place, such as on or next to a bathroom mirror.

6. Properly dispose of at the pMDI after the last dose is dispensed and replace it with a new pMDI.

Spacers and holding chambers. A spacer or a valved holding chamber can reduce oropharyngeal deposition and the need for hand-breath coordination. A spacer is a simple, valveless extension device that adds distance between the pMDI outlet and the patient's mouth. This allows the aerosol plume to expand and the propellants to evaporate before the medication reaches the oropharynx.

Holding chambers allow exhaled aerosol to remain in a chamber and remain available to be inhaled with the next breath. These devices provide less oropharyngeal deposition by retaining larger droplets and increasing respirable drug dosages. A holding chamber minimizes the cold Freon effect and any bad tastes associated with a drug. A valve may be incorporated into the holding chamber to prevent the chamber aerosol from being cleared on exhalation. This allows patients with small tidal volumes to empty the aerosol from the chamber with multiple successive breaths. These valved holding chambers enable infants, small children, and adults who cannot control their breathing pattern or who demonstrate poor hand-breath coordination to be treated effectively with pMDIs.

It is worth mentioning that multiple actuations of one or more drugs placed into a spacer can reduce both the total dose and the respirable dose of drug available for inhalation. The extent of these losses may vary for different drugs and spacer designs. Also, a pMDI drug administered with one type of accessory device may produce differences in the MMAD, GSD, and FPF when used with different accessory devices. Placement of a valve between the pMDI and the chamber and the mouthpiece also can affect drug delivery, because the valve acts as a baffle, reducing the size of particles inhaled. A simple tube spacer may reduce oral deposition by up to 90%, whereas a valved holding chamber can reduce oral deposition by 99%.

Another factor that can affect the performance of spacers and holding chambers is electrostatic charge. Electrostatic charges on the surface of a spacer or holding chamber attract and capture small aerosol particles, reducing the amount of respirable drug available to the lung. With repeated use (20 to 40 puffs), drug builds up on the wall of the chamber and the charge is dissipated, allowing more drug to be inhaled by the patient. Washing the chamber with water (without soap) reestablishes the electrostatic charge, making the device less effective until drug is deposited in the chamber and the static charge is once again reduced.[58] Manufacturers recommend washing spacers/valved holding chambers with soap and water once a week. However, previous research suggests cleaning spacers after each use due to bacterial contamination found with spacers by patients at home. The concentration of soap or detergent is not important because it does not influence aerosol drug delivery to patients; therefore only a few drops is enough for cleaning spacers/valved holding chambers. Although previous research recommended not rinsing off spacers to protect them against electrostatic charge,[58a] not rinsing the detergent off may cause contact dermatitis.

Therefore clinicians should consider using spacers and valved holding chambers that are made of nonelectrostatic material. The use of conductive metal, paper, or nonelectrostatic plastic chambers, or washing the plastic chamber periodically with deionizing detergent (e.g., dilute liquid dish soap) can overcome the loss of fine-particle mass caused by electrostatic charge and increase the inhaled mass from 20% to up to 50% of the emitted dose of the pMDI, even in children.[58] Washing the chamber with conventional dishwashing soap reduces the static charge for up to 30 days. All valved holding chambers and spacers should be regularly cleaned, as recommended by their manufacturer. Use of dilute liquid dishwashing soap, with rinsing, and allowing to air-dry is commonly recommended. Also, clinicians should replace the chamber when the valve stiffens.

Types of spacers. Fig. 6.33 shows examples of several commercially available spacers. Selection of the appropriate spacer should be based on whether the patient requires a small-volume adapter, an open-tube design, a bag reservoir, or a valved holding chamber. More than a dozen different devices, with volumes ranging from 15 to 750 mL, have been developed over the past 30 years.

Proper use of a simple open-tube spacer requires some hand-breath coordination, because a momentary delay between triggering and inhalation of the discharged spray results in a substantial loss of drug and reduced lung delivery. Exhalation into a simple spacer after pMDI actuation clears the aerosol from the device and wastes most of the dose to the atmosphere. This reduction in dose also occurs with small-volume, reverse-flow spacers if no provision is made for "holding" the aerosol in the device. Box 6.8 outlines the proper technique for using a pMDI with a valved holding chamber.

Holding chambers with masks (Fig. 6.34) are available for use in the care of infants, children, and adults who are unable to use a mouthpiece device because of their size, age, or level of hand-breath coordination. Holding chambers are useful in

---

BOX 6.8   Technique for Using a Pressurized Metered-Dose Inhaler With a Valved Holding Chamber

1. Remove the caps from the boot of the pressurized metered-dose inhaler (pMDI) and from the valved holding chamber (VHC). Insert the inhaler into the VHC.
2. Shake the pMDI and chamber.
3. Actuate one dose into the chamber while breathing through the VHC.
4. Take a large breath, and hold it for up to 10 s. If this is not possible, breathe through the VHC for several breaths (for adults, this should involve 1 to 3 tidal breaths; infants can take up to 10 breaths or 30 s with tidal breathing).
5. Repeat actuation at 30- to 60-s intervals.
6. Remove the pMDI from the VHC.
7. Replace the caps on the pMDI and VHC.
8. Store both the pMDI and VHC properly.
9. Periodically wash the VHC in warm, soapy water; rinse it; and allow it to air-dry.

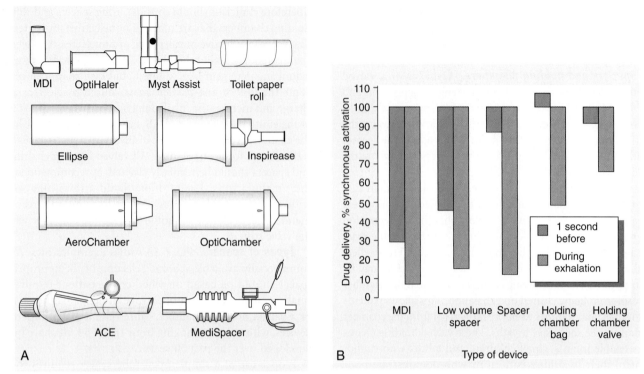

FIGURE 6.33 A, pMDI, low-volume spacers (OptiHaler, Myst Assist), large-volume spacers (toilet paper roll, Ellipse), holding chamber bag (InspirEase), and valved holding chambers (AeroChamber, OptiChamber, ACE, and MediSpacer). B, The percentage of inhaled mass with perfect technique was compared with actuation 1 second before inhalation *(dark blue bar)* and during exhalation *(light blue bar).* Most of the dose is lost with the pMDI and the small-volume spacer. Valved holding chambers gave the highest dose under both conditions. *MDI,* Metered-dose inhaler; *pMDI,* pressurized metered-dose inhaler. (Modified from Wilkes W, Fink JB, Dhand R: Selecting an accessory device with a metered-dose inhaler: variable influence of accessory devices on fine particle dose, throat deposition, and drug delivery with asynchronous actuations from a metered-dose inhaler. *J Aerosol Med* 14:351, 2001.)

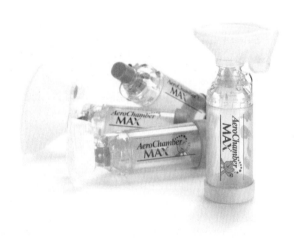

FIGURE 6.34 Mouthpiece and masks are available in a range of sizes for use with valved holding chambers in infants through adults. (Courtesy Trudell Medical International, London, Ontario, Canada.)

the administration of steroids because deposition of the drug in the mouth is largely eliminated, and systemic side effects can be minimized.

Clinicians should choose a spacer that maximizes the delivery efficiency of the aerosol for the individual patient. Differences of twofold to threefold in the amount of drug available at the mouth have been measured among spacers currently used to treat infants. Spacers and holding chambers that use the manufacturer-designed boot that comes with the pMDI are more effective for a wider range of formulations than is a "universal adapter" that fits any pMDI canister. With solution HFA pMDIs, the diameter of the valve stem and actuator orifice is smaller than that of albuterol CFC pMDIs. When the HFA pMDI is used in an actuator designed for use with CFC pMDIs, output is reduced. When these HFA formulations are used with any particular spacer, it is important to know how comparable the available dose and particle size distribution are with the dose and particle size from an existing CFC pMDI.[52] Additional accessory devices for the pMDI include the Vent-Ease MDI adapter (Glaxo), which serves as a mechanical lever system to make actuation of the pMDI easier for patients with arthritic limitations (Clinical Scenario 6.3).

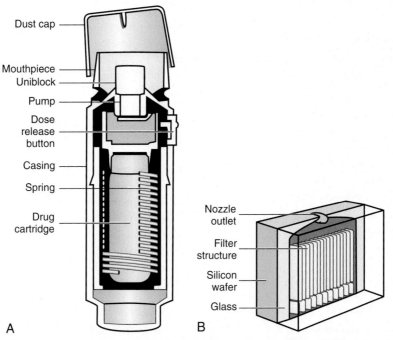

FIGURE 6.35 A, Respimat soft-mist inhaler provides multidose convenience. B, Mechanical energy drives 11 µL of liquid medication through the Uniblock to generate aerosol.

CLINICAL SCENARIO 6.3

You are called to the emergency department to deliver a medicated aerosol to a 6-year-old child who is alert but restless and complains of shortness of breath. The child's mother says that the child has had several "asthma attacks" since 1 year of age, but that all have been mild and this is the first visit to a hospital. The emergency department physician asks you to suggest an appropriate aerosol device. What do you recommend?

See Appendix A for the answer.

Soft-Mist Inhalers (Liquid Metered-Dose Inhalers)

Equipment design and function. The Respimat (Boehringer Ingelheim) is a disposable, multiple-dose, soft-mist inhaler (Fig. 6.35). It uses energy produced by spring compression to squeeze liquid formulation from the collapsible drug container through a proprietary valve generating a low-dose (10 to 15 µL), low-velocity (10 m/sec) spray produced over 1.2 seconds to achieve up to 45% lung deposition.[58b,58c]

Technique, cleaning, and maintenance. To operate the device the patient turns the base of the device to cock a spring, then places the Respimat in the mouth and presses a button to release the drug spray as the user begins a slow, deep inspiration. Although the Respimat requires hand-breath coordination, it produces lower oropharyngeal deposition than standard pMDIs or DPIs. The Respimat has been released in Europe, Canada, and the United States for delivery of ipratropium bromide, tiotropium bromide, and other formulations. The Respimat should be protected from freezing temperature because it has liquid drugs. Also, it is recommended to wipe the mouthpiece of the Respimat with a damp cloth once a week.

Atomizers and Spray Pumps

Hand-bulb atomizers and nasal spray pumps are used to administer sympathomimetic, antimuscarinic, antiinflammatory, and anesthetic aerosols to the upper airway (nasal passages, pharynx, and larynx). These agents are used to manage upper airway inflammation and rhinitis, to provide local anesthesia, and to achieve systemic effects. AARC has developed guidelines for the delivery of drugs to the upper airway.[59]

A nasal spray pump produces an aerosol suspension with a high MMAD and GSD, which are ideal for upper airway deposition. Nasopharyngeal deposition is greatest for particles 20 to 50 µm. Deposition with the hand-bulb atomizer applied to the nose occurs mostly in the anterior nasal passages, with clearance to the nasopharynx. The 100-µL puffs appear to deposit more medication than do 50-µL puffs, and deposition to a greater surface area occurs with a 35-degree spray angle than with a 60-degree angle.

Dry Powder Inhalers

As the name implies, **dry powder inhalers (DPIs)** are aerosol devices that deliver a drug in powder form. DPIs typically are breath-actuated dosing systems. The theory of operation for these devices is that the patient generates the aerosol by drawing air though a dose of finely milled drug powder with sufficient force to disperse and suspend the powder in the air. DPIs are relatively inexpensive, do not need propellants, and do not require the hand-breath coordination needed for pMDIs. Dispersion of the powder into respirable particles depends on the creation of turbulent flow in the inhaler. Turbulent flow is a function of the patient's ability to inhale the powder with a sufficiently high inspiratory flow rate.[60]

Equipment design and function. There are several types of DPIs on the market that can be divided into three categories based on the design of their dose containers:

- *Unit-dose DPIs:* Unit-dose DPIs deliver individual doses of drug from gelatin capsules. The Aerolizer (Merck Schering-Plough) and the HandiHaler (Boehringer Ingelheim) are examples of unit-dose DPIs.
- *Multiple unit–dose DPIs:* Multiple unit–dose DPIs such as Diskhaler (GlaxoSmithKline) have a case of four or eight individual blister packets of drugs on a disk inserted into the inhaler.
- *Multiple-dose DPIs:* The multiple-dose DPIs like the Twisthaler and the Flexhaler (AstraZeneca) have a reservoir powder system preloaded with 120 doses of drug. The Diskus (GlaxoSmithKline) incorporates a tape system that contains up to 60 sealed single doses.

Fig. 6.36 shows the major components of a single-dose DPI and a multidose DPI, and Table 6.3 shows methods to determine doses left in the dry powder inhaler.

Small respirable-sized particles tend to attract each other and aggregate. Passive dry powder dispensing systems use a carrier substance (lactose or glucose) mixed with the small particles of drug to enable the drug powder to disaggregate during inhalation. (Note that reactions to lactose or glucose appear to be fewer than reactions to the surfactants and propellants used in pressurized pMDIs.) The particle size of the dry powder particles of drug ranges from 1 to 3 $\mu\mu$m, but the size of the lactose or glucose particles can range from approximately 20 to 65 μm; therefore most of the carrier (up to 80%) is deposited in the oropharynx.

The performance of DPIs can be affected by the materials used in production and manufacturing. Optimum performance for each type of DPI occurs at a specific inspiratory flow rate. The FPF of respirable drug from existing DPIs ranges from 10% to 60% of the nominal dose. The amount varies with inspiratory flow and device design. The higher the resistance or the greater the flow requirement of a DPI, the more difficult it is for a compromised or young patient to generate inspiratory flow sufficient to obtain the maximum dose of drug. The

high peak inspiratory flow rates required to dispense the drug powder from most passive DPIs (>60 L/min) result in a pharyngeal dose comparable with that received from a typical pMDI without an add-on device. If inhalation is not performed at the optimum inspiratory flow rate for a particular device, the dose of drug dispensed decreases and the particle size of the powder aerosol increases.[60] Finally, it should be evident that ambient humidity can affect drug delivery from DPIs. The emitted dose decreases in a humid environment, likely because of powder clumping. Exposure to humidity can affect dry powder in milliseconds. The higher the level of absolute humidity, the lower the dose emitted.

Despite the foregoing issues, DPIs in general are convenient and easy to use. Newer designs are being developed that provide aerosols with higher FPFs and more reproducible dosing, independent of inspiratory flow rate. For example, passive, or patient-driven, DPIs rely on the patient's inspiratory effort to dispense the dose. The result is differences in lung delivery and clinical response. Active, or powered, DPIs, which disaggregate the powder before inhalation, are independent of patient effort. Active DPIs use an energy source to disaggregate the powder and suspend it into an aerosol, allowing the dose to be suspended independent of the patient's inspiratory flow rates.

New Dry Powder Inhaler Technologies

- *Easyhaler:* The Easyhaler (Orion Corporation), is a DPI that has been developed for use with a range of medications such as albuterol, beclomethasone, formoterol, and budesonide. Although its shape and operation are similar to a pMDI, it is a DPI with a built-in dose counter that provides a red signal in the last 20 doses left in the device. The Easyhaler is currently available in Europe and Canada. Release in the United States is anticipated in the near future.
- *Ellipta:* The Ellipta (GlaxoSmithKline) is a multidose DPI with a double-foil blister strip. Three types of Ellipta are available on the market: (1) Breo Ellipta, (2) Incruse Ellipta, and (3) Anoro Ellipta. Whereas the Breo Ellipta includes a combination of fluticasone furoate and vilanterol, the Incruse Ellipta is used to deliver umeclidinium, a long-acting muscarinic antagonist used for the treatment of

TABLE 6.3   Determining Doses Left in the Dry Powder Inhaler

		Drug Container	Doses	Indicator Type	Meaning of Dose Indicator
Unit-Dose DPI	Aerolizer or Handihaler	Single Capsule	1	None	Check capsule to ensure full dose is inhaled. Repeat to empty capsule
Multiple Unit-Dose DPI	Diskhaler	Dose Blister	4 or 8	None	Inspect visually to confirm use of all blisters
Multiple Dose DPIs	Diskus	Blister strip	60	Red numbers	Red numbers indicate that ≤5 doses are left in DPI.
	Flexhaler	Reservoir	60 or 120	"0"	Marked in intervals of 10 doses, "0" indicates empty.
	Twisthaler	Reservoir	30	"01"	"01" indicates last dose.

DPI, Dry powder inhaler.
From Kacmarek RM, Stoller JK, Heuer AJ: *Egan's fundamentals of respiratory care,* ed 11, St. Louis, 2016, Mosby-Elsevier.

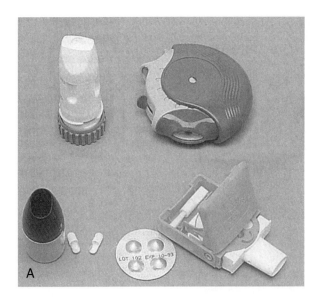

A

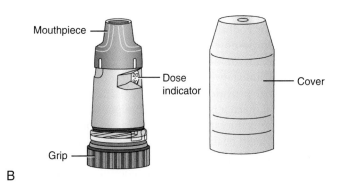

Mouthpiece

Dose indicator

Cover

Grip

B

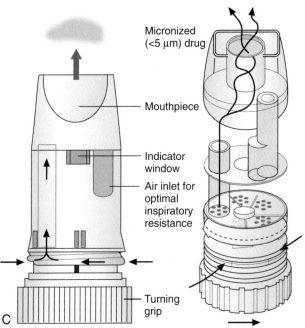

Micronized (<5 μm) drug

Mouthpiece

Indicator window

Air inlet for optimal inspiratory resistance

Turning grip

C

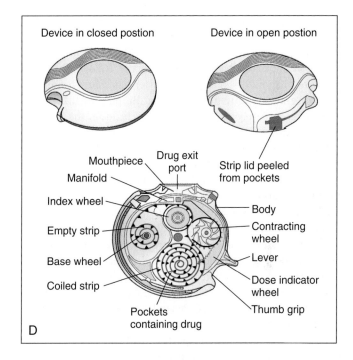

Device in closed postion

Device in open postion

Strip lid peeled from pockets

Mouthpiece

Drug exit port

Manifold

Index wheel

Empty strip

Base wheel

Coiled strip

Pockets containing drug

Body

Contracting wheel

Lever

Dose indicator wheel

Thumb grip

D

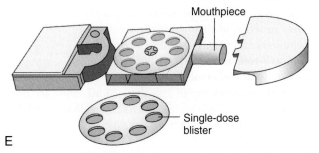

Mouthpiece

Single-dose blister

E

FIGURE 6.36 Dry powder inhalers (A) and diagrams of the Rotahaler (B), Flexhaler (C), Diskus (D), and Diskhaler (E). (A Modified from Albert R, Spiro S, Jett J, editors: *Comprehensive respiratory medicine,* St. Louis, 1999, Mosby. C-E modified from Dhand R, Fink JB: Dry powder inhalers. *Respir Care* 44(9):940-951, 1999.) (From Gardenhire DS: *Rau's respiratory care pharmacology,* ed 8, St. Louis, 2012, Mosby-Elsevier.)

chronic obstructive pulmonary disease (COPD), and the Anoro Ellipta consists of a combination of umeclidinium and vilanterol. Through a three-step technique, patients open the device, inhale, and close after treatment. When the device is opened, the patient hears an auditory feedback that confirms the loading of the dose and advances the number doses left in the dose counter.

- *Podhaler:* The Podhaler (Novartis Pharmaceutical Corporation) is a single-dose reusable DPI that is used to deliver TOBI (tobramycin inhalation powder). Using the Pulmo-Sphere technology with less interparticle cohesive forces, the Podhaler provides light, porous particles. It has an easy-to-use mechanism in which the patient opens the inhaler, inserts the capsule in the device, and inhales. The Podhaler should be disposed of after 7 days of use.

- *Taifun:* The Taifun (Leiras OY) is a multidose DPI with a reservoir that is used to deliver budesonide, salbutamol, formoterol, and fentanyl. It provides uniform and reproducible doses to patients with pulmonary diseases. Currently Taifun is available in Europe.

- *Tudorza Pressair:* As a multidose DPI with both visual and auditory feedback mechanisms, the Tudorza Pressair (Forest Laboratories) is used to deliver aclidinium bromide, a long-acting anticholinergic. If the patient takes the dose completely using a correct technique, the device shows green in the control window as opposed to red, which indicates the incorrect technique. The Tudorza Pressair has a dose counter that reduces by 10 doses and shows a 0 sign, as well as the red mark, when the device is completely empty.

- *Spiromax:* The Spiromax (Teva Pharmaceuticals) is a multidose DPI that delivers albuterol, budesonide/formoterol, and fluticasone/salmeterol in Europe. Like other multidose DPIs, opening the device loads the dose automatically, and it is ready to be inhaled by the patient.

- *Staccato:* Using a thermal aerosol technology, the Staccato (Alexza Pharmaceuticals) generates aerosols by heating a thin film of drug to form aerosols that cools and condenses into 1-to 3-μm diameter particles with inspiration. The Staccato is not sensitive to inspiratory rates and does not require a special breathing technique. It has been approved for delivery of loxapine in the United States.

Technique, cleaning, and maintenance. The most critical factor in the use of a passive DPI is the need for high inspiratory flow. Patients must generate inspiratory flows of at least 40 to 60 L/min to produce a respirable powder aerosol. Because infants, small children (younger than 5 years of age), and those unable to follow instructions cannot develop flow this high, these patient groups cannot use DPIs effectively. Patients with severe airway obstruction also may not be able to achieve the required flow (DPIs therefore are not to be used in the management of acute bronchospasm).

Although hand-breath coordination is not as important with DPIs as it is with pMDIs, exhalation into the device can result in loss of drug delivery to the lung. Some devices also require assembly, which can be cumbersome or difficult for some patients, especially those with arthritis. It is important

---

BOX 6.9 **Technique for Using a Dry Powder Inhaler**

Priming instructions: Before using a new DPI for the first time, check the manufacturer's instructions, and prime the DPI.

Steps for using the DPI:
1. Assemble the apparatus.
2. Load dose based on the manufacturer's instructions.
3. Exhale slowly to functional residual capacity (i.e., quiet exhalation).
4. Exhale away from the mouthpiece.
5. Seal lips around the mouthpiece.
6. Inhale deeply and forcefully (>60 L/min). A breath-hold should be encouraged but is not essential.
7. If more than one dose is required, repeat the previous steps.
8. Monitor adverse effects.
9. Replace the cover on the inhaler.
10. Keep the inhaler clean and dry at all times (following manufacturer's instructions).
11. Keep the device in a dry place at a controlled room temperature (i.e., 20°C to 25°C [68°F to 77°F]). Do not submerge in water.

DPI, Dry powder inhaler.

---

that patients receive demonstrations with their inhalers and have the opportunity to assemble and use the DPI before self-administration. Box 6.9 outlines the basic steps in the use and care of DPIs. Cleaning of DPIs should be done in accordance with the product label, and they should never be submerged in water because moisture in the device will dramatically reduce available dose.

It is important to protect DPIs from humidity and keep them dry. Otherwise, humidity in the environment or exhaled gas may result in improper function of the inhaler and a reduction in aerosol drug delivery. Also, the mouthpiece of the DPI should be wiped with a dry paper towel or cloth before use.

Nebulizers

Nebulizers are aerosol delivery devices generating aerosols from solutions and suspensions. There are two types of nebulizers in terms of their reservoir volume: (1) small-volume nebulizers and (2) large-volume nebulizers.

Small-volume nebulizers. Because nebulizers commonly used at home and in the hospital for drug administration have medication reservoirs of less than 10 mL, they are called small-volume nebulizers (SVNs). SVNs are divided into three categories: (1) jet nebulizers (JNs), (2) USNs, and (3) vibrating mesh nebulizers (VMNs).

Jet Nebulizers

Most modern JNs are powered by high-pressure air or oxygen provided by a portable compressor, compressed-gas cylinder, or 50-psi wall outlet. There are four types of JNs:
- The *JN with a reservoir tube* is a traditional small-volume JN that is commonly used clinically even though it is

inefficient as a result of the release of aerosol to ambient air during exhalation and when the patient is not inhaling. A large-bore reservoir that is attached to the expiratory side of the nebulizer is used to increase inhaled dose while decreasing drug loss during therapy.

- The *JN with collection bag* has a collection bag that is attached to the expiratory side of the nebulizer, which acts as a reservoir by filling with aerosol during continuous nebulization. Thus the patient inhales from the reservoir through a one-way valve and exhales to the atmosphere through an exhalation port.

- Breath-enhanced nebulizers (BENs) generate aerosol continuously, using an inspiratory vent that allows the patient to draw in air through the nebulization chamber containing aerosolized drug. On exhalation the inlet vent closes, and aerosol exits by a one-way valve near the mouthpiece; this process increases the inhaled mass by as much as 50% over standard continuous nebulizers and reduces aerosol waste to the atmosphere. Fig. 6.37 illustrates this principle and gives an example of a BEN.

- Breath-actuated nebulizers (BANs) generate aerosol only during inspiration. This feature eliminates waste of aerosol during exhalation and increases the delivered dose threefold or more over continuous nebulizers and BENs. Breath-synchronized nebulization can increase the inhaled aerosol mass threefold to fourfold over conventional continuous nebulization. Historically this was accomplished with a patient-controlled finger port that directs gas to the nebulizer only during inspiration

(Fig. 6.38). Although this type of system wastes less of the drug being aerosolized, it can quadruple the treatment time and requires good hand-breath coordination.

The AeroEclipse II BAN (Trudell Medical International), shown in Fig. 6.39, is a BAN with a spring-loaded, one-way valve design that draws a jet to the capillary tube during inspiration. Nebulization stops when the patient's inspiratory flow decreases below the threshold. Cessation of negative inspiratory pressure or flow allows the nebulizer baffle to move away from its position directly above the jet orifice, stopping nebulization. The AeroEclipse nebulizer also can be operated manually to synchronize aerosol on inspiration for use with infants and children too small to trigger the device. Although this device has a residual volume similar to that of other JNs, aerosol drug waste and contamination of the environment during the expiratory phase of the breathing cycle are greatly reduced.

A number of factors can affect the performance of these devices, including nebulizer design, gas pressure, gas density, temperature and humidity, and medication characteristics. These factors are explained next.

Nebulizer design. As shown in Fig. 6.40, a typical SVN is powered by a high-pressure stream of gas directed through a restricted orifice known as the jet. The gas stream leaving the jet passes the opening of a capillary tube immersed in solution. Because it produces low lateral pressure at the outlet, the high jet velocity draws the liquid up the capillary tube and into the gas stream, where it is sheared into filaments of liquid that break up into droplets. This primary spray produces a

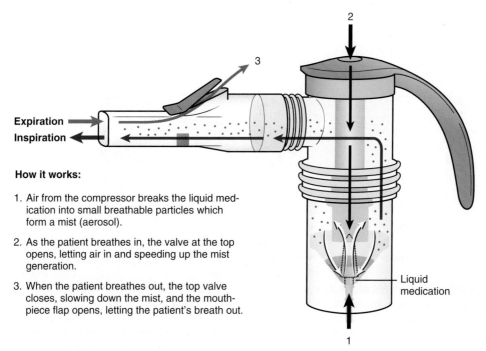

How it works:

1. Air from the compressor breaks the liquid medication into small breathable particles which form a mist (aerosol).

2. As the patient breathes in, the valve at the top opens, letting air in and speeding up the mist generation.

3. When the patient breathes out, the top valve closes, slowing down the mist, and the mouthpiece flap opens, letting the patient's breath out.

FIGURE 6.37 Operating principles of the Sprint breath-enhanced nebulizer. (1) Gas enters through the jet, entrains fluid from the reservoir, and shears droplets into the baffler. (2) During inspiration, gas is inhaled both from the jet and through a valve at the top of the device. (3) During exhalation, gas passes through the valve on the mouthpiece while the jet continues to generate aerosol. (From PARI Respiratory Equipment, Midlothran, VA.)

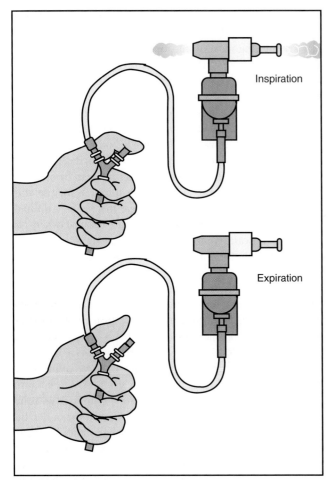

FIGURE 6.38 Use of a finger control to regulate production during inspiration and expiration.

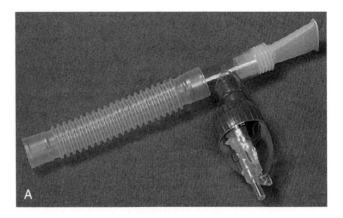

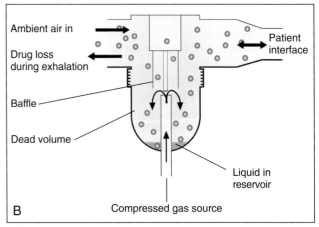

FIGURE 6.40 A, Small-volume jet nebulizer for liquid drug delivery. B, Schematic of a small-volume jet nebulizer.

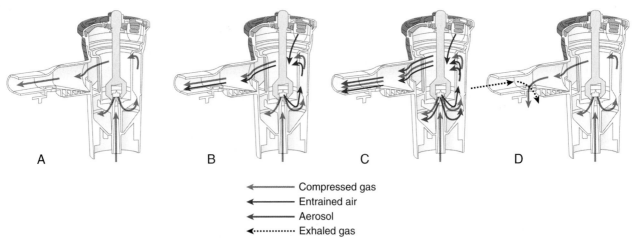

A   B   C   D

← Compressed gas
← Entrained air
← Aerosol
←·············· Exhaled gas

FIGURE 6.39 Diagram of the flow path for the AeroEclipse II BAN, a breath-actuated pneumatic nebulizer. A, Before inhalation the actuator is up, and compressed gas freely circulates with no aerosol produced. B, As the patient inhales, the actuator starts to move down. C, Negative pressure pulls the diaphragm down with the actuator, sealing around the nozzle cover and producing aerosol. D, The patient exhales through a valve in the mouthpiece; as the pressure increases, the diaphragm and actuator move up, stopping aerosol production. (Courtesy Trudell Medical International, London, Ontario, Canada.)

heterodisperse aerosol with droplets that range in size from 0.1 to 500 μm.[61] The droplets are directed against one or more baffles, which can include a sphere or plate placed in line with the jet flow. The internal walls of the nebulizer, the surface of the solution being nebulized, or the internal walls of the delivery system can serve the same purpose. In many designs, droplets that strike the baffles in the SVN return to the medication reservoir to be nebulized again. Drug formulation may circulate through the jet interface more than 30 times before exiting the nebulizer as aerosol.

The medication reservoir is lower than the mouthpiece or patient interface. Consequently, medication can be contaminated by patient-generated secretions or aerosols. The stimulation of using a mouthpiece can result in drooling that enters the mouthpiece and reservoir, contaminating the medication.

Baffles are key elements in the design of SVNs. In JNs, well-designed baffling systems reduce both the MMAD and the GSD of the generated aerosol. Baffling also can occur unintentionally. Unintentional baffles are created by the angles within delivery tubing, by interfaces with other devices outside the aerosol generator, and by the surfaces of the upper airway itself.[62]

Residual drug volume, or dead volume, is the medication that remains in the SVN and cannot be nebulized.[63] The residual volume of a 3-mL dose varies from as little as 0.5 mL to more than 2.2 mL, which can be more than two-thirds of the total dose. It should be obvious that the greater the residual drug volume, the more drug wasted and the less efficient the delivery system. Residual volume also depends on the position of the SVN. Some SVNs stop producing aerosol when tilted as little as 30 degrees from vertical. Increasing the liquid volume in the SVN allows a greater proportion of active medication to be nebulized. For example, in a nebulizer with a residual volume of 1.5 mL, filling the device with 3 mL would leave only 50% of the nebulizer charge (nominal dose) available for nebulization. In contrast, filling the nebulizer with 5 mL would make 3.5 mL (or >70%) of the medication available for nebulization. To date, no significant difference in clinical response has been shown with varying diluent volumes and flow rates.

Continuous nebulization with conventional nebulizers emits aerosol throughout the respiratory cycle. Inhalation is less than 40% of the respiratory cycle; therefore more than 60% of the emitted aerosol is lost to the atmosphere. Lung delivery of 6% to 12% deposition has been measured in adults receiving continuous nebulizer therapy. Deposition in neonates and infants is less than 1%.

Flow. Droplet size and nebulization time are inversely proportional to gas flow through the jet. The higher the flow of gas to the nebulizer, the smaller the particle size generated and the shorter the time required for nebulizing the full dose of the drug. Nebulizers that produce smaller particle sizes by use of baffles, such as one-way valves, may reduce total drug output per minute compared with the same nebulizer without baffling. Consequently, these devices may require more time to deliver a standard dose of medication to the lungs.

Gas source (hospital versus home). The driving pressure supplied to the nebulizer can affect particle size distribution and output. Higher driving pressures (and flows) result in smaller particle sizes, greater aerosol output, and shorter treatment times. A nebulizer that produces an MMAD of 2.5 μm when driven by a gas source of 50 psi at 6 to 10 L/min may produce an MMAD of more than 5 μm when operated on a home compressor (or ventilator), which can develop a pressure of only 10 psi. Using a driving pressure or flow that is too low can result in significantly decreased nebulizer output. Consequently, nebulizers used for home care should be matched to the compressor according to data supplied by the manufacturer so that the specific nebulizer used delivers the desired medications prescribed for the patient. In Europe, equipment manufacturers are required to characterize the performance of their nebulizer and compressor combinations using standardized methods so that consumers can compare the performance characteristics of a nebulizer with a particular compressor. Until such time as similar standards are required in the United States, clinicians should make every effort to determine whether the system prescribed meets these criteria.

Other concerns in the use of disposable nebulizers with compressors at home involve possible performance degradation of the plastic device with multiple uses. One study showed that repeated use did not alter the MMAD or output as long as the nebulizer was cleaned properly.[62] Failure to clean the nebulizer properly can result in degradation of performance as a result of clogging of the Venturi orifice (which reduces the output flow) and the buildup of electrostatic charge in the device (Clinical Scenario 6.4).

Gas density. The density of the driving gas affects both aerosol generation and the delivery of aerosols to the lungs. Lowering the density of a carrier gas reduces the amount of turbulent flow (i.e., lowers the Reynolds number), which results in less aerosol impaction in the upper airways. This phenomenon has been demonstrated with low-density helium–oxygen (heliox) mixtures. The lower the density of a carrier gas, the less aerosol impaction occurs as the gas passes through the upper airways, and the greater the deposition of aerosol in the lungs.[64] Heliox concentrations equal to or greater than 40% have been shown to increase aerosol delivery to obstructed airways and through an ETT by as much as 50%.[65] However,

---

🏃 CLINICAL SCENARIO 6.4

A 75-year-old female patient with chronic obstructive pulmonary disease (COPD) is receiving bronchodilator therapy at home with a small-volume nebulizer (SVN). She reports to the therapist during a home-care visit that her nebulizer does not seem to be working properly and that she has noticed that mist production has decreased since she changed her portable air compressor. Describe the steps you would take to determine whether a problem exists and suggest solutions to remedy the situation.

See Appendix A for the answer.

it is worth noting that when heliox is used to drive a JN at standard flow rates, aerosol output is substantially less than with air or oxygen, and aerosol particles are considerably smaller. (Nebulizers driven with heliox typically require a twofold to threefold increase in flow to produce a comparable aerosol output.)

Humidity and temperature. Humidity and temperature can affect particle size and the concentration of drug remaining in the nebulizer. Evaporation of water and adiabatic expansion of gas can reduce the temperature of an aerosol to as much as 10°C below the ambient temperature. This cooling may increase solution viscosity and reduce the nebulizer output.[66] Aerosol particles entrained into a warm and fully saturated gas stream increase in size. These particles can also coalesce (stick together), further increasing the MMAD and severely compromising the output of respirable particles. How much these particles enlarge depends primarily on the tonicity of the solution. Aerosol particles generated from isotonic solutions probably maintain their size as they enter the respiratory tract; particles generated from hypertonic solutions tend to enlarge, and evaporation can cause hypotonic droplets to shrink in size.

Characteristics of drug formulation. The viscosity and density of a drug formulation affect both output and particle size. Some drugs, such as antibiotics, are so viscous that they cannot be nebulized effectively in standard SVNs. This also is an issue with suspensions in which some aerosolized particles contain no active drug and other, generally larger, particles are required to carry the active medication.

Vibrating Mesh Nebulizers

Mesh nebulizers are electromechanical devices that pump or push liquid through a mesh (aperture plate) to form droplets. Unlike in SVNs, aerosol is emitted at the intended particle size and does not require baffling, or recirculation. VMNs rely on two different operating principles, which are classified as passive and active.[67]

Passive (static) mesh nebulizers use an ultrasonic horn to generate vibrations of 180 kHz, which push liquid through the static mesh to produce aerosol that can be inhaled directly by the patient. The particles range in size from 3 to 6 μm MMAD. The passive vibrating mesh was first introduced on a limited basis in the 1980s and is now available in the Micro-Aire NEU-22V (Omron Healthcare) and the I-neb (Philips Healthcare).

Active mesh nebulizers use a dome-shaped aperture plate containing 1000 to 4000 funnel-shaped (tapered) apertures. The wider inlet of the aperture interfaces with the reservoir of medication, and the narrow outlet determines the size of particles produced. The domed aperture plate is attached to a flat disk, which is attached to a piezoelectric ceramic element that surrounds the aperture plate. Electricity is applied to the vibrational element at a frequency greater than 128 kHz (one-tenth that of an USN), moving the apertures up and down by 1 or 2 μm, creating a micropumping action. As liquid passes through the apertures, it is broken into fine droplets. The exit velocity of the aerosol is slow (<4 m/sec), and the particle size

can range from 2 to 5 μm (MMAD), varying with exit diameter of the aperture of the specific nebulizer. Active vibrating mesh (VM) aerosol generators can nebulize individual drops of solution as small as 5 μL, with as little as 1 μL residual drug. Examples of active VM nebulizers are the Aeroneb Professional (Pro), Solo, and Go nebulizers (Aerogen) and the eFlow Rapid (PARI).

Mesh nebulizers can generate aerosol from a single drop to up to 10 mL of liquid and have residual drug volumes ranging from 0.1 to 0.5 mL, based largely on the design of the medication reservoir feeding the mesh. Unlike JNs and USNs, the mesh acts as a physical barrier between the drug in the medication reservoir and the body of the nebulizer in which the aerosol output is collected. This reduces the risk for condensate, secretions, or exhaled pathogens contaminating the medication in the reservoir.

Mesh nebulizers do not require any propellants or gas and add no gas to the aerosol stream. This makes them attractive for use in closed systems, such as during mechanical ventilation and continuous positive airway pressure, especially with smaller patients. Unlike the USN, piezoelectric components used to vibrate the mesh form the aerosol as the drug passes through the mesh, rather than creating a standing wave in the medication, as happens in a USN. Compared with most USNs, VM technology has lower residual drug volumes, requires less energy, generates less heat, and is more reliable for generation of suspensions and for extended use.

Mesh nebulizers are considerably more expensive than JNs but are similar to USNs (Table 6.4). Mesh nebulizers are small, silent, portable, and compatible with a broad range of drug compounds. Delivery of some suspensions may be less efficient with the VMN, because larger particles (larger than the mesh aperture diameter of 4 to 5 μm) are filtered out and do not reach the patient as aerosol.

Marketed mesh nebulizers for home use (Micro-Aire NEU-22V, Aeroneb Go, and eFlow Rapid) are probably similar in performance to the best of the breath-enhanced/breath-actuated pneumatic nebulizers in terms of inhaled drug mass and particle size. The Aeroneb Pro and Solo were both designed for hospital use and primarily targeted for use during mechanical ventilation. They have been shown in vitro to be more efficient than standard JNs.[68]

The I-neb has been released only as a drug-device combination for use with iloprost (Ventavis) in the treatment of ambulatory patients with primary pulmonary hypertension. A variant of the PARI eFlow nebulizer is distributed with aztreonam (Cayston), an antibiotic used in the treatment of cystic fibrosis (CF).

Ultrasonic Nebulizers

Small-volume ultrasonic nebulizers. A number of small-volume USNs have been marketed for aerosol drug delivery. Unlike the larger units, some of these systems do not use a couplant compartment; the medication is placed directly into the manifold on top of the transducer. The transducer is connected by cable to a power source; often the device is battery powered to increase portability. These devices have no blower;

TABLE 6.4   Comparison of Aerosol Generators Used to Administer Medications to the Lung

	MDI Alone	MDI With VHC	DPI	SVN	USN	VMN
Flow-independent	–	+ + +	–	+ + +	+ + +	+ + +
Volume-independent	–	+ + +	–	+ + +	+ + +	+ + +
Coordination-independent	–	+ + +	+ + +	+ + +	+ + +	+ + +
Low oral deposition	– –	+ + +	– –	+	+	+
Ease of use	+ +	+ + +	+ +	+ + +	+ +	+ + +
Portable	+ + +	+ +	+ + +	+	+ +	+ + +
Quick to administer	+ + +	+ + +	+ + +	+	+ +	+ + +
Cost	+ + +	+ +	+ +	+ +	– –	– –
Low infection risk	+ + +	+ + +	+ + +	– – –	– – –	+
Effective with:						
• Severe asthma	+	+ + +	+	+ + +	+ +	+ + +
• Small children	–	+ + +	– –	+ + +	–	+ + +
• Ventilators	–	+ + + +	– – –	+	+ + +	+ + +
• Unusual medication	– –	– –	– –	+ +	+	+ +

+, Positive characteristic; *–*, negative characteristic.
DPI, Dry powder inhaler; *MDI*, metered-dose inhaler; *MDI with VHC*, metered-dose inhaler with a valved holding chamber; *SVN*, small-volume nebulizer; *USN*, ultrasonic nebulizer; *VMN*, vibrating mesh nebulizer.

the patient's inspiratory flow draws the aerosol from the nebulizer into the lung.

Small-volume USNs have been promoted for administration of a wide variety of formulations, ranging from bronchodilators to antiinflammatory agents and antibiotics.[69] USNs should not be used with suspensions such as budesonide (Pulmicort) because the mean MMAD of the suspension (2.8 µm) may be larger than the droplet produced (see the Pulmicort drug label). Residual drug volume of USNs may be similar to or less than that of jet SVNs. Use of a small-volume USN with low residual volume may increase the available respirable mass for devices with less residual drug volume than SVNs. This may reduce the need for a large amount of diluent to ensure delivery of the drugs. The contained portable power source adds a great deal of convenience in mobility. However, these advantages are offset by relatively high purchase costs and poor reliability.

Some ventilator manufacturers (e.g., Siemens, Medtronic Minimally Invasive Therapies Nellcor Puritan Bennett) have advocated the use of USNs for administration of aerosols during mechanical ventilation. Unlike SVNs, USNs do not add extra gas flow to the ventilator circuit during use. This feature reduces the need to change and reset ventilator and alarm settings during aerosol administration.[59]

Large-volume ultrasonic nebulizers. Large-volume USNs are used mainly for bland aerosol therapy or sputum induction. These devices incorporate air blowers to carry the mist to the patient. Low flow through these large-volume USNs is associated with smaller particles and higher mist density. High flow yields larger particles and less density. Unlike in JNs, the temperature of the solution placed in a USN increases during use. As the temperature increases, the drug concentration increases, as does the likelihood of undesirable side effects.

Large-Volume Nebulizers

A large-volume nebulizer (LVN) is used to provide continuous nebulization. The high-output, extended aerosol respiratory therapy nebulizers are examples of devices designed for this purpose. These nebulizers have a reservoir greater than 200 mL, and they can produce an aerosol with an MMAD of 2.2 to 3.5 µm. Actual output and particle size vary with the pressure and flow at which the nebulizer operates. As was already mentioned, a potential problem with continuous bronchodilator therapy (CBT) is increased drug concentration in the reservoir over time. Therefore patients receiving CBT should be closely monitored for signs of drug toxicity (e.g., tachycardia and tremor).

CBT can be administered with LVNs that can hold 10 to 200 mL, or with SVNs with a continuous feed mechanism to fill the nebulizer (Fig. 6.41). Dose output is based on the output rate of the nebulizer and the concentration of medication placed in the nebulizer. With JNs, changing the rate of gas driving the nebulizer can make small changes in the output rate, but larger changes in output require emptying the reservoir or feed system and using a new concentration. Because output rates for SVNs and LVNs vary between devices of the same model (even within the same lot), accurate delivery can be ensured only by calculation of the actual output of the individual nebulizer and adjustment of the flow as required.

Another special-purpose LVN is the small particle aerosol generator (SPAG), like the one shown in Fig. 6.42. The SPAG (Valeant Pharmaceuticals International) was designed specifically for administration of ribavirin (Virazole) to infants with respiratory syncytial virus infection. The SPAG incorporates a drying chamber with its own flow control to produce a stable aerosol. The SPAG reduces the medical gas source to as low as 26 pounds per square inch gauge (psig) with an adjustable regulator. The regulator is connected to two flowmeters that

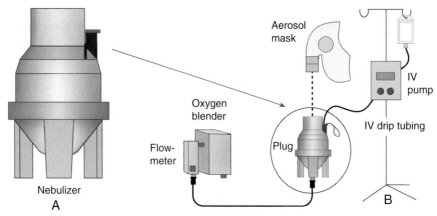

FIGURE 6.41 Intravenous (IV) drip for continuous nebulization. A, Small-volume nebulizer. B, Intravenous drip with blender, flowmeter, and drip. (From Kacmarek RM, Stoller JK, Heuer AJ: *Egan's fundamentals of respiratory care,* ed 10, St. Louis, 2013, Mosby-Elsevier.)

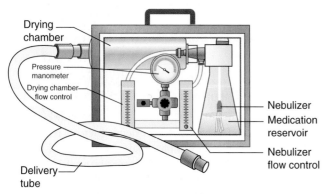

FIGURE 6.42 Small-particle aerosol generator. (From Kacmarek RM, Stoller JK, Heuer AJ: *Egan's fundamentals of respiratory care,* ed 10, St. Louis, 2013, Mosby-Elsevier.)

separately control flow to the nebulizer and the drying chamber. The nebulizer is in the medication reservoir, the fluid surface and wall of which serve as primary baffles. The aerosol enters the long, cylindrical drying chamber where the separate flow of dry gas reduces the particle size by evaporation, creating a monodisperse aerosol with an MMAD of 1.2 to 1.4 μm. Nebulizer flow should be maintained at approximately 7 L/min, with total flow from both flowmeters no lower than 15 L/min. The latest model operates consistently, even with back pressure, and can be used with masks, hoods, tents, or ventilator circuits. It is worth mentioning that when the SPAG is used to deliver ribavirin through a mechanical ventilation circuit, drug precipitation can jam breathing valves or occlude the ventilator circuit. This problem can be prevented by (1) placing a one-way valve between the SPAG and the circuit and (2) filtering out the excess aerosol particles before they reach the exhalation valve.[70]

Patients who come to the emergency department with a severe exacerbation of asthma or acute bronchospasm often have been taking their bronchodilator for 24 to 36 hours without any relief of the symptoms. Giving nebulizer treatments with standard bronchodilator doses and repeating the treatments at increased frequency (up to every 15 minutes) until the symptoms are relieved can require hours of staff time.[71,72]

New Nebulizer Designs

- *Fox:* The Fox (Vectura Group) is an active VMN that controls flow and volume to increase pulmonary deposition in the peripheral and central airways by controlling the time of aerosol release during inhalation therapy. When it releases aerosols in the beginning of inspiration, this results in aerosol deposition in the peripheral airways as opposed to the release of aerosols in the middle of inhalation that leads to aerosol deposition in central airways.
- *Micro:* The Micro (Philips Respironics) is a small, handheld, battery-operated, breath-actuated vibrating mesh liquid inhaler that generates aerosol in a range of specific low inspiratory flows for optimal lung deposition, and inspiratory times ranging from 9 to 20 seconds per breath.
- *Akita:* The Akita2 system (Vectura Group) is a microprocessor-controlled system that integrates a breath-actuated aerosol generator (pneumatic or vibrating mesh) with a separate gas source to control the patient's inspiratory flow. Low inspiratory flows allow for prolonged inspirations, up to 12 seconds. Low inspiratory flow also reduces turbulence in the upper and middle airways, allowing a dramatic increase in aerosol delivered to the lung periphery. Breath parameters are set on the basis of the individual patient's pulmonary function and the intended target area for deposition. The Akita2 has been used in the treatment of patients with CF in Germany and currently is used in research applications for the delivery of specific drug formulations. The Akita2 is the first commercial liquid aerosol delivery system that provides an opportunity for controlled delivery of aerosols to different regions of the lung.
- *I-neb:* The I-neb system and its predecessor the ProDose (Respironics) (Fig. 6.43) are examples of breath-actuated nebulizer (mesh and jet, respectively) with adaptive aerosol delivery (AAD). These devices monitor the pressure changes and inspiratory time for the patient's first three consecutive breaths (see Fig. 6.43).[73] The drug then is aerosolized for 50% of the inspiration during the fourth and all subsequent breaths. When the patient's preestablished dose has been

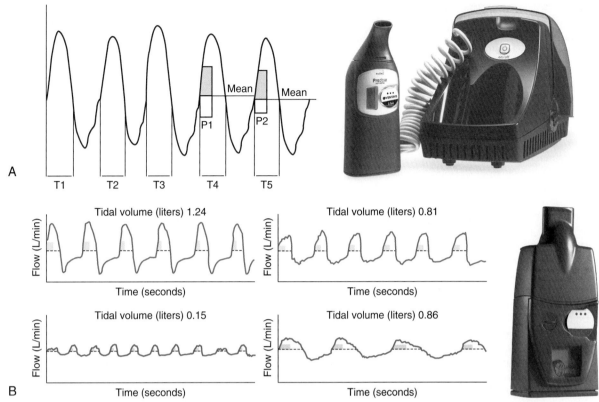

FIGURE 6.43 Adaptive aerosol delivery (AAD) delivers a precise, preset dose with variation between patients. A microprocessor tracks the patient's breathing pattern on a running average of the previous three breaths, generating aerosol for 50% of the predicted inspiration. A, The ProDose uses a compressor and jet nebulizer. B, The I-neb is a handheld unit that uses a vibrating mesh. (From Kacmarek RM, Stoller JK, Heuer AJ: *Egan's fundamentals of respiratory care*, ed 10, St. Louis, 2013, Mosby-Elsevier.)

aerosolized, the system provides an audible signal indicating that treatment should be stopped and the remaining medication discarded. Built-in electronics monitor the patient's treatment schedules and delivered doses. The device is programmed with an externally applied chip that determines the inhaled dose for the specific drug used. By design, these breath-actuated devices are highly efficient at providing emitted aerosol to the lungs; however, the overall efficiency of the dose placed in the nebulizer is considerably less. A unit dose of drug may only need to be partly nebulized to achieve the intended dose, which leaves a large proportion of the drug in the reservoir.

The I-neb (see Fig. 6.43) is a handheld AAD device that uses passive vibrating mesh technology with AAD. The I-neb has been released for delivery of iloprost (Ventavis), a form of inhaled prostacyclin used to treat primary pulmonary hypertension. As a drug-device combination, the I-neb is available only for use with this one drug.

• *Tyvaso:* The Tyvaso Optineb (United Therapeutics Corporation) is a USN that is designed to deliver treprostinil. The device has different parts, and clinicians need to assemble dome, inhalation piece, filters, and mouthpiece. They also need to fill the couplant chamber with water that is placed between the piezo and the medication cup. Using auditory and visual feedback on the patient's inhalation technique, patients take a set number of breaths per treatment at certain intervals during the day. When the therapy is not completed by the patient, the numerical display of the Tyvaso shows the remaining breaths that need to be taken by the patient.

Technique

Box 6.10 outlines the optimum technique for using an SVN for aerosol drug delivery. A slow inspiratory flow optimizes aerosol deposition with an SVN; however, deep breathing and breath-holding during SVN therapy do little to enhance deposition over normal tidal breathing.[74] Because the nose is an efficient filter of particles larger than 5 mm, many clinicians prefer not to use a mask for SVN therapy. As long as the patient is mouth-breathing, little difference in the clinical response is seen between therapy given by mouthpiece and that given by mask. The selection of delivery method (mask or mouthpiece) should be based on the patient's ability, preference, and comfort.

Infection Control Issues

The CDC recommends that nebulizers be cleaned and disinfected (or rinsed with sterile water) and air-dried between uses.[75] Box 6.11 provides some useful recommendations for care of an SVN used in the home care setting.

BOX 6.10 Technique for Using a Small-Volume Nebulizer

1. Assemble the tubing or cable, the nebulizer, and the mouthpiece or mask.
2. Place the prescribed amount of medication in the nebulizer's reservoir.
3. For a pneumatic nebulizer:
   - Connect the tubing to the flowmeter or compressor.
   - Set the flow according to the manufacturer's recommendation (often 6 to 10 L/min).
4. For a vibrating mesh or small ultrasonic nebulizer:
   - Connect a clean nebulizer/medication reservoir to the mask or mouthpiece.
   - Attach the nebulizer/reservoir to the electronic controller.
   - Attach the nebulizer to a power source or make sure the device's battery has a sufficient charge.
5. Instruct the patient to sit in an upright position, as tolerated.
6. Apply the mouthpiece or mask, and encourage the patient to breathe through the mouth. If an artificial airway is used, make sure the nebulizer is positioned appropriately and does not put undue pressure on the airway.
7. Encourage relaxed tidal breathing with low inspiratory flow rates and occasional deep breaths.
8. Operate the nebulizer in an upright position, 45 degrees from vertical.
9. Run the nebulizer until the onset of sputter or until aerosol is no longer produced.
10. At the conclusion of therapy, wash and rinse with sterile water, disinfect, and air-dry the nebulizer/reservoir or dispose of it.
11. Do not submerge the electronic controller or compressor in water or disinfectant.
12. Store the nebulizer in a clean, dry place.

BOX 6.11 Cleaning and Disinfection of Nebulizers for Home Use

- After each use:
  - Disassemble the nebulizer and mouthpiece or mask.
  - Wash them in warm, soapy water.
  - Rinse with tap water.
  - Shake off the excess water.
  - Place the parts on a clean, absorbent towel and allow them to air-dry.
  - Reassemble the nebulizer, and store it in a clean, dry place.
- Once a day:
  - After washing the nebulizer and mouthpiece or mask, place them in a disinfectant solution to soak for 1 h.
  - Rinse with sterile or distilled water.
  - Shake off the excess water, and allow the parts to air-dry.
  - Reassemble the nebulizer, and store it in a clean, dry place.
- Some types of homemade disinfecting solutions:
  - 1 ounce quaternary ammonium compound (QAC) to 1 oz distilled water; discard weekly.
  - 1 part vinegar (5% acetic acid) to 3 parts hot sterile water; discard after each use.
  - 1 teaspoon household chlorine bleach to 1 gal of water; discard after use.

Selecting an Aerosol Drug-Delivery System

Selection of the most appropriate aerosol delivery system requires a knowledge of the advantages and disadvantages of the various systems currently available. Table 6.2 compares the pMDI, DPI, SVN, USN, and VMN delivery systems. Fig. 6.44 compares aerosol distribution for a DPI, pMDI, pMDI with holding chamber, and SVN.

The American College of Chest Physicians (CHEST) commissioned an extensive, evidence-based review of the literature to determine which types of aerosol delivery system were most effective. They concluded that pMDIs, DPIs, and nebulizers all work with comparable clinical results, as long as they are prescribed for the appropriate patients and are used properly.[76]

The AARC has published several clinical practice guidelines to guide practitioners in selecting the best aerosol delivery system for a given clinical situation. Summaries of the various guidelines can be found in Clinical Practice Guidelines. Excerpts from three of these guidelines are included in Clinical Practice Guidelines 6.1 to 6.3.

A number of factors should be considered when selecting the appropriate aerosol delivery device for a particular patient: (1) the available drug formulation, (2) the desired site of deposition, (3) the patient's characteristics (age, acuity of respiratory problem, alertness, and ability to follow instructions), (4) the patient's ability to properly use the device, and (5) the patient's preference.[68]

For administration of maintenance therapy bronchodilators and antiinflammatory agents to adults, a pMDI with a valved holding chamber is the most convenient, versatile, and cost-effective method. DPIs are gaining popularity as equivalents to pMDIs for maintenance therapy with available drugs for patients capable of generating an adequate inspiratory flow. In acute situations, when high or multiple doses are needed, or when adult patients are not able to follow instructions, an SVN or large-volume continuous nebulizer is an alternative.

An adult patient's preference must be considered, because a device that is not favored will not be used. USN and VMNs may be the devices of choice when portability and short duration of therapy is desired; however, cost is often a mitigating factor in device selection. For ambulatory use, compressor-driven nebulizers often are the least-expensive option.

Finally, it is important to state that the effectiveness of aerosol therapy (or any type of self-administered therapy) is greatly influenced by the patient's understanding of the procedure. Nearly all aerosol therapy is self-administered. Interestingly, many patients using aerosol devices report that they did not receive adequate instruction on how to use their equipment. Box 6.12 provides some suggestions for improving the effectiveness of patient education about aerosol therapy.

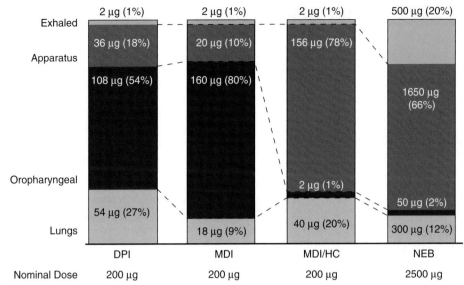

FIGURE 6.44 Distribution of albuterol via nebulizer (NEB), pressurized metered-dose inhaler (MDI), MDI with a holding chamber (electrostatic and nonelectrostatic), and dry powder inhaler (DPI). (From Kacmarek RM, Stoller JK, Heuer AJ: *Egan's fundamentals of respiratory care*, ed 10, St. Louis, 2013, Mosby-Elsevier.)

CLINICAL PRACTICE GUIDELINE 6.1   Selection of an Aerosol Delivery Device

Description

The device selected for administration of a pharmacologically active aerosol to the lower airway should produce particles with an MMAD of 1 to 3 μm. Such devices include pMDIs, pMDIs with accessory devices (e.g., spacers), DPIs, SVNs, LVNs, and USNs. Note that this guideline does not address bland aerosol administration and sputum induction.

Indications

Aerosol delivery devices are needed to deliver aerosolized medications to the lower airways, such as β-adrenergic agents, anticholinergic agents (antimuscarinic), antiinflammatory agents (e.g., corticosteroids), mediator-modifying compounds (e.g., cromolyn sodium), and mucokinetics.

Contraindications

No contraindications exist to the administration of aerosols by inhalation, although contraindications may be posed by the substances being delivered. Package inserts should be consulted for product-specific contraindications.

Hazards and Complications

1. Malfunction of the device or improper technique may result in the delivery of an incorrect dose of medication.
2. Complications of specific pharmacological agents may occur.
3. Cardiotoxic effects of Freon have been reported as idiosyncratic responses that may be a problem with excessive use of an MDI.

4. Freon may harm the environment by its effect on the ozone layer.
5. Repeated exposure to aerosols has been reported to produce asthmatic symptoms in some caregivers.

Monitoring

1. Device performance
2. Device application technique
3. Patient response, including changes in vital signs

Infection Control

1. Standard precautions for body substance isolation must be used.
2. SVNs and LVNs are for single-patient use or should be subjected to high-level disinfection between patients.
3. Published data establishing a safe use period for SVNs and LVNs are lacking; however, SVNs and LVNs probably should be changed or subjected to high-level disinfection at approximately 24-hour intervals.
4. Medications should be handled aseptically. Medications from multidose sources in acute care facilities must be handled aseptically and discarded after 24 hours, unless the manufacturer's recommendations specifically state that medications may be stored longer than 24 hours. Tap water should not be used as a diluent.
5. MDI accessory devices are only for single-patient use. No documented concerns exist about contamination of medication in pMDI canisters. Cleaning of accessory devices is based on aesthetic criteria.

DPI, Dry powder inhaler; *LVN,* large-volume nebulizer; *MDI,* metered-dose inhaler; *MMAD,* mass median aerodynamic diameter; *pMDI,* pressurized metered-dose inhaler; *SVN,* small-volume nebulizer; *USN,* ultrasonic nebulizer.
Modified from the American Association for Respiratory Care: Clinical practice guideline: selection of aerosol delivery device. *Respir Care* 37:891, 1992.

CLINICAL PRACTICE GUIDELINE 6.2   Bland Aerosol Administration

Description

For purposes of this guideline, bland aerosol administration includes the delivery of sterile water or hypotonic, isotonic, or hypertonic saline in aerosol form. Bland aerosol administration may be accompanied by oxygen administration.

Indications

Cool, bland aerosol therapy is indicated primarily for upper airway administration; therefore an MMAD equal to or greater than 5 μm is desirable. The use of hypotonic and hypertonic saline is indicated primarily for inducing sputum specimens; therefore an MMAD of 1 to 5 μm is desirable. Heated bland aerosol is indicated primarily for minimizing humidity deficit when the upper airway has been bypassed; for this purpose an MMAD of 2 to 10 μm is desirable. Specific indications include:

1. Upper airway edema (cool bland aerosol)
2. Laryngotracheobronchitis
3. Subglottic edema
4. Postextubation management of the upper airway
5. Postoperative management of the upper airway
6. Bypassed upper airway
7. Need for sputum specimens

Contraindications

1. Bronchoconstriction
2. History of airway hyperresponsiveness

Hazards and Complications

1. Wheezing or bronchospasm
2. Bronchoconstriction when an artificial airway is used
3. Infection
4. Overhydration
5. Patient discomfort
6. Caregiver exposure to droplet nuclei of *Mycobacterium tuberculosis* or other airborne contagious organisms released through coughing, particularly during sputum induction

Assessment of Need

The presence of one or more of the following may be an indication for administration of a water or isotonic or hypotonic saline aerosol:

1. Stridor
2. Brassy, crouplike cough
3. Hoarseness after extubation
4. Diagnosis of laryngotracheobronchitis or croup
5. Clinical history suggesting upper airway irritation and increased work of breathing (e.g., smoke inhalation)
6. Patient discomfort associated with airway instrumentation or insult
7. Need for sputum induction (e.g., for diagnosis of *Pneumocystis jiroveci* pneumonia or tuberculosis)

Assessment of Outcome

The desired outcomes for administration of water or hypotonic or isotonic saline include:

1. Decreased work of breathing
2. Improved vital signs
3. Decreased stridor
4. Decreased dyspnea
5. Improved arterial blood gas values
6. Improved oxygen saturation, as indicated by pulse oximetry (SpO_2)

The desired outcome for administration of hypertonic saline is a sputum sample adequate for analysis.

Monitoring

The extent of patient monitoring should be determined by the stability and severity of the patient's condition. Monitoring may include:

1. Subjective patient responses of pain, discomfort, dyspnea, or restlessness
2. Heart rate and rhythm
3. Blood pressure
4. Respiratory rate, as well as the breathing pattern and use of accessory respiratory muscles
5. Breath sounds
6. Sputum production quantity, color, consistency, and odor
7. Pulse oximetry (if hypoxemia is suspected)

Modified from Kallstrom TJ, AARC: AARC clinical practice guideline. Bland aerosol administration—2003 revision & update. *Respir Care* 48(5)529-533, 2003.

BOX 6.12   Teaching Patients Psychomotor Skills for Inhaler Use

1. Set aside uninterrupted time to complete the instruction.
2. Perform the demonstration in a suitable environment.
3. Have all necessary equipment and spares close at hand.
4. Engage the patient's attention.
5. Explain verbally what you will do and why.
6. Demonstrate the technique for using the inhaler, naming and explaining each step.
7. Repeat the demonstration without explanation (talking, although necessary in the previous step, interferes with correct timing and inspiratory maneuvers).
8. Repeat again with verbal comments.
9. Have the patient demonstrate the maneuver, including correct identification of inhalers and assembly of the inhaler/spacer combination.
10. Identify problems in performance, and repeat the instruction and patient return demonstration.
11. Ask the patient to verbalize the most important aspects of the procedure and those that are most troublesome.
12. Arrange for follow-up instruction. Assure the patient that some loss of skill over time is typical and can be corrected. Remind the patient to bring inhalers and spacers to every appointment.
13. Provide instruction to family or friends if requested.
14. Review and provide instructional leaflets or videos if available.

Modified from Coates VE: *Education for patients and clients,* London, 1999, Routledge.

CLINICAL PRACTICE GUIDELINE 6.3   Selection of a Device for Aerosol Delivery to the Lung Parenchyma

Description

A device selected for administration of a pharmacologically active aerosol to the lung parenchyma should produce particles with an MMAD of 1 to 3 μm. Such devices include USNs, some LVNs (e.g., the SPAG unit, which is intended only for ribavirin delivery), and some SVNs (e.g., the Circulaire, Respirgard II).

Indications

The indication for selecting a suitable device is the need to deliver a topical medication (in aerosol form) with a site of action in the lung parenchyma or that is intended for systemic absorption. Such medications may include antibiotics, antivirals, antifungals, surfactants, and enzymes.

Contraindications

No contraindications exist to choosing an appropriate device for parenchymal deposition. Contraindications may exist related to the substances being delivered. Package inserts should be consulted for product-specific contraindications to medication delivery.

Hazards and Complications

1. Device malfunction or improper technique may result in delivery of incorrect medication doses.
2. For mechanically ventilated patients, the nebulizer design and the characteristics of the medication may affect ventilator function (e.g., filter obstruction, altered tidal volume, decreased trigger sensitivity) and medication deposition.
3. Aerosols may cause bronchospasm or airway irritation, and complications related to specific pharmacological agents can occur.
4. Exposure to medication should be limited to the patient for whom it has been ordered. Nebulizer medication released into the atmosphere from the nebulizer or the patient may affect health care providers and others near the treatment. For example, awareness has increased of the possible health effects of aerosols such as ribavirin and pentamidine. Anecdotal reports associate symptoms such as conjunctivitis, decreased tolerance of contact lenses, headaches, bronchospasm, shortness of breath, and rashes in health care workers exposed to secondhand aerosols. Similar concerns have arisen concerning health care workers who are pregnant or plan to become pregnant within 8 weeks of administration. The potential exposure effects of aerosolized antibiotics

(which may contribute to the development of resistant organisms), steroids, and bronchodilators are less often discussed. Because the data are incomplete regarding adverse health effects on health care workers and those casually exposed, exposure should be minimized in all situations.

5. The Centers for Disease Control and Prevention recommends that:
   a. Warning signs should be posted in an easy-to-see location to apprise all who enter the treatment area of the potential hazards of exposure. Accidental exposures should be documented and reported according to accepted standards.
   b. Staff members who administer medications must understand the inherent risks of the medication and the procedures for disposing of hazardous waste safely. Department administrators should screen staff members for adverse effects of aerosol exposure and provide alternative assignments for those at high risk for such adverse effects (e.g., pregnant women or those with demonstrated sensitivity to the specific agent).
   c. Filters or filtered scavenger systems should be used to remove aerosols that are not considered safe.
   d. Booths or stalls should be used for sputum induction and administration of aerosolized medications in areas where multiple patients are treated. The booths or stalls should be designed to provide adequate airflow to draw aerosol and droplet nuclei from the patient into an appropriate filtration system, with exhaust directed to an appropriate outside vent. Note that filters, nebulizers, and other contaminated components of the aerosol delivery system used with suspect agents (e.g., pentamidine and ribavirin) should be handled as hazardous waste. If scavenger systems or specially designed booths are not available, clinicians administering these treatments should wear personal protection devices to reduce exposure to the medication residues and body substances. These devices may include fitted respirator masks, goggles, gloves, gowns, and splatter shields.

Monitoring

1. Device and scavenging system performance
2. Device application technique
3. Patient response

LVN, Large-volume nebulizer; *MMAD,* mass median aerodynamic diameter; *SPAG,* small particle aerosol generator; *SVN,* small-volume nebulizer; *USN,* ultrasonic nebulizer.
Modified from the American Association for Respiratory Care: Clinical practice guideline: selection of a device for delivery of aerosol to the lung parenchyma. *Respir Care* 41:647, 1996.

Special Considerations
Aerosol Delivery in Infants and Children

Infants and small children require smaller minute volumes than adults; therefore they inhale a smaller proportion of a continuous nebulizer output.[40] For patients who can tolerate a mask, a medication nebulizer can be attached to an appropriately sized aerosol mask. Because the clinical response is the same to a mouthpiece or close-fitting mask treatment, patient compliance and preference should guide selection of the device. However, aerosol delivery to a patient is substantially reduced when a loosely fitting mask (leak >1 cm) is used rather than a snug mask or mouthpiece.[77]

Blowing the aerosol into the face of an infant or a child is not a good aerosol delivery option for children who will not tolerate mask treatment (e.g., will not wear a close-fitting mask). This "blow-by" technique typically is performed by directing the aerosol from the nebulizer toward the patient's nose and mouth from several inches from the face. Studies suggest that very little drug enters the airway with this method.

It may be more efficient to take the time to condition the patient to tolerate the mask or to deliver medication with a close-fitting mask when the patient is sound asleep.[78] A possible alternative to the blow-by technique is the PediNeb (Westmed), shown in Fig. 6.45. The PediNeb is a pacifier that directs aerosol from a JN toward the infant's nose. No published data are available, in vitro or otherwise, on the effectiveness of this device.

Crying greatly reduces lower airway deposition of aerosol medication. If a mask is not tolerated, other options should be considered. Aerosol hoods and tents have been used for aerosol delivery to small children, with good effect. In infants, a properly fitted hood can deliver a lung dose similar to that obtained with a tightly fitting mask; however, hoods are rarely used for toddlers and older children.

The SootherMask (InspiRx Inc.) is a pediatric mask with a small dead space that aligns aerosols with the naris of the child. Threading the pacifier attached to the mask during therapy

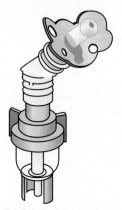

FIGURE 6.45 The PediNeb (Westmed) combines a pacifier with aerosol ports directed at the nares. No data are available to confirm the device's efficacy, and concerns have been raised about high ocular deposition.

improves the face-mask seal and may prevent agitation and crying caused by aerosol therapy (Fig. 6.46). Previous research reported a similar lung deposition with the SootherMask compared with the conventional face mask without a pacifier.[78a] The pacifier in the SootherMask may help calm the children during therapy and improve patient compliance to aerosol treatments.[78a,78b]

Aerosol Delivery With High-Flow Nasal Cannula

Aerosol drug delivery via high-flow nasal cannula (HFNC) has been increasingly popular in clinical practice based on in vitro research and reported aerosol delivery efficiency in adults, young children, and infants.[79-82] For patients who will not tolerate a mask but will tolerate a nasal cannula, aerosol delivery with humidified gas via nasal cannula provides an attractive option. Bhashyam et al.[79] administered aerosol from a VMN (Aeroneb) with 3 L/min of humidified oxygen through three sizes of nasal cannula, reporting inhaled doses ranging from 8% to 29%, with greater delivery associated with the larger cannula (Fig. 6.47). They reported that the 5-μm VMD aerosol exiting the nebulizer was reduced to ≤2 μm when exiting the cannula. Particles of this size should readily pass through the nose and upper airways with little impactive loss. Previous research showed that aerosol drug delivery with synchronized inspiratory positive airway pressure (SiPAP) was lower than HFNC and the bubble continuous positive airway pressure (CPAP) using a spontaneously breathing lung model attached to a low-birth-weight anatomical nasal airway cast.[82a] Delivery efficiency of HFNC was less than 2% but higher than the bubble CPAP. Also, placing the nebulizer at the humidifier increased aerosol deposition in HFNC, SiPAP, and bubble CPAP.[82a]

The size of nasal cannula, type of humidifier, and amount of flow rate used in aerosol therapy influence aerosol deposition.[82] To optimize aerosol delivery, use the lowest flow tolerated while using the largest tolerated ID of nasal cannula.[82] In general, the higher the gas flow, the lower the deposition; however, the higher the inspiratory flow of the patient, the

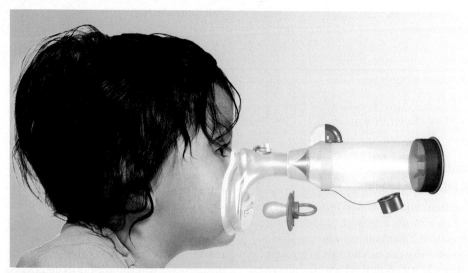

FIGURE 6.46 The SootherMask (InspiRx Inc.). (Reproduced with permission from InspiRx.)

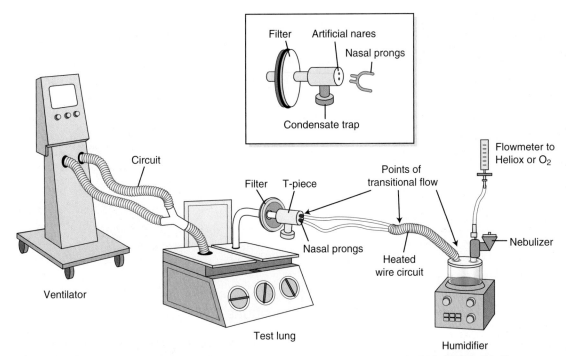

FIGURE 6.47 Aerosol delivery through nasal cannulas. (From Kacmarek RM, Stoller JK, Heuer AJ: *Egan's fundamentals of respiratory care*, ed 10, St. Louis, 2013, Mosby-Elsevier.)

greater proportion of aerosol that is inhaled.[82b] Further in vivo studies are required to confirm the therapeutic benefits of this approach.

Aerosol Delivery in Mechanical Ventilation

Many patients undergoing mechanical ventilation receive aerosolized medications, with variable effects. The following subsections cover issues and techniques to optimize SVN, USN, VMN, and pMDI delivery to patients receiving ventilatory support. For all aerosol systems, HMEs should be considered a barrier to aerosol delivery and should not be placed between the aerosol generator and the patient. Also, active humidification should not be turned off during aerosol administration of standard medications. Up to 40% of aerosol is exhausted to the environment during mechanical ventilation if a protecting filter is not placed in the expiratory limb of the ventilator circuit.[82c]

Use of a Small-Volume Nebulizer During Mechanical Ventilation

Of the four types of JNs described before, only the simple nebulizer can be used with pressurized circuits. Commercial reservoir, breath-enhanced, and breath-actuated nebulizers are not suitable for use in a closed, pressurized system. Aerosols administered by SVN to intubated patients receiving mechanical ventilation tend to be deposited mainly in the tubing of the ventilator circuit and expiratory filter, with a large volume of drug remaining in the nebulizer. Under normal conditions with heated humidification and standard JNs, pulmonary deposition ranges from 1.5% to 3%. When the nebulizer output, humidity level, tidal volume, flow, and I:E ratio are optimized, deposition can increase to as much as 15%. Box

6.13 outlines the optimum technique for drug delivery by SVN to intubated patients undergoing mechanical ventilation. Although in vitro models using dry gas demonstrated up to 40% higher aerosol delivery compared with heated humidity, these effects have not been shown to improve outcomes in patients, whereas the risks associated with administering cold, dry gas through an ETT have been demonstrated. If available with the specific ventilator, breath actuation can increase aerosol delivery by 20% to 50%, depending on placement, but may prolong the administration time by more than threefold.

Although some ventilators compensate for nebulizer gas flow entering the circuit, many do not. The additional flow of gas into the ventilator circuit may change the set flow and delivered volumes, as well as require adjustments to alarm settings both during and after nebulization. Smaller patients are affected to a greater extent when extra flow is added to the ventilator circuit. For example, with infants, 6 L/min of additional gas flow can more than double tidal volumes and inspiratory pressures, thus placing the patient at risk. Consequently, ventilator and alarm parameters should be adjusted to compensate for this gas flow during nebulization and returned to previous settings when nebulizer flow is turned off. This presents the risk for busy clinicians not returning ventilator parameters to pretreatment levels after the treatment is completed. When placing the nebulizer in the ventilator circuit, positive pressure in the circuit can push medication from the reservoir out through the gas inlet. This can be avoided by applying gas flow to the SVN before placing in the circuit. SVNs often are attached to the ventilator circuit with a standard 22-mm (adult) or 15-mm (pediatric) T-adapter, requiring interruption of ventilation and positive pressure

BOX 6.13 Technique for Using a Small-Volume Nebulizer With Mechanical Ventilation

1. Assess the need for medication.
2. Establish the dose needed to compensate for decreased delivery (possibly two to five times the dose given to patients who are not ventilated).
3. Place the prescribed amount of drug in the SVN.
4. Place the SVN in the inspiratory line 12 to 18 in from the patient Y-adapter. Check to make sure the circuit has no leaks.
5. Remove the HME from between the SVN and the patient during the treatment; use an alternative form of humidification.
6. Consider placing a filter in the expiratory limb of the ventilator circuit to avoid loading the expiratory flow transducer with medications.
7. Connect the nebulizer to the nebulizer outlet port of the ventilator.
8. Use the ventilator nebulizer compressor if it meets the flow needs of the nebulizer and cycles on inspiration; otherwise, use continuous flow from an external 50-psi source with continuous gas flow to the nebulizer at 1 to 10 L/min; adjust the volume or pressure limit to compensate for additional flow during treatment.
9. Turn off the flow-by or continuous flow function while nebulizing.
10. Tap the nebulizer periodically until all the medication has been nebulized.
11. Remove the nebulizer from the circuit. Rinse it with sterile water and air dry. Store the nebulizer in a clean bag between treatments or replace between treatments.
12. Check to make sure the ventilator circuit has no leaks. Return the ventilator and alarms to the previous settings.
13. Monitor the patient for an adverse response.
14. Assess the outcome of the treatment.

HME, Heat and moisture exchanger; *SVN,* small-volume nebulizer.

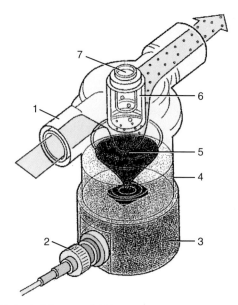

FIGURE 6.48 Maquet SUN 145 ultrasonic nebulizer with power control module. *(1)* Main gas flow connector; *(2)* power cable from ventilator; *(3)* ultrasonic generator; *(4)* couplant cup; *(5)* medication cup; *(6)* T-piece adapter containing baffles; *(7)* injector membrane.

while attaching and removing the SVN to the ventilator circuit. The integrity of the ventilator circuit should be evaluated whenever a nebulizer is inserted or removed to ensure that there are no leaks. Spring-loaded valved T-adapters connect the SVN to the circuit when inserted and seal the circuit when the nebulizer is removed, avoiding lung derecruitment and interruption of ventilation; however, the valve mechanism acts as a baffle, reducing aerosol delivery by up to 40%. Bacterial contamination of ventilator circuits occurs within minutes of attaching to the patient airway, and any condensate or secretions that drain into the nebulizer reservoir contaminate the medication being delivered to the lungs.

Use of an Ultrasonic Nebulizer During Mechanical Ventilation

Aerosol administration by USN may deliver more drug to the lung than SVN during mechanical ventilation, with the benefit of not adding gas into the ventilator circuit. The most efficient placement of the USN is proximal to the patient in the inspiratory limb. Unfortunately, the size and weight of USNs make this positioning difficult, especially with infant ventilators. USNs are operated continuously and are not breath actuated. Two examples of USNs used with controlled (continuous) mandatory ventilation are the SUN 345 (Maquet) and the EasyNeb (Medtronic Minimally Invasive Therapies). The SUN 145 (Fig. 6.48) operates with either an integrated module with the Maquet ventilator or as a stand-alone device. An on/off button turns on the nebulizer for 30 minutes, and a temperature override turns off the nebulizer if it heats beyond a set temperature. (This means that nebulization may be interrupted without warning to the clinician.) The EasyNeb has a stand-alone power/timer box that is designed to be placed on the ventilator. Both nebulizers use a disposable, plastic, single-patient-use medication cup designed to separate medications from the liquid couplant that conducts energy from the vibrational piezoceramic element. Couplant must be maintained at an adequate level to ensure contact between the piezo and the medication in the medication reservoir; the nebulizer top and T-piece should be cleaned and sterilized between patient uses. As with the SVN, the USN medication reservoir is open to and below the ventilator, acting as a condensate collector.

Use of a Vibrating Mesh Nebulizer During Mechanical Ventilation

Aerosol administration by VMN has been reported to deliver greater than 10% deposition in adult, pediatric, and infant models without the addition of gas into the ventilator circuit. The low residual drug volume and small particle size are associated with improved delivery efficiency. Two models of VMN are available. The Aerogen Pro is a multiple-patient-use, autoclavable nebulizer designed to be sterilized between patients. The Aerogen Solo is a single-patient, multiple-dose, disposable nebulizer designed to remain in the ventilator circuit for up to 28 days. The Aerogen Solo has a continuous feed tubing for use with continuous syringe infusion systems. Unlike jet SVNs and USNs, the medication reservoir is above the circuit and separated from the ventilator tubing by the mesh, which reduces the risk for contamination or of contaminated aerosols being introduced into the ventilator circuit. Unlike with the SVN, VM aerosol generation characteristics are the same in air, oxygen, or heliox. Although the VM has 1000 apertures with apertures of 3 to 5 μm, no perceptible leakage occurs, even with heliox, when the nebulizer reservoir is open to the atmosphere. Thus the VMN can be opened and refilled without interrupting ventilation or derecruitment of the lung.

Use of a Pressurized Metered-Dose Inhaler During Mechanical Ventilation

The pMDI with actuator that is provided by the manufacturer cannot be used in a closed, pressurized circuit, because it is open to the atmosphere. Consequently, a third-party adapter is required to use the pMDI canister. In vitro studies have shown that effective aerosol delivery by pMDIs during mechanical ventilation can range from as little as 2% to as much as 98%.[83] Actuator design and placement has a huge impact on drug-delivery efficiency. Actuation with a simple elbow adapter at the airway typically results in the least pulmonary deposition, with most of the aerosol affecting the adapter or tracheal airway. Higher aerosol delivery percentages occur when a spacer or twin nozzle adapter is placed in the inspiratory limb of the ventilator circuit proximal to the patient (Fig. 6.49). These adapters allow the aerosol "plume" to develop (reducing the size of the aerosol) before the bulk of the particles affect the surface of the circuit or ETT. The result is a more stable aerosol mass that can penetrate beyond the artificial airway and be deposited mainly in the lung. This leads to a better clinical response at lower dosages.[84] For medications delivered by pMDI, the amount of drug required to achieve the same therapeutic end point is similar for intubated patients (8%) and nonintubated patients (8% to 11%).[85] In stable COPD patients receiving mechanical ventilation, 4 puffs of albuterol produced as much bronchodilation as 12 or 28 puffs. Differences in response may be a result of the level of airway obstruction, ventilator parameters, and the techniques used for assessing response. During CMV, actuation of pMDIs should be synchronized with the beginning of inspiration. Box 6.14 outlines the optimum technique for drug delivery by pMDI to intubated patients undergoing mechanical ventilation.

Techniques for assessing the response to a bronchodilator in intubated patients undergoing mechanical ventilation differ from those used in the care of spontaneously breathing patients because expiration is passive during mechanical ventilation, and forced expiratory values (peak expiratory flow rate [PEFR], forced vital capacity [FVC], and FEV_1) cannot normally be obtained. For mechanically ventilated patients (1) a change in the differences between peak and plateau pressures (the

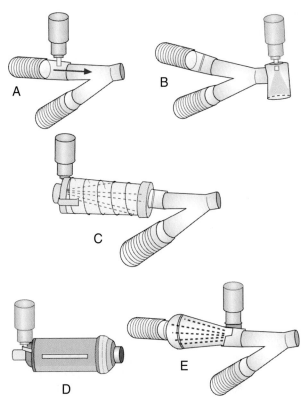

FIGURE 6.49 Devices for adapting a pressurized metered-dose inhaler (pMDI) to a ventilator circuit. A, In-line. B, Elbow. C, Collapsible chamber. D, Rigid chamber. E, Cone-shaped chamber in which aerosol is directed retrograde to gas flow to the patient. (Reproduced with permission from the European Respiratory Society ©. *Breathe* 3(2):128-139, Dec 2006: DOI: 10.1183/18106838.0302.128.)

most reliable indicator of a change in airway resistance during continuous mechanical ventilation) can be measured, (2) auto–positive end-expiratory pressure (auto-PEEP) levels may decrease in response to bronchodilators, and (3) breath-to-breath variations make measurements more reliable when the patient is not actively breathing with the ventilator.

Aerosol Delivery in Noninvasive Positive-Pressure Ventilation

Several studies reported that aerosol drug delivery during noninvasive positive-pressure ventilation (NIV) is feasible and effective in improving bronchospasm.[86-90] Factors influencing aerosol drug delivery during NIV include the type of circuit used, the position of the aerosol generator in relation to the leak port, and the type of aerosol generators and interface used during the treatment.[91-93] When a leak port is present in a single-limb circuit, placement of the aerosol generator should be between the leak and the patient. When the leak port is integrated into the mask, aerosol delivery is reduced.[92,93] When NIV is delivered through a conventional ventilator circuit and mask with no leak, aerosol methods used with continuous mechanical ventilation apply. Parameters impact delivery and response to bronchodilators during NIV, with higher peak inspiratory pressure associated with greater deposition and

BOX 6.14   Technique for Using a Pressurized Metered-Dose Inhaler With Mechanical Ventilation

1. Assess the need for medication.
2. Establish the ventilator dose of four puffs (for bronchodilators with a standard dose of two to four puffs) with heated humidity for stable patients with COPD. Higher doses may be required to treat an acute exacerbation.
3. Adjust the ventilator:
   - Leave the humidifier on (remove the HME from between the pMDI and the patient).
   - To optimize delivery: Ensure a tidal volume of 400 mL or higher (for adults). Reduce the peak inspiratory flow rate as tolerated. Use ramp or sine wave flow patterns. Increase the T_I/T_{TOT} to 0.3 or greater. Turn off continuous flow through the circuit.
4. Shake the pMDI, and warm it to hand temperature.
5. Place the pMDI in the chamber or other type of adapter in the ventilator circuit's inspiratory limb at the Y or between the elbow and the endotracheal tube. Use an adapter that has been shown in vitro to deliver greater than 10% of the dose.
6. Actuate the pMDI at the beginning of inspiration.
7. Wait 15 s or longer between actuations (the inhaler need not be shaken between puffs up to a total of eight actuations).
8. If the patient can take a spontaneous breath equal to or greater than 500 mL, coordinate actuation with the beginning of a deep, spontaneous breath, and encourage the patient to hold the breath for 4 to 10 s.
9. After administering the total dose, collapse or remove the chamber from the circuit, replace the HME, and return all ventilator parameters to pretreatment settings. A small-volume adapter may be left in line as long as it does not create a leak or pool condensate.
10. Monitor the patient for an adverse response.
11. Assess the outcome of the treatment.

COPD, Chronic obstructive pulmonary disease; *HME*, heat and moisture exchanger; *pMDI*, pressurized metered-dose inhaler; T_I/T_{TOT}, ratio of inspiratory time to total breathing cycle time.

changes in FEV_1 as opposed to an increase in expiratory pressure decreasing aerosol delivery.[91] Percentage of drug delivery is lower with JN than with pMDI or VMN, but the amount of drug delivered with the mesh nebulizer is greater than with either a JN or a pMDI.[93,94] Galindo-Filho and colleagues reported that radiolabeled aerosol deposition to healthy adults with VMN was 5.5% versus JN at 1.5% ($p = .005$).[94a]

Aerosol Delivery During Intrapulmonary Percussive Ventilation and High-Flow Oscillatory Ventilation

Intrapulmonary percussive ventilation (IPV) provides high-frequency oscillation of the airway while administering aerosol using an integrated nebulizer (Percussionaire). Reychler et al.[95] compared aerosol administration during IPV with administration with a standard JN. The MMAD was smaller with IPV than with the JN (0.2 μm vs. 1.89 μm), and the FPF was also lower (16.2% vs. 67.5%). However, the lung dose was similar

(2.49% with IPV vs. 4.2% with the JN alone). The authors concluded that IPV was too variable and thus too unpredictable to recommend for drug delivery to the lung.

During high-frequency oscillatory ventilation (HFOV) with the Sensormedics 3100A and B ventilators (Becton, Dickinson and Company), aerosol delivery can be difficult because of the high continuous flows (20 to 60 L/min) that pass through the ventilator circuit, diluting and scavenging aerosol. Fang et al. compared use of a VMN (Aeroneb or JN during HFOV placed before the humidifier [distal] and between the circuit and ETT [proximal]). The inhaled drug delivered by JN was 0% to 3% at the proximal position, whereas the VMN was 8.6% to 22.7% at the proximal position ($p < .01$). Aerosol delivery during HFOV was greater with adult settings than pediatric and infant settings with VMN and JN (22.7%, 8.6%, and 17.4%, respectively; $p < .01$). Placement of either nebulizer at the distal position resulted in negligible drug mass (<0.5%).[96]

Factors That Affect Aerosol Delivery During Mechanical Ventilation

In vitro testing has helped to identify a number of factors that can optimize the efficiency of aerosol delivery during mechanical ventilation. These include the nebulizer type, the nebulizer's position in the ventilator circuit, continuous flow in the circuit, the inspiratory flow rate, the I:E ratio, humidity, and gas density.[97]

Nebulizer type and position. Ari et al.[98] studied SVNs, USNs, pMDIs, and VMNs in an adult ventilator with no continuous or bias flow under both wet and dry conditions. Aerosol generators were placed either between the ventilator circuit and the patient's airway or in the inspiratory limb of the ventilator circuit at 6 in from the Y, or 6 in from the ventilator and before the heated humidifier under wet conditions. JNs, operating continuously, delivered more aerosol particles when placed closer to the ventilator, where the aerosol tubing acts as a reservoir. In contrast, all the aerosol generators that do not add gas flow into the ventilator circuit appear to be most efficient when placed in the inspiratory limb, 6 in from the Y. With the addition of continuous bias or trigger flow in the ventilator circuit, aerosol generators placed at the ventilator may be more efficient. In contrast, during infant ventilation with or without bias flow, placement of the VMN proximal to the patient is more effective than placement at the humidifier.[99]

The inspiratory flow rate and I:E ratio can affect aerosol delivery. The lower the flow and the longer the inspiratory time, the greater the amount of aerosol delivered. Inspiratory flow has been shown, using pMDIs, to be the more important variable. Deposition increased twofold at 40 L/min compared with 80 L/min, whereas a difference of less than 25% was seen in the I:E ratio (between 1:1 and 1:3) at either inspiratory flow. Flow patterns can make a significant but small difference, with descending ramp wave patterns providing higher efficiency than square wave patterns at the same peak flow.

Tidal volumes seem to be an issue only when the delivered volume is not sufficient to move the aerosol from the generator to the end of the patient airway in a single breath. A 6-ft adult circuit has an internal volume of 600 mL. Consequently, an aerosol generated at the ventilator would not reach the patient with a 500-mL tidal volume. Additional flow in the circuit could drive the aerosol down the inspiratory limb and improve efficiency.

Classic in vitro models of mechanical ventilation have demonstrated up to a 50% reduction in aerosol delivery with heated/humidified versus dry ventilator circuits. This difference may be partly a result of a limitation of the model used. Adding a simulation of exhaled humidity has been shown to reduce the difference between wet and dry circuits. In general, it is not a good idea to subject a patient with a bypassed upper airway to dry, cold gas, which may precipitate bronchospasm and changes in the airways, just to increase aerosol deposition. It is far better to increase the dose than to turn off the humidifier.

Gas density has been demonstrated to make a substantial difference in aerosol delivery. Heliox mixtures in the ventilator circuit in concentrations greater than 50% have been demonstrated in vitro to increase aerosol delivery with SVNs, VMNs, and pMDIs by up to 50%. Controlling the heliox concentration is easier when a pMDI, USN, or VM aerosol generator is used.

Controlling Environmental Contamination

Nebulized drugs that escape from the nebulizer into the atmosphere or are exhaled by the patient can be inhaled by anyone in the vicinity of the treatment. The risk associated with this environmental exposure is clear, and it can arise with a variety of drugs. Pentamidine and ribavirin both have been associated with health risks to health care providers, even with the use of filters on the exhalation ports of nebulizers, containment and scavenger systems, high-efficiency particulate air (HEPA) filter hoods, and ventilation systems.

Continuous pneumatic nebulizers (standard SVNs) produce the greatest amount of secondhand aerosol, and most of the aerosol produced (up to 60%) passes directly into the environment. The Respirgard II nebulizer (Carefusion), which was developed for administration of pentamidine, added one-way valves and an expiratory filter to contain aerosol that is exhaled and not inhaled (Fig. 6.50). BANs and pMDIs offer another alternative, because these devices tend to generate less secondhand aerosol. A study that surveyed respiratory therapists found that they were more than twice as likely as physical therapists to develop asthmalike symptoms during the course of their careers. The authors associated this increased incidence of asthmalike symptoms with the administration of ribavirin and exposure to glutaraldehyde.[100] Over the years there have been anecdotal reports of respiratory care clinicians who developed a sensitivity to secondhand aerosol from bronchodilators. Further research is required to provide a more thorough understanding of the hazards of secondhand exposure to aerosols in the clinical setting.

During mechanical ventilation, aerosols generated by the nebulizer or exhaled by the infected patient can pass through the expiratory circuit of the ventilator and be ultimately released into the ambient air. Ari et al.[101] estimated that

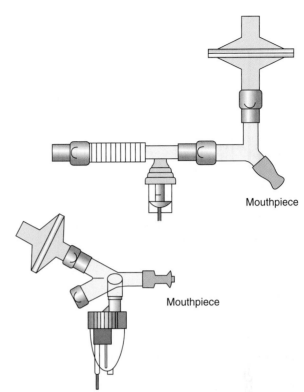

Mouthpiece

Mouthpiece

FIGURE 6.50 Nebulizers using a combination of one-way valves and filters collect exhaled aerosol and reduce secondhand aerosol exposure.

unfiltered aerosol escaping from the expiratory valve of a ventilator was greater than 160-fold compared to when a filter was used in the expiratory limb. Aerosol antibiotics passing through the ventilator can settle on surfaces in low concentrations, presenting a risk for contributing to the prevalence of antibiotic-resistant bacteria. Patients commonly generate aerosols during mechanical ventilation, which can infect other patients, visitors, and health care providers. Consequently, use of expiratory filters on mechanical filters is highly recommended.

Patients with infectious diseases, such as tuberculosis (TB) or severe acute respiratory syndrome (SARS), require respiratory isolation. It is imperative that caregivers protect themselves and their patients when working with infected patients. A variety of techniques are available for protecting caregivers and patients from environmental exposure during aerosol drug therapy. As was already mentioned, the greatest occupational risk for exposure to secondhand aerosols has been associated with administration of ribavirin and pentamidine. Conjunctivitis, headaches, bronchospasm, shortness of breath, and rashes have been reported among those administering these drugs.[102] These problems can be reduced by treating patients receiving aerosolized ribavirin or pentamidine in a private room, booth, or tent, or at a special station designed to minimize environmental contamination.

Negative-pressure rooms. When ribavirin or pentamidine is administered in a private room, the room should be equipped for negative-pressure ventilation with adequate air exchanges (at least six per hour) to clear the room of residual aerosols

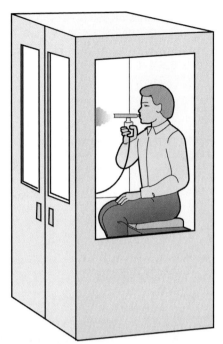

FIGURE 6.51 An environmental chamber for aerosol delivery to patients filters all exhaled gas through a high-efficiency particulate air (HEPA) filter.

CLINICAL SCENARIO 6.5

The medical director of the respiratory care department asks you to design a protocol for administering aerosolized pentamidine. Describe the protective measure that should be taken to ensure safe delivery of this drug.
See Appendix A for the answer.

before the next treatment. HEPA filters should be used to filter room or tent exhaust, or the aerosol should be scavenged to the outside.

Booths and stations. Booths or stations should be used for sputum induction and aerosolized medication treatments given in any area where more than one patient is treated. The area should be designed to provide adequate airflow to draw aerosol and droplet nuclei from the patient into an appropriate filtration system or an exhaust system directly to the outside. Booths and stations should be adequately cleaned between patients.

A variety of booths and specially designed stations are available for delivery of pentamidine or ribavirin. The Emerson containment booth (Fig. 6.51) is an example of a system that completely isolates the patient during aerosol administration. All gas is drawn through a prefilter and a HEPA filter. In areas where proper air exchanges do not exist, devices such as the Enviracaire (Honeywell) have been used to provide local exhaust ventilation through a HEPA filter medium. Few data exist to support the efficacy of these devices, although they are enjoying increasing popularity in the home environment.

The AeroStar Aerosol Protection Cart (Respiratory Safety Systems) is a portable patient isolation station for administration of hazardous aerosolized medication. It can be used during sputum induction and for pentamidine treatment. The patient compartment is collapsible and has a swing-out counter and three polycarbonate walls. Captured aerosols are removed with a HEPA filter. A prefilter is used to retain larger dust particles and to prevent early loading of the more expensive HEPA filter (Clinical Scenario 6.5).

Filters and nebulizers used in treatments with pentamidine and ribavirin should be treated as hazardous wastes and disposed of accordingly. Goggles, gloves, and gowns should be used as splatter shields and to reduce exposure to medication residues and body substances. The staff should be screened for adverse effects of exposure to the aerosol medication. The risks and safety procedures should be reviewed regularly.

In addition to the risks associated with administration of aerosol medication, the risk for TB transmission has become a great concern because of an increase in case numbers and the development of multidrug-resistant strains of the organism. TB is transmitted in the form of droplet nuclei (0.3 to 0.6 μm) that carry TB bacilli. Patients with known or suspected TB need private rooms with negative-pressure ventilation that exhausts to the outside. If environmental isolation is not possible or the health care worker must enter the patient's room, personal protective equipment should be used.

Personal protective equipment. Personal protective equipment is recommended when care is provided for any patient with a disease that can be spread by the airborne route.[103] The greatest risks that respiratory therapists encounter usually involve TB or chickenpox. Although environmental controls should be instituted in the care of these patients, standard and airborne precautions should also be implemented. A variety of masks and respirators have been recommended for use when caring for a patient with TB or other respiration-transmitted diseases. Traditional surgical masks, particulate respirators, disposable and reusable HEPA filters, and powered air-purifying respirators (PAPRs) have been used. No data are available determining the most effective and most clinically useful device to protect health care workers and others, although the US Occupational Safety and Health Administration requires specific levels of protection (HEPA and PAPRs).

KEY POINTS

- Conditioning of inhaled and exhaled gas is accomplished primarily by the nose and upper airway. Bypassing the upper airway without providing similar levels of heat and humidity to inhaled gas can cause damage to the respiratory tract.

- The primary goal of humidification is to maintain normal physiological conditions in the lower airways. Gases delivered to the nose and mouth should be conditioned to 20°C to 22°C with 10 mg/L of water vapor (50% RH).

- When being delivered to the trachea, gases should be warmed and humidified to 32°C to 40°C with 36 to 40 mg/L of water vapor (>90% RH).
- A humidifier is a device that adds invisible molecular water to gas.
- Temperature is an important factor affecting humidifier output. The higher the temperature, the greater the water vapor capacity of the delivered gas.
- Bubble, passover, wick, membrane humidifiers, and HMEs are the major types of humidifiers. Active humidifiers incorporate heating devices, as well as a source of water, with reservoir and/or feed systems.
- Most HMEs are passive, capturing both heat and moisture from expired gas and returning it to the patient at approximately 70% efficiency. HMEs are not recommended for use with infants because of issues related to increased mechanical dead space and use of uncuffed ETTs, which allow some exhaled gas to bypass the HME.
- Common problems with humidification systems include condensation, cross-contamination, and ensuring proper conditioning of the inspired gas.
- Bland aerosol therapy with sterile water or saline is used to (1) treat upper airway edema, (2) overcome heat and humidity deficits in patients with tracheal airways, and (3) help obtain sputum specimens.
- LVNs and USNs are used to generate bland aerosols. Delivery systems include a variety of direct airway appliances and mist tents.
- Common problems with bland aerosol therapy are cross-contamination and infection, environmental safety, inadequate mist production, overhydration, bronchospasm, and noise.
- An aerosol is a suspension of solid or liquid particles in gas. In the clinical setting, therapeutic aerosols are made with atomizers or nebulizers.
- The general aim of aerosol drug therapy is delivery of a therapeutic dose of the selected agent to the desired site of action.
- Where aerosol particles are deposited in the respiratory tract depends on their size, shape, and motion and on the physical characteristics of the airways. Key mechanisms causing aerosol deposition include inertial impaction, sedimentation, and Brownian diffusion.
- For targeting aerosols for delivery to the upper airway (nose, larynx, and trachea), particles in the 5- to 50-µm MMAD range are used; 1- to 5-µm particles are used for the lower airways and lung parenchyma (alveolar region).
- The primary hazard of aerosol drug therapy is an adverse reaction to the medication being administered. Other hazards are related to infection control, airway reactivity, and systemic effects of bland aerosols.
- Drug aerosol delivery systems include pMDIs, DPIs, SVNs, LVNs, USNs, VMNs, hand-bulb atomizers, and nasal spray pumps.
- MDIs and DPIs are the preferred method for maintenance delivery of bronchodilators and steroids to spontaneously breathing patients. The effectiveness of this therapy is highly technique dependent.
- Accessory devices, spacers, and holding chambers are used with pMDIs to reduce oropharyngeal deposition of a drug and to overcome problems with poor hand-breath coordination.
- LVNs and SVNs with continuous feed can be used to provide continuous aerosol delivery when traditional dosing strategies are ineffective in controlling severe bronchospasm.
- Small-volume USNs can be used to administer bronchodilators, antiinflammatory agents, and antibiotics.
- Careful, ongoing patient assessment is the key to an effective bronchodilator therapy protocol. Components of the assessment include a patient interview, observation, tests of expiratory airflow, measurement of vital signs, auscultation, blood gas analysis, and oximetry.
- Standard SVNs are less efficient than pMDIs, USNs, or VMNs for aerosol drug delivery during mechanical ventilation. Device selection, proper positioning of the device, and ventilator parameter selection are needed to optimize deposition and achieve the desired clinical outcome. A variety of techniques are available for protecting patients and caregivers from environmental exposure during aerosol drug therapy.

ASSESSMENT QUESTIONS

See Appendix B for the answers.

1. A gas at body temperature and ambient pressure (BTPS) contains:
   a. 10 mg/L of water vapor
   b. 30 mg/L of water vapor
   c. 33.9 mg/L of water vapor
   d. 43.9 mg/L of water vapor

2. If the temperature of a saturated gas decreases, which of the following occurs?
   a. Condensation develops.
   b. Absolute humidity increases.
   c. Relative humidity decreases.
   d. Water vapor pressure increases.

3. If a patient has an artificial airway in place, what should be the minimum level of absolute humidity provided to the patient's airways?
   a. 10 mg/L
   b. 20 mg/L
   c. 30 mg/L
   d. 40 mg/L

4. A sample of room air gas contains 10 mg/L of humidity. What is the relative humidity (RH) of the gas if the room temperature is 25°C (77°F)?
   a. 10%
   b. 22%
   c. 43%
   d. 98%

5. Based on the American Association for Respiratory Care (AARC) Clinical Practice Guideline, the temperature of medical gas delivered through an artificial airway should be:
   a. 20°C to 25°C (68°F to 77°F)
   b. 31°C to 35°C (87.8°F to 95°F)
   c. 36°C to 40°C (96.8°F to 104°F)
   d. Over 45°C (113°F)

6. Which of the following are potential problems that may arise in patients with a tracheostomy who are breathing nonhumidified oxygen at a rate of 6 L/min?
   1. Atelectasis
   2. Destruction of the airway epithelium
   3. Inspissation of secretions
   4. Mucociliary dysfunction
      a. 1 and 3 only
      b. 2 and 4 only
      c. 1, 2, and 3 only
      d. 1, 2, 3, and 4

7. Which of the following is a contraindication to use of a heat and moisture exchanger (HME)?
   a. Minute volume greater than 10 L/min
   b. Minimal secretions
   c. Small tidal volumes
   d. Short-term mechanical ventilation

8. Which of the following is classified as a passive humidifier?
   a. Bubble humidifier
   b. Ultrasonic nebulizer
   c. Wick humidifier
   d. Heat and moisture exchanger

9. Name four types of heating devices that can be used to increase the humidity output of an active humidifier.

10. Which of the following results in increased aerosol deposition?
    a. Large tidal volume
    b. Slow inspiratory flow rate
    c. Decrease in the expiratory peak flow
    d. Short expiratory times

11. The optimum range of aerosol particle sizes that are to be inspired for general deposition through the upper and lower airways is:
    a. 0.1 to 1 μm
    b. 1 to 5 μm
    c. 3 to 10 μm
    d. 5 to 15 μm

12. What is the recommended gas flow rate to operate a small-volume nebulizer (SVN)?
    a. 1 L/min
    b. 6 to 8 L/min
    c. 10 L/min
    d. 15 L/min or more

13. What is the most important factor influencing aerosol deposition from a metered-dose inhaler (MDI)?
    a. Tidal volume
    b. Inspiratory flow rate
    c. Respiratory rate
    d. Breath-hold

14. The active drug component of a typical pressurized metered-dose inhaler (pMDI) accounts for what percentage of the total content of the mixture in the device?
    a. Less than 1%
    b. 10%
    c. 25%
    d. 60%

15. List six factors that can affect the performance of an SVN.

REFERENCES

1. Kapadia F, Shelley M: Normal mechanisms of humidification. *Probl Respir Care* 4:395, 1991.
2. Primiano F, Montague F, Saidel G: Measurement system for water vapor and temperature dynamics. *J Appl Physiol* 56:1679-1685, 1984.
3. Shelley M, Lloyd G, Park G: A review of the mechanisms and the methods of humidification of inspired gas. *Intensive Care Med* 14:1-9, 1988.
4. Ingelstedt S: Studies on the conditioning of air in the respiratory tract. *Acta Otolaryngol* 131(suppl):1, 1956.
5. Chalon J, Loew D, Malbranche J: Effects of dry air and subsequent humidification on tracheobronchial ciliated epithelium. *Anesthesiology* 37:338-343, 1972.
6. Marfatia S, Donahoe P, Henderson W: Effect of dry and humidified gases on the respiratory epithelium in rabbits. *J Pediatr Surg* 10:583-592, 1975.
7. American Association for Respiratory Care: Clinical practice guideline: humidification during mechanical ventilation. *Respir Care* 37:887-890, 1992.
8. Chatburn R, Primiano F: A rational basis for humidity therapy. *Respir Care* 32:249, 1987.
9. Anderson S, Herbring B, Widman B: Accidental profound hypothermia. *Br J Anaesth* 42:653-655, 1970.
10. Weinberg A: Hypothermia. *Ann Emerg Med* 22:370-377, 1993.
11. Chen T: The effect of heated humidifier in the prevention of intra-operative hypothermia. *Acta Anaesthesiol Sin* 32:27-30, 1994.
12. Giesbrecht G, Younes M: Exercise and cold-induced asthma. *Can J Appl Physiol* 20:300-314, 1995.
13. American Society for Testing and Materials (ASTM): *Standard specification for humidifiers for medical use (F1690)*, Conshohocken, PA, 1996, ASTM.
14. Gray H: Humidifiers. *Probl Respir Care* 4:423, 1991.
15. Klein E: Performance characteristics of conventional prototype humidifiers and nebulizers. *Chest* 64:690-696, 1973.
16. Darin J, Broadwell J, MacDonell R: An evaluation of water-vapor output from four brands of unheated, prefilled bubble humidifiers. *Respir Care* 7:41-50, 1982.
17. Kallstrom T, AARC: AARC Clinical practice guideline: bland aerosol administration—2003 revision and update. *Respir Care* 5:529-533, 2003.
18. Hill T, Sorbello J: Humidity outputs of large-reservoir nebulizers. *Respir Care* 32:225-260, 1987.

19. Mercer T, Goddard R, Flores R: Output characteristics of several commercial nebulizers. *Ann Allergy* 23:314-326, 1965.

20. Khajotia R: Induced sputum and cytological diagnosis of lung cancer. *Lancet* 338:976-977, 1991.

21. Gershman N: Comparison of two methods of collecting induced sputum in asthmatic subjects. *Eur Respir J* 9:2448-2453, 1996.

22. Gilmour I, Boyle M, Streifel A: Humidifiers kill bacteria. *Anesthesiology* 75:498, 1991.

23. Fink J: Extending ventilator circuit change interval beyond two days reduces the likelihood of ventilator associated pneumonia (VAP). *Chest* 113:405-411, 1998.

24. Craven D, Goularte T, Make B: Contaminated condensate in mechanical ventilator circuits: a risk factor for nosocomial pneumonia. *Am Rev Respir Dis* 129:625-628, 1984.

24a. Chiumello D, Pelosi P, Park G, et al.: In vitro and in vivo evaluation of a new active heat moisture exchanger. *Crit Care* 8(5):R281-R288, 2004.

24b. Davies MW, Dunster KR, Cartwright DW: Inspired gas temperature in ventilated neonates. *Pediatr Pulmonol* 38(1):50-54, 2004.

24c. Lellouche F, Maggiore SM, Lyazidi A, et al.: Water content of delivered gases during non-invasive ventilation in healthy subjects. *Intensive Care Med* 35(6):987-995, 2009.

24d. Prat G, Renault A, Tonnelier JM, et al.: Influence of the humidification device during acute respiratory distress syndrome. *Intensive Care Med* 29(12):2211-2215, 2003.

25. International Organization for Standardization: *Heat and moisture exchangers for use in humidifying respired gases in humans (ISO 9360)*, Geneva, 1992, International Organization for Standardization.

26. Shelly M: Inspired gas conditioning. *Respir Care* 37:1070-1080, 1992.

27. Branson R, Davis K: Evaluation of 21 passive humidifiers according to the ISO 9360 standard: moisture output, deadspace, and flow resistance. *Respir Care* 41:736, 1996.

27a. Lemmens HJM, Brock-Utne JG: Heat-and-moisture exchanger devices: Are they doing what they are supposed to do? *Anesth Analg* 98:382-385, 2004.

28. Ploysongsang Y, Branson RD, Rashkin MC, et al.: Effect of flowrate and duration of use on the pressure drop across six artificial noses. *Respir Care* 34:902-907, 1989.

29. Inui D, Oto J, Nishimura M: Effect of heat and moisture exchanger (HME) positioning on inspiratory gas humidification 2007, www.biomedcentral.com/1471-2466/6/19.

30. Lacherade JC, Auburtin M, Cerf C, et al.: Impact of humidification systems on ventilator-associated pneumonia, a randomized multicenter trial. *Am J Respir Crit Care Med* 17:1276-1282, 2005.

31. Prasad K, Chen L: Complications related to the use of heat and moisture exchangers. *Anesthesiology* 72:958, 1990. [Erratum: *Anesthesiology* 73(2):372, 1900.]

32. Nishida T: Performance of heated humidifiers with a heated wire according to ventilatory settings. *J Aerosol Med* 14:43-51, 2001.

33. Williams R: Relationship between the humidity and temperature of inspired gas and the function of the airway mucosa. *Crit Care Med* 24:1920-1929, 1996.

34. Kollef M: Mechanical ventilation with or without 7-day circuit changes: a randomized controlled study. *Ann Intern Med* 123:168-174, 1995.

35. Beydon L: Correlation between simple clinical parameters and the in vitro humidification characteristics of filter heat and moisture exchangers. *Chest* 112:739-744, 1997.

36. Fulmer JD, Snider DL: American College of Chest Physicians/National Heart, Lung, and Blood Institute National Conference on Oxygen Therapy. *Heart Lung* 13(5):550-562, 1984.

37. Branson R, Chatburn R: Humidification during mechanical ventilation [editorial]. *Respir Care* 38:461, 1993.

38. Dolovich MA, MacIntyre NR, Anderson PJ, et al.: Consensus statement: aerosols and delivery devices. American Association for Respiratory Care. *Respir Care* 45:589-596, 2000.

39. Kim C: Methods of calculating lung delivery and deposition of aerosol particles. *Respir Care* 45(6):695-711, 2000.

40. Dolovich M: Assessing nebulizer performance. *Respir Care* 47:1290-1301, 2002.

41. Newhouse M, Dolovich M: Aerosol therapy in children. In Chermick V, Mellins R, editors: *Basic mechanisms of pediatric respiratory disease: cellular and integrative*, Toronto, ON, 1991, Decker.

42. Pierce A, Sanford J, Thomas G: Long-term evaluation of inhalation therapy equipment and the occurrence of necrotizing pneumonia. *N Engl J Med* 282:528-531, 1970.

43. Wojnarowski C: Comparison of bronchial challenge with ultrasonic nebulized distilled water and hypertonic saline in children with mild-to-moderate asthma. *Eur Respir J* 9:1896-1901, 1996.

44. Ari A, Restrepo RD: Aerosol delivery device selection for spontaneously breathing patients: 2012. *Respir Care* 57:613-626, 2012.

45. Glick R: Drug reconcentration in aerosol generators. *Inhal Ther* 15:179, 1970.

46. Ari A, Fink J, Harwood R, et al.: Secondhand aerosol exposure during mechanical ventilation with and without expiratory filters: an in-vitro study. *Respir Care* 55:1566, 2010.

47. Carnathan B, Martin B, Colice G: Second hand (S)-albuterol: RT exposure risk following racemic albuterol. *Respir Care* 46:1084, 2001.

48. Dimich-Ward H, Wymer ML, Chan-Yeung M: Respiratory health survey of respiratory therapists. *Chest* 126:1048-1053, 2004.

49. Ari A, Hess D, Myers TR, et al.: *A guide to aerosol delivery devices for respiratory therapists*, Dallas, TX, 2009, American Association for Respiratory Care.

50. American Association for Respiratory Care: Aerosol consensus conference statement—1991. *Respir Care* 36:916-921, 1991.

51. Dolovich M, Ruffin R, Corr D: Clinical evaluation of a simple demand inhalation MDI aerosol delivery device. *Chest* 84:36-41, 1983.

52. Fink J: Metered-dose inhalers, dry powder inhalers and transitions. *Respir Care* 45:623-635, 2000.

53. Newman S: Aerosol generators and delivery systems. *Respir Care* 36:939-951, 1991.

54. Fink JB, Rubin BK: Problems with inhaler use: a call for improved clinician and patient education. *Respir Care* 50:1360, 2005.

55. Fink JB, Dhand R, Grychowski J, et al.: Reconciling in vitro and in vivo measurements of aerosol delivery from a metered-dose inhaler during mechanical ventilation and

defining efficiency-enhancing factors. *Am J Respir Crit Care Med* 159:63-68, 1999.

56. Chhabra SK: A comparison of "closed" and "open" mouth techniques of inhalation of a salbutamol metered-dose inhaler. *J Asthma* 31:123-125, 1994.

56a. Slader C, Bosnic-Anticevich S, Reddel H: Lack of awareness of need to clean CFC-free metered-dose inhalers. *J Asthma* 41(3):367-373, 2004.

57. Hampson N, Mueller M: Reduction in patient timing errors using a breath-activated metered dose inhaler *Chest* 106:462, 1994.

58. Wildhaber JH, Janssens HM, Pierart F, et al.: High-percentage lung delivery in children from detergent-treated spacers. *Pediatr Pulmonol* 29:389-393, 2000.

58a. Hess DR: Aerosol delivery devices in the treatment of asthma. *Respir Care* 53(6):699-723, 2008.

58b. Fink J, Hodder R: Adherence and inhaler devices in COPD. *Respir Ther* 6:28-33, 2011.

58c. Watts AB, McConville JT, Williams RO: Current therapies and technological advances in aqueous aerosol drug delivery. *Drug Dev Ind Pharm* 34(9):913-922, 2008.

59. American Association for Respiratory Care: Clinical practice guideline: delivery of aerosols to the upper airway. *Respir Care* 39:803, 1994.

60. Dhand R, Fink J: Dry powder inhalers. *Respir Care* 44:940, 1999.

61. Nerbrink O, Dahlback M, Hansson H: Why do medical nebulizers differ in their output and particle characteristics? *J Aerosol Med* 7:259-276, 1994.

62. Dennis J, Hendrick D: Design characteristics for drug nebulizers. *J Med Eng Technol* 16:63-68, 1992.

63. Hess D, Fisher D, Williams P, et al.: Medication nebulizer performance. Effects of diluent volume, nebulizer flow, and nebulizer brand. *Chest* 110:498-505, 1996.

64. Goode ML, Fink JB, Dhand R, et al.: Improvement in aerosol delivery with helium-oxygen mixtures during mechanical ventilation. *Am J Respir Crit Care Med* 163:109-114, 2001.

65. Hess DR, Fink JB, Venkataraman ST, et al.: The history and physics of heliox. *Respir Care* 51:608-612, 2006.

66. Phipps P, Gonda I: Droplets produced by medical nebulizers. Some factors affecting their size and solute concentration. *Chest* 97:1327-1332, 1990.

67. Dhand R: Nebulizers that use a vibrating mesh or plate with multiple apertures to generate aerosol. *Respir Care* 47:1406-1416, 2002.

68. Vecellio L: The mesh nebulizer: a recent technical innovation for aerosol delivery. *Breathe* 2:253, 2006.

69. Thomas SH, O'Doherty MJ, Page CJ, et al.: Delivery of ultrasonic nebulized aerosols to a lung model during mechanical ventilation. *Am Rev Respir Dis* 148:872-877, 1993.

70. Kacmarek R, Kratochvil J: Evaluation of a double-enclosure double-vacuum unit scavenging system for ribavirin administration. *Respir Care* 37:37-45, 1992.

71. National Asthma Education and Prevention Program: *Expert Panel III: Guidelines for the diagnosis and management of asthma 2007*, Bethesda, MD, 2007, National Institutes of Health.

72. Fink J, Dhand R: Bronchodilator resuscitation in the emergency department, part 2: dosing. *Respir Care* 45:497, 2000.

73. Denyer J, Nikander K, Smith N: Adaptive aerosol delivery (AAD) technology. *Expert Opin Drug Deliv* 1:165-176, 2004.

74. Zainuddin B, Tolfree S, Short M: Influence of breathing pattern on lung deposition and bronchodilator response to nebulized salbutamol in patients with stable asthma. *Thorax* 43:987-991, 1988.

75. Oie S, Kamiya A: Bacterial contamination of aerosol solutions containing antibiotics. *Microbios* 82:109-113, 1995.

76. Dolovich MB, Ahrens RC, Hess DR, et al.: Device selection and outcomes of aerosol therapy: evidence-based guidelines: American College of Chest Physicians/American College of Asthma, Allergy, and Immunology. *Chest* 127:335-371, 2005.

77. Rubin B, Fink J: Aerosol therapy for children. *Respir Care Clin North Am* 7:100, 2001.

78. Janssens H, Tiddens H: Aerosol therapy: the special needs of young children. *Paediatr Respir Rev* 7:S83-S85, 2006.

78a. Amirav I, Luder A, Chleechel A, et al.: Lung aerosol deposition in suckling infants. *Arch Dis Child* 97(6):497-501, 2012.

78b. Amirav I, Newhouse MT, Luder A, et al.: Feasibility of aerosol drug delivery to sleeping infants: a prospective observational study. *BMJ Open* 4:e004124, 2014.

79. Bhashyam AR, Wolf MT, Marcinkowski AL, et al.: Aerosol delivery through nasal cannulas: an in vitro study. *J Aerosol Med Pulm Drug Deliv* 21(2):181-188, 2008.

80. Ari A, Harwood R, Sheard M, et al.: In vitro comparison of heliox and oxygen in aerosol delivery using pediatric high flow nasal cannula. *Pediatr Pulmonol* 46(8):795-801, 2011.

81. Dailey P, Walsh K, Fink J, et al.: Aerosol delivery through adult high flow nasal cannula: an in-vitro comparison with heliox and oxygen. *Respir Care* 54:1522, 2009.

82. Ari A, Roark S, Lucrecia L, et al.: Influence of nasal cannula, flow rate and humidifier in aerosol drug delivery during high flow nasal oxygen administration in a simulated neonatal lung model. *Respir Care* 55:1576, 2010.

82a. Sunbul FS, Fink JB, Harwood R, et al.: Comparison of HFNC, bubble CPAP and SiPAP on aerosol delivery in neonates: An in-vitro study. *Pediatr Pulmonol* 50:1099-1106, 2015.

82b. Reminiac F, Laurent Vecellio L, Ronan MacLoughlin RM, et al.: Nasal high flow nebulization in infants and toddlers: An in vitro and in vivo scintigraphic study. *Pediatr Pulmonol* 2016. doi: 10.1002/ppul.23509. [Epub ahead of print].

82c. Ari A, Fink JB: Aerosol drug delivery during mechanical ventilation: Devices, selection, delivery technique, and evaluation of clinical response to Therapy. *Clin Pulmonary Med* 22(2):79-86, 2015.

83. Dhand R: Aerosol therapy with metered-dose inhalers during mechanical ventilation: the need for in-vitro tests. *Respir Care* 43:699-702, 1998.

84. Dhand R, Tobin MJ: Bronchodilator delivery with metered-dose inhalers in mechanically-ventilated patients. *Eur Respir J* 9:585-595, 1996.

85. Fink J, Dhand R, Duarte A, et al.: Aerosol delivery from a metered-dose inhaler during mechanical ventilation. An in-vitro model. *Am J Respir Crit Care Med* 154:382-387, 1996.

86. Hess DR: The mask for noninvasive ventilation: principles of design and effects on aerosol delivery. *J Aerosol Med* 20:S85, 2007.

87. Pollack C, Fleisch K, Dowsey K: Treatment of acute bronchospasm with β-adrenergic agonist aerosols delivered by a nasal bilevel positive airway pressure circuit. *Ann Emerg Med* 26:552-557, 1995.

88. Nava S, Karakurt S, Rampulla C, et al.: Salbutamol delivery during non-invasive mechanical ventilation in patients with chronic obstructive pulmonary disease: a randomized, controlled study. *Intensive Care Med* 27:1627-1635, 2001.

89. Fauroux B, Itti E, Pigeot J, et al.: Optimization of aerosol deposition by pressure support in children with cystic fibrosis: an experimental and clinical study. *Am J Respir Crit Care Med* 162:2265-2271, 2000.

90. Dhand R, Dolovich M, Chipps B, et al.: The role of nebulized therapy in the management of COPD: evidence and recommendations. *COPD* 9:58, 2012.

91. Chatmongkolchart S, Schettino G, Dillman C, et al.: In vitro evaluation of aerosol bronchodilator delivery during noninvasive positive pressure ventilation: effect of ventilator settings and nebulizer position. *Crit Care Med* 30:2515-2519, 2002.

92. Branconnier M, Hess D: Albuterol delivery during noninvasive ventilation. *Respir Care* 50:1649, 2005.

93. Abdelrahim ME, Plant P, Chrystyn H: In-vitro characterisation of the nebulised dose during non-invasive ventilation. *J Pharm Pharmacol* 62:966-972, 2010.

94. AlQuaimi M, Fink J, Harwood R, et al.: Efficiency of aerosol devices during noninvasive positive pressure ventilation in a simulated adult lung model. *Respir Care* 56:1632, 2011.

94a. Galindo-Filho VC, Ramos ME, Rattes CS, et al: Radioaerosol pulmonary deposition using mesh and jet nebulizers during noninvasive ventilation in healthy subjects. *Respir Care* 60(9):1238-1246, 2015.

95. Reychler G, Wallemacq P, Rodenstein DO, et al.: Comparison of lung deposition of amikacin by intrapulmonary percussive ventilation and jet nebulization by urinary monitoring. *J Aerosol Med* 19:199-207, 2006.

96. Fang T, Lin H, Chiu S, et al.: Aerosol delivery using jet nebulizer and vibrating mesh nebulizer during high frequency oscillatory ventilation: an in vitro comparison. *J Aerosol Med Pulm Drug Deliv* 29: 447-453, 2016.

97. Ari A, Fink JB: Factors affecting bronchodilator delivery in mechanically ventilated adults. *Nurs Crit Care* 15(4):192-204, 2010.

98. Ari A, Areabi H, Fink JB: Evaluation of position of aerosol device in two different ventilator circuits during mechanical ventilation. *Respir Care* 55(7):837-844, 2010.

99. DiBlasi R, Crotwell D, Shen S, et al.: Iloprost drug delivery during infant conventional and high-frequency oscillatory ventilation. *Pulm Circ* 6(1):63-69, 2016.

100. Christiani DC, Kern DG: Asthma risk and occupation as a respiratory therapist. *Am Rev Respir Dis* 148(3):671-674, 1993.

101. Ari A, Fink J, Harwood R, et al.: Secondhand aerosol exposure during mechanical ventilation with and without expiratory filters: an in-vitro study. *Ind J Resp Care* 5(1):677-682, 2016.

102. Harrison R: Reproductive risk assessment with occupational exposure to ribavirin aerosol. *Pediatr Infect Dis J* 9:S1025, 1990.

103. Garner J: Guideline for isolation precautions in hospitals. *Infect Control Hosp Epidemiol* 17:53-58, 1996. [Erratum: *Infect Control Hosp Epidemiol* 17(4):214, 1996.]

INTERNET RESOURCES

Humidity

American College of Chest Physicians: Patient Instruction for Inhaled Devices: http://www.chestnet.org/patients/guides/inhaledDevices.php

Humidity and Humidification Lecture: http://www.usyd.edu.au/anaes/lectures/humidity_clt/humidity.html

Infoplease.com: http://www.infoplease.com/ce6/weather/A0824520.html

Humidity calculator: http://www.bom.gov.au/lam/humiditycalc.shtml

Relative humidity: http://en.wikipedia.org/wiki/Relative_humidity

Relative humidity: http://www.fphcare.com/humidification/relative_humidity.asp

Virtual Hospital: http://www.vh.org

Aerosol

The Aerosol Society: http://www.aerosol-soc.org.uk/index.asp

American Association of Aerosol Research: https://www.aaar.org

Guide to Aerosol Delivery Devices: http://www.aarc.org/education/aerosol_devices/aerosol_delivery_guide.pdf

American Association for Respiratory Care (AARC) Clinical Practice Guideline for aerosol therapy: http://www.rcjournal.com/cpgs/Journal of Aerosol Medicine: http://www.liebertonline.com/loi/jam

American College of Chest Physicians: Patient Instruction for Inhaled Devices: http://www.chestnet.org/patients/guides/inhaledDevices.php

American College of Chest Physicians (ACCP) Patient Education Guides: http://www.chestnet.org/patients/guides/

International Society of Aerosol in Medicine: http://www.isam.org/

RDD Online: http://www.rddonline.com/education/index.asp

Total Ozone Mapping Spectrometer: http://toms.gsfc.nasa.gov/aerosols/aerosols.html

7

Lung Expansion Therapy and Airway Clearance Devices

Lung expansion or hyperinflation therapy and airway secretion clearance techniques are an integral part of respiratory care. The primary indication for lung expansion therapy and airway clearance techniques is to prevent or reverse atelectasis. If left untreated, atelectasis can result in pulmonary shunting, hypoxemia, hypercapnia, and, ultimately, respiratory failure. Factors that contribute to the development of atelectasis include retained secretions, altered breathing pattern, pain associated with surgery and trauma, chronic obstructive and restrictive pulmonary diseases, prolonged immobilization in a supine position, and increased intra-abdominal pressure.

Various strategies and devices are used to help patients achieve and maintain optimum lung function. The most common strategies involve deep-breathing exercises, directed coughing, chest physiotherapy (CPT), postural drainage, endotracheal suctioning, and medical aerosol therapy. The devices most often used by respiratory therapists for this type of therapy include incentive spirometers, intermittent positive-pressure breathing (IPPB) devices, chest wall percussors, high-frequency oscillation devices, and mechanical insufflation–exsufflation devices.

Selection of the appropriate device should be based on the patient's ability to perform the assigned therapy. Continuation of therapy or changes in therapeutic goals should be determined by frequent assessment of the patient's status through physical assessment and review of laboratory test values.

The American Association for Respiratory Care (AARC) released an updated Clinical Practice Guideline in 2013 on the effectiveness of nonpharmacological airway clearance therapies in hospitalized patients.[1] This Clinical Practice Guideline provides several recommendations for the use of airway clearance techniques in hospitalized adult and pediatric patients without cystic fibrosis, adult and pediatric patients with neuromuscular disease, respiratory muscle weakness, or impaired cough, and postoperative adult and pediatric patients. The recommendations were based on the consensus of a committee that relied on a systematic review of the literature and clinical experience.[1,2] A summary of these recommendations is provided in Clinical Practice Guideline 7.1. It is important to state that these recommendations are based on *low-level*

CLINICAL PRACTICE GUIDELINE 7.1
Effectiveness of Nonpharmacologic Airway Clearance Therapies in Hospitalized Patients

Recommendations for Hospitalized Adult and Pediatric Patients Without Cystic Fibrosis

1. Chest physiotherapy is not recommended for the routine treatment of uncomplicated pneumonia.
2. Airway clearance therapy is not recommended for routine use in patients with chronic obstructive pulmonary disease.
3. Airway clearance therapy may be considered in patients with COPD with symptomatic secretion retention, guided by patient preference, toleration, and effectiveness of therapy.
4. Airway clearance therapy is not recommended if the patient is able to mobilize secretions with cough, but instruction in effective cough technique (e.g. forced exhalation technique) may be useful.

Recommendations for Adult and Pediatric Patients With Neuromuscular Disease, Respiratory Muscle Weakness, or Impaired Cough

1. Cough assist techniques should be used in patients with neuromuscular diseases, particularly when peak cough flow is <270 L/min.
2. Chest physiotherapy, positive expiratory pressure, and intrapulmonary percussive ventilation, and high-frequency chest wall compression cannot be recommended due to insufficient evidence.

Recommendation for Postoperative Adults and Pediatric Patients

1. Incentive spirometry is not recommended for routine, prophylactic use in postoperative patients.
2. Early mobility and ambulation is recommended to reduce postoperative complication and promote airway clearance.
3. Airway clearance therapy is not recommended for routine postoperative care.

COPD, Chronic obstructive pulmonary disease.
Modified from American Association for Respiratory Care: AARC clinical practice guideline: effectiveness of nonpharmacologic airway clearance therapies in hospitalized patients. *Respir Care* 58:2187-2193, 2013.

---

evidence due to the lack of *high-level* clinical evidence in the medical literature. Furthermore, these guidelines do not include the use of airway clearance therapies in patients with cystic fibrosis. Lester and Flume[3] have previously provided a summary of the guidelines for airway clearance therapy.

I. INCENTIVE SPIROMETERS

Incentive spirometry (IS) is a lung expansion technique designed to mimic natural sighing or yawning by encouraging the patient to take slow, deep breaths.[4] It is a simple and relatively safe method of preventing and treating atelectasis in alert patients who are predisposed to shallow breathing (e.g., patients recovering from thoracic or upper abdominal surgery, patients with chronic obstructive pulmonary disease [COPD] who are recovering from surgery, and patients who are immobilized or confined to bed).[5] The only contraindication to IS involves patients who are confused, uncooperative, unable to deep-breathe effectively (i.e., the vital capacity is <10 mL/kg or the inspiratory capacity is less than one-third of the predicted value), or are unable to be instructed or supervised to ensure appropriate use of the device.[4,5]

Although commercially produced incentive spirometers have been available for approximately two decades, the concept of sustained maximum inspiration (SMI) has been used since the latter part of the 19th century. Before the introduction of incentive spirometers, clinicians used devices and techniques such as blow-bottles, blow-gloves, and carbon dioxide–induced hyperventilation to accomplish the goal of having the patient take deep breaths to prevent atelectasis.

The principle of IS is based on the idea that the patient is encouraged to achieve a preset volume or flow, which is determined from predicted values or baseline measurements. Commercially available incentive spirometers are classified as either *volume-displacement* or *flow-dependent* devices. With volume-displacement devices, the volume of air the patient inspires during an SMI is measured and displayed. In contrast, flow-dependent devices measure the inspiratory flow the patient achieves during an SMI effort. Volume displacement can be derived with these latter devices by multiplying the flow achieved by the amount of time the flow is maintained.

The efficacy of using IS remains controversial because of the lack of prospective studies to demonstrate that it is superior to other hyperexpansion methods that rely on natural deep-breathing exercises. Indeed, evidence suggests that deep breathing alone—without an incentive spirometer—can be beneficial for preventing or reversing pulmonary complications in some postoperative patients.[6-8]

The effectiveness of IS ultimately depends on patient selection, as well as proper instruction and supervision during the training period. The advantage of using an incentive spirometer may be related to the fact that patients receive immediate visual feedback about whether they are achieving the prescribed goal (Clinical Scenario 7.1). Furthermore, many patients can perform the treatment regimen without the direct supervision of a respiratory therapist after they have demonstrated mastery of the technique, which allows a cost-effective approach to

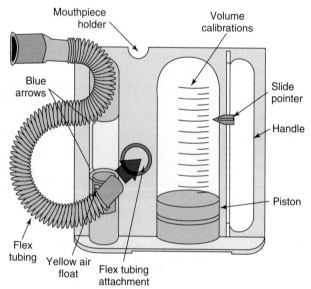

FIGURE 7.1 Voldyne 5000 Volumetric Exerciser. (Teleflex/Hudson RCI, Morrisville, NC.)

lung expansion therapy. Clinical Practice Guideline 7.2 summarizes the Clinical Practice Guideline for incentive spirometry established by the AARC.[4]

Volume-Displacement Devices

Fig. 7.1 is a schematic of a volume-displacement incentive spirometer. The operational principle is simple: the patient inhales air through a mouthpiece and corrugated tubing attached to a plastic bellows. The volume of air displaced is indicated on a scale located on the device enclosure. After the patient has achieved the maximum volume, the individual is instructed to hold this volume constant for 3 to 5 seconds.

Commercially available incentive spirometers for adults typically have a total volume capacity of approximately 4 L, and those for children have a volume capacity of approximately 2 L. The Voldyne 5000 Volumetric Exerciser (Teleflex/Hudson RCI) shown in Fig. 7.1 consists of a movable piston in a clear cylinder. As the patient inhales, the piston rises and the inspired volume is indicated on a scale engraved on the side of the cylinder. A flow indicator is included as a visual aid to encourage the patient to take slow, deep breaths.

Clinical trials involving IS suggest that patients should perform a minimum of 10 breaths per session every 1 to 2 hours while awake.[4] Note that the respiratory therapist does

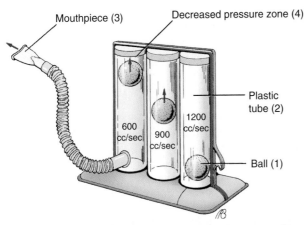

FIGURE 7.2 Flow-dependent incentive spirometer. (From Eubanks DH, Bone RC: *Comprehensive respiratory care,* St. Louis, 1985, Mosby.)

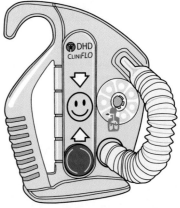

FIGURE 7.3 CliniFLO Low-Flow Breathing Exerciser incentive spirometer.

not have to be present for each performance, and patients should be encouraged to perform this therapy independently.

Most incentive spirometers are designed for single-patient use; multiple-use devices are available, but they are rarely used anymore. Single-patient devices usually are made of plastic and can be discarded after the patient has completed the course of therapy.

Flow-Dependent Devices

Fig. 7.2 shows an example of a flow-dependent incentive spirometer, which consists of a mouthpiece and corrugated tubing connected to a manifold composed of three flow tubes containing lightweight plastic balls. As the patient inhales through the mouthpiece, negative pressure is created within the tubes, causing them to rise. The device is designed so that the number of balls and the level to which they rise depend on the flow achieved. At lower flows the first ball rises to a level that depends on the magnitude of the flow. As the inspiratory flow increases, the second ball rises, followed by the third ball. The flow achieved by the patient can be estimated based on the manufacturer's specifications. For example, with the Hudson RCI TriFlo II incentive spirometer (Teleflex), the patient must achieve a flow of 600 mL/s to raise the first ball. A flow of 900 mL/s is required to raise the second ball, and a flow of 1200 mL/s must be generated to raise the third ball. As with volume-displacement incentive spirometers, it is important that the patient perform a maximum sustained inspiration.

The CliniFLO incentive spirometer (Smiths Medical; Fig. 7.3) consists of a single plastic tube containing an indicator that rises as the patient makes an inspiratory effort. An adjustable volume selector can be used to vary the patient effort necessary to attain the desired inspiratory capacity. The Clini-FLO contains an oxygen port that allows the clinician to provide supplemental oxygen if necessary. The Hudson/Teleflex Medical Hu1750 (lung volume exerciser) (Teleflex/Hudson RCI; (Fig. 7.4) uses a different type of design: The patient inhales through a mouthpiece and corrugated tubing connected to a dual-chamber device. The two chambers of this

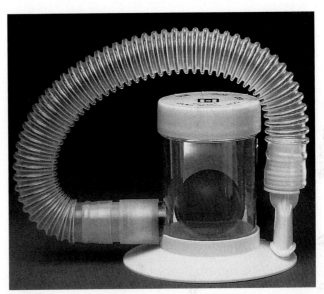

FIGURE 7.4 LVE (lung volume exerciser) incentive spirometer. (Courtesy Teleflex/Hudson RCI, Morrisville, NC.)

device are arranged in series. The ball in the inner chamber rises when the patient achieves a flow that equals the inspiratory flow selected by the operator. Inspiratory flows vary from 200 mL/s to 1200 mL/s.

II. INTERMITTENT POSITIVE-PRESSURE BREATHING DEVICES

IPPB is a short-term therapeutic modality that involves the delivery of inspiratory positive pressure to spontaneously breathing patients. Since its introduction in 1947, IPPB has been used for a variety of purposes, including short-term ventilatory support and lung expansion therapy, and as an aid in the delivery of aerosolized medications.[9,10] Over the past three decades, the effectiveness of IPPB as a therapeutic modality has been questioned rigorously, resulting in a reassessment of the indications for its prescription. The AARC produced a Clinical Practice Guideline in 1993 and a revised version in 2003 to provide a rational basis for prescribing and administering IPPB treatments (Clinical Practice Guideline 7.3 summarizes

CLINICAL PRACTICE GUIDELINE 7.3 Intermittent Positive-Pressure Breathing

Indications

1. The need to improve lung expansion, particularly for patients who demonstrate clinically important atelectasis when other forms of therapy, such as incentive spirometry, chest physiotherapy (CPT), deep-breathing exercises, and positive airway pressure (PAP), are unsuccessful. It may also be useful for patients who cannot cooperate with standard lung expansion techniques.
2. Inability to clear secretions adequately because of pathology that severely limits the patient's ability to ventilate or cough effectively.
3. As an alternative to endotracheal intubation and continuous ventilatory support for patients requiring short-term ventilatory support. Devices specifically designed to deliver noninvasive positive-pressure ventilation (NIV) should also be considered.
4. To deliver aerosolized medications to patients fatigued as a result of respiratory muscle weakness. Note that this guideline does not address aerosol delivery for patients on long-term mechanical ventilation. It may also be used to deliver aerosolized medications to patients unable to use a metered-dose inhaler (MDI).
5. IPPB may reduce the sensation of dyspnea and its associated discomfort during nebulizer therapy in patients with severe hyperinflation.

Contraindications

1. Untreated tension pneumothorax
2. Elevated intracranial pressure (>15 mm Hg)
3. Hemodynamic instability
4. Recent facial, oral, or skull surgery
5. Tracheoesophageal fistula
6. Recent esophageal surgery
7. Active hemoptysis
8. Nausea
9. Air swallowing
10. Active, untreated tuberculosis
11. Radiographic evidence of a bleb
12. Hiccups

Hazards

1. Increased airway resistance and work of breathing
2. Barotrauma, pneumothorax
3. Nosocomial infection
4. Hypocarbia (hypocapnia)
5. Hemoptysis
6. Hyperoxia when oxygen is the gas source
7. Gastric distention
8. Impaction of secretions associated with inadequately humidified gas mixture
9. Psychological dependence
10. Impeded venous return
11. Exacerbation of hypoxemia
12. Hypoventilation or hyperventilation
13. Increased mismatch of ventilation and perfusion
14. Air trapping, auto–positive end-expiratory pressure, overdistended alveoli

Assessment of Need

1. Presence of clinically significant atelectasis.
2. Reduced pulmonary function: forced vital capacity (FVC) <70% of predicted; maximum voluntary ventilation (MVV) <50% of predicted; or vital capacity (VC) <10 mL/kg of predicted, precluding an effective cough.
3. Neuromuscular disorders or kyphoscoliosis associated with reduced lung volumes.
4. Fatigue or respiratory muscle weakness with impending respiratory failure.
5. Based on proven therapeutic efficacy, variety of medications, and cost-effectiveness, the MDI with a spacing device or holding chamber should be the first method considered for administration of aerosol therapy.
6. If effective, the patient's preference for a positive-pressure device should be honored.
7. IPPB may be indicated for patients who are at risk for the development of atelectasis and are unable or unwilling to perform deep-breathing exercises without assistance.

Assessment of Outcomes

1. A minimum delivered tidal volume of at least one-third of the predicted inspiratory capacity ($\frac{1}{3} \times 50$ mL/kg) has been suggested (e.g., 1200 mL for a 70-kg individual).
2. Increase in forced expiratory volume in 1 second (FEV_1) or peak expiratory flow (PEF).
3. Improved cough with treatment, leading to better clearance of secretions.
4. Improvements in chest radiographs.
5. Improved breath sounds.
6. Favorable patient response.

Monitoring

1. Machine performance: trigger sensitivity, peak pressure, flow setting, fractional inspired oxygen (F_IO_2), inspiratory time, expiratory time, plateau pressure, positive end-expiratory pressure
2. Respiratory rate
3. Delivered tidal volume
4. Patient's subjective response to therapy
5. Sputum production (quantity, color, consistency)
6. Skin color
7. Breath sounds
8. Blood pressure
9. Arterial hemoglobin saturation by pulse oximetry if hypoxemia is suspected
10. Intracranial pressure (ICP) in patients for whom it is of critical importance
11. Chest radiograph

IPPB, Intermittent positive-pressure breathing.
Modified from the American Association for Respiratory Care: AARC clinical practice guideline: intermittent positive pressure breathing—2003 revisions and update. *Respir Care* 438:540, 2003.

this guideline).[10,11] Although it has been suggested that noninvasive positive-pressure ventilation (NIV) may be considered a form of IPPB, the current Clinical Practice Guideline does not provide guidance on this therapeutic modality.[11]

In the critical care setting, IPPB can be used every 1 to 6 hours as tolerated. In these cases the IPPB order should be reevaluated at least daily. Continuation or discontinuation of the order should be based on the assessment outcomes for the patient obtained during each treatment session. When it is prescribed in the general-care setting, IPPB typically is ordered two to four times daily and usually is determined by the patient's response to therapy. In these cases, therapy should be reevaluated at least every 72 hours or with any change in the patient's health status. Similarly, patients receiving IPPB therapy in the home should be reevaluated periodically and with any change in health status.[11]

It should be recognized that although IPPB is not the therapy of choice when other modalities can be used for aerosol delivery or lung expansion in spontaneously breathing patients, it can be potentially beneficial when IS, CPT, deep-breathing exercises, and positive airway pressure (PAP) techniques have been unsuccessful (Clinical Scenario 7.2).

IPPB can be administered with any device that can deliver intermittent positive pressure to the airway (e.g., conventional mechanical ventilators or manual resuscitators), but it historically has been administered using specially designed electrically and pneumatically powered ventilators.[12] These IPPB machines usually are categorized as patient-triggered, pressure- and time-limited, and pressure- or flow-cycled mechanical ventilators. Regardless of the manufacturer, all IPPB machines require a 45- to 55-pounds-per-square-inch gauge (psig) gas source, such as a compressed-gas cylinder, a bulk air or oxygen system, or an air compressor. Furthermore, they all incorporate control valves that begin inspiration when a negative pressure is generated by the patient and terminate it when a preset pressure or flow is achieved. The amount of negative pressure (i.e., patient effort) required to initiate inspiration depends on the sensitivity of the device, which may be fixed or adjustable. The pressure that must be achieved to end inspiration, and thus initiate exhalation, typically can be adjusted to as high as 60 cm H_2O.[10,11]

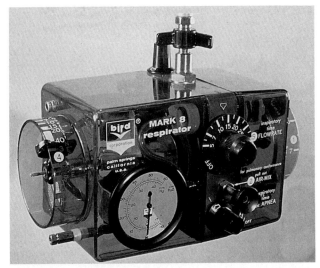

FIGURE 7.5 Bird Mark 8 ventilator. (Courtesy CareFusion, Critical Care Division, Palm Springs, CA.)

Machines manufactured by Medtronic Minimally Invasive Therapies Puritan Bennett and Bird Products (CareFusion) historically have been the most widely used devices for IPPB therapy. A relatively recent advance in IPPB equipment is the introduction of a single-use, disposable device by Vortran Medical Technology. A brief description of these devices follows.

Puritan Bennett and Bird Devices

Medtronic Minimally Invasive Therapies Puritan Bennett manufactured pneumatically and electrically powered IPPB machines. The tank ventilator (TV), pedestal ventilator (PV), and pedestal respirator (PR) series are pneumatically powered IPPB machines; the air-powered (AP) series of ventilators are electrically powered. The PR-1 and PR-2 models are the most commonly used pneumatically powered IPPB devices. The AP-4 and AP-5 models are the most commonly used electrically powered IPPB machines.

The prototype Bird ventilator is the Mark 7 (CareFusion), which was designed and developed by Forrest M. Bird, founder of the Bird Corporation. Bird subsequently introduced the Mark 8, which functions similarly to the Mark 7 but can provide a flow of source gas during the expiratory phase, thus allowing the operator to apply a negative expiratory pressure. Subsequent generations of Bird ventilators (i.e., Bird Mark 8, 10, and 14 series) that were introduced beginning in the late 1970s provided additional capabilities.

Bird IPPB devices are classified as pneumatically powered ventilators. They can be time, pressure, or manually triggered and time or pressure cycled. The tidal volume delivered to the patient can be adjusted by manipulating the peak inspiratory pressure.[12] Fig. 7.5 illustrates the major components of the prototype Bird Mark 8 ventilator. Additional information about the theory of operation of Puritan-Bennett and Bird IPPB devices can be found on the Evolve website.

Vortran (IPPB) Device

The Vortran IPPB (Vortran Medical Technology) device provides short-term, pressure-triggered, pressure-cycled,

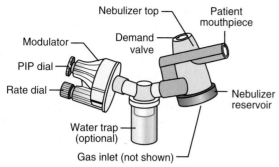

FIGURE 7.6 Major components of the Vortran intermittent positive-pressure breathing device. *PIP,* Peak inspiratory pressure. (Redrawn from Vortran Medical Technology: *Vortran IPPB user's guide,* Sacramento, CA, 2005, Vortran.)

TABLE 7.1   Estimated Tidal Volume (mL) Delivered at Various Flows and Inspiratory Times

Flow (L/min)	INSPIRATORY TIME (SECONDS)					
	0.5	1	1.5	2	2.5	3
15	125	250	375	500	625	750
20	167	333	500	667	833	1000
25	208	417	625	833	1042	1250
30	250	500	750	1000	1250	1500
35	292	583	875	1167	1458	1750
40	333	667	1000	1333	1667	2000

From Vortran Medical Technology: *Vortran IPPB user's guide,* Sacramento, CA, 2005, Vortran.

constant-flow ventilatory support in combination with aerosol delivery.[13] The primary advantage of this device is that it is relatively compact and inexpensive compared with conventional IPPB devices. Also, Vortran IPPB units are single-patient, multiple-use devices, which reduces the incidence of nosocomial infections from cross-contamination.

The major components of the Vortran IPPB device include a pressure modulator coupled with a nebulizer (Fig. 7.6). The unit runs on a continuous flow of gas of up to 40 L/min. (Flows of 40 L/min are automatically achieved when the unit is connected to a 50-psig source gas; flows of 15 to 40 L/min can be achieved by connecting the system to a 50-psig source gas using a standard hospital flowmeter.) Peak inspiratory pressures can be adjusted between 20 and 50 cm H_2O, and the device can produce a positive end-expiratory pressure (PEEP) of 2 to 5 cm H_2O (the manufacturer reports that the set PEEP typically is one-tenth of the peak pressure). The inspiratory time and rate can be adjusted over a wide range (i.e., 8 to 20 breaths per minute). As Table 7.1 shows, the estimated delivered tidal volume depends on the flow and the inspiratory time.

The device's nebulizer, which provides the continuous flow of gas and a patient demand valve, can hold 20 mL of solution for nebulization. The nebulizer is also equipped with an air entrainment valve, which allows the patient to entrain

additional air through the nebulizer. (Note that the fractional inspired oxygen [F_1O_2] will vary with the amount of room air entrained by the patient through the nebulizer.)

Recent studies demonstrate that the Vortran IPPB device can achieve inspiratory flows and tidal volumes comparable with those produced by conventional IPPB units. Furthermore, this device offers an alternative for the delivery of IPPB to hospitalized and home-care patients. It is important to recognize that the Vortran IPPB device's modulator is similar to that of a pop-off valve. The device is *not* equipped with a redundant pop-off valve and should not be used with patients with endotracheal or tracheostomy tubes. It should be cautiously used when IPPB is administered with a mask.

III. POSITIVE AIRWAY PRESSURE DEVICES

PAP techniques, which include continuous positive airway pressure (CPAP), expiratory positive airway pressure (EPAP), and positive expiratory pressure (PEP), are airway adjuncts that can be used to enhance bronchial hygiene therapy by reducing air trapping in susceptible patients. As such, these techniques have been shown to be quite effective in mobilizing retained secretions, preventing or reversing atelectasis, and optimizing the delivery of bronchodilators to patients with cystic fibrosis and chronic bronchitis. The AARC produced a Clinical Practice Guideline for PAP adjuncts to bronchial hygiene therapy in 1993, which provided guidance on the use of PAP therapy[14] (see Clinical Practice Guideline 7.4). Clinicians are also encouraged to review Clinical Practice Guideline 7.1 for a summary of the effectiveness of PAP therapy and other nonpharmacological airways clearance therapies in hospitalized patients.[1]

Continuous Positive Airway Pressure

CPAP therapy involves the application of positive pressure to a patient's airways throughout the respiratory cycle (i.e., the airway pressure is consistently maintained between 5 and 20 cm H_2O during both inspiration and expiration). It is accomplished by having the patient breathe from a pressurized circuit that incorporates a threshold resistor in the expiratory limb.

Fig. 7.7 shows four types of threshold resistors: underwater seal resistors, weighted-ball resistors, spring-loaded valve resistors, and magnetic valve resistors.[15] With underwater seal resistors, tubing attached to the expiratory port of the circuit is submerged under a column of water. The level of CPAP is determined by the height of the column. Weighted-ball resistors consist of a specially milled steel ball placed over a calibrated orifice, which is attached directly above the expiratory port of the circuit. It is important that the balls are maintained in a vertical position to ensure consistent pressure. Spring-loaded valve resistors rely on a spring to hold a disk or diaphragm down over the expiratory port of the circuit. Magnetic valve resistors contain a bar magnet that attracts a ferromagnetic disk seated on the expiratory port of the circuit. The amount of pressure required to separate the disk from the magnet is determined by the distance between them (i.e., the greater the distance between the magnet and the disk, the lower the pressure required to open the expiratory port and thus the lower the level of CPAP).

All these valves operate on the principle that the level of PAP generated within the circuit depends on the amount of resistance that must be overcome to allow gas to exit the exhalation valve. The main advantage of threshold resistors is that they provide predictable, quantifiable, and constant force during expiration that is independent of the flow achieved by the patient during exhalation.[15]

Expiratory Positive Airway Pressure

EPAP is another method of delivering PAP to spontaneously breathing patients. EPAP differs from CPAP because it involves the creation of PAP only during expiration. With EPAP, the patient generates a subatmospheric pressure on inspiration and then exhales against a threshold expiratory resistance similar to that described for CPAP devices. Airway pressures during EPAP can be set at 10 to 20 cm H_2O.

Positive Expiratory Pressure

PEP has received considerable attention during the past 10 years, especially in the management of patients with cystic fibrosis. The rationale for performing PEP therapy is similar to that for the use of CPAP and EPAP, except that PEP seems to be less cumbersome and more manageable for patients.

Fig. 7.8A shows a prototype device that can be used for PEP therapy. The device includes a mouthpiece (or ventilation mask), a T-piece assembly with a one-way valve, a series of fixed orifice resistors (or an adjustable orifice resistor), and a pressure manometer. The theory of operation of these PEP devices is that the patient exhales against a fixed resistance, creating a back pressure that in turn helps maintain airway patency in patients who experience airway closure (e.g., bronchiectasis). The TheraPEP device (Smiths Medical; see Fig. 7.8B) provides a series of fixed orifices that can be used to accommodate patients over a wide range of lung capacities. The amount of PAP generated with the fixed-orifice resistor varies with the size of the orifice and the level of expiratory flow produced by the patient. For example, for any given expiratory flow, the smaller the resistor's orifice, the greater the expiratory pressure generated. Similarly, for a given orifice size, the higher the expiratory flow, the greater the expiratory pressure generated. For this reason the patient must be encouraged to achieve a flow high enough to maintain expiratory pressure at 10 to 20 cm H_2O. Notice that bronchodilator therapy with a metered-dose inhaler (MDI) or small-volume nebulizer (SVN) can be performed simultaneously by attaching these devices to the inspiratory port of the mask or mouthpiece. The AeroPEP (Monaghan Medical) is a specially designed device with a pressurized MDI, a valved holding chamber, and a fixed-orifice resistor for simultaneously administering aerosol therapy and PEP.

Box 7.1 presents the procedure for performing PEP therapy. Several factors should be considered when a therapeutic regimen is created using these devices. The level of resistance chosen should allow the patient to achieve the therapeutic goal of

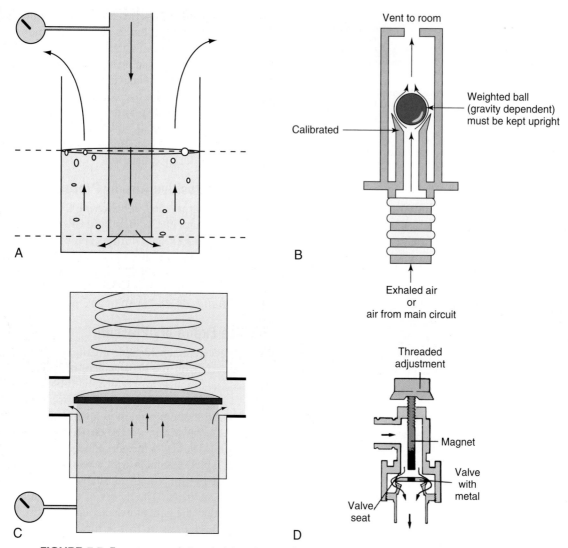

FIGURE 7.7 Four types of threshold resistors. A, Underwater seal resistor. B, Weighted-ball resistor. C, Spring-loaded valve resistor. D, Magnetic valve resistor. (A and C redrawn from Burton GG, Hodkin JE, Ward JJ: *Respiratory care: a guide to clinical practice,* ed 4, Philadelphia, 1997, JB Lippincott. B redrawn from Pilbeam SP: *Mechanical ventilation: physiological and clinical applications,* ed 2, St. Louis, 1992, Mosby. D from Spearman CB, Sanders GH: Physical principles and functional designs of ventilators. In Kirby RR, Smith RA, Desautels DA, editors: *Mechanical ventilation,* New York, 1985, Churchill Livingstone.)

generating PEP of 10 to 20 cm H_2O with a ratio of inspiratory time to expiratory time (I:E ratio) of 1:3 or 1:4. The patient should perform 10 to 20 breaths through the device, then perform a series of 2 or 3 huff coughs to clear loosened secretions. This cycle should be repeated 5 to 10 times during a 15- to 20-minute session. Finally, the patient should be encouraged to learn to self-administer this therapy, although more than one session may be required to ensure patient proficiency in the use of these devices.

IV. CHEST PHYSIOTHERAPY DEVICES

CPT is a collection of techniques to help clear airway secretions and improve the distribution of ventilation in patients with chronic respiratory diseases (e.g., cystic fibrosis). Historically these techniques have included breathing exercises, directed coughing, postural drainage, and chest percussion. Newer techniques involving the delivery of high-frequency oscillations to the lungs and chest wall are receiving increased interest as alternative methods for clearance of airway secretions.

Percussion and vibration, both of which involve the application of mechanical energy to the chest wall and lungs, provide a means of loosening retained secretions from the walls of the tracheobronchial tract. After they are loosened, the secretions can be coughed up and expectorated, or they can be removed by suctioning.

Percussion can be accomplished using either the hands or various mechanical or electrical devices. For this discussion, chest percussors have been divided into three categories:

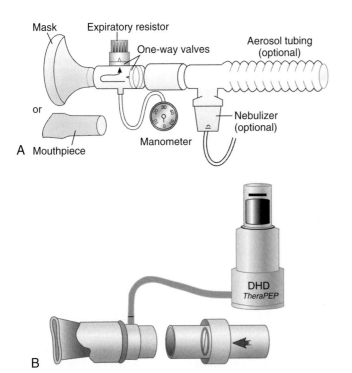

FIGURE 7.8 A, Prototype positive expiratory pressure (PEP) device. B, TheraPEP device. (Courtesy Smiths Medical, Dublin, OH.)

BOX 7.1 **Procedure for Performing Positive Expiratory Pressure Therapy**

1. The mask is applied tightly but comfortably over the patient's nose and mouth. When a mouthpiece is used, the patient is instructed to form a tight seal around the mouthpiece.
2. The patient is instructed to inspire through the one-way valve to a volume that is greater than the normal tidal volume, but not to the total lung capacity.
3. At the end of inspiration the patient is encouraged to actively but not forcefully exhale to functional residual capacity (FRC) to achieve an airway pressure of 10 to 20 cm H_2O.
4. The patient should perform 10 to 20 breaths through the device, then perform a series of 2 or 3 huff coughs to clear loosened secretions.
5. This cycle should be repeated 5 to 10 times during a 15- to 20-minute session.

manual percussors, pneumatically powered devices, and electrically powered devices. Devices that produce vibrations to the lungs and chest wall are discussed separately in the section on high-frequency oscillation devices.

Manual Percussors

The traditional method of administering CPT involves cupping the hand (as if scooping water from a basin) and clapping on the patient's chest wall. Although this technique is quite effective in most cases, it can be tiring for the person administering the therapy and somewhat painful for the patient (if performed by someone inexperienced in CPT). As a result of these potential problems, several companies have produced

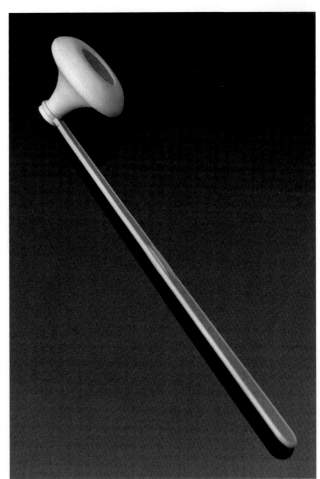

FIGURE 7.9 A manual percussor. (Courtesy Smiths Medical, Dublin, OH.)

some simple manual percussors that are fairly inexpensive and easy to use. Fig. 7.9 shows a typical manual percussor made by Smiths Medical. This device is made of soft vinyl and is formed to the shape of the palm. It is available in neonatal, pediatric, and adult sizes.

Pneumatically Powered Devices

Pneumatically powered percussors are driven by a compressed-air or oxygen source that operates at 45 to 55 psig. Although devices may differ in the number of accessories provided, each device usually comprises a high-pressure hose, a body with controls for varying the frequency and force of percussive strokes, and a remote head with a concave applicator. The Fluid Flo pneumatically powered percussor shown in Fig. 7.10 (Med Systems) is designed for adult patients. The Mercury MJ pneumatically powered percussor (Mercury Enterprises, Inc,) is a device designed for use with pediatric and adult patients.

Electrically Powered Percussors

Most electrically powered percussors are powered by electrical outputs of 110 V of alternating current, although some units are battery powered. Several of the more common units available in the United States are produced by General Physiotherapy (the Vibramatic/Multimatic, the Flimm Fighter, and the Neo-Cussor) and Medtronic Minimally Invasive Therapies-Nellcor Puritan Bennett (Vibrator/Percussor). Most units typically have a variable control switch for setting the frequency of percussions and can be used for both adult and pediatric patients.

Each system, however, has unique features. The Vibramatic/Multimatic (Fig. 7.11) produces two directional forces: one produces a stroking action that operates perpendicular to the chest wall to loosen mucus attached to the tracheobronchial tubes, and the other operates parallel to the chest wall and moves the mucus toward the central airways. The Flimm Fighter is designed primarily for home use. It comes with a foam pad and a Velcro belt to allow self-application of the device. The Neo-Cussor is a battery-operated device that uses a disposable applicator and is specifically designed for use with neonates and pediatric patients. The Vibrator/Percussor allows for independent control of frequency and stroke intensity.

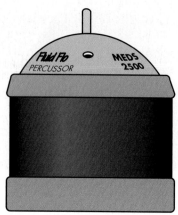

FIGURE 7.10 Fluid Flo pneumatic percussor. (Courtesy Med Systems, San Diego, CA.)

V. HIGH-FREQUENCY OSCILLATION DEVICES

Administration of high-frequency oscillations to the lungs via the airway opening or through the chest wall is quite effective in mobilizing secretions in select patient groups. Although the mechanism of action of these devices is uncertain, several factors are thought to enhance clearance of airway secretions. Some of these factors may include reducing the viscoelasticity of sputum through sheering forces generated during the oscillations, transient changes in airflow that occur during the inspiratory and expiratory phases of each oscillation, and redistribution of lung volume to airways partially obstructed by mucus.[16]

The most commonly used devices for delivering high-frequency oscillation therapy include intrapulmonary percussive ventilation (IPV), vibratory PEP (e.g., Flutter valve, Acapella, and Quake), and high-frequency chest compressions (e.g., the Vest [Hill-Rom] and the Hayek RTX). IPV devices, Flutter valves, Acapella, and Quake devices transmit high-frequency oscillation via the airway opening, whereas the Vest and the Hayek RTX produce vibration of the chest wall by delivering high-frequency oscillations to the external chest wall.

Intrapulmonary Percussive Ventilation

IPV, a form of oscillator therapy, was introduced by Forrest Bird in 1979 as an adjunct technique for mobilizing airway secretions.[17] It involves the delivery of high-frequency percussive breaths into the patient's airways instead of applying percussions to the outside of the chest wall, as in standard CPT techniques (Clinical Scenario 7.3).

The Percussionaire Intrapulmonary Percussive Ventilator (IPV-1) (Percussionaire) is the prototype IPV device (Fig. 7.12). It is manually cycled and can provide pressure- or flow-targeted breaths. Inspiration can be triggered manually by

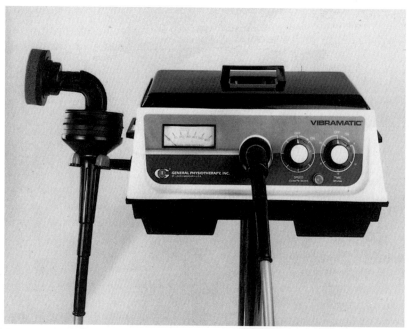

FIGURE 7.11 Vibramatic/Multimatic electrically powered percussor. (Courtesy General Physiotherapy, St. Louis, MO.)

selecting a push button control on the nebulizer (i.e., the patient typically is instructed to trigger inspiration by depressing the button for 5 to 10 seconds). Alternately, the therapist can trigger the percussive cycle by pressing the inspiration button on the control panel. Expiration is manually cycled by releasing the inspiratory control button.

The Percussionaire is powered by a 25- to 50-psi compressed-gas source. Fig. 7.13 shows gas flow through the IPV-1 unit. Gas enters the unit and passes through a filter before flowing into a pressure regulator, which reduces the pressure to a value preset by the operator. From there, gas flows to (1) an oscillator cartridge and a Phasitron, which increases and decreases air pressures; (2) a nebulizer; and (3) a remote control. Gas travels from the Phasitron outlet through small-bore tubing to the Phasitron unit, which contains a sliding Venturi (Fig.

7.14).[17] The Venturi slides forward during the impact phase, and a burst of air travels into the Venturi orifice, which in turn entrains room air (i.e., for each unit of gas that passes through the Venturi, four units of air are entrained). This enhanced burst of gas then passes through the mouthpiece to the patient. After the injection phase the Venturi slides back, and the expiratory valve simultaneously opens, allowing the patient to passively exhale.

The nebulizer receives high-pressure gas from the internal regulator via the small-bore tubing connected to the front of the unit. Air flows through the jet, past the nebulizer, creating an area of reduced pressure that draws medication from the reservoir. A high-pressure gas at the top of the jet meets the

---

CLINICAL SCENARIO 7.3

A 22-year-old man previously diagnosed with cystic fibrosis is admitted to the emergency department after a recent history of upper respiratory infection. A physical examination reveals that the patient is alert and cooperative; his respiratory rate is 40 breaths/min. Coarse, wet breath sounds are heard over all lung fields. He reports producing copious amounts of purulent, foul-smelling sputum for the past 3 days. His heart rate is 110 beats/min, and his oral temperature is 38.9°C (102°F). The arterial blood pressure is 150/100; the maximum inspiratory pressure (MIP) is −50 cm H_2O; and the pulse oximetry oxygen saturation (SpO_2) is 90%. Chest radiographs show bilateral pneumonia.

The pulmonology resident suggests using intermittent positive-pressure breathing (IPPB) treatments. Do you agree with this suggestion?

See Appendix A for the answer.

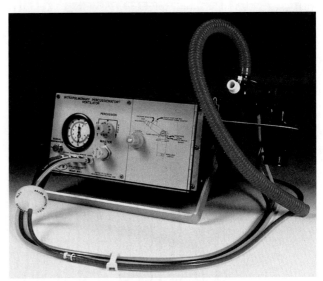

FIGURE 7.12 Percussionaire Intrapulmonary Percussive Ventilator (IPV-1). (Courtesy Percussionaire, Sandpoint, ID.)

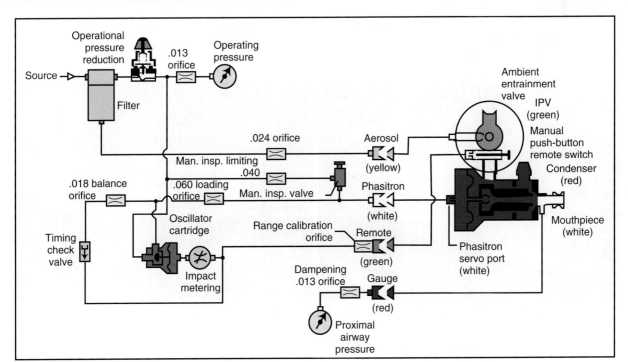

FIGURE 7.13 Gas flow through the IPV-1. (Courtesy Percussionaire, Sandpoint, ID.)

stream of medication, creating a mist that is delivered to the circuit. Note that the entrainment post of the Venturi is connected to the nebulizer by large-bore aerosol tubing, allowing the patient to receive the mist during the percussive phase of operation.

The Percussionaire can deliver percussive pressures of 25 to 40 cm H_2O at approximately 100 to 300 cycles per minute, or 1.7 to 5 Hz (Fig. 7.15). The effectiveness of IPV therapy, compared with traditional CPT techniques, is still under investigation. It has been suggested that IPV may provide another potentially useful method of improving sputum mobilization in certain patients (e.g., those with cystic fibrosis or chronic bronchitis). Although a study by Deakins and Chatburn[18] provided encouraging results for this type of therapy for the treatment of atelectasis in pediatric patients compared with conventional CPT techniques, additional studies are needed to more clearly define the appropriate indications and contraindications for IPV therapy.

Flutter Valve Therapy

The concept of "flutter" mucus clearance therapy was first introduced by Freitag et al.[19] The appeal for this device undoubtedly is influenced by its simplicity of design and by the fact that it is relatively easy for patients to use. The **Flutter valve** (Aptalis Pharma US, Inc) consists of a pipe-shaped apparatus with a steel ball in a bowl covered by a perforated cap (Fig. 7.16). The steel ball creates a PEP (similar to a PEP device) that helps prevent early airway closure, and the internal dimensions of the pipe allow the steel ball to "flutter," resulting

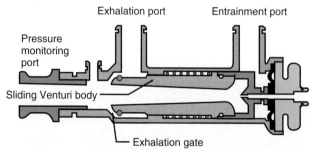

FIGURE 7.14 Phasitron unit used in the IPV-1. (Courtesy Percussionaire, Sandpoint, ID.)

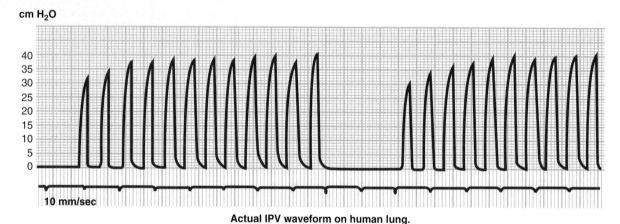

Actual IPV waveform on human lung.

FIGURE 7.15 Pressure waveform generated during operation of the IPV-1. (Courtesy Percussionaire, Sandpoint, ID.)

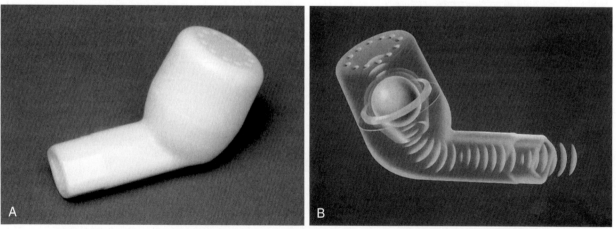

FIGURE 7.16 A, Flutter device. B, During exhalation, the position of the steel ball is the result of an equilibrium between the pressure of the exhaled gas, the force of gravity on the ball, and the angle of the cone where the contact with the ball occurs. As the steel ball rolls and bounces up and down, it creates oscillation in the airway. (Courtesy Aptalis Pharma US, Inc., Birmingham, AL. Used with permission.)

BOX 7.2   Procedure for Administering Flutter Valve Therapy

1. Assess whether Flutter valve therapy is indicated and design a treatment program.
   a. Bring the equipment to the bedside and provide initial therapy, adjusting the pressure settings to meet the patient's needs.
   b. After the initial treatment or patient training, communicate the treatment plan to the patient's physician and nurse and provide instruction to the nursing staff, if required.
2. Explain that Flutter therapy is used to reexpand lung tissue and help mobilize secretions. Patients should be taught to huff cough.
3. Instruct the patient to:
   a. Sit comfortably.
   b. Take in a breath that is larger than normal but that does not fill the lungs completely.
   c. Seal the lips firmly around the Flutter device mouthpiece and exhale actively but not forcefully, holding the Flutter valve at an angle that produces maximum oscillation.
   d. Perform 10 to 20 breaths.
   e. Remove the Flutter mouthpiece and perform 2 or 3 huff coughs and then rest as needed.
   f. Repeat this cycle 4 to 8 times, not to exceed 20 minutes.
4. Evaluate the patient for the ability to self-administer the therapy.
5. When appropriate, teach the patient to self-administer Flutter therapy. Observe the patient conduct the self-administration on several occasions to ensure proper Flutter technique before allowing the patient to self-administer without supervision.
6. When patients are also receiving bronchodilator aerosol, administer in conjunction with Flutter therapy by administering the bronchodilator immediately before the Flutter breaths.
7. If the Flutter device becomes visibly soiled, rinse it with sterile water and shake and air-dry. Leave the device within reach at the patient's bedside.
8. Send the Flutter device home with the patient.
9. In the patient's medical record, document the procedures performed (including the device, number of breaths per treatment, and frequency), the patient's response to therapy, the patient teaching provided, and the patient's ability to self-administer the treatment.

From Fink JB: High-frequency oscillation of the airway and chest wall. *Respir Care* 47:799, 2002.

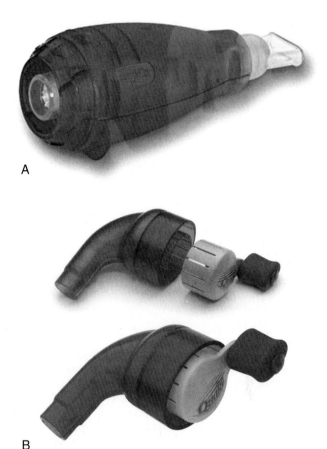

FIGURE 7.17 A, Acapella positive expiratory pressure (PEP) device. B, Quake PEP device. (A Courtesy Smiths Medical, Carlsbad, CA. B Courtesy Thayer Medical, Tucson, AZ.)

in the creation of a series of high-frequency oscillations that are transmitted to the lung through the airway opening.

Box 7.2 summarizes the protocol for administering Flutter valve therapy. A number of studies have demonstrated that this therapy is a viable alternative to standard CPT techniques in select patient groups.[16] Further in vivo studies involving greater numbers and more diverse patient groups are required to better determine the effectiveness of Flutter valve therapy devices compared with other airway clearance techniques involving PAP.

The Acapella (Smiths Medical) (Fig. 7.17A) uses a counterweighted plug and magnet to create the expiratory resistance.

Unlike the Flutter valve, which the patient must use while seated upright or standing, the Acapella can be used in the upright or supine position, according to the manufacturer.[20]

The Quake (Thayer Medical; see Fig. 7.17B) consists of two barrels with matching slots that fit snugly over each other. When these slots are aligned, the patient can inhale and exhale freely through the device. When the slots are not aligned, back-pressure is created because the patient's continuous breath is prevented from escaping. This design allows the patient to create the ideal frequency and percussive pressure by manually rotating the outer barrel at the ideal rate while breathing through the device. The faster a patient rotates the handle, the greater the frequency and lower the pressure; the slower the handle rotation, the lower the frequency and greater the pressure. Box 7.3 provides a summary of the instructions for using the Quake.

High-Frequency Chest Wall Oscillation Devices

The Vest and the Hayek RTX oscillator can be used to deliver high-frequency external chest wall oscillations. The Vest was developed by Warwick and colleagues. As Fig. 7.18 shows, it consists of a nonstretchable, inflatable vest that extends over the entire torso area down to the iliac crest.[16] Chest wall vibrations are delivered to the vest through a series of pressure pulses produced by an air compressor connected to the vest

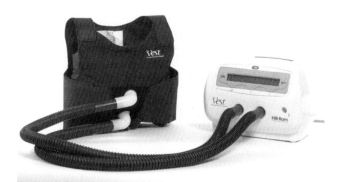

FIGURE 7.18 The Vest airway clearance system. (Courtesy Advanced Respiratory, St. Paul, MN.)

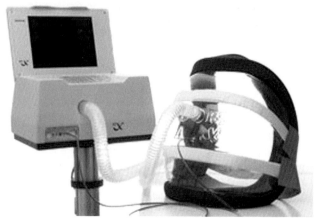

FIGURE 7.19 Hayek RTX. (Courtesy United Hayek Industries, London, UK.)

BOX 7.3 Procedure for Using the Quake Device

1. The Quake can be used while the patient is sitting, standing, or lying down.
2. The patient is instructed to inhale deeply then place their lips on the Quake mouthpiece and begin rotating the Quake's handle as they exhale at a slightly faster rate than normal.
3. The patient should continue rotating the handle while inhaling and repeating the exhalation cycle.
4. The patient should keep their cheeks rigid as they exhale so that the percussive effect is transmitted to the lungs rather than to their mouth.
5. Repeat step 2 three to six times while actively suppressing the desire to cough during these cycles. If this does not trigger a productive cough, the patient should be instructed to perform a huff cough to force the secretions from the airways.
6. The device can be cleaned by hand using warm household dishwashing detergent or by placing it on the top rack of a dishwasher for a complete cycle. To ensure proper cleaning, the inner gray barrel must be disassembled from the outer blue body.

From Thayer Medical, Tucson, AZ, www.thayermedical.com.

---

by a vacuum hose. A remote control switch also is available to start and stop the device. The patient can adjust the intensity and frequency of the pressure pulses to achieve pressures ranging from approximately 25 to 40 mm Hg over a frequency range of 5 to 25 Hz, respectively.

The Hayek RTX (Fig. 7.19) is technically classified as an electrically powered noninvasive ventilator, high-frequency chest wall oscillator, and assist cough device. It consists of a power unit with cathode-ray tube (CRT) screen, control keyboard, and flexible chest cuirass with disposable foam seal that is applied over the anterior chest wall and abdomen from the upper part of the sternum to below the umbilicus. The Hayek RTX is designed to deliver negative and positive pressures to the chest wall to control or assist both phases of the respiratory cycle, and to provide high-frequency chest wall oscillation (HFCWO) to patients from <1 to 180 kg. The negative pressure delivered during the inspiratory portion of the cycle causes the chest wall and lungs to expand, whereas the positive pressure can produce or assist with expiration. The pressure differential between the negative and positive pressure settings used for normal respiratory rates influences the tidal volume delivered. The frequency of oscillations, the I:E ratio, and the inspiratory and expiratory pressures are controlled by a microprocessor, which can be programmed by the respiratory therapist according to the patient's needs. The frequency of oscillations in ventilation mode can range from 6 to 1200 cycles per minute, and the I:E ratio can be varied from 1:6 to 6:1. Inspiratory and expiratory pressures of −50 to 50 cm H_2O can be achieved.

In secretion clearance mode the Hayek RTX delivers timed cycles of HFCWO in a range from 240 to 1200 cycles per minute for durations from 1 to 99 minutes, with a typical duration for treatments set for 3 to 4 minutes. The RTX then automatically cycles into the assisted cough mode after a treatment to produce a strong inspiratory phase from −20 to −35 at I:E ratios of 4:1 to 6:1 with a positive phase of +15 to +25. Assisted cough duration can be set from 1 to 99 minutes but is usually set for 2 to 3 minutes. Each time the RTX cycles between HFCWO and assisted cough is considered one cycle of treatment; it can be set to repeat up to 20 cycles, with typical treatment consisting of 4 to 6 cycles for treatments of 20 to 30 minutes in duration.

Several therapeutic regimens have been suggested to improve the efficacy of high-frequency oscillations for clearing airway secretions.[3] However, more studies are required to determine the best method of using these devices.[22]

VI. MECHANICAL INSUFFLATION–EXSUFFLATION

The purpose of the mechanical insufflation–exsufflation device is to replace or augment cough clearance in individuals with respiratory muscle weakness or paralysis (e.g., neuromuscular disease).[21] The original device, which was produced during the polio epidemic in the 1950s, consisted of a vacuum cleaner motor that was designed to produce either a positive or negative pressure across the airway opening. The popularity of these devices declined in the years after the polio epidemic, and it was not until the early 1990s that Philips Respironics (formerly J.H. Emerson Co.) decided to redesign the device (originally called the In-Exsufflator) and market it as the CoughAssist. The redesigned device can generate positive pressures of 30 to 50 cm H_2O on inspiration for 1 to 3 seconds. The pressure is then reversed to −10 to −50 cm H_2O during exhalation, generating a mean expiratory flow of 7.5 L/s (Fig. 7.20).[3] Treatments can be administered via face mask or tracheal airway. Use of the device has increased considerably since the redesign, but its use is directed primarily to individuals with Duchenne muscular dystrophy and spinal muscular atrophy.[22]

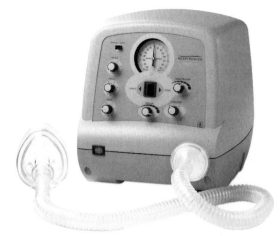

FIGURE 7.20 CoughAssist mechanical insufflation–exsufflation device. (Courtesy Philips Respironics, Murrysville, PA.)

KEY POINTS

- The primary indications for lung expansion therapy are to prevent and treat atelectasis. One of the most important ways to accomplish this goal is to maintain effective clearance of airway secretions with lung inflation therapy.
- A variety of strategies and devices have been used to accomplish airway clearance. The most commonly used techniques involve IS, IPPB, PAP, and CPT/postural drainage.
- Devices that provide high-frequency oscillations to the lungs and chest wall are receiving increased attention as viable alternatives to traditional bronchial hygiene techniques.

- Selection of the appropriate device and therapeutic modality should be based on the patient's ability to perform the procedure and on the therapeutic goals. Evaluation of the effectiveness of therapy should be based on the history and physical findings, chest radiographs, and a review of laboratory test results (e.g., arterial blood gas levels).
- It is important to recognize that additional clinical studies will be required to determine the effect of using nonpharmacological airway clearance therapies on long-term outcomes, such as health-related quality of life, hospitalization length of stay, and mortality rates of patients with acute and chronic lung diseases.

ASSESSMENT QUESTIONS

See Appendix B for the answers.

1. What is the primary indication for lung inflation therapy?
   1. To prevent atelectasis
   2. To prevent hypoxemia
   3. To reverse hypercapnia
   4. To reduce pulmonary shunting
      a. 1 only
      b. 1 and 2 only
      c. 2 and 3 only
      d. 1, 2, 3, and 4

2. Incentive spirometry (IS) is indicated for patients who are predisposed to develop atelectasis. List four medical conditions for which IS is indicated.

3. You are asked to show an adult patient how to properly use a TriFlo incentive spirometer. Although the patient appears to be following your instructions, she is unable to achieve the prescribed goal that you have established for her. Briefly describe several factors that could cause this problem.

4. Which of the following parameters is used to set the therapeutic goal for a patient using a volume-displacement incentive spirometer?

   a. Total lung capacity
   b. Inspiratory capacity
   c. Inspiratory reserve volume
   d. Expiratory reserve volume

5. You are asked to suggest a lung inflation therapy for a 55-year-old man who is 72 inches tall and weighs 85 kg. He has just undergone a cholecystectomy, and his chest radiograph shows right middle lobe atelectasis. He has a 10-pack-per-year history of smoking cigarettes, and his preoperative pulmonary function studies showed that his vital capacity was 20 mL/kg. He is alert and cooperative but complains of some upper abdominal pain when taking a deep breath. What modality would you suggest?

6. Which of the following are contraindications to the administration of intermittent positive-pressure breathing (IPPB)?
   1. Active hemoptysis
   2. Nausea
   3. Intracranial pressure >15 mm Hg
   4. Recent esophageal surgery
      a. 1 and 3 only
      b. 2 and 3 only
      c. 1, 2, and 3 only
      d. 1, 2, 3, and 4

7. The American Association for Respiratory Care (AARC) Clinical Practice Guideline for IPPB states that this form of therapy is a viable lung expansion technique for patients with reduced lung function. Which of the following findings from a patient suggest that IPPB is warranted?
   1. Forced vital capacity (FVC) = 50% predicted
   2. Forced expiratory volume in 1 second (FEV$_1$) = 70% predicted
   3. Maximum voluntary ventilation (MVV) < 50% predicted
   4. Vital capacity (VC) = 15 mL/kg
   a. 1 only
   b. 4 only
   c. 2 and 3 only
   d. 1 and 3 only

8. You can adjust the tidal volume delivered by a Bird Mark 7 ventilator by manipulating which of the following parameters? (Hint: See Evolve website for additional information about the Bird Mark 7 ventilator).
   a. Inspiratory time
   b. Inspiratory flow
   c. Peak inspiratory pressure
   d. Trigger sensitivity

9. According to the manufacturer, what is the flow of gas from a Vortran IPPB device connected directly to a 50-psig gas source?
   a. 10 L/min
   b. 25 L/min
   c. 40 L/min
   d. The flow varies as the amount of gas entrained by the patient changes.

10. What types of percussive pressure does the Percussionaire IPV device deliver?
    a. 10 to 20 cm H$_2$O
    b. 25 to 40 cm H$_2$O
    c. 50 to 100 cm H$_2$O
    d. >200 cm H$_2$O

11. Name two types of commercially available threshold resistors that are used to administer continuous positive airway pressure (CPAP).

12. Which of the following are considered positive outcomes to positive expiratory pressure (PEP) therapy?
    1. Increased sputum production
    2. Increased respiratory rate
    3. Resolution of hypoxemia
    4. Diminished breath sounds become adventitious sounds that can be auscultated over the larger airways.
    a. 1 only
    b. 1 and 3 only
    c. 2 and 3 only
    d. 1, 3, and 4 only

13. The function of the steel ball in the Flutter device is to:
    a. Help prevent early airway closure
    b. Provide high-frequency oscillation
    c. Create a positive expiratory pressure
    d. All of the above

14. The Vest is used to:
    a. Provide positive pressure on exhalation
    b. Keep infants' core temperature stable
    c. Oscillate the chest wall to promote secretion clearance
    d. Provide biofeedback in the teaching of diaphragmatic breathing

15. Mechanical insufflation–exsufflation therapy has been shown to be most effective in patients with:
    a. Croup
    b. Duchenne muscular dystrophy
    c. Asthma
    d. Acute respiratory distress syndrome

REFERENCES

1. Strickland SL, Rubin BK, Drescher MA, et al.: AARC clinical practice guideline: effectiveness of nonpharmacologic airway clearance therapies in hospitalized patients. *Respir Care* 58(12):2187-2193, 2013.
2. Andrews J, Sathe A, Krishnaswami S, et al.: Nonpharmacologic airways clearance techniques in hospitalized patients: a systematic review. *Respir Care* 58(12):2160-2186, 2013.
3. Lester MK, Flume PA: Airway clearance therapy guidelines and implementation. *Respir Care* 52(10):733-750, 2009.
4. Restrepo RD, Wettstein R, Wittnebel L, et al.: American Association for Respiratory Care: AARC clinical practice guideline: incentive spirometry. *Respir Care* 56(10):1600-1604, 2011.
5. Kacmarek RM, Stoller JK, Heuer AH: *Egan's fundamentals of respiratory care*, ed 10, St. Louis, 2012, Elsevier-Mosby.
6. Gooselink R, Schever K, Cops P, et al.: Incentive spirometry does not enhance recovery after thoracic surgery. *Crit Care Med* 29:679-683, 2000.
7. Overend TJ, Anderson CM, Lucy SD, et al.: The effect of incentive spirometry on postoperative pulmonary complications: a systematic review. *Chest* 120:971-978, 2001.
8. Craven JL, Evans GA, Davenport PJ, et al.: The evaluation of incentive spirometry in the management of postoperative pulmonary complications. *Br J Surg* 61:793-797, 1974.
9. Petz TJ: Physiologic effects of IPPB, blow bottles, and incentive spirometry. *Curr Rev Respir Ther* 1:107-111, 1979.
10. American Association for Respiratory Care: AARC clinical practice guideline: intermittent positive pressure breathing (IPPB). *Respir Care* 38:1189-1195, 1993.
11. American Association for Respiratory Care: AARC clinical practice guideline: intermittent positive pressure breathing—2003 revisions and update. *Respir Care* 48:540-546, 2003.
12. McPherson SP: *Respiratory care equipment*, ed 5, St. Louis, 1995, Mosby.
13. Vortran Medical Technology: *Vortran IPPB user's guide*, Sacramento, CA, 2005, Vortran.

14. American Association for Respiratory Care: AARC clinical practice guideline: use of positive airway pressure adjuncts to bronchial hygiene therapy. *Respir Care* 38:516-521, 1993.

15. Cairo JM: *Pilbeam's mechanical ventilation*, ed 6, St. Louis, 2016, Elsevier.

16. Fink JB, Mahlmeister MJ: High-frequency oscillation of the airway and chest wall. *Respir Care* 47:797-807, 2002.

17. Percussionaire: *Operator's manual for the Percussionaire intrapulmonary percussive ventilation (IPV-1) unit*, Sandpoint, ID, 1990, Percussionaire.

18. Deakins K, Chatburn R: A comparison of intrapulmonary percussive ventilation and conventional chest physiotherapy for the treatment of atelectasis in the pediatric patient. *Respir Care* 47:1162-1167, 2002.

19. Freitag L, Long WM, Kim CS, et al.: Removal of excessive bronchial secretions by asymmetrical high-frequency oscillations. *J Appl Physiol* 67:614-619, 1989.

20. Volsko TA, DiFiore J, Chatburn RL: Performance comparison of two oscillating positive expiratory pressure devices: Acapella versus Flutter. *Respir Care* 48:124-130, 2003.

21. Scherer TA, Barandun J, Martinez E, et al.: Effect of high-frequency oral airway and chest wall oscillations and conventional chest physical therapy on expectoration in patients with stable cystic fibrosis. *Chest* 113:1019-1027, 1998.

22. McCool FD, Rosen MJ: Nonpharmacologic airway clearance therapies: ACCP evidence-based clinical practice guidelines. *Chest* 129; 250S-259S, 2006.

SECTION IV

Assessment

Assessment of Pulmonary Function

OBJECTIVES

Upon completion of this chapter, you will be able to:

1. Identify three types of volume-collecting spirometers.
2. Explain the operational theory of thermal flowmeters.
3. Name three types of pneumotachometers.
4. Describe three types of body plethysmographs.
5. Compare the nitrogen washout and the helium dilution techniques for measuring functional residual capacity and residual volume.
6. Discuss the standards for lung function testing established by the American Thoracic Society and the European Respiratory Society.
7. Explain the operational theories of strain gauge, variable inductance, and variable capacitance pressure transducers.
8. Describe various conditions that interfere with the operation of impedance pneumographs.
9. List and describe measured and derived variables commonly used to assess respiratory mechanics.
10. Compare the operational principles of the two types of oxygen analyzers used in the clinical setting.
11. Describe two techniques for monitoring nitrogen oxides in the clinical setting.
12. Identify the components of a normal capnogram.
13. Assess an abnormal capnogram and suggest possible pathophysiological processes that could contribute to the contour of the carbon dioxide waveform.
14. Compare closed-circuit and open-circuit indirect calorimeters.
15. Calculate energy expenditure using measurements obtained during indirect calorimetry.
16. Explain how indirect calorimetry can be used to determine substrate utilization patterns in healthy individuals and in those with cardiopulmonary dysfunctions.

OUTLINE

KEY TERMS

accuracy
airway resistance (R_{aw})
ammonia
anemometers
aneroid manometer
auto–positive end-expiratory
   pressure (auto-PEEP)
bell factor
body plethysmography
capnogram

chemiluminescence monitoring
closed-circuit method
dead space ventilation
Doppler effect
dry rolling seal spirometers
electrical impedance
electrochemical
electrochemical monitoring
electromechanical transducer
energy expenditure (EE)

Fleisch pneumotachograph
functional residual capacity
   (FRC)
galvanic analyzer
Haldane transformation
indirect calorimetry
inert gas techniques
kymograph
lung and chest wall compliance
mainstream capnograph

maximum voluntary ventilation
(MVV)
metabolic carts
minute ventilation ($\dot{V}_E$)
Monel screen
open-circuit method
P_{100} ($P_{0.1}$)
paramagnetic
peak flowmeters
peak inspiratory pressure (PIP)

plateau pressure (P_{plat})
pneumotachographs
polarographic
precision
quenching
Raman effect
repeatability
reproducibility
residual volume (RV)

respiratory system compliance
sidestream capnograph
spirogram
Stead-Wells spirometer
thermal flowmeters
total lung capacity (TLC)
vital capacity (VC)
Wheatstone bridge
work of breathing

Respiration is the exchange of oxygen and carbon dioxide between an organism and its environment. Normal gas exchange in humans requires efficiently functioning chest bellows and lungs, an alveolar-capillary network in which ventilation and blood flow are evenly matched, intact systemic circulation for transporting oxygen from the lungs to the tissues and carbon dioxide from the tissues to the lungs, and integrated neural and chemical control mechanisms that regulate pH, oxygen, and carbon dioxide levels in the blood.[1] If any of these processes fails, hypoxia, hypercapnia, and, ultimately, respiratory and cardiovascular failure may result.

Advances in microprocessor technology have significantly improved our ability to evaluate a patient's respiratory function, both in the laboratory and at the bedside. This chapter discusses the devices and techniques commonly used by respiratory therapists to assess the respiratory system mechanics, gas exchange, and metabolic function of patients with cardiopulmonary disease.

I. RESPIRATORY SYSTEM MECHANICS

Ventilation can be defined as the movement of air between the atmosphere and the lungs. Gas flow into and out of the respiratory system is influenced by the pressure gradient between the airway opening and the alveoli and the impedance offered by the lungs and the chest wall. Respiratory muscular effort or the force generated by a mechanical ventilator establishes the pressure gradient between the atmosphere and the alveoli. The impedance to airflow results from the elastic and frictional forces offered by the lungs and thorax.[2]

The mechanics of breathing can be assessed by measuring the air volume exchanged during ventilation, the gas flow into and out of the lungs, and the pressure that must be generated to achieve a given volume or flow during breathing. Derived variables (e.g., airway resistance [R_{aw}], lung and chest wall compliance, and work of breathing) can be calculated using these three measurements.

The usefulness of respiratory mechanics measurements ultimately depends on the accuracy and precision of the equipment used. Accuracy can be explained as how closely a measured value is related to the true (correct) value of the quantity measured. The accuracy of any instrument depends on its linearity and frequency response, its sensitivity to environmental conditions, and how well it is calibrated.[3] The accuracy of mechanics measurements is also influenced by patient cooperation while the test is performed. In most cases, patient cooperation depends on a firm understanding of how the test is to be performed. If the technologist does not properly instruct patients in how to perform the test, the results can be severely affected. Precision is the expression of an instrument's ability to reproduce a measurement (i.e., repeatability). The precision of a measuring device can be quantified by calculating the standard deviation of repeated measurements made by the device.[3]

Volume and Flow Measurements

A spirometer is a device for measuring volume or flow changes at the airway opening. Therefore spirometers generally are classified by whether they measure lung volume changes or airflow. Volume-displacement devices measure the volumes of exhaled and inhaled gas into an expandable container by noting the amount of displacement that occurs. Typical examples of volume-displacement devices include water-sealed spirometers, bellows spirometers, and dry rolling seal spirometers. Flow-sensing devices measure airflow by using thermal, or "hot wire," anemometers, turbine flowmeters, and differential pressure pneumotachographs.

Flow can be determined when using volume-displacement devices by dividing the volume change relative to the time interval of the measurement (flow in L/s = volume measured in L/time measured in seconds). Volume can be determined when using flow-sensing devices by integrating the flow relative to time (volume in L = flow measured in L/s × time measured in seconds). It is worth mentioning that modern pulmonary function systems rely on solid-state circuits and computer software to accomplish these calculations, thus relieving the therapist from having to perform them manually.

Water-Sealed Spirometers

As Fig. 8.1 shows, a water-sealed spirometer (commonly referred to as a "Collins spirometer" after Warren E. Collins, who designed and manufactured the original device) consists of a bell that is sealed from the atmosphere by water. The patient is connected to the bell in rebreathing fashion by a breathing circuit, which includes inspiratory and expiratory tubing. The circuit is equipped with one-way valves to minimize dead space and a carbon dioxide absorber (i.e., soda lime) to remove exhaled CO_2. The bell, which is made of metal (usually aluminum), is suspended by a chain-and-pulley mechanism with a weight that counterbalances the weight of the bell. (The counterweight minimizes the effects of gravity acting on the metal bell.) A pen attached to the chain-and-pulley mechanism records bell movements on a separate, motor-driven rotating drum called a kymograph. As patients exhale into the system, the bell moves upward, and the attached pen moves proportionately downward on graph paper, creating a spirogram. Inhalation causes the bell to move downward and the pen to move upward. The rotating drum can be set to move at a constant speed (32, 160, or 1920 mm/min), allowing the

operator to measure volume changes relative to time. The slower speeds (32 and 160 mm/min) are used for measuring tidal volume, minute ventilation ($\dot{V}_E$), and maximum voluntary ventilation (MVV). The slower speeds are also used for specialized measurements (e.g., the diffusion capacity of carbon monoxide [D_LCO]). The fastest speed (1920 mm/min) is used for recording volume changes during forced vital capacity (FVC) maneuvers. Notice that the volume of gas is measured under ambient temperature and pressure, saturated (ATPS) conditions and must therefore be converted to body temperature and ambient pressure, saturated (BTPS) before reporting the data.

Two bell sizes are available: 9 L and 13.5 L. The volume of the bell determines how many millimeters the pen moves when a given volume is displaced. For example, a 9-L bell moves 1 mm for every 20.93 mL of gas displaced, and a 13.45-L bell moves 1 mm for every 41.73 mL of gas displaced. (Note that the number of milliliters of gas that must be displaced to cause the kymograph pen to move 1 mm is called the bell factor.) The total gas volume displaced during a breath is calculated by multiplying the number of millimeters the pen is displaced on the spirogram by the bell factor for the spirometer.

The Stead-Wells spirometer (Fig. 8.2) is similar in design to the original Collins water-sealed spirometer, except that a plastic bell is used instead of the metal one; this eliminates the need for a counterweight, because the bell weighs less. A more recent version of the Stead-Wells spirometers uses a dry seal in place of the water-sealed design. (The next section on dry rolling seal spirometers provides more details about the mechanism used with these latter devices.)

Stead-Wells spirometers show excellent frequency response characteristics, especially when recording rapid-breathing

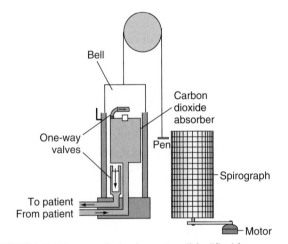

FIGURE 8.1 Water-sealed spirometer. (Modified from materials provided by Collins Medical, Braintree, MA.)

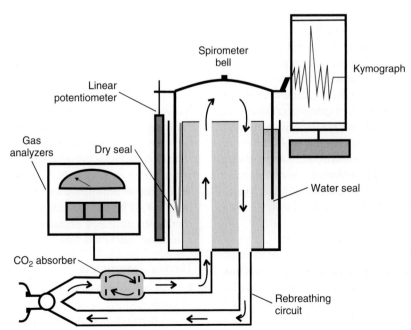

FIGURE 8.2 Stead-Wells spirometer. (From Mottram C: *Ruppel's manual of pulmonary function testing*, ed 10, St. Louis, 2012, Mosby.)

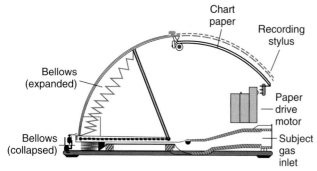

FIGURE 8.3 Wedge-bellows spirometer. (Modified from material provided by Vitalograph, Shawnee Mission, KS.)

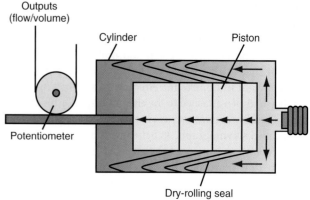

FIGURE 8.4 Dry rolling seal spirometer. (Courtesy Datex-Ohmeda, Madison, WI.)

maneuvers such as FVC, timed expiratory volume measurements (e.g., forced expiratory volume in 1 second [FEV_1]), and MVV. Stead-Wells spirometers are available in 7-, 10-, and 14-L bell sizes. The pen recorder for the Stead-Wells spirometer is attached directly to the bell; consequently, as the bell moves upward during exhalation, the pen inscribes on the spirogram in an upward motion. Conversely, the bell and pen move downward during inhalation.

Water-sealed and Stead-Wells spirometers that are currently used for clinical pulmonary function measurements are equipped with potentiometers that produce analog voltage signals. The voltage produced is proportional to the volume displacement measured as the patient breathes into and out of the spirometer. The measured analog DC voltage signal can be used to drive a strip chart recorder or converted to a digital signal, which can be stored and processed by a computer.[3] (Note that flow can be determined if the spirometer's potentiometer simultaneously measures the speed of the volume displacement.)

The most common problem encountered with water-sealed and dry-sealed spirometers involves leaks that occur in the bell or breathing circuit. Raising the bell and then occluding the patient connection to the device can accomplish detection of a leak. The height of the bell will gradually decrease because of the pull of gravity on the bell if a leak is present. Maintenance of these devices typically involves routine draining of the water well and replacement with sterile water. Chemical absorbers must also be checked and replaced on a routine basis. Infection control practices require the replacement of breathing circuit (tubing and mouthpieces) after each patient. Some systems allow for the placement of a low-resistance bacterial filter to protect those parts of the circuit that are not changed after patient use.[3]

Bellows Spirometers

With bellows or wedge spirometers, exhaled gases are collected into an expandable bellows (Fig. 8.3). Air entering the bellows causes the free wall of the bellows to move outward and inward, and its displacement is directly related to the volume of air exhaled and inhaled, respectively. Bellows-type spirometers can be mounted either horizontally or vertically. The mounting determines the movement of the bellows. In horizontally

mounted devices, the bellows moves in a horizontal plane, whereas vertically mounted devices move in a vertical plane. Wedge-type spirometers expand and contract in a fanlike motion. Volume changes can be recorded by attaching a pen recorder or a potentiometer to the free wall of the bellows.

The bellows usually is constructed of silicone rubber or plastic, and several different designs are currently available. These designs differ in that the free wall can move horizontally, vertically, and/or diagonally. Because the frequency response of these devices is good, they can be used to measure lung volume changes during rapid-breathing maneuvers (e.g., FVC, FEV_1, and MVV). Volume and flow measurements are obtained under ATPS conditions and must be converted to BTPS before reporting patient data.

Dry Rolling Seal Spirometers

Dry rolling seal spirometers consist of a cylinder containing a lightweight aluminum piston that is mounted horizontally in the canister and sealed to it with a rolling, diaphragmlike plastic seal. (In the case of a dry-seal Stead-Wells spirometer, the bell, which is used in place of the aluminum cylinder, is mounted vertically.) As Fig. 8.4 shows, gas entering the cylinder displaces the piston. The large surface area of the piston minimizes the mechanical resistance to movement and gives these devices good frequency response characteristics. A pen recorder or linear or rotary potentiometer attached to the cylinder shaft detects the piston's movement and registers the signal on an output display (e.g., graph paper or an oscilloscope). In those devices that use a potentiometer, the volume displacement produces a DC voltage output for volume and flow.[3] As with other volume displacement devices, measurements are obtained under ATPS conditions and must be converted to BTPS before reporting patient data.

Thermal Flowmeters

Fig. 8.5 is a schematic of a thermal, or hot wire, anemometer. These devices use sensors that are temperature-sensitive, resistive elements (e.g., thermistor beads or heated wires). Thermal flowmeters operate on the principle that as gas passes over the thermistor bead or the heated wire, the sensor cools and its resistance changes in proportion to the gas flow past it. Note that the amount of cooling depends on the viscosity and the thermal conductivity of the gas measured. With thermistor beads, cooling increases resistance, whereas with a heated platinum wire, cooling decreases resistance. The wire is typically heated above 37°C (98.6°F) and protected by a low-resistance screen to prevent moisture accumulation and debris impaction on the wire. The gas flow can be calculated because the amount of power needed to maintain the temperature of the heating element above the temperature (e.g., 37°C) is related to the velocity of the gas flow. Actually, the signal is related to the log of the velocity of gas flow and therefore must be linearized.[3] Thermal flowmeters are unidirectional devices and cannot be used for measuring bidirectional flows during breathing. It is important to recognize that the density and viscosity of the gas being measured can affect the accuracy and precision of the flow measurement. Correction factors for various gases can be applied through computer software.[3] Note that most heated-wire flowmeters meet the American Thoracic Society/European Respiratory Society (ATS/ERS) recommendations for accuracy and precision, which are discussed later in this chapter. Clinical Scenario 8.1 presents a decision-making problem involving a thermal flowmeter spirometer.

Turbine Flowmeters

Turbine flowmeters (Fig. 8.6) use a rotating vane or turbine to measure gas flow. As gas flows through the device, the vane turns at a rate dependent on the flow rate of the gas. The flow rate can be measured by counting the number of times the vane turns, which can be done mechanically (by linking the vane to a needle attached to a calibrated display) or electronically (by using a light beam that is interrupted each time the vane turns).

Turbine flowmeters (e.g., handheld respirometers) usually are accurate for flows of 3 to 300 L/min. They are portable and easy to use, but they are slow to respond to flow changes because of inertia (low-frequency response). Some turbine devices, such as those found in commercially available

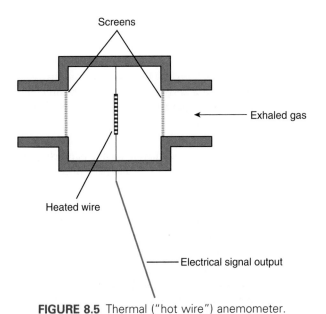

FIGURE 8.5 Thermal ("hot wire") anemometer.

CLINICAL SCENARIO 8.1

You are asked to perform bedside simple spirometry on a patient receiving bronchodilator therapy. You connect the mouthpiece to the measuring device (a heated-wire [thermal] flowmeter) and instruct the patient to breathe in deeply and exhale forcefully into the mouthpiece. When the patient does this, you notice that the digital display fails to register a reading of estimated volume. What could cause this type of problem? See Appendix A for the answer.

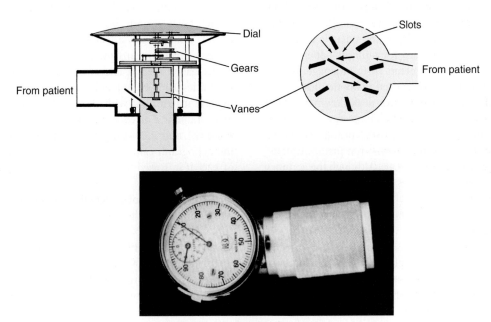

FIGURE 8.6 Turbine flowmeter.

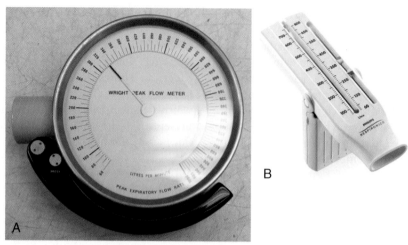

FIGURE 8.7 A, Wright peak flowmeter. B, Commercially available disposable peak flowmeter. (B courtesy Respironics/HealthScan, Cedar Grove, NJ.)

metabolic carts, use a bias flow of gas to keep the turbine constantly turning, thereby reducing the inertia of the vane. These devices are good for measuring unidirectional flow, but they are inaccurate for measuring bidirectional flows.[2]

Some **peak flowmeters** operate by measuring the gas flow against a rotating vane. The operating mechanism consists of a pivoted vane with an attached needle indicator. Air resistance and a calibrated spring oppose the rotation of the vane. During a forced exhalation the vane and the indicator needle rotate until the maximum available flow is reached. Because the indicator needle attached to the vane is spring loaded, it maintains the measurement of peak expiratory flow (PEF) until it is mechanically reset.

Peak flowmeters typically are calibrated in liters per minute. The Wright Peak Flow Meter (Fig. 8.7A), designed by B.M. Wright, can measure flows of 60 to 1000 L/min with an accuracy of ±10 L/min. Its reproducibility is within ±2 L/min. Because of its wide range, it can be used to measure peak flows for both pediatric and adult patients. Reusable and disposable mouthpieces are available in pediatric and adult sizes, so these devices can be used for multiple patients.[3]

Increased use of peak flowmeters in the management of individuals with asthma has prompted many medical device manufacturers to market inexpensive peak flowmeters that are durable and easy to use (Fig. 8.7B). These expendable units are constructed of plastic and operate with a piston-and-spring mechanism. Exhaled air pushes against the piston, causing the needle to move on a calibrated scale. Although the accuracy and reproducibility of these devices are similar to nonexpendable peak flowmeters, they typically operate over a slightly narrower range of flows (80 to 800 L/min).

Pneumotachographs

Fig. 8.8 shows several different types of pneumotachographs (also referred to as pneumotachometers), including a Fleisch-type pneumotachograph, a screen pneumotachograph, a variable orifice pneumotachograph, and an ultrasonic pneumotachograph. All these devices, except the ultrasonic

pneumotachograph, operate on the principle that gas flow through them is proportional to the pressure drop that occurs as the gas flows across a known resistance. Ultrasonic pneumotachographs rely on the **Doppler effect** to quantify the airflow velocity.

The **Fleisch pneumotachograph** (see Fig. 8.8A) uses a bundle of brass capillary tubes arranged in a parallel manner to create the known resistance. A differential pressure transducer monitors the pressures before and after the resistance and converts the difference into a flow signal. (With unidirectional flow, a single pressure measurement is required.) A heater is attached to raise the temperature of the entering gas and prevent moisture condensation on the capillary tubes. It is important to recognize that the accumulation of moisture on the capillary tubes can change their resistance, and this alters the accuracy of the device.

Fleisch pneumotachographs are most accurate when the gas flow is smooth, or laminar. Turbulent airflow, which occurs at high flows or with obstructions or bends in the breathing circuit, can adversely affect the accuracy of airflow measurements. Turbulent airflow can also be caused by increases in the gas viscosity. Therefore compensating for different viscosities is important, either mathematically or by calibrating the instrument with the gas mixture breathed during measurement. For example, room air has a viscosity of 184 poise (P), and 100% oxygen has a viscosity of 206 P. A pneumotachograph calibrated with room air will show an error of 12% if it is used to measure airflow in a patient breathing 100% oxygen.[4]

Ceramic pneumotachographs are similar in design to Fleisch pneumotachographs, except that they use ceramic material containing a number of parallel channels to create the fixed resistance. The ceramic channels smooth the air flowing through them and provide a constant resistance to airflow. A heating element is incorporated into the design. The temperature of the gas mixture flowing through these devices tends to equilibrate with the temperature of the ceramic material because of the high heat capacity of the ceramic. In addition, moisture

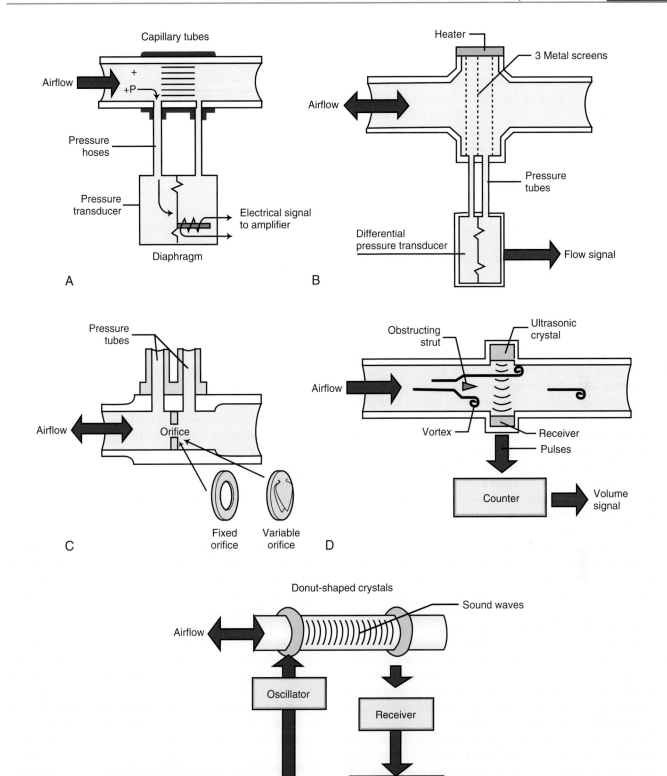

FIGURE 8.8 Pneumotachographs. A, Fleisch-type device. B, Screen-type device. C, Variable orifice device. D, Vortex ultrasonic device. E, Nonvortex device. (Redrawn from Sullivan WJ, Peters GM, Enright PL: Pneumotachography: theory and clinical application. *Respir Care* 29:736, 1984.)

that condenses during breathing tends to be absorbed by the porous ceramic material rather than occluding the tubes.[4]

Screen pneumotachographs (or Silverman pneumotachographs; see Fig. 8.8B) use a series of fine-mesh screens to create a fixed resistance. Most of these devices use a stainless steel (Monel) screen with a mesh size of 400 wires/in.[4] When a triple-screen configuration is used, the center screen acts as the main resistive element, and the two outer screens smooth the airflow and protect the inner screen from particulate matter.[4] Similar to Fleisch-type devices, a heating element is incorporated to prevent water condensation on the metal screens.

Some screen devices use fibrous material, which looks like a paper filter, instead of metal screens to create the known resistance. These devices operate at ambient temperature and therefore do not require a heating element. The main advantage of these devices is that they are inexpensive and disposable, which allows patients to have their own peak flowmeter, reducing the risk for cross-contamination. The disadvantages are that they are unidirectional devices, and accuracy varies by device.[4,5] It is also worth mentioning that moisture absorbed by the paper filter can severely affect the device's accuracy.

Variable orifice pneumotachographs (see Fig. 8.8C) are disposable, bidirectional, flow-measuring devices that use a variable area, flexible obstruction for measuring flow as a function of the pressure differential generated by the obstruction. They contain minimum dead space (approximately 10 mL) and can measure flows from 1.2 to 180 L/min.[2] Note that although the flow-pressure characteristics of variable orifice pneumotachographs are nonlinear (i.e., not proportional at very low and high flows), this discrepancy can be compensated for electronically.

Vortex ultrasonic flowmeters (see Fig. 8.8D) use struts to create a partial obstruction to gas flow. As gases flow past these struts, whirlpools, or vortices, are produced. The frequency at which these whirlpools are produced is related to gas flow through the struts. An ultrasonic transmitter perpendicular to the flow produces sound waves that are modulated by the frequency of the vortices. The extent of modulation related to actual flow is then determined.[6] Vortex ultrasonic flowmeters are not affected by the viscosity, density, or temperature of the gas being measured. They are unidirectional devices and therefore cannot measure inspiratory and expiratory flow simultaneously.[2]

Nonvortex ultrasonic flowmeters (see Fig. 8.8E) estimate airflow by projecting pulsed sound waves along the longitudinal axis of the flowmeter (i.e., parallel to the gas flow instead of across it). The theory is that the speed of the ultrasonic wave transmission is influenced by the rate of gas flow through the device. Nonvortex ultrasonic flowmeters are not affected by moisture or the viscosity of the gas being breathed and can be used to measure bidirectional flows.

Point-of-Care (Office) Spirometers

Advances in solid-state electronics during the past 20 years have made it possible for clinicians to obtain accurate and reliable spirometric data at the bedside or in the physician's office. These spirometers are typically classified as screening devices and therefore typically provide measurements of FVC and timed FEV_t.

Portable spirometers fall into two categories: spirometers that consist of a stand-alone computer with a permanently attached pneumotachometer, and spirometers that are PC-based devices, which include a detachable pneumotachometer that connects to a laptop computer via a serial connection port or a USB (Universal Serial Bus).[6] Fig. 8.9 shows several examples of commonly used portable spirometers.[3] Technical requirements for the use of these devices have been provided by the National Lung Health Education Program (NLHEP; Box 8.1).[6] These portable spirometers are ideal for office spirometry because they are low-cost, small devices that are relatively easy to use. They have improved calibration checks and an improved quality-assurance program. It is important to recognize that portable office spirometers have limitations and should not be used for diagnostic testing, surveillance for occupational lung disease, disability evaluations, or research purposes.[5,6] Box 8.1 provides the NLHEP recommendations for portable office spirometers.

Measurement of Residual Volume

Vital capacity (VC) and its subdivisions can be measured in the pulmonary function laboratory with any of the aforementioned spirometers. Measurements of residual volume (RV), functional residual capacity (FRC), and total lung capacity (TLC) are obtained using body plethysmography and inert gas techniques, such as nitrogen washout and helium dilution.[6-8]

Body Plethysmography

A body plethysmograph (or "body box") is a rigidly walled, airtight enclosure (Fig. 8.10). A number of variables can be

---

BOX 8.1   National Lung Health Education Program Spirometer Recommendations

- Office spirometers must meet or exceed current ATS/ERS minimum standards.
- Office spirometers should only report FEV_1, FEV_6, and FEV_1/FEV_6 ratio.
- Measurement end-of-test should be terminated at 6 seconds (FEV_6).
- National Health and Nutrition Examination Survey (NHANES) III reference set should be used for determining lower limits of normal (LLN).
- Automated maneuver acceptability/repeatability messages should be displayed and reported.
- Airway obstruction is determined when FEV_1/FEV_6 and FEV_1 are below respective LLNs.
- Display/printout of spirograms and flow-volume curves is optional.
- Office spirometers should include easy-to-understand educational materials.
- Simple means of checking calibration should be included.

ATS/ERS, American Thoracic Society/European Respiratory Society; *FEV*, forced expiratory volume.
From Mottram C: *Ruppel's manual of pulmonary function testing*, ed 10, St. Louis, 2012, Elsevier-Mosby.

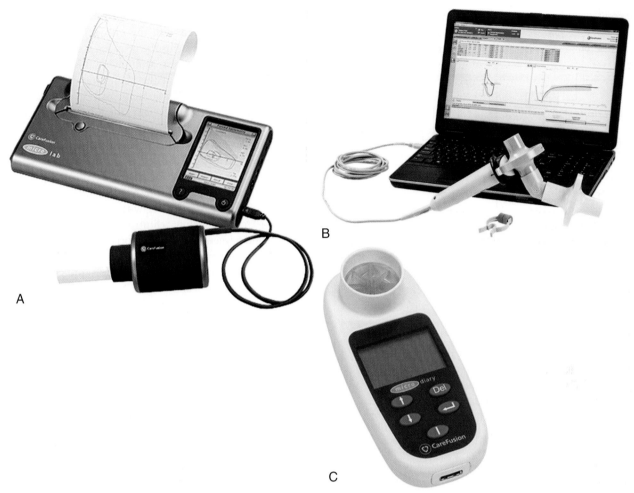

FIGURE 8.9 Various types of point-of-care (office) spirometers. A, MicroLab spirometer. B, Vmax Vyntus SPIRO. C, Micro Diary. (Courtesy Becton, Dickinson and Company, Franklin Lakes, NJ.)

measured with a body plethysmograph, but FRC and R_{aw} are by far the most common measurements obtained with these devices. Airway conductance (G_{aw}), which is the reciprocal of R_{aw}, and specific airway conductance (sG_{aw}; or, conductance per unit of lung volume) are calculated variables that also are routinely reported.

Two types of body plethysmographs are usually described: constant-volume chamber (variable-pressure) devices and constant-pressure chamber (volume-displacement) devices. Thoracic volume changes can be determined by measuring changes in pressure within a constant-volume chamber device or by measuring changes in volume within a constant-pressure chamber. Changes in a patient's thoracic volume can also be obtained by measuring changes in airflow into and out of a constant-pressure chamber.[8]

Constant-volume chamber (variable-pressure) devices are the most common plethysmographs. With these devices the patient sits in the enclosure, which has a pressure transducer within the wall of the device, and breathes through a mouthpiece connected to an assembly containing an electronic shutter and a differential pressure pneumotachometer. Mouth pressure and box pressure changes measured during tidal breathing and panting maneuvers performed by the patient at the end

of a quiet expiration are displayed on an oscilloscope and directed to a microprocessor unit that calculates the FRC from empirically derived pressure–volume relationships.[3,7,8] (Note that the reference pressure–volume relationships are empirically derived using an electronically driven piston to deliver known volumes into the enclosure. Pressure changes associated with a known volume change are recorded in the system's microprocessor and used to calculate the FRC.) The microprocessor corrects for variations in ambient temperature and pressure from data entered manually by the technologist.

The FRC is calculated using the following relationship:

$$V_{FRC} = (\Delta V \div \Delta P) \times P_B - P_{H2O}$$

where ΔV and ΔP are the box volume and alveolar pressure changes measured during the panting maneuver, P_B is the ambient barometric pressure, and P_{H2O} is the water vapor pressure (assume 47 mm Hg for 37°C). The V_{FRC} is then corrected for the volume displaced from the box by the patient.[8]

R_{aw} is derived from two separate maneuvers. In the first maneuver the patient pants while the mouth shutter is open so that flow changes ($\dot{V}$) can be measured. In the second part of the measurement, the pulmouth shutter is closed at the patient's end-expiratory or FRC level, and the patient is instructed to

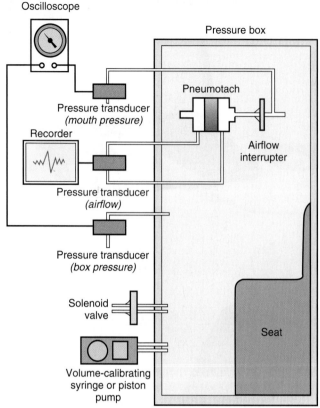

FIGURE 8.10 Schematic of a constant-volume (pressure) plethysmograph. (Redrawn from Miller WF, Scacci R, Gast LR: *Laboratory evaluation of pulmonary function*, Philadelphia, 1987, JB Lippincott.)

continue panting while maintaining an open glottis. This maneuver provides a measure of the driving pressure that is used to move air into the lungs (i.e., P_{mo}). It is important to recognize that airflow and mouth pressure measurements are recorded separately and therefore must be related to changes in the plethysmograph, or box pressure, to ensure accurate readings. The R_{aw} ultimately is derived using the following relationship:

$$R_{aw} = P_{mo} \div \dot{V}$$

Inert Gas Techniques

Nitrogen washout tests are performed with the equipment shown in Fig. 8.11, including a spirometer with a rapidly responding nitrogen analyzer, a source of 100% oxygen, a nonrebreathing valve, and the appropriate tubing.[3,7,9] The FRC is determined by initiating the test at the end of a quiet expiration. (The RV is calculated by subtracting the expiratory reserve volume [ERV] from the FRC. The ERV can be determined by simple spirometry.) The patient inspires 100% oxygen and exhales into the spirometer through the nonrebreathing valve. The patient continues to breathe the 100% oxygen until the exhaled nitrogen concentration is less than 1.5%. The nitrogen volume present in the lungs at the beginning of the test (i.e., FRC) can be determined by first measuring the total volume of exhaled gas and then multiplying this

volume by the percentage of nitrogen in the mixed expired air, which is measured with the nitrogen analyzer.[8,10] The resultant volume represents the nitrogen volume in the lungs at the beginning of the test. Multiplying this volume by 1.25 allows the lung volume at the beginning of the test to be determined. (The correction factor of 1.25 is used because the room air that filled the patient's lungs before the test began contains approximately 80% nitrogen.) Remember that the resultant volume is measured under ATPS conditions and must be converted to BTPS.

Fig. 8.12 is a schematic illustrating the breathing circuit of a device used for helium dilution tests. Note that this type of device contains a spirometer with a thermal conductivity analyzer (for measuring helium), a mixing fan, a source of helium and oxygen, and the appropriate tubing for a rebreathing breathing circuit.[3,8] The FRC is measured while the patient breathes into and out of a reservoir containing known concentrations of helium and oxygen. As the patient breathes into and out of the system, the added volume of air from the patient's lungs dilutes the helium concentration. The end point of the test is reached when the helium percentage remains steady for 2 minutes, indicating that the helium is equilibrated between the spirometer and the patient's lungs. The FRC volume is calculated as

$$FRC = (He_{mL} \div He_{final}) - (He_{mL} \div He_{initial}) - Vrb - Vcorr$$

where He_{mL} is the number of milliliters of helium added to the system, $He_{initial}$ is the helium concentration at the beginning of the test, He_{final} is the helium concentration at the end of the test, Vrb is the apparatus dead space, and $Vcorr$ is a correction volume for the amount of helium theoretically absorbed by the body, respiratory quotient (RQ) changes, and changes in nitrogen in the circuit.[3,8]

It is important to recognize that inert gas techniques can measure gas volumes only in communicating airways (i.e., airways that are open between the mouth and the alveoli), whereas body plethysmography measures all the volume in the thorax (i.e., thoracic lung volume). Therefore inert gas measurements of FRC for patients with chronic obstructive pulmonary distress and severe air trapping are lower than FRC measurements from body plethysmography.

Lung Function Testing Standards

Since 1979 the American Thoracic Society (ATS) has provided a series of standardization documents on instruments and techniques used during spirometric testing. The initial goal of these recommendations was to improve the performance characteristics of spirometers and to reduce the variability of laboratory testing.[11,12] During the 1990s the ATS widened the scope of its recommendations to include guidelines for the selection of reference values, the performance of spirometry, and the quality control of spirometers, as well as minimal recommendations for monitoring devices.[13,14]

Comparable documents have been released by the European Respiratory Society (ERS) during the past 25 years, beginning with the European Community for Coal and Steel document on standardized lung function testing.[15] The European

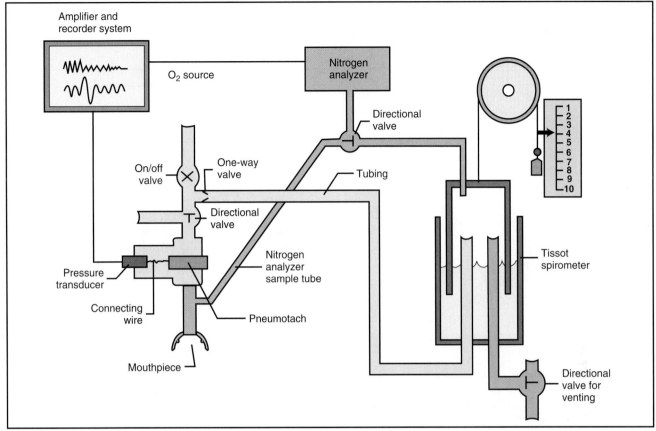

FIGURE 8.11 Breathing circuit for performing nitrogen washout test. (Redrawn from Miller WF, Scacci R, Gast LR: *Laboratory evaluation of pulmonary function*, Philadelphia, 1987, JB Lippincott.)

documents were similar to those released by the ATS except that the ERS standards provided guidance for measuring lung volumes and did not include separate recommendations for monitoring devices.

In 2000 the ATS and the ERS came together in a millennium project to issue a set of unified standards for lung function tests.[16] The result of this collaborative effort was a series of documents published in 2005 that provides guidance on measurement and interpretation of spirometry, diffusing capacity, and lung volume tests.[8,10,17,18] The most notable items addressed in these updated standards relate to terminology, infection control, and reporting of data. Although the standards for spirometry and lung volume measurements are comparable with those in earlier published statements, some noteworthy changes were made. For example, the repeatability standard for FEV_1 was changed from 200 mL to 150 mL.[10] Notice that the term *repeatability* is used in place of **reproducibility**. Repeatability is a measure of the closeness of agreement for a series of successive measurements of the same variable when they are recorded under identical conditions over a period of time (i.e., methodology, instrument, location).[10] Reproducibility describes the closeness of agreement of successive measurements of a variable when the conditions have changed (e.g., measurement of the FEV_1 before and after administration of a bronchodilator).

It is important to recognize that the updated standards do not include separate recommendations for monitoring devices. Table 8.1 summarizes the updated standards for equipment used in spirometry. The complete set of standards has been published in the *European Respiratory Journal* and also can be downloaded from the ATS website (https://www.thoracic.org).

Quality Control

Attention to quality control for laboratory equipment is essential for ensuring the accuracy of pulmonary function measurements. An effective quality control program includes documentation of daily and quarterly calibration checks, repairs, and other alterations that may be required to return malfunctioning equipment to acceptable operation, and dates of computer software and hardware updates.[17] Table 8.2 provides a summary of the components of a typical quality control program.

Calibration checks of a spirometer can be accomplished with a 3-L calibrated syringe. Notice that calibration involves establishing a relationship between sensor-determined values of flow and volume with the actual flow and volume; calibration checks are used to validate that the device is within the calibration limits.[17] Daily calibration checks of the volume-measuring capability and the presence of leaks usually involve a single discharge of a 3-L syringe into the device. More

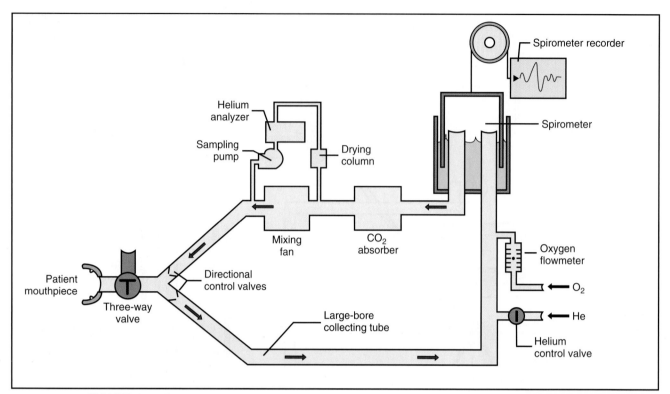

FIGURE 8.12 Breathing circuit for performing helium dilution tests. (Redrawn from Miller WF, Scacci R, Gast LR: *Laboratory evaluation of pulmonary function*, Philadelphia, 1987, JB Lippincott.)

extensive calibration checks over the entire volume range of the spirometer should be conducted intermittently (e.g., every 3 months). The linearity of a volume-measuring device can be determined by injecting a series of consecutive 1-L samples of air and comparing the observed volume with the corresponding accumulative volume.[17] Daily calibration checks of flow-measuring spirometers should include injecting 3-L discharges from the calibration syringe using flows varying from 0.5 to 12 L/s. Weekly volume calibration checks of flow-measuring spirometers should be performed to verify the linearity of these devices. This can be accomplished by injecting 3-L discharges of air into the device at low, medium, and high flows.

It is important to recognize that daily calibration checks help define the day-to-day laboratory variability.[17,18] More frequent checks are required when the equipment is used for industrial surveys or other circumstances in which large numbers of individuals are being tested.

Impedance Plethysmography

Impedance plethysmographs estimate lung volume changes by measuring the changes in electrical impedance between two electrodes placed on the chest wall. **Electrical impedance**, which is in opposition to the flow of an alternating current, is determined by the resistance and capacitance of the circuit through which the current must pass. In the case of lung volume measurements, changes in chest wall impedance are caused by variations in the amount of blood, bone, and tissue present. Therefore, as the chest wall expands during inspiration, the thoracic blood volume increases. Conversely, as the lungs deflate during expiration, the thoracic blood volume decreases, and its electrical impedance decreases. Note that the contributions of air to electrical impedance are minimal.

The electrodes used in impedance plethysmography are similar to the standard electrocardiograph electrodes and are placed in the midclavicular line at the level of the manubrium. A constant high-frequency (100 kHz), low-amplitude electrical current is passed between the two electrodes, and the return voltage is used to calculate the impedance. Variations in impedance measured during the respiratory cycle are demodulated and displayed as a waveform. The respiratory rate is extrapolated from a four- to breath-breath average.[19]

Impedance pneumography is most often used in home apnea monitoring units (Fig. 8.13). Each unit contains adjustable low and high respiratory rate alarms. The sensitivity of the monitor can be adjusted by the operator to prevent false alarms because of changes in impedance caused by movement instead of by changes in respiration.

It has been suggested that bradycardia and upper airway obstruction may cause these monitors to fail to recognize apnea.[20,21] In the case of bradycardia, cardiac oscillations and intrathoracic blood volume changes cause an increase in impedance, which is sensed as part of the respiratory cycle. Continued respiratory efforts in the presence of upper airway obstruction are sensed as normal respiratory efforts.

TABLE 8.1 Range and Accuracy Recommendations Specified for Forced Expiratory Maneuvers

Test	Range/Accuracy (BTPS)	Flow Range L s⁻¹	Time(s)	Resistance and Back Pressure	Test Signal
VC	0.5 to 8 L, ± 3% of reading or ± 0.050 L, whichever is greater	0 to 14	30		3-L Calibration syringe
FVC	0.5 to 8 L, ± 3% of reading or ± 0.050 L, whichever is greater	0 to 14	15	< 1.5 cm H_2O L⁻¹ s⁻¹ $(0.15$ kPa L⁻¹ s⁻¹)	24 ATS waveforms, 3-L calibration syringe
FEV_1	0.5 to 8 L, ± 3% of reading or ± 0.050 L, whichever is greater	0 to 14	1	< 1.5 cm H_2O L⁻¹ s⁻¹ $(0.15$ kPa L⁻¹ s⁻¹)	24 ATS waveforms
Time zero	The time point from which all FEV_1 measurements are taken			Back extrapolation	
PEF	Accuracy ± 10% of reading or ± 0.30 L s⁻¹ (20 L min⁻¹), whichever is greater, repeatability: ± 5% of reading or ± 0.15 L s⁻¹ (10 L min⁻¹), whichever is greater	0 to 14		Mean resistance at 200, 400, 600 L min⁻¹ (3.3, 6.7, 10 L s⁻¹) must be < 2.5 cm H_2O L⁻¹ s⁻¹ $(0.25$ kPa L⁻¹ s⁻¹)	26 ATS flow waveforms
Instantaneous flows (except PEF)	Accuracy, ± 5% of reading or ± 0.200 L s⁻¹, whichever is greater	0 to 14		< 1.5 cm H_2O L⁻¹ s⁻¹ $(0.15$ kPa L⁻¹ s⁻¹)	Data from manufacturers
$FEF_{25\%-75\%}$	7.0 L s⁻¹, ± 5% of reading or ± 0.200 L s⁻¹, whichever is greater	± 14	15	Same as FEV_1	24 ATS waveforms
MVV	250 L min⁻¹ at V_T of 2 L within ± 10% of reading or ± 15 L min⁻¹, whichever is greater	± 14 (± 3%)	12 to 15	< 1.5 cm H_2O L⁻¹ s⁻¹ $(0.15$ kPa L⁻¹ s⁻¹)	Sine wave pump

ATS, American Thoracic Society; *BTPS,* body temperature and ambient pressure saturated with water vapor; *FEF₂₅%-₇₅%,* mean forced expiratory flow between 25% and 75% of FVC; *FEV₁,* forced expiratory volume in 1 second; *FVC,* forced vital capacity; *MVV,* maximum voluntary ventilation; *PEF,* peak expiratory flow; *VC,* vital capacity; *V_T,* tidal volume.
From Miller MR, Hankinson J, Brusasco V, et al.: Standardisation of spirometry. *Eur Resp J* 26:319-338, 2005.

TABLE 8.2 Key Aspects of Quality Control for Pulmonary Function Testing Equipment

Test	Minimum Interval	Action
Volume	Daily	Calibration check with a 3-L syringe
Leak	Daily	3 cm H_2O (0.3 kPa) constant pressure for 1 minute
Volume linearity	Quarterly	1-L increments with a calibrating syringe measured over entire volume range
Flow linearity	Weekly	Test at least three different flow ranges
Time	Quarterly	Mechanical recorder check with stopwatch
Software	New versions	Log installation date and perform test using "known" subject

From Miller MR, Hankinson J, Brusasco V, et al.: Standardisation of spirometry. *Eur Resp J* 26:319-338, 2005.

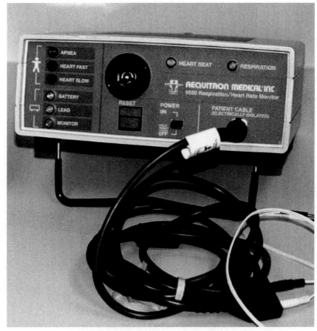

FIGURE 8.13 Apnea monitor.

Respiratory Inductive Plethysmography

Respiratory inductive plethysmography is based on the principle developed by Konno and Mead[22] that the respiratory system moves with 2 degrees of freedom; that is, it consists of two moving parts: the rib cage and the abdomen. During inspiration the rib cage moves outward as the lungs expand in the thorax. Simultaneously, the abdomen is displaced outward by the downward movement of the diaphragm. Because the two compartments are arranged in a series, the sum of the two displacements can be used to calculate the volume of air inspired (Fig. 8.14).

The respiratory inductive plethysmograph consists of two elastic cloth bands into which insulated polytetrafluoroethylene wire has been sewn in a sinusoidal pattern.[23] One band is placed around the rib cage, and the other is placed around the abdomen. The wires of the two bands are connected to an oscillator, which provides a 20-mV alternating current voltage at a frequency of 300 kHz. Changes in the cross-sectional diameter of the wire caused by changes in the rib cage or abdominal diameter alter the oscillatory frequencies as a function of changes in self-inductance.[20] The frequency alterations are processed and converted to analog voltages, which are displayed on an oscilloscope or with a pen recorder.

The clinical indices most often reported from respiratory inductive plethysmography are the tidal volume (V_T) and respiratory rate. The total compartmental displacement (TCD; or, the sum of rib cage plus abdominal movements) can be expressed as TCD/V_T. The percentage of the total displacement (i.e., V_T) contributed by rib cage (RC) movement is expressed as % RC/V_T.

Respiratory inductive plethysmography has been used extensively in research on respiratory muscle function. It has also been used clinically as a means of monitoring the breathing patterns of patients in sleep laboratories, in pulmonary function laboratories, and in intensive care units (ICUs). In the ICU it has been used primarily to identify the uncoordinated thoracoabdominal movements associated with respiratory muscle fatigue or failure.

Pressure Measurements

In Chapter 1, several simple devices that can be used to measure pressure (e.g., U-shaped tubes and mercury barometers) were described. These devices are effective in measuring constant or slowly changing pressures (e.g., atmospheric pressure) but are limited in their ability to measure dynamic pressures. Pressure changes such as those that occur during breathing can be measured with an aneroid manometer or an electromechanical transducer.

An aneroid manometer (Fig. 8.15) consists of a vacuum chamber with a flexible cover or diaphragm that flexes when pressure is applied to it. This flexing motion is translated into a pressure measurement via a lever system attached to a calibrated scale. The Bourdon gauge, which consists of a coiled tube with a needle attached to a calibrated scale by a gear mechanism (see Chapter 1), is a variation of this concept. As the pressure in the Bourdon tube increases, its force tends to straighten the tube, causing the attached needle to become

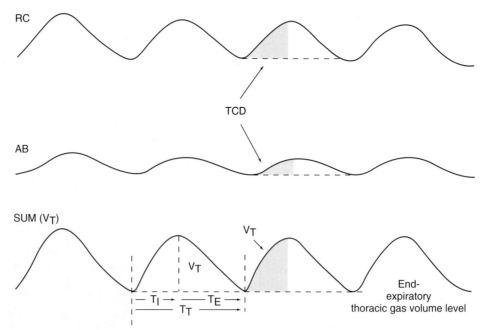

FIGURE 8.14 Idealized respiratory inductive plethysmography tracing showing rib cage *(RC)*, abdominal *(AB)*, and total compartment displacement *(TCD)*. Note that RC and AB motions are in synchrony. TCD equals the sum of RC and AB. Inspiratory time *(T$_I$)*, expiratory time *(T$_E$)*, and total respiratory time *(T$_T$)* are marked on the TCD tracing. *V$_T$*, Tidal volume. (From Branson R, Campbell RS: Impedance pneumography, apnea monitoring, and respiratory inductive plethysmography. In Kacmarek RM, Hess D, Stoller JK, editors: *Monitoring in respiratory care*, St. Louis, 1993, Mosby.)

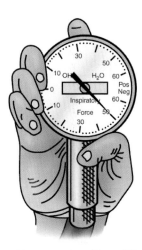

FIGURE 8.15 Aneroid manometer. (From Pilbeam SP: *Mechanical ventilation: physiological and clinical applications*, ed 3, St. Louis, 1998, Mosby.)

displaced. The amount of displacement is measured on the calibrated scale.

Aneroid manometers can be used to obtain instantaneous pressure measurements, such as maximum inspiratory and expiratory pressures. The pressure is displayed relative to atmospheric pressure or as gauge pressure (pounds per square inch gauge [psig]). Thus a gauge pressure of 5 mm Hg measured at sea level (1 atmosphere [atm] = 760 mm Hg) corresponds to an absolute pressure of 765 mm Hg. Although aneroid manometers can measure a wide range of pressures, their frequency response is low.

Electromechanical transducers generally are classified as strain gauge devices, variable inductance devices, or variable capacitance devices.[3] Strain gauge pressure transducers (Fig. 8.16A) use sensors consisting of a metal wire or semiconductor incorporated into a Wheatstone bridge circuit. When pressure is applied to the sensor, the wire or semiconductor elongates, causing its electrical resistance to increase. The increased resistance reduces the output voltage by an amount that is proportional to the applied pressure.

The variable inductance transducer (see Fig. 8.16B) consists of a stainless steel diaphragm positioned between two coils. When the diaphragm is not flexed, the inductance of the two coils is equal. The diaphragm flexes when pressure is applied, changing the inductance between the two coils by an amount proportional to the applied pressure.

The variable capacitance transducer (see Fig. 8.16C) operates similarly to the variable inductance device, except that the diaphragm of the capacitance device constitutes one plate of a capacitor. The other half of the plate is a stationary electrode. Displacement of the diaphragm alters the capacitance of the device and changes the output voltage in a manner that is proportional to the applied pressure.[3]

Strain gauge and variable inductance pressure transducers are commonly used for measuring respiratory and cardiovascular pressures. These devices respond quickly to pressure changes and thus have good frequency response characteristics over a wide range of pressures. They usually are quite stable, being relatively insensitive to vibration and shock.[3] Variable capacitance transducers are large, bulky, very sensitive to vibration, and have poor frequency response compared with strain gauge and variable inductance types of transducers.

Bedside Measurement of Respiratory Mechanics

Current mechanical ventilators have microprocessor units incorporated into their designs for measuring bedside respiratory mechanics, especially during mechanical ventilation. "Stand-alone" units, like the monitor shown in Fig. 8.17, have also been used for obtaining respiratory mechanics measurements. These systems are rarely used today, having been replaced by monitors that are incorporated into current generation mechanical ventilators.

Respiratory system mechanics measurements typically include lung volumes and flows, peak inspiratory pressure (PIP), mean airway pressure ($P_{\overline{aw}}$), plateau pressure (P_{plat}), and intrapleural pressure, which can be approximated by measuring the esophageal pressure. Pneumotachographs are used to measure airflow and airway pressures. Intrapleural pressures are obtained using an electronic transducer attached to the proximal end of a catheter inserted into the esophagus (i.e., esophageal pressure). Esophageal pressures have been shown to be approximately equal to intrapleural pressure. (Triple-lumen catheters, which are multifunctional, may be used for measuring esophageal pressures, as well as for gastric suctioning and feeding.)

Esophageal balloon catheters are relatively thin small-lumen devices that have small holes at the distal end of the catheter. A balloon, which is incorporated into the design of the catheter, covers the distal end of the catheter to prevent the holes from becoming occluded with esophageal tissue or secretions. Correct positioning of the catheter is important to obtain accurate esophageal pressure measurements. The catheter can be inserted nasally or orally to approximately 35 to 40 cm from the airway opening, which places the catheter in the lower third of the esophagus. Alternatively, the catheter can be positioned using the pressure measurements detected as the catheter is inserted. For example, when the catheter enters the stomach, a positive pressure is recorded. Therefore, after the pressure becomes positive, the catheter can be positioned correctly by retracting it until the pressure returns to a negative value. Cardiac oscillations will also be evident on the pressure tracing. The catheter then can be anchored to the nose with surgical tape.

Airflow and pressure measurements are relayed to the system's microprocessor and displayed on a cathode ray tube. The system can display real-time tracings of airway pressure, tidal volume, and airflow measured at the mouth (Fig. 8.18). The microprocessor unit can also provide flow-volume, pressure-volume, and pressure-flow plots, along with calculations of R_{aw}; patient-ventilator compliance; intrinsic, or auto–positive end-expiratory pressure (auto-PEEP); P100 (P0.1); and work of breathing.

Clinical Applications of Respiratory Mechanics Measurements

Respiratory mechanics data can provide valuable information about the ventilatory capacity of a patient with cardiopulmonary

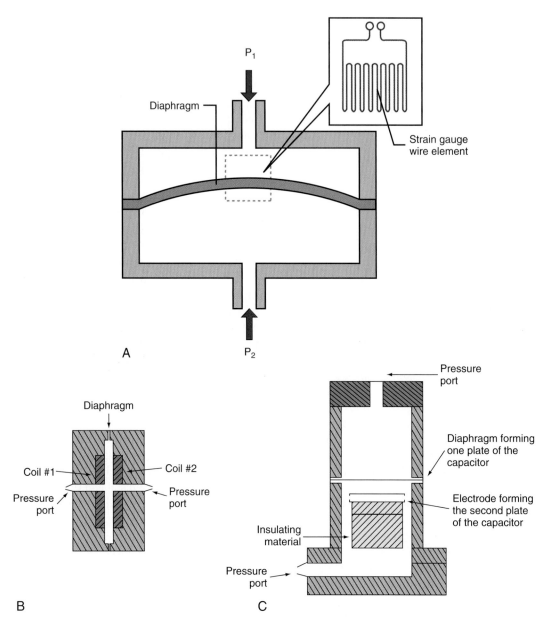

FIGURE 8.16 Electromechanical transducers. A, Strain gauge device. B, Variable inductance device. C, Variable capacitance device. (B and C Courtesy Snow M: Instrumentation. In Clause JL, editor: *Pulmonary function testing guidelines and controversies*, New York, 1992, Academic Press.)

disease. These data generally are divided into two categories: measured and derived variables. Measured variables include lung volumes and capacities, airflow, and airway and intrapleural pressures. Airway resistance, respiratory system compliance, and work of breathing are derived variables that can be calculated from volume, flow, and pressure measurements.[23,24]

Box 8.2 lists some of the more common respiratory mechanics measurements used by clinicians.

Lung Volume Measurements

Laboratory measurements of lung volumes focus on the standard subdivisions shown in Fig. 8.19. As previously stated, simple spirometers can measure three of the four standard lung volumes (i.e., V_T, inspiratory reserve volume [IRV], and

ERV) and therefore the VC and inspiratory capacity (IC). They also can measure all the dynamic lung volumes, including FVC, FEV_1, forced expiratory flow from 25% to 75% of the vital capacity ($FEF_{25\%-75\%}$), and peak flows. The RV, FRC, and TLC cannot be measured with simple spirometry; they require specialized equipment and procedures, such as body plethysmography and inert gas techniques. Simple spirometry routinely is used to diagnose individuals suspected of having a pulmonary dysfunction, to monitor the effectiveness of therapeutic interventions used to treat patients with pulmonary disease, for disability evaluations, and for public health screenings. (Box 8.3 lists the indications for spirometry.) Full lung volume tests usually are reserved for patients who have abnormal spirometry results.[10] Table 8.3 describes the characteristic

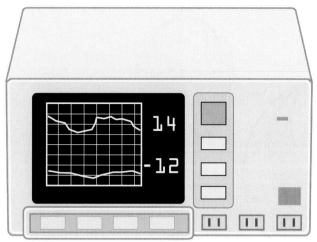

FIGURE 8.17 Bedside respiratory mechanics monitor.

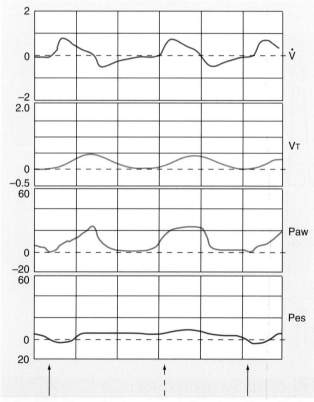

FIGURE 8.18 Real-time tracings of airway pressure (*Paw*), tidal volume (*V_T*), and airflow (*P_{es}*) at the mouth recorded during mechanical ventilation. (From MacIntyre NR, Gropper C: Monitoring ventilatory function. II. Respiratory system mechanics and muscle function. In Levine RL, Fromm RE, editors: *Critical care monitoring: from prehospital to ICU*, St. Louis, 1995, Mosby.)

BOX 8.2   Respiratory Mechanics Measurements

Standard Lung Volumes and Capacities
- Tidal volume (V_T or TV)
- Inspiratory reserve volume (IRV)
- Residual volume (RV)
- Total lung capacity (TLC)
- Vital capacity (VC)
- Functional residual capacity (FRC)
- Inspiratory capacity (IC)

Dynamic Lung Volumes (Flows)
- Forced vital capacity (FVC)
- Forced expiratory volume in 1 second (FEV_1)
- Forced expiratory flow from 25% to 75% of the vital capacity ($FEF_{25\%-75\%}$)
- Peak expiratory flow (PEF)

Minute Ventilation
- Minute volume ($\dot{V}_E$, $\dot{V}_I$, or MV)
- Breathing frequency (f_B)

Respiratory Pressures
- Maximum inspiratory pressure (MIP)
- Maximum expiratory pressure (MEP)
- Peak airway inspiratory pressure (PIP)
- Plateau pressure (P_{plat})

BOX 8.3   Indications for Spirometry

Diagnostic Purposes
- To evaluate symptoms, signs, or abnormal laboratory test results
- To measure the effect of disease on pulmonary function
- To screen individuals at risk for having pulmonary disease
- To assess preoperative risk
- To assess prognosis
- To assess health status before beginning strenuous physical activity programs

Monitoring
- To assess therapeutic intervention
- To describe the course of diseases that affect lung function
- To monitor individuals exposed to injurious agents
- To monitor for adverse reactions to drugs with known pulmonary toxicity

Disability/Impairment Evaluations
- To assess patients as part of a rehabilitation program
- To assess risks as part of an insurance evaluation
- To assess individuals for legal reasons

Public Health
- Epidemiological surveys
- Derivation of reference equations
- Clinical research

Modified from Miller MR, Hankinson J, Brusasco V, et al.: Standardisation of spirometry. *Eur Resp J* 26:319-338, 2005.

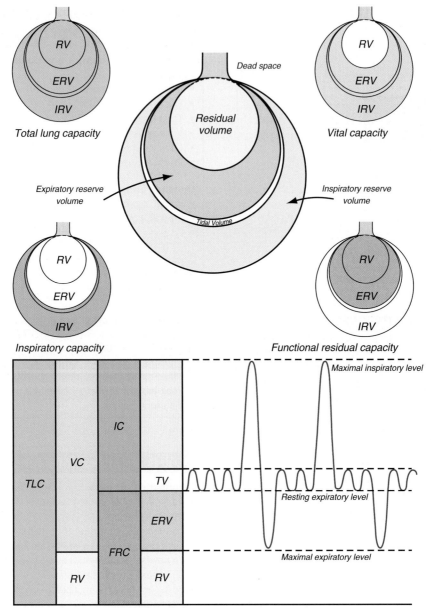

FIGURE 8.19 Standard lung volumes and capacities. *ERV,* Expiratory reserve volume; *FRC,* functional residual capacity; *IC,* inspiratory capacity; *IRV,* inspiratory reserve volume; *RV,* residual volume; *TLC,* total lung capacity; *TV,* tidal volume; *VC,* vital capacity. (From Comroe J: *The lung,* ed 3, Chicago, 1986, Mosby.)

lung volume changes associated with obstructive and restrictive pulmonary disorders, and Clinical Scenario 8.2 presents a case related to lung volume measurements in a patient with chronic obstructive pulmonary disease (COPD).

At the bedside the most commonly measured lung volume is the expired minute volume. In spontaneously breathing patients, the minute volume usually is measured with a hand-held respirometer. For mechanically ventilated patients, the minute volume can be measured by attaching a spirometer to the exhalation valve of the ventilator. In most recently made ventilators, a flow transducer is incorporated into the system design to give continual updates of the V_T and the minute volume. (Note that the minute volume can be calculated based on 5 to 10 breaths and extrapolated to a minute volume value.)

CLINICAL SCENARIO 8.2

The following lung volume measurements were obtained from a 65-year-old man whose chief complaint is shortness of breath on exertion, which has increased significantly during the past year. He has a 40-pack-year history of cigarette smoking (i.e., he smoked 2 packs of cigarettes per day for 20 years). FVC is 60% of predicted, FEV_1 is 50% of predicted, $FEF_{25\%-75\%}$ is 40% of predicted, FEV_1/VC is 60% of predicted, RV is 140% of predicted, and FRC is 150% of predicted. Interpret these results.

See Appendix A for the answer.

$FEF_{25\%-75\%}$, Forced expiratory flow from 25% to 75% of the vital capacity; FEV_1, forced expiratory volume in 1 second; *FRC,* functional residual capacity; *FVC,* forced vital capacity; *RV,* residual volume; *VC,* vital capacity.

TABLE 8.3 Static and Dynamic Lung Volume Changes Associated With Obstructive and Restrictive Pulmonary Disease

	Obstructive Pulmonary Disease	Restrictive Pulmonary Disease
TLC	Increased	Decreased
FRC	Increased	Normal or decreased
VC	Normal or decreased	Decreased
FEV$_1$	Decreased	Decreased
FEV$_1$/VC	Decreased	Normal
FEF$_{25\%-75\%}$	Decreased	Normal
MVV	Decreased	Decreased in severe disease

FEF$_{25\%-75\%}$, Forced expiratory flow from 25% to 75% of the vital capacity; *FEV$_1$*, forced expiratory volume in 1 second; *FEV$_1$/VC*, ratio of forced expiratory volume in 1 second to vital capacity; *FRC*, functional residual capacity; *MVV*, maximum voluntary ventilation; *TLC*, total lung capacity; *VC*, vital capacity.

Minute ventilation expresses the patient's ventilatory needs in liters per minute. The metabolic demands of the tissues and the level of alveolar ventilation influence the minute ventilation required. For example, elevated minute volumes are associated with increased metabolic rates such as during exercise and/or reductions in effective ventilation (i.e., decreased alveolar ventilation or increased dead space ventilation).

Monitoring of dynamic lung volumes can also alert the clinician to significant changes in a patient's R$_{aw}$. PEF measurements are routinely monitored at the bedside to assess the effectiveness of bronchodilator therapy. The same devices can be used at home by asthma patients to monitor daily variations in R$_{aw}$ and thus guide therapeutic interventions.[14] (Clinical Practice Guideline 8.1 summarizes the American Association for Respiratory Care [AARC] Clinical Practice Guideline for assessing the response to a bronchodilator at the point of care.)

Airflow measurements during mechanical ventilation can signal changes in the resistance and compliance of the patient-ventilator system. For example, high-frequency ripples on the inspiratory flow tracing can indicate turbulent flow caused by secretions in the airway or water in the ventilator circuit.[24] Expiratory flow limitations should be suspected if the decay in expiratory flow is linear rather than exponential.[7]

Airway Pressures

The most common airway pressure measurements made on spontaneously breathing patients are the maximum inspiratory pressure (MIP) and maximum expiratory pressure (MEP), peak inspiratory pressure (PIP), P$_{\overline{aw}}$, and static pressure, or plateau pressure (Pplat).

Maximum Inspiratory and Expiratory Pressures

The MIP is obtained by measuring the maximum sustained pressure patients achieve while making a forceful inspiration starting at the RV. The MEP is recorded while the patient makes a forceful effort starting at the TLC. The MIP and MEP are easily obtained from spontaneously breathing patients with an aneroid manometer such as that shown in Fig. 8.15. The MIP normally is −60 to −100 cm H$_2$O, and the MEP is 80 to 100 cm H$_2$O.

Peak Inspiratory Pressure, Mean Airway Pressure, and Plateau Pressure

The PIP, P$_{\overline{aw}}$, and P$_{plat}$ are measured during mechanical ventilation. Instantaneous PIP is the PIP generated during a tidal breath. The PIP can be derived from continuous recordings of airway pressure, which can be made during the breathing cycle using a strain gauge transducer.

P$_{\overline{aw}}$, which is an estimate of the P$_{alv}$, is determined by the PIP, fraction of time that the inspiratory phase lasts (T$_I$/T$_{tot}$), and level of positive end-expiratory pressure (PEEP).[24] The mean airway pressure can be calculated as

$$P_{\overline{aw}} = 0.5 \times [(PIP - PEEP) \times (T_I/T_{tot})] + PEEP$$

The P$_{\overline{aw}}$ during pressure-controlled ventilation, the airway pressure waveform, is a rectangular (square) waveform. During volume-controlled ventilation the airway pressure waveform appears as an ascending (triangular) waveform.

It is important to note that the P$_{\overline{aw}}$ is not a true reflection of the P$_{alv}$ if the inspiratory airway resistance (R$_I$) and the expiratory airway resistance (R$_E$) are different (e.g., as occurs during bronchospasm).[24] The P$_{\overline{aw}}$ can be calculated in these instances using the following formula:

$$P_{alv} = P_{\overline{aw}} + (\dot{V}_E/60) \times (R_E - R_I)$$

Notice that $\dot{V}_E$ is the expired minute ventilation.

The P$_{plat}$ represents the amount of pressure needed to maintain the V$_T$ in the patient's lungs during a period when gas flow is absent. It is determined by the compliance of the lungs and the chest wall during full ventilatory support. The P$_{plat}$ is measured during mechanical ventilation by temporarily occluding the expiratory valve of the ventilator for 0.2 to 0.5 sec at the end of a tidal inspiration and noting the new pressure level. In most newer ventilators a manual control is incorporated into the ventilator circuit to operate an inflation-hold shutter valve, which closes at the end of inspiration.[24,25]

Fig. 8.20 shows a tracing of the measurement of the PIP and P$_{plat}$. Note that the PIP is greater than the P$_{plat}$; however, remember that the PIP is a dynamic measurement, and the P$_{plat}$ is measured under static conditions. The PIP represents the total force that must be applied to overcome the elastic and frictional forces offered by the patient-ventilator system, whereas the P$_{plat}$ represents that portion of the total pressure required to overcome only elastic forces.

Increases in the elastance of the respiratory system (i.e., decreases in compliance of the lung or chest wall) increase both the PIP and P$_{plat}$. Elevated R$_{aw}$ increases the peak airway pressure but does not affect the P$_{plat}$.

Airway Resistance

R$_{aw}$ is the opposition to airflow from nonelastic forces of the lung. Expiratory airway resistance can be calculated by

CLINICAL PRACTICE GUIDELINE 8.1 Assessing the Response to Bronchodilator Therapy at the Point of Care

Indications
1. To confirm appropriateness of therapy
2. To individualize patient's dose per treatment or frequency of administration
3. To help determine the patient's status during acute and long-term pharmacological therapy
4. To determine the need for change of therapy

Contraindications
In cases of acute severe distress, some assessment maneuvers may be contraindicated or should be postponed until therapy and supportive measures have been instituted.

Hazards and Complications
Forced exhalations may be associated with bronchoconstriction, airway collapse, and paroxysmal coughing with or without syncope.

Limitations of Methodology
1. Cost and accessibility.
2. Patient's inability to perform FVC or PEF maneuvers.
3. Accuracy and reproducibility of peak flowmeters vary among models and units; therefore results from the same device should be compared for consistency and accuracy.
4. The measurement of peak flows is an effort-dependent test. The patient should be encouraged to perform the maneuver vigorously. Three trials are desirable; report the best of the three peak flows measured.

5. An artificial airway increases resistance and may limit inspiratory and expiratory flows.

Resources
1. Equipment may include portable laboratory spirometer, peak flowmeter, stethoscope, and pulse oximeter. Spirometers and peak flowmeters should meet ATS standards.
2. Personnel performing the tests should be licensed or credentialed respiratory care practitioners or individuals with equivalent knowledge.
3. The patient or family caregiver providing maintenance therapy must demonstrate an ability to monitor and measure the response to the bronchodilator, use proper technique for administering medication and using the devices, modify doses and frequency as prescribed and instructed in response to adverse reactions or increased severity of symptoms, and appropriately communicate the severity of symptoms to the physician.

Monitoring
The following observations can assist the clinician in assessing the patient's response to bronchodilator therapy:
1. Patient's general appearance, use of accessory muscles, and sputum volume and consistency
2. Patient's vital signs and FVC, FEV_1, PEF, and pulse oximetry measurements
3. In ventilator patients, peak inspiratory pressure (PIP), plateau pressure (P_{plat}), increased inspiratory/expiratory flows (F-V loops), and decreased auto-PEEP

ATS, American Thoracic Society; *auto-PEEP*, auto–positive end-expiratory pressure; *FVC*, forced vital capacity; FEV_1, forced expiratory volume in 1 second; *PEF*, peak expiratory flow.
Modified from the American Association for Respiratory Care: AARC clinical practice guideline: capnography. *Respir Care* 40:1300, 1995.

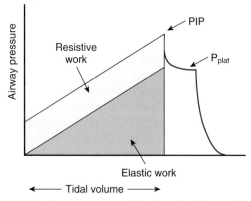

FIGURE 8.20 Airway pressure tracing showing peak airway pressure and plateau pressure (P_{plat}). *PIP*, Peak inspiratory pressure.

subtracting the P_{plat} from the PIP and dividing the resultant pressure by the airflow.

$$R_{aw} = PIP - P_{Plat}/\dot{V}_E$$

Inspiratory airway resistance can be calculated as

$$R_{aw} = PIP - P_{Plat}/\dot{V}_I$$

R_{aw} resistance averages 2 to 5 cm H_2O/L/s in a healthy spontaneously breathing adult. It is determined primarily by the caliber of the airway (according to Poiseuille's law, a twofold decrease in the airway diameter results in a 16-fold increase in R_{aw}). Thus retention of secretions, peribronchiolar edema, and bronchoconstriction associated with asthma result in increased R_{aw}. Smoke inhalation can also cause severe bronchoconstriction. Conversely, bronchodilation causes a reduction in airway resistance, such as occurs after administration of a bronchodilator (see Clinical Practice Guideline 8.1).

Respiratory System Compliance

Respiratory system compliance can be defined simply as the distensibility of the lungs and the chest wall. Lung-thorax compliance (C_{RS}) can be determined by dividing the V_T by the P_{plat} − PEEP. The normal compliance of the respiratory system averages 0.05 to 0.1 L/cm H_2O.

Pathological conditions (e.g., pulmonary interstitial fibrosis, atelectasis, and pulmonary vascular engorgement) reduce the compliance of the pulmonary parenchyma, resulting in increases in both the P_{plat} and PIP (i.e., decreasing lung compliance). Conditions such as kyphoscoliosis and myasthenia gravis increase the PIP and P_{plat} by reducing chest wall compliance.[22]

TABLE 8.4 Measurements of Lung Mechanics Used to Assess Ventilatory Function in Mechanically Ventilated Patients With Obstructive and Restrictive Pulmonary Diseases

Variable	Description	Measuring Technique
Effective compliance (C_{eff})	The reciprocal of the elastic property of the patient-ventilator system (in mL/cm H_2O)	Mandatory (i.e., passive inspiration expiration) breath (V_T); end-inspiratory pause of at least 1 second (P_{plat}); corrected for tubing compression. Calculation: $C_{eff} = V_T/(P_{plat} - \text{Total PEEP})$
Inspiratory resistance	Inspiratory resistive component of patient-ventilator system impedance (cm H_2O × sec × L^{-1})	Mandatory (i.e., passive inspiration and expiration) breath (V_T) with fixed constant flow over fixed time (T_i); end-inspiratory pause as described for C_{eff}. Calculation: $R_1 = \dfrac{P_{peak} - P_{plate}}{V_T/T_i}$
Expiratory resistance	Expiratory resistive component of the patient-ventilator system (cm H_2O × sec × L^{-1})	Mandatory (i.e., passive inspiration and expiration) breath (V_T); end-inspiratory pause as described for C_{eff}. Calculation: $R_E = \dfrac{P_{plat} - \text{Total PEEP}}{\text{Flow at onset of exhalation}}$
Mean airway pressure	Average airway pressure over a respiratory cycle	Mean airway pressure should be reported over a time period that includes a representative number of machine- and patient-cycled breaths.
Maximum inspiratory pressure	Maximum negative inspiratory pressure generated by patient against closed circuit	One-way valve allowing expiration; 15 to 20 seconds.
Intrinsic positive end-expiratory pressure (auto-PEEP)	Positive end-expiratory alveolar pressure resulting from inadequate expiratory time, dynamic airway collapse, or both	Auto-PEEP measurement is clinically important but may be difficult during spontaneous or assisted breathing. It is recommended that the ventilator be equipped with an expiratory hold control to facilitate manual determination of auto-PEEP by airway occlusion as close to the proximal airway as possible; circuit pressures should stabilize during the expiratory hold. Measurement reflects total PEEP but tends to underestimate the intrinsic component because of pressure equilibration in compliant circuitry.

PEEP, Positive end-expiratory pressure; *P_{plat}*, plateau pressure; *V_T*, tidal volume.
From MacIntyre NR, Gropper C: Monitoring ventilatory function. II. Respiratory system mechanics and muscle function. In Levine RL, Fromm RE, editors: *Critical care monitoring: from prehospital to ICU*, St. Louis, 1995, Mosby.

Work of Breathing

In normal, healthy individuals the work of breathing constitutes only approximately 2% to 5% of total oxygen consumption; normal work of breathing is approximately 0.3 to 0.7 J/L. The work of breathing can rise sharply with pathological pulmonary conditions that lead to increases in R_{aw} or decreases in respiratory system compliance (i.e., decreases in lung compliance [C_L] or chest wall compliance [C_{CW}]), and thus increased oxygen consumption.

Although there has been an increased interest in using work of breathing measurements in clinical practice, the technique for manually obtaining and calculating work of breathing is somewhat difficult to master and limited in use. (The work of breathing feature is available on a limited number of ICU mechanical ventilators [e.g., Puritan-Bennett 840]). The most practical uses proposed have been in establishing optimum levels of pressure-support ventilation, determining the work of breathing for various forms of ventilatory support, and

evaluating a patient's ability to be liberated from mechanical ventilation.

Table 8.4 summarizes the lung mechanics measurements used to assess patients receiving ventilatory support.

II. MEASUREMENT OF INSPIRED OXYGEN

Oxygen Analyzers

Two types of analyzers generally are used for measuring the oxygen concentration in inspired gases: electrochemical analyzers (including polarographic and galvanic devices) and electrical analyzers. A brief discussion of paramagnetic analyzers is included for historical purposes (Historical Note 8.1).

Electrochemical Analyzers

Electrochemical analyzers are the most commonly used oxygen analyzers. They generally are classified as galvanic or polarographic devices.

HISTORICAL NOTE 8.1   **Paramagnetic Oxygen Analyzers**

The paramagnetic oxygen analyzer was first described by Pauling et al.[26] in 1946. The device operates on the principle that oxygen is a paramagnetic gas and the other respired gases (e.g., nitrogen and carbon dioxide) are diamagnetic. Therefore the paramagnetic oxygen molecules align themselves with the strongest part of a heterogeneous magnetic field. Because the diamagnetic nitrogen and carbon dioxide molecules are repelled by the magnetic field, they tend to be found in the weaker part of a magnetic field.

The Beckman D-2 oxygen analyzer is an example of a device that uses the physical principle of paramagnetism to measure oxygen concentration. With this device a glass dumbbell filled with nitrogen is suspended on a quartz string and held in place by two magnets. The dumbbell and the magnets are enclosed within a sample chamber. When oxygen is introduced into this chamber, it is attracted to the magnetic field, which causes the dumbbell to rotate slightly. The amount of rotation depends on the concentration of the oxygen introduced into the chamber. The oxygen concentration can be measured because a mirror attached to the dumbbell reflects a light focused on it onto a translucent scale. The scale is calibrated to display both partial pressures (in mm Hg) and the percentage of oxygen concentration.

A **galvanic analyzer** uses an oxygen-mediated chemical reaction to generate an electrical current. A gold cathode and a lead anode are immersed in a potassium hydroxide bath (Fig. 8.21A). The gas sample is separated from the bath by a semipermeable membrane that usually is made of polytetrafluoroethylene (Teflon). As oxygen diffuses across the membrane into the hydroxide solution, it reacts with water and free electrons from the gold cathode to form hydroxyl ions (OH^-). The OH^- ions diffuse toward the lead (Pb) anode, forming lead oxide (PbO_2), water, and free electrons. The flow of the electrons produces a current that can be measured with an ammeter, and the amount of current flow detected is directly related to the oxygen concentration. (Note that galvanic oxygen analyzers do not have to be "turned on." They continually read 21% oxygen when the sensor is exposed to room air; therefore it is important to keep the sensor capped to prolong its life.)

Polarographic analyzers also use an oxygen-mediated chemical reaction to create current flow, but they differ slightly in design from galvanic devices (see Fig. 8.21B). Polarographic analyzers contain a platinum cathode and a silver anode immersed in a potassium hydroxide bath. Also, they typically use a 9V battery to polarize the silver anode, resulting in an improved response time because the OH^- ions are attracted to the difference in electrical charge. The reaction formula basically is similar to that of galvanic analyzers, but the reaction time is faster.

Galvanic and polarographic analyzers can be used for intermittent or continuous monitoring of the fractional inspired oxygen (F_IO_2) and can be used with flammable gases during anesthesia. Because they respond to changes in partial pressure, readings can be affected by changes in ambient pressure,

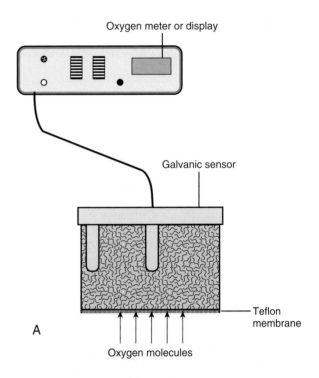

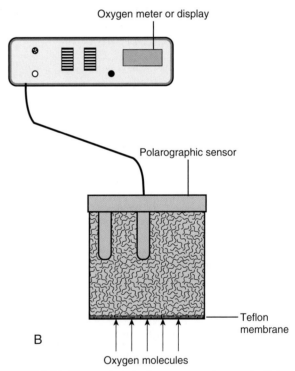

FIGURE 8.21 Electrochemical oxygen analyzers. A, Galvanic device. B, Polarographic device.

as may occur during mechanical ventilation or at high altitudes. Although galvanic analyzers have a slower response time than polarographic analyzers, they do not require an external power supply, and their electrodes may last longer.

Commercially available galvanic analyzers are made by Teledyne, Hudson, Biomarine, and Ohmeda. Polarographic oxygen analyzers are available from SensorMedics/Viasys

Healthcare, Hudson-Ventronics, Instrumentation Laboratory, IMI, Teledyne, and Critikon.

Electrical Analyzers

Electrical analyzers operate on the principle of thermal conductivity and use an electronic device called a *Wheatstone bridge* (Fig. 8.22). Two parallel wires receive current flow from an external power source, usually a battery. One of these wires, which serves as the reference, is exposed to room air. The other wire is located in the sample chamber and is exposed to the gas being analyzed. If the sample gas contains a higher oxygen-to-nitrogen ratio than room air, the sample wire cools, and its resistance decreases because oxygen is a better conductor of heat than nitrogen. Consequently, current flow increases through the sample wire compared with the reference wire. An ammeter detects the change in current flow and relates it to the oxygen concentration.

The primary advantage of an electrical analyzer is that it compares the oxygen concentration of an unknown gas with ambient air. Therefore it is responsive to changes in the percentage of oxygen instead of partial pressure, and it is unaffected by changes in pressure (e.g., those that occur with altitude changes). However, several problems can occur with these devices. For example, the Wheatstone bridge can generate significant amounts of heat and therefore is dangerous to use in the presence of flammable gases. Also, contaminant gases can dissipate heat at rates different from those of oxygen and

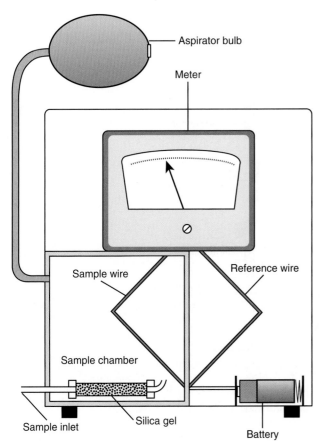

FIGURE 8.22 Electrical oxygen analyzer showing Wheatstone bridge circuit.

nitrogen; therefore, if gases other than oxygen and nitrogen are present, the F_IO_2 levels may be erroneous.

III. MEASUREMENT OF NITROGEN OXIDES

As was discussed in Chapter 4, nitric oxide (NO) is a simple, diatomic molecule that can cause vasodilation, macrophage cytotoxicity, and platelet adhesion.[27] NO has been used to successfully treat pulmonary hypertension in neonates and to improve gas exchange in critically ill patients.[28,29]

Because of the potential for pulmonary toxicity induced by high levels of NO and nitrogen dioxide (NO_2), it is important to monitor the concentration of these molecules when NO is used clinically. Body et al.[29] provided an excellent review of NO measurement. Two types of monitoring systems are routinely used when NO is administered: chemiluminescence monitoring and electrochemical monitoring.

Chemiluminescence Monitoring

Chemiluminescence monitoring involves the quantification of gas-specific photoemission.[27] Gases sampled by the chemiluminescence monitor react with ozone (O_3) to produce NO_2 with an electron in an unstable, excited state (NO_2^* is the chemical symbol indicating that it is an excited chemical state of NO_2). Because this unstable molecule decays to its lower energy (ground) state, photons are emitted with energies in the wavelength range of 600 to 3000 nanometers (nm).[27] Photon emissions are measured by photomultiplier tubes and electronically converted into a displayable signal.

NO_2 levels can be measured indirectly by converting NO_2 to NO with a catalytic or chemical converter and then by measuring the NO concentration as described previously.[29] Thermal catalytic converters, which are made of stainless steel, operate at temperatures of 600°C (1112°F) to 800°C (1472°F).[29] Chemical converters rely on molybdenum and carbon to convert NO_2 to NO. Although chemical converters must be replenished periodically, they can be used at lower temperatures and are more stable than catalytic converters. They are also less affected by interference from other gases.

Measuring the total concentration of nitrogen oxides and subtracting the NO concentration can be used to determine the NO_2 concentration. Fig. 8.23 shows the schematics of two types of commercially available chemiluminescence nitrogen oxide monitors. A single–reaction chamber model (Fig. 8.23A) is used to measure NO and NO_2. This system operates on the principle that the NO_2 converter is switched into the sample line at 10- to 30-second intervals. A dual–reaction chamber device (Fig. 8.23B) uses two separate chambers to measure NO and NO_2, and a single photomultiplier tube measures the outputs of both chambers.

The accuracy of a chemiluminescence monitor can be altered either by variations in the sample gas composition or by interference with the operation of the photomultiplier tubes. Variations in the composition of the sample gas can result from quenching of excited states of NO_2, false identification of contaminant gases (e.g., NO_2), and alterations in the viscosity of the sample gas by background gases. Quenching

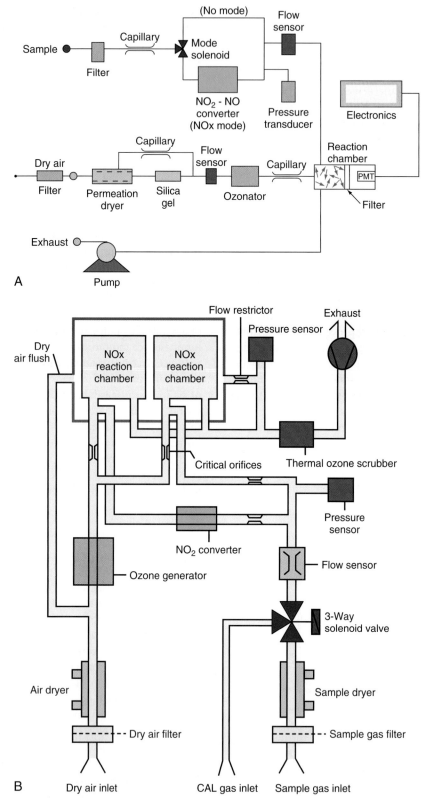

FIGURE 8.23 Schematic illustrating two types of chemiluminescence nitrogen oxide monitors. A, Single-reaction chamber chemiluminescence device. B, Dual-reaction chamber chemiluminescence device. *CAL,* Calibration gas; *PMT,* photomultiplier tube. (From Body S, Hartigan PM, Shernan SK, et al.: Nitric oxide: delivery, measurement, and clinical application. *J Cardiothorac Vasc Anesth* 9:748, 1995.)

occurs when NO_2 is converted to ground state NO_2 by inadvertent collisions of the former gases with other background gases, such as oxygen, carbon dioxide, and water.[27] Ammonia (NH_2) and nitrous oxide (N_2O) are two gases that can be falsely identified as NO_2. Increases in the viscosity of the sample gas (such as can occur with high percentages of oxygen) reduce the gas flow into the reaction chamber, thus reducing the number of NO molecules entering the chamber. Inaccuracies caused by photomultiplier tube interference generally are associated with photon emissions from contaminating gases in the sample reaction chamber and with thermal fluctuations.

Electrochemical Monitoring

Electrochemical monitoring is based on a principle similar to that used with polarographic (Clark) electrodes; that is, gases diffusing across a semipermeable membrane react with an electrolyte solution, generating a current flow between two polarized electrodes as electrons are liberated or consumed.[27]

An electrochemical NO analyzer (Fig. 8.24) consists of three electrodes (a sensing electrode, a counter electrode, and a reference electrode) immersed in an electrolyte solution that contains a highly conductive concentrated acid or alkali solution. The electrodes are separated from the gas sample to be analyzed by a semipermeable membrane. NO and NO_2 from

the unknown gas sample diffuse across a semipermeable membrane and react with the electrolyte solution near the sensing electrode, generating electrons in the following oxidation reaction:

$$NO + 2H_2O \rightarrow HNO_3 + 3H^+ + 3e^-$$

The electrons generated are consumed at the counter-electrode through the reduction of oxygen, or

$$O_2 + 4H^+ + 4e^- \rightarrow 2H_2O$$

Balancing the equations at both electrodes yields the following equation:

$$4NO + 2H_2O + 3O_2 \rightarrow 4HNO_3$$

NO_2 can be measured by electrochemical analysis using a similar principle. In this series of reactions, NO_2 is reduced to NO at the sensing electrode, and H_2O is oxidized at the counterelectrode, or

$$NO_2 + 2H^+ + 2e^- \rightarrow NO + H_2O$$

$$2H_2O \rightarrow 4H + 4e^- + O_2$$

The accuracy of NO/NO_2 electrochemical monitors can be altered by increases in ambient pressure (as occur with positive-pressure ventilation) and also by the presence of background

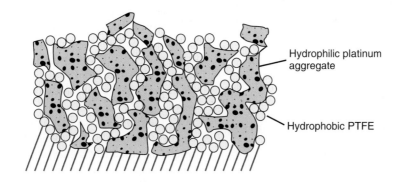

Hydrophilic platinum aggregate

Hydrophobic PTFE

A   PTFE backing tape membrane

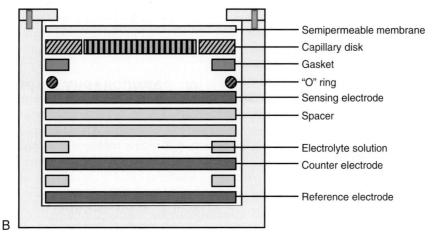

B

Semipermeable membrane
Capillary disk
Gasket
"O" ring
Sensing electrode
Spacer
Electrolyte solution
Counter electrode
Reference electrode

FIGURE 8.24 Schematic of an electrochemical nitrogen oxide monitor. *PTFE,* Polytetrafluoroethylene. (From Body S, Hartigan PM, Shernan SK, et al.: Nitric oxide: delivery, measurement, and clinical application, *J Cardiothorac Vasc Anesth* 9:748, 1995.)

BOX 8.4   Proposed Standards for Nitric Oxide and Nitrogen Dioxide Monitoring Devices[a]

Monitoring Range
1 ppm NO lower limit; no upper limit specified
1 to 5 ppm NO_2

Accuracy[b]
≤20 ppm NO; ±20% of NO concentration, or 0.5 ppm, which-
    ever is greater.
>20 ppm NO; ±10% of NO concentration
±20% of NO_2 concentration

Response Time
10% to 90% of full signal response time <30 seconds

Alarms
Audible and visual alarms: for NO, an upper-level alarm able
    to be sent from 2 ppm NO to maximum signal; for NO_2,
    an upper-level alarm able to be sent from 2 ppm NO_2 to
    maximum signal.

Other Considerations
Electrical safety (IEC601-1)
Electromagnetic compatibility and immunity (IEC601-1-2)
Environmental protection (temperature, humidity, and spill
    resistance)
Environmental pollution
Software safety (IEC601-1-4)

[a]The US Food and Drug Administration (FDA) has proposed these standards.
[b]The stated accuracy must be present in the following background gases: 0 and 5 ppm NO_2 (for NO monitoring); 0, 10, and 40 ppm NO (for NO_2 monitoring); 21%, 60%, and 95% oxygen and 0%, 50%, and 100% relative humidity. If the monitoring device is placed within the ventilator circuit and subject to lung inflation pressures, the accuracy must be maintained over a pressure range of −15 to 100 cm H_2O.
Modified from Body SC, Hartigan PM: Manufacture and measurement of nitrogen oxides. *Respir Care Clin N Am* 3:414, 1997.

TABLE 8.5   Comparisons of Chemiluminescence and Electrochemical Monitoring Devices

Factor	Electrochemical Device	Chemiluminescence Device
Cost	$2500 to $5800	$11,00 to $23,000
Ease of use	+ + +	+
Ease of servicing	+ + +	+
Ease of setup	+ + +	+
Accuracy	+	+ + +
Response time	10 to 30 seconds	0.15 to 20 seconds
Measurement range	+ +	+ + +
Size	+ + +	+
O_2% correction required	No	Yes
Ozone production	No	Yes

Modified from Body S, Hartigan PM, Shernan SK, et al.: Nitric oxide: delivery, measurement, and clinical application. *J Cardiothorac Vasc Anesth* 9:748, 1995.

gases (e.g., carbon dioxide [CO_2], carbon monoxide [CO], and NH_2) that have lower oxidation potentials than the sensor potential. The accuracy of these electrochemical monitors is also limited in the clinical setting for NO concentrations less than 0.1 ppm.[30]

Box 8.4 lists the standards set by the US Food and Drug Administration for NO and NO_2 monitoring devices. Table 8.5 compares chemiluminescence and electrochemical nitrogen oxide analyzers.

Exhaled Nitric Oxide Monitoring

As previously stated, nitric oxide has potent dilatory effects on the pulmonary vessels and airways. The synthesis of NO by the body is mediated through a series of enzymes that are referred to as NO synthases (NOS), which exist in constitutive and inducible forms. The constitutive form is associated with endothelial and neural cells; the inducible NOS is particularly seen in epithelial cells. Although both forms of NOS are present in the airways, the expression of the inducible NOS appears to correlate with the level of NO found in exhaled air.

The most common method used to quantify the level of exhaled NO is chemiluminescence. The fraction of exhaled nitric oxide (FeNO) can be detected in exhaled gas in the range of 7.8 to 41.1 parts per billion (ppb).[31] It is important to mention that the concentration of NO can vary with the flow of exhaled air because it is continually formed in the airways. The presence of pathological conditions, as well as the patient's gender, atopic status, smoking habits, and use of medications can affect the level of FeNO measured. Box 8.5 provides a list of factors that have been shown to affect the levels of eNO.

Exhaled NO is currently used as a marker for airway inflammation associated with asthma.[31] Monitoring the level of eNO can also be used to monitor the effectiveness of inhaled corticosteroid in the treatment of asthma patients. Table 8.6 provides an outline for FeNO interpretation.[31]

IV. CAPNOGRAPHY (CAPNOMETRY)

Capnography, or capnometry, is the continuous measurement of CO_2 concentrations at the airway opening during respiration. The term *capnography* is used to describe the technique in which the CO_2 concentration is displayed as a graphic waveform called a capnogram; *capnometry* is the technique in which the CO_2 concentration is displayed as a numeric reading.[28] In both cases the CO_2 concentration can be displayed in millimeters of mercury (i.e., mm Hg), representing the partial pressure, or as a percentage of CO_2.[32]

Several methods are used to measure CO_2, including infrared (IR) spectroscopy, mass spectroscopy, and Raman spectroscopy.

BOX 8.5   **Factors Affecting Exhaled Nitric Oxide Levels**

Conditions Associated With Reductions in Exhaled NO
Systemic hypertension
Pulmonary hypertension
Cystic fibrosis
Sickle cell anemia
Ciliary dyskinesia

Conditions Associated With Elevated Levels of Exhaled NO
Asthma
Bronchiectasis
Airway viral infections
Alveolitis
Allergic rhinitis
Pulmonary sarcoidosis
Chronic bronchitis
Systemic sclerosis
Pneumonia

Courtesy Aerocrine, Solna, Sweden.

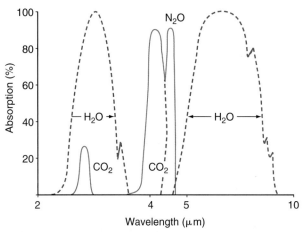

FIGURE 8.25 Infrared absorption spectra for carbon dioxide, nitrous oxide, and water. (From Hess D: Capnometry and capnography: technical aspects, physiological aspects, and clinical applications. *Respir Care* 35:558, 1990.)

TABLE 8.6   **FeNO levels and Inflammation**

FeNO (ppb)	Normal	Elevated	High
Adults	<20-25	20/25-50	>50
Children	<15-20	15/20-35	>35

FeNO, Exhaled NO.
Modified from Dweik RA, Boggs PB, Erzurum SC, et al.: Interpretation of exhaled nitric oxide levels (F$_E$NO) for clinical applications. *Am J Respir Crit Care Med* 184:602-615, 2011.

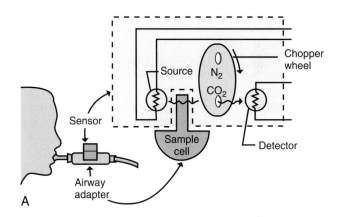

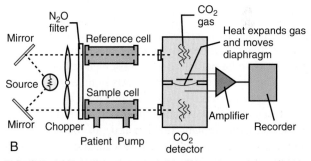

FIGURE 8.26 A, Single-beam nondispersive infrared capnograph. B, Double-beam nondispersive infrared capnograph. (Redrawn from Gravenstein JS, Paulus DA, Hayes TJ: *Capnography in clinical practice*, Boston, 1989, Butterworth.)

IR and Raman spectrometers are portable devices used by individual patients. Mass spectrometers are shared devices that can sample gases from 10 to 12 patients. IR spectroscopy currently is the method of choice in critical care settings, and mass spectroscopy most often is used in surgical suites. The use of Raman spectroscopy for capnography is limited.

Infrared Spectroscopy

IR spectroscopy is based on the principle that molecules containing more than one element absorb IR light in a characteristic manner.[33] Normally, CO_2 maximally absorbs IR radiation at 4.26 μm. The CO_2 concentration of a gas sample can be estimated because the amount of CO_2 in a gas sample is directly related to the amount of IR light absorbed.[34]

The peak CO_2 absorption is very close to the absorption peaks for water and N_2O (Fig. 8.25). Therefore, if water or N_2O is present, the CO_2 readings during IR monitoring can be erroneous. Passing the gas sample through an absorbent (i.e., drying the sample) before it is analyzed can eliminate the effects of water vapor on the measurement. N_2O artifacts can be removed with filters or by using correction factors.[35]

The two types of IR capnographs are a single-beam, negative filter device (Fig. 8.26A) and a double-beam, positive filter capnograph (Fig. 8.26B). With the single-beam device, the

sample gas is directed to a sample chamber that lies between the IR radiation source and a detection chamber. A chopper blade with two transparent cells (one containing CO_2 and the other containing nitrogen) is positioned between the sample chamber and the detector. Gas passing through the sample must pass through the circulating chopper cells before reaching the detection chamber. As the blade turns, two signals are generated, the ratio of which is detected and used to calculate the CO_2 concentration.

CLINICAL SCENARIO 8.3

A patient is being monitored with sidestream capnography. Although no problems were noted during the initial period of monitoring, the capnograph now shows an irregular waveform because the percentage of CO_2 does not rise above 1%. What could cause this?

See Appendix A for the answer.

In the double-beam analyzer, gas is drawn into a sample chamber that contains a cuvette made of sodium chloride and sodium bromide.[33] IR radiation is beamed through the cuvette containing the sample of gas to be analyzed and through a reference chamber containing gas free of CO_2. The CO_2 in the sample chamber absorbs some of the radiation, thereby reducing the amount of radiation reaching the detector. The difference between the radiation transmitted through the sample cell and the radiation transmitted through the reference causes a diaphragm within the detector chamber to move. This movement is converted into an electrical signal, which is amplified and displayed in millimeters of mercury (representing the partial pressure) or a percentage of CO_2.[36]

Clinicians generally classify IR analyzers as sidestream or mainstream devices, depending on the method used to sample gases at the airway. With a sidestream capnograph (Fig. 8.27A), the gas to be analyzed is aspirated from the airway at a flow rate of approximately 500 mL/min through a narrow-bore polyethylene tube and transferred to the sample chamber, which is located in a separate console. With a mainstream capnograph (Fig. 8.27B), analysis is performed at the airway, and gas passes into the sampling chamber, which is attached directly to the endotracheal tube (ETT).

Although sidestream devices are quite reliable, they have a slight delay between sampling and reporting times because of the time required to transport the sample from the airway to the sample chamber. Consequently, these devices may not be appropriate for patients breathing at high rates (e.g., neonates). The plastic tube that transports sample gas from the airway to the analyzer is prone to plugging by water and secretions and therefore can lead to erroneous readings. Contamination with ambient air from leaks in the sample line also is a concern. Clinical Scenario 8.3 illustrates a common problem that occurs with a sidestream capnograph.

Mainstream capnography does not have a delay between sampling and reporting times because the analyzer is attached directly to the ETT. However, these devices add dead space to the airway, which must be quantified to prevent erroneous readings of the partial pressure of CO_2. The additional weight placed on the artificial airway by this type of analyzer increases the possibility of dislodgment or complete extubation. It should also be recognized that because this type of analyzer is directly attached to the airway, it is subject to damage from mishandling (i.e., dropping the device on the floor).

Mass Spectroscopy

Mass spectroscopy is based on the principle that gas molecules can be identified by their mass-to-charge ratio when they are

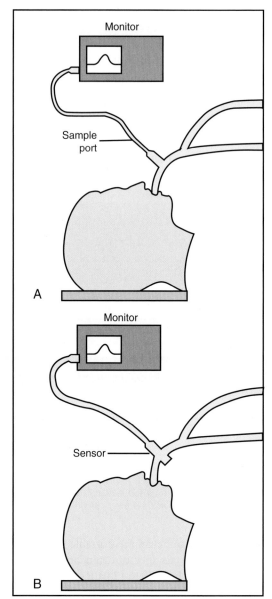

FIGURE 8.27 Classification of capnographs by sampling technique. A, Sidestream capnograph: exhaled gas is extracted through small-bore tubing and transported to a console containing the infrared sensor. B, Mainstream capnograph: exhaled gas is measured at the airway.

passed through a magnetic field (Fig. 8.28). The gas to be analyzed is aspirated into a chamber and ionized by a stream of electrons emitted from a filament. The ionized gas molecules are accelerated and deflected by a magnetic field onto a collector plate. The amount of deflection depends on their mass-to-charge ratio. The gas molecules are then separated according to their mass-to-charge ratio, and as they reach the collector plate, they generate a signal that is picked up by a detector. The strength of the signal, which depends on the number of particles detected, can then be amplified and displayed.[36]

Although mass spectrometers are expensive, they can be used for several patients (i.e., multiplexing in the surgical suite) and can be used to measure gases other than CO_2, including oxygen, nitrogen, and N_2O. This added capacity

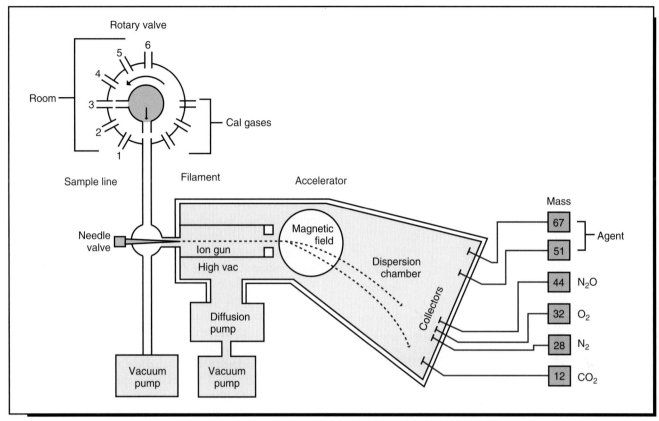

FIGURE 8.28 Schematic of a mass spectrometer. *Cal,* Calibration gases. (Redrawn from Gravenstein JS, Paulus DA, Hayes TJ: *Capnography in clinical practice,* Boston, 1989, Butterworth.)

does have drawbacks, however, because CO_2 and N_2O have the same molecular weight. Therefore separation on the basis of weight alone can lead to erroneous readings. This problem is overcome by ionizing N_2O to N_2O^+ and CO_2 to C^+.[34,37]

Raman Spectroscopy

Raman spectroscopy relies on the Raman effect, which occurs when light interacts with gas molecules to cause rotational or vibrational energy changes in the gas molecules. The light that is emitted from a gas molecule as it relaxes to its original state results in a shift in the wavelength that is characteristic of the molecule being analyzed. For example, monochromatic radiation passed through a gas mixture demonstrates a spectral change that depends on the structure of the individual molecules present in the gas mixture.[37]

Although Raman spectroscopy has been available for some time, its use in clinical medicine is still somewhat limited. Because the accuracy of these devices has been shown to be similar to that of mass spectroscopy, future use of this technology is promising.

Physiological Basis of Capnography

Under normal circumstances, inspired air contains very little CO_2 (approximately 0.3%). Expired air, on the other hand, contains approximately 4% to 6% CO_2. Fig. 8.29 shows an idealized capnogram of a resting individual who is quietly breathing room air. This waveform, which is divided into four phases, reflects the elimination of CO_2 from the lungs during respiration. During phase 1, gas is exhaled from the large conducting airways, which contain essentially no CO_2. In phase 2, some alveolar gas containing CO_2 mixes with gas from the smaller conducting airways, and the CO_2 concentration rises. During phase 3 the CO_2 concentration curve remains relatively constant, as primarily alveolar gas is exhaled (alveolar plateau). (The concentration of CO_2 at the end of the alveolar phase [just before the inspiration begins] is called the *end-tidal PCO_2* [$P_{ET}CO_2$].) On inspiration (phase 4) the concentration falls to zero.

The amount of CO_2 in exhaled air depends on the balance between CO_2 production and the elimination. Production is determined primarily by the metabolic rate, whereas elimination depends on alveolar ventilation, which ultimately is influenced by the ventilation/perfusion ($\dot{V}/\dot{Q}$) ratio of the lungs.

The relationship between the $\dot{V}/\dot{Q}$ and gas exchange (i.e., the partial pressure of alveolar carbon dioxide [P_ACO_2]) therefore can be expressed with $\dot{V}/\dot{Q}$ relationships. Fig. 8.30 shows three $\dot{V}/\dot{Q}$ relationships that can affect the partial pressure of arterial carbon dioxide ($PaCO_2$). In Fig. 8.30A, ventilation and perfusion are equally matched; the $PaCO_2$ and P_ACO_2 are nearly equal. Note that although the $P_{ET}CO_2$ should equal the $PaCO_2$, it actually is approximately 4 to 6 mm Hg lower than the $PaCO_2$. In Fig. 8.30B, ventilation declines relative to perfusion (low $\dot{V}/\dot{Q}$, or shunt). The P_ACO_2 eventually equilibrates with the partial pressure of CO_2 in mixed venous blood. This type of $\dot{V}/\dot{Q}$ relationship can exist throughout the lung in a number of clinical conditions, leading to higher than normal levels of $P_{ET}CO_2$. These conditions include respiratory center depression, muscular paralysis, and COPD. In Fig. 8.30C, ventilation is higher than perfusion (high $\dot{V}/\dot{Q}$, or dead space ventilation). Physiological dead space ventilation increases, and the P_ACO_2 approaches inspired air (0 mm Hg). Decreased $P_{ET}CO_2$ levels are found with this type of $\dot{V}/\dot{Q}$ relationship in patients with pulmonary embolism, excessive PEEP (mechanical or intrinsic), and any disorder involving pulmonary hypoperfusion.

Clinical Applications of Capnography

Capnography can be used both for spontaneously breathing patients and for those who are mechanically ventilated. Because capnography has been used primarily with mechanically ventilated patients, the AARC has prepared a guideline for the use of capnography to monitor such patients.[31] Clinical Practice Guideline 8.2 summarizes the key points of this guideline.

Capnogram contours. In mechanically ventilated patients, capnography can be used to detect increases in dead space ventilation, hyperventilation and hypoventilation, apnea (periodic breathing), inadequate neuromuscular blockade in pharmacologically paralyzed patients, and CO_2 rebreathing. It also can be used to monitor gas exchange during cardiopulmonary resuscitation (CPR). Fig. 8.31 shows various capnogram contours characteristic of several common situations.

When physiological dead space increases, as in COPD, phase 3 becomes indistinguishable (see Fig. 8.31A). Hyperventilation is characterized by a reduction in the $PaCO_2$ and therefore in the $P_{ET}CO_2$ (see Fig. 8.31B). Conversely, hypoventilation is associated with elevated levels of $PaCO_2$ and $P_{ET}CO_2$ (see Fig. 8.31B). Fig. 8.31C shows a capnogram from a patient demonstrating Cheyne-Stokes breathing. During bradypnea, phase 3 typically shows cardiac oscillations that result from the transferal of the beating heart motion to the conducting airways (see Fig. 8.31D). Rebreathing of exhaled gas is recognized because the capnogram does not return to baseline (see Fig. 8.31E). Fig. 8.31F shows a capnogram demonstrating the characteristic phase 3 "curare cleft" that can occur when a patient is receiving insufficient neuromuscular blockade.[34,36]

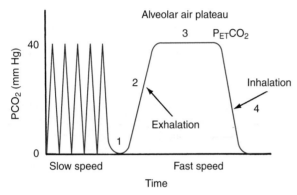

FIGURE 8.29 Idealized capnogram of a resting individual breathing room air. *1,* Exhaled gas from conducting airways; *2,* mixture of conducting airways and alveolar air; *3,* alveolar plateau; *4,* inspired air (0.3% CO_2). *PCO_2,* Partial pressure of carbon dioxide; *$P_{ET}CO_2$,* partial pressure of end-tidal carbon dioxide. (From Cairo JM: *Pilbeam's mechanical ventilation: physiological and clinical applications,* ed 5, St. Louis, 2012, Mosby-Elsevier.)

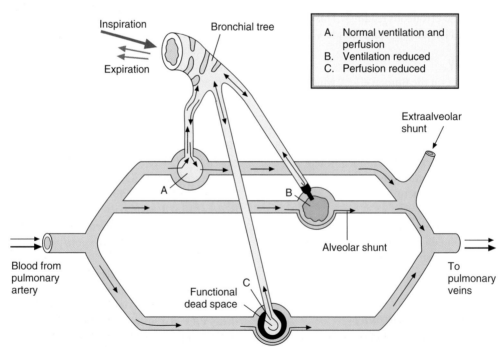

FIGURE 8.30 Ventilation/perfusion ($\dot{V}/\dot{Q}$) relationships. *A,* Normal $\dot{V}/\dot{Q}$; *B,* low $\dot{V}/\dot{Q}$; *C.* high $\dot{V}/\dot{Q}$. (Modified from Despopoulos A, Sibernagl S: *Color atlas of physiology,* ed 4, New York, 1991, Thieme.)

CLINICAL PRACTICE GUIDELINE 8.2   Capnography/Capnometry During Mechanical Ventilation

Indications

Based on current evidence, capnography is useful for:

1. Verification of artificial airway placement.
2. As an adjunct to determine whether tracheal rather than esophageal intubation has been achieved.
3. Monitoring of effective ventilation through a supraglottic airway such as a laryngeal mask airway.
4. Evaluating the efficiency and quality of chest compressions during cardiopulmonary resuscitation (CPR).
5. Detecting inadvertent airway intubation during gastric insertion.
6. Assessment of pulmonary circulation and respiratory status.
7. Optimization of mechanical ventilation by allowing for continuous monitoring of the integrity of the patient-ventilator circuit interface.
8. Monitoring of the severity of pulmonary disease and evaluating the response to therapeutic interventions, particularly those intended to improve the effectiveness of ventilation.
9. Measuring the volume of CO_2 eliminated to assess metabolic rate and alveolar ventilation.

Contraindications

No absolute contraindications to capnography in mechanically ventilated adult patients have been established.

Hazards and Complications

1. The composition of the respiratory gas may affect the capnogram, depending on the measurement technique used.
2. The presence of high airways resistance, respiratory rate, and inspiratory time-to-expiratory time (I:E) ratio may decrease the accuracy of a measurement obtained by a sidestream capnograph compared with a mainstream capnograph.
3. Secretions and condensate may contaminate a capnograph monitor. Additionally, using a sampling tube or obstruction of the sampling chamber can lead to unreliable results.
4. Use of filters between the patient airway and the capnograph's sampling line may lead to artificially low $P_{ET}CO_2$ readings.
5. Various conditions can lead to false-negative results, such as when a low cardiac output is present. Negative confirmation

of ETT placement can occur if it is placed in the esophagus or if it is placed in an airway if there is poor or absent pulmonary blood flow.

6. False-positive readings can result with colorimetric CO_2 detectors if contaminated with acidic or CO_2-filled gastric contents or intratracheal medications (e.g., epinephrine). A transient rise in $P_{ET}CO_2$ can occur after administration of sodium bicarbonate.
7. Elimination and detection of CO_2 can be dramatically reduced in patients with severe airway obstruction or pulmonary edema.
8. Inaccurate measurements of exhaled CO_2 may be caused by leaks in the ventilator circuit, the tracheal tube cuff, or mask, and if a bronchopleural fistula is present. Dialysis and extracorporeal life support can also affect the accuracy of expired CO_2 measurements.

Recommendations

1. Continuous waveform capnography is recommended in addition to clinical assessment as the most reliable method of confirming and monitoring correct placement of an ETT.
2. If waveform capnography is not available, a nonwaveform exhaled CO_2 monitor in addition to clinical assessment is suggested as the initial method for confirming correct tube placement in a patient in cardiac arrest.
3. $P_{ET}CO_2$ is suggested as a method to guide ventilator management.
4. Continuous capnometry during transport of a mechanically ventilated patient is suggested.
5. Capnography is suggested to identify abnormalities of exhaled air flow.
6. Volumetric capnography is suggested to assess CO_2 elimination and volume of distribution-to-tidal volume ratio (V_D/V_T) to optimize mechanical ventilation.
7. Quantitative waveform capnography is suggested in intubated patients to monitor CPR quality, optimize chest compressions, and detect the return of spontaneous circulation during chest compressions or when rhythm check reveals an organized rhythm.

ETT, Endotracheal tube; $P_{ET}CO_2$, partial pressure of end-tidal carbon dioxide.
Modified from the American Association for Respiratory Care: AARC clinical practice guideline: capnography during mechanical ventilation 2011. *Respir Care* 56(4):503-509, 2011.

Capnography also can be used to detect cessation of pulmonary blood flow, as occurs with pulmonary embolism and during cardiac arrest.[28,30,32] A number of investigators have advocated the use of capnography as an adjunct to CPR. Laboratory studies suggest that capnography can be used as an indication of the progress and success of CPR. These studies demonstrated that the $P_{ET}CO_2$ increases as $\dot{V}/\dot{Q}$ is restored to normal.[33,34]

In addition, capnography can be used during CPR to detect accidental esophageal intubation.[32,36] The gastric partial pressure of carbon dioxide (PCO_2) generally is equal to room air. Therefore failure to detect the characteristic changes in the CO_2 concentration during ventilation may indicate esophageal intubation. However, low perfusion of the lungs is also associated with a low $P_{ET}CO_2$ and should not be

confused with esophageal intubation. Also, the gastric PCO_2 may be elevated after mouth-to-mouth breathing or ingestion of a carbonated beverage.

Arterial to maximum end-expiratory PCO_2 difference. The arterial to end-tidal partial pressure of carbon dioxide (a-et PCO_2) for tidal breathing should be negligible (essentially zero). It becomes elevated in patients with COPD, left-heart failure, and pulmonary embolism because of an increase in physiological dead space.[32-34,36]

Another technique that can be used to further evaluate the severity of disease is to compare the $PaCO_2$ measurements with the maximum expired PCO_2 measurements (the arterial to maximum expiratory PCO_2 gradient).[37,38] With this technique the expired PCO_2 recorded at the end of a maximum exhalation to RV is compared with the $PaCO_2$. Normally, the

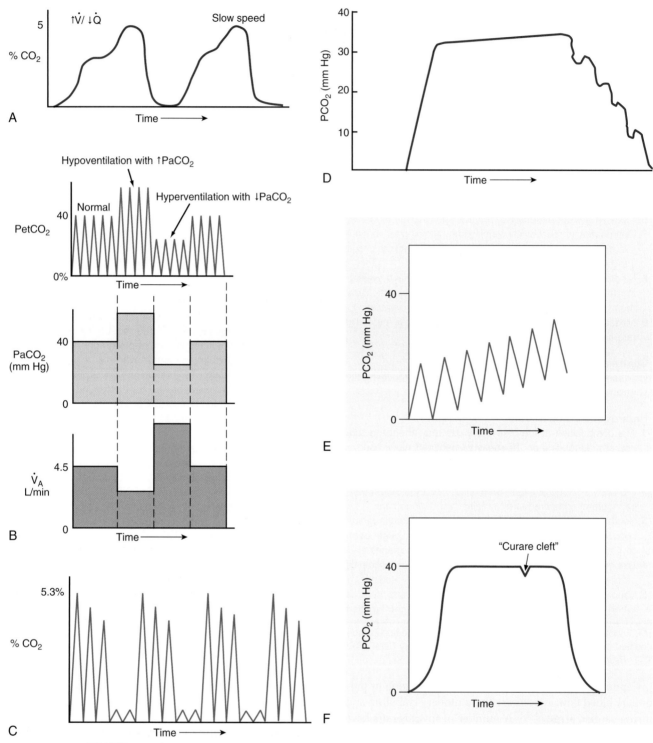

FIGURE 8.31 Capnogram contours associated with various breathing patterns. A, Chronic obstructive pulmonary disease (COPD). B, Hyperventilation and hypoventilation. C, Cheyne-Stokes breathing. D, Cardiac oscillations. E, Rebreathing of exhaled gases. F, Curare cleft. *PaCO2*, Partial pressure of alveolar carbon dioxide; $P_{ET}CO_2$, partial pressure of end-tidal carbon dioxide; $\dot{Q}$, perfusion; $\dot{V}$, ventilation; $\dot{V}_A$, alveolar ventilation. (From Cairo JM: *Pilbeam's mechanical ventilation: physiological and clinical applications*, ed 6, St. Louis, 2016, Mosby-Elsevier.)

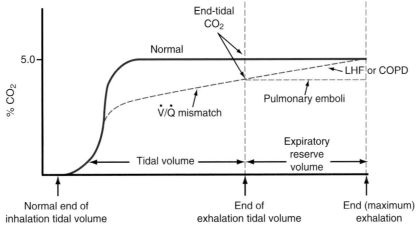

FIGURE 8.32 Capnogram illustrating exhaled CO_2 at the end of a quiet expiration and after a maximum expiration. The difference between these two values can be used to assess ventilation/perfusion ($\dot{V}/\dot{Q}$) relationships. A patient with chronic obstructive pulmonary disease (COPD) typically has an end-tidal carbon dioxide value less than that measured after a maximum expiration. In patients suspected of having a pulmonary embolus, the end-tidal and maximum expiratory CO_2 measurements are nearly equal. *LHF*, Left-heart failure. (Compiled from Darin J: Capnography. *Curr Rev Respir Ther* 3:146, 1981; Erickson L, Wollmer P, Olsson CG, et al.: Diagnosis of pulmonary embolism based upon alveolar dead space analysis. *Chest* 96:357, 1989; and Hatle CJ, Rokseth R: The arterial to end-expiratory carbon dioxide tension gradient in acute pulmonary embolism and other cardiopulmonary diseases. *Chest* 66:352, 1974.)

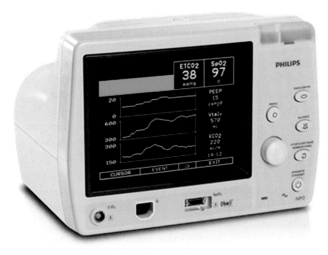

FIGURE 8.33 Volumetric capnograph. (Courtesy Philips North America Corporation, Andover, MA.)

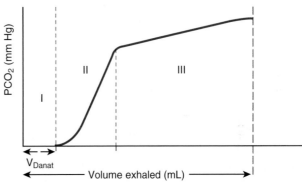

FIGURE 8.34 Single-breath CO_2 (SBCO₂) curve. The horizontal axis of the graph represents the expiratory/inspiratory volume; the vertical axis is the partial pressure of CO_2 in mm Hg. See text for description of the graph. V_{Danat}, Anatomical dead space. (From Cairo JM: *Pilbeam's mechanical ventilation: physiological and clinical applications*, ed 6, St. Louis, 2016, Mosby-Elsevier.)

difference between these two values is minimal. Interestingly, patients with COPD and left-heart failure do not show an arterial to maximum expiration PCO_2 difference, whereas patients with pulmonary embolism do show an increased gradient (Fig. 8.32).

Volumetric capnography. End-tidal CO_2 monitoring tracks exhaled CO_2 plotted over time; volumetric capnometry tracks exhaled CO_2 plotted relative to exhaled volume. The Philips NM3 (Philips North America Corporation) is an example of a capnometer that can provide this type of monitoring (Fig. 8.33).

Single-breath carbon dioxide curve. The single-breath CO_2 (SBCO₂) curve is produced by the integration of airway

flow and CO_2 concentration and is presented on a breath-to-breath basis. As shown in Fig. 8.34, this type of graph can provide information on anatomical dead space, alveolar dead space (when the $PaCO_2$ is known), and CO_2 elimination ($\dot{V}CO_2$) for each breath.

The SBCO₂ curve is divided into three phases:
- *Phase I:* The first part of the curve represents the volume exhaled from the anatomical dead space that is free of CO_2 (i.e., fraction of expired carbon dioxide [F_ECO_2] = 0).
- *Phase II:* The second part of the curve shows a rapid rise in F_ECO_2, which represents the transition between airway and alveolar exhaled gas.

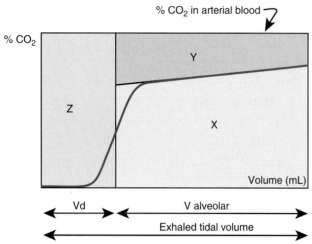

FIGURE 8.35 Graph of exhaled volume (*x* axis) versus % CO_2 (*y* axis). A horizontal line drawn at the top of the curve represents the % CO_2 in arterial blood. Three distinct regions are illustrated: Area X represents actual CO_2 exhaled in one breath; area Y is the amount of CO_2 not eliminated because of alveolar dead space; and area Z is the amount of CO_2 not eliminated because of anatomical dead space. $V_{alveolar}$, Alveolar volume; V_d, dead space volume. (Redrawn from material from Respironics, Murrysville, PA.)

- *Phase III:* The third phase is referred to as the *alveolar plateau*, which typically has a positive slope. The slope represents a rising $P_A CO_2$; the alveoli empty at different rates because of the anatomy of the lung and the various time constants of different units. (*Note:* Perfusion from the pulmonary artery maintains a relatively constant rate of flow past the alveoli. Although the blood is constantly delivering CO_2 to the alveoli, the alveoli get smaller during exhalation. Consequently, the CO_2 level increases in relation to a shrinking volume.)

If a horizontal line is drawn at the top of the curve to represent the percentage of carbon dioxide (% CO_2) in arterial blood, four distinct regions of the curve are established (Fig. 8.35).

Area X represents the actual amount of CO_2 exhaled in the breath, assuming that no exhaled air is rebreathed. In other words, the area under the SBCO$_2$ curve is the volume of CO_2 in a single breath. Adding all the single breaths in a minute gives the $\dot{V}CO_2$, the same results that would occur if exhaled gas were collected using a Douglas bag. Area Y represents the amount of CO_2 that is *not* eliminated because of alveolar dead space (i.e., ventilated alveoli that are poorly perfused or receive no perfusion at all). Area Z represents the amount of CO_2 that was *not* eliminated because of anatomical dead space.

This type of graphic analysis, along with direct measurement of the $PaCO_2$, can provide insight to some important physiological parameters. The ratios of the areas created in the SBCO$_2$ curve can provide the same result as the relationship seen in the Enghoff-modified Bohr equation:

$$[PaCO_2 - P_{\bar{E}}CO_2]PaCO_2 = (Y + Z)(X + Y + Z)$$

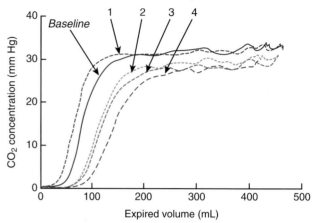

FIGURE 8.36 Changes in volumetric CO_2 tracing in an experimental model when pulmonary artery blood flow was progressively restricted. Note that phase II shifts to the right as perfusion decreases. (From Cairo JM: *Pilbeam's mechanical ventilation: physiological and clinical applications*, ed 5, St. Louis, 2012, Mosby-Elsevier.)

where $PaCO_2$ is the arterial partial pressure of carbon dioxide and $P_{\bar{E}}CO_2$ is the mixed expired partial pressure for CO_2. (*Note:* X, Y, and Z have been defined previously.)

Four major factors influence the $PaCO_2$: CO_2 production, perfusion of the lungs, diffusion, and ventilation. The balance of these four components represents the total transport and elimination of CO_2. It should be apparent that altering any one of the four without a compensatory change in the other three factors results in changes in the $PaCO_2$ and the volume of CO_2 eliminated through the lungs.[38] For example, $\dot{V}CO_2$ increases in patients with sepsis, fever, severe burns, and trauma and during increased work of breathing, in which the respiratory muscles produce additional CO_2 (i.e., conditions that can increase the volume of CO_2 produced are related to increases in metabolism). Therefore, if the metabolism increases and ventilation does not, the $PaCO_2$ rises, and the amount of CO_2 exhaled during the SBCO$_2$ increases.

Fig. 8.36 shows changes in the volumetric CO_2 tracing that occur in an experimental model in which the pulmonary artery blood flow was progressively restricted. Volume and metabolism remain constant, and overall CO_2 production ($\dot{V}CO_2$) remains stable. As perfusion to the lung is progressively reduced (represented by curves 1 to 4), the phase II curve shifts to the right, showing increased dead space in the system. In this case, physiological dead space increased. Notice that the area under the curves progressively decreases because less CO_2 is exhaled per breath. This is a simple explanation for a complex series of events. As the clinician becomes more familiar with the monitoring technique and applies physiological principles, the two parameters provide a valuable assessment tool.[39,40]

Single-breath carbon dioxide loop of inspiration and exhalation. When the SBCO$_2$ graph includes both inspiration and exhalation, a loop is produced (Fig. 8.37). The net volume of CO_2 exhaled in one breath is the area between the exhaled

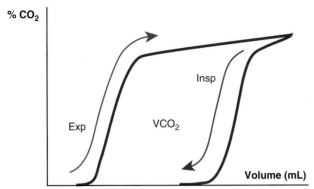

FIGURE 8.37 Single-breath CO_2 (SBCO$_2$) curve recorded during inspiration and expiration. % CO_2, Percentage of carbon dioxide; $\dot{V}CO_2$, carbon dioxide elimination; *exp*, expiration; *insp*, inspiration. (Courtesy Teb Tabor, Paris, France.)

and inhaled CO_2 of this loop. Often the inspiratory portion of the curve is negligible. The net CO_2 in one breath is the difference between the amount of CO_2 inhaled and the amount exhaled.

Trending CO_2 production and alveolar minute ventilation over time. As mentioned earlier, the Philips NM3 monitor can trend data over time. The display for this purpose reports the CO_2 produced each minute ($\dot{V}CO_2$) rather than SBCO$_2$ curves. Trended data can be used for monitoring a variety of clinical procedures. For example, during a recruitment maneuver in a patient with acute respiratory distress syndrome (ARDS), trended CO_2 data will reveal a transient rise in CO_2 when previously closed alveoli are reopened. This tool can also be used in weaning patients. For example, if the patient's respiratory rate increases during a spontaneous breathing trial (SBT), monitoring of the $\dot{V}CO_2$ can help determine whether the patient's metabolic rate is increasing, thus working the respiratory muscles, or a change in dead space is affecting the patient's ability to be weaned.

Trending of CO_2 can also be useful for noting the time lag that can occur in CO_2 removal as a result of CO_2 stores (CO_2 bound in the cells or through bicarbonate or bound in the blood). With large stores the time lag is long, whereas when stores are small, the time lag is short. For example, suppose the alveolar ventilation increases. As a result, $PaCO_2$ decreases, and the stores of CO_2 also start to decrease; however, this second part takes time. In this situation, if alveolar ventilation ($\dot{V}_A$) increases, the SBCO$_2$ increases and the $PaCO_2$ decreases initially. After a slight delay, because the production of CO_2 remains constant, the $PaCO_2$ remains low, and the monitored exhaled $\dot{V}CO_2$ returns to baseline, indicating that a balance has returned (Clinical Scenario 8.4).[37]

V. INDIRECT CALORIMETRY AND METABOLIC MONITORING

Clinicians have historically relied on equations derived by Harris and Benedict[41] in 1919 to estimate an individual's energy requirements. These formulae can be appropriate for normal individuals and patients who are not critically ill, but

---

> ### CLINICAL SCENARIO 8.4
>
> Volumetric capnography tracings for a patient being mechanically ventilated with 5 cm H_2O of PEEP have demonstrated a progressive decrease in phase II after the PEEP was increased to 10 cm H_2O. Describe the significance of this finding.
>   See Appendix A for the answer.

PEEP, Positive end-expiratory pressure.

> ### BOX 8.6   Formulae Used During Indirect Calorimetry
>
> **Energy Expenditure**
> ***Weir Equation[46]***
>
> $$EE = [3.941(\dot{V}O_2) + 1.106(\dot{V}CO_2)]1.44 - 12.17(UN)$$
>
> ***Modified Weir Equation***
>
> $$EE = [3.9(\dot{V}O_2) + 1.1(\dot{V}CO_2)] \times 1.44$$
>
> **Substrate Utilization[47]**
> ***Carbohydrates***
>
> $$dS = 4.115(\dot{V}CO_2) - 2.909(\dot{V}O_2) - 2.539(UN)$$
>
> ***Fats***
>
> $$dF = 1.689(\dot{V}O_2 - \dot{V}CO_2) - 1.943(UN)$$
>
> ***Proteins***
>
> $$dP = 6.25(UN)$$

dS, dF, and *dP* represent grams of carbohydrate, fat, and protein, respectively, for a fasting individual.
EE, Energy expenditure; *UN*, urinary nitrogen.

their usefulness may be limited for some critically ill patients. Kinney[42] derived correction factors to compensate for the increased energy demands in critically ill patients (e.g., those with burns or bone fractures), but these factors are of limited help when a patient has multiple conditions simultaneously (e.g., sepsis and ARDS).

Advances in microprocessor technology have made it relatively easy for respiratory therapists to measure accurately the energy needs and substrate utilization patterns of hospitalized patients. The technique used to accomplish this task is called *indirect calorimetry*. See Clinical Practice Guideline 8.3 for more information on metabolic measurement using indirect calorimetry during mechanical ventilation.

Indirect Calorimetry

Indirect calorimetry is based on the theory that all of a person's energy is derived from the oxidation of carbohydrates, fats, and proteins and that the ratio of CO_2 produced to oxygen consumed (i.e., the RQ, or $\dot{V}CO_2/\dot{V}O_2$) is characteristic of the fuel burned.[43] Energy expenditure (EE) is calculated from $\dot{V}O_2$ and $\dot{V}CO_2$ measurements using the Weir equation, and substrate utilization patterns can be determined using equations such as those derived by Burszein et al.[44] and Consolazio et al.[45] Box 8.6 summarizes these equations.

CLINICAL PRACTICE GUIDELINE 8.3   Metabolic Measurements Using Indirect Calorimetry During Mechanical Ventilation—2004 Revision and Update

Indications

1. In patients with known nutritional deficits or derangements. Multiple nutritional risk and stress factors that may considerably skew prediction by the Harris-Benedict equation include:
   a. Neurological trauma
   b. Paralysis
   c. COPD
   d. Acute pancreatitis
   e. Cancer with residual tumor burden
   f. Multiple trauma
   g. Amputations
   h. Patients in whom height and weight cannot be accurately obtained
   i. Patients who fail to respond adequately to estimated nutritional needs
   j. Patients who require long-term acute care
   k. Severe sepsis
   l. Extremely obese patients
   m. Severely hypermetabolic or hypometabolic patients
2. When patients fail attempts at liberation from mechanical ventilation to measure the O_2 cost of breathing and the components of ventilation.
3. When the need exists to assess oxygen consumption ($\dot{V}O_2$) to evaluate the hemodynamic support of mechanically ventilated patients.
4. To measure cardiac output by the Fick methods.
5. To determine the cause or causes of increased ventilatory requirements.

Contraindications

When a specific indication is present, no contraindications to performing a metabolic measurement using indirect calorimetry exist unless short-term disconnection of ventilatory support for connection of measurement lines results in hypoxemia, bradycardia, or other adverse effects.

Hazards and Complications

1. Closed-circuit calorimeters may cause a reduction in alveolar ventilation as a result of increased compressible volume of the breathing circuit.
2. Closed-circuit calorimeters may reduce the trigger sensitivity of the ventilator and result in increased work of breathing for the patient.
3. Short-term disconnection of the patient from the ventilator for connection of the indirect calorimetry apparatus may result in hypoxemia, bradycardia, and patient discomfort.
4. Inappropriate calibration or system setup may result in erroneous readings, causing incorrect patient management.
5. Isolation valves may increase circuit resistance and cause increased work of breathing and/or dynamic hyperinflation.
6. Inspiratory reservoirs may cause a reduction in alveolar ventilation as a result of increased compressible volume of the breathing circuit.
7. Manipulation of the ventilator circuit may cause leaks that may lower alveolar ventilation.

COPD, Chronic obstructive pulmonary disease.
Modified from American Association for Respiratory Care: AARC clinical practice guideline: metabolic measurements using indirect calorimetry during mechanical ventilation—2004 revision and update. *Respir Care* 49:107, 2004.

Indirect calorimeters generally are classified according to their method of determining the $\dot{V}O_2$. Two methods usually are described: the closed-circuit method and the open-circuit method. With the closed-circuit method, the patient breathes into and out of a container prefilled with oxygen. Oxygen consumption is determined by simply measuring the oxygen volume used by the patient. With the open-circuit method, the volumes of inspired and expired gases are measured, as well as the fractional concentrations of oxygen in each. The $\dot{V}O_2$ is then determined by calculating the difference between the amount of oxygen in inspired gas ($\dot{V}_I \times F_IO_2$) and the amount of oxygen in expired gas ($\dot{V}_E \times F_EO_2$ [fraction of expired oxygen]).

Closed-Circuit Calorimeters

With closed-circuit devices, oxygen consumption can be determined by measuring either the oxygen volume removed from the device or the oxygen volume that must be added to the system to maintain the original oxygen volume.

Fig. 8.38 illustrates a closed-circuit system in which the $\dot{V}O_2$ is determined by measuring the amount of oxygen removed from a reservoir over time. The system consists of a breathing circuit connected to a spirometer that is prefilled with oxygen. The patient's exhaled gases are directed to a mixing chamber,

then through a CO_2 absorber, and back to the spirometer. CO_2 production ($\dot{V}CO_2$) can be measured by incorporating the CO_2 analyzer positioned between the mixing chamber and the CO_2 absorber. Closed-circuit calorimeters can be used both for spontaneously breathing and for mechanically ventilated patients.

Oxygen consumption is determined by measuring the oxygen volume removed from the spirometer. Thus the volume of oxygen removed can be determined by measuring the change in the end-expiratory level. (Oxygen consumption is expressed in milliliters per minute.) The F_ECO_2 is determined by aspirating a sample of the mixed expired gas (from the mixing chamber) into the CO_2 analyzer between the mixing chamber and the spirometer. CO_2 production, which is expressed in milliliters per minute, is calculated by multiplying the fractional concentration of mixed expired CO_2 (F_ECO_2) by the minute ventilation ($\dot{V}_E$).

Another variation of the closed-circuit technique for estimating oxygen consumption involves measuring the oxygen volume that must be replenished while the patient removes oxygen from the reservoir. This system consists of a breathing circuit, a bellows containing oxygen, a CO_2 absorber, and an ultrasonic transducer to monitor the bellows position. As the patient breathes into and out of the bellows, the oxygen used

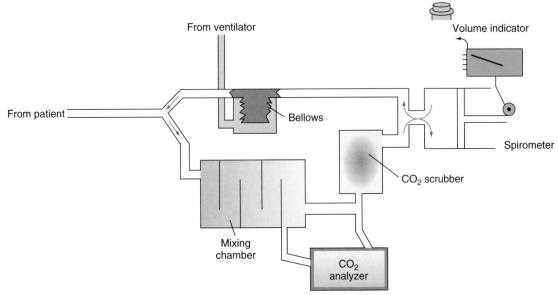

FIGURE 8.38 Closed-circuit indirect calorimeters. Oxygen consumption is estimated by measuring the amount of oxygen used from a reservoir. (From Branson RD: The measurement of energy expenditure: instrumentation, practical considerations, and clinical applications. *Respir Care* 35:640, 1990.)

by the patient is replaced on demand by an external oxygen supply. The amount of oxygen that must be added to the system is a measure of oxygen consumption. These systems can be used for spontaneously breathing and for mechanically ventilated patients.

Open-Circuit Calorimeters

Open-circuit calorimeters use mixing chambers, dilution techniques, and breath-by-breath measurements to determine oxygen consumption. With mixing chambers, expired gases are directed into a collecting chamber containing baffles to ensure adequate mixing of gases. A vacuum attached to the chamber aspirates a sample of the mixed expired gas and directs it into the oxygen and CO_2 analyzers. After they are analyzed, the gases are returned to the mixing chamber, and the entire volume of the mixing chamber is routed through a volume- or flow-sensing device.

Dilution systems also use a mixing chamber, but they use a bias flow of room air to dilute the gas sample and move it through the system. The amounts of oxygen and CO_2 exhaled are calculated by multiplying the fractional concentrations of oxygen and CO_2 by the total flow through the system, which usually is approximately 40 L/min.

Breath-by-breath devices measure the volume and fractional concentrations of oxygen and CO_2 in each breath. The amount of oxygen and CO_2 in inspired and mixed expired gases actually is determined by averaging the volumes and concentrations of several breaths. The number of breaths to be averaged can be preselected by the technologist or preset by the manufacturer.

Fig. 8.39 is a schematic of an open-circuit indirect calorimeter. A flow- or volume-sensing device is used to measure the inspired and expired gas volumes, a polarographic analyzer

is used to measure the fractional concentrations of oxygen, and a nondispersive IR analyzer is used to measure the fractional concentration of CO_2. Because changes in ambient temperature and pressure can affect gas concentrations, a sensor for measuring the ambient temperature and barometric pressure of the gases analyzed also is incorporated into the system.

Although open-circuit devices can be used for both spontaneously breathing and mechanically ventilated patients, special problems can arise when these systems are used with mechanically ventilated patients. Some of these problems include fluctuations in the F_1O_2 level, separation of the patient's inspired and expired gases from the continuous gas flow from the ventilator, and handling of water vapor.[45] Problems with fluctuations in the F_1O_2 level can be alleviated to some extent by using air/oxygen blenders or premixed gases. Beyond F_1O_2 levels of 0.5 to 0.6, most systems are unreliable because of the Haldane transformation and should be viewed skeptically. Inspired and expired gases can be separated using isolation valves supplied by the manufacturer of the metabolic monitor. Water vapor is always a problem when continuous measurements are performed on ventilator patients, but the difficulty is accentuated when cascade humidifiers are used to supply humidity to the patient. Replacement of these humidifiers with artificial noses may help minimize the problem.

Practical Applications of Indirect Calorimetry

Spontaneously breathing patients, breathing room air, can be connected to an indirect calorimetry system by breathing through a mouthpiece or mask attached to a nonrebreathing valve. Specially designed canopies and hoods can also be used for spontaneously breathing patients who are not receiving ventilatory support.

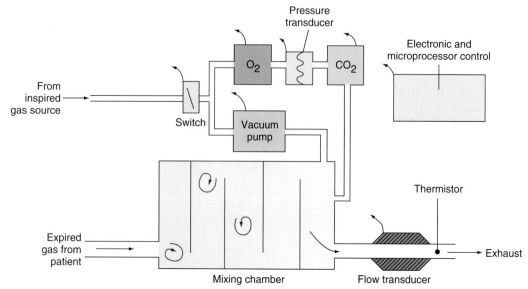

FIGURE 8.39 Open-circuit indirect calorimeter. Oxygen consumption and CO_2 production are estimated by multiplying the minute ventilation by the fractional concentration of oxygen and CO_2 during inspiration and expiration. (From Branson RD: The measurement of energy expenditure: instrumentation, practical considerations, and clinical applications. *Respir Care* 35:640, 1990.)

Patients with ETTs or tracheostomy tubes (TTs) can be connected to the system if the nonrebreathing valve is placed directly onto the airway opening and expired gases are routed into the system. It is important to inflate the cuffs of ETTs and TTs when inspired and exhaled gases are to be measured, because failure to do so results in loss of expired air around the tube and erroneous measurements of $\dot{V}O_2$ and $\dot{V}CO_2$. For patients receiving a continuous flow of gas during ventilatory support, such as occurs when a bias flow is present, an isolation valve must be used to ensure that only the patient's exhaled gases are delivered to the system.

As previously stated, oxygen consumption and CO_2 production are calculated by comparing the fractional concentrations of oxygen and CO_2 of inspired and expired air. When the patient is breathing room air, however, it is reasonable to assume that the fractional concentration of inspired oxygen is 20.9%, and the fractional concentration of inspired CO_2 is 0.3%. For patients receiving enriched oxygen mixtures, the fractional concentration of inspired oxygen must be measured by the system. Fluctuations in the F_IO_2 can be caused by air leaks in the patient-ventilator/metabolic monitoring system (e.g., incompetent ETT cuffs, chest tubes, bronchopleural fistulas) and by varying gas volumes and pressure demands, as occur during intermittent mandatory ventilation and the use of high levels of PEEP (i.e., >10 to 12 cm H_2O). Unstable air-oxygen blending systems in the ventilator circuit may also contribute to unstable F_IO_2 levels. In addition, clinical studies have demonstrated that currently available systems cannot provide accurate and reproducible $\dot{V}O_2$ measurements for patients breathing F_IO_2 at levels greater than 0.5. Box 8.7 summarizes the conditions that should be observed when indirect calorimetry measurements are made (see Clinical Scenario 8.5).

BOX 8.7 **Conditions for Obtaining Indirect Calorimetry Measurements**

1. The patient should be at rest and in a supine position for at least 30 minutes before the measurement is made.
2. The room temperature should be 20°C to 25°C (68°F to 77°F).
3. The patient should remain relaxed during the measurement (i.e., no voluntary physical activity).
4. Measurements should be recorded for 15 to 30 minutes or until the $\dot{V}O_2$ and $\dot{V}CO_2$ vary by less than 5%.

CLINICAL SCENARIO 8.5

While obtaining indirect calorimetric measurements from a mechanically ventilated patient receiving an F_IO_2 of 0.6, you notice that her $\dot{V}O_2$ continually varies from 250 to 800 mL/min over a 10-minute period. Briefly describe several possible causes for these erratic measurements.

See Appendix A for the answer.

F_IO_2, Fractional inspired oxygen; *$\dot{V}O_2$,* oxygen consumption.

Metabolic Monitoring

The main advantage of using indirect calorimetry instead of prediction equations (e.g., the Harris and Benedict equations) is that indirect calorimetry can provide actual measurements of a patient's caloric needs. Indeed, modern ICU ventilators typically have sensors and transducers incorporated into their design along with microprocessors that allow for instantaneous measurements and trending data for $\dot{V}O_2$, $\dot{V}CO_2$, RQ, and EE of patients receiving mechanical ventilation. Combined with nitrogen excretion measurements, indirect calorimetry can also provide information about substrate utilization, giving the clinician valuable insight into the types of substrates the patient is using to generate energy.

Energy Expenditure

EE typically is expressed in kilocalories per day (kcal/day) or relative to an individual's body surface area (kcal/h/m²). A normal, healthy adult uses 1500 to 3000 kcal/day, or approximately 30 to 40 kcal/h/m².[43,44]

Many factors can influence the metabolic rate, including the type and rate of food ingested, the time of day of the measurement, the patient's activity level, and whether the patient is recovering from infection, surgery, or trauma.

Prolonged starvation is associated with a decreased metabolic rate. Eating raises the metabolic rate through a mechanism called *specific dynamic action*. Specific dynamic action is thought to be related to the digestion and absorption of food.[45] EE shows diurnal variation (i.e., it is usually higher in the morning than in the evening), which may be related to the variations in hormone levels that naturally occur daily.[46] Changes in activity are a well-recognized factor that can alter the metabolic rate. Fig. 8.40 shows how changes in physical activity can affect EE in a hospitalized patient. Note that sleep is associated with a reduction in the metabolic rate, and even the slightest exertion is associated with an increase in the metabolic rate. Fever,

as can occur with bacterial and viral infections, also can have a profound effect on the metabolic rate. For example, an increase in body temperature of 0.6°C (1°F) causes a 10% increase in the metabolic rate. Burns, long-bone fractures, and surgery can increase the metabolic rate by as much as 200%.[43]

Substrate Utilization Patterns

The substrate utilization pattern comprises the proportions of carbohydrates, fats, and proteins that contribute to the total energy metabolism. As was previously stated, the percentage of the total energy that a substrate contributes can be determined using the RQ. Remember that the RQ is the ratio of $\dot{V}CO_2$ to $\dot{V}O_2$. RQ can vary from approximately 0.67 to 1.2. Table 8.7 shows the RQs for various foods. When pure fat is

TABLE 8.7   Variations in the Respiratory Quotient

Substrate	Respiratory Quotient
Carbohydrate oxidation	1.0
Fat oxidation	0.7
Protein oxidation	0.8
Lipogenesis	>1.0

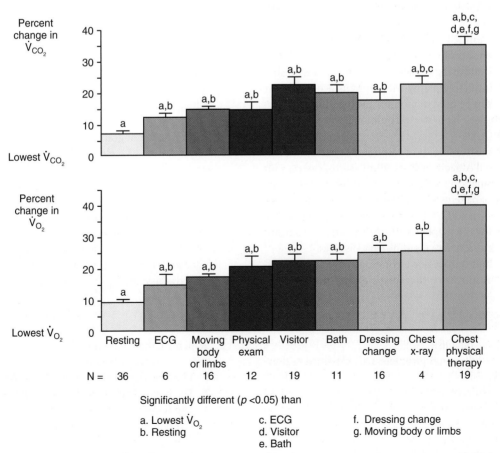

Significantly different (*p* <0.05) than
a. Lowest $\dot{V}_{O_2}$ c. ECG f. Dressing change
b. Resting d. Visitor g. Moving body or limbs
e. Bath

FIGURE 8.40 Variations in oxygen consumption ($\dot{V}O_2$) and carbon dioxide production ($\dot{V}CO_2$) (expressed as percent change) associated with diagnostic and therapeutic interactions in a patient in the intensive care unit. *ECG,* Electrocardiogram. (From Weismann C, Kemper MC, Damask M: The effects of routine interactions on metabolic rate. *Chest* 86:815, 1984.)

burned, the RQ is 0.7. The RQ for pure carbohydrate is 1, and the RQ for protein is approximately 0.8. RQs greater than 1 are associated with lipogenesis (fat synthesis), metabolic acidosis, and hyperventilation. RQs less than 0.7 are associated with ketosis.

Healthy adults who consume a typical American diet derive 45% to 50% of their calories from carbohydrates, 35% to 40% from lipids, and 10% to 15% from proteins. The resultant RQ ranges from 0.8 to 0.85.[45] Under normal conditions, proteins normally contribute only minor amounts to energy metabolism. Note that the percentage of protein used represents the normal turnover rate for replenishing structural and functional proteins in the body. Proteins may contribute significantly to EE, however, in cases of starvation. For this reason, a nonprotein RQ usually is reported to indicate the contribution to RQ made by carbohydrates and lipids.

Substrate utilization is determined by the types of substrates ingested and an individual's ability to use various types of foods. For example, eating a large amount of glucose raises the RQ to approximately 1, which suggests that carbohydrates are providing most of the EE. Prolonged starvation lowers the RQ to approximately 0.7, indicating that the individual is relying almost completely on fats for energy. Many systemic diseases adversely affect an individual's ability to use various types of substrates. For example, several studies have shown that patients with severe sepsis have RQs of approximately 0.7 because of their reliance on lipid metabolism for energy and an inability to use carbohydrates.[47]

KEY POINTS

- Spirometers generally are classified as volume-collecting or flow-sensing devices. Common examples of volume-collecting devices include water-sealed spirometers, bellows spirometers, and dry rolling seal devices. The most commonly used flow-sensing devices include thermal and turbine flowmeters and pneumotachographs.
- Variable orifice pneumotachographs and vortex ultrasonic flowmeters are relatively low-cost pneumotachometers that can provide valuable bedside measurements of respiratory mechanics.
- The ATS/ERS unified standards for lung function testing provide guidance on the measurement and interpretation of spirometry, diffusing capacity, and lung volume tests.
- Respiratory inductive plethysmography is a noninvasive method that can be used to monitor the breathing patterns of patients in sleep laboratories, pulmonary function laboratories, and ICUs.
- Noninvasive measurements of respiratory system mechanics, such as vital capacity and its subdivisions, can provide valuable information that can be used in the diagnosis and management of patients with cardiopulmonary dysfunctions.
- Measurements of FRC, RV, and TLC can provide valuable information for the management of patients with chronic obstructive and restrictive pulmonary diseases.
- Advances in microprocessor technology have significantly improved a respiratory therapist's ability to assess the ventilatory function of mechanically ventilated patients. Evaluation of R_{aw}, respiratory system compliance, and work of breathing studies can provide information that can assist the management of these patients.
- Accurate measurements of the inspired oxygen concentration are essential for successful management of hypoxemic patients.
- Chemiluminescence and electrochemical monitoring are routinely used when NO is administered to prevent the potential toxic effects induced by high levels of NO and NO_2.
- Capnography is a simple, noninvasive method for monitoring the ventilatory status of spontaneously and mechanically ventilated patients. The contour of the capnograph can be evaluated to detect dead space ventilation, hyperventilation and hypoventilation, apnea, and periodic breathing.
- Volumetric capnography is a useful method for noninvasively assessing CO_2 elimination, which can be used to help wean patients from mechanical ventilatory support.
- Indirect calorimetry allows clinicians to obtain actual measurements of a patient's caloric needs rather than relying on prediction equations. Although prediction equations can provide useful estimates of metabolic requirements for normal, healthy individuals, they may underestimate the caloric and substrate needs of patients afflicted with multiple organ dysfunction.

ASSESSMENT QUESTIONS

See Appendix B for the answers.

1. Which of the following spirometers are classified as flow-sensing devices?
   1. Wright respirometers
   2. Hot wire anemometers
   3. Dry rolling seal spirometers
   4. Stead-Wells spirometers
      a. 1 and 2 only
      b. 2 and 3 only
      c. 2 and 4 only
      d. 1, 2, and 3 only

2. Which of the following can influence the accuracy of spirometer measurements?
   1. The linearity and frequency response of the device
   2. The device's sensitivity to environmental conditions
   3. The frequency of calibration
   4. The presence of an obstructive or restrictive pulmonary disease
      a. 1 and 2 only
      b. 2 and 3 only
      c. 1, 2, and 3 only
      d. 1, 2, 3, and 4

3. According to American Thoracic Society/European Respiratory Society (ATS/ERS) standards, spirometers used to measure vital capacity should have an accuracy range (in body temperature and ambient pressure, saturated [BTPS]) of:
   a. 0.5 to 5 L +/− 10% of the reading or 50 mL, whichever is greater
   b. 0.5 to 6 L +/− 5% of the reading or 50 mL, whichever is greater
   c. 0.5 to 8 L +/− 3% of the reading or 50 mL, whichever is greater
   d. 0.5 to 12 L +/− 3% of the reading or 50 mL, whichever is greater

4. Which of the following is considered the primary criterion for identifying the end of a successful nitrogen washout test?
   a. Patient becomes fatigued
   b. Exhaled nitrogen concentration is less than 1.5%
   c. Nitrogen percentage remains stable for 2 minutes
   d. Exhaled volume equals the functional residual capacity (FRC)

5. Which of the following can cause erroneous measurements with impedance pneumography?
   1. Sinus tachycardia
   2. Upper airway obstruction
   3. Central apnea
   4. Tachypnea
      a. 1 only
      b. 2 only
      c. 2 and 3 only
      d. 1, 2, and 3 only

6. Which of the following lung volumes cannot be measured by simple spirometry?
   1. Vital capacity (VC)
   2. Residual volume (RV)
   3. Total lung capacity (TLC)
   4. Inspiratory capacity (IC)
      a. 1 and 2 only
      b. 2 and 3 only
      c. 3 and 4 only
      d. 1, 3, and 4 only

7. Maximum inspiratory pressures (MIPs) normally are:
   a. −20 to −40 cm H_2O
   b. −50 to −80 cm H_2O
   c. −60 to −100 cm H_2O
   d. −150 to −200 cm H_2O

8. Which of the following measurements is considered a good indicator of a patient's effort during a forced vital capacity (FVC) maneuver?
   a. Forced expiratory volume in 1 second (FEV_1)
   b. Peak expiratory flow (PEF)
   c. FEV_1/FVC
   d. Forced expiratory flow from 25% to 75% of the vital capacity ($FEF_{25\%-75\%}$)

9. Lack of a definitive phase 3 on a capnogram most often is associated with:
   a. Insufficient neuromuscular blockade
   b. Cardiac oscillations

c. $\dot{V}/\dot{Q}$ imbalances, such as occur with patients with emphysema or chronic bronchitis
   d. Rebreathing of exhaled gases

10. How many kilocalories of energy per day should a typical healthy adult ingest to maintain energy balance?
    a. 500 to 1000
    b. 900 to 1200
    c. 1200 to 1800
    d. 1500 to 3000

11. You notice that the FRC measured on a patient with chronic obstructive pulmonary disease (COPD) with the nitrogen washout technique is different from that measured with body plethysmography. In fact, the volume measured with the body box is approximately 500 mL greater than the FRC measured with nitrogen washout. Why might this difference exist?
    a. Trapped gas in the lungs
    b. Ventilation-perfusion mismatch
    c. Elevated CO level in the patient's blood
    d. Severe hypercapnia

12. Which of the following analyzers are typically used to measure exhaled NO?
    1. Chemiluminescence analyzer
    2. Paramagnetic analyzer
    3. Electrochemical analyzer
    4. Capnography
       a. 1 only
       b. 2 only
       c. 1 and 3 only
       d. 1, 2, and 3 only

13. A patient receiving mechanical ventilatory support via an endotracheal tube (ETT) is being monitored for oxygen consumption. Which of the following could lead to an erroneous measurement?
    1. The patient appears agitated
    2. The measurement is performed immediately after the patient receives a physical therapy treatment
    3. The fractional inspired oxygen (F_1O_2) is 0.8
    4. The patient's ETT cuff is inflated to seal the airway
       a. 1 and 2 only
       b. 2 and 3 only
       c. 1, 2, and 3 only
       d. 1, 2, 3, and 4

14. The only source of nutrition administered to a patient is D5W (i.e., 5% dextrose in water). What would you expect to find when measuring the respiratory quotient (RQ)?
    a. 0.7 to 0.75
    b. 0.8 to 0.85
    c. 0.9 to 0.95
    d. 1

15. Which of the following patient conditions would you expect to be hypermetabolic (elevated $\dot{V}O_2$)?
    a. Starvation
    b. Fever
    c. Sedation
    d. Hypothermia

REFERENCES

1. Wasserman K, et al.: *Principles of exercise testing and interpretation*, Philadelphia, 1994, Lea & Febiger.

2. East TD: What makes noninvasive monitoring tick?: a review of basic engineering principles. *Respir Care* 35:500, 1990.

3. Mottram C: *Ruppel's manual of pulmonary function testing*, ed 10, St. Louis, 2012, Elsevier-Mosby.

4. Sullivan WJ, Peters GM, Enright PL: Pneumotachography: theory and clinical application. *Respir Care* 29:736, 1984.

5. Ferguson GT, Enright PL, Buist AS, et al.: Office spirometry for lung health assessment in adults: a consensus statement from the National Lung Health Education Program. *Chest* 117:1146-1161, 2000.

6. American Association for Respiratory Care: AARC clinical practice guideline: body plethysmography. *Respir Care* 46:506, 2001.

7. American Association for Respiratory Care: AARC clinical practice guideline: static lung volumes—2001 revision and update. *Respir Care* 46:531, 2001.

8. Wanger J, Clausen JL, Coates A, et al.: Standardization of the measurement of lung volumes. *Eur Respir J* 26:511, 2005.

9. Kacmarek RM, Hess D, Stoller JK: *Monitoring in respiratory care*, St. Louis, 1993, Mosby.

10. Miller MR, Crapo R, Hankinson J, et al.: General considerations for lung function testing. *Eur Respir J* 26:153, 2005.

11. American Thoracic Society: Snowbird workshop on standardization of spirometry. *Am Rev Respir Dis* 119:831, 1979.

12. American Thoracic Society: Standardization of spirometry—1987 update. *Am Rev Respir Dis* 136:1285, 1987.

13. American Thoracic Society: Lung function testing: selection of reference values and interpretation. *Am Rev Respir Dis* 144:1202, 1991.

14. American Thoracic Society: Standardization of spirometry—1994 update. *Am Rev Respir Dis* 152:1107, 1995.

15. Quanjer PH, editor: Standardized lung function testing: report of the Working Party on Standardization of Lung Function Test, European Community of Coal and Steel. *Bull Eur Physiopathol Respir* 5:1, 1983.

16. Brusasco V, Crapo R, Viegi G: Coming together: the ATS/ERS consensus on clinical pulmonary function testing. *Eur Respir J* 26:1, 2005.

17. Miller MR, Hankinson J, Brusasco V, et al.: Standardization of spirometry. *Eur Respir J* 26:319, 2005.

18. MacIntyre N, Crapo RO, Viegi G, et al.: Standardization of the single-breath determination of carbon monoxide uptake in the lung. *Eur Respir J* 26:720, 2005.

19. Branson RD, Campbell RS: Impedance pneumography, apnea monitoring, and respiratory inductive plethysmography. In Kacmarek RM, Hess D, Stoller JK, editors: *Monitoring in respiratory care*, St. Louis, 1993, Mosby.

20. Southhall DP, et al.: Undetected episodes of prolonged apnea and severe bradycardia in preterm infants. *Pediatrics* 72:541, 1983.

21. Wayburton D, Stork AR, Taeusch HW: Apnea monitoring in infants with upper airway obstruction. *Pediatrics* 60:742, 1967.

22. Konno K, Mead J: Measurement of the separate changes of rib cage and abdomen during breathing. *J Appl Physiol* 22:407, 1967.

23. Pellegrino R, Viegi G, Brusasco V, et al.: Interpretative strategies for lung function tests. *Eur Respir J* 26:948, 2005.

24. Hess DR: Mechanics in mechanically ventilated patients. *Respir Care* 59(11):1773-1794, 2014.

25. Osborne JJ, Wilson RM: Monitoring the mechanical properties of the lung. In Spence AA, editor: *Respiratory monitoring in the intensive care unit*, New York, 1980, Churchill Livingstone.

26. Pauling L, Wood RE, Sturdivant JH: Oxygen meter. *J Am Chem Soc* 68:795, 1946.

27. Etches PC, et al.: Clinical monitoring of inhaled nitric oxide: comparison of chemiluminescence and electrochemical sensors. *Biomed Instrum Technol* 29:134, 1995.

28. Miller CC: Chemiluminescence analysis and nitrogen dioxide measurement. *Lancet* 34:300, 1994.

29. Body S, Hartigan PM, Shernan SK, et al.: Nitric oxide: delivery, measurement, and clinical application. *J Cardiothorac Vasc Anesth* 9:748, 1995.

30. Purtz E, Hess D, Kacmarek R: Evaluation of electrochemical nitric oxide and nitrogen dioxide analyzers suitable for use during mechanical ventilation. *J Clin Monit* 13:25, 1997.

31. Dweik RA, Boggs PB, Erzurum SC, et al.: Interpretation of exhaled nitric oxide levels (F_ENO) for clinical applications. *Am J Respir Crit Care Med* 184:602-615, 2011.

32. American Association for Respiratory Care: AARC clinical practice guideline: capnography. *Respir Care* 40:1321, 1995.

33. Stock MC: Capnography for adults. *Crit Care Clin* 11:219, 1995.

34. Walsh BK, Crotwell DN, Restrepo RD: Capnography/capnometry during mechanical ventilation 2011. *Respir Care* 56(4):503-509, 2011.

35. Kennel EM, Andrews RW, Wollman H: Correction factors for nitrous oxide in the infrared analysis of carbon dioxide. *Anesthesiology* 39:441, 1973.

36. Gravenstein JS, Paulus DA, Hayes TJ: *Capnography in clinical practice*, Boston, 1989, Butterworth.

37. Cairo JM: *Pilbeam's mechanical ventilation*, ed 6, St. Louis, 2016, Elsevier.

38. Davis PD, Parbrook GD, Kenny GNC: *Basic physics and measurement in anesthesia*, ed 4, Oxford, 1995, Butterworth-Heinemann.

39. Taskar V, Larsson A, Wetterberg T, et al.: Dynamics of carbon dioxide elimination following ventilator resetting. *Chest* 108:196, 1995.

40. Gravenstein JS, Jaffe MB, Paulus DA: *Capnography: clinical aspects—carbon dioxide over time and volume*, Cambridge, UK, 2004, Cambridge University Press.

41. Harris JA, Benedict F: *Standard basal metabolism constants for physiologists and clinicians: a biometric study of basal metabolism in man*, Philadelphia, 1919, JB Lippincott.

42. Kinney JM: The application of indirect calorimetry in clinical studies: assessment of energy metabolism in health and disease. In Kinney JM, editor: *Report of the first Ross conference on medical research*, Columbus, Ohio, 1980, Ross Laboratories.

43. Ferrannini E: The theoretical basis of indirect calorimetry: a review. *Metabolism* 37:287, 1987.

44. Burszein P, et al.: Utilization of protein, carbohydrate, and fat in fasting and postabsorptive subjects. *Am J Clin Nutr* 33:998, 1980.

45. Consolazio CJ, Johnson RE, Pecora LJ: *Physiological measurements of metabolic function in man*, New York, 1963, McGraw-Hill.

46. Weir JB: New method for calculating metabolic rate with special reference to protein metabolism. *J Physiol* 109:1, 1949.

47. Branson RD, Lacey J, Berry S: Indirect calorimetry and nutritional monitoring. In Levine RL, Fromm RE, editors: *Critical care monitoring*, St. Louis, 1995, Mosby.

Assessment of Cardiovascular Function

OBJECTIVES

Upon completion of this chapter you will be able to:

1. Explain the principles of electrocardiography.
2. Identify the major components of an electrocardiograph.
3. Demonstrate the correct placement of electrodes on a patient to obtain a 12-lead electrocardiogram.
4. Explain the various waves, complexes, and intervals that appear on a normal electrocardiogram.
5. List and describe the most common arrhythmias encountered in clinical electrocardiography.
6. Describe the pressure, volume, and flow events that occur in the heart and major blood vessels during a typical cardiac cycle.
7. Explain the principle of operation of various noninvasive and invasive devices routinely used to obtain blood pressure measurements.
8. Describe various invasive and noninvasive methods used to measure cardiac output.
9. Interpret hemodynamic measurements obtained from patients in a critical care setting.

OUTLINE

KEY TERMS

atrial fibrillation
atrial flutter
atrial premature depolarizations
automaticity
cardiac cycle
cardiac work
conductivity
excitability
floating electrodes
heart blocks
impedance cardiography
impedance plethysmography
incisura
isovolumetric contraction

isovolumetric relaxation
junctional escape rhythm
Korotkoff sounds
murmurs
normal sinus rhythm
oscillometry
paroxysmal atrial tachycardia (PAT)
phonocardiogram
premature ventricular beats
premature ventricular depolarizations
pulmonary vascular resistance (PVR)
relative refractory period

sinus arrhythmia
sinus bradycardia
sinus tachycardia
sphygmomanometer
systemic vascular resistance (SVR)
ventricular asystole
ventricular diastole
ventricular fibrillation
ventricular systole
ventricular tachycardia
volume conductor
Wolff-Parkinson-White (WPW) syndrome

Successful management of patients with cardiovascular and pulmonary dysfunctions requires a working knowledge of cardiovascular physiology. This knowledge can be applied clinically to quantify various aspects of cardiovascular function with techniques such as electrocardiography and hemodynamic monitoring. This chapter provides an overview of evidence-based standards for the most common noninvasive and invasive devices and techniques used by respiratory therapists to assess cardiovascular function.

Electrocardiography is used in the acute care setting during cardiopulmonary resuscitation (CPR), for preoperative screening, and in the diagnosis and treatment of individuals with unstable angina, myocardial infarction, and heart failure. It also is routinely used as part of the annual assessment of individuals who are involved in high-risk occupations and in sports.[1] Electrocardiography can provide valuable information that can be used to monitor patients who are being treated with various drugs for the management of cardiovascular dysfunction.

Respiratory therapists are often called upon to obtain hemodynamic measurements to assist in the diagnosis and treatment of patients with cardiovascular and pulmonary dysfunctions. These measurements when coupled with effective therapeutic interventions can provide valuable information that can be used in the management of critically ill patients (e.g., advanced cardiac life support [ACLS]).

I. PRINCIPLES OF ELECTROCARDIOGRAPHY

Electrophysiology of the Heart

Contraction of cardiac muscle provides the energy required to propel blood through the circulation. Under normal circumstances, each heartbeat is initiated by specialized pacemaker cells of the heart, which have the property of rhythmic, spontaneous electrical activity. When these specialized pacemaker cells depolarize (i.e., become electrically activated), they cause other electrically excitable cells of the heart to depolarize, resulting in simultaneous electrical activation of the right and left atria, followed by simultaneous electrical activation of the right and left ventricles.[2]

To fully appreciate this ability of cardiac cells to initiate and conduct electrical impulses, three important aspects of the electrophysiology of the heart must be considered: excitability, automaticity, and conductivity. *Excitability* may be defined as the ability of a cell to respond to an electrical stimulus. *Automaticity* is the ability of certain specialized cells of the heart to depolarize spontaneously. These specialized cells, which are located at the sinoatrial (SA) and atrioventricular (AV) nodes, can initiate action potentials in the absence of nerve impulses from the central nervous system. *Conductivity* is the ability of cardiac tissue to propagate an action potential.

The following sections present a brief discussion of the cellular events that occur during a heartbeat. This information provides a foundation for the study of electrocardiography and for identifying abnormalities of the electrical activity of the heart. We therefore begin our discussion of electrocardiography with a brief description of the basic electrophysiological properties of the heart.

Cardiac Action Potentials

As with other excitable tissue, cardiac cells can depolarize, rapidly initiating an action potential, and then repolarize. In muscle cells, action potentials are responsible for the initiation of muscle contraction. Once an excitable cell is depolarized either by a propagated wave of excitation originally initiated by pacemaker cells or by artificial stimulation, it may reach a critical level, called its *threshold potential*, and an action potential occurs.[2]

Most of the excitable cardiac cells, including atrial and ventricular muscle cells, and the specialized conducting cells, such as Purkinje fibers, have action potentials like the one shown in Fig. 9.1A. Pacemaker cells, including those of the SA node and AV node, have a slightly different type of action potential (see Fig. 9.1B). The latter type of action potential is discussed in the section on pacemaker cell action potentials.

Fig. 9.1A shows that action potential begins when the cell membrane of the excitable cell is exposed to a depolarizing current and eventually reaches its excitation threshold potential.

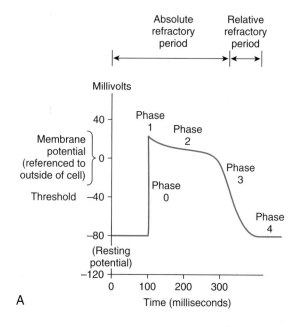

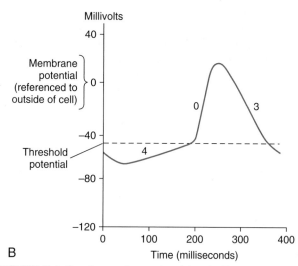

FIGURE 9.1 Cardiac action potentials. A, Fast-type action potentials, such as those seen in atrial and ventricular muscle and His-Purkinje fibers. B, Slow-type action potentials characteristic of nodal tissue, such as the sinoatrial (SA) node and atrioventricular (AV) node.

The initial phase of this type of action potential (at the point where the cell reaches its threshold potential), referred to as *phase 0*, consists of a rapid upstroke or depolarization. This change in membrane potential to a more positive value occurs because of a rapid influx of sodium ions into the cell. (At the peak of phase 0, the inside of the cell actually becomes positive relative to the outside of the cell.) The increased conductance of sodium into the cell during this phase of the action potential is thought to occur as a result of activation of the so-called *fast* sodium channels in the cell membrane.[2] After several milliseconds, these sodium channels become inactivated and close. They remain closed until the cell reaches its resting membrane potential. During phase 1, the cell undergoes a partial repolarization, in which the membrane potential falls from a value of approximately 20 millivolts (mV) to a value of approximately 0 mV. It is thought that this partial repolarization results from a countercurrent flow of potassium out of the cell and to a decrease in sodium conductance into the cell with closure of the fast sodium gates. At this time, a series of slow calcium and sodium channels opens, and a plateau phase 2 is established. Phase 2 lasts approximately 200 to 300 milliseconds (msec). Phase 3 of the action potential begins when the myocardial cell starts to repolarize and return toward the negative resting membrane potential, or phase 4 of the action potential. This repolarization occurs because the membrane becomes more permeable to potassium ions, allowing a greater number of these charged ions to move outside of the cell, and inactivation of the slow channels for calcium and sodium. The increased efflux of positive potassium ions at the same time as the decreased influx of sodium and calcium ions results in restoration of the negative resting membrane potential.[2]

The period from the beginning of phase 0 to the middle of phase 3 is referred to as the absolute or effective refractory period, because regardless of the strength of the stimulus, the myocyte cannot be depolarized again. A relative refractory period follows immediately after the absolute refractory period (this period begins during the middle of phase 3 and lasts until the beginning of phase 4). During the relative refractory period, the myocyte can be depolarized again by a stronger than normal stimulus; however, the amplitude and duration of these action potentials are considerably reduced.

Pacemaker Action Potentials

As was mentioned previously, pacemaker cells of the SA and AV nodes normally have action potentials that differ from those of other excitable cells of the heart. As shown in Fig. 9.1B, the resting membrane potential and threshold potential of pacemaker cells are less negative than those of other excitable myocardial cells. Phase 0 of pacemaker cells is slower than the action potentials of atrial, ventricular, and Purkinje fiber myocardial cells. (Because the slope of phase 0 of the pacemaker cell's action potential is less than those of the atrial, ventricular, and Purkinje fiber action potentials, the former often are referred to as *slow* action potentials, whereas the latter are called *fast* action potentials.) In addition, pacemaker cells do not have a prolonged phase 2, or plateau (i.e., the action potential for these cells includes only phases 0, 3, and 4). The most important difference between the *slow* and *fast* action potentials is the rate at which pacemaker cells can elicit a spontaneous action potential during phase 4. It is thought that this ability of pacemaker cells to discharge automatically results from a progressive decrease in permeability of the cell membrane to potassium ions while the permeability of the membrane to sodium remains unchanged. As a result, the inside of the cell progressively depolarizes (i.e., phase 4, diastolic depolarization). When the threshold is reached, the action potential occurs. Although the frequency of discharge (i.e., the heart rate) is influenced primarily by the decrease in permeability of the membrane to potassium, the amplitude of the slow action potential is determined by the influx of

calcium into the cell. Under normal conditions the SA node discharges approximately 60 to 100 times per minute, whereas the AV node discharges 40 to 60 times per minute. Although other myocardial cells, such as Purkinje fiber cells, can also discharge spontaneously, their discharge rate is so low (15 to 40 times per minute) that they do not normally act as pacemaker cells.

The heart rate can be increased by anything that increases the rate of spontaneous depolarization. That is, anything that increases the slope of the phase 4 diastolic depolarization raises the resting membrane potential (i.e., makes it less negative) or decreases the threshold potential. Conversely, the heart rate is decreased by anything that decreases the rate of spontaneous phase 4 depolarization, whether by decreasing the slope of phase 4, hyperpolarizing the resting membrane potential (making the resting membrane potential more negative), or raising the threshold potential.

Although it has been stated that the heart can initiate impulses in the absence of inputs from the central nervous system, it should be apparent that an individual's heart rate changes dramatically with alterations in the level of activation of the autonomic nervous system (i.e., sympathetic vs. parasympathetic control). Norepinephrine and epinephrine, which mediate sympathetic control, can increase the heart rate by increasing the slope of the phase 4 diastolic depolarization, decreasing the threshold potential, or hypopolarizing the resting membrane potential; acetylcholine, which mediates parasympathetic control, can decrease the heart rate by decreasing the slope of the phase 4 depolarization, increasing the threshold potential, or hyperpolarizing the resting membrane potential. It is important to understand that pacemaker cells receive continuous input from both divisions of the autonomic nervous system. Therefore the heart rate can be increased by an increase in sympathetic stimulation or by a decrease in parasympathetic activity. Conversely, it can be decreased by an increase in parasympathetic stimulation or by a decrease in sympathetic tone.

Conduction Pathways of the Heart

As was stated previously, conductivity is the ability of the heart to propagate impulses throughout the heart. This property of conductivity is remarkably consistent under normal circumstances. Depolarization of the SA node, which is located at the bifurcation of the superior vena cava and the right atrium, initiates the heartbeat by triggering a wave of excitation that spreads throughout the right and left atria as it moves toward the AV node. (*Note:* The SA node normally is considered the pacemaker of the heart because it has the highest rate of automatic discharge.) As shown in Fig. 9.2, the movement of electrical impulses between the SA and AV nodes occurs through a series of high-speed internodal conduction pathways, referred to as the anterior, middle, and posterior *internodal pathways*. Impulses travel to the left atrium via a branch of the anterior internodal pathway, which is called the *Bachmann bundle*.[2]

As the impulse travels through the AV node, a 100-msec delay occurs in conduction. This important delay allows the

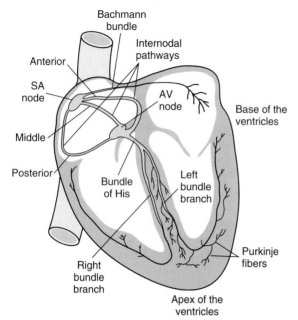

FIGURE 9.2 Electrical conduction system of the heart. *SA,* Sinoatrial.

atria to become fully depolarized and contract before ventricular excitation begins, thus allowing the atrial contraction and emptying (i.e., "atrial kick") to contribute optimally to ventricular filling. After the delay and depolarization of the AV node, the wave of excitation spreads to the muscle cells of the ventricles via a specialized high-speed conduction system that starts at the *bundle of His* and then splits into the right and left bundle branches. The bundle branches ultimately divide into a complex network of specialized conducting fibers, the *Purkinje fibers,* located beneath the surface of the endocardium. Excitation of the ventricular muscle cells finally occurs as impulses travel cell to cell from the inner endocardial surface to the outer epicardial surface and from the apex to the base of the heart. Repolarization of the ventricles normally occurs from epicardium to endocardium; that is, in the opposite direction of depolarization. Repolarization of the ventricles also usually begins in the apex of the heart and travels toward the base.

The Electrocardiograph

The electrocardiogram (ECG) is a graphic representation of electrical voltages generated by cardiac tissue. Because the heart can be considered an electrical generator within a volume conductor, electrical potentials measured at various points on the body surface can be related to electrical impulses traveling through the heart. (Although the term *volume conductor* sometimes is difficult to understand, it can best be explained in the following manner: The heart is surrounded by tissues that contain ions, which can conduct electrical impulses generated in the heart to the body surface, where these electrical signals can be detected by electrodes placed on the skin.) The electrical activity measured by the ECG is not directly comparable with the action potentials of any individual cell but rather represents *summed* information from

many cells at any instant. Therefore the potential difference determined actually shows the resolved direction, or vector, with respect to a particular frame of reference, of the movement of a wave of depolarization as it travels within the heart.

Fig. 9.3 shows the major components of an electrocardiograph. Electrodes placed on the patient's skin act as transducers to convert ionic potentials into electrical impulses. These electrical impulses are then transmitted to an amplifier before being registered on an output display, such as a graphic recorder or an ECG monitor.

The electrocardiograph is wired in such a way that two or more electrodes are connected together to form an ECG lead. Each ECG lead will have an electrode that is designated as the positive or sensing electrode and one or more leads that form the negative or reference electrode. With this configuration a wave or vector of depolarization traveling toward the sensing or positive electrode results in an upward deflection on the recording paper or monitor. Conversely, a wave of depolarization moving away from the sensing electrode results in a downward deflection on the recording paper or monitor.

Most, if not all, electrocardiography machines currently used in the clinical setting use computerized systems for recording and storing digital data, along with proprietary software, which can provide nearly instantaneous interpretation of ECGs.[1] The following sections provide evidence-based guidelines that should be used during the electrocardiography procedure. Several aspects of electrocardiography are considered, including standard methods for recording ECGs, selective criteria that can be used to define a "normal" ECG, and a clinically relevant approach to the analysis of ECGs to facilitate recognition of abnormalities in cardiac electrical activity.

Electrodes

A variety of electrodes have been used in clinical electrocardiography, including plate electrodes, suction-cup electrodes, floating electrodes, and tab electrodes. Plate and suction-cup electrodes, which are made of silver, nickel, or a similar alloy with high conductivity, were the original electrodes used in the development of electrocardiography. A thin coat of conduction jelly or electrolyte paste, which reduced the impedance of the skin–electrode interface, was applied evenly to the electrode before the electrode was attached to the body surface. Although both plate and suction-cup electrodes provided accurate and reliable results, they are rarely if ever used in clinical electrocardiography.

Current ECG technology relies on disposable floating electrodes. Floating electrodes consist of a silver–silver chloride electrode embedded in a plastic housing (Fig. 9.4). The surface of the electrode is covered with a conductive gel or paste. The entire electrode assembly can be attached to the skin with a double-sided ring, which adheres to the patient's skin and to the plastic housing of the electrode. These pregelled electrodes are referred to as "floating" electrodes because the only conductive path between the electrode and the patient's skin is the electrolyte gel or paste. Floating electrodes are typically used for long-term monitoring and for ECG recordings during exercise testing. Electrodes can be connected to the lead cables

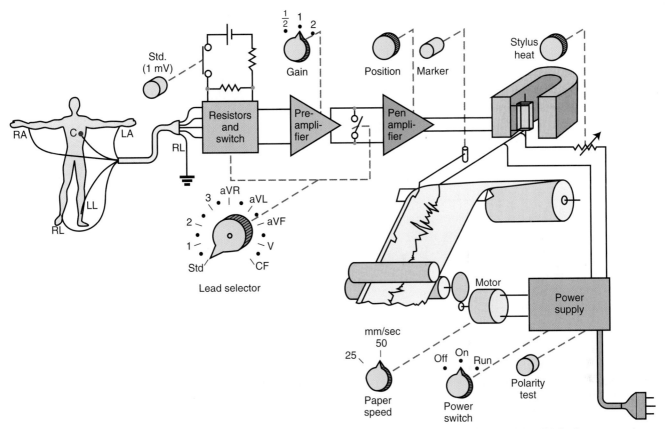

FIGURE 9.3 Major components of an electrocardiograph. (Modified from Cromwell L, Weibell FJ, Pfeiffer EA: *Biomedical instrumentation and measurements,* ed 2, ©1980. Reprinted by permission of Pearson Education, Inc., New York, New York.)

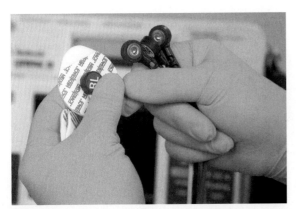

FIGURE 9.4 Floating electrode used in electrocardiogram monitoring. (From Aehlert B: *ECGs made easy,* ed 5, St. Louis, 2013, Mosby-Elsevier.)

of the electrocardiograph by a snap, which is incorporated into the plastic housing of the electrode.

Tab electrodes are made of plastic that is coated with a silver chloride adhesive gel. These electrodes offer effective adhesion and can be used to obtain high-quality traces. They are attached to the ECG lead cables via an alligator clamp mechanism. Tab electrodes are hypoallergenic and usually easy to remove. They are routinely used for obtaining ECGs in emergency departments and in general care situations (e.g., preoperative ECGs).

Lead Configurations

The standard ECG has 12 leads: three standard limb leads, three augmented limb leads, and six precordial or chest leads. The standard limb leads plus the augmented limb leads are oriented in a hexaxial arrangement that gives information about the frontal plane of the heart (i.e., the frontal plane of the heart is divided into six different angles). The chest leads provide information about electrical activity of the heart when it is observed in the horizontal plane. Fig. 9.5 shows electrode placement for a standard 12-lead ECG.

The standard limb leads, which are designated leads I, II, and III, form an equilateral triangle, often referred to as the *Einthoven triangle* (Fig. 9.6). These leads are *bipolar*, having one positive electrode and one negative electrode. In lead I the right arm is negative, and the left arm is positive. In lead II the right arm is negative, and the left leg is positive. In lead III the left arm is negative, and the left leg is positive. In all the standard limb leads, the right leg electrode serves as a ground. Notice that the limb electrodes may be attached to the torso rather than on the arms (i.e., *Mason-Liker* lead configurations).[3]

The augmented leads, which are designated leads aVR, aVL, and aVF, are all *unipolar*; that is, each lead is arranged such that each one of the three limb electrodes is designated as the positive electrode, whereas the other two are taken together to be zero or the reference electrode. For example, in lead aVR

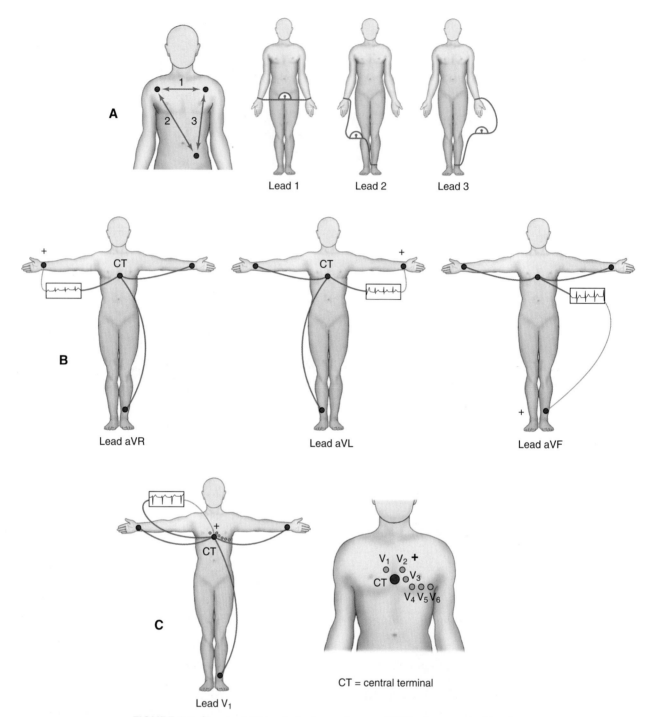

FIGURE 9.5 Standard 12-lead electrocardiogram (ECG) placement of leads.

the right arm is the positive electrode, and the left arm and left leg electrodes constitute the zero reference. In lead aVL the left arm is positive, and the right arm and left leg, taken together, are the zero reference. For lead aVF the left leg is positive, and the right arm and left arm, taken together, are the reference. The term *augmented* is applied to these electrodes because the waveforms generated with these lead configurations typically are electronically amplified one and one-half times the recorded amplitude before being displayed.[3]

The precordial or chest leads V_1 to V_6 are *unipolar* leads arranged on the surface of the chest. In these leads the positive

or exploring electrode is located at a standard position on the chest (see Fig. 9.5); the three limb electrodes are averaged together to create a reference, or the central terminal, which in this case would be located at the center of the thoracic cavity. In special cases, additional precordial leads may be used, including leads V_7, V_8, V_9, and V_3R, V_4R, V_5R, V_6R, V_7R, V_8R, and V_9R. Note that V_7 is located in the fifth intercostal space at the posterior axillary line.[4] Leads V_8 and V_9 are located at the angle of the scapula, over the spine at the level of V_3 and V_4. V_3R through V_9R are placed on the right side of the chest in a position oriented similarly to those of V_3 through

Standard limb leads

Augmented leads

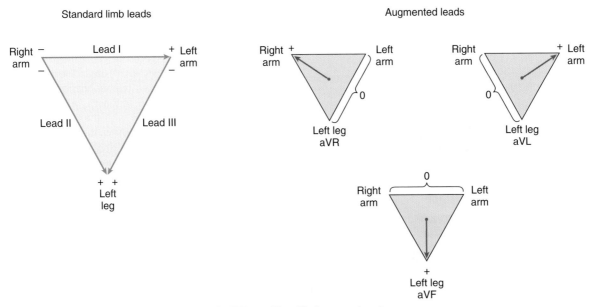

FIGURE 9.6 The Einthoven triangle.

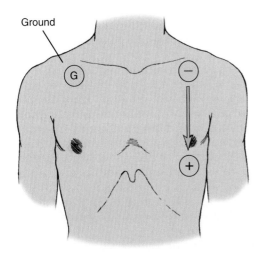

FIGURE 9.7 Electrode placement for modified chest leads (MCL3).

TABLE 9.1 American Heart Association Standards for Electrode Placement		
Location	**Inscription**	**Color**
Right arm	RA	White
Left arm	LA	Black
Right leg	RL	Green
Left leg	LL	Red
Chest	V_1 to V_6	Brown

Compiled from American Heart Association website (http://www.heart.org), accessed May 20, 2016.

V_9.[3] V_3R through V_9R are often used in cases where right ventricular hypertrophy is suspected.

During clinical exercise testing, modified chest leads (MCLs) often are used to monitor patients with suspected arrhythmias. These leads include a positive electrode in the V_3 or V_5 position and a negative electrode placed on the left shoulder or forehead. For example, with the MCL3 lead, the positive electrode is at the V_3 position (Fig. 9.7).[4] Table 9.1 provides a summary of the American Heart Association (AHA) standards for electrode placement.

Electrocardiographic Recorders

The typical ECG recorder includes a differential amplifier with filtering circuits and an output display, such as a strip chart recorder or an ECG monitor. The differential amplifier and filtering circuits serve to increase the power output of the electrical signals detected by the surface electrodes and to remove extraneous electrical interference. Electrical interference, or "noise," can be caused by action potentials generated by skeletal muscle (electromyographic interference), fluorescent lights, and television and radio signals, as well as by other electrical monitoring devices attached to the patient.[5] A special circuit that allows a 1-mV standardization voltage to be introduced into the system also is included in the central processing unit so that the output display can be calibrated.

Modern microprocessor-controlled systems can automatically digitally record and analyze a standard 12-lead ECG or allow the technician to manually record selected ECG leads (Fig. 9.8). As discussed later in this chapter, automated analysis of ECGs depends on precise signal acquisition and processing; the accurate identification and measurements of waves, complexes, and intervals; and applying these findings to an appropriate diagnostic classification.[1]

Most electrocardiographs are equipped with direct-writing recorders to provide hard-copy ECG records, as well as computer data storage and graphic displays for long-term monitoring. For direct-writing strip chart recorders, the ECG is inscribed on a moving sheet of heat-sensitive paper with an electrically heated stylus. The paper upon which the ECG is recorded is ruled in lines 1 mm apart, both vertically and

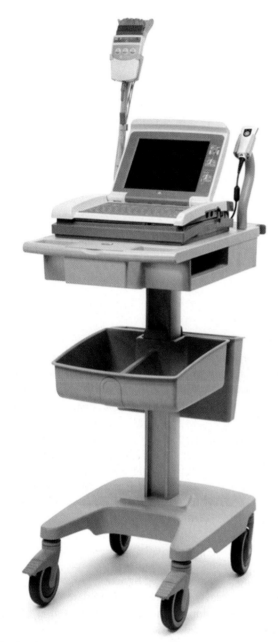

FIGURE 9.8 Modern microprocessor-controlled electrocardiograph. (Courtesy GE Healthcare, Milwaukee, WI.)

horizontally. As discussed in the next subsection, when properly standardized, the amplitude and duration of waves, complexes, and intervals can be determined from the ECG. Box 9.1 provides a standard protocol for recording a 12-lead ECG.

The Normal Electrocardiogram

Fig. 9.9 shows the various waves, complexes, and intervals normally seen on an ECG.[6] (The ECG waveform shown in this figure is derived from lead II. Note that the amplitude of each of the waves varies, depending on the lead examined and the vectors of depolarization and repolarization.) It is important to understand that all ECGs are standardized; that is, ECGs are recorded on paper that is ruled in millimeters in the horizontal and vertical planes. Notice that the graph has

heavy lines every fifth millimeter, both in the horizontal and vertical directions. When an ECG is recorded, the paper speed is set at 25 mm/s, the equivalent of 1500 mm/min. As such, time is recorded on the *x* axis, with each millimeter representing 0.04 seconds and 0.2 seconds between each heavy vertical line. Marks often are seen at 75-mm intervals along the top

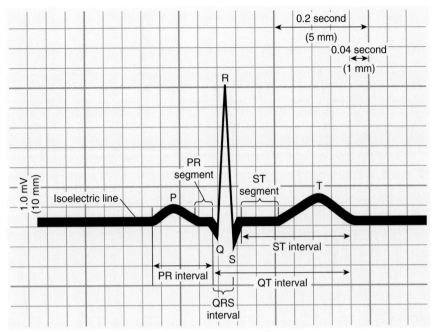

FIGURE 9.9 Normal electrocardiogram showing waves, complexes, and intervals.

of the strip, corresponding to 3-second intervals. ECGs also are calibrated so that each millimeter on the y axis is equal to 0.1 mV. Therefore a 10-mm deflection vertically equals 1 mV.

Waves, Complexes, and Intervals

P wave. The P wave represents depolarization of the atria. As was discussed previously, atrial depolarization normally begins at the SA node and travels from right to left and toward the AV node. The P wave is upward in leads I, II, aVF, and V_3 to V_6. It usually is inverted in leads aVR, V_1, and sometimes V_2. The P wave normally is 0.1 to 0.3 mV in amplitude and 0.06 to 0.1 second in duration. Atrial disease is associated with a prolongation of the P wave to greater than 0.1 second.

PR interval. The PR interval, which is the time interval between the beginning of the P wave and the beginning of the QRS complex, represents the conduction time required for an impulse initiated in the atria to travel through the AV node. It normally ranges from 0.12 to 0.2 second in duration. The PR segment, which occurs between the end of the P wave and the beginning of the QRS complex, corresponds to the 0.1-second delay that occurs as the cardiac impulse travels through the AV node. Because the delay occurs after the atrial muscle mass has depolarized completely, the PR segment is on the line of zero potential, which is called the *isoelectric line.* Blocks in conduction through the AV node, which are discussed in greater detail later, may result in either prolonged PR intervals or P waves that are not followed by QRS complexes. These are called first-degree, second-degree, and third-degree AV blocks. Shortening of the PR interval is associated with pre-excitation syndrome (see Wolff-Parkinson-White syndrome later in this chapter) and with atrial impulses initiated low in the atria near the AV node.

QRS complexes. The QRS complex represents ventricular depolarization. A Q wave is a downward deflection that

precedes the upward deflection of an R wave; an S wave is a downward deflection following an R wave. Fig. 9.10 shows several types of QRS complexes that may be seen in ECGs. Under normal circumstances the QRS duration is approximately 0.1 second because the high-speed conduction system of the bundle of His, left and right bundle branches, and the Purkinje fiber system allow rapid and complete depolarization of the ventricles. Prolonged QRS durations and abnormal-appearing QRS complexes indicate ventricular muscle cell-to-muscle cell conduction caused either by blocks in the high-speed conduction pathway or by initiation of ventricular depolarization by an ectopic focus. An ectopic beat typically is defined as electrical activation of the heart outside of the normal pacemaker cells (i.e., SA node). The QRS vector normally is upward in leads I, II, aVL, and V_5 and V_6. It usually is downward in leads aVR and V_1.

ST segment. After the ventricles are completely depolarized, an ST segment appears on the ECG. The ventricles stay completely depolarized for a substantial interval, as noted in the discussion of the phase 2 plateau in the section on cardiac action potentials. The ST segment, which is measured from the end of the QRS complex to the beginning of the T wave, falls on the isoelectric line. ST segments above and below the isoelectric line may be seen during myocardial injury as a result of "currents of injury" caused by ions moving into and out of injured cardiac cells. The *J point,* which is the junction between the QRS complex and ST segment, often is used as a reference for describing alterations in the ST segment.

T wave. The T wave represents ventricular repolarization. It usually is upright in all leads except aVR. At first this may seem odd because repolarization is the opposite of depolarization; however, as was noted previously, repolarization usually occurs in a direction opposite to that of depolarization. The T wave usually is rounded, and its amplitude is less than

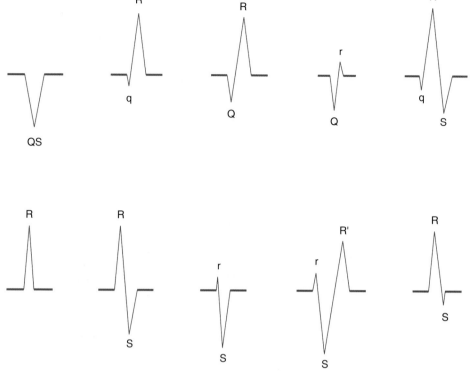

FIGURE 9.10 Types of QRS complexes. (From Phalen T, Aehlert B: *The 12-lead ECG in acute coronary syndromes*, ed 3, St. Louis, 2011, Mosby-Elsevier.)

0.5 mV in the limb leads and less than 1 mV in the precordial leads. It typically is 0.1 to 0.2 seconds in duration.

Repolarization is an energy-dependent phenomenon that is mainly a function of the movement of potassium ions. Any situation compromising the energy state, such as myocardial ischemia, injury, or infarction, therefore can affect this potassium balance of the heart, resulting in altered T waves. Tall T waves may suggest myocardial infarction, potassium excess, coronary ischemia, or ventricular overload. Inversion of T waves is related to coronary ischemia and injury. T-wave inversion occurs in these situations if the T wave originally was upright. If the individual initially demonstrated inverted T waves, ischemia and injury produce an upright T wave. This sometimes is referred to as *pseudonormalization* of the T wave.[6]

Atrial repolarization is not usually visible in the ECG because it does not represent much electrical activity and it usually occurs during ventricular depolarization.

QT interval. The QT interval is measured from the beginning of the QRS complex to the end of the T wave. It represents the time required for ventricular depolarization and repolarization to occur and also approximates the time of ventricular systole. For heart rates of 60 to 100 beats/min, the QT interval is approximately 0.4 seconds. Note that the QT interval varies inversely with the heart rate. Slowing the heart rate lengthens the QT interval, whereas increasing the heart rate shortens the QT interval. The QT interval can be prolonged in congestive heart failure and myocardial infarction, during the administration of antiarrhythmic drugs (e.g., quinidine) and some antibiotics (e.g., erythromycin, fluoroquinolones), and in

electrolyte disturbances (i.e., hypocalcemia and hypomagnesemia). The QT interval is shortened by digitalis, hypercalcemia, and hyperkalemia.[7]

U wave. The U wave follows the T wave and precedes the succeeding P wave. It is thought to represent remnants of ventricular repolarization or repolarization of the papillary muscles. The amplitude and duration of U waves are considerably less than those of the T wave; however, the polarity of the U wave normally is in the same direction as the preceding T wave. When present, U wave amplitude is made more prominent by hypokalemia and bradycardia.[7]

Interpretation of Electrocardiograms

Alterations in the initiation and conduction of electrical impulses through the heart can result in abnormal cardiac rhythms, or arrhythmias (also called *dysrhythmias*). A typical interpretation of an ECG contains information about the effective atrial and ventricular rates, an estimation of the mean ventricular electrical axis, and the presence of arrhythmias. The following subsections present basic techniques for interpreting ECGs.

Determination of the Heart Rate

Fig. 9.11 shows a practical method for determining the heart rate from an ECG. To calculate the heart rate, count the number of cardiac cycles during a 6-second interval and multiply this number by 10. This can be easily accomplished because most ECG paper has vertical markings on the top of the paper corresponding to 3-second intervals when the paper speed is

CLINICAL SCENARIO 9.1

The ECG shown here was obtained from a healthy 20-year-old woman during a maximum exercise effort. Calculate her effective ventricular heart rate.

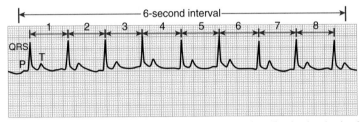

See Appendix A for the answer.

ECG, Electrocardiogram.

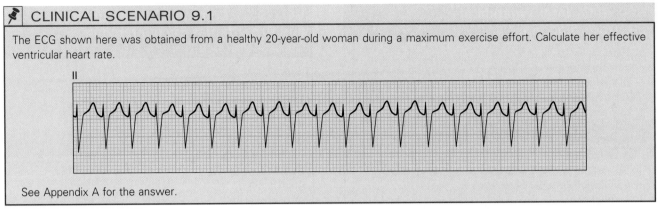

FIGURE 9.11 Determination of the heart rate. (From Huszar RJ: *Basic dysrhythmias: interpretation and management,* ed 3, St. Louis, 2002, Mosby.)

25 mm/s Alternatively, if the patient's heart rate is fairly constant, you can calculate the effective ventricular rate by counting the number of millimeters between two successive R waves (i.e., the R-R interval) and dividing this number into 1500 (25 mm/s = 1500 mm/min). The atrial rate can be calculated similarly by dividing the P-P interval or the number of millimeters between two successive P waves into 1500. Test your ability to calculate the heart rate using the ECG shown in Clinical Scenario 9.1.

Mean electrical axis. As was discussed previously, the mean ventricular axis of the heart represents the average direction and magnitude of the electrical activity of the heart. Fig. 9.12 shows a method for determining the mean ventricular axis. Ordinarily, the frontal plane electrical axis is determined from the standard limb leads. In healthy subjects the mean ventricular axis is between −30 and 105 degrees because of the anatomical position of the heart in the thorax and because the muscle mass of the left ventricle is approximately three times greater than that of the right ventricle. The axis rotates more to the left in normal subjects during expiration and when a subject lies down because the diaphragm rises. Rotation to the right occurs during inspiration and when a subject assumes an upright position. Chronic changes in the mean ventricular axis of the heart occur in pathological conditions, such as left or right ventricular hypertrophy and myocardial infarction and during interventricular conduction delays or bundle-branch blocks.

Pattern Regularity

Identifying abnormal rhythms can be challenging to even an experienced clinician. The following is a list of questions that can be used to determine whether an abnormal rhythm is

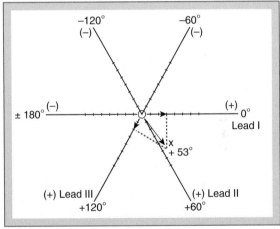

FIGURE 9.12 Simplified method of calculating the mean ventricular axis. The amplitude of the QRS complexes is plotted on the lead I and lead III axes, respectively. The axis is established by determining the resolved vector for these two values.

present. First, are P waves present? Is each QRS complex preceded by a P wave (i.e., is there a 1:1 relationship between the number of P waves and the number of QRS complexes present)? Do the P waves have the same contour, or do they vary from beat to beat? Is the time interval between the initiation of the P wave and the QRS complex less than 0.2 second? Furthermore, does the PR interval have a repeatable value or does it continually vary? The contour of the QRS complexes should be noted. Is the QRS interval less than 0.1 second? If the QRS complexes are prolonged, do the QRS complexes show any abnormal notching? Next, the examiner should look at the contour of the T wave. Is it peaked, depressed, or inverted?

BOX 9.2   Interpretation of Electrocardiograms

I. Rate
   a. Atrial rate
   b. Ventricular rate
II. Rhythm (Supraventricular Versus Ventricular Rhythm)
   a. Presence of P waves
   b. Measurement of the PR interval
   c. QRS duration
   d. QT duration
   e. Presence of premature atrial or ventricular beats
III. Conduction Disturbances
   a. AV blocks
   b. Intraventricular (bundle-branch) blocks
IV. Mean Ventricular Electrical Axis
   a. Chamber enlargement (hypertrophy)
V. Ischemia and Infarction
   a. ST-segment displacement
   b. T-wave changes
   c. Abnormal Q waves
VI. Miscellaneous Findings
   a. Drug effects
   b. Electrolyte disturbances

AV, Atrioventricular.

BOX 9.3   Common Cardiac Rhythms and Arrhythmias Encountered in Clinical Practice

Supraventricular Rhythms
Sinus rhythms
   Normal sinus rhythm
   Sinus tachycardia
   Sinus bradycardia
   Respiratory sinus arrhythmia

Atrial Tachycardia
Atrial flutter
Atrial fibrillation
Junctional (nodal) rhythms

Ventricular Rhythms
Ventricular tachycardia
Ventricular fibrillation
Wolff-Parkinson-White syndrome

Heart Blocks
Intraventricular (bundle-branch) blocks
Atrioventricular blocks
   First degree
   Second degree (Mobitz I and Mobitz II)
   Third degree (complete)

Abnormal Beats
Premature atrial beats
Premature junctional beats
Premature ventricular beats

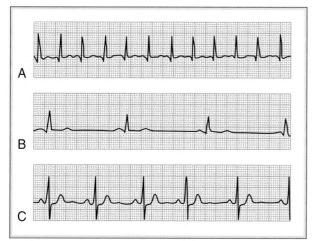

FIGURE 9.13 Sinus rhythms. A, Sinus tachycardia. B, Sinus bradycardia. C, Respiratory sinus arrhythmia.

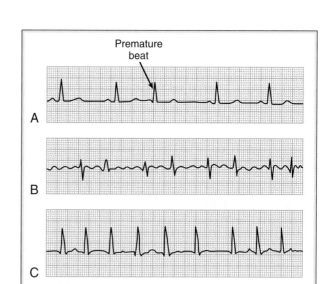

FIGURE 9.14 Supraventricular arrhythmias. A, Atrial premature depolarizations. B, Atrial flutter. C, Atrial fibrillation.

Finally, the position of the ST segment should be evaluated. Is it elevated or depressed below the isoelectric line by 2 mm for 0.08 second or greater? Box 9.2 summarizes various criteria that can be used to identify common arrhythmias encountered in clinical practice. More details about the pathophysiology of the various types of arrhythmias described can be found in the references at the end of this chapter. Box 9.3 lists the most common rhythms and arrhythmias encountered in clinical medicine. Examples of each may be found in Figs. 9.13 to 9.22. Also note that unless stated otherwise, each of the arrhythmias shown is illustrated using lead II.

Sinus rhythms. Remember that under normal circumstances, the heart rate is determined by the number of times the SA node depolarizes per minute. In healthy subjects, if the resting

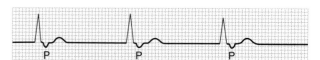

FIGURE 9.15 Junctional rhythm.

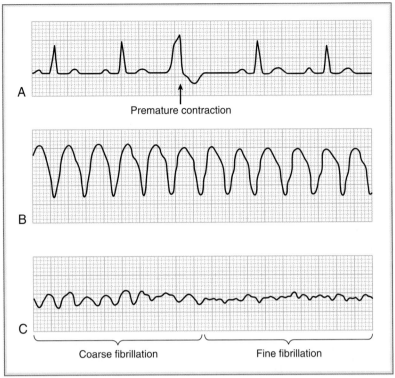

FIGURE 9.16 Ventricular arrhythmias. A, Premature ventricular beats. B, Ventricular tachycardia. C, Ventricular fibrillation.

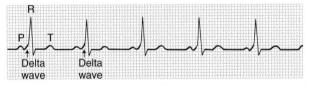

FIGURE 9.17 Electrocardiographic tracing from a patient with Wolff-Parkinson-White syndrome.

heart rate is 60 to 100 beats/min and each QRS complex is preceded by a normally appearing P wave, the rhythm is referred to as a normal sinus rhythm.

In sinus tachycardia (see Fig. 9.13A), the SA node remains the source of cardiac excitation, but the ventricular rate exceeds 100 beats/min. Stimulation of the sympathetic branch of the autonomic nervous system, as occurs with the administration of sympathomimetic amines (e.g., isoproterenol or epinephrine) or drugs that block parasympathetic impulses to the heart (e.g., atropine), causes considerable increases in the heart rate. Sinus tachycardia can also result from exertion, ingestion of large amounts of caffeine or nicotine, fever, anemia, hypoxemia, hypotension, myocardial ischemia, thyrotoxicosis, pulmonary emboli, and congestive heart failure.

Sinus bradycardia (see Fig. 9.13B) refers to a heart rate of less than 60 beats/min. Again, each QRS complex is preceded by a P wave. This rhythm is caused by increased vagal tone, as occurs during carotid sinus massage and after the administration of β-adrenergic blocking agents (e.g., propranolol). Clinically, sinus bradycardia most often is associated with hypothermia, eye surgery, increased intracranial pressure, cervical and mediastinal tumors, vomiting, myxedema, and

vasovagal syncope. (Note that well-trained athletes may demonstrate sinus bradycardia because of an improved ventricular stroke volume. It is not uncommon for these individuals to have resting heart rates as low as 40 beats/min.)

The term sinus arrhythmia (see Fig. 9.13C) is used to describe a regular acceleration of the heart rate during inspiration followed by a slowing of the heart rate during expiration. It should be noted that although these variations in the heart rate may be quite exaggerated, all QRS complexes have a normal duration and they are all preceded by P waves. Also, the PR interval is of normal duration. Sinus arrhythmias are common findings in children and young adults. (It has been suggested that sinus arrhythmias result from the lung inflation reflex or from activation of the Bainbridge reflex; inspiration causes a reduction in intrathoracic pressure, an increase in venous return, and a consequent stretching of the atria, which ultimately leads to an increase in the heart rate. Conversely, during expiration, intrathoracic pressure rises, atrial filling declines, and the heart rate slows.)

Supraventricular arrhythmias. Supraventricular arrhythmias include atrial premature contraction, atrial flutter, atrial fibrillation (see Fig. 9.14), and junctional rhythm (see Fig. 9.15).

Atrial premature depolarizations are ectopic beats that can originate in any part of the atria. The terms *atrial premature contractions, premature atrial beats,* and *atrial extrasystole* are used synonymously in discussions of these arrhythmias. These beats are characterized by P waves that come before the next expected sinus depolarization. Because the atrial premature beat may cause depolarization of the SA node, the interval between the premature P wave and the next normal sinus P

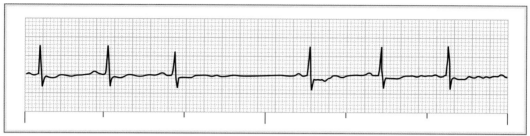

FIGURE 9.18 Sinoatrial (SA) conduction block.

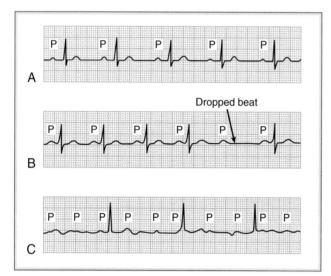

FIGURE 9.19 Atrioventricular (AV) blocks. A, First-degree block. B, Second-degree (Mobitz II) block. C, Third-degree block.

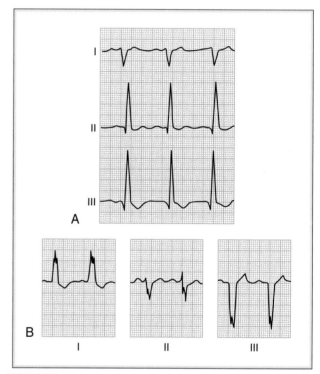

FIGURE 9.20 Intraventricular (bundle-branch) blocks. A, Right bundle-branch block. B, Left bundle-branch block.

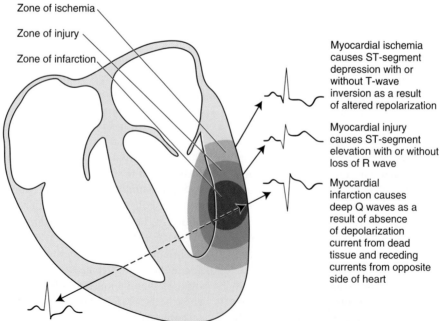

Zone of ischemia
Zone of injury
Zone of infarction

Myocardial ischemia causes ST-segment depression with or without T-wave inversion as a result of altered repolarization

Myocardial injury causes ST-segment elevation with or without loss of R wave

Myocardial infarction causes deep Q waves as a result of absence of depolarization current from dead tissue and receding currents from opposite side of heart

FIGURE 9.21 Electrocardiogram changes associated with myocardial ischemia, injury, and infarction.

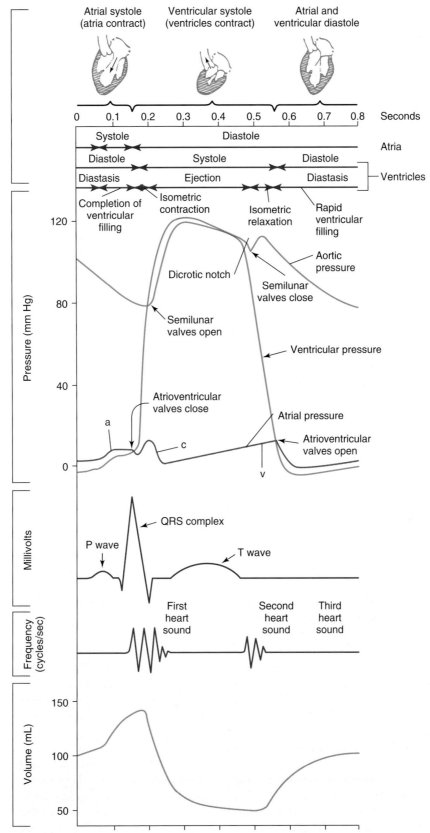

FIGURE 9.22 Pressure, ECG, phonocardiography, and ventricular volume changes occurring during a typical cardiac cycle for a normal healthy individual. (From Cairo JM: *Pilbeam's mechanical ventilation,* ed 5, St. Louis, 2012, Mosby.)

wave is equal to or slightly longer than the usual P-P interval. The configuration of the P wave of an atrial premature beat varies, depending on the site of the ectopy and the lead examined. For example, in lead II, if the impulse is generated high in the atria, the P wave has a normal upright appearance. However, if the focus is low in the atria, the P wave appears inverted because its axis is directed superiorly.

Atrial tachycardia usually involves atrial rates of 150 to 250 beats/min. It can be caused by a number of agents, including stimulants such as caffeine, tobacco, and alcohol; sympathomimetic drugs; hypoxia; elevation of atrial pressure; and digitalis intoxication.

Paroxysmal atrial tachycardia (PAT) is a distinct clinical syndrome characterized by repeated episodes of atrial tachycardia that have an abrupt onset and last a few seconds to many hours. The genesis of this type of arrhythmia is a premature atrial depolarization with a prolonged AV conduction time.[2,6] The prolonged AV conduction time permits the impulse to be reflected back into the atrium (i.e., reentry), resulting in the production of this type of supraventricular tachycardia. Vagal stimulation, caused by gagging, carotid sinus massage, face immersion, or the Valsalva maneuver, often is helpful for determining the underlying rhythm because these maneuvers generally convert PAT to a normal sinus rhythm. Although PAT can be well tolerated in healthy young adults, it can cause serious problems in elderly patients with other forms of heart disease, such as coronary atherosclerosis and valvular stenosis. In the latter group of patients, PAT can lead to myocardial ischemia, infarction, or pulmonary edema.

In atrial flutter the atrial rate is regular and ranges from 250 to 350 beats/min. The ventricular rate typically is approximately 125 to 150 beats/min, and it is regular if a constant degree of AV block is present. Atrial flutter waves (F waves) replace the normal P waves, giving the ECG a characteristic "sawtooth" or "picket fence" appearance.

As with atrial flutter, atrial fibrillation is characterized by gross irregularities in both atrial and ventricular depolarization. The atrial rate usually is 400 to 700 beats/min but generally cannot be quantified. P waves are replaced by fibrillatory waves, which vary in size and shape and are irregular in rhythm. As a result, an undulation of the baseline can be seen on the ECG. The ventricular rate is 120 to 200 beats/min. Note that this ventricular rate occurs because, as a result of the inherent refractoriness of the AV node, not every atrial depolarization that reaches the AV node is transmitted. Therefore only depolarizations that arrive at a period when the AV node is not refractory and that have sufficient strength are transmitted into the ventricles.

Atrial fibrillation may occur intermittently or as a chronic arrhythmia, in which case it is the result of some underlying form of heart disease, such as mitral stenosis, thyrotoxicosis, chronic pericarditis, and congestive heart failure. It also is a common finding in patients recovering from a myocardial infarction, particularly during exercise. However, it may occur paroxysmally in individuals with no apparent heart disease.

Junctional rhythms (see Fig. 9.15) are impulses that originate in or near the AV node. The P wave may precede, coincide with, or follow the QRS, depending on the relative conduction times from the impulse's site of origin in the AV node to the atria and ventricles. Impulses generated high in the AV node are likely to be associated with a P wave that occurs before the QRS complex, whereas impulses generated low in the AV node result in a P wave that follows the QRS complex. Note that because of the retrograde transmission of the impulse into the atria, the P wave appears inverted in the ECG leads that face the left side of the heart (e.g., leads II, III, and aVF), whereas it appears upright in the leads that face the right side of the heart (e.g., leads aVR and V_1).

Junctional rates may vary from 40 to 60 beats/min to well over 100 beats/min. In the case of slower heart rates, the junctional rhythm may serve as an escape mechanism to protect ventricular function. This phenomenon occurs when the SA node either fails to depolarize or impulses generated by the SA node or atria fail to be conducted to the AV node. If the AV node is not depolarized within 1 to 1.5 seconds, it initiates an impulse called an *escape beat.* A series of these beats therefore is called a junctional escape rhythm. Junctional rates greater than 100 beats/min can occur because of an inherent instability in the AV node caused by ischemia or a toxin. This type of junctional rhythm is referred to as *junctional tachycardia.*

Ventricular rhythms. Ventricular arrhythmias include premature ventricular beats, ventricular tachycardia, and ventricular fibrillation (see Fig. 9.16). Premature ventricular beats (PVBs), which are often called *premature ventricular contractions (PVCs),* occur when ectopic impulses originate in the ventricles before the normal sequence of depolarization beginning at the SA node. PVBs are characterized by the absence of P waves and the presence of wide QRS complexes (longer than 0.12 second in duration) that result from sequential activation of the two ventricles rather than the usual simultaneous activation. (Also, remember that the QRS duration is prolonged as a result of cell-to-cell conduction rather than through the normal high-speed conduction pathways in the His-Purkinje system.) Because this type of abnormal depolarization affects repolarization, T waves also are affected (i.e., inverted T waves).

In some instances, ectopic beats originating in the ventricles are conducted to the AV node and into the atria, resulting in inverted P waves. However, in most cases this does not occur, and the impulses generated in the ventricles are blocked from entering the atria; the SA node therefore is unaffected by the abnormal impulse. Consequently, the SA node continues to fire at its own inherent rate. Because the ventricles are refractory to any stimuli after activation, they typically show a "compensatory pause" between the generation of the PVB and the next normally conducted depolarization. This can be seen on an ECG by noting that the duration of two cardiac cycles (including the PVB) is the same as the duration of two normal cycles.

Premature ventricular depolarizations may occur alone or as multiples. *Ventricular bigeminy* refers to a rhythm in which every other beat is a PVB. *Ventricular trigeminy* is the presence of a PVB on every third beat. Ventricular tachycardia exists when three or more PVBs occur in succession at a rate in excess of 100 beats/min. Usually during ventricular tachycardia, AV dissociation occurs; this simply means that the atria depolarize at a rate independent of the ventricular rate. P waves may be discernible between successive QRS complexes in ventricular tachycardia, but they generally are hard to find. Occasionally an impulse originating in the SA node reaches the AV node and ventricles during an interval when the ventricles are not in a refractory period. The SA node depolarization therefore is conducted into the ventricles, resulting in the production of a normal QRS complex or a "captured" beat.

PVBs can occur in normal, healthy subjects who ingest large amounts of caffeine, alcohol, or tobacco, or who are experiencing abnormally high levels of physical or mental stress. Ventricular tachycardia usually is associated with myocardial ischemia and infarction, excessive adrenergic stimulation, and digitalis toxicity. Premature ventricular depolarization that occurs during the T wave (i.e., during the ventricle's vulnerable period or supernormal period, which occurs immediately after the relative refractory period) may cause ventricular tachycardia and possibly even ventricular fibrillation.

In ventricular fibrillation, no effective ventricular contractions occur, and consequently there is no cardiac output. The ECG can show "coarse" or "fine" fibrillatory waves, which replace the normal PQRST waves. The terms *coarse* and *fine* refer to the amplitude of the fibrillatory waves. Ventricular fibrillation should be treated immediately with CPR, including the establishment of a patent airway so that the patient can be ventilated either by mouth-to-mouth methods or with a self-inflating (bag-valve-mask) resuscitator, external chest-wall compressions, pharmacological agents to maintain circulation, and electrical defibrillation. Coarse fibrillatory waves usually indicate that cardiovascular collapse has occurred recently and thus may respond to prompt defibrillation. Fine fibrillatory waves usually indicate that some time has elapsed since the onset of fibrillation and that the success rate for resuscitation may be significantly reduced.

Wolff-Parkinson-White (WPW) syndrome is an unusual rhythm that results from the presence of an abnormal route of conduction that bypasses the AV nodes as the impulse travels from the atria to the ventricles.[6] In most cases this abnormal route is attributed to a group of muscle fibers called the *bundle of Kent*. (It should be noted that other bypass tracts between the atria and the ventricles can also cause WPW preexcitation syndrome.) WPW syndrome is characterized by the presence of a P wave with an abnormally short PR interval. Probably the most ominous sign of WPW syndrome is the presence of an early, slurred upstroke of the QRS wave, often referred to as a *delta wave*. The QRS complex is prolonged, not because of a delay as the impulse travels through the ventricles, but because it started earlier than usual (preexcitation). Fig. 9.17 shows a typical ECG tracing from a patient with WPW syndrome.

Ventricular asystole is the complete absence of any ventricular electrical activity and thus the absence of ventricular

contractions. Ventricular asystole typically occurs after ventricular fibrillation; however, it may occur as a primary event during cardiac arrest.

Heart blocks. Heart blocks, or abnormal conduction delays, may occur anywhere in the heart when the refractory period at a certain point in the conduction path is prolonged. Generally, heart blocks are divided into three categories: (1) SA blocks, (2) AV blocks, and (3) intraventricular (bundle-branch) blocks.

Sinoatrial blocks. SA blocks (see Fig. 9.18) occur when the impulse generated at the SA node is blocked before it can enter the atrial muscle. Typically, the ECG shows a sudden loss of P waves resulting from the absence of atrial depolarization. The contour of the QRS complex is normal, but the R-R intervals usually are prolonged, indicating the presence of a junctional escape rhythm. Transient SA blocks usually do not produce symptoms; prolonged SA blocks can cause dizziness and syncope, particularly if the escape rhythm is slow.

AV blocks. AV blocks occur when impulses generated at the SA node are abnormally prolonged or blocked in or near the AV node. Clinically, AV blocks are classified as first-degree, second-degree, or third-degree blocks. Fig. 9.19 shows ECGs demonstrating each of these conduction delays.

A first-degree AV block is characterized by prolongation of the PR interval (i.e., longer than 0.2 second), although every impulse does result in ventricular depolarization. Patients with a first-degree AV block generally are asymptomatic if they do not demonstrate any other cardiovascular problems.

A second-degree AV block occurs when some of the impulses generated at the SA node fail to pass through the AV node into the ventricles. The ECG shows characteristic "dropped" beats (i.e., the P wave is not followed by a QRS complex), resulting from failure to conduct every impulse from the atria to the ventricles. A second-degree AV block may be further described as a Mobitz type I block or a Mobitz type II block. In a Mobitz type I block, progressive prolongation of the PR interval occurs until at some point a QRS complex does not follow the P wave. In a Mobitz type II AV block, the PR interval does not show the progressive lengthening before the dropped beat.

Mobitz type I blocks usually are associated with blockage of the atrial impulses at the level of the atrial–AV node junction. They often are the result of increased parasympathetic tone or of the effects of drugs (e.g., digitalis or propranolol). Mobitz type II blocks typically occur below the level of the AV node, at the junction of the AV node and the bundle of His. Mobitz type II blocks are most often associated with an organic lesion in the conduction pathway. Mobitz type I blocks usually do not require treatment, whereas Mobitz type II blocks typically require the insertion of a permanent artificial pacemaker.

A third-degree AV block often is referred to as a *complete AV block*, because a complete dissociation of atrial and ventricular conduction occurs. The SA node continues to depolarize at a normal or elevated rate, but the ventricles "escape" to a slower rate. The ECG shows an atrial rate completely dissociated from the ventricular rate. Treatment of third-degree AV blocks usually requires the insertion of an artificial pacemaker if the ventricular rate is too low to permit normal activity.

Intraventricular blocks. Intraventricular blocks, also called *bundle-branch blocks,* occur when impulses are delayed or blocked in either the right or left branches of the Purkinje fiber system. The hallmark of this type of conduction delay is a prolongation of the QRS complex, because distal to the blockage, ventricular excitation must occur by cell-to-cell conduction.

In a right bundle-branch block (see Fig. 9.20A), the QRS complex shows a characteristic rSR′ pattern in the right precordial leads (i.e., leads V_1, V_2, and V_3) and a prolonged, deep S wave in the left precordial leads (leads V_4, V_5, and V_6). Vector analysis of ECGs from patients with a right bundle-branch block shows that the mean ventricular axis is shifted to the right (greater than 90 degrees) as a result of the delayed cell-to-cell conduction through the right ventricle. Right bundle-branch blocks are associated with hypertensive cardiac disease, cardiac tumors, rheumatic heart disease, pulmonary emboli, and congenital cardiac defects.

Left bundle-branch blocks (see Fig. 9.20B) are characterized by the absence of Q waves in the left limb leads (i.e., leads I and aVL) and in the left precordial leads (i.e., leads V_4, V_5, and V_6). The QRS complexes in the left precordial leads show an rsR′ configuration. The mean ventricular axis is shifted to the left in this type of block (less than 30 degrees). Although left bundle-branch blocks are less common than right bundle-branch blocks, they are almost always indicative of coronary artery disease or systemic hypertension. (Other possible causes include aortic stenosis, myocarditis, and congenital cardiac disease.)

Myocardial ischemia and infarction. If coronary blood flow is severely limited, as occurs with atherosclerosis or as a result of obstruction secondary to thromboembolism, the heart's oxygen demand exceeds its oxygen delivery, and myocardial ischemia results. The inability of the coronary circulation to provide blood flow sufficient to meet the increased metabolic demands of the myocardium is manifested in the ECG.

As shown in Fig. 9.21, three types of ECG changes are associated with myocardial ischemia, injury, and infarction: T-wave inversion, ST-segment elevation and depression, and abnormal Q waves. T-wave inversion occurs during periods of transient ischemia. Transient ischemia affects repolarization waves before any other on the ECG because this period represents the most energy-sensitive activity of the heart.

ST-segment alterations occur if ischemia progresses to injury. During myocardial injury the cardiac cell membrane, or sarcolemma, is unable to maintain its integrity, and ions continue to stream into and out of the myocardial cells. These so-called currents of injury are responsible for depression or elevation of the ST segment.

If cardiac tissue is deprived of blood for a prolonged period, the tissue dies, leading to a myocardial infarction (MI). The most characteristic finding in MI is the presence of abnormal Q waves. The abnormal Q waves are most notable on the left precordial leads in MIs that involve the left anterior descending and circumflex branches of the left coronary artery. These Q waves occur because of a lack of counterbalancing electrical forces on the affected side; as a result, the unaffected side demonstrates the predominant electrical forces. Consequently, a downward deflected (Q) wave, rather than an upright (R) wave, appears on the ECG.

Both clinical research and basic research have provided valuable information about localizing MIs by electrocardiography. Table 9.2 lists the common electrocardiographic changes associated with inadequate blood flow to various arteries supplying the heart.[6] A note of caution is appropriate concerning ECG findings associated with MI. Abnormal T waves, ST-segment amplitude, and Q waves can occur with other serious cardiac disorders. For example, T-wave changes and ST-segment displacements (elevation or depression) are associated with pericarditis as well as myocardial ischemia, injury, and infarction (Clinical Scenario 9.2).

II. HEMODYNAMIC MONITORING

Hemodynamic measurements provide valuable information about the mechanical function of the cardiovascular system. To fully appreciate the significance of these measurements, it is important to recognize that the cardiovascular system is essentially a hydraulic system that consists of a pump that propels liquid (i.e., blood) through a series of branched tubes or blood vessels (i.e., arteries, capillaries, and veins) to supply the various organ systems of the body.

A functional description of any hydraulic system requires simultaneous evaluation of a variety of parameters, so that a reasonable estimate can be made of the system's performance characteristics.[8] Therefore the amount of force the heart must generate to propel the blood through the circulation depends on the impedance offered by the blood vessels. As such, measurements of intracardiac and intravascular pressures and cardiac output, along with computation of vascular resistance, can provide fundamental information about the mechanical properties of the cardiovascular system and its ability to perform under varying conditions.

Technological advances in the design of sensors, recording devices, and data analysis systems have greatly improved the ability to obtain accurate and reliable data that can be used in the diagnosis and treatment of patients with various types of cardiopulmonary dysfunction. Indeed, advances in solid-state electronics present possibilities for the future that were previously unimaginable.

Before the various devices routinely used to obtain hemodynamic measurements are described, a review of some basic physical principles as they apply to the heart and circulation is warranted.

The Cardiac Cycle

An appropriate place to begin the discussion of hemodynamics is to describe the pressure, volume, and flow events that occur in the heart and great vessels during a single heartbeat, or cardiac cycle. Fig. 9.22 shows these events as they occur in the left heart chambers and the aorta.[9] The cardiac cycle

TABLE 9.2   Localization of Acute Myocardial Infarction

Anterior Infarcts

Anterolateral (occlusion of the anterior interventricular branch of the left coronary artery)	Deep Q waves in precordial leads V_3 to V_5 Loss of R waves in the left precordial leads (V_4 and V_5) ST-segment elevation in lead I; ST-segment depression in lead III
Anteroseptal (occlusion of the right division of the interventricular branch of the coronary artery)	Deep Q wave in precordial leads V_2 and V_3 Normal QRS complexes in limb leads I, II, and III ST-segment depression in limb lead II
Apical (occlusion of the terminal portions of the anterior interventricular branch of the left coronary artery)	Loss of R waves with deep Q waves in limb lead I and in precordial leads V_3 and V_4 ST-segment elevation in lead I; ST-segment depression in lead III
Anterobasal (occlusion of a branch of the circumflex artery)	Small Q wave in limb lead I; large Q waves in precordial lead V_6 ST-segment elevation in leads I and V_6 T-wave inversion in leads I and V_6

Posterior Infarcts

Posteroseptal (occlusion of the right coronary artery)	ST-segment depression in precordial leads V_3 and V_4
Posteroinferior (occlusion of the posterior interventricular branch of the right coronary artery)	Large Q waves in limb leads II and III and aVF ST-segment depression in leads I, V_3, and V_4; ST-segment elevation in lead aVF
Posterolateral (occlusion of the circumflex artery)	Q waves in leads aVL and V_6 ST-segment elevation and T-wave inversion in limb leads II, III, and aVL

CLINICAL SCENARIO 9.2

A 45-year-old man is admitted to the emergency department complaining of shortness of breath and angina. The patient appears diaphoretic and cyanotic. The 12-lead electrocardiogram shown here was obtained on admission. What are the most significant electrocardiographic findings?

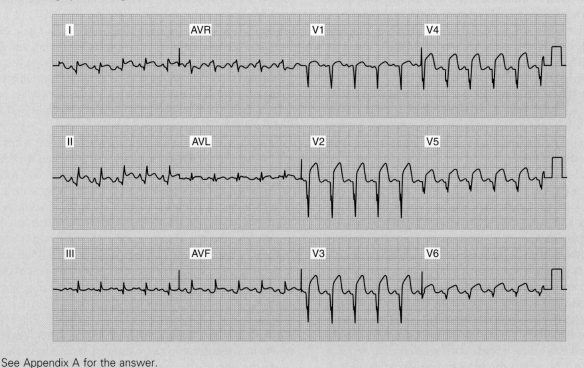

See Appendix A for the answer.

---

typically is divided into two periods, a *systolic period,* during which the heart muscle is contracting and ejecting blood, and a *diastolic period,* during which the heart is relaxing and filling with blood. As shown in Fig. 9.22, the cardiac cycle can be further divided into ventricular and atrial events.

Ventricular Events

Ventricular systole begins with a period of isovolumetric contraction, which follows the peak of the R wave on the ECG. During this period of contraction, ventricular muscle fibers shorten, but the volume of blood in the ventricle remains constant. The volume remains constant because the AV valves (i.e., mitral and tricuspid valves) and the semilunar valves (aortic and pulmonary valves) are closed. (Although the term *isometric contraction* often is used to describe this period, this is not a true isometric contraction, because some of the fibers shorten and others increase in length.[2]) During this period the left ventricular pressure increases from 0 to approximately 80 mm Hg, and the right ventricular pressure increases from 0 to approximately 12 mm Hg.

As the ventricular muscle fibers continue to shorten and the left ventricle pressure exceeds the aortic diastolic pressure (approximately 80 mm Hg) and the right ventricle pressure exceeds the pulmonary artery diastolic pressure (approximately 12 mm Hg), a period of ejection occurs, and blood flows rapidly out of the ventricles as the semilunar valves open. At this point in the cycle, the pressures in the aorta and pulmonary artery increase from their diastolic values toward their peak systolic pressures (approximately 120 mm Hg and 25 mm Hg, respectively). A longer phase, in which the ejection of blood is considerably reduced, immediately follows this period of rapid ejection and lasts until the pressures in the aorta and pulmonary artery decrease to approximately 80 mm Hg and 15 mm Hg, respectively. The rapid ejection period can be distinguished from the reduced ejection period by the contour of the aortic and pulmonary artery flow curves. During the rapid ejection period, the volume flow from the ventricle decreases sharply after the first third of the ejection. During the final two-thirds of ejection, corresponding to the period of reduced ejection, the flow curve tapers. Thus blood flow into the aortic and pulmonary artery increases dramatically during the early period of ejection and gradually decreases during the latter stage of ejection. Notice that the pressures in the ventricles are higher than the pressures in the great vessels during the first third of ejection, whereas the reverse is true during the following two-thirds of ventricular systole. Although it may not be apparent, the point of peak ejection occurs when the ventricular and aortic or pulmonary artery pressure tracings intersect.[2]

A period of ventricular diastole begins with closure of the aortic and pulmonary valve and can be identified by the presence of an incisura on the descending limb of the aortic or pulmonary artery pressure tracings. (This incisura, which is a small negative deflection on the aortic and pulmonary artery tracing, is thought to be associated with a transient reversal of flow that results from elastic recoil of these vessels after ventricular systole, which forces the blood to push against the respective semilunar valve.) The period between the closure of the semilunar valves and the opening of the AV valves is called isovolumetric relaxation, because the pressure in the ventricle falls dramatically, whereas the volume of the ventricle remains constant. As was described for isovolumetric contraction, the AV and semilunar valves are closed during isovolumetric relaxation. The aortic pressure gradually returns to its resting or diastolic value. This gradual decrease in pressure results from the inertia of blood flowing from the heart and to the elastic recoil of the aorta, which propels the blood through the systemic circulation even after ventricular systole

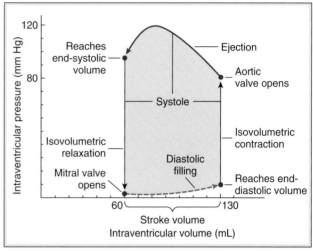

FIGURE 9.23 Pressure–volume graph illustrating changes during a normal cardiac cycle.

has concluded. Upon opening of the AV valves, which occurs as the ventricular pressure drops below the atrial pressure, rapid ventricular filling begins. This rapid filling period typically occurs during the first third of ventricular filling, and it is followed by a longer period of reduced filling, or diastasis. Fig. 9.23 shows another way to illustrate the pressure–volume changes that occur during each cardiac cycle. Although it may not be apparent, these changes are expressed independent of time and thus appear as a pressure-volume loop, with ventricular volume expressed on the abscissa, or *x* axis, and intraventricular pressure plotted on the ordinate, or *y* axis. Note that although the contours of the pressure, volume, and flow tracings for the left and right heart chambers, the aorta, and pulmonary artery are similar, there is a considerable difference in the magnitude of their values.

Atrial Events

Atrial systole begins immediately after the P wave, which, as mentioned previously, is associated with atrial depolarization on the ECG. Atrial systole is indicated on the atrial pressure tracing as an *"a" wave*. Under normal circumstances, ventricular filling occurs mainly during the period of atrial diastole, when the AV valves are open between the atria and ventricles. Atrial systole (i.e., the "atrial kick" mentioned previously) occurs just before the beginning of ventricular systole. Contraction of the atria normally contributes only a small amount of blood to ventricular filling. However, it can contribute a significant amount of blood to ventricular filling if the heart rate is increased and the period of diastasis is reduced. This occurs during ventricular tachycardia, because the higher heart rate results in a reduction in the volume of blood that passively enters the ventricle during atrial diastole.

The next important wave on the atrial pressure tracing is the *"c" wave*, which occurs at the beginning of atrial diastole. This wave coincides with the period of ventricular systole and is associated with a transient increase in atrial pressure as the pressure in the ventricle increases and forces the closed AV valves backward into the atrial chamber. It should be noted that the pressures in the two atria are normally only slightly higher than the ventricular pressures, indicating that minimal resistance exists between these two chambers when the valves are open. The atrial pressure wave shows a slight increase during atrial filling when the AV valves are closed and can be seen as a "v" wave. After the valves open, the pressure in the ventricle falls below the atrial pressure, and the atrial pressure tracing drops sharply as blood flows from the atria into the ventricles, initiating the period of ventricular filling.

Heart and Lung Sounds

Four heart sounds usually are associated with the various ventricular and atrial events of the cardiac cycle (see Fig. 9.22). The first heart sound, typically designated S_1, occurs at the onset of ventricular contraction and is associated with closure of the AV valves and opening of the semilunar valves. It is a relatively low-pitched, high-intensity sound that is best heard over the apex of the heart. It has the longest duration of the four heart sounds. The second heart sound (S_2) occurs at the beginning of ventricular relaxation and is associated with closure of the semilunar valves and opening of the AV valves. It has a higher pitch and a lower intensity than the first heart sound. The third heart sound (S_3) occurs during early ventricular filling and normally is characterized as a low-intensity, low-frequency sound. The fourth heart sound (S_4) occurs during atrial contraction. It also is a low-intensity, low-pitched sound. Under normal circumstances, only the first two heart sounds are audible through a stethoscope. The third and fourth heart sounds are not typically heard with a stethoscope but can be amplified and recorded graphically as a phonocardiogram.

The relationship between ventricular systole and diastole can be correlated with these various heart sounds by simply recognizing that ventricular systole occurs between S_1 and S_2 and ventricular diastole occurs during the period from S_2 to the next S_1. This division of the cardiac cycle based on heart sounds can be very useful when describing murmurs or abnormal heart sounds, which are associated with the generation of turbulent blood flow resulting from abnormal mechanical function of the heart, such as occurs when a valve fails to open or close properly. Clinicians typically describe a murmur as being a systolic murmur or a diastolic murmur, depending on when it is heard relative to S_1 and S_2. Test yourself on this principle by determining whether a stiff, calcified aortic valve causes a systolic or diastolic murmur.

Pressure Measurements

As stated in Chapter 1, pressure (P) may be defined as the force (F) exerted per unit area (A) or

$$P = F/A$$

where pressure can be measured in pounds per square inch (lb/in^2), dynes per square centimeter (dynes/cm^2), millimeters of mercury (mm Hg), centimeters of water (cm H$_2$O), or kilopascals (kPa). You might also remember that a variety of devices can be used to measure atmospheric pressures, most notably the mercury barometer and the aneroid barometer.

This chapter focuses on the pressure-measuring devices routinely used to determine intravascular and intracardiac pressures.

Noninvasive Measurement of Arterial Blood Pressure

The simplest and most widely used technique for measuring arterial blood pressure involves the Riva-Rocci sphygmomanometer. This device consists of an aneroid manometer connected by rubber tubing to a cuff, which can be inflated with a hand bulb. Deflation of the cuff is accomplished with a pressure control valve, which is attached to the tubing that connects the hand bulb to the inflatable cuff.

For blood pressure measurement, the deflated cuff is wrapped snugly around the patient's arm so that the bottom edge of the cuff is approximately 2 to 3 cm above the antecubital fossa. Selecting the appropriate-size cuff is important, because using a cuff that is too big or too small can seriously affect the accuracy of the measurement. The width of the cuff should be approximately 40% to 50% of the circumference of the patient's arm. The length of the cuff should be approximately 80% to 100% of the patient's humerus. For example, the standard blood pressure cuff used for adults is 5 inches wide and approximately 8 to 10 inches long. Pediatric cuffs are available for children younger than 5 years of age. These cuffs typically range from 1.5 to 3 inches wide and 3 to 6 inches long.[9-11] The measurements should be taken on an arm that is not being used for the infusion of fluids or drugs, because inflation of the cuff can obstruct the blood vessel and slow the infusion of the fluids.

While palpating the radial artery in the arm used for measurement, the examiner inflates the cuff to a pressure approximately 30 mm Hg above the pressure at which the radial pulse disappears. A stethoscope is placed over the brachial artery, and the cuff is gradually deflated at a rate of approximately 3 to 5 mm Hg/s. The pressure at which a tapping sound is first heard as the cuff is deflated is the systolic pressure. The pressure at which these sounds become inaudible during cuff deflation is the diastolic pressure. The tapping sounds heard with the aid of the stethoscope are called Korotkoff sounds; these are attributed to turbulent blood flow that occurs when blood is forced through a partially occluded artery.[9,11] As the diameter of the vessel becomes larger with deflation of the compression cuff, blood flow becomes more laminar, and the turbulence that caused the tapping sound essentially disappears.

Automated blood pressure measurement systems (Fig. 9.24) operate on similar principles. These systems are particularly convenient when frequent determinations of blood pressure are required, such as during surgical procedures or in the intensive care unit.[10] Automated blood pressure measurement systems use electricity in the form of either a 110-V, 60-Hz alternating current or a battery as the power source. As with the manual systems, the automated devices can be attached to different-sized disposable cuffs. A microphone or ultrasound transducer attached to the cuff is used instead of the stethoscope to detect pressure pulsations that occur as the blood is forced through the partially occluded blood vessel during cuff deflation.

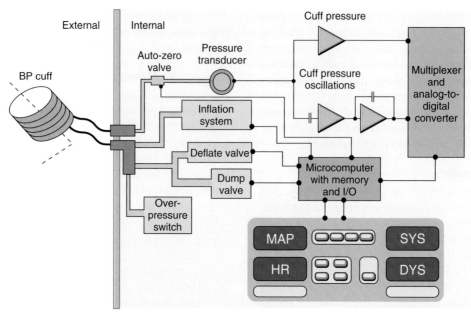

FIGURE 9.24 Automated blood pressure (BP) measurement system. *DYS,* Diastolic pressure; *HR,* heart rate; *I/O,* input/output transfer; *MAP,* mean arterial pressure; *SYS,* systolic pressure. (Courtesy VIASYS, a brand of CareFusion, Yorba Linda, CA.)

Most automated blood pressure devices operate on the principle of oscillometry. When the system is first activated, the cuff is inflated to a preset pressure and held constant for a period of pressure stabilization (e.g., 160 mm Hg). The system then determines whether pressure oscillations are present and records the pressures as the cuff is deflated in a stepwise manner to atmospheric pressure (Fig. 9.25). If oscillations are sensed during the period of pressure stabilization, indicating that the initial cuff pressure was less than the patient s peak systolic pressure, the system increases the inflation pressure on the next cycle. Conversely, the system decreases the inflation pressure on the next cycle if the inflation pressure was too high.

The systolic and diastolic blood pressures, along with the mean arterial blood pressure, can be recorded graphically on an oscilloscope or registered on a light-emitting diode (LED) display. The system automatically zeros itself periodically by opening the transducer to the atmosphere. The systolic pressure corresponds to the point where the cuff oscillations begin to increase, whereas the diastolic pressure occurs at the point where oscillations begin to decrease. The mean arterial pressure corresponds with the point of maximum oscillation.

Automated systems can automatically determine the maximum inflation pressure in the cuff, the cuff inflation time, and the cuff deflation rate by relying on a specially designed control circuit. These circuits are also designed to automatically reject oscillation artifacts that can interfere with the accuracy of the measurements. Audible and visual alarm systems are available on all systems. In many systems the alarms are set at default values but can be manually adjusted by the operator.[11] In several commercially available systems, the alarms are automatically set around the initial readings of the patient's peak systolic, diastolic, and mean arterial pressures.

Although automated noninvasive blood pressure monitors are considered to be a safe alternative to invasive monitoring, several complications can occur when they are used. Complications are associated with prolonged excessive inflation and inappropriate placement of the cuff over a joint. These can include petechiae and ecchymosis, limb edema, venous stasis, peripheral neuropathy, and thrombophlebitis.

The most common errors in determining the arterial blood pressure with both manual sphygmomanometers and automated blood pressure monitoring systems are failure to use the proper size cuff, improper positioning of the cuff, excessively rapid cuff deflation, and motion artifacts. For example, an undersized cuff causes falsely elevated readings, whereas an oversized cuff results in underestimated readings. Mechanical problems, such as a defective pressure control valve or old, porous connecting tubing, also can lead to erroneous results. Improper cuff placement, such as moving it more peripherally away from the level of the heart, typically results in an abnormally high reading for the systolic pressure and an erroneously low diastolic pressure. The most common problem encountered with deflation of the cuff occurs in automated systems that fail to deflate because of obstruction of the cuff vent. This problem may also cause an erroneous zero setting, resulting in lower than actual pressure readings. Motion artifacts caused by patient shivering, tremors, convulsions, or simply by restless movements can affect the measurement. Although most automated systems can reject these extraneous signals, they occasionally fail to do so and therefore provide misleading information.

Invasive Measurement of Arterial Blood Pressure

Invasive measurements, which allow for determination of intravascular and intracardiac pressures, require insertion of fluid-filled catheters into the vascular space. For arterial blood

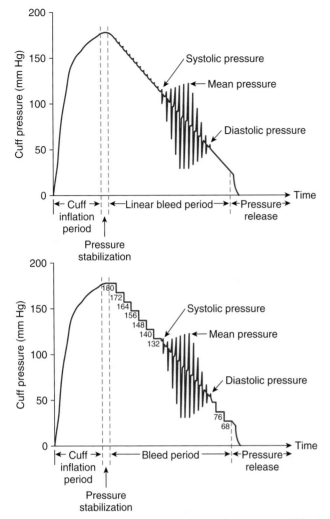

FIGURE 9.25 Pressure oscillation method for automated blood pressure measurement. (Courtesy Medtronic Minimally Invasive Therapies [formerly Tyco Healthcare], Boulder, CO.)

pressure measurements, a catheter made of polytetrafluoroethylene (PTFE, or as it is more commonly known, Teflon) is inserted into a peripheral artery, such as the radial, brachial, or dorsalis pedis artery. Although the radial artery in the nondominant hand is generally considered the preferred site for most applications, the insertion site should be chosen based on assessment of the integrity of the vessel and the presence of adequate collateral circulation. This can be accomplished using the modified Allen test (see Chapter 10).

Box 9.4 lists the equipment required for arterial cannulation. Box 9.5 summarizes the technique for inserting and maintaining an indwelling arterial line catheter.[12] The accuracy of the displayed arterial pressure tracing can be affected by the integrity of the various components of the monitoring system, including the compliance of the arterial catheter, extension tubing, stopcocks, flush devices, pressure transducer, amplifier, and recorder. Table 9.3 is a guide for troubleshooting arterial monitoring systems.[13] The most often cited complications associated with peripheral artery cannulation include bleeding at the insertion site, arterial thrombosis and embolization, limb ischemia, and localized infection. Technical issues

---

BOX 9.4 Equipment Required for Invasive Arterial Monitoring

Cannulation
Teflon intravascular catheter
Guidewire (for use with femoral arterial cannulation)
1% Lidocaine solution
Suture material

Monitoring
Fluid-filled noncompliant tubing with stopcocks
Disposable transducer and dome
Constant flush solution
Connecting cable
Monitor with amplifier
Oscilloscope for displaying arterial waveforms
Direct writing recorder

From Clermon G, Theodore AC: Arterial catheterization techniques for invasive monitoring, https://www.uptodate.com, accessed May 15, 2016.

BOX 9.5 Technique for Insertion and Maintenance of an Indwelling Arterial Line Catheter

1. Identify arterial pulse by palpation.
2. Perform the Allen test before radial artery cannulation to ensure adequate collateral circulation in the limb that will be cannulated. Ischemic complications are lowest when the ulnar artery refill time is less than 5 seconds. Immobilize the wrist on a padded arm board.
3. Sterile technique must be used during insertion (antiseptic preparation, gloves, drapes).
4. Local anesthesia with lidocaine should be considered to avoid pain to the patient in which a percutaneous needle puncture is used. Administering local anesthesia is mandatory in cases where a skin nick (i.e., dermatotomy) is used. (Note that a dermatotomy may be used to avoid skin plug, which can occlude the insertion needle and damage the catheter.)
5. Catheter insertion can be performed using a separate-guidewire approach, the integral-guidewire approach, or the direct puncture approach (Fig. 9.26).
6. Once the catheter is inserted and a patent line is assured, the catheter should be secured with a suture or with a sutureless fixation device.
7. Use a continuous flush system with normal saline solution containing heparin.
8. Assess daily to detect any evidence of inflammation or ischemia in the distal extremity. Remove catheter if there is evidence of distal ischemia, local infection, persistently damped pressure tracing, or difficulty with blood withdrawal.
9. Limit cannulation to 4 to 5 days at one site.

From Clermon G, Theodore AC: Arterial catheterization techniques for invasive monitoring, https://www.uptodate.com, accessed May 15, 2016.

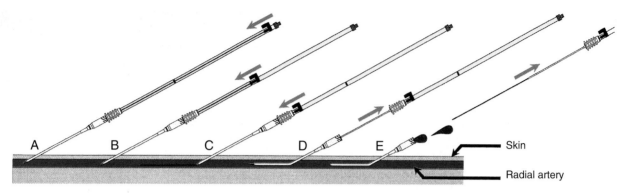

FIGURE 9.26 Percutaneous cannulation of radial artery by a modified Seldinger technique using a catheter-over-needle device with integral guidewire. A, Tab is used to advance guidewire into needle after artery is punctured. B, Tip of guidewire is at the level of the needle orifice once tab reaches marker. C, Guidewire is advanced into artery. D, Catheter is advanced over needle and guidewire into artery. E, Needle and guidewire are removed. (From Kruse J, Fink M, Carlson R: *Saunders manual of critical care medicine*, Philadelphia, 2003, Saunders-Elsevier.)

BOX 9.6   Recommendations for Optimizing Arterial Blood Pressure Monitoring

1. Recommended frequency of dynamic response validation
   A. At least once every 8 hours
   B. After each "opening" of the system such as for zeroing, blood drawing, or changing of tubing
   C. Whenever the pressure waveform appears to be "damped" or otherwise distorted
2. Steps to optimizing dynamic response
   A. Select monitoring "kits" that are simple with a minimum amount of pressure tubing and noncompliant tubing, flush device and transducers
   B. Remove all air bubbles during setup, especially near the transducer. Air bubbles in the side ports of three-way stopcocks are invisible and can be troublesome. Eliminate them by fluid filling all the ports of the stopcock
   C. Minimize the potential for clot formation at the catheter tip by using a continuous flush system. Ascertain that there is not a clot in the catheter by "fast flushing" and, if necessary, aspirate blood from the catheter
   D. Eliminate kinks in the catheter or tubing
   E. Eliminate long lengths (>60 cm) or compliant interconnecting tubing
   F. Use low-volume displacement transducers and continuous flush devices
   G. When all of the above steps have been taken and the system has a natural frequency >7.5 Hz, use of a damping adjustment device is indicated

From Gardner RM: Direct arterial pressure monitoring. *Curr Anaesth Crit Care* 1:239-246, 1990.

that can lead to erroneous measurements include tubing disconnection, air bubbles in the catheter transducer, and arterial thrombosis on the catheter tip or against the catheter wall. Proper transducer calibration is essential for accurate measurements. Box 9.6 describes the procedure that can be used to optimize arterial blood pressure monitoring.

Right-Heart Catheterization

Right-heart pressure measurements are obtained by inserting a catheter into a peripheral vein and slowly guiding it into the right atrium, right ventricle, and ultimately the pulmonary artery with the aid of fluoroscopy or real-time pressure measurements. A significant improvement in right-heart catheterization, including fewer complications and the ability to perform this procedure at the bedside, came with the balloon-tipped, flow-directed pulmonary artery catheter introduced by Swan and Ganz in 1970.[12]

The standard balloon flotation catheter (Fig. 9.27) is a multiple-lumen catheter constructed of Teflon. Adult and pediatric catheters are available. The standard adult catheter is 110 cm long and comes in size 5 or 7 French (Fr) (the French number divided by 3.14, or π, is the external diameter of the catheter in millimeters).[2] Pediatric catheters are 60 cm long and available in either 4 or 5 Fr. All catheters are marked at 10-cm increments. The Swan-Ganz catheter, as it is commonly called, has an inflatable balloon attached to the tip of the catheter with multiple lumens that can be attached to pressure manometers or used for the injection of fluids.

In standard balloon flotation catheters, one lumen connects to a balloon at the tip of the catheter. A second lumen runs the length of the catheter and terminates at a port at the distal end of the catheter. The second lumen's distal port can be used to monitor pulmonary artery systolic and diastolic pressures, as well as pulmonary artery occlusion pressure (PAOP; this pressure is also often referred to as the *pulmonary artery wedge pressure*). It can also be used to obtain mixed venous blood samples when the catheter's distal end is positioned in the pulmonary artery. A third lumen runs to a proximal port 30 cm from the tip of the catheter. When the catheter is placed properly, this proximal port is located in the area of the right atrium and thus can be used to monitor the central venous pressure (CVP). Specially designed thermodilution catheters have a fourth lumen, which contains electrical wires that connect a thermistor located approximately 2 cm from the tip of the catheter to a cardiac output computer.

TABLE 9.3   Troubleshooting Guide for Arterial Monitoring Systems

Problem	Cause	Prevention/Intervention
Blood backup in: catheter, transducer, flush device	Disconnection or leak in pressure system Low pressure (<300 mm Hg) in pressure bag	Return stopcock to proper position Check connections frequently for tightness and leaks Keep pressure bag inflated and flush solution replenished
Air bubbles in: catheter, transducer, device	Inadequate setup of pressurized flush system Improper position of stopcocks Leaks or cracks in catheter or flush system	Careful setup of continuous flush system (CFS) to avoid microbubbles Remove bubbles through stopcock if flush possible by placing the opening in a superior position and "tapping" the flush device so that air bubbles escape out the open stopcock port If there is a stopcock on the transducer dome, simply open the one-way stopcock on the side port and flush fluid and bubbles out of the system Transducers without side ports may require sterile disassembly to remove air bubbles
Pressure stays >200 mm Hg when fast flush released	Broken flush device	Replace flush device
"Pegging" on the top of oscilloscope	Clot on catheter tip or tip against vessel wall (occlusion at tip)	Withdraw catheter 1 to 2 cm Irrigate catheter
Pressure <200 mm Hg when fast flush released	Not enough pressure or fluid in flush bag	Check for adequate pressure and solution in flush bag
Cannot aspirate blood	Catheter against vessel wall Clot in catheter or at tip	Aspirate clot if possible Do not force flush catheter If catheter irrigates easily, flush with syringe Withdraw catheter 1 to 2 cm Maintain continuous flush with heparinized solution Look at catheter for kinks
Cannot irrigate catheter	Catheter clotted or kinked Stopcock turned incorrectly	Check catheter for kinks Check position of stopcocks If catheter clotted, replace Do not force flush clotted catheter, aspirate clot if possible
Tracing off top scale of oscilloscope	Stopcock mispositioned Catheter clotted Wrong scale on monitor Improper zero of monitor	Check stopcock position (see above) Change scale on monitor Check monitor zero
Cannot zero	Wrong monitor channel Bad pressure transducer Bad monitor Improper stopcock position	Select proper monitor channel Replace transducer Replace monitor Check position of stopcocks
No waveform on monitor or strip recorder	Transducer not connected to catheter Monitor off, bad zero Catheter clotted Faulty transducer	Check monitor and stopcock position Turn on and check monitor Aspirate clot from catheter Check and replace transducer
Damp dressings around connects or catheter insertion site	Loose connections Cracked connections Worn connections Infiltration of fluid from vessel or site	Check plumbing connections Check catheter hub and catheter Check insertion site
Questionable low- or high-pressure readings	Improper zero Change in transducer position	Rezero and check transducer position (hydrostatic) Check transducer calibration
Decreased or absent distal pulse or extremity cool and discolored	Thrombosis of artery	Check distal circulation frequently Remove catheter immediately Embolectomy if necessary
Bleeding at insertion site	Coagulation problems Blood leak around catheter	Apply pressure at insertion site Apply pressure dressing or sandbag insertion site
Poor dynamic response	See Box 9.6	See Box 9.6

From Gardner RM, Chapman RH: Trouble-shooting pressure monitoring systems: when do the numbers lie? In Fallat RJ, Luce JM, editors: *Cardiopulmonary critical care management*, New York, 1987, Churchill Livingstone, pp. 145-163.

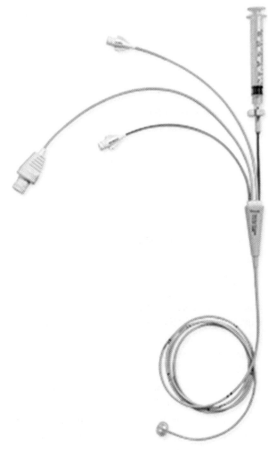

FIGURE 9.27 Balloon-tipped, flow-directed (Swan-Ganz) right-heart catheter. (Courtesy Edwards-American Hospital Supply, Santa Ana, CA.)

(Thermodilution cardiac output measurements are discussed in the section on cardiac output measurements.) Additional features are available with newer catheters for more advanced applications. These additional features include capabilities that allow for (1) temporary right atrial and/or ventricular transvenous pacing, (2) angiographic catheters that are designed for high-pressure dye injections used in radiographic examination, (3) continuous fiberoptic mixed venous oximetry ($S\bar{v}O_2$), and (4) continuous cardiac output measurements. The catheter is introduced percutaneously into a peripheral vein, such as the antecubital, subclavian, internal or external jugular, or femoral vein. Surgical cutdown may be necessary if the antecubital route is used. The catheter is advanced using fluoroscopy or with the aid of continuous pressure monitoring and electrocardiography until the tip of the catheter enters the intrathoracic vessels. Alternatively, the distance required to enter the intrathoracic vessels can be ascertained by noting the 10-cm marks on the catheter. If the catheter is introduced through the antecubital route, this distance is approximately 40 to 50 cm. The distance for the femoral route is approximately 30 to 40 cm, and it is 10 to 15 cm if the internal jugular route is chosen.

After the catheter is positioned in the intrathoracic vessels, the balloon is inflated with a small volume of air (approximately 0.8 mL). (Carbon dioxide [CO_2] sometimes is used to inflate the balloon, because if the balloon should rupture, the CO_2 is absorbed by the tissues rather than causing an air embolism.) The balloon on the tip of the catheter is carried by the blood (like a sail being pushed by the wind) into the ventricle and then to the pulmonary artery. It can be further advanced and wedged into a small pulmonary artery for measurement of the PAOP. The PAOP can be used as an estimate of the left atrial pressure and thus preload of the left ventricle (i.e., the left ventricular end-diastolic pressure [LVEDP], which is not easily measured in the critical care setting). Deflation of the balloon after it is wedged in a small pulmonary artery typically causes the catheter to drift backward into the main pulmonary artery. Fig. 9.28 shows a typical pressure tracing for a healthy adult during right-heart catheterization with a Swan-Ganz catheter.

Box 9.7 summarizes the most common problems encountered during right-heart catheterization. (Clinical Scenario 9.3 presents an exercise involving right-heart catheterization.) It generally has been accepted that the number of critical incidences and problems associated with the use of balloon flotation catheters in critical care medicine has been relatively low in light of the number of catheterizations that have been performed during the past 30 years. However, recent editorials and articles appearing in the medical literature have raised questions regarding the risk-benefit ratio when this procedure

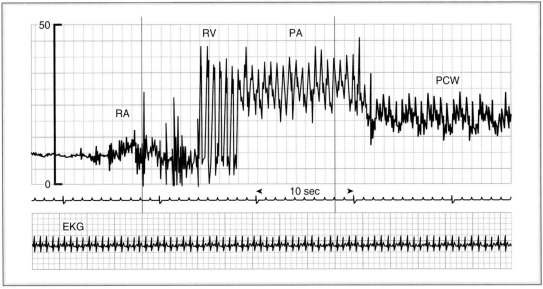

FIGURE 9.28 Pressure tracing obtained during a typical right-heart catheterization in a healthy adult. *EKG,* Electrocardiogram; *PA,* pulmonary artery; *PCW,* pulmonary capillary wedge; *RA,* right atrium; *RV,* right ventricle. (Redrawn from Grossman W: *Cardiac catheterization and angiography,* ed 3, Philadelphia, 1986, Lea & Febiger.)

CLINICAL SCENARIO 9.3

A number of factors can lead to inaccurate pressure measurements during right-heart catheterization with a balloon flotation catheter. Briefly describe how each of the following conditions would adversely affect these measurements:

1. Hypovolemic patient is ventilated with positive end-expiratory pressure.
2. Therapist is unable to obtain a PAOP measurement.
3. Attending physician notes that the pressure tracings are erratic and difficult to decipher.

See Appendix A for the answer.

PAOP, Pulmonary artery occlusion pressure.

is used in critically ill patients. A special commission established by the American College of Chest Physicians, the American Society of Anesthesiologists, and the American Thoracic Society was formed in 2001 to address these issues. A final report from the commission proposed and ultimately succeeded in implementing an educational program to better prepare clinicians using this technology.[14]

Left-Heart Catheterization

Left-heart catheterization, which involves placing a catheter into the aorta, left ventricle, and left atrium, requires a retrograde approach in which the catheter is inserted into a peripheral artery (usually the brachial or femoral artery) under fluoroscopic guidance.[15] A transseptal approach also can be used. In the transseptal technique a specially designed catheter containing a retractable needle is introduced into a peripheral vein and positioned in the right atrium.[15] The clinician then extends the needle and punctures the interatrial septum, establishing a communication between the distal tip of the catheter or needle, which lies within the left atrium, and the proximal opening of the catheter, which can be attached to a

pressure transducer. Left-heart catheterizations are performed in specially designed cardiac catheterization laboratories, whereas right-heart catheterization can be performed either in a cardiac catheterization laboratory or at the bedside in the intensive care unit. Specific information on the procedures for left-heart catheterization can be found in the references at the end of this chapter.

Pressure Transducers

A transducer can be defined simply as a sensor that converts one form of energy into another form. A pressure transducer is an electromechanical device that converts a pressure signal into an electrical signal, which can be recorded or displayed on some type of output device. The number and variety of pressure transducers available for clinical practice have increased during recent years. The principles upon which these devices are based are the electrical properties of resistance, capacitance, and inductance.

Fig. 9.29 shows the three types of electromechanical transducers.[16] A resistance transducer (see Fig. 9.29A) consists of a thin metal diaphragm attached to four wires, forming a Wheatstone bridge. Recall from Chapter 1 that a Wheatstone bridge is an electronic circuit consisting of four resistors connected in parallel. One branch of the circuit contains two resistors (R1 + R2) that form a fixed resistance, and the second branch of the circuit is made up of two resistors (R3 + R4) that form a variable resistance. As pressure is applied to the metal diaphragm, the attached wires are stretched, changing their length and diameter and their electrical resistance. This change in electrical resistance changes the output voltage by an amount that is proportional to the applied pressure.

The variable capacitance transducer (see Fig. 9.29B) also uses a flexible diaphragm to sense pressure changes. In this type of device a thin metal diaphragm is linked to an electrode,

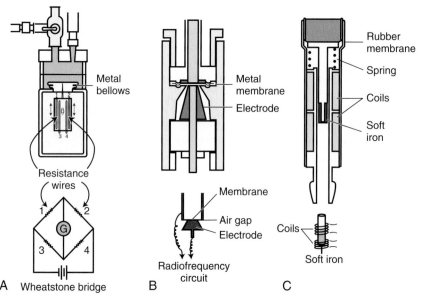

FIGURE 9.29 Electromechanical pressure transducers. A, Resistive transducer. B, Variable capacitance transducer. C, Variable inductance transducer.

forming a capacitor. Notice that when the diaphragm is not flexed, a small gap of air exists between the diaphragm and the electrode. As pressure is applied to the diaphragm, the gap narrows and ultimately causes the capacitor to discharge. As with the resistance transducer, the output voltage is directly proportional to the movement of the diaphragm and thus the pressure applied to it.

A variable inductance transducer (see Fig. 9.29C) consists of a stainless steel diaphragm attached to a soft iron core positioned between two coils. The application of pressure to the diaphragm results in downward displacement of the iron core, ultimately causing a change in the inductance of the two coils. The change in inductance caused by the movement of the iron core between the two coils is proportional to the applied pressure.

Strain gauge and variable inductance pressure transducers are the most frequently used devices because they can respond quickly to pressure changes. They both have good frequency response characteristics over a wide range of pressures. These devices are also quite stable and relatively insensitive to vibration and shock.[17] Variable capacitance transducers are usually large, bulky, and very sensitive to vibrations. They also have poor frequency response characteristics compared with strain gauge and variable inductance transducers.

Cardiac Output Measurements

Historically, invasive techniques involving right-heart catheterization have been the preferred method of determining cardiac output in clinical medicine. The direct Fick method, which is based on a principle formulated by Adolph Fick, has served as the gold standard for cardiac output measurements for more than a century. The development of thermistors and the thermodilution technique for measuring cardiac output have largely supplanted the use of the Fick method in clinical medicine during the past 20 years. More recent advances in the development of noninvasive technologies, which are based on impedance plethysmography and the Doppler effect, may very well prove to be the methods of choice for measuring cardiac output in critically ill patients because of their accuracy and safety.

Noninvasive methods of measuring cardiac output, such as impedance plethysmography and the indirect Fick method, currently are available but are not routinely used by most critical care clinicians for cardiac output determinations. It is reasonable to assume, however, that clinicians will gain more confidence in these techniques and recognize their value in critical care medicine because they can provide another means of assessing the cardiopulmonary status of patients with minimal risk.[17]

Invasive Techniques

Direct Fick method. The Fick principle states that the total uptake of a substance by an organ ($\dot{V}_x$) is directly related to the blood flow through the organ ($\dot{Q}$) and the arteriovenous concentration or content difference of the substance across the organ ($Ca_x - Cv_x$), or

$$\dot{V}O_2 = \dot{Q} \times (CaO_2 - C\overline{v}O_2) \qquad \text{Equation 9.1}$$

We can determine the output of the right ventricle (i.e., pulmonary blood flow) by simultaneously measuring the total uptake of oxygen by the lungs, or oxygen consumption ($\dot{V}O_2$), and the arteriovenous oxygen content difference between arterial blood (CaO_2) and mixed venous blood ($C\overline{v}O_2$). Oxygen consumption is determined from measurements of the volumes and oxygen concentrations of a patient's inspired and expired gases, whereas the arteriovenous oxygen difference is determined by measuring the oxygen content of arterial blood obtained from a peripheral artery and that of a mixed venous sample obtained from the pulmonary artery. The cardiac output can by derived by simply applying Eq. 9.2:

$$\dot{Q} = \dot{V}O_2 \div (CaO_2 - C\overline{v}O_2) \qquad \textbf{Equation 9.2}$$

Clinical Scenario 9.4 presents a scenario for testing yourself on the calculation of cardiac output using the Fick method.

Indicator dilution methods. The indicator dilution method of determining cardiac output, also known as the *Stewart-Hamilton dye dilution technique,* is commonly used to measure cardiac output during cardiac catheterization because of its accuracy and simplicity.[15] A known amount of dye (e.g., indocyanine green or Evans blue) is injected into a peripheral vein. The passage of dye through the pulmonary artery and its appearance and changing concentration in the arterial blood are recorded by continuously passing samples of arterial blood obtained from an indwelling radial, brachial, or femoral arterial line through a densitometer, which determines the concentrations of the dye in the blood. The results are recorded as time–concentration curves, which can be displayed on an

oscilloscope and digitally processed to determine the cardiac output using the relationship shown in Eq. 9.3:

$$\dot{Q} = I/C_o \qquad \textbf{Equation 9.3}$$

where $\dot{Q}$ is the cardiac output, I is the total amount of dye injected (measured in milligrams per minute), and C_o is the average concentration of dye in the first pass through the circulation (measured in milligrams per liter). As shown in Fig. 9.30, if the first-pass curve is extrapolated with regard to time (dashed line), the effects of recirculation can be eliminated and the cardiac output can be calculated by integrating the area under the curve.

Several factors must be considered when this technique is used. Cardiac output determinations are adversely affected in patients with intracardiac shunts and also in patients with low cardiac output. With low cardiac output the downslope of the time–concentration curve may be prolonged because the dye moves more slowly past the detector; this makes it difficult to differentiate recirculated dye from the dye that appears in the first-pass sample.

The thermodilution technique of determining cardiac output is another variation of the indicator dilution method. For the thermodilution technique, approximately 10 mL of cold (or room temperature) sterile 0.9% saline or 5% dextrose is injected through the proximal port of an indwelling balloon-tipped, flow-directed catheter, and a small thermistor at the tip of the catheter senses changes in the temperature of the blood. A cardiac output computer, which is connected to the catheter through electrical contacts, calculates the cardiac output by relying on temperature relationships (similar to the time–concentration relationships mentioned with the dye dilution technique) that occur as the injected fluid changes the temperature of the blood sensed by the catheter's thermistor.

The thermodilution technique is widely used in the critical care setting. The advantage of this technique is that it does not require monitoring of arterial blood samples; measurements require only small volumes of injectate (e.g., cold normal saline), and therefore multiple determinations are possible and there is essentially no problem with recirculation. Inaccuracies can occur in patients with tricuspid valve insufficiency

---

CLINICAL SCENARIO 9.4

The data shown here were obtained from a 70-year-old male patient who is being treated for congestive heart failure. Calculate his cardiac output.

pHa	7.32
PaCO$_2$	50 mm Hg
PaO$_2$	60 mm Hg
HCO$_3^-$	26 mm Hg
SaO$_2$	92%
P$\overline{v}$O$_2$	30 mm Hg
S$\overline{v}$O$_2$	60%
$\dot{V}$O$_2$	200 mL/min
$\dot{V}$CO$_2$	180 mL/min
Temperature	37°C (98.6°F)
$\overline{P}$	750 mm Hg
Hb	12 gm%

See Appendix A for the answer.

Hb, Hemoglobin; *HCO$_3^-$*, bicarbonate; $\overline{P}$, barometric pressure; *PaCO$_2$*, partial pressure of carbon dioxide in the arteries; *PaO$_2$*, partial pressure of oxygen in the arteries; *pHa*, pH of arterial blood; *P$\overline{v}$O$_2$*, partial pressure of oxygen in the mixed venous blood; *SaO$_2$*, arterial oxygen saturation; *S$\overline{v}$O$_2$*, mixed venous oxygen saturation; *$\dot{V}$CO$_2$*, carbon dioxide production per minute; *$\dot{V}$O$_2$*, oxygen consumption per minute.

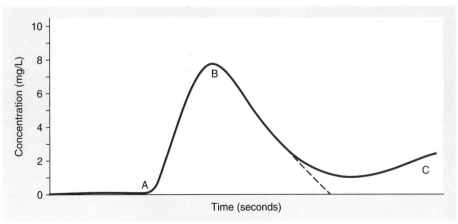

FIGURE 9.30 Indicator dilution curve.

and intracardiac shunts. Measurements are also affected by a low cardiac output. When cardiac output is measured in mechanically ventilated patients, the normal saline should be injected during the end-expiration portion of the ventilatory cycle to ensure that consistent measurements are obtained.

Noninvasive Techniques

Impedance plethysmography. Impedance plethysmography, as it is used in cardiac output measurements, is based on the principle that changes in blood volume associated with pulsations of blood as it passes through a blood vessel cause changes in the electrical impedance, or resistance, of the tissue surrounding the blood vessel.[17] This electrical impedance can be measured by passing a small amount of alternating current through the body segment in question. The amount of alternating electrical current is small enough that the patient does not feel it. An important application of this principle is the diagnosis of deep vein thrombosis.

Impedance cardiography, a variation of impedance plethysmography, can be used to measure cardiac output. A series of two pairs of electrodes is placed on the thorax (Fig. 9.31). The assumption is that changes in bioimpedance that occur with changes in the thoracic blood volume during ventricular systole and diastole can be used to calculate beat-to-beat changes in stroke volume and thus cardiac output. Electrical voltage signals sensed by the measuring electrodes are processed, along with a simultaneous recording of the patient's ECG, and an impedance cardiograph curve is derived. Different points on the impedance cardiograph curve can be labeled and used to calculate variables such as stroke volume and systolic time intervals.

Studies have demonstrated that cardiac output measurements made with thoracic electrical bioimpedance correlate with those obtained by thermodilution and the direct Fick method.[17] The potential uses for impedance cardiography include screening for cardiac disease, pacemaker adjustments, long-term continuous monitoring of cardiac output during surgery and in the intensive care unit, noninvasive

hemodynamic measurements during cardiopulmonary stress testing, and monitoring of the effects of pharmacological interventions.

Transesophageal doppler. Transesophageal Doppler (TED) ultrasonography was first described by Side and Gosling in 1971 and refined by a number of investigators over the following 30 years.[17,18] It is based on the Doppler effect, which describes an apparent change in the frequency of an ultrasonic wave detected downstream of the source of the wave. The change in frequency (Δf) that is detected is directly proportional to the relative velocity between the emitted wave and the received wave, or

$$V = \frac{\Delta f \times c}{2f_T} \times \cos\theta$$

where c is the velocity of the ultrasound waves in body tissue and f_T is the transmitted frequency. The cosine of the angle between the Doppler beam and the blood flow ($\cos\theta$) is a correction factor to adjust the angle of insonation.[18]

Modern TED devices use 4-MHz continuous-wave or 5-MHz pulse-wave Doppler signals that are insonated at angles of 45 to 60 degrees.[17] Table 9.4 provides information about two currently available TED devices. Fig. 9.32 illustrates an esophageal probe in situ.[18] Notice that the probe is inserted via the nose or mouth and positioned in the esophagus in the midthorax at the level of the fifth to sixth thoracic vertebra, which corresponds to the level where the esophagus and descending aorta are approximately parallel. In this position it is possible to determine the descending aortic blood flow

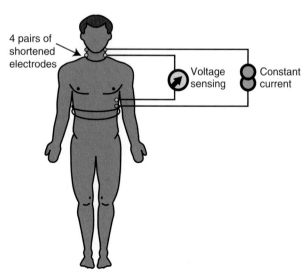

FIGURE 9.31 Impedance cardiograph.

4 pairs of shortened electrodes

Voltage sensing

Constant current

TABLE 9.4	Technical Details of Two Transesophageal Doppler (TED) Devices	
Device	**CardioQ**	**Hemosonic 100**
Manufacturer	Deltex Medical, Chichester, UK	Arrow International, Reading, PA
Doppler mode	Continuous-wave Doppler	Pulsed wave Doppler
Frequency	4 MHz	5 MHz
Angle of insonation	45°	60°
M-mode	None	10 MHz
Probe diameter	14-17 Fr (4.7-5.7 mm), single use	20 Fr (6.7 mm), reusable
Unit dimensions	320 × 250 × 170 mm; 6 kg	300 × 250 × 200 mm; 4 kg
Translation of flow measurement into cardiac output	Nomogram (based on patient's age, weight, and height)	Determination of aortic diameter through M-mode aortography

From Schober P, Loer SA, Schwarte LA: Perioperative hemodynamic monitoring with transesophageal Doppler technology. *Anesth Analg* 109(2):340-353, 2009.

(i.e., cardiac output) by calculating the velocity of erythrocytes passing through an ultrasonic beam emitted into the descending aorta. Fig. 9.33 illustrates a typical velocity-time graph generated during a TED measurement. The systolic portion of the plot is triangular, whereas the base represents the systolic ejection time. The cycle time is calculated as the time interval on the plot between two succeeding flow curves, and the area under the triangular plot represents the stroke volume. Cardiac output is determined by multiplying the stroke distance derived from the triangular plot by the aortic cross-sectional area. It is important to mention that the cardiac output calculation depends on the algorithm used by the manufacturer. For

example, the CardioQ device (Deltex Medical) derives the cardiac output using a nomogram based on the patient's age, height, and weight, whereas the HemoSonic 100 (Arrow International) measures the aortic cross-sectional area via a 10-MHz M-mode ultrasound probe.

TED has been shown to be a safe and relatively quick method for assessing cardiac output in critically ill patients. There are several contraindications for the use of TED devices and conditions in which these devices may give inaccurate data (Box 9.8). Potential complications associated with TED include trauma to the buccal cavity, transient vagal response during probe insertion, epistaxis, esophageal perforation, and endobronchial probe misplacement.[18-23] Endobronchial tube placement can also lead to aspiration of gastric fluid caused by a compromise of the seal of the endobronchial tube cuff.

Indirect fick method. As might be surmised from the name of this technique, the indirect Fick method is based on the Fick principle, which was described previously. In the indirect technique, however, cardiac output is determined through continuous measurements of CO_2 production rather than through oxygen consumption. Arterial and mixed venous oxygen differences are replaced by noninvasive measurements of arterial CO_2 content and mixed venous CO_2 content, respectively.[18] CO_2 production is obtained from continuous measurements of the mixed expired CO_2 (F_ECO_2) and the expired minute ventilation ($\dot{V}_E$). The arterial CO_2 content is calculated from measurements of the partial pressure of the end-tidal CO_2 ($P_{ET}CO_2$) (to approximate the partial pressure of CO_2 in the arteries [$PaCO_2$]); the mixed venous CO_2 content is derived from measurements of the partial pressure of mixed expired CO_2 ($P\overline{v}CO_2$) when the patient intermittently rebreathes a 10% CO_2 mixture (at 10- to 15-second intervals). Cardiac output therefore is calculated as shown in Eq. 9.4:

$$\dot{Q} = \dot{V}CO_2/(P_{\overline{v}}CO_2 - P_{ET}CO_2) \qquad \textbf{Equation 9.4}$$

Results indicate that the indirect Fick technique may prove to be useful for measuring cardiac output in most patients; however, more studies are required to determine the accuracy of this technique in critically ill patients.

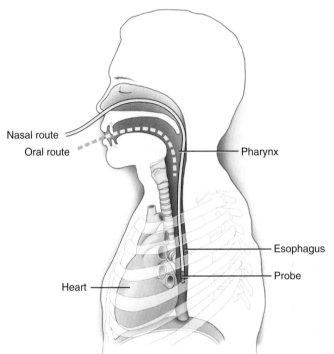

FIGURE 9.32 An esophageal probe in situ. The probe is inserted via the oral or nasal route and positioned at the midthoracic level between the fifth and sixth thoracic vertebrae.

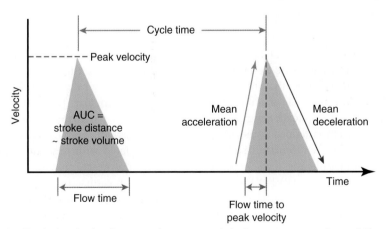

FIGURE 9.33 Typical velocity-time graph generated during a transesophageal Doppler (TED) measurement. *AUC,* Area under the curve. (From Schober P, Loer SA, Schwarte LA: Perioperative hemodynamic monitoring with transesophageal Doppler technology. *Anesth Analg* 109[2]:340-353, 2009.)

BOX 9.8   Contraindications for the Use of Transesophageal Doppler Devices and Conditions in Which the Device May Potentially Produce Inaccurate Readings

Contraindications

1. Local esophageal or oropharyngeal pathology
   Malformations, esophageal varices, tumors
   Strictures
   Esophagitis
   Recent esophageal or upper airway surgery
2. Systemic pathology increasing the risk for local tissue damage or bleeding
   Long-term corticosteroid treatment
   Severe bleeding disorders
3. Specific pathology depending on the route of probe insertion
   Craniofacial trauma or basilar skull fracture for nasal route

Conditions in Which the Device May Potentially Give Inaccurate Readings

1. Conditions potentially resulting in turbulent aortic blood flow
   Aortic coarctation
   Severe aortic stenosis
   Intraaortic balloon counterpulsation
2. Conditions potentially resulting in major deviations of the insonation angle
   Severe scoliosis
   Operative manipulations of the anatomical relationship between esophagus and aorta
3. Conditions potentially resulting in altered distribution of blood flow
   Aortic cross-clamping neuraxial anesthesia
   Severe aortic insufficiency
4. Conditions restricting free access to patient's head
   Head and neck surgery

Modified from Schober P, Loer SA, Schwarte LA: Perioperative hemodynamic monitoring with transesophageal Doppler technology. *Anesth Analg* 109(2):340-353, 2009.

Interpretation of Hemodynamic Profiles

Interpreting hemodynamic data is a fairly straightforward task. However, using this information in the management of patients can be considerably more challenging for even the most skilled clinician. It is reasonable to state that the hemodynamic profile ultimately focuses on the factors that influence cardiac output, namely, the heart rate, preload, contractility, and afterload. Preload, which typically is defined as the filling pressure of the ventricle at the end of ventricular diastole, is estimated by measuring the end-diastolic pressures. As such, the right ventricular end-diastolic pressure (RVEDP) is used as an indicator of the right ventricular preload, and the LVEDP is used to estimate the left ventricular preload. Because both of these intracardiac pressures are difficult to measure in the critical care setting, clinicians rely on measurements of the CVP to estimate the RVEDP and measurements of the PAOP to estimate the LVEDP.

Contractility, which is related to the force the ventricle generates during each cardiac cycle, can be estimated using the ejection fraction (EF) or the ratio of the stroke volume to the ventricular end-diastolic volume. The ventricular afterload is the resistance the ventricle must overcome to eject blood and is estimated from calculations of systemic resistance and the pulmonary vascular resistance.

The information that follows in this section is meant to provide an overview of basic measurements obtained in a standard hemodynamic profile. It is not our purpose to provide an extensive analysis of the various factors and conditions that can influence a patient's hemodynamic status. A number of excellent references related to hemodynamic monitoring in clinical practice are listed at the end of this chapter for readers interested in obtaining more detailed information about this area of clinical physiology.

Cardiac Output

Cardiac output is the volume of blood pumped by the heart each minute; it usually is expressed in liters or milliliters per minute. Cardiac output can be calculated by multiplying the heart rate by the stroke volume, which is the volume of blood pumped by the heart per beat (measured in liters or milliliters per beat). Alternatively, cardiac output can be measured using one of the techniques described in the previous section of this chapter on cardiac output determinations.

In many cases the cardiac output and the stroke volume may be expressed relative to the patient's body surface area (BSA), which can be easily obtained using a Dubois chart. This indexing technique allows the clinician to compare an individual's cardiac output or stroke output with that of normal healthy individuals of the same weight and height (the BSA is calculated using these two anthropometric values). The cardiac index (CI) is calculated by dividing the cardiac output by the BSA as shown in Eq. 9.5:

$$\text{Cardiac Index} = \dot{Q}/\text{BSA} \qquad \textbf{Equation 9.5}$$

Similarly, the stroke index is calculated by dividing the stroke volume by the BSA as shown in Eq. 9.6:

$$\text{Stroke Index} = \text{SV}/\text{BSA} \qquad \textbf{Equation 9.6}$$

The normal CI for an adult is approximately 3.5 L/min/m^2. The stroke index normally ranges from 40 to 50 mL/beat/m^2. Cardiac output can be reduced by decreases in either the heart rate or stroke volume. Decreases in the effective ventricular rate usually are associated with an increase in parasympathetic tone or with various types of bradyarrhythmias. Decreases in stroke volume typically are associated with reductions in the preload or contractility of the heart, or with an abnormally high afterload. Increases in cardiac output are associated with increases in the heart rate or stroke volume. Tachycardia associated with an increase in sympathetic tone or a decrease in parasympathetic tone increases cardiac output. Increases in stroke volume are associated with increases in preload and contractility and with reductions in afterload. Note that profound increases in the heart rate actually can reduce cardiac output by reducing the ventricular filling time and the resultant ventricular preload.

Mixed Venous Oxygen Saturation

If the $\dot{V}O_2$ and cardiac output remain constant, then the difference between the arterial oxygen content and the mixed venous oxygen content also remains constant. Mixed venous oxygen values decline when arterial oxygenation is decreased. They also decrease when cardiac output is reduced. With a reduced cardiac output, more time is available for the extraction of oxygen from blood delivered to the tissues. Reductions in $S\overline{v}O_2$ are also associated with increases in metabolic rate in patients with limited cardiac output. Mixed venous oxygen values can be higher than normal in patients with histotoxic hypoxia (e.g., cyanide poisoning) and in situations where intrapulmonary shunting occurs, (i.e., ventilation/perfusion mismatching).

With recent advances in fiberoptic reflectance oximetry, continuous recordings of $S\overline{v}O_2$ can be obtained. Reflectance oximetry technology has been incorporated into specialized balloon-flotation catheters that are used for right-heart catheterization. Although the potential for this type of monitoring is promising, more studies are required to delineate more clearly the indications for its use in critical care.

Oxygen Delivery

Oxygen delivery (DO_2) is the product of cardiac output and arterial oxygen content. It represents the total amount of oxygen that is carried in the blood to the tissues each minute. Under normal circumstances, DO_2 is approximately 1000 mL/min or approximately 550 to 650 mL/min/m^2.

DO_2 is increased in situations in which cardiac output or arterial oxygen content is elevated. A reduced DO_2 indicates a decrease in cardiac output or arterial oxygen content.[9] For example, DO_2 is increased in hyperdynamic states (increased cardiac output) such as septic shock. Conversely, DO_2 is decreased after hemorrhage in which there is a decrease in arterial oxygen content.

Shunt Fraction

A *shunt* is defined as that portion of the cardiac output that does not participate in gas exchange with alveolar air (i.e., *perfusion without ventilation*). Shunts are usually identified as anatomical shunts, intrapulmonary shunts, and physiological shunts, with the last being the sum of anatomical and intrapulmonary shunts.

Normal anatomical shunts exist because venous blood that would ideally return to the right side of the heart (deoxygenated blood) drains into vessels served by the left side of the heart (oxygenated blood). This venous admixture includes deoxygenated blood from bronchial veins, pleural veins, and thebesian veins, and it typically represents only approximately 2% to 3% of the normal cardiac output. Abnormal anatomical shunts can occur when blood is allowed to bypass the pulmonary circulation and enter directly into the left atrium or left ventricle, as occurs with atrial and ventricular septal wall defects.

Intrapulmonary shunts occur when blood passes through pulmonary capillaries that are not ventilated. Shuntlike states can exist in either poorly ventilated alveolar units that are well perfused or in alveolar-capillary units where oxygen diffusion is impaired. Intrapulmonary shunts can be caused by disorders such as atelectasis, pulmonary edema, pneumonia, pneumothorax, complete airway obstruction, consolidation of the lung, acute respiratory distress syndrome, and, on rare occasions, by arterial-to-venous fistulas.

The total shunt fraction or, more specifically, *physiological shunt*, can be determined by the following classic shunt equation:

$$\dot{Q}s/\dot{Q}_T = (CcO_2 - CaO_2)/(CcO_2 - C\overline{v}O_2)$$

where $\dot{Q}_s$ is the shunted portion of the cardiac output, $\dot{Q}_T$ is total cardiac output, CcO_2 is the content of oxygen of the pulmonary end-capillary after oxygenation of the blood, CaO_2 is the arterial O_2 content, and $C\overline{v}O_2$ is the mixed venous oxygen content (i.e., pulmonary capillary blood before oxygenation). CcO_2 is calculated based on the assumption that pulmonary end-capillary partial pressure of oxygen (PO_2) is the same as partial pressure of alveolar oxygen (P_AO_2). Mixed venous blood can be obtained from a pulmonary artery catheter. As discussed later in this text, calculation of shunt fraction can be useful in the differential diagnosis of hypoxemia.

Vascular Resistance

Vascular resistance represents the impedance, or opposition to blood flow, offered by the systemic or pulmonary vascular beds. It influences the force the ventricular muscle must generate during cardiac contractions (remember that $\Delta P = \dot{Q} \times R$). It has been reported historically as dyne sec cm^{-5}; however, more recent publications have used the units of mm Hg/L/min. In this text we use the units of dyne sec cm^{-5}.

Vascular resistance usually is described as systemic vascular resistance (SVR) or pulmonary vascular resistance (PVR). A simple way to think of these calculations is to understand that *ΔP* represents the pressure gradient across the vascular bed, and *Q̇* is the blood flow through the vascular bed. Thus the SVR can be calculated as shown in Eq. 9.7:

$$\text{SVR} = (\text{MAP} - \text{MRAP/SBF})80 \qquad \textbf{Equation 9.7}$$

where *MAP* is the mean arterial pressure (expressed in mm Hg), *MRAP* is the mean right atrial pressure (also expressed in mm Hg), and *SBF* is the systemic blood flow, or cardiac output. Clinicians routinely multiply the equation by 80 to convert the units of mm Hg/L/min to dyne sec cm^{-5}.

Similarly, the PVR is calculated as shown in Eq. 9.8:

$$\text{PVR} = (\text{MPAP} - \text{MLAP/PBF})80 \qquad \textbf{Equation 9.8}$$

where *MPAP* is the mean pulmonary artery pressure, *MLAP* is the mean left atrial pressure (both measured in mm Hg), and *PBF* is the pulmonary blood flow, or cardiac output (expressed in L/min). Note that PAOP can be used in place of MLAP.

The normal SVR ranges from 900 to 1500 dyne sec cm^{-5}, and the PVR ranges from 100 to 250 dyne sec cm^{-5}. A variety of factors can influence vascular resistance, most importantly, the caliber of the blood vessels and the viscosity of the blood. Remember that $R = 8 \eta l/\pi r^4$, where in this case η is the viscosity of the blood, l is length, and r is the radius of the vessel. Thus the SVR can be increased in left ventricular failure and hypovolemia because of the vasoconstriction that results from stimulation of the baroreceptor reflex. The SVR may also be increased by an increase in blood viscosity, as occurs in polycythemia. The SVR is reduced by systemic vasodilation, such as occurs with moderate hypoxemia or after administration of pharmacological agents such as nitroglycerin and hydralazine.

The PVR can increase significantly during periods of alveolar hypoxia or when high intraalveolar pressures are generated, such as during positive-pressure ventilation. A low cardiac output can increase the PVR by causing derecruitment of pulmonary vessels. The PVR is reduced by administration of pulmonary vasodilator drugs, such as tolazoline and prostacyclin.

Ejection Fraction

The EF is a derived variable that provides an estimate of ventricular contractility. It is calculated by dividing the stroke volume by the end-diastolic volume. The EF shows a positive correlation with CI in most cases, and it is a valuable measurement in the prognosis of heart failure.[9] Note that the correlation between EF and CI may be inaccurate in cases of mitral regurgitation. EFs of 0.5 to 0.7 are considered normal for healthy adults. EFs lower than 0.30 are associated with compromised cardiovascular function and imminent heart failure.

Cardiac Work

In Chapter 1 we defined *work* as the product of a force acting on an object to move it a certain distance. In calculations of cardiac work, the pressure generated by the heart during a ventricular contraction is used to quantify the amount of force developed, and the distance traveled is replaced with the volume of blood pumped by the heart, either as cardiac output or more often as stroke volume. The amount of work performed by each ventricle during the cardiac cycle can be quantified by applying Eqs. 9.9 and 9.10:

$$LSW = MAP \times SV \times 0.0136 \qquad \textbf{Equation 9.9}$$

$$RSW = MPAP \times SV \times 0.0136 \qquad \textbf{Equation 9.10}$$

where *LSW* is the left ventricular stroke work, *RSW* is the right ventricular stroke work, *MAP* is the mean arterial pressure, *MPAP* is the mean pulmonary artery pressure, *SV* is the stroke volume, and 0.0136 is a factor for converting mL–mm Hg to gram–meters. In most clinical situations, stroke work measurements are indexed to the BSA by dividing the LSW or RSW by the patient's BSA. Therefore the left ventricular stroke work index (LSWI) and right ventricular stroke work index (RSWI) are calculated as shown in Eqs. 9.11 and 9.12:

$$LSWI = LSW/BSA \qquad \textbf{Equation 9.11}$$

$$RSWI = RSW/BSA \qquad \textbf{Equation 9.12}$$

The LSWI normally ranges from 50 to 62 g-m/m^2/beat, and the RSWI from 5 to 10 g-m/m^2/beat. It should be apparent from these equations that conditions that increase the stroke volume or mean pressure generated by the ventricles increase the amount of work the ventricle must perform.

KEY POINTS

- The assessment of cardiovascular function is an integral part of the management of patients with cardiopulmonary dysfunction.
- Conventional electrocardiography provides valuable information about the electrophysiological properties of the heart: excitability, rhythmicity, and conductivity.
- The standard 12-lead ECG comprises three sets of leads: standard limb leads, augmented limb leads, and precordial or chest leads. Analysis of these three sets of leads provides an electronic view of the heart both from a frontal and a horizontal perspective.
- A number of waves, complexes, and intervals should be quantified in the analysis of typical ECG waveforms. These include the P, QRS, and T waves; the PR interval; the QT interval; and the ST segment.
- Interpretation of the ECG should focus on three major factors: atrial and ventricular rates, the presence of abnormal rhythms or arrhythmias, and calculation of the mean electrical axis.
- Hemodynamic monitoring provides valuable information about the mechanical function of the cardiovascular system. Noninvasive measurements of arterial blood pressure and heart sounds can give the clinician an overview of cardiovascular function. The most common invasive techniques use vascular and cardiac catheterization to assess pressure, volume, and flow events that occur during the cardiac cycle.
- Interpretation of the hemodynamic profile should focus on quantifying cardiac output, vascular resistance, and cardiac work.

ASSESSMENT QUESTIONS

See Appendix B for the answers.

1. Which of the following correctly describes the permeability characteristics of the membrane potential for a ventricular myocyte during phase 0 (depolarization)?
   a. $Na^+ > K^+$
   b. $Ca^{++} > Na^+$
   c. $Ca^+ > K^+$
   d. $Na^+ = K^+$

2. Which of the following statements is true concerning nodal tissue action potentials?
   a. The action potential demonstrates five phases, like ventricular myocytes.
   b. The amplitude of this type of action potential is the same as an action potential for a ventricular myocyte.
   c. The threshold potential for this type of tissue is more negative than the threshold potentials for a ventricular myocyte.
   d. The slope of phase 4 of the sinoatrial (SA) node is greater than that of the ventricular myocyte.

3. For the lead aVF configuration, the positive electrode is placed on the:
   a. Right arm
   b. Left arm
   c. Right leg
   d. Left leg

4. A patient's electrocardiogram (ECG) tracing shows an R-R interval of 15 mm. What is this patient's effective heart rate?
   a. 50 beats/min
   b. 75 beats/min
   c. 100 beats/min
   d. 150 beats/min

5. Which of the following electrocardiographic leads provides information related to the horizontal plane of the heart?
   a. Lead I
   b. Lead III
   c. Lead V_4
   d. Lead aVR

6. The last structure of the heart to depolarize is the:
   a. Left bundle branch
   b. Apex
   c. Endocardial surface of the right ventricle
   d. Epicardial surface of the base of the left ventricle

7. Which of the following is *not* characteristic of a respiratory sinus arrhythmia?
   a. The SA node is the pacemaker of the heart.
   b. The R-R interval is constant.
   c. A P wave precedes every QRS.
   d. The heart rate varies throughout the respiratory cycle.

8. The heart rate of an individual who demonstrates sinus tachycardia typically shows a ventricular rate of:
   a. Less than 60 beats/min
   b. 40 to 60 beats/min
   c. 60 to 100 beats/min
   d. Greater than 100 beats/min

9. For a person with a mean ventricular axis of 90 degrees, the amplitude of the QRS typically is greatest (upstroke) in which of the following leads?
   a. Lead I
   b. Lead III
   c. Lead aVF
   d. Lead V_3

10. Which of the following rhythms is characterized by the presence of delta waves on the ECG?
    a. First-degree atrioventricular (AV) block
    b. Bundle-branch block
    c. Wolff-Parkinson-White (WPW) syndrome
    d. Atrial fibrillation

11. Which of the following rhythms is characterized by a constant PR interval with intermittent loss of a QRS complex?
    a. Intraventricular conduction delay
    b. Second-degree (Mobitz I) AV block
    c. Second-degree (Mobitz II) AV block
    d. Respiratory sinus arrhythmia

12. Which of the following statements is true concerning ventricular action potentials?
    a. The action potential demonstrates three phases (phases 0, 3, and 4).
    b. The amplitude of this type of action potential typically is approximately 60 mV.
    c. The threshold potential for this type of tissue is more negative than the threshold potentials for a nodal myocyte.
    d. The slope of phase 4 of the SA node is greater than that of the SA node myocyte.

13. During a normal cardiac cycle:
    1. The first heart sound is associated with atrial contraction
    2. The period of isovolumetric contraction follows closure of the semilunar valves
    3. The dicrotic notch of the aortic pressure tracing is associated with closure of the aortic and pulmonary valves
    4. The pressure in the left ventricle is higher than aortic pressure during the period of maximum ejection
    a. 1 and 2 only
    b. 3 and 4 only
    c. 1, 3, and 4 only
    d. 1, 2, 3, and 4

14. An increase in right ventricular preload can be estimated clinically by measuring:
    a. Left ventricular end-diastolic pressure (LVEDP)
    b. Right ventricular end-diastolic pressure (RVEDP)
    c. Pulmonary artery occlusion pressure (PAOP)
    d. Mean pulmonary artery pressure (MPAP)

15. A 30-year-old woman has a stroke index of 50 mL/beat/m^2. If her body surface area (BSA) is 2 m^2 and her heart rate is 60 beats/min, what is her cardiac output in liters per minute?
    a. 3.4 L/min
    b. 4 L/min
    c. 5.6 L/min
    d. 6 L/min

REFERENCES

1. Kligfield P, Gettes LS, Bailey JJ, et al.: Recommendations for the standardization and interpretation of the electrocardiogram: Part I: the electrocardiogram and its technology. A scientific statement from the American Heart Association Electrocardiography and Arrhythmias Committee, Council on Clinical Cardiology; the American College of Cardiology Foundation; and the Heart Rhythm Society. *J Am Coll Cardiol* 49(10):1109-1127, 2007.
2. Katz AM: *Physiology of the heart*, ed 5, Philadelphia, 2010, Lippincott Williams & Wilkins.
3. Scheidt S: *Basic electrocardiography*, West Caldwell, NJ, 1989, CIBA-GEIGY.
4. Cromwell L, Weibell FJ, Pfeiffer EA: *Biomedical instrumentation and measurements*, ed 2, Englewood Cliffs, NJ, 1980, Prentice-Hall.
5. Zywietz C, Willems JL: Stability of ECG amplitude measurements in systematic noise tests: results and recommendations from the CSE project. *J Electrocardiol* 20(suppl):61-66, 1987.
6. Scheidt S: *Interactive electrocardiography*, New York, 2000, Novartis.
7. Hall JE: *Guyton and Hall textbook of medical physiology*, ed 13, Philadelphia, 2015, Saunders.
8. Fishman AP, Richards DW: *Circulation of the blood*, Bethesda, MD, 1982, American Physiological Society.
9. Heuer AJ, Scanlon CL: *Clinical assessment in respiratory care*, ed 7, St. Louis, 2014, Mosby Elsevier.
10. Parbrook GD, Kenny GNC, Davis PD: *Basic physics and measurement in anaesthesia*, New York, 1999, Butterworth-Heinemann.
11. Perloff D, Grim C, Flack J, et al.: Human blood pressure determination by sphygmomanometry. *Circulation* 88:2460-2670, 1993.
12. Swan HJC, Ganz W, Forrester J, et al.: Catheterization of the heart in man with the use of a flow-directed balloon tipped catheter. *N Engl J Med* 75:83, 1975.
13. Gardner RM: Direct arterial pressure monitoring. *Curr Anaesth Crit Care* 1:239-246, 1990.
14. American Society of Anesthesiologists Task Force on Pulmonary Artery Catheterization: Practice guidelines for pulmonary artery catheterization. *Anesthesiology* 99:988-1014, 2003.
15. Baim DS, Grossman W: *Grossman's cardiac catheterization, angiography, and intervention*, ed 6, Philadelphia, 2000, Lippincott Williams & Wilkins.
16. Rushmer RF: *Structure and function of the cardiovascular system*, ed 2, Philadelphia, 1976, WB Saunders.
17. Side CD, Gossling RG: Non-surgical assessment of cardiac function. *Nature* 22:561-571, 1971.
18. Durbin CG: Noninvasive hemodynamic measurements. *Respir Care* 35:709, 1990.
19. Schober P, Loer SA, Schwarte LA: Perioperative hemodynamic monitoring with transesophageal Doppler technology. *Anesth Analg* 109(2):340-353, 2009.
20. Stawicki SP, Hoff WS, Cipolla I, et al.: Use of noninvasive esophageal echo-Doppler system in the ICU: a practical experience. *J Trauma* 59(2):506-507, 2005.
21. Iregui MG, Prentice D, Sherman G, et al.: Physicians' estimates of cardiac index and intravascular volume based on clinical assessment versus transesophageal Doppler measurements obtained by critical care nurses. *Am J Crit Care* 12:336-342, 2003.
22. Chandan GS, Hull JM: Incorrectly placed oesophageal Doppler probe. *Anaesthesia* 59:723, 2004.
23. Moxon D, Pinder M, van Heerden PV, et al.: Clinical evaluation of the HemoSonic monitor in cardiac surgical patients in the ICU. *Anaesth Intensive Care* 31:408-411, 2003.

Blood Gas Monitoring

OBJECTIVES

Upon completion of this chapter you will be able to:

1. Describe how to perform and evaluate the modified Allen test.
2. Identify various sites used to obtain samples for blood gas analysis.
3. Label the components of a modern, in vitro blood gas analyzer.
4. Compare the operational principles of the pH, partial pressure of carbon dioxide (PCO_2), and partial pressure of oxygen (PO_2) electrodes.
5. Apply values for the PO_2 at which 50% saturation of hemoglobin (P_{50}) occurs, as well as bicarbonate, buffer base, and base excess in the interpretation of arterial blood gases.
6. Explain the operational principle of CO-oximetry.
7. Name the components of a quality assurance program for blood gas analysis.
8. Compare the effects of hyperthermia and hypothermia on arterial blood gases.
9. Discuss advantages of point-of-care blood gas analysis and potential disadvantages associated with this method of blood gas testing.
10. Describe physiological and technical factors that can affect pulse oximeter readings.
11. Identify preanalytic factors that can influence transcutaneous PO_2 and PCO_2 measurements.
12. State criteria for identifying four types of acid–base disorders.

OUTLINE

KEY TERMS

absorbance sensors
actual bicarbonate
modified Allen test
amperometric
base excess/deficit
buffer base
capillary blood gas (CBG)
central processing unit (CPU)
Clark electrode
Clinical Laboratory Improvement Amendments of 1988 (CLIA-88)
electrochemical sensors
electrodes
fetal hemoglobin (HbF)
fluorescent sensors

fractional hemoglobin saturation
functional hemoglobin saturation
glucose oxidase
half-cells
Henderson-Hasselbalch equation
hyperbilirubinemia
in vitro
in vivo
invasive
Levy-Jennings charts
light-emitting diodes (LEDs)
microcuvette
Nernst equation
noninvasive
one-point calibration

optical plethysmography
optical shunting
oxygen content (O_2ct)
palpebral conjunctiva
partial pressure of carbon dioxide in arterial blood ($PaCO_2$)
partial pressure of oxygen in arterial blood (PaO_2)
pH
photoplethysmography
point-of-care (POC) testing
potentiometric
quality assurance (QA)
quality control (QC)
Sanz electrode

servo-controlled	standard bicarbonate	three-point calibration
Siggaard-Andersen alignment	sulfhemoglobin (sulfHb)	total hemoglobin (THb)
nomogram	temperature correction	two-point calibration

Measurements of arterial blood gases (ABGs) and pH are used extensively in the diagnosis and treatment of patients with acute and chronic illnesses. This is most evident in the management of critically ill patients, for whom ABG analysis can provide valuable information, such as acid–base status, ventilatory function, and oxygenation status.

Blood gas techniques generally are classified as invasive or noninvasive. Invasive blood gas analysis, which involves direct exposure of a sample of blood to a series of electrochemical sensors or electrodes, is considered the gold standard for measuring the hydrogen ion concentration (pH), partial pressure of carbon dioxide (PCO_2), and partial pressure of oxygen (PO_2) in the arterial blood. Until recently, invasive blood gas analysis could provide only intermittent in vitro measurements of a patient's blood gas and acid–base status; however, the development of fiberoptic catheters has extended the possibilities of in vivo blood gas monitoring by allowing for real-time determinations of the pH of arterial blood (pHa), partial pressure of carbon dioxide in the arteries ($PaCO_2$), and partial pressure of oxygen in arterial blood (PaO_2).

Noninvasive techniques, which include pulse oximetry and transcutaneous monitoring, do not require blood samples and are performed with sensors placed on the surface of the body. Because pulse oximetry and transcutaneous monitoring can provide continuous estimates of blood gas levels with minimal risk to the patient, they are indispensable tools in the management of patients with unstable ventilatory and oxygenation status. Appropriate use of noninvasive monitoring can significantly reduce the need for more expensive invasive blood gas analysis.

This chapter describes the various devices and techniques commonly used to determine ABGs and pH. Some basic principles to ensure an understanding of how blood gas measurements can be used to assess a patient's acid–base and respiratory status are presented. You should remember, however, that ABGs must be interpreted in the context of other clinical indices, including other laboratory tests (e.g., hematology and electrolytes), chest radiographs, the patient's history, and the physical examination findings. Interpreting blood gas values without considering other clinical findings can lead to serious mistakes and ultimately harm the patient.

I. INVASIVE BLOOD GAS ANALYSIS

Invasive blood gas analysis can be performed in a variety of settings, including hospitals, clinics, physicians' offices, and extended care facilities. The primary indications for invasive blood gas analysis are to quantify a patient's response to a diagnostic or therapeutic intervention and to monitor the severity and progression of a documented disease process.[1]

The American Association for Respiratory Care (AARC) has published a series of Clinical Practice Guidelines for ABG and hemoximetry analysis to help ensure that these tests are performed in a safe and standardized manner.[1-3] Besides providing information related to obtaining blood samples, the guidelines also list the indications, contraindications, hazards, and complications of ABG analysis. The AARC Clinical Practice Guideline for blood gas analysis and hemoximetry[2] is summarized in Clinical Practice Guideline 10.1.

Health care professionals who perform blood gas analysis should understand patient assessment techniques and the relationship of the patient's history, physical findings, and various cardiopulmonary dysfunctions. Therefore individuals who perform blood gas analysis should be formally trained in respiratory therapy, pulmonary function testing, clinical laboratory sciences, nursing, medicine, or osteopathy.[1,2] Periodic reevaluation of these individuals should focus on all aspects of blood gas analysis, including the proper technique for obtaining blood samples, postsampling care of the puncture site, and safe handling of blood, needles, and syringes.[1,2]

II. SAMPLING TECHNIQUES AND COLLECTION DEVICES

Specimens for ABG analysis can be drawn from a peripheral artery by means of a percutaneous needle puncture or from an indwelling intravascular cannula. Venous blood gases (VBGs) can be obtained from a central venous line. Although some evidence suggests that VBG samples are comparable to ABG samples when assessing pH, PCO_2, and HCO_2 in a clinical setting, VBG samples obtained from a central line should be used as a surrogate for an ABG only in specific clinical circumstances.[2] Mixed venous blood samples can be obtained with a flow-directed (Swan-Ganz) intracardiac catheter. For percutaneous sampling, blood most often is drawn from the radial, brachial, or femoral artery or the dorsalis pedis artery of the foot.[3-5] Capillary blood samples from an earlobe or the side of the heel may be substituted when arterial blood cannot be obtained. As is discussed later in the chapter, capillary blood gas (CBG) values may vary considerably from ABG values.

In the case of percutaneous puncture of the radial artery, a modified Allen test should always be performed before the sample is obtained (Fig. 10.1).[4,5] For this test the patient clenches the fist to force blood from the hand. While the fist is formed, pressure is applied to the radial and ulnar arteries. The patient then is instructed to release the fist; the hand should appear blanched. When pressure on the ulnar artery is released, blood should return to the hand, causing the palm to blush and indicating that the ulnar artery is patent. If the

CLINICAL PRACTICE GUIDELINE 10.1 Blood Gas Analysis and Hemoximetry

Setting

1. Hospital laboratories
2. Hospital emergency areas
3. Patient care area
4. Clinical laboratory
5. Laboratory in physician's office
6. Interfacility critical care transport
7. Pulmonary diagnostic laboratory
8. Operating room suite
9. Cardiac catheterization laboratory
10. Postmortem examination

Indications

1. Evaluate the adequacy of a patient's ventilatory (P_aCO_2), acid–base (pH), or oxygenation (P_aO_2 and oxyhemoglobin saturation) status, oxygen-carrying capacity (P_aO_2 and hemoglobin saturation, total hemoglobin, and dyshemoglobin saturations); and intrapulmonary shunt.
2. Quantify a patient's response to therapeutic intervention (supplemental oxygen administration and mechanical ventilation) and/or diagnostic evaluation (exercise desaturation).
3. The need to assess early goal-directed therapy using central venous saturation in patients with sepsis, septic shock, and after major surgery.
4. Monitor the severity and progression of documented disease processes.
5. The need to assess the circulatory response (e.g., assessing central venous/arterial PCO_2 difference during severe hemorrhage shock, during cardiopulmonary resuscitation, and after cardiopulmonary bypass).

Contraindications

1. Improperly functioning analyzer or an analyzer that has not had its functional status validated by analysis of commercially prepared quality control products or tonometered whole blood, or participation in a proficiency testing program.
2. A specimen that has not been properly anticoagulated.
3. A sample that contains visible air bubbles.
4. A sample that has been stored in a plastic syringe at room temperature for longer than 30 minutes, stored at room temperature for longer than 5 min for a shunt study, or stored at room temperature in the presence of an elevated leukocyte or platelet count.
5. Sample is submitted without adequate background information, including patient's name or other unique identifier (e.g., medical record number, birth date or age, date and time of sampling), location of the patient, name and signature of the requesting physician or authorized individual, clinical indication and tests to be performed, sample source (arterial line, central venous catheter, peripheral artery), respiratory rate, fractional inspired oxygen (F_IO_2), ventilator settings (tidal volume, respiratory rate, mode, F_IO_2), body temperature, activity level, and working diagnosis. (Note that verbal requests must be supported by written authorization within 30 days [unless local regulations specify a different time frame]). Sample is submitted without the signature or initials of the person who obtained the sample.

Hazards and Complications

1. Infection of the specimen handler from blood containing human immunodeficiency virus (HIV), hepatitis C, or other blood-borne pathogens.

2. Inappropriate medical treatment of the patient based on improperly analyzed blood sample or from analysis of an unacceptable specimen, or from incorrect reporting of results.
3. In the case of samples received from a contaminated (isolation) room, cross-contamination of areas of the hospital or handlers of the sample.
4. Improperly identified patient.

Limitations of Procedure and Validation of Results

1. Sample clotting as a result of improper anticoagulation or improper mixing.
2. Sample contaminated with air, improper anticoagulant or anticoagulant concentration, saline or other fluids, inadvertent sampling of systemic venous blood.
3. Delay in sample analysis.
4. Incomplete clearance of analyzer calibration gases and previous waste or flushing solution or solutions.
5. Hyperlipidemia (interference with electrode membranes).
6. Failure to obtain an adequate sample size for the type of anticoagulant and/or the sample requirements of the analyzer.
7. Possible error in calculation of derived variables (e.g., calculated oxyhemoglobin saturation may be overestimated in the presence of carboxyhemoglobin and methemoglobin, and with changes in diphosphoglycerate [2,3-DPG] concentrations).
8. The presence of excess fetal hemoglobin (i.e., the blood gas analyzer will assume that the fetal hemoglobin is adult hemoglobin resulting in calculations showing underestimated oxygen saturations).
9. Inappropriate sample site for the analyte being assessed (e.g., arterialized capillary samples and central venous samples may be adequate to assess pH and PCO_2 in hemodynamically stable patients but underestimate the patient's oxygenation).
10. Possible erroneous temperature-corrected results because of errors in measurement of the patient's temperature. The laboratory should have a defined procedure for temperature correction of measured results. If the temperature-corrected results are reported, the report should be clearly labeled and the results at 37°C should be reported.
11. Hemodilution or altered osmolality when measuring hematocrit using conductometry sensor technology.
12. Analytic procedure conforms to recommended established guidelines and follows the manufacturer's recommendations.
13. Results of pH–blood gas analysis fall within the calibration range of the analyzer and quality control product range.
14. Laboratory procedures and personnel are in compliance with quality control and recognized proficiency testing programs.
15. Questionable results should be reanalyzed (preferably on a separate analyzer), and an additional sample should be obtained if the discrepancy cannot be resolved. *Note:* The results of the analysis of the discarded sample should be documented, and the reason for discarding the sample should be given.

Assessment of Need

1. A valid indication in the patient to be tested supports the need for sampling and analysis.

Continued

CLINICAL PRACTICE GUIDELINE 10.1 **Blood Gas Analysis and Hemoximetry—cont'd**	
Infection Control 1. Staff, supervisors, and physician-directors associated with the pulmonary laboratory should be knowledgeable about the "Guidelines for Isolation Precautions in Hospitals," published by the Centers for Disease Control and Prevention (CDC) and the Hospital Infection Control Practices Advisory Committee (HICPAC).	2. The manager and medical director of the laboratory should maintain communication and cooperation with the institution's infection control service and the personnel health service to help ensure consistency and thoroughness in complying with the institution's policies related to immunization, postexposure prophylaxis, and community-related illnesses and exposures.

2,3-DPG, 2,3-Diphosphoglycerate; *PaCO₂,* partial pressure of carbon dioxide in the arteries; *PaO₂,* partial pressure of oxygen in the arteries; *PCO₂,* partial pressure of carbon dioxide; *pH,* hydrogen ion concentration.
Modified from the American Association of Respiratory Care: Clinical practice guideline: blood gas analysis and hemoximetry: 2013. *Respir Care* 58:1694-1703, 2013.

CLINICAL SCENARIO 10.1

How would a large air bubble affect the PCO_2 and PO_2 of an arterial blood sample taken from a normal healthy person breathing room air?
  See Appendix A for the answer.

PCO₂, Partial pressure of carbon dioxide; *PO₂,* partial pressure of oxygen.

CLINICAL SCENARIO 10.2

A CBG sample is obtained from a 2-day-old infant in apparent respiratory distress. The results indicate respiratory alkalosis (high pH, low PCO_2) and apparent hypoxemia (low PO_2). How would you interpret these findings?
  See Appendix A for the answer.

CBG, Capillary blood gas; *PCO₂,* partial pressure of carbon dioxide; *pH,* hydrogen ion concentration; *PO₂,* partial pressure of oxygen.

palm does not blush, the ulnar artery is either absent or partially or totally occluded. Another sampling site, such as the brachial artery, should be chosen if the modified Allen test is negative. Note that a similar test can be performed when blood is obtained from the dorsal artery of the foot. Pressure is applied directly over the artery to occlude it, and then pressure is applied to the nail of the big toe, causing it to blanch. When pressure on the big toe is released, color returns to the toe if the collateral circulation is sufficient from the posterior tibial and lateral plantar arteries.[6]

After tests have shown that sufficient collateral circulation is present, the site should be prepared for puncture. It should be cleaned with 70% isopropyl alcohol or another suitable antiseptic solution.[7] In some cases anesthetization of the puncture site may be necessary, which can be accomplished by injecting a local anesthetic such as 2% lidocaine HCl.[1,4,5] Proper administration of the anesthetic can alleviate some of the pain associated with the procedure and reduce the patient's anxiety.

Samples to be analyzed should be obtained with a small-gauge needle (23 to 25 gauge) attached to a plastic syringe of low diffusibility containing an anticoagulant (sodium or lithium heparin, 1000 U/mL) (Fig. 10.2).[1,2] For infants, 25- to 26-gauge scalp vein needles can be used to collect arterial samples. The blood should be drawn anaerobically to prevent contamination by room air. Room air that is inadvertently drawn into the syringe should be removed before analysis because contamination with room air can lead to erroneous results and ultimately compromise patient care. Clinical Scenario 10.1 gives an example of this type of problem in the clinical setting.

After blood has been withdrawn and the needle removed, direct pressure should be applied to the puncture site to prevent the formation of a hematoma. For adult patients with

indwelling cannulas, 1 to 2 mL of blood should be removed and discarded before blood is removed for analysis. For infants the discarded volume typically is only approximately 0.2 to 0.5 mL. (Remember that the volume of blood removed and discarded should be minimal; this is particularly important in neonates.) After the blood sample to be analyzed has been removed, the cannula should be flushed with several milliliters of normal saline to prevent blood coagulation in the cannula and loss of a functioning indwelling line.

As mentioned previously, CBG samples may be substituted for arterial blood samples in certain situations.[8] CBGs most often are used in pediatric patients, especially in the neonatal intensive care unit, to avoid multiple arterial sticks.[6,9,10] The site should be warmed before the sample is obtained to increase perfusion to the area (i.e., "arterializing"). "Arterialized" capillary samples actually contain a combination of arterial and venous blood and therefore may not be equivalent to an arterial blood sample.[10,11] The correlation between capillary and arterial pH and PCO_2 measurements is better than the correlation between capillary and arterial PO_2 measurements. Consequently, CBGs more often are used to discern acid–base status rather than to assess a patient's oxygenation status. Table 10.1 presents accepted normal blood gas values. Clinical Scenario 10.2 shows how CBGs can be used in clinical decision making.

Personnel responsible for performing blood gas analysis should understand that they are dealing with a potential biohazard and should take appropriate precautions when performing these tests.[12,13] Such precautions include wearing gloves, protective eyewear (goggles), and other barriers deemed necessary to prevent exposure. Needles used for blood sampling should be recapped with the one-handed "scoop" technique, or they can be removed after being inserted into a cork or similar device to shield the sharp end. Unused blood samples,

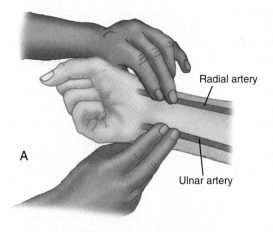

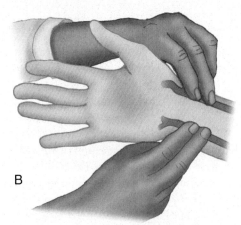

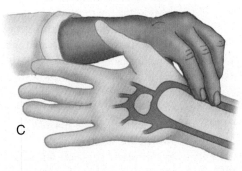

FIGURE 10.1 Modified Allen test. A, The hand is clenched into a tight fist, and pressure is applied to the radial and ulnar arteries. B, The hand is opened (but not fully extended), and the palm and fingers are blanched. C, Pressure on the ulnar artery is removed, which should result in flushing of the entire hand. (From Kacmarek RM, Stoller JK, Heuer AJ: *Egan's fundamentals of respiratory care*, ed 10, St. Louis, 2013, Mosby.)

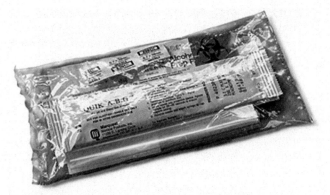

FIGURE 10.2 Commercially available blood gas kit. (Courtesy Marquest Medical Products, Vital Signs, Newark, NJ.)

TABLE 10.1 Normal Blood Values for a Healthy Adult	
Parameter	**Value**
pHa	7.40 ± 0.05
PaCO₂	40 ± 5 mm Hg
PaO₂	80-100 mm Hg
HCO₃⁻	24 ± 2 mEq/L
Base excess	±2 mEq/L
SaO₂	95% to 100%
pHv̄ [a]	7.35 ± 0.05
Pv̄CO₂ [a]	40-55 mm Hg
Pv̄O₂ [a]	35-40 mm Hg
Sv̄O₂ [a]	70% to 75%
HbCO	<1.5%
MetHb	<1.5%
THb	12-18 g/dL
Lactate	0.7-2.1 mEq/L
P₅₀	27 ± 2 mm Hg

[a]Mixed venous blood gases are obtained from samples of blood drawn from a balloon flotation catheter inserted into the pulmonary artery.

HbCO, Carboxyhemoglobin; *HCO₃⁻,* bicarbonate; *MetHb,* methemoglobin; *P₅₀,* partial pressure of oxygen at which hemoglobin is 50% saturated; *PaCO₂,* partial pressure of carbon dioxide in the arteries; *PaO₂,* partial pressure of oxygen in the arteries; *pHa,* hydrogen ion concentration of arterial blood; *pHv̄,* hydrogen ion concentration of mixed venous blood; *Pv̄CO₂,* partial pressure of carbon dioxide in mixed venous blood; *Pv̄O₂,* partial pressure of oxygen in mixed venous blood; *SaO₂,* arterial oxygen saturation; *Sv̄O₂,* mixed venous oxygen saturation; *THb,* total hemoglobin.

needles, and other "sharps" should be discarded in appropriately marked containers. (See Chapter 2 for a full discussion of infection control principles in respiratory care.)

Specimens should be transported to the blood gas laboratory and analyzed as soon as possible after obtaining a blood specimen because blood cells remain metabolically active in vitro; therefore prolonged delay between obtaining and analyzing a specimen (longer than 5 minutes) can lead to erroneous results (i.e., a reduction in PO₂ and a rise in PCO₂). This problem is particularly evident in patients with high leukocyte counts.[4,5] Chilling the specimen to below 5°C (41°F) by placing the syringe in ice water can reduce the metabolic rate of the white blood cells, minimizing this problematic effect.

III. MODERN IN VITRO BLOOD GAS ANALYZERS

Modern in vitro blood gas analyzers (Fig. 10.3) have three electrodes for determining the pH, PCO₂, and PO₂ of a blood

TABLE 10.2 Normal Values for Derived Blood Gas Variables

Variable	Symbol	Normal Values
Oxyhemoglobin	O_2Hb	≥95%
Carboxyhemoglobin	HbCO	<1.5%
Methemoglobin	MetHb	<1.5%
Deoxygenated Hb	HHb	<2%
Sulfhemoglobin	SulfHb	<1%
Total Hb	THb	Males: 15.8 ± 2 g/dL
		Females: 14 ± 2 g/dL
Partial pressure of oxygen at 50% saturation	P_{50}	27 ± 2 mm Hg

TABLE 10.3 Hydrogen Ion–pH Relationships

pH	[H$^+$][a]
7.80	16
7.70	20
7.60	26
7.50	32
7.40	40
7.30	50
7.20	63
7.10	80
7.00	100
6.90	125
6.80	160

[a]Reported in nanomoles per liter.

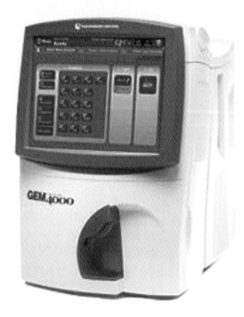

FIGURE 10.3 Modern in vitro blood gas analyzer. (GEM, courtesy Instrumentation Laboratories, Bedford, MA.)

sample. They also have a **central processing unit (CPU)** for data management and outputs for displaying measured and derived variables. Many of these systems may also have sensors for providing hemoglobin (Hb), oxyhemoglobin, carboxyhemoglobin, and methemoglobin measurements, along with serum electrolyte and blood glucose measurements. Table 10.2 lists the normal values for the derived variables commonly recorded during blood gas analysis. Unlike early blood gas analyzers, which were cumbersome to operate and required large amounts of blood to make accurate measurements, modern analyzers are fully automated, self-calibrating devices that can analyze blood samples as small as 50 to 100 μL.

pH and Hydrogen Ion Concentration

S.P.L. Sorenson introduced the term *pH* as a shorthand way to express the hydrogen ion activity of solutions.[14,15] It is defined as the negative logarithm (base 10) of the hydrogen ion concentration, or

$$pH = -\log_{10}[H^+]$$

For example, a hydrogen ion concentration of 0.0000007 mol/L, or 1×10^{-7} mol/L, can be expressed as a pH of 7. Although scientific efforts have increased to express hydrogen ion concentrations in Système International d'Unités (SI) units (i.e., nanomoles per liter [nmol/L]), the concept of pH is still recognized as a convenient and useful way of discussing a patient's clinical acid–base status.[15,16] Table 10.3 shows the relationship between hydrogen ion concentration and pH. Note that the pH decreases as the hydrogen ion concentration increases, and vice versa. Despite the fact that hydrogen ion activity is not exactly equal to the hydrogen ion concentration, these two terms are interchangeable for practical purposes in clinical situations.

In general chemistry textbooks the pH scale is described as ranging from 1 to 14, with a pH of 7 representing universal neutrality. (Neutrality is defined as the pH of pure water, which contains 1×10^{-7} mol/L of hydrogen ions and 1×10^{-7} mol/L of hydroxyl ions.) A solution with a pH less than 7 is acidic, and a solution with a pH higher than 7 is alkaline. Although the pHa can vary from 6.9 to 7.8, it normally ranges (± 2 standard deviations [SD]) from 7.35 to 7.45, with a mean pH of 7.4. For interpretative purposes, a blood pH less than 7.4 is considered acidic, and a blood pH higher than 7.4 is alkaline.

pH Electrode

The standard pH electrode, which sometimes is called the Sanz electrode, is composed of two half-cells connected by a potassium chloride (KCl) bridge (Fig. 10.4).[17] One of the cells, the measurement half-cell, has a special glass membrane that is permeable to hydrogen ions (H$^+$). The measuring electrode is made of silver–silver chloride (Ag/AgCl) and immersed in a phosphate buffer solution with a pH of 6.84. The second cell, the reference half-cell, is composed of mercury–mercurous chloride (Hg/HgO$_2$) (calomel) and is immersed in a solution of saturated KCl.

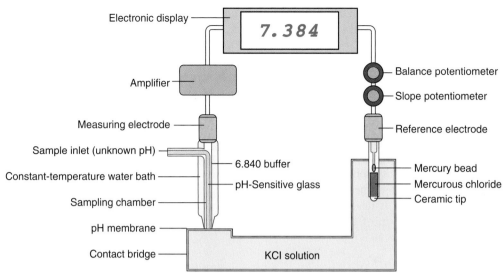

FIGURE 10.4 Schematic of the pH electrode. (From Hess DR, MacIntyre NR, Mishoe SC, et al.: *Respiratory care: principles and practice*, St. Louis, 2002, WB Saunders.)

According to the Nernst equation, the electrical potential generated as H^+ ions pass through the glass membrane (EH^+) is a logarithmic function of the ratio of hydrogen ion concentration across the membrane, or

$$EH^+ = (RT/F) + \ln[(H_o^+)/(H_i^+)]$$

where R is the gas constant, F is Faraday's constant, T is the absolute temperature in Kelvin, H_o^+ is the hydrogen ion concentration outside the membrane, and H_i^+ is the hydrogen ion concentration inside the membrane. If you consider that at body temperature (37°C [98.6°F], or 310 K) the quantity (RT/F) is 61.5 mV, then the equation becomes

$$EH^+ = 0.0615 \times \log_{10}[H^+] \; or$$

$$EH^+ = 0.0615 \times pH$$

Therefore a voltage of 61.5 mV is developed for every pH unit difference between the sample and the measuring electrode, which is constant (6.84). Consider the following example: A voltage difference of 30.75 mV is measured when a sample is analyzed. This voltage difference equals 0.5 pH units (30.75 ÷ 61.5 = 0.5). The resultant pH can be calculated as 6.84 + 0.5 = 7.34.

It should be apparent that these devices are quite sensitive and therefore are adversely affected by changes in the permeability of the glass membrane, such as can occur when the electrode is damaged or coated with protein. As is discussed later in this chapter, an effective quality assurance program can prevent these types of problems.

Partial Pressures of Carbon Dioxide and Oxygen

As was discussed in Chapter 1, the partial pressure a gas exerts in a gas mixture is calculated by multiplying the fractional concentration of the gas by the total pressure of the gas mixture. For example, if oxygen makes up approximately 21% of the atmosphere and the barometric pressure is 760 mm Hg, the

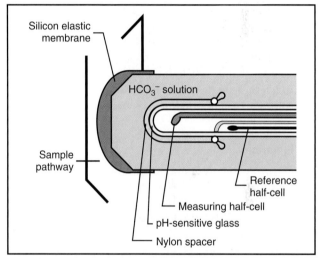

FIGURE 10.5 Stowe-Severinghaus PCO_2 electrode. (Redrawn from Shapiro BA, Peruzzi WT, Templin R: *Clinical application of blood gases*, ed 5, St. Louis, 1994, Mosby.)

PO_2 in room air is 0.21 × 760 mm Hg, or approximately 159 mm Hg.

The $PaCO_2$, which is regulated primarily by the respiratory system, can vary from 10 to above 100 mm Hg. People breathing room air at sea level typically have a $PaCO_2$ of 35 to 45 mm Hg (the mean is 40 mm Hg; the range represents ± 2 SD). The PaO_2 can range from 30 to 600 mm Hg, depending on the fractional concentration of inspired oxygen. For healthy people breathing room air at sea level, the PaO_2 usually is 80 to 100 mm Hg.

PCO_2 Electrode

The PCO_2 electrode was first described by Stowe in 1957 and later refined by Severinghaus and Bradley[18]; consequently, the standard PCO_2 electrode is commonly called the *Stowe-Severinghaus electrode* (Fig. 10.5). It is basically a pH electrode covered with a carbon dioxide–permeable Teflon or silicone (Silastic) membrane. A bicarbonate-buffered solution is held between the Teflon (or Silastic) membrane and the pH glass electrode by a nylon spacer. Carbon dioxide from the blood diffuses across the semipermeable Teflon (or Silastic) membrane and reacts with the water to form carbonic acid, which dissociates into hydrogen ions and bicarbonate. The reaction can be written as

$$CO_2 + H_2O \rightarrow H_2CO_3 \rightarrow H^+ + HCO_3^-$$

H^+ ions from the bicarbonate-buffered solution then diffuse across the glass electrode, and the pH of the solution is measured as described earlier. The pH is related to the PCO_2 by using the following modification of the Henderson-Hasselbalch equation:

$$pH = pK + \log(HCO_3^- / PCO_2)$$

Thus the PCO_2 is determined as a function of the change in pH of the bicarbonate solution (i.e., the pH changes by 0.1 unit for every 10-mm Hg increase in PCO_2).

The most common problems encountered with PCO_2 electrodes involve interference with the diffusion of CO_2 across the Teflon (or Silastic) membrane and the H^+ ions across the glass membrane (e.g., worn or cracked electrodes, protein deposits). If the bicarbonate solution dehydrates between the Teflon (or Silastic) membrane and the pH glass electrode, erroneous data can result. As with the pH electrode, these problems can be minimized by an effective quality assurance program.

PO₂ Electrode

The PO_2 in blood is most commonly measured using the Clark electrode.[17] As Fig. 10.6 shows, the Clark electrode consists of a negatively charged platinum electrode (cathode) and a positively charged Ag/AgCl reference electrode (anode) immersed in a phosphate–KCl buffer, the pH of which can range from 7 to 10, depending on the manufacturer. The cathode and anode are connected by a KCl bridge. An external voltage is applied to the platinum electrode, creating a small potential difference of approximately 0.5 to 0.6 mV between it and the anode. (Because an external polarizing voltage is applied to create this potential difference, the Clark electrode is called a *polarographic electrode*.) The active surface of the electrode is separated from the blood to be analyzed by a

polyethylene or polypropylene membrane that is permeable to oxygen.

Fig. 10.7 illustrates the principle of PO_2 measurement. Oxygen from the blood sample diffuses across the semipermeable plastic membrane into the KCl solution and reacts with the platinum cathode, altering the conductivity of the electrolyte solution. Specifically, the platinum cathode donates electrons, which reduce oxygen to produce hydroxyl ions:

$$O_2 + 2H_2O + 4e^- \rightarrow 4OH^-$$

The electrons donated by the cathode are derived from oxidation of Ag at the anode:

$$4g \rightarrow 4g^+ + 4e^-$$

$$Ag^+ + Cl^- \rightarrow AgCl$$

The volume of oxygen reduced at the cathode is directly proportional to the number of electrons used in the reaction. Therefore the amount of oxygen diffusing across the membrane into the electrolyte solution can be determined by measuring the current change that occurs between the anode and the cathode when the electrode is exposed to a blood sample containing oxygen. Because the PO_2 is determined by measuring current changes that occur as oxygen is reduced, this technique is an example of an amperometric measurement; determinations of pH and PCO_2 as described before are examples of potentiometric measurements (i.e., they are based on voltage changes).

The electrical output of the Clark electrode, and thus its sensitivity for measuring PO_2, can be altered by several factors, including protein buildup, cracked electrodes, and loss of electrolyte. When blood samples are analyzed, the consumption of oxygen by the electrode leads to an underestimation of the PO_2 in a blood sample by 2% to 6%. This phenomenon,

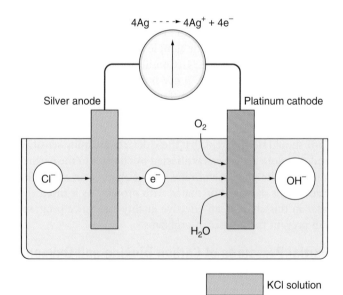

FIGURE 10.7 Principles of PO_2 measurements. See text for discussion. (From Shapiro BA, Peruzzi WT, Templin R: *Clinical application of blood gases*, ed 5, St. Louis, 1994, Mosby.)

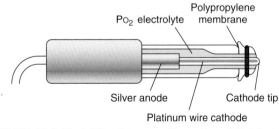

FIGURE 10.6 Clark PO_2 electrode. (From Hess DR, MacIntyre NR, Mishoe SC, et al.: *Respiratory care: principles and practice*, St. Louis, 2002, WB Saunders.)

which has been called the *blood gas factor*, is a result of the slow rate of oxygen diffusion in fluids (i.e., oxygen consumed by the electrode is not replaced by oxygen from the blood).[19] The magnitude of the blood gas factor depends on the diameter of the cathode and the thickness of the membrane between the sample and the cathode. Exposure of the PO_2 electrode to nitrous oxide and halothane (gaseous anesthetic agents) may also alter its electronic output by increasing the production of peroxide ions.[16]

Derived Variables

Several variables can be calculated from the measurements of pH, $PaCO_2$, and PaO_2. The oxygen saturation (O_2SAT) of Hb, the PO_2 at which Hb is 50% saturated (P_{50}), bicarbonate, buffer base, and base excess/deficit are examples of derived variables. Although most modern blood gas analyzers have computer software that automatically calculates these variables, they can also be determined using formulae or nomograms that incorporate accepted constants. Note, however, that these derived variables are calculated and not measured. As such, they may be inaccurate compared with actual measurements because they may not necessarily account for all confounding factors. For example, calculations of O_2SAT of Hb do not account for the presence of dyshemoglobins, such as carboxyhemoglobin and methemoglobin.

Oxygen Saturation of Hemoglobin

The percentage of available Hb that is saturated with oxygen can be calculated by using an equation empirically derived from the oxyhemoglobin saturation curve. These calculations do not account for all of the variables (e.g., the actual $PaCO_2$ or the presence of dyshemoglobins) that can affect this value and therefore can lead to erroneous conclusions about the level of oxyhemoglobin saturation. Direct measurement of oxyhemoglobin saturation is discussed along with oximetry later in this chapter. Directly measured values are more reliable and should be used instead of a derived O_2SAT value when decisions are made about a patient's oxygenation status. Notice that although the calculated and the measured O_2SAT are identical in many cases, this is not always true.

P_{50} Determinations

P_{50} is a convenient way of describing Hb affinity for oxygen because it identifies the PO_2 in millimeters of mercury (mm Hg) when Hb is 50% saturated with oxygen. It is determined by equilibrating a blood sample with various oxygen concentrations at 37°C, which can be accomplished with a tonometer connected to a series of certified gas mixtures. (The P_{50} measurements are standardized for a pH of 7.4, a $PaCO_2$ of 40 mm Hg, and a temperature of 37°C.[17,19]) As Fig. 10.8 shows, alterations in Hb affinity for oxygen are associated with

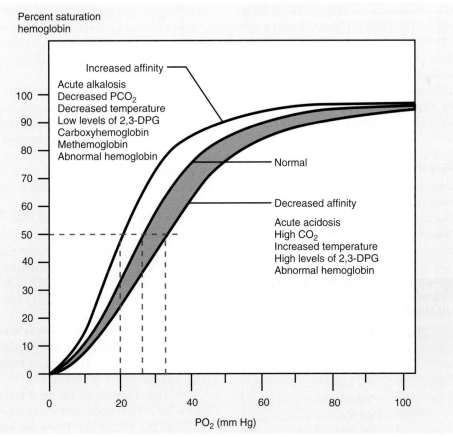

FIGURE 10.8 Effects of changes in pH, PCO_2, and 2,3-diphosphoglycerate (2,3-DPG) on the oxyhemoglobin dissociation curve. (Redrawn from Lane EE, Walker JF: *Clinical arterial blood gas analysis*, St. Louis, 1987, Mosby.)

shifting of the oxyhemoglobin dissociation curve. It is well established that the affinity of hemoglobin A (HbA, or normal adult Hb) for oxygen (and thus the P_{50}) can be altered by changes in the pH, PCO_2, temperature, and concentration of 2,3-diphosphoglycerate (2,3-DPG) in arterial blood. The presence of fetal hemoglobin (HbF) and carboxyhemoglobin (HbCO) can also alter the oxyhemoglobin curve. P_{50} determinations are not routinely performed, but they can be helpful in diagnosing and managing hypoxemia associated with various types of hemoglobinopathies.

Bicarbonate, Buffer Base, and Base Excess

The actual bicarbonate is the concentration of bicarbonate (HCO_3^-) in the plasma of anaerobically drawn blood.[15] It is derived from measurements of pH and $PaCO_2$ using the Henderson-Hasselbalch equation. (Note that the standard bicarbonate is also derived from the Henderson-Hasselbalch equation, but it represents the HCO_3^- concentration in a fully oxygenated plasma sample measured at a temperature of 37°C and a $PaCO_2$ of 40 mm Hg.) Plasma HCO_3^- levels normally range from 22 to 26 mmol/L. The HCO_3^- level becomes elevated in metabolic alkalosis and chronic respiratory acidosis and reduced in metabolic acidosis and chronic respiratory alkalosis.

The buffer base represents the sum of all the anion buffers in the blood, including HCO_3^-, Hb, inorganic phosphate, and negatively charged proteins.[17] The buffer base usually ranges from 44 to 48 mmol/L. The base excess/deficit is the number of millimoles of strong acid required to titrate a blood sample to a pH of 7.4 at a PCO_2 of 40 mm Hg. Theoretically, the buffer base and the base excess are not affected by changes in respiratory function; therefore they can be used to identify nonrespiratory disturbances in acid–base status. Fig. 10.9 is a Siggaard-Andersen alignment nomogram for calculating the actual and standard HCO_3^-, buffer base, and base excess concentrations.

Whole-Blood Analysis: Electrolytes and Glucose

Many blood gas analyzers incorporate sensors for measuring electrolytes (e.g., sodium [Na^+], potassium [K^+], chloride [Cl^-], calcium [Ca^{++}]) and metabolites (e.g., glucose). Table 10.4 presents the normal values for plasma electrolytes. The sensors

used for electrolyte measurements are ion-selective electrodes, but those used to measure glucose are coated with an enzyme called glucose oxidase. Electrolytes are determined by potentiometric measurements, but metabolites are determined by amperometric measurements.

The typical electrolyte sensor is composed of a measuring half-cell and an external reference half-cell, which form a complete electrochemical cell. The measuring half-cell is made of a Ag/AgCl wire that is surrounded by an electrolyte-specific solution. For example, the electrolyte solution used in the sodium and chloride sensors contains a fixed concentration of sodium and chloride, the potassium sensor electrolyte contains a fixed concentration of potassium, and the calcium electrolyte contains a fixed concentration of calcium. The electrolyte solution is separated from the sample solution by an ion-selective membrane, and as the sample comes in contact with the membrane, a transmembrane potential develops across the membrane because of the exchange of ions across it. The potential developed across the membrane is compared with the constant potential of the external reference sensor, and the magnitude of the potential difference is proportional to the ion activity of the sample.

A glucose sensor consists of four electrodes:
- The measuring electrode, made of platinum and glucose oxidase, which is enclosed in a binder.
- A second reference electrode, which is composed of Ag/AgCl.
- A "counter" electrode, composed of platinum, which ensures that a constant polarizing voltage is applied to the sensor.
- A second "counter" electrode, which does not contain the enzyme glucose oxidase, to quantify interfering substances in the sample.

As the sample contacts the measuring electrode, glucose oxidase on the surface of the electrode converts the glucose in the sample to hydrogen peroxide and gluconic acid. The polarizing voltage applied to the electrode causes the hydrogen peroxide to oxidize, resulting in the loss of electrons. The loss of electrons causes current flow to be directly proportional to the glucose concentration of the sample.

Quality Assurance of Blood Gas Analyzers

The Joint Commission (TJC), the Centers for Medicare and Medicaid Services (formerly the Health Care Financing Administration), and the College of American Pathologists (CAP) have published standards that clinical blood gas laboratories must follow to ensure the accuracy and reliability of blood gas measurements. These standards, which are based on recommendations from the Clinical Laboratory Improvement Amendments of 1988 (CLIA-88), require routine calibrations of instruments, as well as programs to assess quality control (QC) and quality assurance (QA).[2,20,21]

Calibration standards for most blood gas analyzers are buffers for pH electrodes and specially prepared gases for the PCO_2 and PO_2 electrodes.[22] (Note that buffers and calibration gases must be clearly labeled with reference values and defined confidence limits.) Verification of the instrument's calibration may vary according to the regulatory agency under which the

TABLE 10.4	Normal Values for Plasma Electrolytes	
Parameter	**Symbol**	**Normal Values (mEq/L)**
Sodium	Na^+	136-145
Potassium	K^+	3.5-5.0
Total calcium	Ca^{++}	4.5-5.25
Magnesium	Mg^{++}	1.7-2.1
Chloride	Cl^-	98-106
Glucose	Glu	80-120 (fasting) 100-140 (postprandial)
Phosphorus	PO_4^-	1.2-2.3

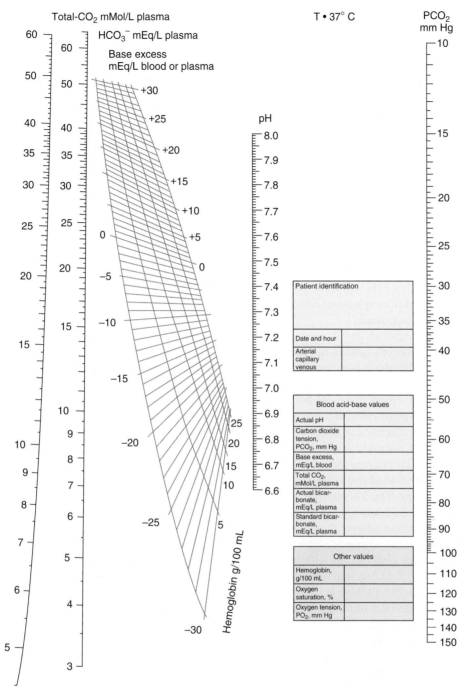

FIGURE 10.9 Siggaard-Andersen alignment nomogram. A line is drawn between the pH and PCO_2, and the actual HCO_3^- is read directly at the intersection of this line. BE_b is Hb dependent and can be read at the intersection of the constructed line and the patient's Hb value. Standard HCO_3^- can be determined by constructing another line through the BE-Hb point and the PCO_2 of 40 mm Hg, and by reading the HCO_3^- scale. Buffer base (BB) can be computed from the equation $BB = 41.7 + (0.42 \times Hb) + BE$. BE_{ECF} is calculated similarly to BE_b, but the BE_{ECF} is read off at the intersection of the constructed line and one-third of the patient's Hb value. *BE*, Base excess; *BE_b*, blood base excess; *BE_{ECF}*, extracellular base excess; *PO_2*, partial pressure of oxygen. (Modified from Siggaard-Andersen O: Arterial blood gas analyzers. In Burton G, Hodgkin JE, Ward JJ, editors: *Respiratory care: a guide to clinical practice*, ed 4, Philadelphia, 1997, JB Lippincott.)

laboratory is accredited or licensed (e.g., CAP, TJC).[2] Generally, every instrument in operation must undergo routine one- and two-point calibrations, which should include high and low pH, PCO_2, and PO_2 values. The one-point calibration involves adjusting the electronic output to a single, known standard. With two-point calibrations, the electrode's electronic output is adjusted to two known standards. A one-point calibration should be performed before an unknown sample is analyzed, unless the analyzer is programmed to perform a one-point calibration automatically at regular intervals (e.g., every 20 to 30 minutes). A two-point calibration usually is performed at least three times daily, usually every 8 hours. In many cases, analyzers can be programmed to perform a two-point calibration at predetermined intervals. A three-point calibration should be performed every 6 months, or whenever an electrode is replaced. Three-point calibrations involve adding a third standard that is intermediate to the other standards to ensure linearity of the electrode response. A fourth level may be required if samples containing high O_2 levels are analyzed with the instrument.[2]

The National Institute of Standards and Technology (NIST) and the International Federation of Clinical Chemistry (IFCC) have established standards for the calibration of blood gas electrodes. A nearly normal pH buffer (pH = 7.384) is used for one-point calibrations; a second, lower pH buffer (pH = 6.84) is analyzed in the two-point calibration to ensure that the electronic output of the electrode is linear over a wide range of pH levels. The PCO_2 electrode is calibrated with two gas concentrations: a 5% CO_2 mixture for establishing the lower end of CO_2 levels encountered and a 10% CO_2 mixture for the high end of the range. The 5% mixture is used for one-point calibrations, but both mixtures are used in the two-point calibration to establish a linear slope for the electrode's electronic output. The PO_2 electrode is also calibrated with two gas mixtures, usually a gas mixture with 0% O_2 and another with 12% or 20% O_2.[17] The accuracy of oxygen electrodes may vary by as much as 20% for high PO_2 levels because of the lack of linearity between electronic output and oxygen

tensions above 150 mm Hg. It has been suggested that this problem can be minimized by using additional calibration gases with higher concentrations of oxygen (i.e., >20% O_2).

QC may be defined as a system that includes analysis of control samples (with a known pH, PCO_2, and PO_2), assessment of the measurements against defined limits, identification of problems, and specification of corrective actions. Internal QC can be accomplished by periodic analysis of commercial products with known pH, PCO_2, and PO_2 values. QC materials include human or bovine whole blood samples that have been tonometered to exact gas tensions or commercially prepared aqueous buffers and perfluorocarbon emulsions that have been equilibrated with a series of known PCO_2 and PO_2 values by the manufacturer. Although tonometry remains the gold standard for QC of PCO_2 and PO_2 electrodes, most laboratories use commercially prepared QC systems for biosafety and convenience. It should be mentioned, however, that commercially prepared controls provide information on the instrument's precision—not the accuracy of the data. (Remember that *precision* refers to the reproducibility of repeat measurements, and *accuracy* relates to how close the measurement is to the correct value.) Also, commercial controls are susceptible to variations in room storage temperature and do not reflect temperature and protein errors in blood gas analyzers.[17]

Regardless of the type of QC material used to assess an instrument's performance, the results should be recorded in a manner that allows the operator to detect changes in the operation of the blood gas analyzer. The most common method of recording QC data involves the use of Levy-Jennings charts (Fig. 10.10). These charts allow the operator to detect trends and shifts in electrode performance, which helps prevent problems associated with reporting of inaccurate data because of analyzer malfunction. For example, a trend (see Fig. 10.10A) typically is associated with protein buildup on an electrode membrane or an electrode that is nearing the end of its life expectancy. A shift (see Fig. 10.10B) can be caused by a tear in the electrode membrane or loss of the electrolyte that bathes the electrode.

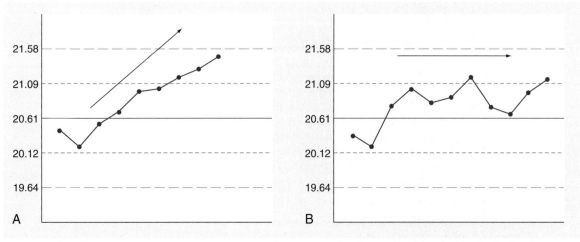

FIGURE 10.10 Levy-Jennings charts showing two types of electrode performance findings. A, Trend. B, Shift.

QA involves testing the proficiency of both personnel and equipment, providing a dynamic process of identification, evaluation, and resolution of problems that affect blood gas measurements.[22] CAP and the American Thoracic Society (ATS) currently offer two proficiency testing programs that provide a means of assessing blind samples (periodically) and the technical competence of laboratory personnel, and a means of reporting the variability of individual blood gas analyzers.

Proficiency testing materials usually include a series of unknown samples with target values that have been established by previously identified reference laboratories. At regular intervals throughout the year (i.e., a minimum of three times per year), all participating laboratories analyze unknown samples (typically three to five samples are used) and forward their results to the sponsoring organization, collating the results from all laboratories. The criteria for acceptable results are defined, and the laboratory personnel are notified of their laboratory's performance. (Generally, an acceptable pH is within ± 0.04 of the target value; PCO_2 values must be ± 3 mm Hg or ± 8% of the target value, whichever is greater; and PO_2 values must be within ± 3 SD.[17,19]) An unsatisfactory performance, which is failure to achieve any of the target values at a single event, necessitates that remedial action be taken and documented. Unsuccessful performance, which is associated with failure to achieve the target values for an analyte in two consecutive events or in two of three consecutive events, can result in the placement of sanctions on the laboratory.[9-17,19,20] These sanctions can cause the laboratory to lose revenue because of suspension of Medicare and Medicaid reimbursement. The laboratory can be reinstated only through additional staff training, increased QC procedures, and reapplication with evidence that the problems have been corrected.

Temperature Correction of Blood Gases

With most modern blood gas analyzers, the blood sample is heated and maintained at a constant temperature of 37°C during analysis. Temperature correction refers to the application of mathematical formulae to adjust blood gas tensions to more accurately reflect the patient's core temperature (i.e., the temperature in the artery from which the blood sample was obtained). Whether these temperature corrections are necessary or even desirable is the subject of considerable debate. Those who favor temperature correction point out that corrected results are a true reflection of the individual's oxygenation and acid–base status. According to Mohler et al.,[23] the PaO_2 changes approximately 7% for each degree Celsius; the $PaCO_2$ changes approximately 4% per degree Celsius; and the pH changes by 0.0146 per degree Celsius. Proponents of reporting blood gases at 37°C believe that pH and $PaCO_2$ values standardized to a body temperature of 37°C reliably reflect the in vivo acid–base status of the patient and that correction of pH and $PaCO_2$ does not affect the calculated HCO_3^-.[17] Furthermore, acid–base nomograms are typically calculated for 37°C, and considerable errors occur if temperature-corrected blood gas data are used with these nomograms. Although all commercial blood gas analyzers

contain solid-state circuitry that can easily perform temperature corrections, most laboratories still report blood gases at 37°C because of the lack of consensus on the topic.

In vivo Blood Gas Monitors

As was previously mentioned, recent advances in fiberoptic technology have made it possible to obtain continuous in vivo ABG and pH measurements. A typical in vivo blood gas monitor has one or more optical sensors that are embedded in a gas- or ion-permeable polymer matrix. The sensors are connected to a CPU by a fiberoptic cable. The fiberoptic sensor is inserted into the intravascular space through an indwelling 20-gauge cannula. Light of a specific wavelength and intensity from the CPU is transmitted along the fiber to a microcuvette containing a fluorescent dye. The incident light striking the microcuvette is modified in proportion to the PO_2, PCO_2, or pH level of the blood, which is in contact with the microcuvette. The modified light is then transmitted back to the monitor through either the same optical path or a second fiber parallel to the fiber carrying the incident light.[24] Fig. 10.11 shows an alternative extraarterial blood gas monitor. In this case the blood gas sensor is located in series with the arterial catheter.

Optical blood gas sensors generally are categorized by how they modify the initial optical signal; they are classified as either absorbance or fluorescent sensors.[17] With absorbance sensors, when light of a known wavelength and intensity is transmitted down the fiber and through the microcuvette, a fraction of the incident light is absorbed, and the remaining light is transmitted. The concentration of the analyte can be determined by measuring the intensity of the light striking the photodetector, because the amount of light transmitted

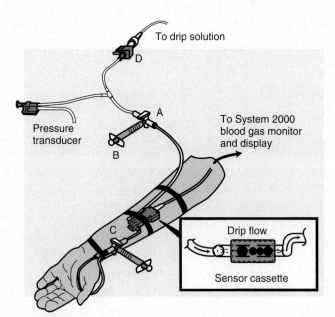

FIGURE 10.11 Fiberoptic blood gas monitor. (Redrawn from Shapiro BA, Peruzzi WT, Templin R, et al.: Clinical performance of a blood gas monitor: a prospective, multicenter trial. *Crit Care Med* 21:487, 1993.)

is proportional to the concentration of the analyte in question (i.e., the pH, PCO_2, or PO_2).

Fluorescent sensors use dyes that fluoresce when they are struck by light in the ultraviolet or nearly ultraviolet visible range. Light from the monitor is transmitted to the microcuvette containing the dye. The dye absorbs the light energy of the optical excitation signal and emits a fluorescent signal that is returned to the monitor along the fiberoptic cable. The concentration of the analyte in question can be measured by determining the ratio of fluorescent light emitted to the original excitation light signal. The pH, PCO_2, or PO_2 of arterial blood can be determined by using sensing fibers containing dye systems that are analyte specific (i.e., most commercially available systems contain three analyte-specific sensing fibers).

Fluorescent sensors currently in use can measure pH values from 6.8 to 7.8, PCO_2 values from 10 to 100 mm Hg, and PO_2 values from 20 to 600 mm Hg. Compared with in vitro blood gas analysis, intraarterial blood gas monitoring systems are comparable for pH, but the correlation may not be as good for PCO_2 and PO_2 measurements.[24]

Calibration of Intraarterial Blood Gas Monitors

Intraarterial blood gas monitoring systems must be calibrated before insertion into a patient by immersion of the sensor in a buffer containing known pH, PCO_2, and PO_2 values. In vivo calibrations are complicated and subject to error, because adjustment must be made using single-point measurements from laboratory (in vitro) ABG analysis.

In many cases, temperature corrections may be required because the sensor may be in a peripheral artery, where the measured temperature may not equal the patient's core temperature. Temperature corrections usually are accomplished by combining a temperature-measuring thermocouple with the analyte-specific sensor. By measuring the sensor's temperature, the pH or blood gas value may then be displayed as measured or corrected to 37°C (or some other user-entered patient temperature).

Point-of-Care Testing

Point-of-care (POC) testing is testing that is done outside the main hospital laboratory. POC testing typically involves the use of portable devices that can be located at or near the point of patient care. As such, these devices are not only portable but also lightweight (total weight is approximately 1 pound); this allows in vitro ABG and pH measurements to be made in the emergency department, intensive care unit, physician's office, or a transport vehicle.[25] Fig. 10.12 shows a typical POC blood gas analyzer. POC devices usually are battery powered but can be powered by a standard AC electrical outlet. The system uses solid-state sensors, which rely on spectrophotometric, fluorescence technology, infrared spectroscopy, or thin-film electrodes that have been fabricated onto silicone chips. The microelectrodes are incorporated into a single-use disposable cartridge that also contains calibration reagents, a sampling stylus, and a waste container. (*Note:* Some POC devices use cartridges that allow for a fixed number of analyses.) In addition to the standard blood gas cartridges,

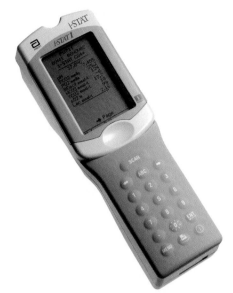

FIGURE 10.12 Point-of-care (POC) blood gas analyzer. (Courtesy i-Stat Corp., East Windsor, NJ.)

several modules are available for the analysis of electrolytes (e.g., sodium, potassium, and chloride), lactates, blood urea nitrogen (BUN), glucose, and hematocrit. The results are shown on a liquid crystal display.

Measurements can typically be made on blood samples of less than 1 mL in 60 to 120 seconds. Manufacturers of POC devices state that these devices are accurate over a wide range of pH, $PaCO_2$, and PaO_2 values. For example, the manufacturer of i-STAT (Abbott Point of Care) states that its device has a range of 6.8 to 8 for pH, 10 to 100 torr (mm Hg) for $PaCO_2$, and 5 to 800 (mm Hg) for PaO_2. The use of these devices is growing, especially as a replacement for "stat" laboratory services. Table 10.5 compares four commercial POC blood gas analyzers currently available.[25] Box 10.1 summarizes the potential advantages and disadvantages of POC testing. It is important to mention that POC devices require QA monitoring.

IV. CO-OXIMETRY

An oximeter is a device that can measure the oxyhemoglobin saturation of arterial, venous, mixed venous, or intracardiac blood. Two types of oximeters are routinely used in respiratory care: CO-oximeters and pulse oximeters. A CO-oximeter can provide simultaneous in vitro measurements of various Hb gases, including oxyhemoglobin (O_2Hb), HbCO, methemoglobin (metHb), sulfhemoglobin (sulfHb), and HbF, using whole-blood samples. Pulse oximeters are noninvasive devices that provide only measurements of arterial O_2Hb saturation. Pulse oximeters are discussed in detail in the section on noninvasive assessment of ABGs.

Oximeters operate on the principle of spectrophotometry, which is based on the relative transmission or absorption of portions of the light spectrum.[26] The various forms of Hb mentioned previously can be identified because each form has its own absorption spectrum. (Fig. 10.13 shows the light spectra for each type of Hb.) The concentration of a certain

TABLE 10.5	Comparison of Four Point-of-Care Blood Gas Analyzers			
	i-STAT	**EPOC**	**OPTI CCA-TS**	**ABL90 FLEX**
Dimensions (H × W × D/Weight)	9.25 × 3 × 2.85 in/22.4 oz	3 × 3.4 × 8.5 in/1.5 lb	4.7 × 14.2 × 9 in/12 lb (10 lb without battery)	17.7 × 9.8 × 11.4 in/24 lb
Specimen types suitable for device	Whole blood, capillary, mixed venous, arterial, venous	Whole blood, capillary, mixed venous, arterial, venous	Whole blood, plasma, serum	Whole blood, capillary, mixed venous, arterial, venous
Sample size for complete panel of analyte results	96 µL blood gas, 65 µL electrolytes	92 µL	125 µL	65 µL
Parameters (measured)	pH, PCO_2, PO_2 Hct, Na, K, Cl, Ca, lactate, glucose, tCO_2	pH, PCO_2, PO_2 Hct, Na, K, Cl, Ca, lactate, glucose, creatinine	pH, PCO_2, PO_2 Hct, THb, O_2SAT, Na, K, Cl, Ca, lactate, glucose, BUN	pH, PCO_2, PO_2 Hct, THb, O_2SAT, Na, K, Cl, Ca, lactate, glucose, O_2Hb, HbCo, MetHb, HHb
Parameters (calculated)	Hb, Hct, O_2SAT, BE, tCO_2, HCO_3^-	Hb, Hct, tCO_2, O_2SAT, BE, BE(ecf), BE(act), BB, AGAP, HCO_3^-	Hb, Hct, tCO_2, O_2SAT, O_2ct, BE, BE(ecf), BE(act), BB, AGAP, stdHCO$_3^-$, P_{50}, Ca	Hb, Hct, tCO_2, HCO_3^-
Analytic method	Electrochemical	Potentiometric/ amperometric/ Conductometric	Optical fluorescence and reflectance	Potentiometric/optical fluorescence/ spectrophotometric analysis

i-STAT (Abbott Point of Care); epoc (Alere); OPTI CCA-TS (Opti Medical Systems); ABL90 (Radiometer America).
AGAP, Anion gap; *BB,* buffer base; *BE,* base excess; *BE(act),* actual base excess; *BE(ecf),* extracellular base excess; *BUN,* blood urea nitrogen; *Ca,* calcium; *Cl,* chloride; *HbCO,* carboxyhemoglobin; *HCO$_3^-$,* bicarbonate; *Hct,* hematocrit; *HHb,* reduced hemoglobin; *K,* potassium; *MetHb,* methemoglobin; *Na,* sodium; *O$_2$ct,* oxygen content; *O$_2$Hb,* oxyhemoglobin; *O$_2$SAT,* oxygen saturation; *P$_{50}$,* partial pressure of oxygen at which hemoglobin is 50% saturated; *PCO$_2$,* partial pressure of carbon dioxide; *pH,* hydrogen ion concentration; *PO$_2$,* partial pressure of oxygen; *O$_2$SAT,* oxygen saturation; *stdHCO$_3$,* standard bicarbonate;*tCO2,* total CO$_2$; *THb,* total hemoglobin.
Data modified from CAP Today (An interactive guide to laboratory software and instrumentation) http://www.captodayonline.com/ productguides/instruments/in-vitro-blood-gas-analyzers-may-2016.html.

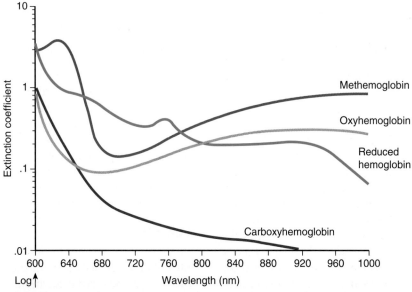

FIGURE 10.13 Absorption spectra for various species of hemoglobin (Hb).

Hb type can be determined using the Beer-Lambert law, which states that the transmission of a specific wavelength of light through a solution is a logarithmic function of the concentration of the absorbing species in the solution.[17,27]

The operating principle of a typical CO-oximeter is fairly straightforward. A blood sample is heated to 37°C and hemolyzed (either chemically or by high-frequency vibrations), creating a translucent solution. The solution is placed in a cuvette, which is positioned between a light source and a condenser and two photodetectors. A series of monochromatic light beams are simultaneously directed through the cuvette containing the sample of blood and through a blank solution (containing no Hb).[17] The condenser lens system focuses the light passing through the sample cuvette onto a photodetector, which generates an electric current proportional to the intensity of the transmitted light and inversely proportional to the amount of light absorbed by the sample. The light passing through the blank solution is simultaneously focused onto a reference photodetector, which generates an electric current proportional to the light transmitted through the blank solution. The absorbance of the blank solution is then subtracted from the absorbances of the blood sample, and the resultant values are used to calculate the concentration of each type of Hb in the blood sample. Table 10.1 shows the normal concentrations of the various Hb types.

Although blood can contain six different types of Hb, most commercially available CO-oximeters provide measurements of only four types: O_2Hb, deoxyhemoglobin, metHb, and HbCO. sulfHb and HbF are not usually determined by CO-oximetry, although the manufacturer Radiometer America has introduced a CO-oximetry procedure to determine HbF. Although these results are different from reference methods, such as radioimmunoassay and chromatographic procedures, CO-oximeter analysis of HbF has been deemed clinically acceptable. Other reported values may include total hemoglobin (THb) and oxygen content (O_2ct).

A number of factors can interfere with CO-oximetry measurements. Incompletely hemolyzed red blood cells, lipids, or air bubbles in the sample can scatter some of the incident light, producing erroneous measurements.[28,29] The presence of bilirubin (>20 mg/dL of whole blood) or intravenous dyes (particularly methylene blue and indocyanine green) can also alter measurements because they absorb near-infrared (NIR) and infrared (IR) light. Absorbance of light by these substances lowers the actual O_2Hb measured. The presence of HbF can also lead to false HbCO readings. Oxygenated HbF produces a 4% to 7% false HbCO level; reduced HbF yields a 0.2% to 1.5% false HbCO level.[17]

Calibration of CO-Oximeters

CO-oximeters should be routinely calibrated with solutions supplied by the manufacturer. These solutions typically are dye-based propylene glycol solutions that allow only for the calibration of THb. Determination of the various forms of Hb is accomplished by relating the relative absorbances recorded at the wavelengths tested. That is, the percentage of a particular Hb type reported is derived from absorbance ratios at predetermined wavelengths.

V. NONINVASIVE ASSESSMENT OF ARTERIAL BLOOD GASES

Noninvasive blood gas monitoring has become a standard practice in respiratory care and anesthesiology. The importance of these devices in the management of patients with cardiopulmonary dysfunctions cannot be overstated. In just 30 years, pulse oximeters and transcutaneous pH, PCO_2, and PO_2 monitors have gone from expensive, bulky units to compact, affordable devices that can provide both continuous and intermittent pH, PCO_2, and PO_2 measurements that are reliable and accurate.

Pulse Oximetry

Pulse oximetry provides continuous, noninvasive measurements of the arterial O_2SAT and pulse rate via a sensor placed over a digit, the earlobe, forehead, or the bridge of the nose. The sensor measures the absorption of selected wavelengths of light beamed through the tissue. Advances in microprocessor technology, coupled with improvements in the quality of light-emitting diodes (LEDs) and photoelectric sensors, have greatly improved the accuracy and reliability of these devices. Most clinicians now consider pulse oximetry an indispensable tool for monitoring the oxygenation status of patients at risk for hypoxemia.

Theory of Operation

Pulse oximetry is based on the principles of spectrophotometry and photoplethysmography.[30-32] As with CO-oximeters, pulse oximeters use spectrophotometry to determine the amount of Hb (and deoxyhemoglobin) in a blood sample. O_2Hb and deoxygenated Hb are differentiated by shining two wavelengths of light (660 and 940 nm) through the sampling site. As Fig. 10.13 shows, at a wavelength of 660 nm (red light), deoxygenated Hb absorbs more light than O_2Hb. Conversely, O_2Hb absorbs more light at 940 nm (IR light) than deoxygenated Hb.

Photoplethysmography, or optical plethysmography, estimates the heart rate by measuring cyclic changes in light transmission through the sampling site during each cardiac cycle. That is, as the blood volume in the finger, toe, or earlobe increases during ventricular systole, light absorption increases and transmitted light decreases. Conversely, as blood volume decreases during diastole, absorbency decreases and transmitted light increases. Fig. 10.14 shows the pulsatile and nonpulsatile components of a typical pulse oximetry signal.

The percentage of O_2Hb in a sample can be determined by first calculating the ratio of absorbencies for pulsatile and nonpulsatile flow at the two specified wavelengths, or

$$Red/Infrared = \frac{Pulsatile_{660nm}/Nonpulsatile_{660nm}}{Pulsatile_{940nm}/Nonpulsatile_{940nm}}$$

This ratio is then applied to an algorithm that relates the ratios of these two absorbencies to the O_2Hb saturation.[32]

As mentioned previously, four types of Hb can be measured by oximetry: reduced or deoxygenated Hb (HHb), O_2Hb, HbCO, and metHb. Two terms often used to describe O_2Hb saturation determinations are *fractional* and *functional saturations*. The fractional hemoglobin saturation is calculated by dividing the amount of O_2Hb by the amount of all four types of Hb present, or

$$Fractional\ O_2Hb = O_2Hb \div [HHb + O_2Hb + HbCO + metHb]$$

The functional hemoglobin saturation is calculated by dividing the O_2Hb concentration by the concentration of Hb capable of carrying oxygen. It may be written as

$$Functional\ O_2Hb = O_2Hb \div [HHb + O_2Hb]$$

Although laboratory CO-oximeters measure all four types of Hb by using a series of wavelengths of light to identify each species, pulse oximeters use only two wavelengths to quantify the amount of O_2Hb and HHb present. Therefore laboratory CO-oximeters can report the fractional O_2Hb saturation, and pulse oximeters can estimate the functional O_2Hb saturation.

Physiological and Technical Considerations

It is important to recognize that both physiological and technical factors can influence the accuracy of pulse oximetry measurements.[33]

Low perfusion states. The accuracy of a pulse oximetry reading depends on identification of an arterial pulse; therefore many conditions can interfere with proper pulse oximeter function. Hypovolemia, peripheral vasoconstriction from drugs or hypothermia, and heart–lung bypass (i.e., extracorporeal membrane oxygenation) are associated with a diminished pulsatile signal, resulting in an intermittent or absent oxygen saturation pulse oximetry (SpO_2) reading.[30] Some oximeters compensate for the weak signal associated with low perfusion states by increasing the signal output. The problem with this approach is that augmenting the signal also causes an increase in the signal-to-noise ratio, which can result in high levels of background noise that can contribute to erroneous results. A simpler approach is to reposition the oximeter sensor in an area of higher perfusion. For example, placing the oximeter probe on the ear instead of the finger may alleviate some of the problems associated with reductions in peripheral perfusion.

Dysfunctional hemoglobins. High levels of dysfunctional hemoglobins (i.e., HbCO and metHb) can adversely affect O_2Hb measurement by pulse oximetry.[30] High HbCO levels

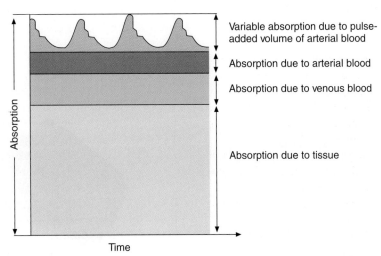

FIGURE 10.14 Pulsatile and nonpulsatile components of a typical pulse oximetry signal. (From McGough EK, Boysen PG: Benefits and limits of pulse oximetry in the ICU, *J Crit Ill* 4:23, 1989.)

can alter SpO_2 measurements because O_2Hb and $HbCO$ have similar absorption coefficients for red light (660 nm); however, $HbCO$ is relatively transparent to IR light (940 nm). Accordingly, significant levels of $HbCO$, as occur in carbon monoxide poisoning, lead to an overestimation of SpO_2.[30] (See Clinical Scenario 10.3 for a decision-making problem involving pulse oximetry.)

Methemoglobinemia, a complication associated with certain types of drugs (e.g., nitrites, benzocaine [a local anesthetic], and dapsone [an antibiotic used to treat malaria and *Pneumocystis carinii*]), can lead to erroneous SpO_2 values because metHb absorbs both red and IR light.[30] Methemoglobinemia is also associated with nitrate poisoning. If enough metHb is present to dominate all pulsatile absorption, the pulse oximeter will measure a red-to-IR ratio of 1:1, corresponding to an SpO_2 of approximately 85%. Consequently, the pulse oximeter reading will overestimate or underestimate the true O_2Hb saturation.[30]

Dyes. Intravascular dyes can adversely affect SpO_2 values by absorbing a portion of the incident light emitted by the pulse oximeter diodes. Injection of methylene blue and indigo carmine during cardiac catheterization causes a false drop in SpO_2; indocyanine green has been shown to have little effect on pulse oximeter readings.[33]

Dark nail polish (particularly blue and black nail polish) can severely affect SpO_2 readings. Some have suggested that nail polish may affect pulse oximetry values by causing the shunting of light around the finger periphery.[34,35] In **optical shunting**, transmitted light never comes in contact with the vascular bed; therefore SpO_2 values can be erroneously high or low, depending on whether this light is pulsatile. This problem can be alleviated to a large extent by placing the device over the lateral aspects of the digit instead of over the nail. Theoretically, skin pigmentation should not affect pulse oximeter readings; however, in practice, SpO_2 readings are inconsistent for patients with dark pigmentation, possibly because of optical shunting.[36] **Hyperbilirubinemia**, a yellow discoloration of the skin associated with hepatic dysfunction, does not seem to affect pulse oximetry readings.[17]

Ambient light. Fluorescent lights and other external light sources (e.g., heat lamps, fiberoptic light sources, and surgical lamps) have been shown to adversely affect heart rate and SpO_2 readings.[37] Most commercially available pulse oximeters attempt to compensate for this interference by continually cycling the transmitted red and IR light on and off at a rate of approximately 480 cycles per second. In this process the pulse oximeter cycles in three modes:

1. Red light on, IR off
2. IR on, red light off
3. Red light and IR off

By using this sequence, ambient light interference can be determined when both red and IR light sources are off. Subtracting any light measured during phase 3 from that measured during phases 1 and 2 provides a means of minimizing ambient light interference.

Calibration of Pulse Oximeters

Pulse oximeters are calibrated by manufacturers with data obtained from studies of healthy humans. Specifically, SpO_2 levels are compared with invasive hemoximetry oxygen saturations (SaO_2) measured simultaneously while each individual breathes several gas mixtures of different fractional inspired oxygen (F_IO_2). Therefore the accuracy and reliability of a pulse oximeter ultimately depend on the initial calibration algorithm programmed into the device by the manufacturer. Generally, pulse oximeters are accurate for oxygen saturations higher than 80%. Pulse oximeter saturations lower than 80% are questionable and should be confirmed with ABG analysis and hemoximetry.

Clinical Applications of Pulse Oximetry

Pulse oximetry probes are available in neonatal, pediatric, and adult sizes. Advances in LED and solid-state technology have led to the miniaturization of pulse oximeters and the manufacture of handheld devices (Fig. 10.15). The response time

---

⚲ CLINICAL SCENARIO 10.3

Assessment of a patient admitted to the emergency department after exposure to an enclosed fire included evaluation of SpO_2 and ABGs. The results, obtained while the patient was breathing room air, were SpO_2 = 98%, pH = 7.38, $PaCO_2$ = 35 mm Hg, PaO_2 = 95 mm Hg, and SaO_2 = 97%. What is your interpretation of these findings?

See Appendix A for the answer.

ABG, Arterial blood gas; *pH,* hydrogen ion concentration; *PaCO₂,* partial pressure of carbon dioxide in the arteries; *PaO₂,* partial pressure of oxygen in the arteries; *SaO₂,* arterial oxygen saturation; *SpO₂,* oxygen saturation as measured using pulse oximetry.

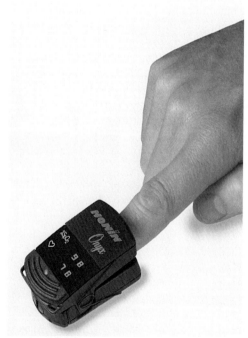

FIGURE 10.15 Handheld pulse oximeter. (Courtesy Nonin Medical, Plymouth, MN.)

of a pulse oximeter (i.e., how long it takes for a change in central circulation [left-heart PO_2] to be detected by the pulse oximeter) depends on the location of the probe. Probes placed on fingers show a delay of 12 seconds or longer compared with a probe placed on the earlobe. Probes placed on the toe show an even greater lag time for detecting PO_2 changes.

Pulse oximetry is well recognized as an early warning system for detecting hypoxemia of patients with unstable oxygenation status. It can provide a continuous display of O_2SAT, which can be used to monitor the oxygenation status of patients during surgery, mechanical ventilation, or bronchoscopy. It also can provide intermittent measurements of SpO_2, which can be useful, for example, in the management of home care patients.

Although pulse oximetry can be quite effective for adjusting oxygen therapy in hospitalized patients, its use in prescribing oxygen therapy for home care patients is questionable. Therefore caution should be exercised when pulse oximeter readings are used to prescribe oxygen therapy. Carlin et al.[38] demonstrated that the use of only pulse oximetry measurements could disqualify a significant number of patients applying for reimbursement for oxygen therapy. The guidelines established by the Centers for Medicare and Medicaid Services for qualifying for oxygen therapy require that the patient demonstrate a PaO_2 less than or equal to 55 torr (mm Hg) or a saturation less than or equal to 85%.[39] Because any of the physiological or technical problems discussed previously can significantly affect pulse oximetry measurements, it is wise to use invasive ABG analysis to establish the need for oxygen therapy for chronically ill patients.

Clinical Practice Guideline 10.2 summarizes the AARC Clinical Practice Guideline for pulse oximetry, which provides valuable information to ensure that SpO_2 values are valid.

Transcutaneous Monitoring

Transcutaneous monitoring provides another method of indirect ABG assessment. Unlike pulse oximetry, which relies on spectrophotometric analysis, transcutaneous monitoring uses modified blood gas electrodes to measure the oxygen and carbon dioxide tension at the skin surface.[18,40,41] The conjunctival PO_2 electrode, a modification of the standard transcutaneous PO_2 ($PtcO_2$) electrode, measures the PO_2 of the palpebral conjunctiva surrounding the eyeball.

Transcutaneous PO_2

Fig. 10.16A is a schematic of a $PtcO_2$ electrode, which consists of a servo-controlled, heated (Clark) polarographic electrode connected to a CPU.[40,41] The electrode is covered with a Teflon membrane, and the entire electrode assembly attaches to the skin surface with a double-sided adhesive ring. The electrode is heated to 42°C to 45°C (107.6°F to 113°F) to produce capillary vasodilation below the surface of the electrode. Heating improves gas diffusion across the skin, because it increases local blood flow at the site of the electrode and alters the structure of the stratum corneum. The stratum corneum has been described as a mixture of fibrinous tissue within a lipid and protein matrix. It has been suggested that heating the skin

---

CLINICAL PRACTICE GUIDELINE 10.2
Pulse Oximetry

Indications
Based on current evidence, pulse oximetry is useful for:
1. Monitoring arterial O_2Hb saturation
2. Quantifying the arterial O_2Hb saturation response to therapeutic intervention
3. Monitoring arterial O_2Hb saturation during bronchoscopy

Contraindications
Pulse oximetry may not be appropriate when ongoing measurements of pH, $PaCO_2$, and THb are required. The presence of abnormal hemoglobins may be a relative contraindication.

Limitations
A number of factors, agents, and situations may affect readings and limit the precision and performance of pulse oximetry, including:
1. Motion artifacts
2. Abnormal hemoglobins (especially HbCO and metHb)
3. Intravascular dyes
4. Exposure of the measuring sensor to ambient light sources
5. Low perfusion states
6. Skin pigmentation
7. Nail polish
8. Low O_2Hb saturations (i.e., <83%)

Monitoring
The following information should be recorded during pulse oximetry:
1. Probe type; measurement site and date and time of measurement; and patient position and activity level
2. F_IO_2 and mode of supplemental oxygen delivery
3. ABG measurements and CO-oximetry results that may have been made simultaneously
4. Clinical appearance of the patient (e.g., cyanotic, skin temperature)
5. Agreement between pulse oximeter heart rate and heart rate determined by palpation or electrocardiogram recordings

ABG, Arterial blood gas; F_IO_2, fractional inspired oxygen; HbCO, carboxyhemoglobin; metHb, methemoglobin; O_2Hb, oxyhemoglobin; $PaCO_2$, partial pressure of carbon dioxide in the arteries; pH, hydrogen ion concentration; THb, total hemoglobin.
Modified from the American Association for Respiratory Care: Clinical practice guideline: pulse oximetry. *Respir Care* 36:1406, 1991.

---

to temperatures greater than 41°C (105.8°F melts the lipid layer, thus enhancing gas diffusion through the skin.[42]

The ratio of $PtcO_2$ to PaO_2 measured by hemoximetry (the $PtcO_2/PaO_2$ index) has been shown to be good for neonatal use, but it often is unreliable for critically ill adults.[43,44] Decreases in peripheral perfusion caused by reductions in cardiac output or increases in peripheral (cutaneous) resistance can significantly affect the accuracy of $PtcO_2$ measurements.[44,45] Current data indicate that when the cardiac index is greater than 2.2 L/min/m², the $PtcO_2/PaO_2$ index is 0.5, but when the cardiac index is less than 1.5 L/min/m², the $PtcO_2/PaO_2$ index is only 0.1.[46] Therefore hypoperfusion of the skin caused by

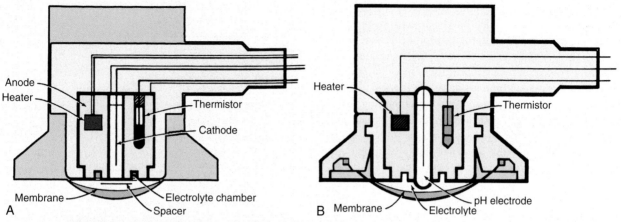

FIGURE 10.16 Transcutaneous electrodes. A, PtcO$_2$. B, PtcCO$_2$. (From Novametrix Medical Systems, Wallingford, CT.)

pathological states (e.g., septic shock, hemorrhage, heart failure) or by increased vascular resistance (e.g., hypothermia or pharmacological intervention) can lead to erroneous data. Because the PtcO$_2$ is influenced by blood flow to the tissues, as well as by oxygen use by the tissues, changes in the PtcO$_2$ may be an early indicator of vascular compromise or shock. In fact, many PtcO$_2$ monitors display the power supplied to the electrode heater as a way of identifying perfusion problems at the site.

Transcutaneous PCO$_2$

The standard transcutaneous carbon dioxide (PtcCO$_2$) electrode is a modified Stowe-Severinghaus blood gas electrode composed of pH-sensitive glass with a Ag/AgCl electrode (see Fig. 10.16B). As with the PtcO$_2$ electrode, the PtcCO$_2$ electrode is heated to 42°C to 45°C. PtcCO$_2$ values are slightly higher than the PaCO$_2$ value, primarily because of the higher metabolic rate at the site of the electrode caused by heating the skin. Most commercial instruments incorporate correction factors into their system's software to remove the discrepancy between the PtcCO$_2$ and PaCO$_2$.

Technical Considerations for Transcutaneous Monitoring

Clinical Practice Guideline 10.3 presents guidelines for transcutaneous monitoring. This guideline updates a previous guideline that was published in 1994.[45,46] The current guideline describes a number of factors that should be considered when using transcutaneous monitoring, including the indications, hazards and complications, and equipment, as well as device limitations and validation of results.

Several points related to the use of transcutaneous monitoring deserve attention:

1. PtcO$_2$ is an indirect measurement of PaO$_2$ and does not reflect oxygen delivery or oxygen content. It is important to recognize that assessment of oxygen delivery also requires knowledge of hemoglobin concentration and cardiac output.[46]
2. Transcutaneous signals are adversely affected by improper placement of the electrode on the patient's skin. Trapped air bubbles and leaks in the fixation device or damaged membranes can produce erroneous results. It is important to ensure that the site is cleaned with an alcohol swab. When hair is present, the site should be shaved to ensure good contact between the electrode and the skin. Before the electrode is attached to the patient, a drop of electrolyte gel or deionized water should be placed on the electrode's surface to enhance gas diffusion between the skin and the electrode.
2. PtcO$_2$ monitors are calibrated with two-point calibration in which room air (PO$_2$ of approximately 150 mm Hg) is the high PO$_2$ of the calibration, and an electronic zeroing of the system is the low PO$_2$ of the calibration. The PtcCO$_2$ electrodes are also calibrated with a two-point calibration procedure. In this case a 5% CO$_2$ calibration gas and a 10% CO$_2$ calibration gas are used for low and high calibration points, respectively. Electrodes should be calibrated before initial use on a patient. Manufacturers typically suggest calibration of an electrode each time it is repositioned.
3. Transcutaneous electrodes are bathed with a small amount of electrolyte solution, which can easily evaporate because heat is applied to the electrode. Loss of electrolyte either through evaporation or leakage from a torn membrane can adversely affect operation of the electrode. The electrolyte and the sensor's membrane should be checked regularly and changed weekly or whenever a signal drift during calibration is noticed. Because Ag can deposit on the cathode, the electrode should be periodically cleaned according to the manufacturer's recommendations.
4. When PtcO$_2$ and PCO$_2$ readings are reported, the date and time of the measurement, the patient's activity level and body position, the site of electrode placement, and the electrode temperature should be noted. The inspired oxygen concentration and the type of equipment used to deliver supplemental oxygen should always be included. The clinical appearance of the patient, including assessment of peripheral perfusion (i.e., pallor, skin temperature), is important data to note. When invasive ABG measurements are available, they are recorded for comparison with PtcO$_2$ and PtcCO$_2$ readings.[45,47]

CLINICAL PRACTICE GUIDELINE 10.3   Transcutaneous Blood Gas Monitoring of Carbon Dioxide and Oxygen: 2012

Indications
1. Monitoring the adequacy of arterial oxygenation and/or ventilation
2. Quantifying a patient's response to diagnostic and therapeutic interventions
3. $PtcO_2/F_IO_2$ can be used as an early indicator of hypoperfusion and mortality[48,49]
4. Tissue perfusion status and revascularization in wound care and peripheral arterial occlusive disease

Contraindications
Relative contraindications to transcutaneous monitoring may be poor skin integrity and adhesive allergy.

Hazards/Complications
1. False-negative or false-positive results may lead to inappropriate treatment (e.g., $PtcO_2$ can underestimates PaO_2, and $PtcCO_2$ can overestimates $PaCO_2$)
2. Tissue injury at the measurement site (e.g., blisters, burns, skin tears)

Limitations
The following factors may increase the discrepancy between arterial and transcutaneous values:
1. Hyperoxemia (PaO_2 >100 mm Hg)
2. Hypoperfused state (e.g., shock)
3. Improper electrode placement
4. Vasoactive drugs
5. Skin factors (skinfold thickness or presence of edema)

Validation
ABG values should be compared with transcutaneous readings taken at the time of arterial sampling to validate the transcutaneous values. The validations should be performed when transcutaneous monitoring is initiated and periodically as dictated by the patient's clinical state.

Assurance of Consistency of Care
1. High- and low-limit alarms are set appropriately
2. Appropriate electrode temperature is set
3. Systematic electrode site change occurs
4. Manufacturer's recommendations for maintenance, operation, and safety are followed

Monitoring
The following information should be recorded at regular intervals (e.g., 1 to 4 h):
1. Date and time of measurement
2. Patient position, respiratory rate, activity level, F_IO_2, mode of ventilatory support and settings
3. Electrode placement site, electrode temperature, time of placement, results of simultaneously obtained in vitro ABG analysis
4. Clinical appearance of the patient, including perfusion, pallor, and skin temperature

Infection Control
Standard precautions are recommended for all patients. The device probe should be cleaned between patient applications according to the manufacturer's recommendations. The external portion of the monitor should be cleaned according to the manufacturer's recommendations whenever the device remains in a patient's room for a prolonged period or if it becomes soiled or contaminated with potentially transmissible organisms.

ABG, Arterial blood gas; *F_IO_2*, fractional inspired oxygen; *$PaCO_2$*, partial pressure of carbon dioxide in the arteries; *PaO_2*, partial pressure of oxygen in the arteries; *$PtcCO_2$*, transcutaneous partial pressure of carbon dioxide; *$PtcO_2$*, transcutaneous partial pressure of oxygen.
Modified from Restrepo RD, Hirst KR, Wittnebel L, et al.: AARC clinical practice guideline: transcutaneous monitoring of carbon dioxide and oxygen: 2012. *Respir Care* 57:1955-1962, 2012.

Burns are probably the most common problem that clinicians encounter during transcutaneous monitoring, because the site of measurement must be heated to 42°C to 45°C. Repositioning the sensor every 4 to 6 hours can minimize this problem. For transcutaneous monitoring of neonates, the sensor should be repositioned more often.

VI. INTERPRETATION OF BLOOD GAS RESULTS

As stated previously, ABG values can provide important information about a patient's acid–base, ventilatory, and oxygenation status. Blood gas analysis is also an integral part of more sophisticated procedures, such as cardiopulmonary and hemodynamic monitoring. It is beyond the scope of this book to discuss fully the interpretive value of blood gas measurements. Therefore a framework for ABG interpretation is provided here, but the titles of several texts and monographs on blood gas analysis are listed at the end of the chapter.

Acid–Base Status

Acid–base disorders can be categorized as either acidosis or alkalosis. Acidosis is associated with an increase in the plasma hydrogen ion concentration and a fall in the pH. Alkalosis is associated with a decrease in plasma hydrogen ion concentration and a rise in pH. The Henderson-Hasselbalch equation can be used to describe how changes in HCO_3^- and $PaCO_2$ can be used to determine whether a metabolic, a respiratory, or a combined acid–base disorder is present. Consider these equations:

$$pH = pKa + \log(HCO_3^-)/(PaCO_2 \times 0.03) \text{ } or$$

$$pH - (HCO_3^-)/(PaCO_2)$$

Acute decreases in HCO_3^- and increases in $PaCO_2$ are associated with decreases in pH and metabolic and respiratory acidosis, respectively. Conversely, acute increases in HCO_3^- and decreases in $PaCO_2$ are associated with increases in pH and metabolic and respiratory alkalosis, respectively. If only one of the parameters changes and the other stays within normal limits, the problem can be classified as an acute or uncompensated acid–base disorder. For example, a reduced pH with an increase in $PaCO_2$ and a normal HCO_3^- indicates an acute or uncompensated respiratory acidosis. If the reduced pH is associated with a decreased HCO_3^- and a normal $PaCO_2$, an acute or uncompensated metabolic acidosis is suggested. Note that a mixed acidosis or mixed alkalosis is also an uncompensated event. In the case of a mixed acidosis, the pH is less than 7.35 with the $PaCO_2$ greater than 45 mm Hg and the HCO_3^- less than 22 mEq/L. A mixed alkalosis is characterized by a pH greater than 7.45, a PCO_2 less than 35 mm Hg, and an HCO_3^- greater than 26 mEq/L. With compensated acid–base disorders, both the $PaCO_2$ and HCO_3^- are out of their normal range of values. The interpretation of ABG values can therefore be an arduous task, particularly when one is trying to differentiate the source of the acid–base disturbance and the compensatory response. The following is offered as one method that can be used to interpret ABG measurements when compensation occurs. First, look at the pH and determine whether an acidosis or alkalosis is present. To determine the primary disorder, look at the $PaCO_2$ to decide whether a respiratory problem could have caused the altered pH. Next, look at the HCO_3^- to determine whether a metabolic disorder is responsible for the altered pH. After the origin of the acid–base disorder has been established, compensation can be discerned by examining whether the other variable has also changed. Consider the following situation: If a patient's pH is below 7.4, then the original problem could be caused by an increase in the $PaCO_2$ (i.e., respiratory acidosis) or a decrease in HCO_3^- (i.e., metabolic acidosis). The compensation for a respiratory acidosis would be a rise in HCO_3^-, whereas the compensation for a metabolic acidosis would be a reduction in the $PaCO_2$. The converse of this situation would follow the same line of logic. If the patient's pH is greater than 7.4, then the original problem could be caused by a reduction in the $PaCO_2$ (i.e., respiratory alkalosis) or an increase in HCO_3^- (i.e., metabolic alkalosis). The compensation for a respiratory alkalosis is loss of HCO_3^-, whereas the compensation for a metabolic alkalosis is CO_2 retention.

The level of compensation usually is described as partially compensated or fully compensated. If the pH is within the range of normal limits, the acid–base disorder is fully compensated. If not, it is partially compensated. For example, a respiratory acidosis is associated with a decreased pH and an increased $PaCO_2$. If HCO_3^- also has increased, there is evidence of metabolic compensation. If the pH is between 7.35 and 7.4, this is interpreted as a fully compensated respiratory acidosis. Table 10.6 summarizes the pH, $PaCO_2$, and HCO_3^- findings associated with various types of acid–base disturbances.

Ventilatory Status

A patient's ventilatory status can be assessed by looking at the $PaCO_2$. An increase in $PaCO_2$ is associated with hypoventilation and a respiratory acidosis. Conversely, a decrease in $PaCO_2$ is associated with hyperventilation and a respiratory alkalosis. As a general rule, a $PaCO_2$ greater than 50 mm Hg is classified as ventilatory failure and often is used as a criterion for initiating mechanical ventilatory support. Note that changes

TABLE 10.6 pH, $PaCO_2$, and HCO_3^- Findings for Various Acid–Base Disturbances

	pH	$PaCO_2$ (mm Hg)	HCO_3^-
Respiratory Acidosis			
Acute	<7.35	>45	Normal
Partly compensated	<7.35	>45	>26
Compensated	>7.35 <7.40	>45	>26
Respiratory Alkalosis			
Acute	>7.45	<35	Normal
Partly compensated	>7.45	<35	<22
Compensated	<7.45 >7.40	<35	<22
Metabolic Acidosis			
Acute	<7.35	Normal	<22
Partly compensated	<7.35	<35	<22
Compensated	>7.35 <7.40	<35	<22
Metabolic Alkalosis			
Acute	>7.45	Normal	>26
Partly compensated	>7.45	>45	>26
Compensated	<7.45 >7.40	>45	>26

HCO_3^-, Bicarbonate; $PaCO_2$, partial pressure of carbon dioxide in the arteries; pH, hydrogen ion concentration.
From Harwood R: *Exam review and study guide for perinatal/pediatric respiratory care*, Philadelphia, 1999, FA Davis.

in the $PaCO_2$ must be interpreted relative to the patient's clinical condition. For example, patients with chronic obstructive pulmonary disease often demonstrate chronic ventilatory failure (e.g., a $PaCO_2$ >50 mm Hg with a pH within normal limits). Therefore acute ventilatory failure is said to exist in patients with chronic obstructive pulmonary disease only if the $PaCO_2$ increases well above 50 mm Hg and the pH is below 7.3.

Oxygenation Status

A patient's oxygenation status can be evaluated by looking at the PaO_2 or the SaO_2. The relationship between these two values can then be illustrated graphically with an O_2Hb dissociation curve (Fig. 10.17). Note that a PaO_2 of 45 mm Hg is associated with an SaO_2 of approximately 80%, a PaO_2 of approximately 60 mm Hg corresponds to an SaO_2 of 90%, and a PaO_2 of 75 mm Hg is equivalent to an SaO_2 of 95%. For interpretative purposes, a PaO_2 of 60 to 80 mm Hg is classified as mild hypoxemia, a PaO_2 of 40 to 60 mm Hg is classified as moderate hypoxemia, and a PaO_2 less than 40 mm Hg is classified as severe hypoxemia. Table 10.7 provides PaO_2 ranges for evaluating a patient's oxygenation status.

Box 10.2 lists examples of conditions and disease states associated with various acid–base disorders. As mentioned previously, blood gas measurements are meaningful only when they are interpreted in the context of other clinical findings. Interpretation of ABGs without other supporting clinical data can be misleading and lead to potentially harmful decisions in patient management.

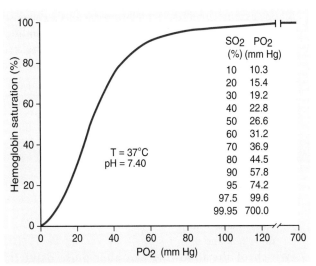

FIGURE 10.17 Oxyhemoglobin (O₂Hb) dissociation curve. *PO₂*, Partial pressure of oxygen; *O₂SAT*, oxygen saturation. (From Lane EE, Walker JF: *Clinical arterial blood gas analysis*, St. Louis, 1987, Mosby.)

SO₂ (%)	PO₂ (mm Hg)
10	10.3
20	15.4
30	19.2
40	22.8
50	26.6
60	31.2
70	36.9
80	44.5
90	57.8
95	74.2
97.5	99.6
99.95	700.0

TABLE 10.7   Criteria for Classifying Hypoxemia Using PaO₂ Measurements

Hypoxemia	PaO₂
Room Air Inspired; Patient Younger Than 60 Years of Age	
Mild[a]	<80 mm Hg
Moderate	<60 mm Hg
Severe[a]	<40 mm Hg
Supplemental Oxygen Inspired; Patient Younger Than 60 Years of Age	
Uncorrected	Less than room air acceptable limit
Corrected	Within the room air acceptable limit; <100 mm Hg
Excessively corrected	>100 mm Hg

[a]Subtract 1 mm Hg of oxygen to limits of mild and moderate hypoxemia for each year older than age 60. A PaO₂ of 40 mm Hg indicates severe hypoxemia in any patient at any age.
PaO₂, Partial pressure of oxygen in the arteries.
Modified from Shapiro BA, Peruzzi WT, Templin R: *Clinical application of blood gases*, ed 4, Chicago, 1989, Mosby.

BOX 10.2   Examples of Disease States Associated With Various Types of Acid–Base Disorders

Metabolic Acidosis
Diabetes mellitus
Diarrhea
Methanol ingestion
Renal dysfunction
Salicylate intoxication

Metabolic Alkalosis
Administration of excessive amounts of bicarbonate
Diuretic therapy
Ingestion of excessive amounts of antacids
Nasogastric suctioning
Vomiting

Respiratory Acidosis
Acute airway obstruction
Ingestion of excessive amounts of sedatives, opiates, and other respiratory depressants
Neuromuscular disorders
Pneumothorax
Restrictive pulmonary disease

Respiratory Alkalosis
Anxiety
Encephalitis
Excessive mechanical ventilatory support
Progesterone

KEY POINTS

- Blood gas analysis is an integral part of the management of patients with cardiopulmonary dysfunctions.
- Modern in vitro blood gas analyzers are fully automated systems that require only small amounts of blood for analysis and can provide intermittent measurements of pH, PaCO₂, and PaO₂, which give valuable information about a patient's acid–base, ventilatory, and oxygenation status.
- Many blood gas analyzers also allow for determinations of plasma electrolytes and metabolites, such as sodium, potassium, calcium, and glucose.
- Noninvasive devices, including pulse oximetry and transcutaneous monitoring, are an alternative to the standard in vitro blood gas analysis and allow for continuous blood gas surveillance.
- Pulse oximetry is based on the principles of spectrophotometry and photoplethysmography. Pulse oximeters use spectrophotometry to determine the amount of Hb (and deoxyhemoglobin) in a blood sample, and photoplethysmography estimates the heart rate by measuring cyclic changes in light transmission through the sampling site during each cardiac cycle.
- A number of factors can influence the accuracy of pulse oximetry measurements, including the level of perfusion, the presence of dysfunctional hemoglobins, dyes, and interference from ambient light.
- Generally, pulse oximeters are accurate for oxygen saturations higher than 80%. Pulse oximeter saturations lower than 80% are questionable and should be confirmed with ABG analysis and hemoximetry.
- Transcutaneous monitoring is a noninvasive method for estimating the arterial oxygen and carbon dioxide tensions. It uses modified blood gas electrodes to measure oxygen and carbon dioxide tensions at the skin surface.

- POC blood gas analyzers are cost-effective devices that can provide accurate and reliable blood gas analysis at the bedside.
- Blood gas measurements should be interpreted relative to other clinical indices, including the history and physical examination findings, chest radiographs, and other clinical laboratory tests.

- Blood gas abnormalities generally are classified as acidosis or alkalosis. Careful interpretation of blood gas findings can identify the cause of the problem as being associated with a respiratory, metabolic, or mixed respiratory and metabolic condition.

ASSESSMENT QUESTIONS

See Appendix B for the answers.

1. Which of the following are current safety requirements for protection of the therapist during drawing of an arterial blood gas (ABG) sample?
   1. Gloves
   2. Gown
   3. Protective eyewear (goggles)
   4. Shoe covers
   a. 1 and 3 only
   b. 2 and 3 only
   c. 2 and 4 only
   d. 1, 2, and 3 only

2. A positive Allen test indicates the presence of:
   a. An occluded radial artery
   b. A patent ulnar artery
   c. Inadequate arterial oxygenation to the hand
   d. Inadequate collateral circulation to the hand

3. The site most often used for sampling of arterial blood in adults is which of the following arteries?
   a. Brachial artery
   b. Dorsalis pedis artery
   c. Radial artery
   d. Femoral artery

4. Interpret the following ABG findings:
   pH = 7.50 PaO_2 = 60 mm Hg
   $PaCO_2$ = 30 mm Hg HCO_3^- = 24 mEq/L
   a. Acute metabolic alkalosis with mild hypoxemia
   b. Chronic metabolic acidosis with moderate hypoxemia
   c. Acute respiratory alkalosis with mild hypoxemia
   d. Chronic respiratory alkalosis with moderate hypoxemia

5. Which of the following conditions is associated with an acute respiratory acidosis?
   a. Barbiturate intoxication
   b. Excessive ingestion of antacids
   c. Emphysema
   d. Anxiety

6. A patient is admitted to the emergency department after a motor vehicle accident. In your initial assessment, you find that he is pale and his pulse is weak. You are unable to obtain a steady pulse oximeter reading. Which of the following is the most probable cause of the erratic pulse oximetry readings?
   1. Poor perfusion state
   2. Increased levels of carboxyhemoglobin (HbCO)
   3. Low partial pressure of oxygen in the arteries (PaO_2)

4. Anemia
   a. 1 only
   b. 1 and 2 only
   c. 1, 2, and 3 only
   d. 1, 2, 3, and 4

7. Which of the following can alter pulse oximetry readings?
   1. Low perfusion states, such as hypovolemic shock
   2. Dark blue nail polish
   3. Methemoglobinemia
   4. Hyperbilirubinemia
   a. 1 and 3 only
   b. 2 and 3 only
   c. 2 and 4 only
   d. 1, 2, and 3 only

8. A patient's P_{50} (the PO_2 at which Hb is 50% saturated) is 37 mm Hg. Which of the following conditions could be responsible?
   1. Hypercarbia
   2. Decreased plasma levels of 2,3-diphosphoglycerate (2,3-DPG)
   3. Acute acidosis
   4. Carbon monoxide poisoning
   a. 1 and 3 only
   b. 2 and 3 only
   c. 2 and 4 only
   d. 1, 2, and 4 only

9. To function effectively, the reference pH electrode must be bathed in which of the following solutions?
   a. 1% Sodium bicarbonate
   b. Saturated potassium chloride
   c. 5% Hydrochloric acid
   d. 0.9% Sodium chloride

10. While assessing the Levy-Jennings graphs for partial pressure of carbon dioxide in the arterial blood (PCO_2) values, you notice that the results for the last five quality assessment (QA) tests have increased progressively. Which of the following is the most likely cause of this finding?
    a. A leak in the electrode membrane
    b. Protein buildup on the electrode
    c. A damaged wire
    d. This is a normal membrane function.

11. Which of the following is *not* an anion buffer?
    a. Hemoglobin
    b. Inorganic phosphate
    c. Bicarbonate
    d. Organic calcium

12. According to Clinical Laboratory Improvement Amendments (CLIA) standards, laboratory instruments used in the hospital for blood sample testing should undergo three-point calibrations at least:
    a. Daily
    b. Weekly
    c. Monthly
    d. Every 6 months

13. Compare the processes of quality control (QC) and QA.

14. Arterial blood was obtained from a patient after open heart surgery. The patient's temperature is 35°C (95°F), and the measured PaO_2 is 80 mm Hg before temperature correction. The patient's actual PaO_2 is approximately:
    a. 70 mm Hg
    b. 80 mm Hg
    c. 90 mm Hg
    d. It cannot be determined from the information provided.

15. What are the consequences of maintaining the temperature of the transcutaneous PO_2 ($PtcO_2$) probe at 48°C (118.4°F)?
    a. Thermal injury
    b. Low $PtcO_2$ readings
    c. Fire hazard
    d. Malignant hyperthermia

16. Which of the following calculated variables derived from transcutaneous monitoring has been shown to be an early marker of hypoperfusion and mortality?
    a. $PtcCO_2$
    b. $PtcO_2$
    c. $PtcO_2/F_IO_2$
    d. $PtcCO_2/F_IO_2$

17. Which of the following tests is indicated for detecting carbon monoxide poisoning?
    a. Pulse oximetry
    b. ABGs
    c. CO-oximetry
    d. $PtcO_2$

REFERENCES

1. American Association of Respiratory Care: Clinical practice guideline: sampling for arterial blood gas analysis. *Respir Care* 37:913, 1992.
2. American Association of Respiratory Care: Clinical practice guideline: blood gas analysis and hemoximetry: 2013. *Respir Care* 58(10):1694-1703, 2013.
3. Browning JA, Kaiser DL, Durbin CG: The effect of guidelines on the appropriate use of arterial blood gas analysis in the intensive care unit. *Respir Care* 34:269, 1989.
4. Bruck E, et al.: Percutaneous collection of arterial blood for laboratory analysis. *National Committee for Clinical Laboratory Standards*, H11A 5:39, 1985.
5. National Committee for Clinical Laboratory Standards: *Procedures for the collection of diagnostic blood specimens by skin puncture*, ed 3, Villanova, PA, 1992.
6. Koch G, Wendel H: Comparison of pH, carbon dioxide tension, standard bicarbonate, and oxygen tension in capillary blood and in arterial blood during the neonatal period. *Acta Paediatr Scand* 56:10, 1967.
7. Burritt MF, Fallon KD: Blood gas preanalytical considerations: specimen collection, calibration, and controls. *National Committee for Clinical Laboratory Standards*, C27-T 9:685, 1989.
8. Ehrmeyer S, Laessig RH: Measurement of the proficiency of pH and blood gas analyses by interlaboratory proficiency testing. *J Med Tech* 2:33, 1985.
9. Duc GV, Cumarasamy N: Digital arteriolar oxygen tension as a guide to oxygen therapy of the newborn. *Biol Neonate* 24:134, 1974.
10. McLain BI, Evans J, Dear PFR: Comparison of capillary and arterial blood gas measurements in neonates. *Arch Dis Child* 63:743, 1988.
11. Desai SD, et al.: A comparison between arterial and arterialized capillary blood in infants. *S Afr Med J* 41:13, 1967.
12. Centers for Disease Control: Update: universal precautions for prevention of transmission of human immunodeficiency virus, hepatitis B virus, and other bloodborne pathogens in healthcare settings. *MMWR Morb Mortal Wkly Rep* 37:377, 1988.
13. Department of Labor, Occupational Safety and Health Administration: Occupational exposure to bloodborne pathogens, 29 CFRR Part 1910.1030. *Fed Regist* 1991.
14. Moran RF, et al.: Oxygen content, hemoglobin oxygen, "saturation," and related quantities in blood: terminology, measurement, and reporting. *National Committee for Clinical Laboratory Standards*, C25-P 10:1, 1990.
15. Davenport HW: *The ABC of acid-base chemistry*, ed 3, Chicago, 1975, University of Chicago Press.
16. Brensilver JM, Goldberger E: *A primer of water and acid-base syndromes*, ed 8, Philadelphia, 1996, FA Davis.
17. Shapiro BA, Peruzzi WT, Kozlowski-Templin R: *Clinical application of blood gases*, ed 5, St. Louis, 1994, Mosby.
18. Severinghaus JS, Bradley FA: Electrodes for blood PO_2 and PCO_2 determination. *J Appl Physiol* 13:515, 1958.
19. National Committee for Clinical Laboratory Standards: *Clinical laboratory technical procedure manual*, ed 2, Pub GP2-A2, Rosemont, IL, 1992, Villanova.
20. Clinical Laboratory Improvement Amendments of 1988: Final rule, subpart H. *Fed Regist* 1992.
21. Medicare, Medicaid, and CLIA Programs: CLIA-88 continuance of approval of the Joint Commission on Accreditation of Healthcare Organizations (JCAHO) as an accrediting organization. *Fed Regist* 67:65585, 2002.
22. Hansen JE, et al.: Assessing precision and accuracy in blood gas proficiency testing. *Am Rev Respir Dis* 141:1190, 1990.
23. Mohler JG, et al.: Blood gases. In Clausen JL, editor: *Pulmonary function testing: guidelines and controversies*, New York, 1982, Academic Press.
24. Barker SJ, Hyatt J: Continuous measurement of intraarterial pH, $PaCO_2$, and PaO_2 in the operating room. *Anesth Analg* 73:43, 1991.
25. MacIntyre NR, et al.: Accuracy and precision of a point-of-care blood gas analyzer incorporating optode. *Respir Care* 41:800, 1996.
26. Brown LJ: A new instrument for the simultaneous measurement of total hemoglobin, % oxyhemoglobin,

% carboxyhemoglobin, % methemoglobin, and oxygen content in whole blood. *IEEE Trans Biomed Eng* 27:132, 1980.

27. Falholt W: Blood oxygen saturation determinations by spectrophotometry. *Scand J Clin Lab Invest* 15:67, 1963.

28. Severinghaus JW, Astrup PB: History of blood gas analysis. VI. Oximetry. *J Clin Monit* 2:270, 1986.

29. Nillson NJ: Oximetry. *Physiol Rev* 40:1, 1960.

30. Tremper KK, Barker SJ: Pulse oximetry. *Anesthesiology* 70:98, 1989.

31. Yang K, Brown SD, Gutierrez G: Noninvasive assessment of blood gases. In Levine RL, Fromm RE, editors: *Critical care monitoring: from pre-hospital to ICU*, St. Louis, 1995, Mosby.

32. Pilbeam S: *Mechanical ventilation*, ed 3, St. Louis, 1998, Mosby.

33. Scheller MS, Unger RJ, Kelner MJ: Effects of intravenously administered dyes on pulse oximetry readings. *Anesthesiology* 65:550, 1986.

34. Cote CJ, et al.: The effect of nail polish on pulse oximetry. *Anesth Analg* 67:685, 1988.

35. Rubin AS: Nail polish color can affect pulse oximeter saturation. *Anesthesiology* 68:825, 1988.

36. Emery JR: Skin pigmentation as an influence on the accuracy of pulse oximetry. *J Perinatol* 7:329, 1987.

37. Amar D, et al.: Fluorescent light interferes with pulse oximetry. *J Clin Monit* 5:135, 1989.

38. Carlin BW, Claussen JL, Ries AL: The use of cutaneous oximetry in the prescription of long-term oxygen therapy. *Chest* 94:239, 1988.

39. Kacmarek RM, Hess D, Stoller JK: *Monitoring in respiratory care*, St. Louis, 1993, Mosby.

40. Lubbers DW: Theory and development of transcutaneous oxygen pressure measurement. *Int Anesthesiol Clin* 25:31, 1987.

41. Severinghaus JS, Stafford M, Bradley FA: Transcutaneous PO_2 electrode design, calibration, and temperature gradient problems. *Acta Anaesthesiol Scand Suppl* 68:118, 1978.

42. Baecjert P, et al.: Is pulse oximetry reliable in detecting hypoxemia in the neonate? *Adv Exp Med Biol* 220:165, 1987.

43. Reed RL, et al.: Correlation of hemodynamic variables with transcutaneous PO_2 measurements in critically ill patients. *J Trauma* 25:1045, 1985.

44. Lubbers DW: Theoretical basis of transcutaneous blood gas measurements. *Crit Care Med* 9:721, 1981.

45. American Association of Respiratory Care: Clinical practice guideline: transcutaneous blood gas monitoring for neonatal and pediatric patients. *Respir Care* 39:1176-1179, 1994.

46. Restrepo RD, Hirst KR, Wittnebel L, et al.: AARC clinical practice guideline: transcutaneous monitoring of carbon dioxide and oxygen: 2012. *Respir Care* 57:1955-1962, 2012.

47. Wahr JA, Tremper KK: Non-invasive oxygen monitoring techniques. *Crit Care Clin* 11:199, 1995.

48. Shoemaker WC, Wo CC, Lu Demetriades D, et al.: Early physiologic patterns in acute illness and accidents: toward a concept of circulatory dysfunction and shock based on invasive and noninvasive hemodynamic monitoring. *New Horiz* 4(4):395-412, 1996.

49. Martin M, Matthew Martina CB, Bayard D, et al.: Continuous noninvasive monitoring of cardiac performance and tissue perfusion in pediatric trauma patients. *J Pediatr Surg* 40:1957-1963, 2005

Sleep Diagnostics

OBJECTIVES

Upon completion of this chapter, you will be able to:

1. Describe the various stages of sleep in adults and children.
2. Discuss the physiological effects of sleep on cardiopulmonary function in healthy individuals.
3. List the measurements most commonly recorded during polysomnography.
4. Summarize the clinical and laboratory criteria used to diagnose obstructive, central, and mixed apnea.

5. Describe various strategies that can be used to monitor arterial oxygen saturation, nasal-oral airflow, and respiratory effort of patients with obstructive sleep apnea syndrome.
6. Explain the physiological consequences of obstructive sleep apnea.
7. Name several common diseases associated with central sleep apnea.

OUTLINE

KEY TERMS

alpha waves
apnea/hypopnea index (AHI)
apnea index (AI)
arousal responses
arousal threshold
beta waves
central sleep apnea
Cheyne-Stokes respiration

circadian cycle
collodion
delta waves
disconjugate
epoch
Holter monitoring
inion
International 10-20 EEG system

K-complexes
mixed sleep apnea
nasion
obstructive sleep apnea (OSA)
polysomnography
sleep spindles
theta waves

The effect of sleep on breathing has received considerable attention during the past 50 years. Much of this attention relates to an increased awareness of sleep-related disorders and improved technology for assessing neurological and cardiopulmonary functions during sleep. The physiological effect of sleep on breathing is normally of little consequence in healthy individuals. Its effect on patients with altered respiratory function (i.e., those afflicted with chronic pulmonary diseases) can be profound, however, and lead to significant consequences.

I. PHYSIOLOGY OF SLEEP

Sleep is part of a cyclic phenomenon (i.e., the circadian cycle) controlled by an endogenous pacemaker that remains active even in an isolated environment free of time cues.[1] Sleep in itself is a nonhomogenous phenomenon consisting of two distinct states: non–rapid eye movement (NREM) sleep and rapid eye movement (REM) sleep. As seen in Table 11.1, these states can be defined by electrographic and behavioral criteria such as brain wave activity, oculomotor activity, responsiveness to external stimuli, and muscle tone.[2,3]

The American Academy of Sleep Medicine (AASM) proposed an updated scoring system in 2007 for identifying the various stages of sleep. The updated AASM system is significantly different from an earlier sleep scoring system developed by Rechtschaffen and Kales (R&K scoring system) that has been widely used since 1968. In addition to changing the rules for staging sleep, the updated *AASM Scoring Manual* also provides recommendations for equipment and techniques used to monitor physiological function during sleep.[2,3] It is important to be aware of the differences in these two systems, particularly when reviewing the medical literature on sleep-related disorders.

TABLE 11.1   Behavioral and Electrographic Characteristics of Sleep-Awake States

Characteristics	SLEEP-AWAKE STATE		
	Awake (Stage W)	Non–REM Sleep (Stages N1, N2, N3)	REM Sleep (Stage R)
Eyelids	Open or closed	Closed	Closed
Eye movements	Slow or rapid	Slow or absent	Rapid[a]
Responsiveness to external stimuli	Simple or complex	Simple	Often absent
Electroencephalogram	Low-amplitude voltage, high-frequency	High-amplitude voltage, low-frequency	Low-amplitude voltage, high-frequency
Electromyogram	High-level tonic activity	Lower-level tonic activity	Muscle twitching interspersed with periods of muscle atonia[a]

[a]REM sleep includes a phasic and tonic component. Eye movement and muscle activity can vary considerably for each component. See text for additional details.

REM, Rapid eye movement.

Modified from Phillipson EA: Sleep disorders. In Murray JF, Nadel JA: *Textbook of respiratory medicine,* ed 3, Philadelphia, 1994, WB Saunders.

Stage W (wakefulness) is characterized by the presence of an alpha rhythm on electroencephalogram (EEG) and electrooculogram (EOG) (Fig. 11.1A). NREM sleep, or quiet sleep, consists of a series of stages that are thought to represent progressively deeper levels of sleep. At sleep onset (NREM stage N1), normal sleepers can be easily aroused because they alternate between wakefulness and sleep. The EEG shows alpha waves and beta waves, which are present during wakefulness and diminish as the sleeper's EEG converts to a rhythm in which *low-amplitude, mixed-frequency (LAMF) waves* make up more than 50% of the epoch (see Fig. 11.1B). (*Note:* Alpha waves are rhythmic waves that occur at a frequency of 8 to 13 cycles per second, whereas beta waves occur at frequencies of 14 to 80 cycles per second.[4]) Skeletal muscle tone changes only slightly from waking levels; eye movements throughout NREM sleep are slow, rolling, pendulous, and disconjugate.[5]

Stage N1 sleep lasts for only a brief time and is followed by a transition to stage N2 sleep, which is identified by the appearance of sleep spindles and K-complexes on the sleeper's EEG (see Fig. 11.1C). Sleep spindles are waveforms with waxing and waning amplitude that occur at a frequency of 9 to 13 cycles per second. K-complexes are large, vertical, slow waves that have an amplitude of at least 75 µV, with an initial negative deflection.[5] Arousal thresholds (i.e., the level of stimuli required to change to a "lighter" stage of sleep or wakefulness) are higher in stage N2 than those in stage N1.

The deepest stage of NREM sleep (stage N3) is referred to as *slow-wave sleep* (SWS) because of the presence of large delta waves that appear when the sleeper enters this stage (see Fig. 11.1D). Delta waves include all electroencephalographic waves with a frequency of less than 3.5 cycles per second.[5] (*Note:* Stage N3 has replaced the R&K scoring system designation in which two stages [stages 3 and 4] were used to identify the deepest level of NREM sleep. Separating SWS into two stages required clinicians to make a somewhat arbitrary decision because the two stages showed only minor differences in the EEG findings. For example, most clinicians defined the beginning of stage 3 as the period in which slow waves constitute

from 20% to 50% of the electroencephalographic recording. Stage 4, on the other hand, was identified by the presence of slow waves for at least 50% of the electroencephalographic recording.[2,5]) The arousal threshold during stage N3 is considerably higher than that during stages N1 and N2 of NREM sleep.

After approximately 70 to 100 minutes of NREM sleep, the normal sleeper enters REM (stage R) sleep. REM sleep is characterized by rapid eye movement, muscle atonia, cortical activation, and low-voltage desynchronization on the person's EEG.[2] Studies have demonstrated that stage R has a phasic and tonic component. During the phasic component there is increased eye movement, pupillary dilation, skeletal muscle twitching, and increased heart and respiratory rates. In contrast, the tonic component is characterized by muscle atonia and decreased eye movements. Cortical activation during stage R is evidenced by an increase in low-voltage waves on the EEG, with a burst of theta waves (see Fig. 11.1E). Theta waves have a sawtooth appearance and occur at a frequency of 4 to 7 cycles per second.[4,5]

It is generally accepted that dreaming occurs during REM sleep because sleepers who awaken after dreaming during REM sleep can recall their dreams. Although dreaming does occur during NREM sleep, those dreams are usually not remembered. The arousal threshold (i.e., skeletal muscle tone) during REM sleep varies and may actually be absent. (It is interesting that if the arousal stimulus is incorporated into the dream content, arousal is less likely.[5])

During a typical night of sleep, a normal adult sleeper cycles between NREM sleep and REM sleep approximately every 90 to 120 minutes.[1] NREM sleep (stages N2 and N3 or S2-S4 in the R&K scoring system) is most prominent during the first half of the night and decreases as the night progresses. REM sleep, on the other hand, becomes longer and more intense throughout the sleep period, with the longest and most intense REM sleep occurring in the early morning hours.

Fig. 11.2 illustrates the average amount of time that a healthy adult spends in each sleep stage. Normally, four to six

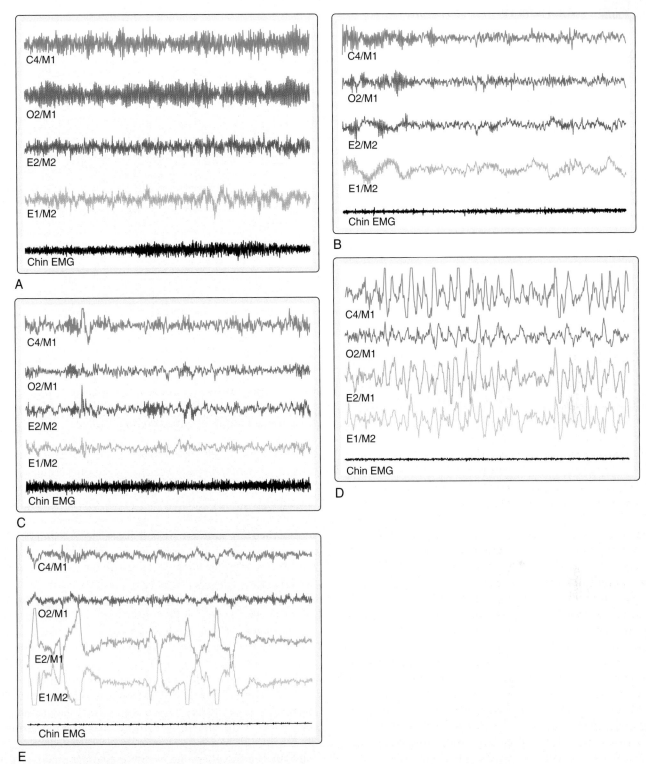

FIGURE 11.1 A, Stage W. Stage W demonstrates a classic wake pattern, with alpha rhythm in the electroencephalogram (EEG) and electrooculogram (EOG). The chin electromyogram (EMG) shows normal muscle tone associated with relaxed wakefulness. B, Stage N1 sleep. Stage N1 is characterized by the disappearance of alpha rhythm, replaced by low-voltage, mixed-frequency EEG. The chin EMG remains tonic, although it can become slightly reduced with sleep onset. C, Stage N2 sleep. Stage N2 is characterized by low-voltage background EEG activity and the presence of sleep spindles and K-complexes, absence of eye movements, and tonic EMG activity. Chin EMG activity shows normal muscle tone. D, Stage N3 sleep. Stage N3 (slow-wave sleep) is characterized by high-amplitude slow waves. In this example the high-amplitude slow waves make up greater than 50% of the sleep epoch. E, Rapid eye movement (REM) sleep. Stage R is characterized by relatively low-voltage, mixed-frequency EEG activity, with a burst of rapid, saccadic, conjugate eye movements; chin muscle tone significantly decreased from that found with waking and non–rapid eye movement (NREM) sleep level. (From Butkov N: *Atlas of clinical polysomnography*, ed 2, Medford, OR, 2011, Synapse Media.)

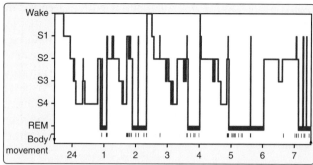

FIGURE 11.2 Sleep-stage distribution in normal healthy adults. (See also Ohayon M, Carskadon MA, Guilleminault C, et al.: Meta-analysis of quantitative sleep parameters from childhood to old age in healthy individuals: developing normative sleep values across the human lifespan. *Sleep* 27:1255-1273, 2004.) *REM*, Rapid eye movement. (From Kryger MH, Roth T, Dement WC: *Principles and practice of sleep medicine*, ed 5, St. Louis, 2011, Elsevier-Saunders.)

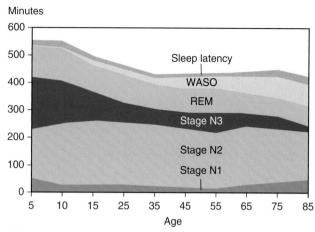

FIGURE 11.3 Changes in sleep with age. *REM*, Rapid eye movement; *WASO*, wake time after sleep onset. (From Ohayon M. Carskadon MA, Guilleminault C, et al.: Meta-analysis of quantitative sleep parameters from childhood to old age in healthy individuals: developing normative sleep values across the human lifespan. *Sleep* 27:1255-1273, 2004.)

TABLE 11.2	**Sleep Distribution for a Healthy Person**
Stage	**Percentage of Total Recording Time**
W	Less than 5%
N1	2% to 5%
N2	45% to 55%
N3	13% to 23%
R	20% to 25%

cycles of sleep stages occur per night. Although there are variations among sleepers, these averages are a good approximation of the time distribution for NREM sleep, REM sleep, and wakefulness during a typical night of sleep (Table 11.2).

The adult stages of NREM sleep and REM sleep are not easily identified at birth by means of standard electroencephalographic, electromyographic, and electrooculographic analysis. Although similarities exist between the sleep states that occur in newborns and those in adults, sleep stages during the neonatal period are generally categorized as active sleep, quiet sleep, and intermediate sleep. Active sleep is comparable with REM sleep; quiet and intermediate sleep states have many of the same characteristics of NREM sleep. It is worth noting that infants enter active sleep first instead of entering into quiet sleep as adults do. Between 2 and 6 months of age, infant sleep becomes more predictable. It is important to mention that NREM sleep becomes more prominent as brain structure and function achieve a level that can support high-voltage SWS.[1,2] Infants typically begin to exhibit the classic sleep stages seen in adults by 6 months of age (i.e., presence of sleep spindles, K-complexes, and delta waves).

As mentioned previously, sleep-state distribution for healthy adult sleepers during a typical 8-hour period of sleep usually involves both NREM sleep and REM sleep states alternating cyclically every 90 to 120 minutes, with periods of REM sleep lasting from 10 to 30 minutes. In contrast, infants spend considerably more time in REM sleep than do adult sleepers

(i.e., during various stages in development, infants may spend as much as 75% of their sleep in REM).[1,5] Fig. 11.3 illustrates the changes in sleep patterns that occur with age (Box 11.1).

Effect of Sleep on Breathing

Table 11.3 summarizes the effects of sleep on breathing. As the sleeper passes through the various stages of NREM sleep, there is a progressive reduction in chemosensitivity and respiratory drive. The reduction in respiratory drive that occurs during the early stages of NREM sleep (stages N1 and N2) predisposes the person to apneic periods (i.e., Cheyne-Stokes respiration) when fluctuating between being awake and asleep. With the establishment of NREM SWS (stage N3), nonrespiratory inputs are minimized and minute ventilation is regulated by metabolic control. Minute ventilation decreases by 1 to 2 L/min when compared with wakefulness. As a consequence, the partial pressure of arterial carbon dioxide ($PaCO_2$) rises by 2 mm Hg to 8 mm Hg, and the partial pressure of oxygen in the arteries (PaO_2) decreases by 5 mm Hg to 10 mm Hg.

As the sleeper enters into REM sleep, breathing becomes irregular as the ventilatory response to chemical and mechanical respiratory stimuli is further reduced and even transiently abolished. Skeletal muscle activity, along with activity in the intercostal and accessory muscles of respiration, is decreased, and the upper airway muscles are inhibited. This inhibition leads to an increase in upper airway resistance, whereas inhibition of the intercostal and accessory muscles is associated with diminished thoracoabdominal coupling and short periods of central apnea for durations of 10 to 20 seconds. $PaCO_2$ and PaO_2 levels are variable, but they are generally similar to those in the latter stages of NREM sleep.

Effect of Sleep on Cardiovascular Function

Fig. 11.4 shows the effects of sleep on cardiovascular function. In most individuals, both heart rate and blood pressure are generally reduced during sleep. Reductions in heart rate average

It is generally accepted that the amount of sleep that an individual requires is influenced by their age. Infants typically require approximately 16 hours per day, and teenagers need 8 or 9 hours per night on average. For most adults, 7 to 8 hours per night seems to be sufficient, although some people require only approximately 5 hours per day, whereas others require as much as 10 hours of sleep each day. Slow-wave sleep (SWS) is quantitatively and qualitatively different in young children when compared with adults.[2] For example, SWS is maximal in young children and decreases with age. The greatest decrease in SWS occurs during an individual's teenage years (i.e., ≈40% reduction in SWS).[2] Furthermore, arousal thresholds for young children in their first sleep cycle are markedly increased when compared with adult sleepers. As a person ages (i.e., older than 60 years of age), sleep occurs for shorter periods and SWS significantly decreases, particularly in men. What may not be obvious is that older individuals continue to need approximately the same amount of sleep that they required in early adulthood. Consequently, the total amount of time that an older person spends sleeping and napping during the day increases so that the person can achieve an adequate amount of sleep. Interestingly, the amount of REM sleep that a person achieves, when measured as a percentage of their total sleep time, remains fairly constant into old age.[2]

Certain conditions can also influence the amount of sleep that we require. For example, we have an increased need for sleep while recovering from an acute illness, such as a cold or the flu. Women in their first trimester of pregnancy often need several more hours of sleep than usual. The amount of sleep a person needs also increases when there has been a deprivation of sleep in previous days. Getting too little sleep creates a "sleep debt" that ultimately must be repaid. Although we may think that we can adapt to getting less sleep than we need, sleep deprivation can severely alter a person's judgment, reaction time, and other neurological functions.

approximately 5 to 10 beats/min during NREM sleep and up to 15 beats/min during REM sleep. Blood pressure shows a moderate decrease of 10 to 15 mm Hg during NREM sleep. Alterations in heart rate seen during sleep seem to parallel sleep-related alterations in blood pressure. These variations are especially evident during REM sleep, when arterial blood pressure fluctuates to a greater extent than it does during NREM sleep.[5] Changes in blood pressure during REM sleep are characterized as intermittent sharp increases in mean arterial pressure that are superimposed on a relatively hypotensive state.

Cardiac output is usually only slightly reduced during NREM sleep when compared with the waking state. The reduction in cardiac output, however, is more pronounced during REM sleep (i.e., an approximately 10% reduction).[5] Changes in cardiac output that are seen during sleep are not accompanied by changes in stroke volume, which tends to remain similar to values measured while the person is in a quiet, awake state.[5]

II. DIAGNOSIS OF SLEEP APNEA

The ability to wake from sleep or to rouse to a lighter stage of sleep requires the activation of higher neurological centers (i.e., the reticular activating system and cortex).[2] Such activation results in an immediate increase in respiratory drive, activation of the upper airway dilator muscles, stimulation of the cough reflex, and initiation of behavioral responses—specifically, increases in skeletal muscle tone.[2,4] If these arousal responses do not occur, sleep apnea or alveolar hypoventilation can result.

The current standard for clinical practice for confirming the diagnosis of sleep apnea is based on information derived from a patient history, a physical examination, and from laboratory polysomnography (PSG) studies that focus on sleep structure and cardiorespiratory function.[6] The medical history and physical examination provide information that can be used to determine whether patients are at risk for sleep apnea and whether they demonstrate the common symptoms

TABLE 11.3 **Physiological Effects of Sleep on Respiration**			
Feature	**Sleep Stages N1 and N2**	**Sleep Stage N3**	**REM Sleep (Stage R)**
Pattern of breathing	Periodic	Stable	Irregular
Apneas	Short, central	Rare	Short, central
PaCO₂	Variable	↑ 2 to 8 mm Hg above wakefulness	Variable, similar to stage N3
Rib cage muscles	Active	Active	Inhibited
Diaphragm	Active	Active	Active
Upper airway muscles	Active	Active	Inhibited
Chemoresponsiveness	↓ Compared with wakefulness	↓ Compared with stages N1, N2	↓ Compared with stage N3
Arousability to respiratory stimuli	Low thresholds	Low thresholds	High thresholds

PaCO₂, Partial pressure of arterial carbon dioxide; *REM*, rapid eye movement.
From Bradley T, Phillipson EA: Sleep disorders. In *Murray and Nadel's textbook of respiratory medicine*, ed 3, Philadelphia, 2000, Saunders-Elsevier.

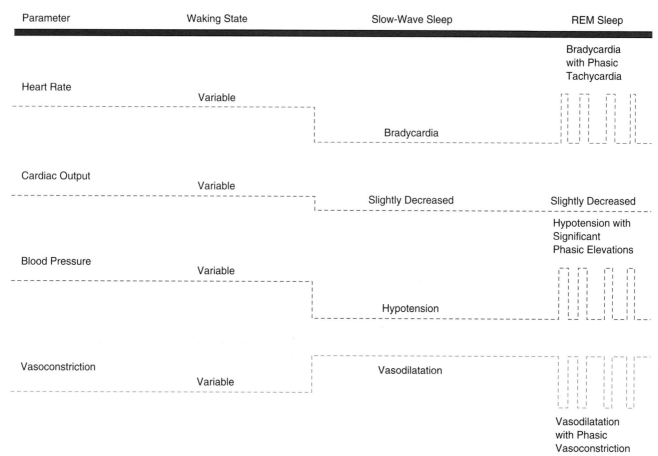

Parameter	Waking State	Slow-Wave Sleep	REM Sleep

Heart Rate — Variable — Bradycardia — Bradycardia with Phasic Tachycardia

Cardiac Output — Variable — Slightly Decreased — Slightly Decreased

Blood Pressure — Variable — Hypotension — Hypotension with Significant Phasic Elevations

Vasoconstriction — Variable — Vasodilatation — Vasodilatation with Phasic Vasoconstriction

FIGURE 11.4 The effects of sleep on cardiovascular function in awake and sleep states. *REM*, Rapid eye movement. (Redrawn from Sheldon SH, Spire JP, Levy HB: *Pediatric sleep medicine,* Philadelphia, 1992, WB Saunders.)

and signs associated with various sleep-related disorders. PSG includes, but is not limited to, audio/visual monitoring, electroencephalography, electrooculography, and electromyography, as well as measurements of cardiorespiratory function, including heart rate, pulse oximetry, end-tidal carbon dioxide (CO_2), oral-nasal airflow, and nasal pressure.

Polysomnography

Although a patient history and a physical examination can provide evidence that a patient may be afflicted with sleep apnea, the data may be equivocal and thus lead the clinician to underestimate or overestimate the severity of the patient's sleep-disordered breathing. For this reason, overnight PSG of patients suspected of having sleep apnea should be performed to ensure a definitive diagnosis.

Table 11.4 summarizes the various laboratory procedures that can be used to investigate physiological function during sleep. Although screening tests can provide valuable information about cardiopulmonary function during sleep, they do not allow for sleep staging and quantification of patient arousal or awakening during the course of the study. It is generally accepted that laboratory PSG is the gold standard for identifying the type and severity of sleep apnea. As previously mentioned, PSG typically includes all-night audio/video

monitoring of the patient, as well as recordings of EEGs, EOGs, electromyograms (EMGs), respiratory status, and electrocardiograms (ECGs).

Although in-laboratory PSG has proven to be accurate with low failure rate, the expenses associated with these studies (e.g., presence of a qualified technical staff) have led many clinicians to advocate for the use of portable monitoring (PM) as a more cost-effective alternative.[6] The available literature suggests that PM provides accurate and reliable data for selected populations when compared with PSG (e.g., PM is acceptable for diagnosis of patients with a high probability of having moderate to severe obstructive sleep apnea [OSA]).[6] A task force of the AASM has provided a series of recommendations outlining the indication for PM for the diagnosis of OSA.[3] A typical PM study would include measurements of pulse rate, oxygen saturation, airflow, and chest wall impedance. The following sections include a brief discussion of the various physiological measurements obtained during PSG. More information regarding the diagnosis of OSA is provided later in this chapter.

Electrocardiography

Cardiac activity, including heart rate and rhythm, is usually monitored with at least two electrocardiographic leads (e.g., lead II and a modified chest lead). It is important to recognize that monitoring two electrocardiographic leads can provide only limited information about the electrical activity of the heart. If more information about the patient's ECG is required, a 12-lead ECG or Holter monitoring may be indicated.

TABLE 11.4 Physiological Measurements Recorded During Polysomnography

Type of Test	Variable Measured	Technique
Standard PSG	EEG	Surface electrodes
	EOG	Surface electrodes
	EMG	Surface electrodes
	Breathing pattern	Surface electrodes; oral-nasal airflow, nasal pressure
	SaO_2, P_ACO_2	Ear oximeter, pulse oximetry, end-tidal CO_2
	ECG	Standard electrodes
	Body position	Videotaping
Special Procedures	Arterial blood gases	Arterial catheter
	Systemic blood pressure	Arterial catheter or automated blood pressure cuff
	Diaphragm EMG	Esophageal or surface electrode
	Esophageal pH	Esophageal electrodes
	Intrapleural pressure	Esophageal catheter

ECG, Electrocardiogram; *EEG,* electroencephalogram; *EMG,* electromyogram; *EOG,* electrooculogram; *P_ACO_2,* partial pressure of alveolar carbon dioxide; *PSG,* polysomnography; *SaO_2,* arterial oxygen saturation.

Electroencephalography

An EEG is a recording of fluctuations in the electric potentials of cortical neurons. These electric potentials are transmitted from the cortex through the coverings of the brain to the scalp, where electrodes placed at various points on the scalp are used to sense the sum of the potentials in the underlying cortex. EEGs provide valuable information on the integrity of the central nervous system and form the basis for identifying the various sleep stages that the patient enters during the sleep study.

To ensure that the information is meaningful and can be compared with that of different laboratories, a standardized system for electrode placement is used to record EEGs during sleep studies. The standard electroencephalographic montage used for PSG is based on the International 10-20 EEG system.[5,7] As Fig. 11.5 illustrates, electrodes are placed at selected points on the patient's skull that represent 10% to 20% of the total distance between the specified landmarks on the head. The landmarks that are used include the nasion (the indentation between the forehead and the nose), the inion (the ridge at the back of the skull), and two preauricular points (indentations in front of the tragus cartilage). Each electrode is designated relative to a particular area of the brain (e.g., F [frontal], T [temporal], O [occipital], C [central], A [auricular], M [mastoid] Z [midline or "zero line"]).[8] Numbers are assigned to each electrode depending on whether the electrode is placed on the right (even) or left (odd) side of the midline.

EEG recordings can be obtained using two different approaches. EEG measurements can be obtained by recording voltage differences between an exploring electrode and a reference electrode (e.g., the reference electrode is placed on the mastoid process) or by recording the voltage difference between two exploring electrodes placed on the patient's skull.

For scoring sleep studies, the AASM has presented an update to recommended EEG montage used in the diagnosis of sleep-related disorders.[8-10] EEG signals recorded from the frontal

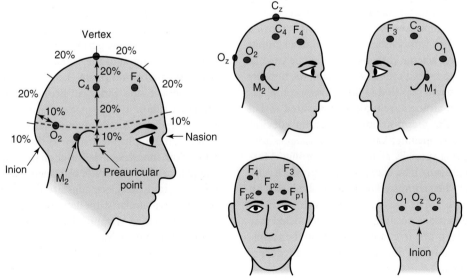

FIGURE 11.5 A standard polysomnographic electroencephalogram (EEG) montage. (From Berry RM: *Fundamentals of sleep medicine*, ed 5, Philadelphia, 2012, Saunders-Elsevier.)

portions of the brain are best for visual scoring of EEGs rather than the central placements recommended in the standard montage because K-complexes and delta waves are maximized in the frontal plane.[2] (EEG signals obtained from the C3/A2 or C4/A1 position are used in the suggested montage in the standard manual for recording sleep spindles, K-complexes, and delta waves.) EEG analysis of occipital signals provides the best opportunities to identify alpha rhythms that occur at sleep onset.[8,10]

Note that modified electroencephalographic recordings that are typically used to determine sleep stages may not enable the identification of seizure disorders; therefore, in cases in which seizures are suspected, more elaborate electroencephalographic recordings, as well as a neurological consultation, may be necessary. It is important to recognize that there is still considerable debate about the various approaches to scoring EEGs.

To place electrodes properly, the technologist should first mark where the electrodes are to be placed on the skull. It is important to recognize that improper placement of these electrodes can severely affect the validity of the sleep study and lead to erroneous data. The scalp should be cleaned with alcohol to minimize electrical impedance. The cup-shaped electrodes are filled with conductive paste or jelly and affixed to the scalp with cotton or gauze. The electrodes can be affixed to the scalp with tape or glue, or they can be anchored to the scalp by placing a piece of gauze soaked in collodion over the electrode (note that the gauze can be dried with compressed air after it has been positioned over the electrode). After the electrodes are affixed to the patient, the electrode wires are then plugged into a junction box, which is coupled to the polygraph recorder.

Respiratory Activity

Assessment of respiratory activity during sleep usually involves measuring oxygen saturation, end-tidal CO_2, nasal-oral airflow, and respiratory effort.[11] Oxygen saturation and end-tidal CO_2 can be easily measured using pulse oximetry and capnography, respectively. The pulse oximeter probe is placed on an earlobe, finger, or toe, and partial pressure of end-tidal carbon dioxide ($P_{ET}CO_2$) can be obtained with sensors attached to nasal prongs or a mask. (Indwelling arterial catheters can also be used to assess arterial blood gases, but the risks outweigh the benefits of using this approach and may lead to unnecessary complications.) Nasal and oral airflows are typically measured with a pneumotachograph (e.g., thermistor or thermocouple device) positioned at the airway opening. Alternatively, nasal pressures can be measured using specially adapted nasal prongs. Measurements of nasal pressure have been shown to produce valid estimates of airflow when compared with those obtained with a pneumotachograph.[10] The most common problems with these devices relate to probe position (i.e., the technician may have to reposition the probe frequently and adjust the amplifier sensitivity, thus disturbing the patient's sleep and reducing the validity of the study).

Respiratory effort can be determined by analyzing recordings of rib cage and abdominal movements, by measuring intrapleural pressure changes, or by measuring airflow at the airway opening with a pneumotachograph. A variety of devices and techniques are available for measuring rib cage and abdominal movements, including strain gauge or piezoelectric belts placed around the chest or abdomen, respiratory inductive plethysmography, and impedance pneumography. Intrapleural pressure changes can be measured with an esophageal balloon catheter positioned in the upper third of the esophagus that is connected to a standard strain gauge pressure transducer.

Remember that although all of these techniques can provide measurements of respiratory effort, techniques that restrict patient movement can compromise test results. Techniques that make the patient uncomfortable can ultimately decrease patient compliance during the study.

Electromyography

Skeletal muscle activity can be estimated during sleep by recording submentalis electromyographic signals with surface electrodes similar to those used for ECGs. Electromyographic signals are derived from a pair of electrodes arranged to record submentalis muscle activity. An electrode placed midline but 1 cm above the mandible's inferior edge is referenced to another electrode placed 2 cm below and 2 cm to the right (or left).[11] A reference electrode is also attached laterally. The submentalis electromyographic signal recorded from these electrodes is used to detect activation of the muscles that expand the upper airways (e.g., the genioglossus and the geniohyoid).[12]

Electromyographic signals recorded from the intercostal muscles can also be used to assess respiratory movements, which is a rather cumbersome technique considering the alternative methods of measuring respiratory activity that were discussed in the previous section.

Electrooculography

The recording of eye movements during sleep allows the clinician to differentiate NREM sleep states from REM sleep states. The EOG is a record of the standing voltage between the cornea and the retina of the eye and represents a standard for assessing eye movements during sleep. In the original electrooculography electrode placements, electrodes were placed on the skin surface in the periorbital region, specifically approximately 1 cm lateral to the outer canthi of the eyes and offset from the horizontal plane (i.e., 1 cm above the horizontal plane on one side and 1 cm below the horizontal plane on the other side).

The updated AASM manual changed the placement of electrooculography electrodes so that they are placed above and below the eyes at the level of the outer canthi, and the lateral part of the electrode placement has been removed. The left and right eye electrodes are designated as E1 and E2, respectively; similarly, the left and right mastoid electrodes are designated as M1 and M2, respectively. (The AASM recommends using E1-M2 and E2-M2 derivations where M2 is used as the reference electrode.) The E1 electrode is positioned 1 cm below the left outer canthus (Fig. 11.6), and the E2 electrode is positioned 1 cm above the right outer canthus. With this configuration the horizontal, vertical, and oblique

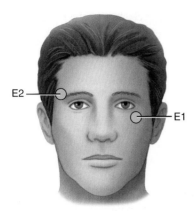

FIGURE 11.6 Placement of electrooculogram (EOG) electrodes.

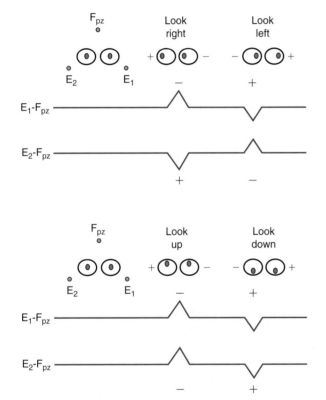

FIGURE 11.7 Electrooculogram electrode placement. (From Berry RM: *Fundamentals of sleep medicine,* ed 5 Philadelphia, 2012, Saunders-Elsevier.)

movements of the eye can be detected. Fig. 11.7 shows how these movements are recorded. Note that the height or depth of the deflection depends on the movement of the eyes relative to the fixed electrodes and is described as being either *right-of-center* (ROC) or *left-of-center* (LOC).

Calibration of Polysomnography Signals

An initial calibration of the PSG equipment should be performed before the electrodes are placed on the patient; for accurate calibration the manufacturer's recommendations should be followed closely. (*Note:* Check the user's manual for details on calibrating various channels.) After the electrodes and sensors are affixed to the patient, a pre sleep calibration should be performed. This calibration lets the technician determine whether all of the electrodes and sensors are positioned properly, whether the amplifier settings are appropriate for retrieving meaningful data, and whether there are any recording device malfunctions (e.g., the chart recorder is functioning improperly). Calibration also provides a series of baseline references for awake measurements. Documenting all calibrations is essential because if calibration is performed inadequately, the test results are ultimately invalid.

III. PATHOPHYSIOLOGY OF SLEEP APNEA

Sleep apnea has been defined as repeated episodes of complete airflow cessation for longer than 10 seconds.[10] *Hypopnea,* in contrast, is usually defined as a reduction in airflow by 50% or more for 10 seconds, with some residual airflow and a physiological consequence (e.g., arterial oxygen desaturation).[13,14] To compare the frequency of apnea with that of hypopnea during a sleep study, an apnea index (AI) or an apnea/hypopnea index (AHI) is usually calculated. The AI is the number of apneic periods observed divided by the total number of hours of sleep; the AHI consists of both apneic and hypopnea episodes per hour of sleep. Normative data on asymptomatic individuals from the study by Guilleminault and Dement[13] suggest that males average approximately seven apnea/hypopnea episodes per 8 hours of sleep, whereas females average only approximately two episodes per 8 hours of sleep.

Sleep apnea syndrome is present if apnea occurs in excess of five times per hour of sleep.[10,13,14] As such, three types of sleep apnea are generally described: obstructive sleep apnea (OSA), central sleep apnea, and mixed sleep apnea. OSA is characterized by the lack of airflow resulting from occlusion of the upper airways despite continued respiratory efforts. Central sleep apnea is characterized by the absence of airflow and respiratory efforts. Mixed sleep apnea has characteristics of both central sleep apnea and OSA, with the central event usually preceding the obstructive event.

Obstructive Sleep Apnea

Obstructive sleep apnea is present if a person has an AHI greater than 5 times per hour with associated symptoms or an AHI greater than 15 times per hour without associated symptoms.[10] In OSA, patients experience an increased AHI resulting from a reduction in airflow at the airway opening because of partial or complete occlusion of the upper airway. A number of anatomical and physiological factors can contribute to the incidence of OSA. These factors include upper airway anatomy, the ability of the upper airway dilator muscles to respond to respiratory challenges during sleep, arousal threshold, and the integrity of the respiratory control system.[15,16] Occlusion of the upper airway may occur with posterior movements of the tongue and palate. As these structures move posteriorly, they become juxtaposed with the posterior pharyngeal wall, resulting in occlusion of the nasopharynx and the oropharynx.[15] Fig. 11.8 shows the sequence of events that typically occur in OSA. Notice that obstruction of the upper airways initiates the primary sequence of events. Then apnea

Underlying Mechanisms   Primary Events

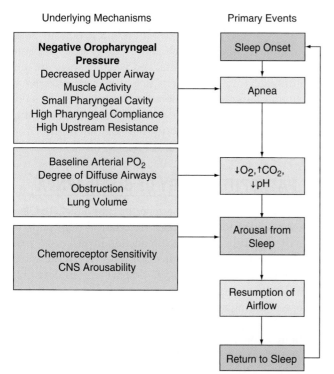

FIGURE 11.8 The primary sequence of events in obstructive sleep apnea (OSA), along with the pathogenic mechanisms that contribute to these events. *CNS,* Central nervous system; *PO₂,* partial pressure of oxygen. (Redrawn from Bradley TD, Phillipson EA: Pathogenesis and pathophysiology of the obstructive sleep apnea syndrome. *Med Clin North Am* 69:1169-1185, 1985.)

and progressive asphyxia develop until there is arousal from sleep, restoration of upper airway patency, and resumption of airflow. With relief from the asphyxia, the person quickly returns to sleep—only to have the sequence of events repeat itself over and over. In fact, the sequence can repeat itself several hundred times per night.[14]

OSA has been associated with several medical conditions, including chronic obstructive pulmonary disease, stroke, heart failure, and idiopathic pulmonary fibrosis. Fig. 11.9 demonstrates the physiological consequences and clinical features of OSA.[15] The physiological consequences of OSA include the development of cardiac arrhythmias, pulmonary and systemic hypertension, acute hypercapnia, cerebral dysfunction, loss of deep sleep, sleep fragmentation, and excessive motor activity. These physiological alterations can in turn result in restless sleep, excessive daytime sleepiness, personality and behavioral changes, intellectual deterioration, right heart failure, and unexplained nocturnal death.[16]

The symptoms most commonly associated with OSA in adult patients include chronic loud snoring, gasping or choking episodes during sleep, excessive daytime sleepiness, morning headaches, and personality and cognitive deterioration related to fatigue from lack of sleep. Box 11.2 contains the clinical definition of OSA.

Patients with an increased incidence of OSA are those who are obese (particularly those with nuchal obesity [i.e., neck size >17 in for men and >16 in for women] and naso-pharyngeal narrowing). Craniofacial and upper airway soft tissue abnormalities can also increase the incidence of OSA. The symptoms of OSA may be worse when patients ingest central nervous system depressants (e.g., sedatives, hypnotics) or consume alcohol, especially when it is ingested close to bedtime. Partial sleep deprivation, which can occur with shift work, may also affect patients with moderate OSA symptoms. Respiratory allergies and environmental factors such as smoking and ascent to altitude can augment the symptoms of patients with mild OSA. The prevalence of OSA is two to three times greater for men than women and is particularly evident in individuals older than the age of 65 years.

Fig. 11.10 shows the key polysomnographic events that occur during the apneic episode of a patient with OSA. Although there is a cessation of airflow, the patient's respiratory efforts continue, as evidenced by movement of the rib cage and the abdomen. The lack of airflow during an OSA episode results in hypoxemia, as evidenced by a fall in oxygen saturation as measured using pulse oximetry (SpO₂).

Patients diagnosed with OSA are typically classified as having mild, moderate, or severe disease.[17] Table 11.5 lists the criteria for diagnosing the severity of OSA in adult patients. Clinical Scenario 11.1 presents the case of a patient with suspected OSA.

The leading causes of OSA in children include tonsillar hypertrophy and obesity. OSA is best identified in these patients by combining phasic oxygen desaturation, hypercarbia, and intermittent paradoxical respiratory efforts. (*Note:* Oxygen desaturation of less than 92% is generally considered abnormal in children, depending on their baseline oxygen saturation.

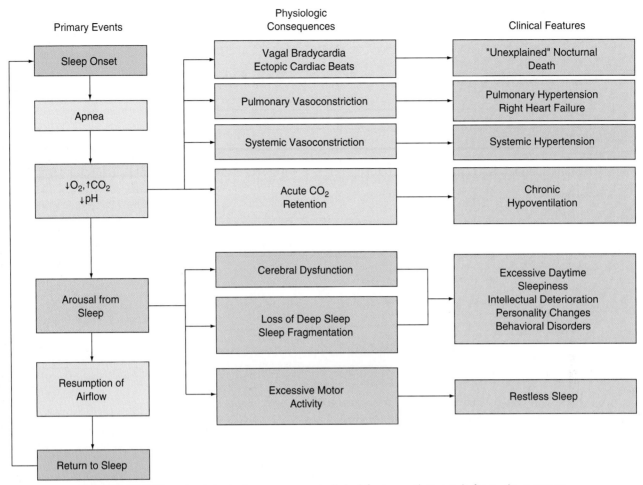

FIGURE 11.9 The physiological response and clinical features that result from sleep apnea. (Redrawn from Phillipson EA: Sleep apnea. *Med Clin North Am* 23:2314-2323, 1982.)

TABLE 11.5 Classifications of the Severity of Obstructive Sleep Apnea

Severity	AHI	Daytime Sleepiness	Sleep Cycles	Comorbidities	Response (Therapy)
Mild	5 to 15	Mild	Preserved	Generally no evidence of cor pulmonale, hypertension, polycythemia	Positive
Moderate	15 to 30	Aware of daytime sleepiness	Sleep cycles	Systemic hypertension may be present; sleep fragmentation	Positive (CPAP/bilevel PAP to treat daytime sleepiness)
Severe	>30	Daytime sleepiness interferes with activities	Oxygen desaturation (<90% for 20% of total sleep time)	Systemic hypertension, heart failure, nocturnal angina, polycythemia, cor pulmonale	Positive (CPAP/bilevel PAP to prevent hypoxemia)

AHI, Apnea/hypopnea index; *CPAP*, continuous positive airway pressure; *PAP*, positive airway pressure.
Adapted from Institute of Clinical Systems Improvement: *Health care guideline: diagnosis and treatment of obstructive sleep apnea*, ed 6, Bloomington, MN, 2008, Institute for Clinical Systems Improvement.

Brief oxygen desaturations of more than 4% occur infrequently in children and thus should be considered abnormal. Measurements of $P_{ET}CO_2$ can also provide evidence of sleep-disordered breathing in children. It has been suggested that $P_{ET}CO_2$ values of greater than 45 mm Hg for at least 60% of the total sleep time or $P_{ET}CO_2$ values greater than 13 mm Hg above baseline values indicate sleep-disordered breathing.[8]) Other criteria that should be noted when diagnosing sleep apnea in children are snoring, frequent arousal, and difficulty breathing while

asleep, as well as failure to thrive, cor pulmonale, or neurobehavioral disturbances.[16-18] Classification of severity of OSA in children (<12 years) differs from the criteria used with adult patients. For example, mild OSA is characterized by AHI of 1 to <5 episodes per hour, moderate OSA is present if 5 to <10 episodes occur per hour, and severe OSA is associated with AHI of >10 episodes per hour.

A variety of devices are available for the treatment of OSA, including positive airway pressure (i.e., continuous positive

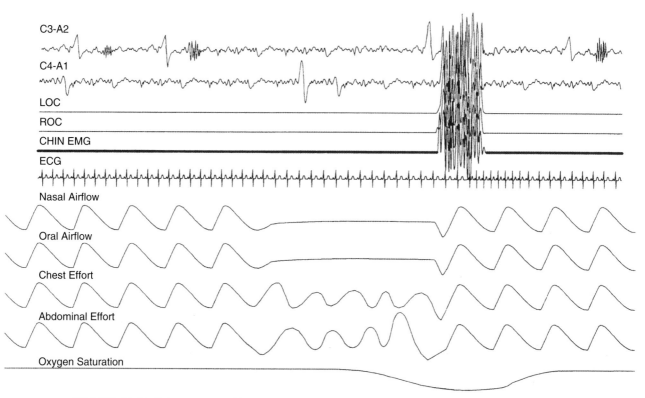

C3-A2

C4-A1

LOC

ROC

CHIN EMG

ECG

Nasal Airflow

Oral Airflow

Chest Effort

Abdominal Effort

Oxygen Saturation

FIGURE 11.10 Polysomnographic tracings of a patient exhibiting obstructive sleep apnea (OSA) during sleep. The patient exhibited constant loud snoring, paradoxical movement of the chest and abdomen, and recurrent complete airway obstructions, leading to oxygen desaturation. *ECG,* Electrocardiogram; *EMG,* electromyogram; *LOC,* left-of-center; *ROC,* right-of-center. (Redrawn from Sheldon SH, Spire JP, Levy HB: *Pediatric sleep medicine,* Philadelphia, 1992, WB Saunders.)

CLINICAL SCENARIO 11.1

Mr. H. is a 62-year-old automobile mechanic with a 60-packs-per-year history of smoking cigarettes. He was referred to the sleep laboratory after he was involved in an automobile accident that occurred when he reportedly fell asleep while driving home from work. He is unaware of any chronic abnormalities with his sleep pattern, but he does acknowledge that he has experienced excessive daytime sleepiness. His wife reports that she has noticed that he snores throughout the night and his sleep has become increasingly restless during the past 6 months. In fact, his wife reports that his snoring has become loud enough to disturb her sleep, and she jokes that if his snoring gets any louder, the neighbor may begin to complain. She also reports that his snoring episodes are more frequent and considerably louder if he has a nightcap (i.e., consumes an alcoholic drink) before going to sleep.

Does this patient demonstrate any history and physical findings that suggest the presence of OSA? Briefly describe a diagnostic strategy to properly diagnose his condition.

See Appendix A for the answer.

airway pressure [CPAP] and bilevel positive airway pressure [bilevel PAP]), oral appliances that can prevent airway occlusion during sleep, as well as surgical procedures to increase the diameter of the airway opening (e.g., repair of deviated nasal septum, tonsillectomy/adenoidectomy, palatal or maxillary expansion).

Box 11.3 provides a summary of the guidelines for the manual titration of PAP therapy for patients with OSA.[19] This guideline also includes suggestions for the use of supplemental oxygen during titration studies along with details regarding split-night studies for adults and children. Chapter 15 provides additional details on noninvasive ventilatory devices used to treat patients with OSA.

Central Sleep Apnea

Central sleep apnea includes several disorders associated with the cessation of respiratory drive and a complete loss of EMG activity in the respiratory muscles. Several mechanisms that have been proposed to account for these alterations involve defects in respiratory control or muscle function, transient fluctuation in respiratory drive, and reflex inhibition of the central respiratory drive.[2] Central sleep apnea is associated with central alveolar hypoventilation, neuromuscular diseases involving the respiratory muscles, and central nervous system diseases, but it can occur secondary to hyperventilation when a person ascends to high altitudes. Central sleep apnea is also a common finding in patients who experience esophageal reflux or upper airway collapse. It is important to mention that only approximately 10% of patients with apnea who are seen in most sleep laboratories have central sleep apnea; thus our knowledge of this disorder is somewhat limited when compared with the information available about OSA.[17]

BOX 11.3   Manual Titration of Optimum Positive Airway Pressure in Patients With Obstructive Sleep Apnea[a]

Indications for Positive Airway Pressure

- PAP is indicated for patients diagnosed with mild, moderate, or severe obstructive sleep apnea (OSA).

Adults ≥12 Years	Mild	Moderate	Severe
Respiratory disturbance index[a]	5 to <15	15 to 30	>30

Children <12 Years	Mild	Moderate	Severe
Respiratory disturbance index[a]	1 to <5	5 to <10	>10

[a]Respiratory disturbance index (RDI) = total apneas, hypopneas, and respiratory effort–related arousals.

Recording Techniques

- PAP titration should be performed using a type 1 attended polysomnography that is performed in an AASM-accredited sleep facility using sensors and data collection parameters identified in the *AASM Manual for the Scoring of Sleep and Associated Events: Rules, Terminology, and Technical Specifications*.
- The results of the polysomnography should be validated, interpreted, and reported by a board-certified sleep physician.

Description and Methodology for Manual PAP Titration

CPAP Titration

Patients <12 Years	Patients ≥12 Years
CPAP minimum = 4 cm H_2O	CPAP minimum = 4 cm H_2O
CPAP maximum = 15 cm H_2O	CPAP maximum = 20 cm H_2O

- Increase pressure by a minimum of 1 cm H_2O with an interval of no less than 5 minutes when the following occur:

Patients <12 Years	Patients ≥12 Years
1 obstructive apnea	2 obstructive apneas
1 hypopnea	3 hypopneas
3 RERAs[a]	5 RERAs[a]
1 min of loud or unambiguous snoring	3 min of loud or unambiguous snoring

[a]Respiratory effort–related arousals (RERAs)—respiratory events characterized by a flattening of the inspiratory airflow profile associates with sleep arousal, when airflow changes do not meet apnea or hypopnea criteria or by changes in the esophageal pressure recording.

Bilevel Positive Airway Pressure

- Use of bilevel PAP is indicated if the patient complains that he or she is uncomfortable or intolerant of high CPAP pressures or when the CPAP level is 15 cm H_2O and respiratory disturbances continue.

Patients <12 Years	Patients ≥12 Years
Minimum IPAP = 8, EPAP = 4 cm H_2O	Minimum IPAP = 8, EPAP = 4 cm H_2O

Patients <12 Years	Patients ≥12 Years
Maximum IPAP = 20 cm H_2O	Maximum IPAP = 30 cm H_2O
Minimum I/E difference = 4 cm H_2O	Minimum I/E difference = 4 cm H_2O
Maximum I/E difference = 10 cm H_2O	Maximum I/E difference = 10 cm H_2O

- Increase pressure by a minimum of 1 cm H_2O with an interval of no less than 5 minutes when the following occur:

Patients <12 Years	Patients ≥12 Years
1 obstructive sleep apnea	2 obstructive sleep apneas

- Increase IPAP by a minimum of 1 cm H_2O with an interval of no less than 5 minutes when the following occur:

Patients <12 Years	Patients ≥12 Years
1 hypopnea	3 hypopneas
3 RERAs	5 RERAs
1 min of loud or unambiguous snoring	3 min of loud or unambiguous snoring

- Indications of optimal titration include:
  - RDI < 5 per hour for a period of at least 15 minutes at the selected pressure and within the manufacturer's acceptable leak limit;
  - SpO_2 > 90% at the selected pressure;
  - Supine REM sleep at the selected pressure is not continually interrupted by spontaneous arousals or awakening.

Technical Documentation

- Polysomnography (PSG) recordings with PAP pressures can be obtained either recorded manually on the record or automatically recorded by a signal from the PAP device. The technologist should include a log of all events, observations, and interventions that occurred during the PSG/PAP titration. The record should also include:
- Beginning and ending pressures
- Pressure or delivery mode changes and rationale
- Body position
- Sleep stage
- Patient behavior (restless, complaints)
- Snoring
- SpO_2
- The reason for changing from one mask or device to another.

Reporting Results

The sleep physician generates the final report with recommendations for PAP pressures during home use after reviewing the preliminary scored data from the PSG/PAP titration study provided by the sleep technologist.

AASM, American Academy of Sleep Medicine; *CPAP*, continuous positive airway pressure; *EPAP*, expiratory positive airway pressure; *I/E*, inspiratory/expiratory; *IPAP*, inspiratory positive airway pressure; *PAP*, positive airway pressure; *REM*, rapid eye movement; SpO_2, oxygen saturation as measured using pulse oximetry.

Modified from the American Association of Sleep Technologists: Sleep technology: technical guideline—summary of AASM clinical guidelines for the manual titration of positive airway pressure in patients with obstructive sleep apnea, Darien, IL, 2012, American Association of Sleep Technologists.

Patients with central sleep apnea typically report gasping for air and shortness of breath upon awakening from a central sleep apneic episode. Depression, as assessed both subjectively and by formal testing, is a common finding among patients with central sleep apnea. It is interesting to note that patients with central sleep apnea do not normally report insomnia and hypersomnolence as do those with OSA. Patients with central sleep apnea typically have a normal body habitus, although obese patients may also exhibit this form of sleep apnea.

Fig. 11.11 shows an example of a polysomnographic tracing for a patient with central sleep apnea. As with OSA, there is a complete cessation of airflow that lasts for 10 seconds or longer. However, in contrast to OSA, airflow cessation is associated with a cessation in respiratory effort and thus no movement of the rib cage or abdomen.

Mixed Sleep Apnea

Most patients who experience central sleep apnea also demonstrate evidence of OSA. In fact, because these two types of apnea typically coexist, most authors define *central sleep apnea* as a condition occurring in individuals in whom more than 55% of the apneic episodes are central in origin. The exact cause of mixed apnea is unclear at this time; nonetheless, it has been suggested that the mechanisms responsible for central sleep apnea and OSA may be related, because several studies have shown that the upper airway muscles behave like respiratory muscles. That is, the upper airway muscles contract and dilate the pharynx when the diaphragm is stimulated.[20,21]

PSG provides clear evidence of the presence of mixed apnea. As Fig. 11.12 shows, airflow cessation is preceded by a central apneic event (i.e., no movement of the rib cage or abdomen). The obstructive component can be ascertained by observing that there is a resumption of respiratory effort, although there is still a cessation of airflow. With arousal from sleep the apneic event ends, and airflow resumes as the airway opens (Clinical Scenario 11.2).

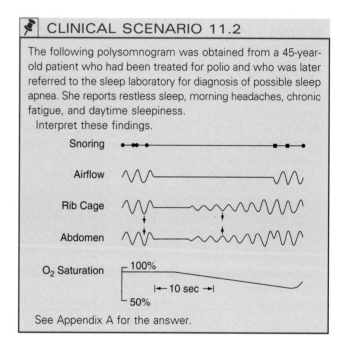

CLINICAL SCENARIO 11.2

The following polysomnogram was obtained from a 45-year-old patient who had been treated for polio and who was later referred to the sleep laboratory for diagnosis of possible sleep apnea. She reports restless sleep, morning headaches, chronic fatigue, and daytime sleepiness.

Interpret these findings.

See Appendix A for the answer.

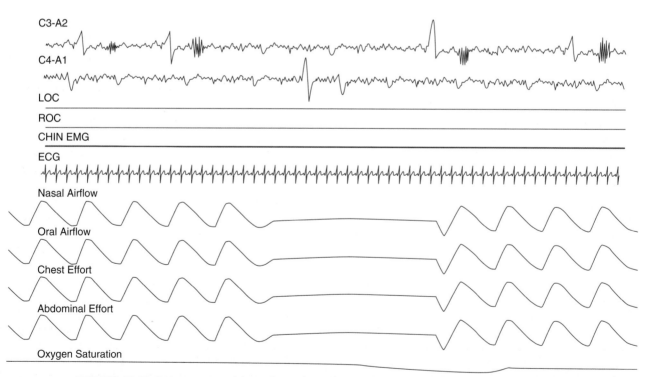

FIGURE 11.11 Polysomnographic tracings of a patient with central sleep apnea. Note that during the apneic episode there is complete cessation of nasal and oral airflow with concomitant absence of respiratory effort (i.e., no movements of chest or abdomen). *ECG,* Electrocardiogram; *EMG,* electromyogram; *LOC,* left-of-center; *ROC,* right-of-center. (Redrawn from Sheldon SH, Spire JP, Levy HB: *Pediatric sleep medicine,* Philadelphia, 1992, WB Saunders.)

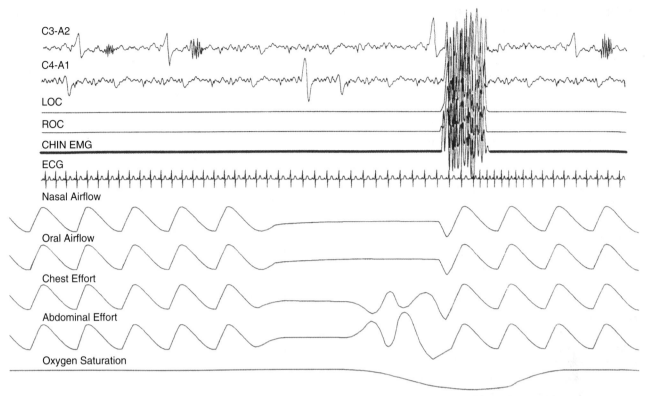

FIGURE 11.12 Polysomnographic tracings from a patient with mixed apnea. There is cessation of airflow at the nose and mouth. Initially there is an absence of respiratory effort (central component), followed by at least two cycles of respiratory effort with continued absence of airflow (obstructive component). Significant oxygen desaturation is also present. *ECG,* Electrocardiogram; *EMG,* electromyogram; *LOC,* left-of-center; *ROC,* right-of-center. (Redrawn from Sheldon SH, Spire JP, Levy HB: *Pediatric sleep medicine,* Philadelphia, 1992, WB Saunders.)

KEY POINTS

- The physiological effects of sleep on breathing are normally of little consequence in healthy individuals. In patients with altered respiratory function, however, sleep can have profound effects on physiological function that—if left untreated—can lead to dire consequences.
- Recent advances in our understanding of sleep structure and the ability to assess cardiopulmonary and neuromuscular function during sleep have greatly improved our ability to recognize and treat sleep-related disorders.
- Three types of sleep apnea have been described: obstructive, central, and mixed.
- Sleep apnea has been defined as repeated episodes of complete airflow cessation for longer than 10 seconds.
- Hypopnea is usually defined as a reduction in airflow by 50% or more for 10 seconds, with some residual airflow and a physiological consequence (e.g., arterial oxygen desaturation).
- To compare the frequency of apnea with that of hypopnea during a sleep study, an AI or an AHI is usually calculated. The AI is the number of apneic periods observed divided by the total number of hours of sleep; the AHI consists of both apneic and hypopnea episodes per hour of sleep.
- OSA is characterized by airflow cessation at the airway opening, even though the patient continues to make respiratory efforts.

- Central sleep apnea involves a complete cessation of respiratory efforts and airflow.
- Mixed apnea includes characteristics of both obstructive apnea and central apnea.
- Patients with mixed apnea typically experience a central apneic component before the obstructive event occurs.
- Diagnosis of sleep apnea is based on clinical findings, including patient history and physical examination, along with the data from laboratory studies.
- Obtaining a complete history and the results of a physical examination is the first step in identifying whether an individual is at risk for sleep apnea.
- Overnight monitoring of arterial blood gases with pulse oximetry and $P_{ET}CO_2$, and PSG is then performed to make a definitive diagnosis of sleep apnea.
- Although there is some controversy about the best strategy to use when attempting to diagnose sleep apnea, it is generally agreed that PSG is the gold standard for evaluating the presence and severity of sleep apnea.
- PSG involves recording various electrogenic potentials (e.g., ECG, EEG, EOG), and respiratory status can also be used to select the most effective management strategy after sleep apnea is identified in a patient.

ASSESSMENT QUESTIONS

See Appendix B for the answers.

1. Which of the following are characteristic findings of stage N2 sleep?
   1. Sleep spindles and K-complexes are seen on an electroencephalogram (EEG).
   2. Slow, pendulous, and disconjugate movements of the eyes.
   3. A relatively low threshold for arousal from sleep.
   4. Adult patients typically enter this stage of sleep after approximately 90 minutes of non–rapid eye movement (NREM) sleep.
      a. 1 and 2 only
      b. 2 and 4 only
      c. 1, 2, and 3 only
      d. 2, 3, and 4 only

2. The classic states of NREM sleep and rapid eye movement (REM) sleep are not easily identified at birth with the use of standard polysomnography (PSG). Briefly describe the structure of sleep for a 2-week-old neonate.

3. Describe the impact of sleep on breathing in a healthy adult.

4. Which of the following changes in cardiovascular function occurs during sleep?
   a. Heart rate increases by approximately 5 to 10 beats/min during NREM sleep.
   b. Blood pressure decreases by as much as 25 mm Hg during REM sleep.
   c. Cardiac output increases only slightly during NREM sleep.
   d. Stroke volume remains constant during NREM sleep and REM sleep.

5. Portable monitoring (PM) of patients with obstructive sleep apnea (OSA) is equivalent to laboratory PSG for all patients. True or False?

6. Sleep apnea is present if the person experiences at least how many apneic events per hour of sleep?
   a. 3
   b. 5
   c. 8
   d. 10

7. List three variables that should be monitored to assess respiratory activity during PSG.

8. Which of the following are typical history and physical findings in patients with OSA?
   1. Chronic loud snoring
   2. Excessive daytime sleepiness
   3. Personality changes
   4. Obesity
      a. 1 and 3 only
      b. 2 and 4 only
      c. 1, 2, and 3 only
      d. 1, 2, 3, and 4

9. Describe the physiological consequences of OSA.

10. Which of the following are associated with central sleep apnea?
    1. Alveolar hypoventilation
    2. Myasthenia gravis
    3. Stroke
    4. Angina pectoris
       a. 1 and 2 only
       b. 2 and 3 only
       c. 1, 2, and 3 only
       d. 1, 3, and 4 only

11. Which of the following conditions will a patient experience during periods of mixed apnea with hypoxemia?
    a. Systemic hypotension
    b. Increased cardiac output
    c. Decreased heart rate
    d. Pulmonary hypertension

12. Which of the following are characteristic findings in children with OSA?
    1. Phasic oxygen desaturation
    2. Hypercarbia
    3. Intermittent paradoxical respiratory efforts
    4. Sinus tachycardia
       a. 1 and 3 only
       b. 2 and 4 only
       c. 1, 2, and 3 only
       d. 1, 2, 3, and 4

13. Which of the following are typical findings for patients with central sleep apnea?
    1. These patients rarely report insomnia.
    2. The patient reports gasping for air upon awakening after an apneic event.
    3. Depression is a common finding in these patients.
    4. Most of these patients are grossly overweight.
       a. 1 and 2 only
       b. 2 and 3 only
       c. 1, 2, and 3 only
       d. 2, 3, and 4 only

14. Define the apnea/hypopnea index (AHI), and describe how normative data for male subjects differ from those for female subjects.

15. Which of the following drugs increase the incidence of OSA?
    1. Ethanol
    2. Sedatives
    3. Tricyclic antidepressants
    4. Hypnotics
       a. 2 and 3 only
       b. 1, 2, and 3 only
       c. 1, 2, and 4 only
       d. 1, 3, and 4 only

REFERENCES

1. Guilleminault C, Dement WC: General physiology of sleep. In Crystal RG, West JB, editors: *The lung: scientific foundations,* New York, 1991, Raven Press.

2. Kryger MH, Roth T, Dement WC: *Principles and practice of sleep medicine,* ed 5, St. Louis, 2011, Elsevier.

3. Iber C, Ancoili-Israel S, Chesson A, et al.: *The AASM manual for the scoring of sleep and associated events: rules, terminology and technical specifications,* Westchester, IL, 2007, American Academy of Sleep Medicine.

4. Guyton AC, Hall JE: *Human physiology and mechanisms of disease,* ed 12, Philadelphia, 2010, Saunders.

5. Sheldon SH, Spire JP, Levy HB: *Pediatric sleep medicine,* Philadelphia, 1992, WB Saunders.

6. Collop NA, Anderson WM, Boehlecke B, et al.: Clinical guidelines for the use of unattended portable monitors in the diagnosis of obstructive sleep apnea in adult patients. *J Clin Sleep Med* 3(7):737-747, 2007.

7. Jasper HH: The ten-twenty system of the International Federation. *Electroencephalogr Clin Neurophysiol* 10:371, 1958.

8. Redland WR, O'Donoghue FJ, Pierce RY, et al.: The 2007 AASM recommendations for EEG electrode placement in polysomnography: impact on sleep and cortical arousal scoring. *Sleep* 34(1):73-81, 2011.

9. Berry RM: *Fundamentals of sleep medicine,* Philadelphia, 2012, Elsevier.

10. Hess DR, MacIntyre NR, Mishoe S, et al.: *Respiratory care: principles and practice,* ed 2, Burlington, MA, 2011, Jones & Bartlett Learning.

11. Berry RB, Budhiraja R, Gottlieb DJ, et al.: Rules for scoring respiratory events in sleep: update of the 2007 AASM manual for the scoring of sleep and associated events. *J Clin Sleep Med* 8(5):597-619, 2012.

12. Kennan S, Hirshkowitz M: Monitoring techniques for evaluating suspected sleep-disordered breathing. In Kryger MH, Roth T, Dement WC, editors: *Principles and practice of sleep medicine,* ed 5, St. Louis, 2011, Elsevier.

13. Guilleminault C, Dement WC: Sleep apnea syndromes and related sleep disorders. In Williams RL, Karacan I, editors: *Sleep disorders: diagnosis and treatment,* New York, 1978, Wiley & Sons.

14. McNicholas WT, Phillipson EA: *Breathing disorders in sleep,* Philadelphia, 2002, WB Saunders.

15. Eckert DJ, Malhotra A: Pathophysiology of adult obstructive sleep apnea. *Proc Am Thorac Soc* 5:144-153, 2008.

16. White DP: Sleep apnea. *Proc Am Thorac Soc* 3:124-128, 2006.

17. Flemons WW: Clinical practice: obstructive sleep apnea. *N Engl J Med* 347:348, 2002.

18. American Academy of Sleep Medicine, Diagnostic Steering Committee: *The international classification of sleep disorders, revised diagnostic and coding manual,* Chicago, IL, 2001, American Academy of Sleep Medicine.

19. American Association of Sleep Technologists: Sleep technology: technical guideline—summary of AASM clinical guidelines for the manual titration of positive airway pressure in patients with obstructive sleep apnea, Darien, IL, 2012, American Association of Sleep Technologists. https://www.aastweb.org/technical-guidelines.

20. Guilleminault C, van den Hoed J, Mitler MM: Clinical overview of the sleep apnea syndromes. In Guilleminault C, Dement WC, editors: *Sleep apnea syndromes,* New York, 1978, Alan R. Liss.

21. Onal E, Lopata M, O'Connor T: Pathogenesis of apneas in hypersomnia—sleep apnea syndrome. *Am Rev Respir Dis* 125:167-174, 1982.

SECTION V

Critical Care and Extended Care Devices

Introduction to Ventilators

Timothy B. Op't Holt

OBJECTIVES

Upon completion of this chapter you will be able to:

1. List the two primary power sources used in mechanical ventilators.
2. Compare and contrast negative-pressure and positive-pressure ventilation.
3. Explain how a closed-loop ventilator system can perform self-adjustment.
4. Define volume-controlled and pressure-controlled ventilation.
6. Name the flow control valve found on most intensive care unit (ICU) ventilators.
7. Explain the two fundamental principles of fluidics.
8. Evaluate available positive end-expiratory pressure (PEEP) valves to determine whether a flow resistor or a threshold resistor is being used.
9. List and describe criteria that can be used to classify various ventilator modes.
10. Describe the four phase variables.
11. Explain how pressure-, flow-, and volume-triggering mechanisms work to begin the inspiratory phase of a breath.
12. Identify the scalars for volume-controlled and pressure-controlled breaths.
13. Identify a pressure-time scalar showing patient triggering.
14. Describe mandatory, spontaneous, and assisted breaths.
15. Describe trigger and synchronization windows.
16. Use the rubrics for classifying trigger and cycle events, determining control variable, and breath sequence.
17. Describe the seven targeting schemes.
18. List examples of modes in each of the seven targeting schemes.
19. List the five common methods of delivering high-frequency ventilation.

OUTLINE

KEY TERMS

adaptive support ventilation (ASV)
adaptive targeting
airway pressure-release ventilation (APRV)
assisted breath
automatic tube compensation (ATC)
baseline pressure
baseline variable

beam deflection
bilevel positive airway pressure (BiPAP, bilevel pressure assist, bilevel pressure support)
breath sequence
chest cuirass
closed-loop system
Coanda effect

continuous mandatory ventilation (CMV)
continuous positive airway pressure (CPAP)
continuous spontaneous ventilation (CSV)
control panel
control variable

cycle variable
direct-drive piston
dual targeting
electrically powered
end-expiratory pause
expiratory hold
external circuit
flip-flop component
flow-control valves
flow resistance
flow triggering
fluidic ventilators
high-frequency jet ventilation
    (HFJV)
high-frequency oscillatory ventila-
    tion (HFOV)
high-frequency ventilation (HFV)
inspiratory hold
inspiratory pause
intermittent mandatory ventilation
    (IMV)
internal circuit
iron lung

limit variable
linear-drive piston
mandatory minute ventilation
    (MMV)
negative-pressure ventilators
neurally adjusted ventilatory assist
    (NAVA)
open-loop system
optimal targeting
patient circuit
patient triggering
peak inspiratory pressure (PIP)
pendelluft
phase variables
plateau pressure (P_{plat})
pneumatically powered
pneumatic circuit
positive end-expiratory pressure
    (PEEP)
pressure-controlled breaths
pressure-controlled inverse ratio
    ventilation (PC-IRV)
pressure-limited ventilation

pressure-regulated volume control
    (PRVC)
pressure-support ventilation (PSV)
pressure triggering
proportional assist ventilation (PAV)
proportional solenoid valves
scalars
separation bubble
servo targeting
set-point targeting
sinusoidal
static compliance
targeting scheme
threshold resistance
time triggering
total cycle time (TCT)
trigger sensitivity
trigger variable
tubing compressibility
user interface
volume-controlled ventilation (VCV)

I. PHYSICAL CHARACTERISTICS OF VENTILATORS

Advances in computer technology continue to be made at a rapid pace. Nowhere is the impact of modern technology more noticeable than in medical devices, particularly mechanical ventilators. A wide variety of mechanical ventilators are available for managing patients of different ages and in various settings. All of these share certain characteristics, as well as important functional properties. This chapter focuses on the physical characteristics of ventilators, method for describing and classifying modes of ventilation, how ventilators deliver breaths, and a separate section on high-frequency ventilation.

Introduction to Ventilators

A ventilator is a medical device that is connected to a pneumatic (gas supply) and/or electrical power source that provides a breath or gas flow to a patient. The operator selects settings on the control panel, sometimes called the user interface or graphical user interface. These settings determine the pattern of gas delivery produced by the ventilator's flow control valves, ultimately providing the breaths the patient receives.

The description of a ventilator begins with a discussion of the physical characteristics of the ventilator (Box 12.1).[1] It then proceeds to a description and classification of predetermined patterns of interaction between a patient and a ventilator, specified as a particular combination of control variable, breath sequence, and targeting schemes for primary and secondary breaths, also referred to as modes. These terms will be defined in a subsequent section of this chapter.

BOX 12.1   Components of a Ventilator

1. Ventilator power source or input power (electric or gas source)
   a. Electrically powered ventilators
   b. Pneumatically powered ventilators
2. Positive- or negative-pressure ventilators
3. Control systems and circuits
   a. Open- and closed-loop systems to control ventilator function
   b. Control panel (user interface)
   c. Pneumatic circuit (internal and patient circuit)
4. Drive mechanisms
   a. Volume displacement, pneumatic designs
   b. Flow-control valves
5. Output (pressure, volume, and flow scalars and loops)

From Cairo JM: *Pilbeam's mechanical ventilation: physiological and clinical applications*, ed 5, St. Louis, 2012, Mosby/Elsevier.

Ventilators typically rely on the same basic components: controls for the breathing pattern, a gas supply, a set of alarms, and a display screen. Once a student or practicing therapist is comfortable with one ventilator, becoming proficient with other ventilators can occur quickly with relatively minimal instruction. The goal of this chapter is to provide a general description of how ventilators work and contemporary terminology; the anatomy of a ventilator-delivered breath is presented, followed by a description of breathing patterns (modes). The operational characteristics of the most commonly used ventilators are described in Chapters 13 to 15.

Power Source—Input Power

Power sources provide the energy to perform the work required to ventilate a patient. Ventilator power sources are typically divided into two categories: pneumatically powered ventilators and electrically powered ventilators.

Pneumatically Powered Ventilators

Pneumatically powered ventilators connect to high-pressure gas sources (35 to 100 pounds per square inch [psi]) and use this pressure to power gas flow to the patient. In general, pneumatically powered ventilators used in an intensive care unit (ICU) rely on two 50-psi gas sources (oxygen and air). Pressure-reducing valves in the ventilator ensure that the airway pressure is lower than the source pressure. In pneumatically powered ventilators, gas flows down a pressure gradient from the wall outlet, through these pressure-reducing valves, and to the patient without the need of a mechanical device such as a piston. Two types of pneumatically powered ventilators are available: pneumatic ventilators and fluidic ventilators.

Pneumatic ventilators may incorporate components such as Venturi devices or air entrainers, needle valves, flexible diaphragms, and spring-loaded valves to perform certain functions. For example, Venturi devices may be used to control an expiratory valve, and a needle valve may control gas flow during inspiration. Most pneumatically powered ventilators, however, rely on microprocessor-controlled proportional solenoid valves to control the flow of gas down its pressure gradient to the patient. Fluidic ventilators use fluidic components that are based on special pneumatic principles. Some transport ventilators and those used in rough environments use the fluidic principle because gas consumption is low and they are not affected by vibration and rough handling.

Electrically Powered Ventilators

Electrically powered ventilators use standard electrical outlets (110 to 220 V alternating current [AC]) to power the internal components. In the United States, standard electrical outlets provide110 V. Higher voltages (e.g., 220 V) are used in other countries. Many ventilators have internal direct current (DC) batteries, which can provide electrical power during patient transport or in the event of a power failure. Some ventilators can also be connected to external DC batteries.

Electrically powered ventilators use electricity to power internal motors for operating air compressors, blowers, pistons, or bellows that provide gas flow to the patient.

Pneumatically Powered Microprocessor-Controlled Ventilators

Ventilator control systems. Ventilator control systems refer to the valves or circuits that regulate gas flow to the patient. Most contemporary ventilators are pneumatically powered and microprocessor controlled. Two 50-psi gas sources provide the pressure to deliver inspiratory gas flow. This gas flow is usually the same gas the patient receives during inspiration. Control of the inspiratory flow waveform is governed by

---

> **BOX 12.2 Types and Examples of Pressure Ventilators**
>
> **Negative-Pressure Ventilators**
> - Iron lung
> - Chest cuirass
>
> **Positive-Pressure Ventilators**
> - Most ventilators in use today are positive-pressure ventilators, such as the Medtronic Minimally Invasive Therapies Puritan Bennett 840, the Servo-i, and the Hamilton G5 ventilators (see Chapter 13)
>
> **Positive-/Negative-Pressure Ventilators**
> - High-frequency oscillators

microprocessor-controlled proportional solenoid valves. For example, the pattern of gas flow may be constant (also known as square), producing a constant-flow scalar, or it may be rapid at the beginning of inspiration and gradually taper, producing a descending ramp scalar (ventilator graphics are presented later in this chapter). These ventilators require both electrical and pneumatic power sources.

Pressure Delivery

A ventilator does all or part of the work of breathing (WOB) for the patient. A ventilator can increase lung volume during inspiration by creating either negative- or positive-pressure gradients. The pressure gradient results in gas flow to produce ventilation (Box 12.2).

Positive-Pressure Ventilators

A pressure gradient must exist for gas flow to occur. During a spontaneous breath, contraction of the inspiratory muscles initiates inspiration (i.e., the diaphragm contracts and descends, and the external intercostal muscles contract). The action of these muscles, especially the diaphragm, results in a decrease in intrapleural and alveolar pressures. This produces a pressure gradient from the mouth, which is at ambient pressure, to the alveoli, which are below ambient pressure, resulting in an increased intrathoracic volume. The pressure gradient is referred to as the transairway pressure (P_{TA}). During expiration, passive relaxation of the respiratory muscles along with chest wall and lung tissue elastic recoil reduces the transairway pressure and volume. Intraalveolar pressure becomes slightly positive (above ambient), and air flows out of the lungs passively.[1]

During positive-pressure ventilation, a supraatmospheric pressure is created at the mouth by mask or artificial airway, and the intraalveolar pressure is ambient at the beginning of the breath. Again, a P_{TA} gradient is created. As a result, air flows into the lungs, expanding them and the chest wall (Fig. 12.1). Expiration during positive pressure ventilation occurs passively (similar to spontaneous breathing) once the supraatmospheric pressure is withdrawn. Positive-pressure ventilation is the most common method of mechanical ventilation.

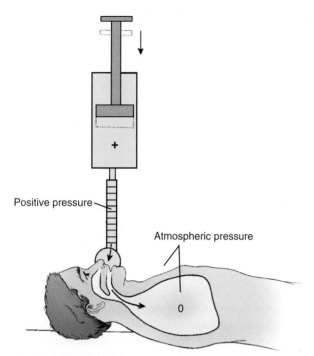

FIGURE 12.1 Application of positive pressure at the airway creates a pressure gradient between the mouth and the alveoli; as a result, gas flows into the lungs. (*Note:* This is a single-circuit ventilator, which is explained later in the chapter.)

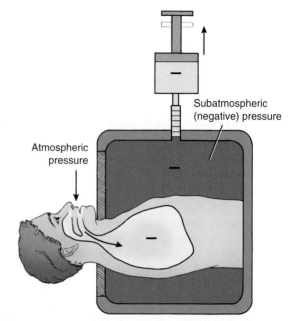

FIGURE 12.2 Application of subatmospheric pressure around the chest wall causes a pressure drop in the alveoli, and air flows into the lungs; this is referred to as *negative-pressure ventilation (NPV)*.

Negative-Pressure Ventilators

Negative-pressure ventilators attempt to mimic normal spontaneous breathing by producing a negative pressure at the body surface during inspiration, which is transmitted across the chest wall to create a negative intraalveolar pressure, allowing air to move into the lungs. During exhalation the negative pressure is withdrawn, and the chest wall pressure is returned to ambient pressure, causing intraalveolar pressure to become slightly positive, which allows air to flow out of the lungs.

Two types of negative-pressure ventilators are typically described: chest cuirass and the tank respirator (or iron lung). In the chest cuirass a negative pressure is created only around the chest. In tank respirators a negative pressure is created around the entire body except for the head (Fig. 12.2). Negative pressure ventilators are rarely used to ventilate patients in the ICU. They are occasionally used in the home as an alternative form of ventilation for ventilator-dependent patients.

Combined-Pressure Devices

The most common example of a combined-pressure device is a high-frequency oscillator. This is a form of high-frequency ventilation (HFV) that produces oscillating gas pressure waveforms at the upper airway. The waveform is a sinusoidal pattern with positive- and negative-pressure oscillations produced at the upper airway by an oscillating device (Fig. 12.3). The section in this chapter on HFV explains oscillator function. Oscillators are used with neonatal, pediatric, and adult patients. Chapter 14, which describes infant and pediatric ventilation,

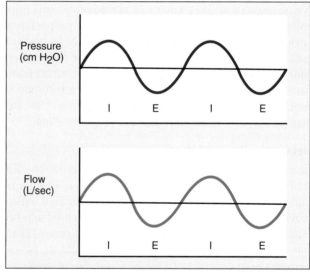

FIGURE 12.3 The sinusoidal waveform produced by an oscillator. *I,* Inspiration; *E,* expiration.

provides an example of a high-frequency oscillator, the CareFusion 3100A.

Control Systems and Circuits
Open-Loop and Closed-Loop Systems

A combination of mechanical, pneumatic, and electronic devices in the ventilator constitutes the control or decision-making functions of the unit. These control systems and circuits, which govern ventilator operation, can create an open-loop system or a closed-loop system.

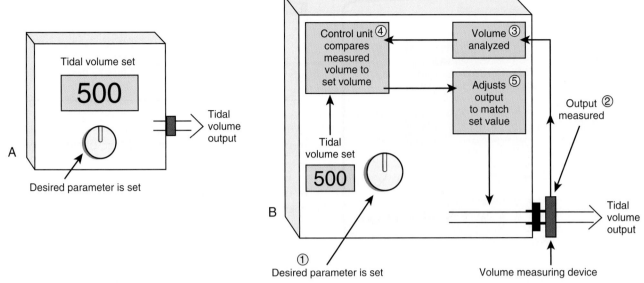

FIGURE 12.4 A, Open-loop system. The path through the device is straight from the control panel to the internal device and out to the patient. No feedback is provided to the ventilator about the output. B, The ventilator "closes the loop" by measuring the gas exhaled by the patient, comparing it to the set value, and feeding this information back to the machine. (See text for further explanation.) (From Cairo JM: *Pilbeam's mechanical ventilation: physiological and clinical applications*, ed 5, St. Louis, 2012, Mosby.)

Ventilators that do not rely on a feedback signal from the patient or circuit to ensure that a set parameter value has been achieved are called *open-loop systems*. For example, when the operator establishes a setting, such as the tidal volume (V_T), the ventilator delivers the set amount of volume to the patient circuit. In reality, this volume might leak into the room and never reach the patient. Unfortunately, an open-loop system cannot discern the difference between the volume actually delivered and the set volume and respond to this difference (Fig. 12.4A).

Closed-loop systems use a microprocessor to control ventilator function.[2] For example, the manufacturer uses a closed-loop program that instructs the ventilator to deliver a specific quantity (e.g., V_T). The control system measures the volume delivered by the ventilator and exhaled by the patient, then makes a comparison and adjusts the volume delivery based on this comparison to deliver the amount of volume set on the control panel. Fig. 12.4B shows an algorithm for a closed-loop system.[1] This type of closed-loop ventilator system is similar to the cruise control mechanism found on most cars. The operator sets the cruise control at a particular speed, and the car then compares the actual speed with the set speed. If the car is moving too slowly, the cruise control accelerates the car to the set speed. The driver does not have to make any adjustments; the cruise control does it automatically. It is referred to as a closed-loop system because it compares the input to the output and "closes the loop" (see Fig. 12.4B). These systems are also called *feedback systems* and *servo-controlled systems*. An example of closed-loop control of a ventilator is in **continuous mandatory ventilation (CMV)** with adaptive targeting. In this breathing pattern, the ventilator is programmed to deliver a certain V_T. However, if compliance

---

CLINICAL SCENARIO 12.1
Open-Loop and Closed-Loop Ventilator Systems

Part I
A respiratory therapist sets a ventilator tidal volume at 650 mL; the peak inspiratory pressure is 8 cm H_2O. The volume measured at the exhalation valve is 500 mL. These measurements occur over the next several breaths with no changes. Is this open-loop or closed-loop logic?

Part II
A respiratory therapist sets the tidal volume at 650 mL. After one breath the exhaled volume measures 500 mL, and the peak pressure is 8 cm H_2O. After a second breath the exhaled volume is 600 mL, and the peak pressure is 14 cm H_2O. After a third breath the exhaled volume is 649 mL, and the peak pressure is 16 cm H_2O. What type of system is this?
See Appendix A for the answers.

---

decreases, so does the V_T. The ventilator measures this decrease in V_T and increases the peak pressure, which in turn increases the V_T back to the initial desired V_T. The ventilator uses the feedback volume signal to increase pressure (Clinical Scenario 12.1, Part II.) Contemporary ventilators have some form of closed-loop control. However, they are not without problems. New modes of ventilation can be introduced on the market with limited patient testing. The manufacturer has only to provide evidence that the mode performs the intended function and that the software has been validated.[3] Clinical Scenario 12.1 provides an exercise to test your understanding of closed- and open-loop systems.

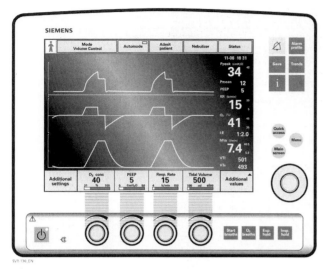

FIGURE 12.5 User interface of the Servo-i ventilator. (Courtesy Maquet, Bridgewater, NJ.)

Control Panel

The control panel, or user interface, is located on the front of most ventilators. It contains the controls by which the operator can adjust all the variables for the chosen mode such as the mandatory rate (f), V_T, pressure above positive end-expiratory pressure (PEEP), and inspiratory time (T_I) (Fig. 12.5). Early-generation ventilators exclusively used knobs to control ventilator parameter values, which led to a plethora of knobs, each of which could control only one parameter. Current ventilators have touchscreen controls, which allow the operator to select a particular breathing pattern using a touchscreen menu or virtual knobs. In the latter case, only those virtual knobs that apply to the parameters for that particular breathing pattern appear. To change the value of a parameter, the operator selects the desired "knob," turns a physical control knob, and then presses a key to accept that parameter value change. For example, if a V_T of 800 mL is desired and the current V_T is 650 mL, the operator touches the V_T icon, turns the physical control knob until it indicates a V_T of 800 mL, then presses the accept key. The ventilator then changes the V_T to 800 mL. This method is common among most contemporary ventilators. Advantages of this system are that the operator sees only those icons applicable to that particular breathing pattern, which eliminates the confusion that might occur when seeing several knobs that do not apply to that breathing pattern; a decrease in the number of moving parts, which may increase the reliability of the ventilator; and the ability to upgrade the ventilator with new breathing patterns or adjuncts by simply downloading the new function to the ventilator's central processing unit. No new hardware is needed. Control panels for many contemporary ventilators are illustrated in Chapters 13 to 15.

Pneumatic Circuit

The pneumatic circuit consists of a series of tubing that directs gas flow both within the ventilator (the internal circuit) and

from the ventilator to the patient (the external or patient circuit).

Internal circuit. The internal circuit conducts gas generated by the power source, passes it through various mechanical or pneumatic mechanisms, and finally directs it to the external circuit. Internal circuits are either single or double circuits (Box 12.3). To use the drive mechanism and the gas delivery valves previously described, the internal circuit must be programmed to manipulate pressure, volume, flow, and time to deliver a breath (inspiration) to the patient. The microprocessor or electronics of the ventilator performs this function. It consists of pneumatic systems such as pressure regulators, entrainment devices, or fluidic components. ICU ventilators tend to use sophisticated devices composed of programmed microprocessors and flow valves controlled by these microprocessors, as described later in this chapter in the section "Flow-Control Valves."

In a single-circuit ventilator, the gas enters the ventilator and goes directly to the patient (Fig. 12.6). This design is common in contemporary ventilators. A double-circuit ventilator consists of two gas sources. One gas source goes to the patient from a bag or bellows, and the other actively compresses the bag or bellows. A double circuit is also called a *bellows* or *"bag-in-a-chamber"* design. The double-circuit design is used in anesthesia machines.

External circuit. The external circuit conducts the gas from the ventilator to the patient and from the patient through an expiratory valve to the room. The external circuit is commonly called the *ventilator circuit* or the *patient circuit* (Fig. 12.7). Fig. 12.7A shows a ventilator circuit with an externally mounted expiratory valve; Fig. 12.7B shows a ventilator circuit with an internally mounted exhalation valve, the most common design used in critical care ventilators today.

In the external circuit, gas flows both through the main inspiratory line to the patient and to the expiratory valve line during inspiration. The expiratory valve line inflates a balloon or puts pressure on a diaphragm during inspiration, closing an orifice through which the patient then exhales when the balloon deflates or when there is a decrease in pressure against the diaphragm. During inspiration the orifice is covered by the balloon or diaphragm. During exhalation, no gas goes through the main inspiratory line or the expiratory valve line. The balloon deflates, and the patient's exhaled volume passes through the open orifice (see Fig. 12.7A, enlarged portion).

Almost all new ventilator circuits use a patient circuit with the exhalation valve mounted inside the machine. These internal valves are usually low-resistance, large-diameter, flexible diaphragms. The advantage of the internal exhalation

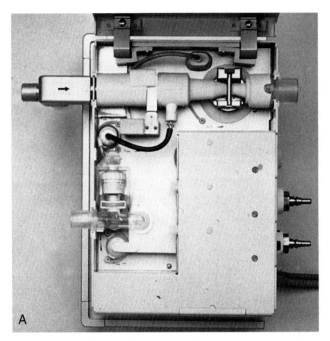

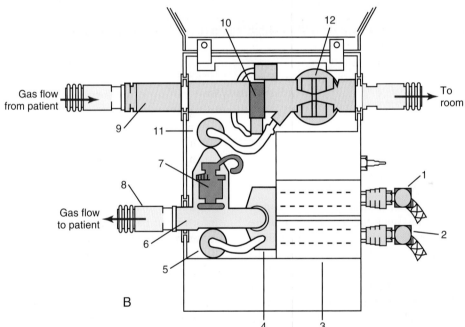

FIGURE 12.6 A, Single-circuit ventilator. B, Air and oxygen (*1* and *2*) are mixed at (*3*), then a flow-control valve in the proximity of (*4*) provides tidal volume (V_T)/pressure/flow to the patient. The exiting gas is measured for pressure (*5*) and enters the inspiratory line (*6*). (*7*) is the housing for the oxygen analyzer, and (*8*) is the main outlet for gas going from the ventilator to the patient. The patient's expired gas passes to the ventilator through the main expiratory connector (*9*), where expiratory gas flows (*10*) and pressure (*11*) are measured.

valve is that it offers little or no resistance to exhalation, which decreases expiratory WOB. The internal exhalation valve is not exposed to the potential damage of the external environment and can be controlled by the ventilator's internal circuit. It operates in a manner similar to that of the externally mounted expiratory valve. During inspiration either gas pressure or a mechanical device pushes the valve over the exhalation orifice. Exhaled gas normally passes through this orifice. During

exhalation the valve is opened, and the patient's exhaled volume can pass through the orifice.

Drive Mechanisms

The power source (gas pressure or electricity), provides the energy to power mechanical devices. This energy and the devices it controls ultimately generate a pressure gradient from the ventilator, through the external circuit, to the patient,

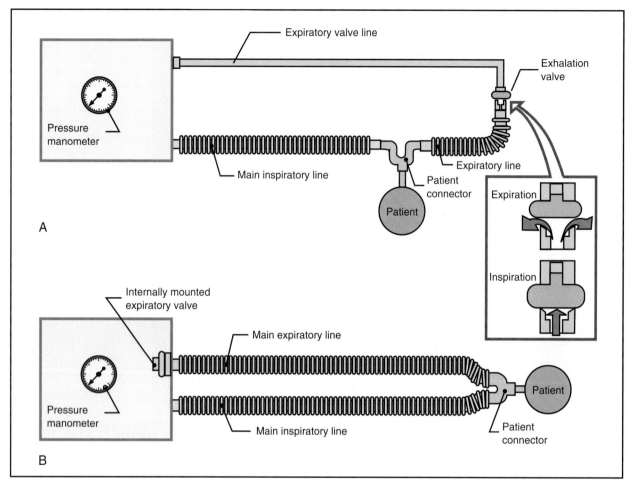

FIGURE 12.7 A, Ventilator circuit with an externally mounted expiratory valve. B, Ventilator circuit with an internally mounted exhalation valve. (See text for further explanation.)

which in turn sets-up the gradient between the opening of the patient's airway pressure (Paw) and the alveoli pressure (P_A) or the P_{TA}, mentioned previously. The pressure gradient provides all or part of the patient's WOB, as defined by the equation of motion, which will be discussed later. The drive mechanism of the ventilator transmits the original energy source (gas, electricity, or both) to direct gas flow to the patient.

From an engineering standpoint, two basic types of drive mechanisms are used in most conventional ventilators: those that control volume delivery and those that control flow delivery.[4-6] For electrically powered ventilators that control volume delivery, compressors, blowers, or volume-displacement devices (such as a piston) are used. For pneumatically powered systems, the power transmission unit utilizes Venturi entrainers, flexible diaphragms, or specially designed pneumatic or fluidic elements. For pneumatically powered, microprocessor-controlled units, the drive mechanism is the source gas pressure from the wall and/or compressor, regulated by flow-control valves (i.e., proportional solenoid valves).

In the past, respiratory therapy students spent a great deal of time studying schematics of ventilator internal circuits because respiratory therapists often were called upon to repair the systems or at least to be able to answer questions about them. More recently, less emphasis has been placed on

respiratory therapists having a working knowledge of this information because they are not typically called upon to repair these devices. The responsibility for repairing ventilators has been assigned to bioengineering technologists and ventilator manufacturer technical support personnel. The following section briefly reviews some examples of volume-displacement devices and flow-control valves.

Compressors or Blowers

Compressors can be driven by pistons, rotating blades (vanes), moving diaphragms, a turbine, or bellows. The most common type of compressor used for ventilators is the rotary compressor or turbine. The rotor acts as a fan, drawing air from the room, compressing it, and directing it through the ventilator's internal circuit. Examples of contemporary ventilators that use an internal rotary device are the CareFusion AVEA ventilator and LTV ventilator (see Chapters 13 and 15).

Volume-Displacement Designs

Some ventilators use volume-displacement devices, including pistons, bellows, or similar "bag-in-a-chamber" mechanisms to deliver a positive-pressure breath.[5] Fig. 12.8 shows an example of a single-circuit piston design. During the backward stroke of the piston, gas is drawn into the piston's cylinder. On the

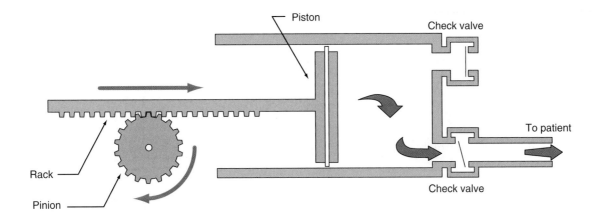

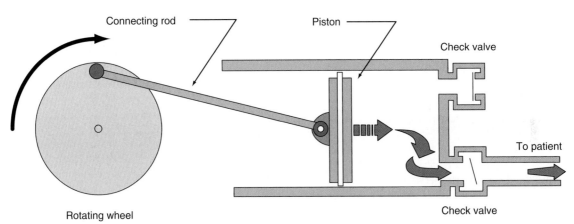

FIGURE 12.8 Piston-driven mechanisms for ventilators. (Redrawn from Dupuis Y: *Ventilators,* ed 2, St. Louis, 1992, Mosby.)

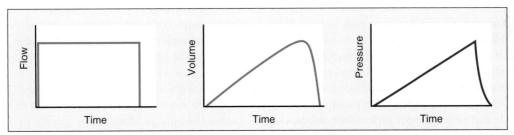

FIGURE 12.9 Flow-time, volume-time, and pressure-time curves generated by a linear-drive piston.

forward stroke of the piston, gas flows out of the cylinder, through the ventilator circuit, and to the patient. Some home care ventilators also use pistons.

Pistons

Two piston designs have been used for ventilators, direct drive and indirect drive. In a **direct-drive piston**, or **linear-drive piston**, gearing connects a motor to a piston rod or arm (see Fig. 12.8). The rod moves the piston forward linearly inside the cylinder housing at a constant rate. This movement produces a constant or rectangular flow scalar to the patient, a linear volume scalar, and a relatively linear ascending ramp pressure scalar (Fig. 12.9). Ventilators that incorporate linear-drive pistons are usually single circuit. Some high-frequency ventilators use direct-drive pistons.

Flow-Control Valves

Most current ICU ventilators use valves that precisely control flow to the patient. In general, high-pressure sources of air and oxygen are mixed and delivered at the desired fraction of inspired oxygen (F_IO_2) to accumulator chambers. These chambers often are similar in shape to medical gas cylinders. They hold approximately 2 to 3 L of gas under pressure and act as reservoirs from which inspired gas for the patient can be withdrawn. The CareFusion AVEA is an example of a ventilator with an accumulator chamber.

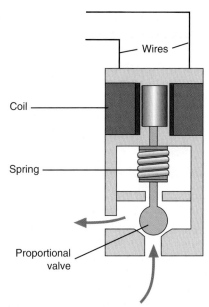

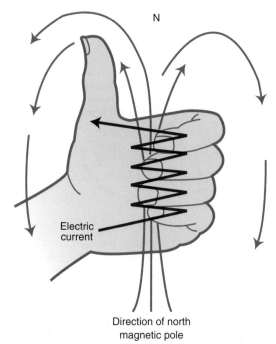

FIGURE 12.10 Proportional solenoid valve. Gas flows upward through the bottom of the valve and out through the side. (See text for description.) (Redrawn from Sanborn WG: Microprocessor-based mechanical ventilation. *Respir Care* 38:72, 1993.)

FIGURE 12.11 A solenoid uses a coil of wire. An electrical current is passed through the coil, generating a magnetic field. The direction of the magnetic field is indicated by the arrows. If you hold your left hand with your thumb pointed up and your fingers slightly curved, the curve of your fingers is the direction of the electrical current through the coil, and your thumb is pointed in the direction of magnetic north. (See text for further explanation.)

Other ventilators, such as the Servo-i (Maquet), take the incoming gas sources individually, regulate their pressures to precise values, and then mix the gases directly without going through an accumulation chamber. This type of system tends to consume less gas during operation than one that uses an accumulator chamber.

Ultimately the gas is sent through one or more valves that control the inspiratory gas flow. These valves can be moved in small, precise increments and at varying rates because their activity is governed by a microprocessor. Because it responds so quickly, a flow-control valve can precisely control the exact pattern of gas and pressure. The more technology has advanced, the faster and more dependable flow valves have become. Three types of flow-controlling valves are typically described: proportional solenoid valves, stepper motors with valves, and digital valves with on/off configurations. Of the three valves mentioned, proportional solenoid valves are used in current ICU ventilators.

Proportional solenoid valves. Proportional solenoid valves control flow by varying the current applied to a plunger that controls the size of an orifice (Fig. 12.10). Commonly this valve has a gate or plunger, a valve seat, an electromagnet, a diaphragm, a spring, two electrical contacts, and an adjustable electric current.

A proportional solenoid valve operates on a basic principle of physics concerning electricity and magnetism. When a current flows through a wire, it creates a magnetic field. Winding a wire into a coil increases the strength of the magnetic field around the wire. Adding an iron rod within the coiled wire further increases the magnetism and produces an electromagnet.

The polarity of an electromagnet can be determined using the left-hand rule (Fig. 12.11). The curved fingers indicate the electric current, and the upward-directed thumb points to the north magnetic pole. When the rod is connected inline in the center of the coiled wire, it moves up and down, depending on the strength of the electric current and the magnetic field it creates. The action of this electromagnet basically describes how solenoid valves operate.[5]

The variation in the amount of current flowing through the coiled wire results in movement of the rod or plunger and causes the plunger to assume a specific position. The term *proportional solenoid valve* is used because the valves move in proportion to the current applied and open a hole or gate a proportional amount. The greater the size of the orifice, the more gas flows through. These proportional solenoid valves are electronically tied to a pneumotachometer that measures the flow and volume that passes across the valve. The valve opens in response to a timer or to a signal from the patient that inspiration is to begin. Once inspiration starts and the valve opens in proportion to the desired flow, it remains open for an operator-set time, then closes when the T_I has elapsed. Because the product of T_I and flow equals V_T, the operator can set an inspiratory flow and a T_I to ensure that a desired volume is delivered to the circuit. A different logic is used for breaths that target pressure.

Examples of ventilators with proportional solenoid valves are the Hamilton G5 (Hamilton Medical), the Dräger Evita (Drägerwerk), and the Maquet Servo-i.

Fluidic Elements in Power Transmission Design

Units that use fluidics, or fluid logic, to deliver gas flow to the patient do not require moving parts or electrical circuits to function. Control is provided solely through fluid dynamics. Fluidic units use air and oxygen as the operating media and have all the same basic functional controls as electrically operated ventilators.[7] The Bio-Med MVP 10 (Bio-Med Devices, Inc.) is an example of a fluidic ventilator.

Because some fluidic ventilators are not disrupted by electromagnetic interference, as is encountered in magnetic resonance imaging (MRI) suites, they can be used in this environment. Of course, they must be constructed of nonferrous metals, such as aluminum. Modifications can also be made to other ventilators to make them MRI compatible.[7]

Fluidic devices operate on two basic physical principles: wall attachment and beam deflection. The principle of wall attachment is commonly called the Coanda effect, a phenomenon that occurs when an air stream (jet stream) is forced through an opening (Historical Note 12.1; Fig. 12.12). The jet exits the opening, creating a localized drop in pressure adjacent to itself. Ambient air is drawn toward the jet stream on all sides as a result of the localized low pressure associated with the rapid movement of the jet through the air (see Fig. 12.12A).

HISTORICAL NOTE 12.1   The Coanda Effect

In 1932 Dr. Henri Coanda, a Romanian aeronautical engineer, first described the "wall attachment" phenomenon. Consequently, this effect now carries his name.

As gas travels faster over a pocket of turbulent air, the increased forward molecular velocity of the gas causes a decreased lateral pressure by the pocket as adjacent molecules are sheared away by the jet stream. The surrounding gas molecules (i.e., those not in the stream) then have a higher pressure, which holds the stream against the wall (see Fig. 12.12).

When a wall is added to one side of the jet stream (see Fig. 12.12B), the entrained gas can enter only from the opposite side. However, a separation bubble (a low-pressure vortex) develops between the wall and the jet stream. The bubble attracts or bends the jet stream toward the wall. The pocket of turbulence forms an air foil, similar to that seen with an airplane wing. When the gas entrained into the bubble from the jet stream equals the amount of air moving from the vortex flow of the bubble back to the jet stream, the attachment is stable.

The second important phenomenon of fluid logic is beam deflection. When a beam or jet of gas is moving through a fluidic device (Fig. 12.13A, P_S to O_2), the direction of the beam can be changed by striking the beam with another jet of gas (see Fig. 12.13B). The second gas jet usually is directed from the side, at a right angle to the main jet stream (see Fig. 12.13B, C_1 to C_2). Note in Fig. 12.13B how this changes the gas output in the device from O_2 to O_1.

The principles of wall attachment and beam deflection can be used to design a host of other devices, which in turn are used in the construction of fluidic ventilators. The nomenclature of fluidics originated in digital electronics, which is the reason many terms (e.g., flip-flop component and *OR/NOR gate*) seem unusual in relation to medical terminology.

Contemporary Drive Mechanisms and Control Valves

For more recently designed ventilators, such as the Servo-i and the Hamilton G5, information from the manufacturers is limited about the specific design of their internal components. This is probably related to the fact that technical support representatives are responsible for the repair of these units.

Additional Devices Used During Patient Ventilation

In addition to the primary drive mechanism of a ventilator, other components are important to its operation. One such component is the expiratory valve.

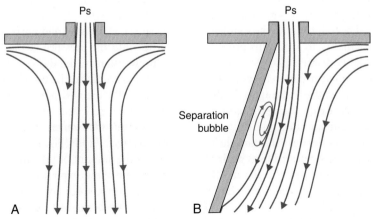

FIGURE 12.12 The Coanda effect (all attachment phenomenon). A, Turbulent jet flow *(P$_s$)* causes a local drop in lateral pressure and draws air inward. B, A wall placed adjacent to the jet stream creates a low-pressure vortex or separation bubble. The gas steam tends to bend toward that wall. (From Dupuis Y: *Ventilators*, ed 2, St. Louis, 1992, Mosby.)

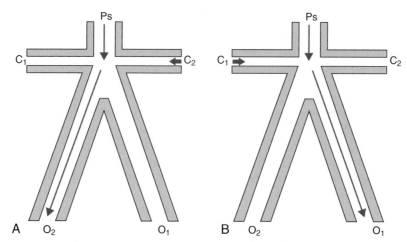

FIGURE 12.13 Diagram of a flip-flop valve illustrating the principle of beam deflection. (See text for explanation.) (From Dupuis Y: *Ventilators*, ed 2, St. Louis, 1992, Mosby.)

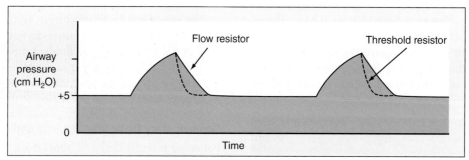

FIGURE 12.14 This airway pressure curve shows a mandatory breath plus positive end-expiratory pressure (PEEP) with two different expiratory flow curves. The solid line indicates pressure with a flow resistor; pressure can vary with flow. The dashed line represents a threshold resistor; flow leaves the lungs rapidly until the set baseline is reached.

Expiratory Valves for Providing Positive End-Expiratory Pressure

Expiratory valves in a ventilator normally close during inspiration, directing gas flow into the patient's lungs. The expiration valve then opens during exhalation, allowing the patient to passively exhale through the valve. Expiratory valves allow unrestricted flow from the patient. Older balloon or diaphragm valves often increased resistance to gas flow when expiratory flow was high or when the patient coughed into the ventilator circuit.[8] Newer ventilator systems try to avoid this problem by using very low-resistance, large-diameter valves.

Besides allowing exhalation to occur passively, with pressures returning to atmospheric, the ventilator can apply positive pressure during exhalation to increase or restore the patient's functional residual capacity (FRC). In certain types of patients, the application of positive pressures during exhalation helps improve oxygenation; this technique is referred to as positive end-expiratory pressure, or PEEP. Use of PEEP elevates the baseline pressure above ambient (zero). Baseline pressure is the pressure sustained during expiration.

When PEEP is selected, it is the threshold-resistive characteristics of the expiratory valve that provide PEEP. The PEEP valve is generally located inside the ventilator housing. Pressure on exhalation can be accomplished in one of two ways:

threshold resistance or flow resistance. Ventilators rely on threshold resistance for the application of PEEP. (*Note:* With flow resistors, expiratory flow is forced through an orifice or a resistor, such as an expiratory retard device like those used in positive expiratory pressure [PEP] masks. The higher the rate of gas flow, the higher the pressure generated. Thus high flows generated during a cough can cause very high pressures in the patient's lungs and airways, which can lead to potential complications.)

Threshold resistors allow expiratory flow to continue unimpeded until the pressure in the circuit equals the threshold value set; that is, the desired PEEP level. A true threshold resistor is unaffected by flow (Fig. 12.14). Current ventilators have PEEP capabilities built into their design and operate through the expiratory valve.

Spring-loaded valves. A spring-loaded valve also may be used to create PEEP (Fig. 12.15). Changing the spring tension adjusts the amount of pressure needed to move the valve off its seat and allows expiration to occur. When the circuit pressure equals the force applied on the valve by the spring, the valve closes. Some of these devices may have flow-resistor characteristics when expiratory flows are high. The CareFusion LTV 1000 is a currently used ventilator with an externally mounted PEEP valve (see Chapter 15). External PEEP valves are also commonly used on manual resuscitation bags.

Diaphragm expiratory valves. Diaphragm expiratory valves commonly incorporate a large-diameter diaphragm to control expiratory gas flow and PEEP. Fig. 12.16 shows the diaphragm valve from a Servo-i ventilator. Fig. 12.17 uses a balloon to illustrate the function of the expiratory valve. During inspiration the ventilator pressurizes the diaphragm (illustrated as a balloon) and closes an expiratory orifice (see Fig. 12.17A). During normal expiration the pressure against the diaphragm (balloon) is released, and the patient's expiratory gas flow continues unimpeded (see Fig. 12.17C). When PEEP is applied, a proportional pressure is held against the diaphragm (balloon) so that the pressure at the end of exhalation is equal to the PEEP value set by the operator (see Fig. 12.17B).

Electromagnetic valves are slightly different from magnetic valves, because solenoids are often used in their construction. In an electromagnetic valve a rheostat is used to regulate the amount of electric current that flows to the solenoid. The solenoid creates a downward force through an actuating shaft. The actuating shaft pushes against a diaphragm, which opposes expiratory gas flow. The stronger the current, the stronger the downward force and the higher the PEEP level. The Maquet Servo-i, Medtronic Minimally Invasive Therapies Puritan Bennett 840, and Hamilton ventilators use an electromagnetic device to control the expiratory diaphragm that controls the level of PEEP in the patient circuit.

Continuous Positive Airway Pressure Devices

Continuous positive airway pressure (CPAP) is very similar to PEEP. CPAP provides positive airway pressure, but it is restricted by definition to use in spontaneously breathing patients. A number of CPAP devices are available for home care to treat sleep apnea (these CPAP machines are described in Chapter 15). CPAP systems are also routinely used for

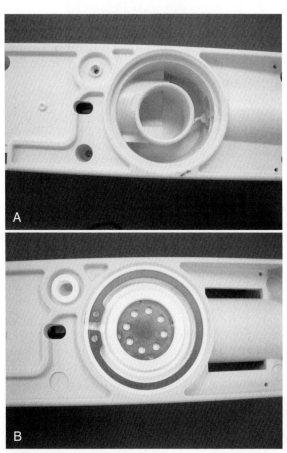

FIGURE 12.16 Diaphragm expiratory valve on the Servo-i ventilator. A, Housing over which the expiratory diaphragm (valve) normally sits. The visible openings represent the channels through which expiratory gas is routed when the diaphragm is in position to allow exhalation. B, Diaphragm in position over the opening.

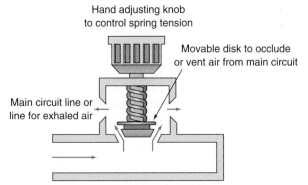

FIGURE 12.15 Spring-loaded positive end-expiratory pressure (PEEP) valve.

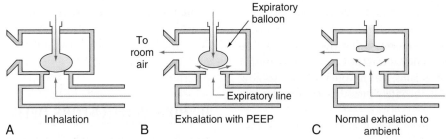

FIGURE 12.17 Functioning of a diaphragm expiratory valve. A, A balloon valve is used to illustrate inspiration; the balloon is fully inflated during inspiration, blocking the expiratory channel. Diaphragm valves function in the same way. B, The expiratory valve (balloon or diaphragm) remains partially pressured during exhalation and closes to keep positive pressure in the circuit at end-exhalation. C, The expiratory valve opens completely to allow unimpeded flow of the exhaled gas. (See text for description.) *PEEP,* Positive end-expiratory pressure.

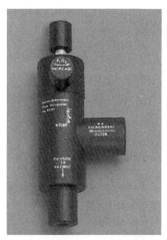

FIGURE 12.18 Downs continuous positive airway pressure (CPAP) generator. (Courtesy Vital Signs Corp., Totowa, NJ.)

neonates with hypoxemic respiratory failure (see Chapter 14). CPAP also is effective for certain types of hospitalized pediatric and adult patients who are able to breathe spontaneously but who need help with oxygenation. Cardiogenic pulmonary edema and hypoxemic respiratory failure are examples of illnesses for which CPAP often is indicated. In general, CPAP is provided using a ventilator or commercially available CPAP device.

In a CPAP device, blended gas at the desired F_IO_2 can be obtained from air and oxygen flowmeters, from a blender, or from a CPAP generator. The gas is warmed and humidified when an artificial airway is in place or if the patient is uncomfortable breathing ambient air. A threshold resistor is attached to the expiratory end of the system. For example, the Downs CPAP generator (Fig. 12.18) is connected to a gas source. A large-bore tube (22 mm) connects the generator with the patient's mask interface (Fig. 12.19). The amount of CPAP is adjusted with a spring-loaded CPAP valve on the mask, as seen in Fig. 12.19. Most valves are spring loaded with fixed pressures (e.g., 5 cm H_2O, 7.5 cm H_2O) although other masks can be adjusted by tightening the spring. For monitoring purposes a pressure manometer can be added to the circuit to monitor circuit pressure.

Ideally, a safety pressure-release valve is incorporated into a CPAP system. The safety pressure-release valve setting is slightly higher than the desired CPAP level. For example, if the CPAP is 10 cm H_2O, the safety pressure release might be set at 15 cm H_2O. If the normal threshold resistor (or, in this case, spring-loaded valve) jams, which would prevent gas flow from exiting the system, the safety pressure-release valve acts as a pop-off valve.

Including a safety pop-in valve is also important in case the source gas is turned off accidentally. A safety pop-in valve provides a source of ambient air for the patient in the event of loss of a source gas. These pop-in valves generally open at a fairly low pressure (−1 to −2 cm H_2O).

Because a variety of problems can occur with a CPAP system, the operator must make sure the safety systems (i.e.,

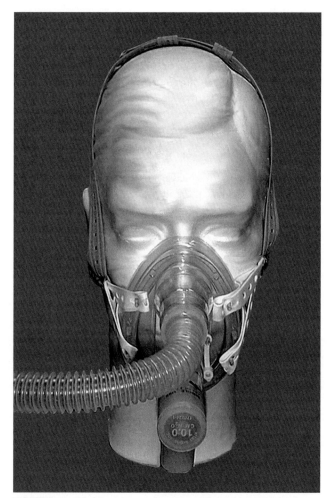

FIGURE 12.19 Model wearing a continuous positive airway pressure (CPAP) mask (spring-loaded valve) connected to a large-bore circuit, which connects to the Downs CPAP generator (see Fig. 12.20). Air flows into the large-bore tubing on the left to the patient. Air exits through the valve mounted on the mask (bottom of the mask). (Courtesy Vital Signs Corp., Totowa, NJ.)

pop-off and pop-in valves) are in place and the patient is monitored. Some potential problems are:

- Inadequate flow to the patient
- Leaks in the system
- Loss of source gas flow
- Jamming or obstruction of the expiratory threshold resistor

Clinical Scenario 12.2 presents some exercises involving problems related to CPAP systems like the one previously described.

II. HOW VENTILATORS DELIVER BREATHS

Perspectives on Ventilator Classification

The use of mechanical ventilators for the treatment of critically ill patients first appeared in the medical literature in the 1950s and 1960s. Mushin et al.[9] subsequently introduced a classification system of mechanical ventilators that was designed to describe how ventilators work on the basis of physical

Troubleshooting Freestanding Continuous Positive Airway Pressure Systems

Problem 1

A patient attached to a freestanding, continuous-flow CPAP system (e.g., the Downs CPAP generator) set at 10 cm H_2O appears to be in distress (e.g., supraclavicular retractions, accessory muscle use, pale and diaphoretic). The operator notices that the manometer drops to -1 cm H_2O during inspiration and rises to 10 cm H_2O during expiration. What do you think is the problem?

Problem 2

The low oxygen saturation alarm is sounding on a patient connected to a continuous-flow CPAP system. The operator notices that the manometer fluctuates around the zero point during both inspiration and expiration. What is the problem?
  See Appendix A for the answers.

CPAP, Continuous positive airway pressure.

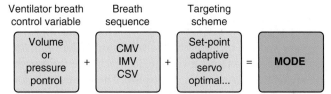

FIGURE 12.20 Classification system uses a defined set of criteria to classify ventilator modes. The system is based on the ventilator breath control variable, the breath sequence, and the targeting scheme.

TABLE 12.1 Ten Basic Maxims for Understanding Ventilator Operation[18]

1. A breath is one cycle of positive flow (inspiration) and negative flow (expiration) defined in terms of the flow versus time curve.
2. A breath is assisted if the ventilator provides some or all of the work of breathing.
3. A ventilator assists breathing using either pressure control or volume control based on the equation of motion for the respiratory system.
4. Breaths are classified according to the criteria that trigger (start) and cycle (stop) inspiration.
5. Trigger and cycle events can be either patient initiated or ventilator initiated.
6. Breaths are classified as spontaneous or mandatory based on both the trigger and cycle events.
7. Ventilators deliver three basic breath sequences: CMV, IMV, and CSV.
8. Ventilators deliver five basic breath patterns: VC-CMV, VC-IMV, PC-CMV, PC-IMV, PC-CSV.
9. Within each ventilatory pattern, there are several types that can be distinguished by their targeting schemes (set-point, dual, biovariable, servo, adaptive, optimal, and intelligent).
10. A mode of ventilation is classified according to its control variable, breath sequence, and targeting schemes.

CMV, Continuous mandatory ventilation; *CSV,* continuous spontaneous ventilation; *IMV,* intermittent mandatory ventilation; *PC,* pressure control; *VC,* volume control.

function. Considerable advances in ventilator technology have occurred during the past 50 years, leading many to advocate for the introduction of an updated classification system.[10-13] Indeed, respiratory therapists and physicians are often perplexed by the names associated with different modes and breath types. Part of this confusion exists because ventilator manufacturers often use different names for a mode that is similar to one that exists on a competitor's ventilator. For example, Autoflow on the Dräger Evita XL (Drägerwerk) ventilator is similar in function to pressure-regulated volume control (PRVC) on the Servo-i (Maquet).

Chatburn and colleagues have provided an updated classification system that addresses many of the concerns expressed by clinicians who work with mechanical ventilators.[4,14-17] As Fig. 12.20 illustrates, this classification system uses a defined set of criteria to classify ventilator modes: (1) the ventilator breath control variable, (2) the breath sequence, and (3) the targeting scheme. For example, does the therapist want to use a ventilatory strategy designed to target a specific volume delivered to the patient, or is the pressure delivered to the patient a greater concern? Are breaths mandatory, spontaneous, or a combination of the two (continuous mandatory ventilation, continuous spontaneous ventilation, or intermittent mandatory ventilation)? What is the relationship between operator inputs and ventilator outputs to achieve a specific ventilator pattern?

Table 12.1 provides a summary of criteria proposed by Chatburn to classify various modes of ventilation.[18] The following is a brief discussion of these criteria.

1. **A breath is one cycle of positive flow (inspiration) and negative flow (expiration) defined in terms of the flow versus time curve.**

   Fig. 12.21 shows a flow versus time curve (scalar), in which the x axis is time and the y axis is flow. Positive flow (inspiration) is indicated as flow above the baseline, whereas negative flow (expiration) is indicated as flow below the baseline. The duration of positive flow is the inspiratory time, and the duration of negative flow is the expiratory time. Although not often set, any pause between the end of inspiratory flow and the onset of expiratory flow is referred to as inspiratory pause or pause time. Inspiratory time includes any inspiratory pause time. From the end of inspiratory flow to the onset of the next inspiration is the expiratory time. There may be a pause from the end of active expiration to the beginning of the next inspiration, called expiratory pause time. The ratio of inspiratory time to expiratory time is the inspiratory:expiratory ratio. The percent of the total cycle time (TCT) that is inspiration is the duty cycle. The sum of the inspiratory and expiratory times is the TCT or ventilatory period. The shape of the

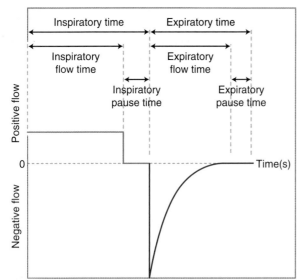

FIGURE 12.21 A flow versus time curve (scalar) for a mechanically delivered breath. Positive flow (inspiration) is indicated as flow above the baseline, whereas negative flow (expiration) is indicated as flow below the baseline. The duration of positive flow is the inspiratory time, and the duration of negative flow is the expiratory time.

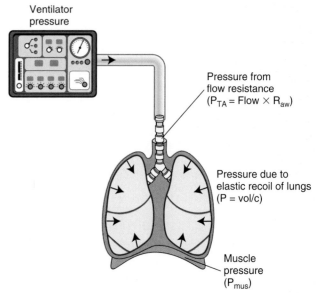

FIGURE 12.22 Model of the equation of motion: Muscle pressure + Ventilator pressure = Elastic recoil pressure + Flow resistance pressure. (See text for description.) P_{TA}, Transairway pressure; R_{aw}, airway resistance.

flow curve defines the pressure and volume curves, which will be described later.

2. **A breath is assisted if the ventilator provides some or all of the work of breathing.**

   An **assisted breath** is one in which the airway pressure rises during inspiration, because the ventilator is providing some or all of the WOB. In some modes, all the breaths are assisted, whereas in others none are. That is, the patient is breathing spontaneously. On an airway pressure curve, the airway pressure (or transairway pressure) rises during the inspiratory time in an assisted breath. If the airway pressure does not rise, then the ventilator is providing flow consistent with the patient's inspiratory effort, as in CPAP, in which pressure does not rise during inspiration. Transrespiratory pressure remains constant throughout the breath.

3. **A ventilator assists breathing using either pressure control or volume control based on the equation of motion for the respiratory system.**

   One approach that can be used to describe the mechanics of breathing during mechanical ventilation involves using a mathematical model that is based on the *equation of motion*. The equation, $P(t) = EV(T) + RV(t)$ states that the pressure needed to inflate the lungs is a function of the lung elastance (elastic resistance or load) plus the airways resistance. During mechanical ventilation, as summarized in Box 12.4 and Fig. 12.22, two forces are available to perform the WOB: the force generated by the ventilator and the force generated by contraction of the patient's respiratory muscles. For a single breath the compliance and resistance of the respiratory system do not change significantly, but the volume, pressure, flow, and time can vary and are regulated by the ventilator.[15] The ventilator may be set to target a volume, in which case the breaths are referred to as volume controlled. The volume and flow are set before inspiration. A flow is set (usually 50 to 70 L/min), followed by a tidal volume. However, the tidal volume setting is actually an inspiratory time setting, because flow × time = volume. The peak pressure varies with tidal volume, compliance, and resistance. In volume control, changes in compliance or resistance will result in a change in airway pressure. Or, the ventilator may be set to control pressure, in which case the breaths are referred to as pressure controlled. A peak pressure above baseline is selected, as is an inspiratory time. Tidal volume varies with the difference between peak and baseline pressure and patient effort. In pressure control, peak pressure remains constant with changes in compliance or resistance.

The first component of defining a mode is to label the mode as either volume or pressure controlled (VC or PC). Some modes are dual controlled. This usually means that assisted breaths are volume or pressure controlled and the spontaneous breaths that occur between assisted breaths are pressure controlled and may be assisted or spontaneous, as in intermittent mandatory ventilation (IMV).

In the case of HFPPV, breaths are time controlled. This means that pressure, volume, and flow are not preset. The only parameters that are set are the inspiratory and expiratory times (which determine rate) and $P_{\overline{aw}}$.

4. **Breaths are classified according to the criteria that trigger (start) and cycle (stop) inspiration.**

Phases of a Breath (Phase Variables)

When the term *breath* is used, it usually refers to inspiration. However, total respiratory cycle must be considered when

---

BOX 12.4 Equation of Motion

The equation of motion is a mathematical model that represents the interaction between the patient and the ventilator during inspiration (and expiration). The simplest version of this equation assumes that the complex respiratory system can be represented by a single resistance, R, representing the airways and the artificial airway (connected in series) and a single elastance, E, representing the lungs and chest wall.

There are two pressures to move gas into the lung, the pressure needed to move gas through the airway (flow resistance pressure) and the pressure to expand the lung and thorax (elastic recoil pressure). These two pressures are provided by the respiratory muscles (muscle pressure) and/or by a ventilator (ventilator pressure).

Equation 1

Muscle pressure + Ventilator pressure
= Elastic recoil pressure + Flow resistance pressure

Or, an abbreviated form can be used:

Equation 2

$$\Delta P_{TR(t)} + \Delta P_{mus(t)} = EV_{(t)} + R\dot{V}_{(t)} + \text{auto-PEEP}$$

Where:

$\Delta P_{TR(t)}$ = the change in transrespiratory pressure difference (i.e., airway opening pressure minus body surface pressure) as a function of time (t), measured relative to end-expiratory airway pressure. This is the pressure generated by a ventilator (Δp_{vent}) during an assisted breath; in other words, the work done on the lungs by the ventilator.

$\Delta P_{mus(t)}$ = ventilator muscle pressure difference as a function of time (t); the theoretical chest wall transmural pressure difference that would produce movements identical to those produced by the ventilator muscles during breathing maneuvers (positive during inspiratory effort, negative during expiratory effort); in other words, the work done on the lungs by the muscles of ventilation. The contribution by the ventilator and muscles of ventilation varies throughout the course of ventilation. Sometimes all the work is done by the ventilator, whereas at other times, the patient carries part of the work.

$V_{(t)}$ = volume change relative to end expiratory volume as a function of time.

$\dot{V}_{(t)}$ = flow as a function of time (t), the first derivative of volume with respect to time.

E = elastance (the reciprocal of compliance; E = 1/C).

auto-PEEP = end-expiratory alveolar pressure above end-expiratory airway pressure.

For the purposes of classifying modes (breathing patterns) in mechanical ventilation the equation is simplified to:

$$P_{vent} = EV + R\dot{V}$$
$$= \frac{cm\ H_2O}{mL} \times mL + cm\ H_2O/mL/min \times mL/min$$

Where P_{vent} is the transrespiratory pressure difference (i.e., airway pressure) generated by the ventilator during an assisted breath.

Or, still further:

Muscle pressure + ventilator pressure
= pressure to overcome elastic resistance
+ pressure to overcome airway resistance

---

defining a breath; that is, the time required for both inspiration (T_I) and expiration (T_E) and the events that occur during that time. This time frame is also called the total cycle time (TCT). A ventilator must be capable of separating a breath into four parts, which proceed as follows (Box 12.5):

1. The trigger variable begins inspiration.
2. The cycle variable ends the inspiratory phase and begins exhalation.
3. The limit variable limits the value for pressure, flow, volume, or time during delivery of inspiration, but it *does not end the breath*. The limit variable is defined by a plateau on the scalar in question. For example, if there is a plateau on the volume scalar, the breath is said to be volume limited. Similarly, if the pressure or flow scalar plateaus during the breath, then the breaths are described as pressure and flow limited, respectively.
4. The baseline variable establishes where the baseline is before a breath is triggered. Usually, the baseline variable is pressure. Pressures and flows can be controlled during exhalation; thus the ventilator is involved in controlling the expiratory phase.

BOX 12.5 Four Phases of a Breath During Mechanical Ventilation and Phase Variables

Breath Phases
1. End of expiration and beginning of inspiration
2. Delivery of inspiration
3. End of inspiration and beginning of expiration
4. Expiratory phase

Phase Variables
Phase variables are controlled by the ventilator and are responsible for each of the four parts of a breath. These variables are:

- *Triggering:* Begins inspiratory gas flow
- *Limiting:* Places a maximum value on a control variable (pressure, volume, flow, or time) during delivery of a breath
- *Cycling:* Ends inspiratory gas flow

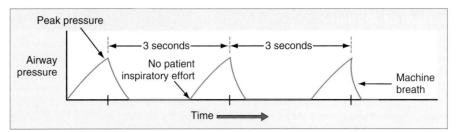

FIGURE 12.23 Time-triggered breaths. (From Cairo JM: *Pilbeam's mechanical ventilation: physiological and clinical applications*, ed 5, St. Louis, 2012, Mosby.)

Beginning of Inspiration: the Trigger Variable

The trigger variable begins the inspiratory phase. Breaths can be time, pressure, flow, or volume triggered.

When a pressure, flow, or volume generated by the patient begins the breath, the patient controls the beginning of inspiration; the umbrella term for these phenomena is patient triggering. Ventilators can be adjusted to sense the patient's inspiratory effort. The control set by the operator is commonly called the *sensitivity setting,* or trigger sensitivity. Pressure and flow are the most common variables used for patient triggering, but volume and neural triggering from the diaphragm can also be used.

The trigger variable should not be confused with the cycle variable. Triggering begins inspiration; cycling (as discussed later) ends inspiration. This difference is mentioned because the term *cycle* historically meant the variable that began the breath, and some journal articles and technical manuals occasionally use this terminology.

Time triggering. As noted, with time triggering the ventilator controls the beginning of inspiration based on the TCT, which in turn controls the set mandatory rate. The breath is mandatory because the ventilator determines that it is time to trigger, based on expiration of TCT (TCT = T_I + T_E or TCT = 60/mandatory rate). A mandatory breath is one that is started or stopped by the ventilator, as opposed to patient respiratory mechanics. For example, if the rate is set at 20 breaths/min as in Fig. 12.23, a breath occurs every 3 seconds. Inspiratory flow starts 3 seconds after the last inspiration, thus providing time triggering.

Pressure triggering. Pressure triggering occurs when the ventilator senses a drop in airway pressure below baseline in the circuit. Pressure triggering usually is set at −0.5 to −1.5 cm H_2O. In other words, the patient must make an inspiratory effort of −0.5 to −1.5 cm H_2O to reduce the airway pressure below baseline to begin inspiration (Fig. 12.24). Baseline pressure is the pressure maintained at the airway at the end of active expiration (expiratory flow is ended) and the pressure from which inspiration begins. (See the discussion of the expiratory phase later in this section under "Expiratory Phase: Baseline Variable.")

Pressure can be measured using pressure transducers or sensors placed at various locations in the ventilator circuit:

- Within the internal ventilator circuit near the point where the main gas flow leaves the unit
- Where expired gas returns to the unit from the patient
- At the proximal airway (near the Y-connector)

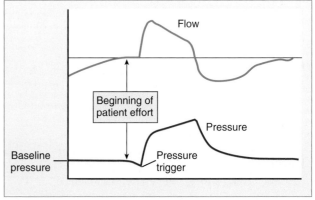

FIGURE 12.24 Pressure-triggered breath. When the pressure drops to the pressure trigger level, the inspiratory flow begins.

📌 **CLINICAL SCENARIO 12.3**
Pressure Triggering

A patient has a baseline pressure of 10 cm H_2O during mechanical ventilation. The trigger sensitivity is set at −1 cm H_2O. At what pressure will the ventilator sense a patient effort and start inspiration?

See Appendix A for the answer.

In the third case a small-bore plastic tubing extends from the ventilator to the patient's Y-connector (Clinical Scenario 12.3). (See Chapter 8 for further information on pressure-monitoring devices.)

Flow triggering. Flow triggering occurs when a drop in flow is detected. In some ventilators a pneumotachometer (see Chapter 8) is located between the ventilator circuit and the artificial airway or patient to measure flow. In others a background flow, also called a *base* or *bias flow,* is set either by the operator or by the ventilator itself (a default value). This flow is present during the expiratory phase. For example, the base flow may be set at approximately 5 to 10 L/min. A flow trigger is also set and can range from approximately 1 to 5 L/min, although this value varies with the type of ventilator used, the patient's size (baby or adult), and inspiratory effort. Most ventilator manufacturers recommend a value or have default values. The ventilator measures the base flow during exhalation. When the flow drops by the amount set on the flow trigger, inspiration begins. For example, if the base flow is set at 7 L/min and the trigger is set at 3 L/min, the ventilator begins inspiration when the expiratory flow is measured at 4 L/min (7 L/min – 3 L/min = 4 L/min). Figs. 12.25 and 12.26 show flow-trigger graphics and a flow-triggering device. Clinical Scenario 12.4 presents a practice problem in flow triggering.

Volume triggering. Volume triggering occurs after the patient has inhaled a specific volume from the circuit. By adjusting the trigger sensitivity, the operator can change the effort required by the patient to begin inspiration.

Fig. 12.27 shows how to determine the type of trigger variable used.

Other triggering mechanisms. Other methods of triggering include the following:
1. Manual triggering, in which the operator activates the "manual breath" or "start breath" control on the ventilator control panel and delivers a mandatory breath based on the set variables.
2. Neural triggering from the electrical activity of the diaphragm, which is called **neurally adjusted ventilatory assist (NAVA)** and is available on the Maquet Servo-i.

Inspiratory Phase

One of the most important ventilator functions is delivery of inspiratory gas flow.

Delivery of inspiratory flow is regulated primarily by a control variable. The three variables the ventilator can control are represented in the equation of motion described earlier—volume, flow, and pressure. The ventilator can control only one of these variables at a time.[7] (*Note:* It is intuitively

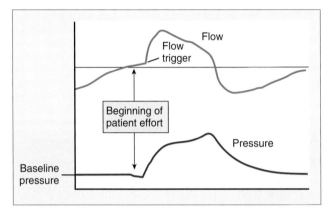

FIGURE 12.25 Flow-triggered breath. When the flow reaches the set flow-trigger level, the inspiratory flow begins.

> ### CLINICAL SCENARIO 12.4
> **Flow Triggering**
>
> The operator decides to use flow triggering for a patient and sets the base flow at 6 L/min and the trigger flow at 2 L/min. The base flow measurement must drop to what value before the ventilator will begin the inspiratory phase?
> See Appendix A for the answer.

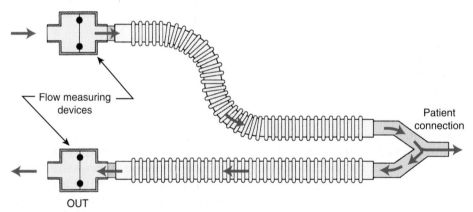

FIGURE 12.26 Schematic of flow triggering, which occurs when the patient makes an inspiratory effort and drops the flow through the patient circuit to the trigger level. (From Dupuis Y: *Ventilators*, ed 2, St. Louis, 1992, Mosby.)

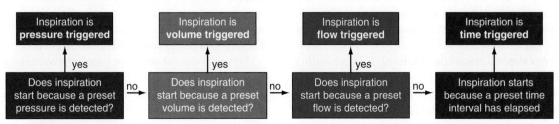

FIGURE 12.27 Criteria for determining the trigger variable during a breath on a mechanical ventilator. The determination is based on observation of the ventilator and ventilator graphics and on previous knowledge. (Modified from Wilkins RL, Stoller JK, Kacmarek RM: *Egan's fundamentals of respiratory care*, ed 9, St. Louis, 2009, Mosby.)

BOX 12.6   Other Names for Volume and Pressure Ventilation

Volume Ventilation
Volume-limited ventilation
Volume-controlled ventilation
Volume-targeted ventilation

Pressure Ventilation
Pressure-limited ventilation
Pressure-controlled ventilation
Pressure-targeted ventilation

CLINICAL SCENARIO 12.5
Breath Variables

Before inspiration the pressure drops to −1 cm H_2O on the pressure manometer, and then inspiratory flow begins. During inspiration the pressure rises to 20 cm H_2O and stays at 20 cm H_2O for 1.2 seconds. Then expiration begins. What are the trigger, limit, and cycle variables?
  See Appendix A for the answer.

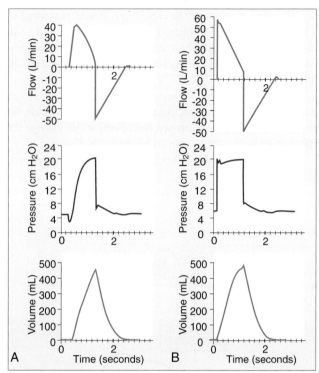

FIGURE 12.28 The effect of rise time, or sloping adjustment, during pressure-support ventilation. The top graph is flow-time, the middle graph is pressure-time, and the bottom graph is volume-time. Breath A, on the left, shows a slow rise time. Breath B, on the right, shows a more rapid rise time. Note how the pressure-time curve is visibly tapered in breath A compared to breath B. Flow is also tapered in breath A when the two are compared. (See text for further explanation.)

understood that time is a part of the equation of motion. However, time generally is not the control variable selected to regulate inspiration.)

In theory, a ventilator that truly controls volume would directly measure volume by using a volume-measuring device such as a bellows or piston.[15] This is the historical definition of volume controlled. Current ventilators do not directly measure volume; however, volume can be controlled indirectly by controlling and measuring flow and time. A volume of gas is simply a flow of gas delivered within a certain time frame. If the flow and the time during which it is delivered are known, the volume can be determined (V_T = Inspiratory Flow × Inspiratory Time). Therefore a volume breath is one in which flow is also controlled (i.e., a flow-controlled breath; Box 12.6).

With pressure-controlled ventilation (PCV), pressure remains constant during inspiration, but the volume and flow delivered may change if the patient's lung characteristics change. See Clinical Scenario 12.5 for a problem related to breath variables.

Because time is not commonly used as a control variable, it was excluded from the previous discussion of these variables. However, when a ventilator delivers a time-controlled breath, pressure, volume, and flow may vary with changes in lung characteristics. Time is constant. Examples of timed breaths are those produced during *high-frequency jet ventilation* (HFJV) and high-frequency oscillation.

Sloping or ramping. Most contemporary ICU ventilators allow the operator to adjust the slope of the pressure and flow curves at the beginning of inspiration, as a function of the percentage of the T_I. This feature, (called *ramping, inspiratory rise time adjustment, rise time, flow acceleration percent, inspiratory rise time percent, slope adjustment,* or *sloping),* allows the operator to vary the flow at the very beginning of inspiration. When no sloping is selected, the ventilator delivers gas

very rapidly at the beginning of inspiration. Flow and pressure rise to their set value as quickly as possible. On the other hand, when the operator uses the sloping or rise time control, pressure and flow delivery are tapered slightly until they reach their maximum value (Fig. 12.28).

With some ventilators, sloping can be used for either pressure-controlled (or targeted) breaths or volume-controlled (or targeted) breaths. Other ventilators allow sloping only with pressure-targeted breaths. Additional information about sloping or ramping is available for selected ventilators reviewed in Chapter 13.

Waveforms and graphics. Monitoring and evaluation of graphic waveforms produced during ventilation are one method of determining the control variable. Although more detailed information about ventilator waveform graphics is available elsewhere,[1] a brief summary is provided here.

Pressure, volume, and flow graphed over time are referred to as *scalars* (i.e., pressure-time, volume-time, and flow-time). The scalars for volume/flow-controlled ventilation, PCV, and a variation of PCV (**continuous spontaneous ventilation** [CSV]) are shown in Fig. 12.29. In Figs. 12.29A, B, and C, the top scalar is volume, the middle scalar is flow, and the bottom scalar is pressure. Fig. 12.29A illustrates the scalars for volume- or flow-controlled CMV. All breaths are time or patient triggered, flow limited, and time cycled. Fig. 12.29B shows the scalars for pressure-controlled CMV. All breaths are time or patient triggered, pressure limited, and time cycled. Fig. 12.29C provides the scalars for CSV. All breaths are patient triggered, pressure limited, and flow cycled. Individually, or in combination, these scalars represent most of the modes to be discussed in this chapter.

Fig. 12.28 illustrates the scalars that are produced during CSV varying with varying rise times. With a slow rise time (see Fig. 12.28A), it takes longer for the pressure scalar to "square-off," if it ever does. With a faster (lower percent) rise time, the pressure scalar "squares-off" quickly (see Fig. 12.28B). Fig. 12.30 shows examples of pressure, volume, and flow scalars produced with several methods of pressure and volume

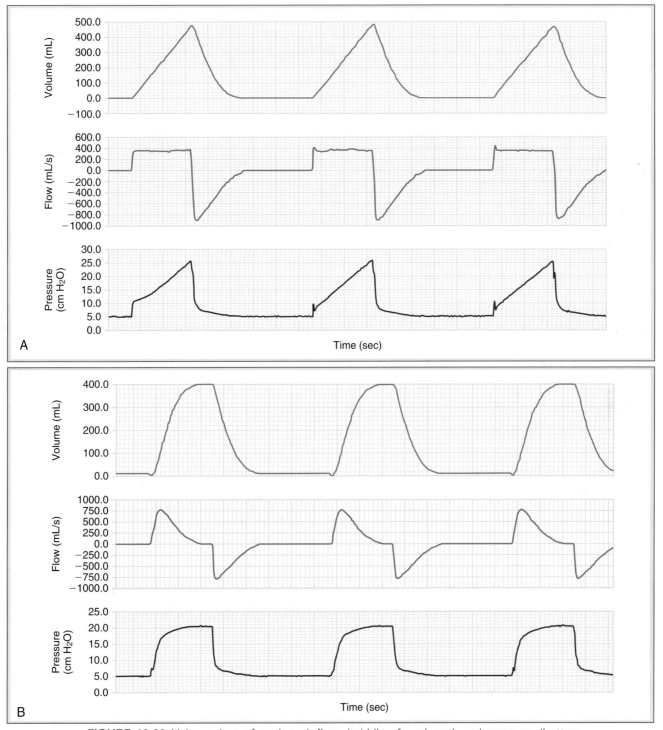

FIGURE 12.29 Volume *(top of each set)*, flow *(middle of each set)*, and pressure *(bottom of each set)* scalars for (A) volume/flow-controlled continuous mandatory ventilation (CMV); (B) pressure-controlled ventilation (PC-CMV); *Continued*

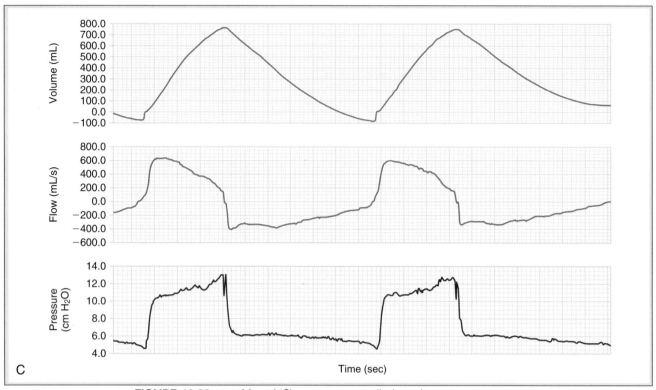

FIGURE 12.29, cont'd and (C) pressure-controlled continuous spontaneous ventilation (PC-CSV or pressure support). See text for details.

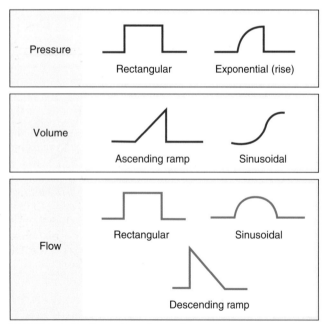

FIGURE 12.30 Examples of waveforms for pressure, volume, and flow. Pressure waveforms usually are the rectangular or rising exponential (similar to an ascending ramp) type. Volume waveforms usually are the ascending ramp or sinusoidal (sine-like) type. Flow waveforms can take various forms; the rectangular, ramp (ascending or descending), sinusoidal, and decaying exponential types are seen most often. (From Cairo: *Pilbeam's mechanical ventilation*, ed 5, St. Louis, 2011, Mosby-Elsevier).

ventilation. The shape of the pressure and volume scalars is dependent on the velocity of flow from moment to moment. A continuous (rectangular) flow tends to produce a linear (ascending ramp) pressure and volume rise. A decelerating (descending ramp) flow produces a "squared" or exponential rise in pressure and volume. Sinusoidal flow is rarely used, except in HFV.

During volume-controlled ventilation (VCV), volume and flow remain constant, while pressure changes with compliance, as shown in Fig. 12.31. During PCV the delivered pressure remains constant, regardless of changes in the patient's lung condition, but volume and flow delivery vary (Fig. 12.32).

Limit variable. As previously discussed, the ventilator controls one of the three primary control variables (pressure, flow, or volume) during inspiration and can also limit the variables. A limit variable has a maximum value that cannot be exceeded during inspiration because the ventilator does not allow it; however, reaching the limit does not end inspiratory flow to the patient. The limit variable reaches a plateau before the end of inspiration. If the pressure reaches a plateau before the end of inspiration during PCV (which is often the case, especially when the T_I is increased), the breath is pressure limited. When a square wave flow is used during VCV, flow plateaus and is the limit variable. Fig. 12.33 provides a simple algorithm for determining the limit variable (Clinical Scenario 12.6).

A breath is considered flow limited if the flow reaches a maximum value before the end of inspiration but does not exceed that value. (When a peak flow is reached and remains constant throughout inspiration, the flow scalar is square, and the breath is flow limited.) Pressure limiting sets a maximum value for pressure, which is not exceeded during inspiration. After the pressure is reached, T_I may continue, but no more pressure (and thus no more volume) is delivered to the patient (Fig. 12.34). Some ventilators have pressure-limited capabilities and use a mode called *time-cycled, **pressure-limited ventilation*** (Clinical Scenario 12.7) (see Chapter 13, CareFusion AVEA ventilator).

Maximum safety pressure/high pressure alarm setting. All ventilators have some type of feature that allows inspiratory pressure to reach but not exceed a maximum value during inspiration. This pressure is usually set by the operator at 10 cm H_2O above the peak pressure reached during inspiration. This particular setting on the control panel can have a variety of names (Box 12.7); the purpose of this feature is to prevent excessive pressure from damaging lung tissue. In most adult ventilators, if there is an obstruction in the ventilator circuit (kinking, cough, secretions), inspiratory flow ends, and the ventilator cycles out of inspiration because the usual peak pressure + 10 cm H_2O is reached. Unfortunately, the labeling used on the control panel of most ventilators includes the term *pressure limit*, which leads to confusion because this feature usually cycles the ventilator out of inspiration (as a safety feature) and does not just limit the pressure allowing the T_I to expire.

A common misconception about PCV is that if a specific pressure is set for the control variable (e.g., 20 cm H_2O), the

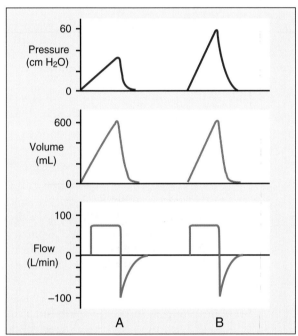

FIGURE 12.31 Example of a patient's lung condition becoming worse during volume-targeted ventilation. The top scalar is pressure, the middle scalar is volume, and the bottom scalar is flow. A, The scalars demonstrate normal pressure, volume, and flow. B, The scalars demonstrate that the patient's lungs have reduced compliance, showing increased pressure delivery while the volume and flow scalars remain constant.

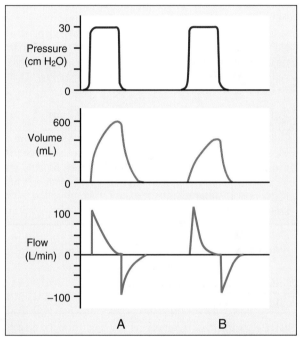

FIGURE 12.32 Examples of scalars for pressure-targeted ventilation. The top scalar is pressure, the middle scalar is volume, and the bottom scalar is flow. A, Breath A scalars demonstrate normal pressure, volume, and flow curves. B, Breath B scalars demonstrate a patient with reduced lung compliance, showing reduced volume delivery. Note that for breath B the flow scalar returns to the zero baseline before exhalation begins. This is an example of a *pause* in pressure at the end of inspiration during pressure ventilation.

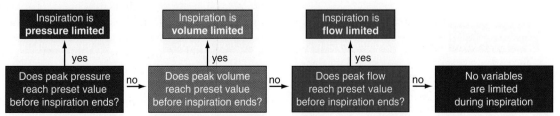

FIGURE 12.33 Criteria for determining the limit variable during a breath on a mechanical ventilator. The determination is based on observation of the ventilator and ventilator graphics and on previous knowledge. (Modified from Chatburn RL, Volsko TA: Mechanical ventilators. In Wilkins RL, Stoller JK, Kacmarek RM: *Egan's fundamentals of respiratory care*, ed 9, St. Louis, 2009, Mosby.)

pressure cannot exceed that value. This is not true. If a patient coughs, the pressure can rise above the set value. It is important to set a safe upper pressure limit during pressure ventilation so that excessively high pressures do not occur. Again, a common upper pressure limit is approximately 10 cm H_2O above the ventilating pressure. In newer ICU ventilators, the active exhalation valve may "float," in which case pressures are less likely to rise with a patient cough.

CLINICAL SCENARIO 12.6
Limit Variables

For volume-controlled ventilation (VCV) with the ventilators currently used in the ICU, the operator sets a volume, inspiratory flow, and mandatory rate. The ventilator does not measure volume. The ventilator calculates and sets the inspiratory time needed to achieve the set volume based on the set variables (volume, flow, and time [rate]). This technically makes them time cycled. The tidal volume control is essentially an inspiratory time control with a label that says Tidal Volume. Think of it this way:

Flow × Inspiratory time = V_T; or L/sec × seconds = L.

Clinicians mistakenly consider these breaths as volume cycled, but because the ventilator neither measures volume nor uses the volume signal to control V_T, these breaths are time cycled. Defend the argument that these ventilators are volume cycled rather than time cycled.

See Appendix A for the answer.

ICU, Intensive care unit; *V_T,* tidal volume.

CLINICAL SCENARIO 12.7
Limit Variables

A respiratory therapist observes the waveforms on the graphic display as an infant is being ventilated. The therapist notices that during inspiration the pressure rises in a linear fashion and then plateaus before cycling into exhalation. The volume scalar resembles the pressure scalar. However, the flow scalar rises rapidly to a constant value and then falls rapidly during inspiration and stays at the baseline flow until the ventilator finally cycles into exhalation. What are the limit and cycle variables for this breath?

See Evolve Resources for the answer.

Termination of the Inspiratory Phase: Cycle Variable

The phase variable measured and used to end inspiration is called the *cycle variable* (Fig. 12.35). A breath can be pressure cycled, time cycled, volume cycled, or flow cycled (Box 12.8).

Pressure cycling. A breath is considered pressure cycled when inspiratory flow ends and expiratory flow begins once a set pressure is reached. Pressure cycling is not a common method used to cycle an ICU ventilator. Contrary to popular belief, breaths that are pressure controlled are not pressure

BOX 12.7   Common Names for Maximum Safety Pressure Control

- Pressure limit
- Upper pressure limit
- Normal pressure limit
- High pressure limit
- Peak/maximum pressure

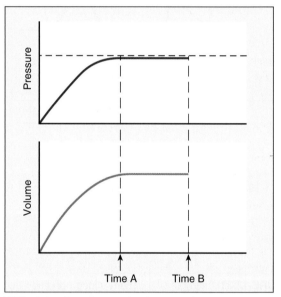

FIGURE 12.34 Pressure and volume scalars illustrate a time-cycled, pressure-limited breath. The pressure peaks and the volume is delivered by time A. The pressure reaches the set limit and stays constant. No more volume enters the patient's lungs after time A. Between A and B, excess pressure is vented. Inspiration ends at time B (time cycled).

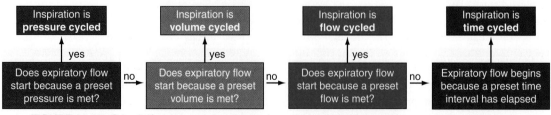

FIGURE 12.35 Criteria for determining the cycle variable during a breath on a mechanical ventilator. The determination is based on observation of the ventilator and ventilator graphics and on previous knowledge. (Modified from Wilkins RL, Stoller JK, Kacmarek RM: *Egan's fundamentals of respiratory care,* ed 9, St. Louis, 2009, Mosby.)

BOX 12.8 Cycling Variables

- *Volume cycling:* The ventilator ends inspiration after a predetermined volume has been reached.
- *Pressure cycling:* The ventilator ends inspiration after a predetermined pressure has been reached.
- *Time cycling:* The ventilator ends inspiration after a predetermined time has elapsed.
- *Flow cycling:* The ventilator ends inspiration after a predetermined flow has been achieved.

BOX 12.9 Tubing Compliance Factor (Compressibility Calculation)

To calculate tubing compliance (C_T), perform the following procedure before connecting the ventilator to the patient:
1. Set the ventilator volume to 100 or 200 mL.
2. Select a low flow setting (e.g., 40 L/min).
3. Set the upper pressure limit to the maximum and the PEEP to zero.
4. Occlude the patient's Y-connector.
5. Manually trigger the ventilator, record the measured PIP, and measure the exhaled volume (V).
   C_T equals the measured volume divided by the measured pressure ($C_T = V/PIP$).

PEEP, Positive end-expiratory pressure; *PIP,* peak inspiratory pressure.

---

cycled. In PCV the set pressure is reached before the end of inspiration (and breaths are therefore pressure limited), so it is actually *time* that cycles pressure-controlled breaths. Presently the only true pressure-cycled breaths are those seen during intermittent positive-pressure breathing (IPPB) using ventilators such as the Mark 7 (CareFusion). The operator of the ventilator sets a peak pressure, and when it is reached, the ventilator cycles into expiration.

The most frequent form of pressure cycling on contemporary ICU ventilators occurs when a ventilator reaches the upper pressure limit (high-pressure limit) that the operator has set above the peak inspiratory pressure (PIP) used to ventilate the patient, as a safety feature. This pressure is usually set at approximately 10 cm H_2O above the peak pressure. This is typically accompanied by a visual and audible alarm, and it is considered an alarm event.

Time cycling. When time is the phase variable used to end inspiration and allow expiratory gas flow to occur, the breath is said to be *time cycled.* The user sets a control called *inspiratory time,* which commonly determines the length of inspiration. In pressure-controlled continuous mandatory ventilation (PC-CMV), the operator sets a T_I, inspiratory pressure above PEEP, and a mandatory rate. By increasing or decreasing the T_I, the inspiratory time-to-expiratory time (I:E) ratio can be decreased or increased, respectively, even to the point of an inverse I:E ratio. In this latter case, the mode is referred to as pressure-controlled inverse ratio ventilation (PC-IRV).

The set T_I can be changed in a few circumstances, depending on the other controls the user sets. First, setting an inspiratory pause (inspiratory hold) instructs the ventilator to deliver inspiration and close both the inspiratory and expiratory valves and "hold" the air in the patient for a fraction of a second (up to 2 seconds) before it opens the expiratory valve and allows expiratory flow to begin. Using inspiratory hold can extend the T_I, depending on the ventilator used and how it is programmed. However, this feature is rarely used because it is uncomfortable for the patient who is triggering breaths.

Second, most ventilators have a maximum time limit for inspiration as a safety feature (e.g., during an assisted continuous spontaneous ventilation pressure-supported breath). If inspiration lasts too long (as in the presence of a leak), the ventilator ends the breath based on a fixed time (e.g., 3 seconds). A pressure support (PS) breath in this instance could not have a T_I longer than 3 seconds.

Volume cycling. During volume ventilation, flow is delivered from the ventilator to the patient circuit and the patient

until a specific volume has been delivered *from the ventilator.* As soon as the volume has been delivered, inspiratory flow ends and exhalation begins. Typically, most current ICU ventilators deliver a specific amount of flow over a certain period of time. Inspiration ends when the calculated V_T, based on the flow and time signals, has been delivered. These breaths are more correctly referred to as volume targeted. The reason for this is that current ventilators do not use volume as a signal to cycle inspiration. Rather, cycling to target a volume is a function of T_I and flow, as described earlier.

Even though the ventilator may measure a specific volume output during volume-cycled ventilation, the amount delivered to the patient may be less. This discrepancy can be caused by leaks in the system or compression of some of the volume in the patient circuit (tubing compressibility). Leaks may occur in the patient circuit, especially where devices are added to the circuit, such as heat and moisture exchangers, filters, humidifiers, sensors tapped into the Y-piece, capnometry devices, and nebulizers. Leaks can also occur around an uncuffed endotracheal tube or through a bronchopleural fistula.

Volume can also be lost due to tubing compressibility. The expansion of the patient circuit can easily be seen when high pressure is generated in a patient circuit during inspiration. The circuit expands during inspiration and returns to its end-expiratory size during exhalation. Part of the V_T delivered from the ventilator contributes to the expansion of the circuit. This amount of volume never reaches the patient. This "lost" volume is important in infants and small children. For this reason, infant patient circuits are much smaller in diameter and are made from a lower compliance plastic and thus expand less.

Most current ICU ventilators (e.g., Medtronic Minimally Invasive Therapies Puritan Bennett 840 and Servo-i) can automatically measure and calculate the loss of volume from tubing compressibility and compensate by increasing actual volume delivery. These ventilators give the operator the option to do this, usually during the new patient setup time of establishing ventilation. Box 12.9 provides an example of how to calculate tubing compliance for a ventilator that does not do so automatically.

CLINICAL SCENARIO 12.8
Calculating Tubing Compliance

Part I

Calculate the C_T of a circuit. The volume was measured at 90 mL during the tubing compliance test, and the PIP was 45 cm H_2O. What is the C_T?

If this circuit is used to ventilate a child with a set tidal volume of 300 mL and a PIP of 20 cm H_2O, how much volume is lost to the circuit? How much of the volume will go to the patient?

Part II

An adult patient circuit has a compliance of 3 mL/cm H_2O. During inspiration, the peak inspiratory pressure reaches 28 cm H_2O. The V_T is set at 640 mL on the ventilator. How much volume is lost to the circuit, and how much will reach the patient?

See Appendix A for the answers.

C_T, Tubing compliance.

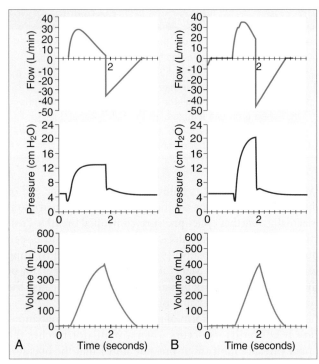

FIGURE 12.36 Effect of changes in expiratory flow trigger (flow drop-off) during pressure-support ventilation. Expiratory flow trigger is set as a small percentage of the peak inspiratory flow (A, *left panel*) and as a greater percentage of the peak inspiratory flow (B, *right panel*). (See text for further explanation.)

Most adult ventilator patient circuits have a tubing compliance factor of 1 to 3 mL/cm H_2O. In other words, for every centimeter of water pressure generated during ventilation of a patient, 1 to 3 mL is lost (compressed) to tubing compliance. For example, if the PIP is 10 cm H_2O and the tubing compliance (C_T) is 2 mL/cm H_2O, the volume lost to the circuit is 10×2 mL/cm H_2O = 20 mL. If the V_T leaving the ventilator is 500 mL, only 480 mL reaches the patient. Clinical Scenario 12.8 provides exercises in determining loss of volume as a result of tubing compressibility.

Flow cycling. Another criterion for terminating inspiration is flow cycling. With flow cycling the ventilator ends inspiration when it measures a specific flow. **Pressure-support ventilation (PSV)** is the most common mode that uses flow cycling.[19,20] During PSV, inspiration ends when the ventilator detects that flow has dropped to some percentage of the peak flow measured during inspiration.

PSV is a patient-triggered, pressure-targeted, flow-cycled mode. Originally, PS breaths ended when gas flow dropped to approximately 25% of the peak inspiratory flow, or when a specific flow was measured, inspiratory flow ended when the inspiratory gas flow decreases to 5 L/min).

Because not all patients have similar breathing patterns, fixed end points do not always synchronize with the patient's breathing pattern. Many of the current ICU ventilators, such as the Medtronic Minimally Invasive Therapies Puritan Bennett 840 and the Maquet Servo-i, allow the operator to adjust the flow termination or "expiratory trigger" point as a percentage of the peak flow of that breath. In some ventilators this feature can be adjusted from 5% to 80% of the peak flow measured during inspiration, but the range varies, depending on the ventilator used. The clinician must carefully adjust the flow cycle value.[21-22]

Fig. 12.36 illustrates two different pressure-supported breaths. In Fig. 12.36A the pressure is set at approximately 13 cm H_2O, the peak flow is approximately 30 L/min, and inspiration ends when the flow drops to approximately 5 L/min (approximately 17% of peak flow). The breath is long enough to reach its set value and produce a pressure plateau. In Fig. 12.36B the pressure is set at approximately 20 cm H_2O, peak flow is approximately 35 L/min, and inspiration ends when flow drops to approximately 20 L/min (approximately 57% of peak flow). Inspiration is short, and a visible pressure plateau does not occur. This feature is usually adjusted to improve patient–ventilator synchrony and comfort.

Inspiratory pause. The T_I can be extended or delayed by keeping the expiratory valve momentarily closed, thus preventing gas flow from leaving the circuit. This maneuver is referred to by several different names, including *inspiratory pause, inflation hold,* and *inspiratory plateau.*

Inspiratory pause can occur in either pressure or volume ventilation. In volume ventilation, it is commonly used to obtain a reading of the **plateau pressure (Pplat)** for estimation of the alveolar pressure and calculation of **static compliance** (C_s = Volume ÷ [P_{plat} − PEEP]) (Box 12.10; Fig. 12.37). It can also be used to extend the T_I for the purpose of increasing the $\overline{P}_{aw}$ and potentially improving a patient's oxygenation.

A control for this function is located on the user interface. The inspiratory pause control enables the operator to select a time ranging from fractions of a second up to approximately 2 seconds.

During PCV an *inspiratory hold pressure* can also be observed when T_I is sufficient to allow the selected pressure to equilibrate with the patient's lungs. In this situation, inflation hold is not actually selected as a parameter on the control panel. Flow

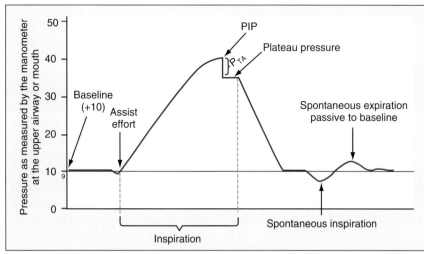

FIGURE 12.37 Volume- or flow-controlled breath with an inspiratory hold provides a pause before expiratory flow begins, allowing estimation of the plateau (alveolar) pressure. For this technique to be performed accurately, the patient cannot be making spontaneous breathing efforts. Also shown are the baseline pressure at a positive end-expiratory pressure (PEEP) of 10 cm H_2O, the transairway pressure (P_{TA}; i.e., the peak inspiratory pressure [PIP] minus the plateau pressure [P_{plat}]; or $P_{TA} = PIP - P_{plat}$), and pressure changes during a spontaneous breath.

BOX 12.10 Peak, Plateau, and Transairway Pressures

As volume is delivered, pressure rises to a peak (PIP) at the end of inspiration. PIP represents the pressure needed to overcome both airflow resistance and compliance.

When an inspiratory pause is selected, the volume is briefly held in the lungs at the end of inspiration, and the pressure reading drops to a plateau. The plateau, or static, reading indicates the pressure needed to overcome the static (lung) compliance alone.

The difference (PIP − P_{plat}) is the P_{TA}, which is the pressure associated with airflow resistance (see Fig. 12.37). This value is used to calculate airway resistance when flow is constant:

$$R_{aw} = P_{TA} \div Flow$$

PIP, Peak inspiratory pressure; *P_{plat},* plateau pressure; *P_{TA},* transairway pressure; *R_{aw},* airway resistance.

BOX 12.11 Positive End-Expiratory Pressure and Continuous Positive Airway Pressure

PEEP is the term most commonly used to value the baseline pressure when mandatory ventilator breaths are delivered from a positive baseline pressure.

CPAP is the term most commonly used to value the positive baseline pressure continuously applied to the airway of a spontaneously breathing patient. Patients doing well on CPAP alone do not require mandatory breaths from a ventilator.

CPAP, Continuous positive airway pressure; *PEEP,* positive end-expiratory pressure.

---

reads zero during this time, before expiratory flow is allowed to begin (see Fig. 12.32B).

A similar phenomenon can be observed with infant ventilators when a pressure-relief valve is used to limit the pressure during inspiration. In this situation the pressure-relief valve opens during the inspiratory phase and allows the pressure in the circuit to be maintained at a constant level. Excessive pressure is vented into the room. The pressure remains constant until the ventilator cycles into expiration (time-cycled ventilation, pressure limited) (see Fig. 12.34).

Expiratory Phase: Baseline Variable

Normally, when inspiratory flow ceases during ventilation, the expiratory valve opens, allowing expiratory flow to begin and the patient exhales passively. The expiratory phase is the time between end inspiration and the start of the next breath.

The baseline variable is the parameter controlled by the ventilator during exhalation. Typically, pressure is the baseline variable.

Baseline pressure. Baseline pressure is the pressure level from which inspiration begins. It generally is sustained throughout the expiratory phase. A zero baseline pressure is equal to atmospheric pressure.

Baseline pressures above zero are commonly called PEEP or CPAP (Box 12.11; see Figs. 12.37 and 12.38).

Positive end-expiratory pressure. PEEP occurs because a resistance, applied during exhalation, limits lung emptying and increases FRC to increase the $P_{\overline{aw}}$ and to improve lung recruitment and oxygenation. The use of PEEP is described elsewhere and is beyond the scope of this text.[1] Increased pressure is accomplished by using a threshold resistance device, which is usually a feature built into the expiratory side of the internal ventilator circuit.

Continuous positive airway pressure. As previously mentioned, CPAP is a technique in which a patient breathes spontaneously at an elevated baseline pressure (see Fig. 12.38). As with PEEP, the expiratory pressure is accomplished with the

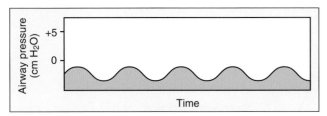

FIGURE 12.38 Pressure scalar for continuous positive airway pressure (CPAP). The patient is breathing spontaneously at higher than ambient pressure.

use of some type of expiratory resistance device, usually a threshold resistor. CPAP can be achieved through a mechanical ventilator or a spontaneous breathing CPAP device, as described earlier in this chapter.

As with PEEP, CPAP can be used to increase the FRC, to increase the $P_{\overline{aw}}$, and to improve lung recruitment and oxygenation. It is also used for the treatment of sleep apnea.

Subambient pressure (negative end-expiratory pressure). Negative pressure during expiration is currently used during high-frequency oscillation (see Fig. 12.3). The ventilator actually creates a pressure drop, drawing air out of the circuit.

Continuous gas flow during exhalation. Ventilators that provide flow triggering to begin inspiration have a flow of gas passing through the circuit throughout expiration, called *base flow* or *bias flow*. In some ventilators this flow does not begin until approximately one-third of the expiratory time has occurred, thus helping prevent resistance to exhalation. Because this bias flow is present in the patient circuit during the remainder of expiration, it provides immediate flow to a patient at the beginning of the next inspiratory effort. Bias flow may be set by the operator or may have default settings for infants, children, and adults.

In current ICU ventilators that use bias flow for flow triggering, the system is designed such that this flow does not increase the baseline pressure. The ventilator's software programming also eliminates this flow in the flow-time scalar so that the baseline flow during exhalation appears to be zero.

Expiratory hold (end-expiratory pause). Expiratory hold or end-expiratory pause is a procedure performed to estimate the pressure in the patient's lung and ventilator circuit caused by trapped air. Air trapping, dynamic hyperinflation (auto-PEEP) can occur when high minute ventilations are used (greater than 10 L/min). Auto-PEEP also occurs in patients with chronic obstructive pulmonary disease (COPD) when airway resistance is high and exhalation takes longer than normal or if the patient is actively exhaling. In these cases, there is not enough time for the patient to exhale completely.

Normally, expiratory flow (the active part of expiration) is finished approximately halfway through the expiratory phase. The second half of expiration is a period with no flow. In other words, the expiratory portion of a flow-time scalar normally shows flow returning to zero during exhalation.

When a patient has air trapping (auto-PEEP), the expiratory flow does not return to zero. A new inspiration begins before the patient has had time to exhale completely. As a result, air remains trapped in the lungs. To be watchful of air

trapping, the operator must be sure the flow scalar returns to zero before the next breath. If it does not (as illustrated by arrow 3 in Fig. 12.39), auto-PEEP is present. The operator then can perform an expiratory pause to determine how much pressure is being trapped.

The expiratory pause maneuver is performed at the end of exhalation after a mandatory breath. For this measurement to be accurate, the patient must not make any spontaneous breathing efforts, or a stable end-expiratory pressure reading cannot be obtained. Activating the expiratory pause control closes both the inspiratory and expiratory valves at the end of expiration and delays delivery of the next mandatory breath. This delay allows time for equilibration of pressures in the circuit and for the operator to obtain a reading of end-expiratory pressure. Current ICU ventilators typically display either the amount of auto-PEEP measured or the total PEEP measured, which can then be compared to the set PEEP value so that the difference can be determined.

A number of ventilator-related maneuvers can be used to decrease the risk for auto-PEEP, including using lower minute ventilation, decreasing T_I, and increasing inspiratory flow, thus allowing more time for exhalation. Using increasing levels of extrinsic (set) PEEP can also be beneficial. Patient-related factors that will decrease auto-PEEP include suctioning, use of bronchodilators and antiinflammatory drugs, and increasing the diameter of the artificial airway.

Time-limited exhalation. Time limiting of exhalation can be used as a safety feature during ventilation. Ventilators can be programmed with a maximum expiratory time so that the patient has an adequate amount of time to exhale. This is especially important for infants, who have very rapid respiratory rates that result in a very short TCT. Stacking of breaths can occur when exhalation is too short, and air trapping (auto-PEEP) can occur.

5. **Trigger and cycle events can be either patient initiated or ventilator initiated.**

Inspiration may be patient triggered or patient cycled by a signal representing patient effort. It is not difficult to understand that inspiration may be triggered by patient effort. But it is more difficult to understand how a breath can be cycled (ended) by a patient effort. The explanation is that in neurally adjusted ventilator assist (NAVA; a technique associated with the Servo-i ventilator), inspiration is cycled by a lack of or decrease in patient effort that is sensed by the diaphragm through a special electrode-laden catheter. A second less frequent mechanism of cycling is via the patient's respiratory mechanics. A decrease in compliance or increase in resistance may increase peak pressure beyond the pressure limit, thereby forcing cycling. Triggering may occur during a trigger window or a synchronization window (Fig. 12.40).

A trigger window is the period that comprises the entire expiratory time, minus a short refractory period required to reduce the risk for a trigger before the current exhalation is complete. A patient trigger effort that occurs during the trigger window starts inspiration. These breaths are defined as patient triggered.

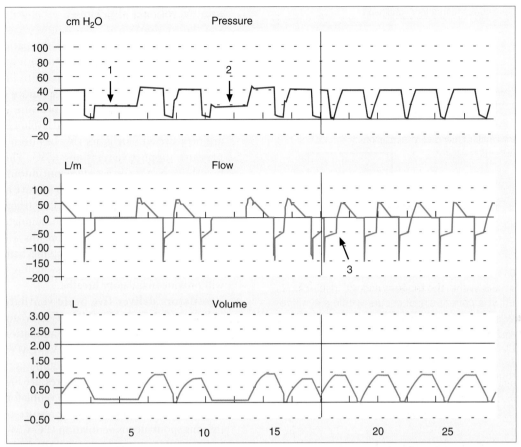

FIGURE 12.39 Pressure, flow, and volume scalars showing the use of end-expiratory pause, allowing the estimation of auto–positive end-expiratory pressure (auto-PEEP) *(arrows 1 and 2)*. Without using a pause, the presence of auto-PEEP can be detected from the flow curve. Flow does not return to zero before the next mandatory breath *(arrow 3)*. (See text for a complete description.) (Redrawn from Nilsestuen JO, Hargett K: Managing the patient-ventilator system using graphic analysis: an overview and introduction to Graphics Corner. *Respir Care* 41:1105, 1996.)

A synchronization window is a short period at the end of an expiratory time or at the end of a preset inspiratory time, during which a patient signal may be used to synchronize a mandatory breath trigger or cycle event to a spontaneous breath (as in IMV). A patient inspiratory effort during an expiratory time synchronization window is classified as a ventilator-initiated mandatory breath because the breath at that time would have been mandatory even in the absence of the patient effort. Likewise, in modes called Airway Pressure Release Ventilation (or similar), if the patient signal occurs, expiration starts and is defined as a machine-cycled event, because the release was already scheduled for that time. A rubric for determining if breaths are patient or machine triggered and patient or machine cycled is presented in Fig. 12.41.

6. **Breaths are classified as spontaneous or mandatory based on both the trigger and cycle events.**

Because the WOB can be accomplished by providing ventilatory support and/or by relying on the patient's efforts to breathe spontaneously, more than one type of breath delivery is possible. If the ventilator initiates the breath, the breath is called a mandatory breath. In this instance, the breath is begun by the ending of a TCT (TCT = T_I + Te). If the breath is ended by the delivery of a set V_T or pressure, the breath is also referred to as a mandatory breath. If the breath is triggered by the patient (usually by pressure or flow) and is then ended by the delivery of a V_T or pressure, it is also a mandatory breath. Mandatory breaths are therefore ended by a set volume or pressure; the patient's lung characteristics are not a factor determining the end of inspiration (Fig. 12.42).

In a spontaneous breath the breath can be initiated only by patient effort, independent of any machine settings for T_I or Te. Then the breath is ended by the patient's lung characteristics (i.e., resistance or compliance of the respiratory system). Thus there can be only two breath types: mandatory and spontaneous. An assisted breath is a breath during which all or part of inspiratory or expiratory flow is generated by the ventilator doing work on the patient. If the airway pressure rises above end-expiratory pressure during inspiration, the breath is assisted. Some ventilatory patterns (modes) can have assisted mandatory breaths; others can have assisted spontaneous breaths, or both. This phenomenon is described in detail in the

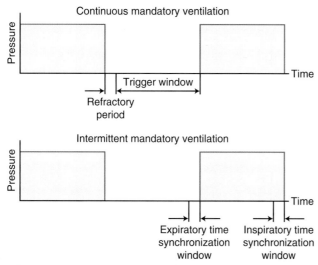

FIGURE 12.40 Trigger and synchronization windows. If a patient signal occurs within the trigger window, inspiration is patient triggered. If a patient signal occurs within a synchronization window, inspiration is ventilator triggered and patient synchronized. In general, a trigger window is used with continuous mandatory ventilation, and a synchronization window is used with intermittent mandatory ventilation. (With permission from Chatburn RL, El-Khatib M, Mireles-Cabodevila E: A taxonomy for mechanical ventilation: 10 fundamental maxims. Respir Care 59(11):1747-1763, 2014.)

section "Descriptions of Commonly Encountered Modes of Ventilation" later.

7. **Ventilators deliver three basic breath sequences: CMV, IMV, and CSV.**

During continuous mandatory ventilation (CMV), breaths are patient (usually by pressure or flow) or time triggered and are time and pressure or volume cycled. Volume-controlled continuous mandatory ventilation (VC-CMV) breaths are volume cycled. PC-CMV breaths are pressure limited and time cycled. They are all assisted breaths; that is, the airway pressure is increased during each breath (see Fig. 12.29). Breaths are usually delivered at a preset mandatory rate, and the rate may be increased by patient triggering. This breath sequence has been referred to in the past as "assist-control."

With intermittent mandatory ventilation (IMV), spontaneous breaths are allowed between mandatory breaths. The mandatory breaths are either volume or pressure controlled, and the spontaneous breaths may be assisted (continuous spontaneous breathing—CSV assisted—i.e., pressure support) or not (CSV unassisted—i.e., CPAP) (Fig. 12.43). The set IMV rate is the number of mandatory breaths per minute and once set, is the maximum mandatory rate. IMV has three variations. The first is as described, when the mandatory rate does not vary, and is the default IMV method for most ventilators. The second is when the spontaneous rate exceeds the set mandatory rate and the mandatory rate decreases. The third is when mandatory breaths are delivered only if the spontaneous minute ventilation falls below an operator-set

minute volume, also known as mandatory minute ventilation (MMV).

The third option is to allow the patient to breathe spontaneously—continuous spontaneous ventilation (CSV). There are two breathing patterns in CSV. The first is when the patient makes an inspiratory effort (flow or pressure trigger) and a preset pressure is delivered to support delivery of an adequate tidal volume. These breaths are flow cycled. For years this has been referred to as pressure support ventilation (PSV). The second CSV breathing pattern is assisted continuous spontaneous ventilation, known as continuous positive airway pressure (CPAP). Breaths are pressure or flow triggered and pressure cycled. In CSV there are no mandatory breaths. If the patient stops breathing, no breaths will be delivered, unless the ventilator has a backup mechanism for recognizing apnea and automatically switching to a mode that will provide mandatory breaths.

8. **Ventilators deliver five basic ventilatory patterns: VC-CMV, PC-CMV, VC-IMV, PC-IMV, and PC-CSV.**

A ventilatory pattern is a combination of a control variable and a breath sequence. VC-CMV consists of all mandatory breaths that are volume cycled. PC-CMV consists of all breaths that are pressure limited and time cycled. IMV modes combine two ventilatory patterns: PC or VC mandatory breaths with pressure-controlled continuous spontaneous ventilation (PC-CSV) that is either assisted (PSV) or unassisted (CPAP). This configuration is sometimes referred to as dual control, particularly when the mandatory breaths are volume controlled and the spontaneous breaths are pressure controlled. PC-CSV consists of all spontaneous breaths that are assisted: pressure limited and flow cycled (PSV), or all spontaneous but not assisted (CPAP). Although there cannot be a VC-CSV ventilator pattern, there are modes that are pressure controlled with spontaneous breaths that are volume targeted, such as volume support mode on the Maquet Servo ventilators. A target tidal volume is set, and the pressure varies with compliance and resistance to achieve the target tidal volume during spontaneous ventilation. It is a modification of PSV.

9. **Within each ventilatory pattern, there are several types that can be distinguished by their targeting schemes (set-point, dual, biovariable, servo, adaptive, optimal, and intelligent).**

By specifying the targeting scheme of a ventilatory pattern, the mode can be defined. When a manufacturer manipulates one of the basic ventilatory patterns by changing the targeting scheme, this changes the mode. The manufacturer may then assign a new mode name. This has led to the plethora of mode names and confusion surrounding modes of ventilation. Establishing uniform criteria for classifying ventilator modes may allow clinicians a better way to interpret the various modes encountered clinically.

A targeting scheme is a model of the relationship between operator inputs and ventilator outputs to achieve a specific ventilatory pattern, usually in the form of a

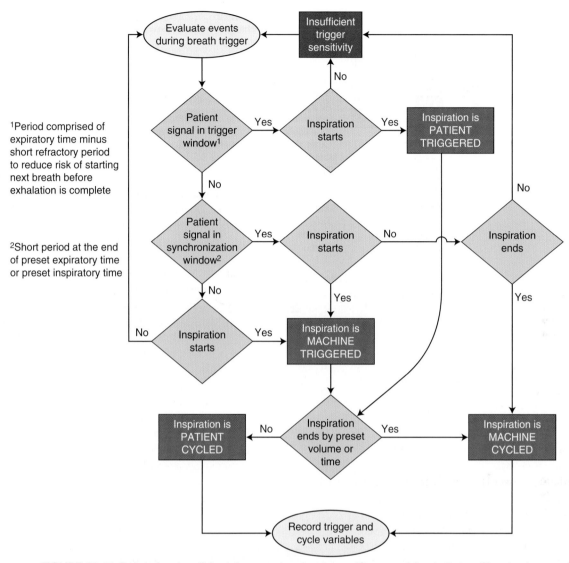

FIGURE 12.41 Rubric for classifying trigger and cycle events. (Courtesy Mandu Press, Cleveland, OH.)

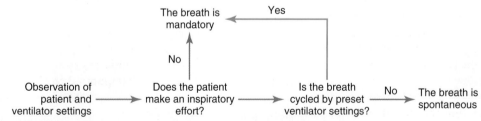

FIGURE 12.42 Determining if a breath is mandatory or spontaneous. Breaths that are time triggered are mandatory. Breaths that are patient triggered and time, volume, or pressure cycled are mandatory. Breaths that are patient triggered and not time, volume, or pressure cycled are spontaneous.

feedback control or closed-loop system. This is defined as use of the ventilator's output as a signal that is compared to the operator-set input such that the difference between the two is used to drive the system toward the desired output. An example is a mode in which compliance and resistance affect the pressure needed to deliver an operator-set tidal volume. The ventilator's output (delivered tidal volume)

is compared to the set tidal volume. If the delivered tidal volume is different than the set tidal volume, the ventilator increases or decreases the delivered pressure to make the delivered tidal volume match the set tidal volume (desired output).

There are seven targeting schemes. In set-point targeting the operator sets all the parameters of the pressure

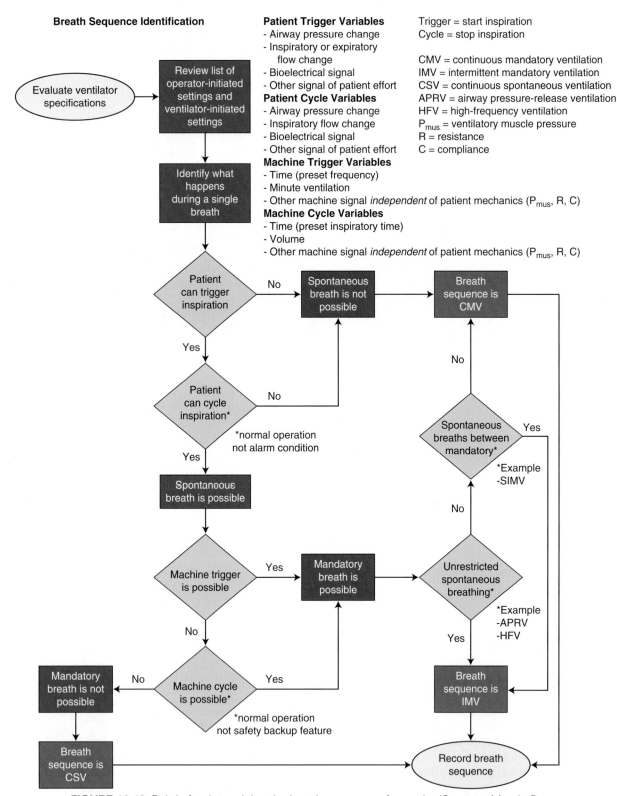

Breath Sequence Identification

Patient Trigger Variables
- Airway pressure change
- Inspiratory or expiratory flow change
- Bioelectrical signal
- Other signal of patient effort

Patient Cycle Variables
- Airway pressure change
- Inspiratory flow change
- Bioelectrical signal
- Other signal of patient effort

Machine Trigger Variables
- Time (preset frequency)
- Minute ventilation
- Other machine signal *independent* of patient mechanics (P_{mus}, R, C)

Machine Cycle Variables
- Time (preset inspiratory time)
- Volume
- Other machine signal *independent* of patient mechanics (P_{mus}, R, C)

Trigger = start inspiration
Cycle = stop inspiration

CMV = continuous mandatory ventilation
IMV = intermittent mandatory ventilation
CSV = continuous spontaneous ventilation
APRV = airway pressure-release ventilation
HFV = high-frequency ventilation
P_{mus} = ventilatory muscle pressure
R = resistance
C = compliance

FIGURE 12.43 Rubric for determining the breath sequence of a mode. (Courtesy Mandu Press, Cleveland, OH.)

waveform (as in pressure-controlled continuous mandatory ventilation) or all the parameters of the volume and flow waveforms (as in volume-controlled continuous mandatory ventilation). There is no feedback from the patient that allows the set parameters to vary; the mode designations are PC-CMV(s) or VC-CMV(s). The lowercase "s" is the tag for set-point targeting.

Dual targeting modes allow the ventilator to switch between pressure and volume control within a single inspiration. Interestingly, the volume control mode on the Maquet Servo-i ventilator is dual control: by adjusting to changing patient conditions to ensure a preset tidal volume or pressure, whichever is deemed more important at the time. In this mode the pressure-controlled breaths are patient triggered (pressure or flow) and flow cycled, which by definition is a spontaneous breath. These are in between mandatory volume-cycled breaths, so this mode is a form of IMV. The designation of the mode is therefore VC-IMVdd.

During biovariable targeting the ventilator automatically sets the inspiratory pressure or tidal volume to mimic the variability observed during normal breathing. The mode referred to as "Variable Pressure Support" on the Dräger Evita Infinity V500 is biovariable because the ventilator automatically adjusts inspiratory pressure or tidal volume randomly. The tag for biovariable targeting is (b), so the mode designation for variable pressure support is PC-CSVb.

In servo targeting the output of the ventilator follows a varying input, usually from the patient, such as inspiratory effort, airway elastance, artificial airway size/type, or an electrical signal from the diaphragm. The operator must know the nature of the varying input to determine how the ventilator will change its output. For example, any ventilator that offers tube compensation will change the amount of pressure support inversely proportionately to the inner diameter of the artificial airway. On the Maquet Servo-i ventilator, the Neurally Adjusted Ventilatory Assist (NAVA) adjunct triggers the ventilator proportionally to an electrical signal from the diaphragm, through a catheter inserted in the esophagus. The tag for servo targeting is (r). The mode designation for this mode is PC-CSVr.

Adaptive targeting allows the operator to set one target (commonly tidal volume), and the ventilator will automatically achieve another target (commonly pressure above PEEP). Several ventilators have a mode that meets these criteria: CMV+autoflow on the Dräger ventilators, PRVC on Maquet ventilators, volume control + on Medtronic Minimally Invasive Therapies ventilators, and adaptive pressure ventilation CMV on the Hamilton ventilators. In each case the operator sets a desired tidal volume, and then the ventilator uses the measured patient compliance and resistance to adapt pressure delivery to match the set tidal volume. Flow is decelerating and variable, so the control variable is pressure. The mode tag for adaptive targeting is (a). The mode designation for these mode names is PC-CMVa.

The optimal targeting scheme automatically adjusts the targets of the ventilator pattern (pressure or volume) to either minimize or maximize some overall performance characteristic (such as WOB). The mode name most commonly associated with optimal targeting is adaptive support ventilation (ASV) on Hamilton ventilators. In ASV the operator sets the patient's ideal body weight in kilograms, and the ventilator uses the Otis WOB formula to determine the best tidal volume and mandatory rate. Breaths are either patient or machine triggered and breaths are either flow or time cycled. The flow-cycled breaths are by definition spontaneous breaths, and the time cycled breaths are mandatory; therefore ASV is a form of IMV. In addition to these breaths having optimal targeting, they also have intelligent targeting. Intelligent targeting is when the ventilator automatically adjusts the targets of the ventilator pattern using artificial intelligence programs, rule-based expert systems (such as the Otis formula), and artificial neural networks. The mode designation for ASV is PC-IMVoi,oi. The reason for having two sets of tags is that the tag for each type of breath (mandatory and spontaneous in IMV) must be specified. Another example of intelligent targeting is Smart Care, found on Dräger ventilators, which has the designation PC-CMVi.

10. **A mode of ventilation is classified according to its control variable, breath sequence, and targeting schemes.**

The reason for using mode designations and tags is that once the control variable is identified (step 1), the breath sequence is determined (VC-CMV, PC-CMV, volume-controlled intermittent mandatory ventilation [VC-IMV], pressure-controlled intermittent mandatory ventilation [PC-IMV], PC-CSV) (step 2), and the tag is determined (s, d, b, r, a, o, i; step 3), then the clinician can classify any mode of ventilation. If the inspiratory pressure is set or if pressure is proportional to inspiratory effort, the control variable is pressure. If the tidal volume and inspiratory flow are set, then volume is the control variable (Fig. 12.44). Breath sequence is identified by using the rubric shown in Fig. 12.43. Targeting schemes are shown in Table 12.2.

Examples of Classifying a Mode

A common mode that has two breath types, some mandatory and some spontaneous, can be used to classify a ventilatory mode. First, using Fig. 12.44, it can be determined that the operator has set the tidal volume and flow for the mandatory breaths. Immediately we should recognize that these breaths are volume controlled. Moving to Fig. 12.43, in step 2 it can be seen that the patient can trigger the mandatory breaths and therefore the patient can cycle the inspiration (i.e., a spontaneous breath is also possible). Breaths may also be cycled by the machine (volume cycling), so there are two breath types, some mandatory and some spontaneous, resulting in the conclusion that the mode is IMV. Moving to Table 12.2, it can be seen that the operator has set all the parameters of the volume and flow waveforms, so the targeting scheme is set-point. This is also the case for the spontaneous breaths, also set-point targeting. The mode designation is then VC-IMVss.

Using another example, the operator has set a tidal volume, but not a flow. Flow is allowed to vary. When the patient triggers the ventilator, the breath is started with a preset pressure (for example, 5 cm H_2O). Therefore the control variable is pressure. Moving on to Fig. 12.43, the patient can trigger inspiration, but a spontaneous breath is not possible. All breaths are therefore mandatory, and the breath sequence is classified as CMV. To determine the targeting scheme, refer to Table 12.2, and note that for each breath the ventilator

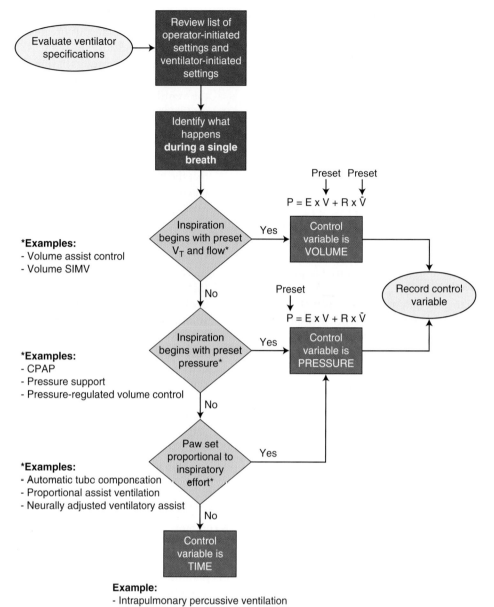

FIGURE 12.44 Rubric for determining the control variable of a mode. *Paw,* Airway pressure; *SIMV,* synchronized intermittent mandatory ventilation; V_T, tidal volume; *P,* pressure; *E,* elastance; *V,* volume; *R,* resistance; $\dot{V}$, inspiratory flow. (Courtesy Mandu Press, Cleveland, OH.)

automatically sets the target pressure between breaths in response to varying patient conditions (in this case airway resistance and compliance) to accomplish the preset tidal volume. The mode designation given this information is PC-CMVa. Manufacturers refer to this mode using a variety of names: pressure-regulated volume control, volume control +, volume control + auto flow, and adaptive pressure ventilation CMV.

III. DESCRIPTIONS OF COMMONLY ENCOUNTERED MODES OF VENTILATION

The following discussion reviews the mode classification and mechanisms of many of the more common modes using each

of the targeting schemes, with the exception of biovariable, which is just emerging as a mode called Variable Pressure Support on the Evita V500 (Dräger).

Continuous Mandatory Ventilation With Set-Point Targeting

Volume-Controlled Continuous Mandatory Ventilation With Set-Point Targeting) and Pressure-Controlled Continuous Mandatory Ventilation With Set-Point Targeting

VC-CMV or PC-CMV with set-point targeting is the delivery of mandatory volume or pressure breaths that are patient or time triggered. VC-CMV breaths are volume cycled, and PC-CMV breaths are time cycled. VC-CMV or PC-CMV are

TABLE 12.2   Targeting Schemes

Name (Abbreviation)	Description	Advantage	Disadvantage	Example Mode Name	Ventilator (Manufacturer)
Set-point (s)	The operator sets all parameters of the pressure waveform (pressure control modes) or volume and flow waveforms (volume control modes).	Simplicity	Changing patient conditions may make settings inappropriate.	Volume control CMV	Evita Infinity V500 (Dräger)
Dual (d)	The ventilator can automatically switch between volume control and pressure control during a single inspiration.	It can adjust to changing patient conditions and ensure either a preset V_T or peak inspiratory pressure, whichever is deemed most important.	It may be complicated to set correctly and may need constant readjustment if not automatically controlled by the ventilator.	Volume control	Servo-i (Maquet)
Servo (r)	The output of the ventilator (pressure/volume/flow) automatically follows a varying input.	Support by the ventilator is proportional to inspiratory effort.	It requires estimates of artificial airway and/or respiratory system mechanical properties.	Proportional assist ventilation plus	Puritan Bennett 840 (Medtronic Minimally Invasive Therapies)
Adaptive (a)	The ventilator automatically sets target(s) between breaths in response to varying patient conditions.	It can maintain stable V_T delivery with pressure control for changing lung mechanics or patient inspiratory effort.	Automatic adjustment may be inappropriate if algorithm assumptions are violated or if they do not match physiology.	Pressure-regulated volume control	Servo-i
Biovariable (b)	The ventilator automatically adjusts the inspiratory pressure or V_T randomly.	It simulates the variability observed during normal breathing and may improve oxygenation or mechanics.	Manually set range of variability may be inappropriate to achieve goals.	Variable pressure support	Evita Infinity V500
Optimal (o)	The ventilator automatically adjusts the targets of the ventilator pattern to either minimize or maximize some overall performance characteristic (e.g., work rate of breathing).	It can adjust to changing lung mechanics or patient inspiratory effort.	Automatic adjustment may be inappropriate if algorithm assumptions are violated or if they do not match physiology.	ASV	G5 (Hamilton Medical)
Intelligent (i)	This is a targeting scheme that uses artificial intelligence programs such as fuzzy logic, rule-based expert systems, and artificial neural networks	It can adjust to changing lung mechanics or patient inspiratory effort.	Automatic adjustment may be inappropriate if algorithm assumptions are violated or if they do not match physiology.	SmartCare/PS IntelliVent-ASV	Evita Infinity V500 S1 (Hamilton Medical)

With permission from Chatburn RL, El-Khatib M, Miriles-Cabodevila E: A taxonomy for mechanical ventilation: ten fundamental maxims. *Respir Care* 59(11):1747-1763, 2014.
V_T, Tidal volume.

used when patients exert enough effort to trigger the ventilator or have no inspiratory effort, as with patients suffering from muscle fatigue, a drug overdose, neurological or neuromuscular disorders, or seizure activities that require sedation and sometimes induced paralysis. Fig. 12.45 shows the pressure, flow, and volume scalars for volume-targeted CMV (see Fig. 12.45A) and for pressure-targeted CMV (see Fig. 12.45B).

Trigger sensitivity should always be set so that if able, the patient may trigger a breath. That is, the ventilator should not be made insensitive to the patient's inspiratory effort by setting a prohibitively low pressure-trigger sensitivity or high flow-trigger sensitivity. This would only serve to increase WOB, which is not generally a goal of mechanical ventilation. If a practitioner wants to eliminate spontaneous breathing, the

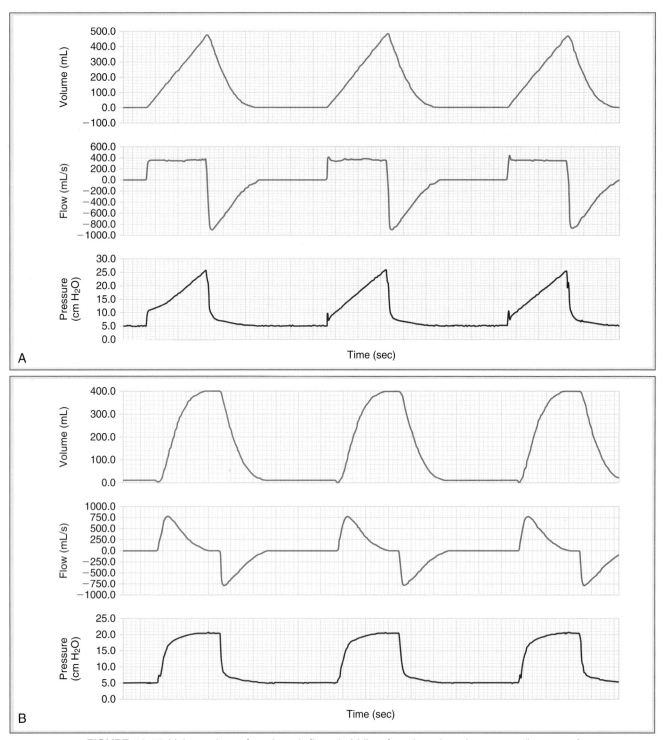

FIGURE 12.45 Volume *(top of each set)*, flow *(middle of each set)*, and pressure *(bottom of each set)* scalars for (A) volume-targeted ventilation with constant flow and (B) pressure-targeted ventilation with a decelerating or ramp flow.

patient must be sedated and paralyzed. Control of the mandatory rate can be provided by any CMV or IMV mode of ventilation once the patient is appropriately sedated. When practitioners in the clinical setting hear the term *control mode* or *assist-control mode* (described in the following section), it may lead to the assumption that volume ventilation is being used. This assumption has come about through the historical development of this breath type. The phrase pressure-controlled ventilation (PCV) is commonly assumed to mean time-triggered ventilation that has pressure as its set-point target. Being specific about the meanings of terms is important so that misunderstandings do not occur.

Modes previously referred to in the clinical setting as assist and assist-control modes should more appropriately be called CMV (either VC-CMV or PC-CMV), in which breaths are mandatory or patient triggered.

In a ventilator, sensing mechanisms are designed to detect a drop in pressure, flow, or volume in the circuit when a patient makes an inspiratory effort. The sensitivity setting determines how easy or how difficult it is for a patient's effort to trigger breath delivery. Operators also set a mandatory breath rate when using patient triggering to ensure that a minimum number of breaths are delivered for patient safety if the patient becomes apneic.

When breaths are patient triggered, the pressure-time scalar shows a downward deflection at the beginning of breath delivery (see Fig. 12.24). Breath intervals may be irregular, but each breath delivers the set volume or pressure to the circuit, regardless of how it was triggered. If the number of patient-triggered breaths drops below the mandatory rate (i.e., if the time between patient-initiated breaths is longer than the ventilator cycle time [60 sec/mandatory rate]), time-triggered breaths occur. Breaths continue at the mandatory rate (time triggered) until the patient's effort is detected before the next TCT interval. Ventilator logic mechanisms can be set to deliver flow in a square, sine, or decelerating ramp pattern, and flow is automatically adjusted to deliver the target V_T within the set T_I.

In PC-CMV, when the breath is triggered, the ventilator produces a rapid inspiratory flow to achieve the set pressure. When the pressure is reached and the lungs fill, the flow decreases (descending ramp). The breath ends when the T_I has passed. Volume delivery varies with the set T_I, the patient's lung characteristics, and whether the patient is actively inspiring (see Fig. 12.45B). For example, when the patient's lungs are stiff, less volume is delivered for the same amount of pressure. As the lungs improve, less pressure is required to deliver the same volume. If the patient actively inspires, the ventilator increases flow delivery to maintain the set pressure, which can increase volume delivery. If the T_I is too short, the ventilator does not have enough time to deliver all the set pressure to the lungs, and the volume may be lower than desired.

Pressure-Controlled Inverse Ratio Ventilation

In its early development, PC-CMV was used with inverse I:E ratios and was termed pressure-controlled inverse ratio ventilation (PC-IRV). PC-IMV is another form of PC-CMVs featuring an increased T_I that makes the I:E ratio inverse: T_I longer than the T_E (Fig. 12.46). Inverse ratios are used to increase the $P_{\overline{aw}}$, with the intent of improving patient oxygenation. PC-IRV has been replaced with the use of PC-IMVs with an inverse I:E ratio, also known as airway pressure release ventilation (APRV), described later.

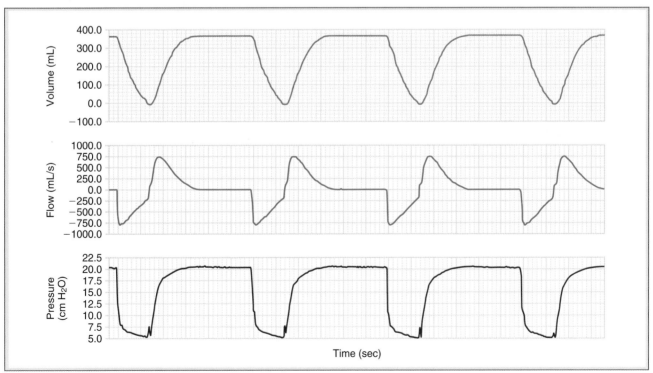

FIGURE 12.46 Volume *(top)*, flow *(middle)*, and pressure *(bottom)* scalars for pressure-controlled inverse ratio ventilation (PC-IRV).

Intermittent Mandatory Ventilation With Set-Point Targeting

Volume-Controlled Intermittent Mandatory Ventilation With Set-Point Targeting and Pressure-Controlled Intermittent Mandatory Ventilation With Set-Point Targeting

- Variations on PC-IMV with set point-targeting (PC-IMVss): all ventilators (PC-IMVss):
  - Airway Pressure Release Ventilation (APRV): Dräger
  - BILEVEL (APRV): Medtronic Minimally Invasive Therapies
  - BIVENT (APRV): Maquet
  - DuoPAP and APRV: Hamilton
  - CareFusion BiPhasic-APRV
  - GE Engström (United Kingdom) Care Station Bilevel Airway Pressure Ventilation (Bilevel)

These modes have the same mode designation (PC-IMVss) because both the mandatory and spontaneous breaths are set-point targeted.

IMV is designed to deliver volume- or pressure-targeted breaths at a mandatory rate (time-triggered, synchronized mandatory breaths). Between mandatory breaths the patient can breathe spontaneously from the ventilator circuit without getting the mandatory V_T or pressure from the ventilator. During this spontaneous breathing period, the patient breathes from the set baseline pressure, which may be ambient pressure or a positive baseline pressure (PEEP/CPAP). Spontaneous breaths can also be augmented by the use of PC-CSVs (i.e., pressure support). Because patients have an opportunity to breathe spontaneously, they must assume part of the WOB. For this reason, IMV is commonly used for patients who can provide part of the ventilatory work. Because there are two breath types in IMV (mandatory and spontaneous), each breath type is classified separately. The mandatory breath types are classified as in VC-CMV or PC-CMV. The spontaneous breaths are classified as PC-CSVs with flow triggering and flow cycling.

During IMV, when the time for a mandatory breath occurs based on the mandatory breath rate, the machine waits briefly for a patient effort (the synchronization window). If the patient triggers the breath (patient effort detected), the ventilator *synchronously* delivers the mandatory breath. If no patient effort is detected, a time-triggered mandatory breath is delivered.

Fig. 12.47 shows the volume, flow, and pressure scalars for volume-controlled intermittent mandatory ventilation (VC-IMV). During IMV with volume ventilation (VC-IMV), mandatory breaths are time or patient triggered, volume targeted, and time cycled. Spontaneous breaths are patient triggered, pressure limited and flow cycled (as shown in Fig. 12.47). During IMV with pressure ventilation (PC-IMV), mandatory breaths are time triggered, pressure targeted, and time cycled, and spontaneous breaths are usually CSV.

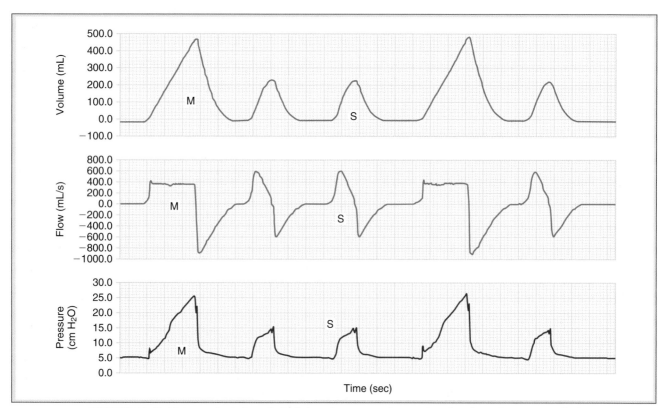

FIGURE 12.47 Volume *(top)*, flow *(middle)*, and pressure *(bottom)* scalars for volume-controlled intermittent mandatory ventilation (IMV) with continuous spontaneous ventilation (VC-IMV + CSV). In pressure-controlled IMV, the mandatory breaths are as in Fig. 12.45B. *M*, Mandatory breath; *S*, spontaneous breath.

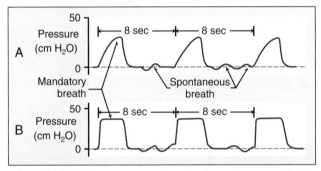

FIGURE 12.48 Pressure-time scalars for volume ventilation (A, *top curve*) and pressure ventilation (B, *bottom curve*) with synchronized intermittent mandatory ventilation (SIMV). (See text for explanation.)

Many commonly used ICU ventilators have controls labeled SIMV (for synchronized IMV) to denote the synchronous nature of coordinating mandatory breaths with spontaneous breaths. It has been suggested that because this is now a built-in feature of all contemporary ventilators, the "S" in SIMV should not be necessary. Box 12.12 outlines how the controls are set for volume- and pressure-targeted breaths in either CMV or IMV ventilation. Fig. 12.48 illustrates the pressure-time scalars for volume controlled (A) and pressure controlled (B) IMV.

When IMV is used for weaning a patient from the ventilator, the mandatory breath rate can be progressively reduced, allowing for more spontaneous breaths from the patient.

Automatic Tube Compensation

Some ventilators offer an adjunct to spontaneous breathing called automatic tube compensation (ATC) to increase inspiratory pressure in proportion to flow to support the resistive load of breathing through the artificial airway. In ATC the operator enters the airway inner diameter into the ATC program. ATC adds a varying input (tube type/size) that the output of the ventilator (level of pressure support) follows to relieve some of the WOB imposed by the tube.

When this is done in addition to any mode, the servo tag (r) is added to the mode designation. In PC-IMV with tube compensation, the mode designation PC-CMVs,sr is used to denote set-point mandatory breaths (no tube compensation) from set-point tube-compensated spontaneous breaths. Current ventilators, such as the Dräger Evita and the Medtronic Minimally Invasive Therapies Puritan Bennett 840, have this adjunct. The unique feature of ATC is that the intratracheal pressure at the carinal end of the artificial airway is used to control flow, as opposed to the pressure monitored at the Y of the ventilator circuit or in the ventilator. This increases the sensitivity of the ventilator to patient effort and decreases WOB. Intratracheal pressure is calculated from the patient's inspiratory flow, circuit pressures and properties of the artificial airway. Scalars are the same as those for CSV (PSV). ATC may be a better choice for patients with a high level of PSV, to reduce WOB and dyssynchrony.[23]

Airway Pressure Release Ventilation

Airway pressure-release ventilation (APRV) is a form of PC-IMVss that provides two levels of CPAP and allows for spontaneous breathing at both levels (Fig. 12.49). It differs from PC-IRV in that the patient breathes spontaneously during time of both high and low pressure, described later. Manufacturers' names for APRV were indicated earlier. This mode was invented by Dr. Christine Stock and Dr. Jay Block in the late 1980s.[24] APRV was introduced as a means of controlling the $P_{\overline{aw}}$ and improving oxygenation in patients with severe lung injuries; it uses inverse I:E ratios.[25]

APRV is a time-triggered, pressure-limited, and time-cycled mode that allows for spontaneous breathing during both the T_{HIGH} and T_{LOW} phases of ventilation. Some ventilators allow CSV (PSV) during the spontaneous breaths. Currently APRV is most frequently used for patients with acute respiratory distress syndrome (ARDS) and acute lung injury. APRV may benefit these patients by reducing the risk for lung injury and providing better ventilation–perfusion matching, cardiac filling, and patient comfort than other modes that do not provide for spontaneous ventilation.[25-28]

The mechanics of APRV provide patients an elevated pressure (referred to as P_{HIGH}) that approximates their P_{plat} or their $P_{\overline{aw}}$ (approximately 20 to 25 cm H_2O) for a time period referred to as T_{HIGH}. P_{HIGH} is periodically released to a lower level (P_{LOW}) for a very brief period (approximately 0.2 to 1 second) called T_{LOW}.[25,26] The settings for APRV are P_{HIGH}, P_{LOW}, T_{HIGH}, and T_{LOW}, rather than the conventional settings such as rate, V_T, f, and flow. The P_{HIGH} increases the $P_{\overline{aw}}$ to improve oxygenation. T_{LOW} allows for ventilation (i.e., exhalation of carbon dioxide). As soon as T_{LOW} is complete, P_{HIGH} is reestablished (see Fig. 12.49).

APRV and bilevel positive airway pressure (BiPAP) are sometimes used interchangeably. Rose and others have provided a systematic review of these two ventilatory strategies.[28,29] It is worth mentioning that BiPAP is often referred to as PSV;

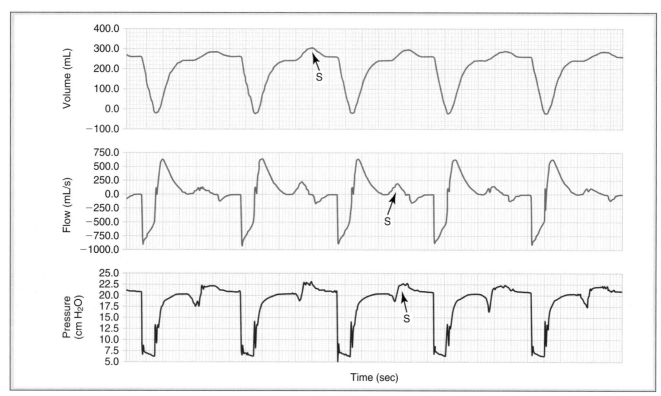

FIGURE 12.49 Volume *(top)*, flow *(middle)*, and pressure *(bottom)* scalars for airway pressure release ventilation (APRV). In this example, P_{HIGH} is 20 cm H_2O, and P_{LOW} is 5 cm H_2O. T_{HIGH} is 2.5 seconds, and T_{LOW} is 0.4 seconds. *S*, Spontaneous breaths.

however, in the updated classification scheme proposed by Chatburn, it is referred to as PC-CSV[18].

Dual-Targeting Modes

Examples of dual-targeting modes:
- CMV with pressure limited ventilation (Dräger): VC-CMVd IMV with pressure limited ventilation (Dräger): VC-IMVd,s
- Volume control (Maquet Servo^i), SIMV volume control: VC-IMVdd
- Automode (Maquet Servo^i): VC-IMVd,a
- Machine Volume: PC-CVMd

In VC-CMV the tidal volume is usually delivered based on a set flow for a set inspiratory time (actually set by the tidal volume control). However, the patient may have an inspiratory demand that is greater than the set tidal volume or flow. In this case, contemporary ventilators may provide additional inspiratory time, volume, or flow to meet this demand and provide a more synchronous breath. This is done by incorporating a flow control valve that responds to this additional patient effort. For example, on the Servo-i a volume-controlled breath is usually delivered within the set inspiratory time. But, if the patient has additional inspiratory effort, the breath changes to pressure controlled and flow cycled to accommodate the extra effort. Because some breaths are mandatory and volume cycled and others are patient triggered and change to pressure controlled and flow cycled, they are PC-CSV breaths. Thus there are two breathing patterns. This results in an IMV pattern with some breaths volume controlled and other breaths

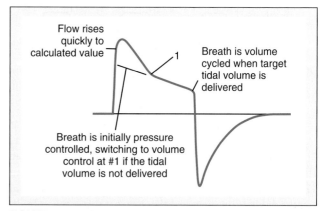

FIGURE 12.50 Flow scalar demonstrating machine volume on CareFusion AVEA ventilator. A dual-target scheme mode. (See text for details.)

pressure controlled, so the mode is classified as VC-IMVdd. In the Carefusion AVEA ventilator, the Machine Volume mode begins as a pressure-controlled breath. If the target V_T is delivered within the calculated T_I with a decelerating flow, the breath cycles into expiration. If the target V_T is not delivered, the ventilator transitions to a constant flow until the target V_T is delivered (Fig. 12.50). The mode is classified as PC-CMVd.

Pressure Limit Ventilation on the Dräger ventilator is an adjunct that can be used to limit peak pressures during volume ventilation. In Pressure Limit Ventilation, breaths are volume targeted. When a breath is triggered, pressure rises to a preset value called P_{MAX} and does not exceed this value. Flow

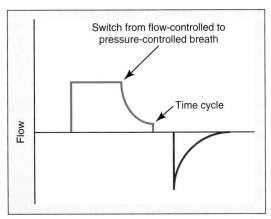

FIGURE 12.51 P$_{MAX}$ on the Dräger Evita ventilators. (See text for details.)

continues throughout the set T$_I$ at P$_{MAX}$, and then it descends to baseline (Fig. 12.51). In this regard the breath begins as volume targeted, then becomes pressure targeted, to limit the peak pressure, hence the name Pressure Limit Ventilation (VC-CMVd and VC-IMVds). There is a complete description of this ventilator mode in Chapter 13 in the section on Dräger ventilators.

Continuous Mandatory Ventilation With Adaptive Targeting

- Pressure Regulated Volume Control (Maquet and Care-Fusion): PC-CMVa
- Autoflow (Dräger): PC-CMVa
- Adaptive Pressure Ventilation (Hamilton): PC-CMVa
- Volume Control+ (Medtronic Minimally Invasive Therapies): PC-CMVa
- Pressure-Controlled Ventilation—Volume Guaranteed (PCV-VG) (GE Engström Carestation): PC-CMVa

These are all adaptive targeting modes that adjust the peak pressure to deliver a target V$_T$. An adaptive targeting mode of ventilation uses one target of the ventilator (in this case pressure) to automatically adjust to another target (in this case V$_T$) as the patient's condition (in this case compliance or resistance) changes. All breaths are mandatory and are patient or time triggered, pressure limited, and automatically adjust the pressure level to achieve the set V$_T$ over several breaths. The scalars are those of PCV (Fig. 12.52). The operator sets a maximum safety pressure and the desired V$_T$. The ventilator gives a test breath and calculates system compliance and resistance. The ventilator determines the pressure needed to deliver the set volume. As it ventilates the patient, the ventilator monitors pressure and volume. It adjusts pressure delivery to accomplish volume delivery in increments of 1 to 3 cm H$_2$O at a time, up to the maximum pressure, which equals the set upper pressure limit minus 5 cm H$_2$O (e.g., Servo-i) or to a maximum pressure limit (e.g., CareFusion AVEA). Pressure delivery can go as low as the set baseline (PEEP level). If the volume cannot be delivered within these parameters, the ventilator sounds an alarm to alert the clinician.

Although this adaptive mode of ventilation targets the set breath delivery, it does not guarantee a constant V$_T$ delivery.

Whether this is a concern depends on the goals of the clinician and the patient's needs. When the patient has an increased effort, the ventilator may not be able to distinguish this from an improvement in compliance and thus reduce its support. Clinicians may find this mode beneficial but should be aware of its limitations.[30,31]

Intelligent Targeting

- Smart Care (Dräger): PC-CSVi

Dräger Smart Care is an intelligent targeting application for PC-CSV that was described earlier as a method of setting the level of CSV according to the patient's spontaneous rate, V$_T$, and end-tidal CO$_2$. Originally, Smart Care was described as a weaning mode, and studies demonstrated that Smart Care predicted ventilator discontinuance at least as well as intensivists, and in some cases recognized patient readiness to undergo a spontaneous breathing trial earlier than intensivists. However, a more recent study in patients being mechanically ventilated for a variety of reasons revealed that weaning time was no different than when experienced critical care nurses managed weaning.[32] Burns et al.[33] have presented a review of closed-loop systems (Adaptive Support, Mandatory Minute Ventilation, and Smart Care).

Volume-Controlled Intermittent Mandatory Ventilation With Adaptive Targeting: Mandatory Minute Ventilation

- Mandatory Minute Volume (Dräger): VC-IMVa,s

Mandatory (or minimum) minute ventilation is a form of volume-targeted adaptive ventilation used in patients who can perform part of the WOB and are progressing toward weaning from mechanical ventilation.[34,35] It is adaptive, in that one target of the ventilator (in this case, rate or pressure support level) is automatically adjusted to achieve another target (in this case, minute ventilation) as the patient's condition (in this case, spontaneous V$_T$ or minute ventilation) changes. It is a form of IMV in that it allows spontaneous breathing between mandatory breaths and may automatically eliminate mandatory breaths if the patient's spontaneous minute ventilation is at or above that set by the operator. MMV guarantees a minimum $\dot{V}_E$ even though the patient's spontaneous ventilation may change. The minimum $\dot{V}_E$ set by the operator in MMV usually is less than the patient's projected spontaneous $\dot{V}_E$. When the measured $\dot{V}_E$ falls below a minimum level, the ventilator increases the pressure, rate, or volume to return the ventilator to the minimum $\dot{V}_E$. MMV is available on the Dräger Evita XL ventilator as MMV and as MMV with Pressure Support (Clinical Scenario 12.9 and Table 12.3).

Pressure-Controlled Intermittent Mandatory Ventilation With Adaptive Targeting

- PRVC-IMV(Maquet): PC-IMVa,s
- PC-IMV + Autoflow (Dräger): a,s
- PC-SIMV + Adaptive Pressure Ventilation (Hamilton): PC-IMVa,s
- PRVC SIMV (CareFusion): PC-IMVa,s
- SIMV—Pressure-Controlled Volume Guarantee (SIMV-PCVG) GE Engström Care Station: PC-IMVa,s

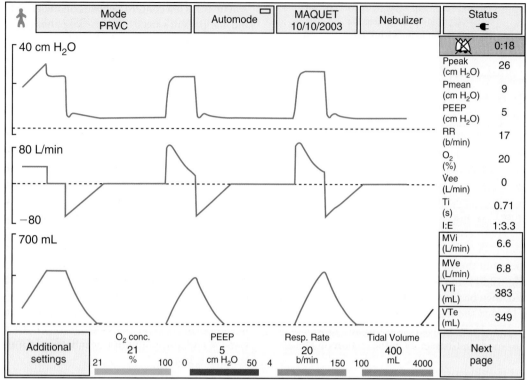

FIGURE 12.52 A screen capture of pressure-regulated volume control (PRVC) in an adult patient on the Servo-i ventilator. The first breath *(left)* is a volume-targeted test breath with an inspiratory hold to measure plateau pressure. The second breath is a pressure-targeted breath with a pressure equal to the measured plateau pressure. Set tidal volume is 400 mL. Measured exhaled tidal volume is approximately 350 mL. Note how the pressure is increased by a few centimeters of H_2O on the third breath for the ventilator to achieve the set tidal volume. *PEEP*, Positive end-expiratory pressure. (From Cairo JM: *Pilbeam's mechanical ventilation: physiological and clinical applications*, ed 5, St. Louis, 2012, Mosby.)

TABLE 12.3 **Constant Minute Ventilation With Changing Alveolar Ventilation**

Tidal Volume (mL)	Dead Space Volume (mL)[a]	Respiratory Rate (breaths/min)	Alveolar Ventilation (L/min)	Minute Ventilation (L/min)
800	150	10	6.50	8.0
667	150	12	6.20	8.0
533	150	15	5.75	8.0
400	150	20	5.00	8.0
250	150	32	3.20	8.0

[a]Assuming a constant anatomical dead space volume of 150 mL, minute ventilation can remain constant while alveolar ventilation decreases, the respiratory rate increases, and the tidal volume (V_T) falls.

CLINICAL SCENARIO 12.9
Mandatory Minute Ventilation

A patient on MMV has a set minute ventilation of 4 L/min and a measured minute ventilation of 6 L/min (spontaneous V_T = 600 mL; spontaneous rate = 10 breaths/min). Over several hours, the patient's V_T drops to 300 mL, and the rate increases to 25 breaths/min. Will the ventilator increase ventilation delivery to reduce the patient's WOB?

See Appendix A for the answer.

MMV, Mandatory minute ventilation; V_T, tidal volume; WOB, work of breathing.

These are all IMV modes with adaptive volume-targeted mandatory breaths and set-point spontaneous breaths. When one describes these modes, the mandatory breaths and spontaneous breaths are classified separately. For mandatory breaths, as compliance and resistance change, peak pressure will vary to maintain the target V_T. The spontaneous breaths are PC-CSV (pressure supported). Specific ventilators capable of providing PC-IMV with adaptive targeting are described in Chapter 13.

Optimal and Intelligent Targeting

- Adaptive Support Ventilation (Hamilton): PCV-IMVoi,oi

ASV is an optimal and intelligent targeted mode of ventilation. This mode is considered an optimal control type because the ventilator target (mandatory rate) is adjusted automatically by the ventilator to optimize another set-point (WOB) based on a model of system behavior (the Otis WOB formula).[36] It is also intelligent because it uses an artificial intelligence program to adjust to changing lung mechanics, in this case, time constant, because it constantly measures compliance and resistance and calculates time constant. It is a mode in which the ventilator determines dynamic compliance ($C_D = V_T/[PIP - PEEP]$) and expiratory time constant (dynamic compliance × airway resistance) for the patient and establishes a respiratory rate and V_T delivery based on monitored and set parameters. Its purpose is to target the respiratory rate and V_T to establish the least amount of work possible for the patient based on lung characteristics.[36] Ultimately, the goal is to facilitate ventilator liberation.[37]

Both mandatory and spontaneous assisted breaths are pressure limited, hence it is an IMV mode. The pressure level is adjusted by the ventilator, based on measured parameters (e.g., expiratory time constant, compliance, pressure, and measured volume), to both minimize the WOB and protect the lung.[36]

The clinician sets the following parameters:
- Patient's ideal body weight (IBW) and the percentage of $\dot{V}_E$ the operator wants the ventilator to supply
- Maximum pressure limit and baseline pressure (PEEP)
- Pressure or flow trigger
- Rise time (pressure ramp)

When the patient is apneic, breaths are time triggered, pressure targeted, and time cycled (PC-CMV). Both the respiratory rate and V_T are calculated to establish the optimum $\dot{V}_E$ based on the patient's IBW and lung mechanics. The maximum pressure limit determines the upper limit of pressure delivery.

When the patient can support some spontaneous breaths, patient-triggered breaths are supported at a calculated pressure using PSV (minimum $P = PEEP + 5$ cm H_2O) (in other words, PC-CSV with a volume target). The difference between the actual number of spontaneous breaths and the calculated number established by the ventilator equals the number of mandatory breaths delivered.

In spontaneously breathing patients with an adequate spontaneous rate, the ventilator adjusts pressure delivery to keep patients in the optimum calculated range for rate and V_T (Fig. 12.53). Table 12.4 presents the ranges for respiratory

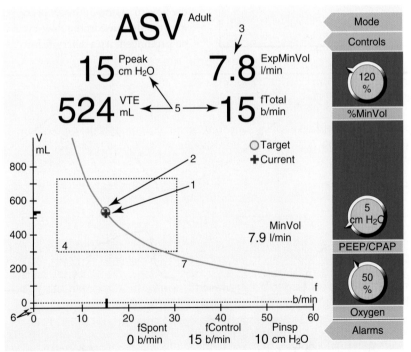

FIGURE 12.53 Adaptive support ventilation (ASV) target graphic window. Scalars for ASV are the same as those for the other pressure-controlled modes. *(1)* Current measured point formed by intersection of measured tidal volume and rate. *(2)* Target point formed by intersection of target tidal volume and target rate (lowest of breathing as determined by the Otis work of breathing formula. The current patient minute volume = target minute volume in this example. *(3)* Numerical value of target minute volume to result in the lowest work of breathing. *(4)* Safety frame in which target point may move. Prevents hyperventilation/hypoventilation, atelectasis, and overdistention. *(5)* Spontaneous ventilatory parameters (patient is presently breathing spontaneously. *(6)* Horizontal axis for rate (f). Vertical axis for tidal volume (V_T). *(7)* Minute volume curve. *CPAP,* Continuous positive airway pressure; *PEEP,* positive end-expiratory pressure. (Courtesy Hamilton Medical, Bonaduz, Switzerland.)

variables in ASV. Chapter 13 provides a more detailed description of ASV and the Hamilton G5 ventilator.

Similar modes are being rapidly designed with the development of each new ventilator. Readers are advised to review literature provided by the manufacturer of the specific ventilator they plan to use to learn more details about the closed-loop modes in use with each unit.

Pressure-Controlled Continuous Spontaneous Ventilation With Set-Point Targeting

Pressure Support Ventilation (All Ventilators): PC-CSVs

PSV, or PC-CSV is a spontaneous breath type that allows the operator to select a pressure to support the patient's WOB. It is patient triggered, pressure limited, and flow cycled (Fig. 12.54).[22] It is also referred to as BiPAP (a trademark of Philips-Respironics). PSV can also be used to support the WOB for spontaneous breaths during IMV/SIMV ventilation. It is important to recognize that PSV is not functional during VC-CMV or PC-CMV, because there are no spontaneous breaths in either mode. Fig. 12.55 shows the scalars for SIMV plus PSV for both volume- and pressure-targeted mandatory breaths.

In PSV, as in PC-CMV and PC-IMV, the ventilator delivers a high flow of gas to the patient when a breath is triggered. As the lungs fill, the flow and the pressure gradient between the machine and the patient decrease. The flow scalar is descending but never decreases to zero during inspiration because ventilators are programmed to measure the drop in flow during inspiration until it reaches a predetermined value. Some ventilators end inspiration when flow drops to 25% of peak flow during inspiration. Most contemporary ventilators provide flow cycling as an adjustable parameter. This allows the operator to change the cycle level (% peak flow) based on the type of patient being ventilated. Terms used to describe this function include *flow trigger* and *% expiratory flow*.

It has been suggested that in the future, new software may be available to automatically adjust the flow-cycling threshold by monitoring such factors as the pulmonary time constant at end-exhalation and the slope of the pressure waveform at end-inspiration. This monitoring may allow adjustment of the flow-cycling threshold by the ventilator.[37-40]

If a leak is present in the system, the ventilator increases the flow to maintain the set pressure. In this situation the flow may not decrease to the flow-cycle value, and inspiration will be prolonged. As a safety feature, ventilators have a backup

TABLE 12.4 Adaptive Support Ventilation in the Hamilton G5	
Parameter	**Range**
Respiratory rate range	5 to 60 breaths/min
Tidal volume range	4.4 to 22 mL/kg
Inspiratory time	0.5 s (or expiratory time constant [RCe]) to 2 × RCe or 3 s

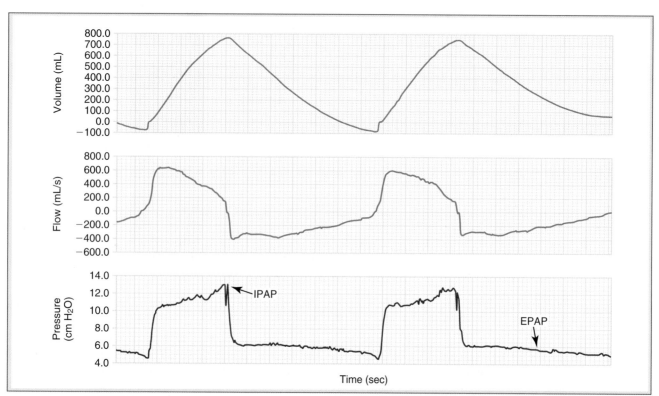

FIGURE 12.54 Volume *(top)*, flow *(middle)*, and pressure *(bottom)* scalars for pressure-controlled continuous spontaneous ventilation (PC-CSV), also known as pressure support ventilation (PSV) and bi-level positive airway pressure (BiPAP). In this example the inspiratory airway pressure (IPAP) is 13 cm H₂O. The expiratory positive airway pressure (EPAP) is 6 cm H₂O.

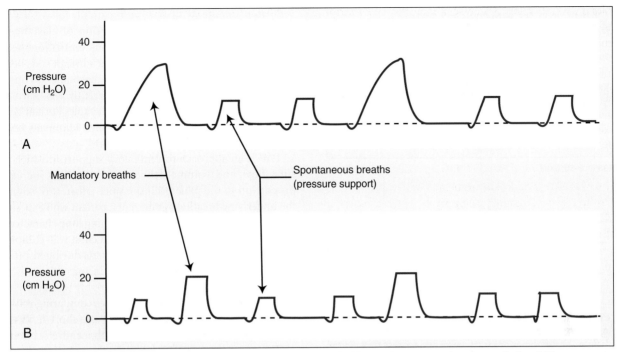

FIGURE 12.55 A, Pressure scalar for volume-controlled intermittent mandatory ventilation (VC-IMV) + continuous spontaneous ventilation (CSV). B, Pressure scalar for pressure-controlled intermittent mandatory ventilation (PC-IMV) + CSV. Note that the CSV breaths demonstrate a constant pressure delivery.

time cycle that usually is a set time between 1 and 5 seconds, depending on the type of ventilator used.

The breath can also be pressure cycled if the pressure begins to rise higher than the set pressure, which might occur if the patient begins to actively exhale or cough. Typically, a PS breath pressure cycles at 2 to 3 cm H_2O above the set pressure. Safety-backup systems are available with a ventilator that provides PSV.

The volume delivery in PSV is determined by three factors: the set pressure, the patient's lung characteristics (resistance and compliance), and the patient's inspiratory effort.

PSV has two common uses. The first is to reduce the patient's WOB when resistance to breathing is increased because of an artificial airway and the ventilatory circuit. The WOB imposed by small endotracheal tubes can be a major contributor to fatigue. A review of Poiseuille's law illustrates the basic theory of pressure support when airway resistance (R_{aw}) is increased (see Chapter 1). Reducing the diameter of the airway significantly increases the resistance to gas flow, which can be a contributing factor to the difficulty of weaning some patients.

When the increased WOB is associated with the artificial airway or the ventilator system, the initial PS level that is set does not have to be very high (a setting of 5 to 10 cm H_2O commonly is used). Another way to estimate the starting pressure level is to calculate the patient's P_{TA}, which is the difference between the peak pressure and the P_{plat} ($P_{TA} = P_{peak} - P_{plat}$). The P_{TA} reflects the pressure generated to overcome the resistance caused by the ventilator circuit, the endotracheal tube, and the patient's airways.[1] The P_{TA} value is a safe starting

BOX 12.13 **Patients Who Are Candidates for Pressure Support Ventilation**

Patients with an artificial airway in place or any of the following conditions:
- Artificial airway smaller than optimum size
- Spontaneous respiratory rates greater than 20 breaths/min (adults)
- Minute ventilation greater than 10 L/min

Patients supported with IMV/SIMV or CPAP (with spontaneous breaths) or any of the following conditions:
- History of COPD
- Evidence of ventilatory muscle weakness requiring ventilatory support
- Spontaneous tidal volume > 5 mL/kg IBW

COPD, Chronic obstructive pulmonary disease; *CPAP,* continuous positive airway pressure; *IBW,* ideal body weight; *IMV,* intermittent mandatory ventilation; *SIMV,* synchronized intermittent mandatory ventilation.

point for PS. The PS level can be adjusted after it is activated to fit the patient's needs.

Box 12.13 lists the types of patients who may benefit from PSV; Clinical Scenarios 12.10 and 12.11 provide exercises demonstrating how PSV is used clinically.

Adaptive Continuous Spontaneous Ventilation

- Volume Support Ventilation (Maquet Servo-i): PC-CSVa
- Proportional volume support (Medtronic Minimally Invasive Therapies): PC-CSVa

CLINICAL SCENARIO 12.10
Pressure-Support Ventilation

A patient has a peak pressure of 24 cm H_2O and a plateau pressure of 18 cm H_2O. What might be an appropriate initial setting for PS in this patient?

Assume that you have initiated pressure support on an 80-kg patient who is spontaneously breathing. What might be an appropriate volume to target with the PS mode?

See Appendix A for the answer.

PS, Pressure support.

CLINICAL SCENARIO 12.11
Pressure-Support Ventilation

If the algorithm (computer program) that controls the ventilator's function determines the cycling criteria in PSV, how would you argue that this breath is classified as a spontaneous breath? Isn't the ventilator determining the cycling time and not the patient?

See Appendix A for the answer.

PSV, Pressure-support ventilation.

Volume-support ventilation (VSV) is a spontaneous ventilatory mode that is available on the Medtronic Minimally Invasive Therapies and Maquet Servo-i ventilators that is similar to PRVC (see Chapter 13). It is patient triggered, pressure limited, and flow cycled. There is no backup rate with VSV; however, the ventilator switches to PRVC if the patient becomes apneic. As with PRVC, the ventilator adjusts the pressure, over several breaths, to achieve the set volume. The scalars for VSV are similar to those seen with PC-CSV. If volume is too low, the pressure is increased. Conversely, the pressure is reduced if the volume is too high. VSV can be used for patients who are ready to be weaned from the ventilator and can breathe spontaneously. Unlike PRVC, it normally is flow cycled when the flow drops to a set percentage of peak flow. It also can be time cycled (if T_I is extended for some reason) or pressure cycled (if the pressure rises too high) It is worth mentioning that some patients may experience difficulty with breath synchrony with VSV.[41,42]

The operator should set appropriate alarms for high and low minute ventilation and high and low rates, as with any mode of ventilation, to be alerted to changes in these parameters.

Pressure-Controlled Continuous Spontaneous Ventilation With Servo Targeting

- Spontaneous Proportional Assist (Medtronic Minimally Invasive Therapies): PC-CSVr

Spontaneous Proportional Assist or **proportional assist ventilation (PAV)** is a method of assisting *spontaneous* ventilation in which the practitioner adjusts the amount of the WOB assumed by the ventilator. PAV provides partial ventilatory support in which the ventilator generates a rapid inspiratory pressure delivery in proportion to the inspiratory effort of the patient.[43] PAV is servo targeted because the output of the ventilator (minute ventilation) automatically follows a varying input (the patient's WOB as a function of elastance and resistance). It is a form of spontaneous ventilation, because all breaths are patient triggered and each breath ends because of changes in the patient's respiratory mechanics, as opposed to a set-point volume or pressure. Currently PAV is available on the Medtronic Minimally Invasive Therapies Puritan Bennett 840 ventilator. (See Chapter 13, Medtronic Minimally Invasive Therapies Puritan Bennett 840, PAV+.)

PAV is an approach to ventilatory support in which pressure, flow, and volume delivery at the airway increase in proportion to the patient's inspiratory effort. PAV augments the underlying breathing pattern of a patient who experiences increased WOB associated with worsening lung characteristics (increasing R_{aw} or decreasing lung and chest wall compliance [C_{LCW}]). The more effort the patient exerts during inspiration, the more pressure and flow the machine provides.

PAV allows patients to reach comfortably whatever ventilatory pattern suits their needs. In studies comparing PSV with PAV, the two modes show comparable safe short-term effects on gas exchange and hemodynamics without adverse effects.[44-48]

The operation of PAV is based on the equation of motion previously described (see Box 12.4). The amount of pressure generated by the patient's own respiratory muscles is used as an index of inspiration effort:

$$P_{mus} = (V \times e) + (Flow \times R) - Paw$$

where P_{mus} is pressure generated by the respiratory muscles, V is volume, e is elastance (1/compliance), R is resistance, and Paw is airway pressure. P_{mus} can be calculated when e and R are known. The signal obtained from these variables can be used as a reference for the amount of pressure the ventilator needs to produce.[46]

Fig. 12.56 shows an example of a device for delivering PAV. A proportional solenoid valve has a gas supply intended for a patient. The valve is connected to the patient through a patient circuit and an artificial airway. Flow through the valve is sensitive to the patient's inspiratory effort. When the patient makes an inspiratory effort, air moves from the valve toward the patient. The valve releases gas to assist the patient's inspiration. The air movement is sensed by a flow-measuring device, which generates flow and volume signals that are sent to a microprocessor. The microprocessor then signals the valve in a positive feedback manner. The greater the patient effort, the greater the gas flow through the valve. A signal from the gain controls supplies current to the valve in proportion to the flow and volume gain signals. The sum of these two signals determines the amount of electric current going to the valve.

Gain controls determine how much pressure will be exerted based on where the gain is set. The gain set for the flow determines how much pressure is generated for each unit of flow (cm $H_2O/L/s$ [i.e., resistance units]). The gain set on the volume signal establishes how much pressure will result for each unit of the volume signal (cm H_2O/L [i.e., elastance units]).[44]

When volume and flow PAVs are used together, they respond to both the elastance (1/C) and resistance (R) components of

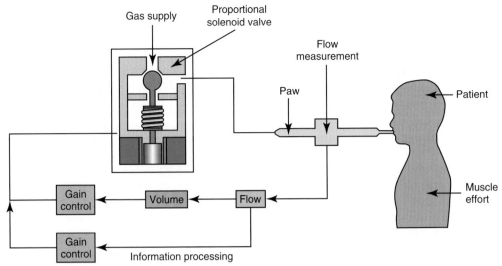

FIGURE 12.56 Simplified diagram of a proportional assist ventilation (PAV) delivery system. A proportional solenoid generates a flow in proportion to the supplied current. The current is determined by the measured rate of volume delivery and gas flow to the patient. The gain controls are set by the operator and determine what portion of patient effort is assisted. *Paw,* Airway pressure.

BOX 12.14 Determining Proportional Assist

Airway pressure using proportional assist can be determined using the following equation:

$$Paw = (f1 \times Volume) + (f2 \times Flow)$$

Where:
Paw is the airway pressure.
f1 is the ventilator-supported load of elastance or the amount of volume assist.
Volume is the ventilating volume.
f2 is the ventilator support for resistance load or the amount of flow assist.
Flow is the flow during ventilation.

---

breathing and help unload the WOB in proportion to patient effort. The greater the volume and flow demand of the patient, the higher the force (pressure) provided by the ventilator.[35,48-51]

For PAV, some of the settings established by the operator include (1) the baseline pressure, (2) the gain for volume (elastance component), and (3) the gain for flow (resistance component). (See Chapter 13, PAV+ in the Medtronic Minimally Invasive Therapies Puritan Bennett 840 ventilator.)

For example, if gain is set at 50% of the patient's elastance and 50% of the resistance, the ventilator will provide half the work performed by the patient required to overcome the forces of elastance and resistance (Box 12.14). If the patient makes no effort, the ventilator does no work. Thus PAV is better suited for patients with abnormalities in resistance and compliance and less suited for those with neuromuscular weakness and chest wall deformities with an inability to generate a strong inspiratory effort.[48,49]

PAV, however, shares a common problem with the conventional partial ventilatory support modes. In mechanically ventilated patients, the respiratory system impedance may change over time. With pressure-limited modes, these changes may result in variation in the amount of assist and volume delivered to the patient by the ventilator. These changes may prevent the synchrony between the ventilator's output and the patient's inspiratory demand.[43,51]

Another difficulty with PAV occurs with excessive unloading. This may result in resonant oscillations and runaway pressures. It is important to determine the appropriate level of unloading that could be applied to clinical practice. The level of resistive unloading should not exceed the resistance of the patient and the artificial airway. The level of elastic unloading most likely should be limited to a level that targets the patient's elastance needs to that of a normal lung.[51] The scalars are those of PC-CSV.

PAV may be used invasively or noninvasively, is recommended for patients who weigh more than 20 kg, and is affected by leaks (when used invasively) and intrinsic PEEP.[52]

In summary, PAV is an alternative mode of ventilation for spontaneously breathing patients. It has been shown to be a safe and effective method of ventilation in a variety of patients compared to PSV. When PAV is used, assessment of the compliance and resistance of the patient and endotracheal tube is important so that levels of unloading that fully compensate for the resistance and compliance levels can be avoided.

- Neurally adjusted ventilatory assist (Servo-i): PC-CSVr

Another example of CSV with servo targeting is neurally adjusted ventilatory assist (NAVA). NAVA is a mode of ventilation based on neural respiratory input. NAVA is available as an option on the Maquet Servo-i ventilator (see Chapter 13). NAVA relies on detection of the electrical activity of the diaphragm (EAdi[a]) to control ventilator function.[53]

---

[a]Medical literature uses the abbreviation *EAdi* for electrical activity of the diaphragm; Maquet, manufacturer of the Servo-i ventilator, uses *Edi* in its literature.

NAVA requires the use of a special nasogastric (NG) tube that is fitted with an electrode array. The catheter is positioned in the esophagus so that the EAdi can be detected by the electrode array. The clinician can use a monitoring screen on the Servo-i during catheter insertion to determine where the electrode array is positioned in the esophagus in relation to the diaphragm. This helps in situating the NG tube correctly so that the sensors can most accurately detect diaphragmatic activity. (NOTE: The NG tube can also be used as a feeding tube.)

A cable connects the electrical array embedded in the NG tube to the EAdi module of the ventilator, which in turn commands the ventilator's functions.

As the diaphragm depolarizes, the electrical signal is captured by the electrode array and transmitted to the EAdi module and the ventilator. The ventilator begins inspiration as soon as the diaphragm begins depolarization. The depth and length of the breath are also established by the diaphragm's electrical activity (i.e., the greater the electrical activity, the deeper the breath). When activity diminishes, inspiratory flow is stopped.

Besides establishing the intensity of diaphragm firing, the ventilator can be programmed to control the level of assistance. The operator sets a level of support proportional to the EAdi (range: 0 to 30 cm $H_2O/\mu V$). For example, if the operator selects 3 cm $H_2O/\mu V$ of muscle activity and the electrode array measures 5 μV (diaphragm depolarization), the potential pressure delivery is 15 cm H_2O. (*Note:* Simple numbers are used here just as an example and do not represent actual readings.) Theoretically, if the activity of the diaphragm increased to 10 μV, the pressure would increase to 30 cm H_2O. However, studies demonstrate that the stretch receptors in the lungs sense the rise in volume with the rise in pressure and signal the brain to reduce the firing of the diaphragm. As a result, a lower pressure and lower volume are delivered than one would expect. Thus the lung is protected from excessive distention.[54]

Just as ventilator triggering and breath limitation are neurally controlled, breath cycling is controlled by the activity of the diaphragm. The breath ends when electrical activity decreases (neural cycling). In addition, if the patient becomes apneic, the ventilator automatically switches to a backup mode of ventilation. Box 12.15 lists the potential benefits of NAVA.

Many patients with a variety of pulmonary disorders may benefit from NAVA as long as the respiratory center, phrenic nerve, and neuromuscular junction are functionally intact and there are no contraindications to or limitations on the use of the NG tube.[54]

NAVA probably represents the first applicable form of assisted ventilation in which the patient's respiratory center controls ventilation. Additional research is needed to verify some of the uses and possible side effects of this mode of ventilation.[55]

IV. HIGH-FREQUENCY VENTILATION

HFV uses mandatory rates higher than normal and tidal volumes lower than normal. HFV generally is defined as any

---

BOX 12.15 Potential Benefits of Neurally Adjusted Ventilatory Assist

- *Reduced WOB:* Fewer patient trigger efforts are missed. Also, intrinsic PEEP does not affect triggering.
- *Improved synchrony:* The patient's neural and diaphragmatic electrical activity control the onset and breath delivery. Synchrony with the ventilator is an important part of unloading the work of the diaphragm during both inspiration and expiration.[53]
- *Reduced need for sedation and/or paralysis:* Allowing the patient basically to control the breathing pattern may reduce the need for sedation.
- *Improvement in ventilation:* Compared to standard methods, ventilation is improved by allowing neural triggering and neurally adjusted ventilator assistance, particularly in patients with severe airflow impairment.[54]
- Potential improvement in synchrony and oxygenation and a reduced incidence of barotrauma in the infant population.[49] Better ventilator regulation in noninvasive ventilation because of the ability of NAVA to ventilate despite variable leaks.[54]

COPD, Chronic obstructive pulmonary disease; *NAVA,* neurally adjusted ventilator assist; *PEEP,* positive end-expiratory pressure; *WOB,* work of breathing.

---

mode of ventilation that provides a mandatory rate of more than 100 breaths (pulses) per minute.[56] For particularly high rates, frequencies are usually given in Hertz (Hz) or cycles per second, with 1 Hz equaling 60 cycles (breaths)/min.

Five basic types of HFV are available:

1. High-frequency positive-pressure ventilation (HFPPV)
2. High-frequency jet ventilation (HFJV)
3. High-frequency oscillatory ventilation (HFOV)
4. High-frequency flow interruption (HFFI)
5. High-frequency percussive ventilation (HFPV)

The two most frequently used forms of HFV are HFJV and HFOV.[57]

High-Frequency Positive-Pressure Ventilation

HFPPV uses a conventional volume- or pressure-limited ventilator with a low-compliance patient circuit. With HFPPV the airway is intermittently pressurized with gas with no air entrainment. Mandatory rates are approximately 60 to 110 breaths/min. As mentioned, breath rates are sometimes given in Hertz (1 Hz = 1 cycle/s). In this case 60 to 100 breaths/min would be 1 to 1.8 Hz.

HFPPV was developed by Sjöstrand[57] in the late 1960s to minimize the cardiovascular side effects of positive-pressure ventilation. Animal studies also showed its effectiveness in eliminating intracranial pressure variations normally associated with breathing, thus providing a better surgical field for microneurosurgical procedures.

Early prototypes used an H-valve assembly in which the circuit was connected to an insufflation catheter attached to the endotracheal tube. The catheter was fitted with either a pneumatic (fluidic) valve (Fig. 12.57) or a rapidly responding exhalation valve (Fig. 12.58).

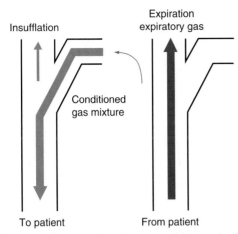

FIGURE 12.57 Pneumatic valve assembly used with high-frequency positive-pressure ventilation (HFPPV) introduces a gas mixture during inspiration. Because of the Coanda effect (see Historical Note 12.1), the gas stream hugs the channel. No air entrainment occurs, and only a small amount of gas leaks from the expiratory limb.

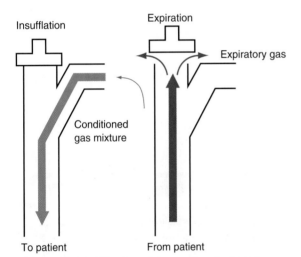

FIGURE 12.58 Modification of the H-valve for high-frequency positive-pressure ventilation (HFPPV) uses an expiratory valve that closes during inspiration to prevent gas leakage.

A problem can occur with HFPPV. The short inspiratory times and high rates may prevent adequate V_T delivery. Breath stacking may develop at these rates, because only passive exhalation occurs.[58,59] That is, when respiratory rates are this rapid, sometimes the air has enough time to enter the lungs but not enough time to leave. Breaths begin to "stack up" in the lungs, resulting in trapped air, which creates auto-PEEP. With other modes of HFV now more popular and the use of other techniques for the management of acute lung injury (e.g., permissive hypercapnia and open lung ventilation), HFPPV is not often used clinically.

High-Frequency Jet Ventilation

In 1977 Klain and Smith[60] developed a method of HFJV that used a percutaneous transtracheal catheter. The catheter was connected to an air source that provided a jet injection of air

controlled by a fluidic logic ventilator. Rates up to 600 breaths/min (10 Hz) were used. Later this technique used a catheter that allowed for air entrainment.

HFJV offers rates of approximately 100 to 600 breaths/min (1.7 to 10 Hz) with a V_T smaller than anatomical dead space volume. (Historical Note 12.2 lists some of the earlier uses of HFJV.) In general, HFJV operates by passing gas from a high-pressure source through a variable regulator that reduces the pressure to the desired working level. The gas then passes through a device, usually a solenoid or a fluidic valve that governs the amount and duration of flow. The gas jet is then delivered through a specially made triple-lumen endotracheal tube (Fig. 12.59A), which is similar to conventional endotracheal tubes except that two additional small lines are added. One is for delivering jet ventilation, and the other is for monitoring distal airway pressures. The jet stream exits the tube at approximately one-third of the tube's length from the distal end. The pressure tube is located at the distal tip of the tube.

If a jet tube is not used, a special jet adapter can be attached to the endotracheal tube (see Fig. 12.59B). Another technique when a special jet tube is not in place is to use a small catheter inserted either through a conventional endotracheal or a tracheostomy tube. Early studies showed that the best position for the jet is close to the proximal end of the trachea near the vocal cords.[60]

High-Frequency Oscillatory Ventilation

High-frequency oscillatory ventilation (HFOV) currently is the most widely used form of HFV in adult patients. However, a recent study has demonstrated poorer outcomes in adults with ARDS when using HFOV.[61] It is most frequently used in neonatal and pediatric patients.

HFOV uses a reciprocating pump to generate an approximation of a sine wave (see Fig. 12.3). Examples of devices that provide this function are reciprocating pumps (usually pistons), diaphragms, and loudspeakers. Although not true oscillators, high-frequency flow interrupters (discussed in the following section) can be used in ventilators to provide a similar effect. These ventilators are called "pseudo-oscillators."

With HFOV, pressure is positive in the airway during the inspiratory phase (forward stroke) and negative during the expiratory phase (return stroke). Therefore both inspiration and expiration are active, and bulk flow rather than jet pulsations is produced. HFOV uses frequencies in the range of 1

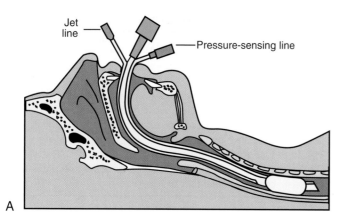

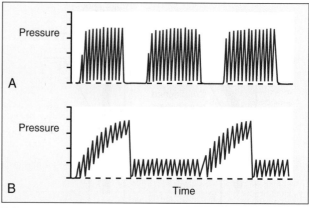

FIGURE 12.60 A, Example of a pressure-time waveform created during high-frequency percussive ventilation (HFPV). B, Example of a pressure-time curve during HFPV superimposed over standard positive-pressure breath delivery.

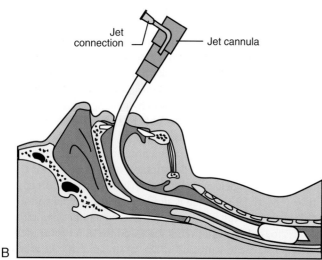

FIGURE 12.59 Diagram of an endotracheal tube used in high-frequency jet ventilation (HFJV) (A) and a jet connection with a jet cannula attached to a standard endotracheal tube (B).

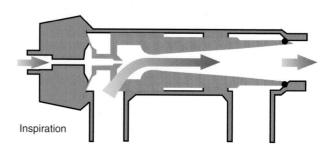

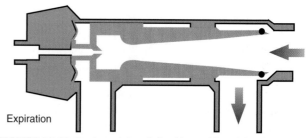

FIGURE 12.61 Design of the sliding Venturi for a high-frequency percussive generator used to provide high-frequency percussive ventilation (HFPV). (See text for explanation.)

to 50 Hz (60 to 3000 cycles/min), and V_T is less than the anatomical dead space volume. Some oscillators have a fixed I:E ratio, and others allow the I:E ratio to be adjusted.

HFOV is one of the most widely used forms of HFV in infants and pediatric patients. An example of an oscillator is the 3100A from CareFusion (see Chapter 14). The 3100A uses a diaphragm-shaped piston that is powered magnetically, much like a stereo speaker. The $P_{\overline{aw}}$ control sets the tension on the diaphragm. Gas is oscillated back and forth by the action of the diaphragm. The amplitude of the wave set by the power control determines the forward and backward excursion of the piston, which helps determine the V_T. In the 3100A, rigid plastic circuits provide the bias flow of warmed and humidified air that is delivered to the patient.

High-Frequency Percussive Ventilation

Forrest M. Bird, a pioneer in ventilatory devices, designed a HFPV device in which he incorporated the beneficial characteristics of both a conventional positive-pressure ventilator and a jet ventilator. It operates in such a way that high-frequency breaths can be provided at ambient pressures. Fig. 12.60A shows the rapid pressure waves representing high-frequency

pulses with pauses following where these pulses are interrupted. High-frequency pulses (100 to 900 cycles/min) can also be superimposed on conventional positive-pressure breaths (5 to 30 cycles/min). In this case the pulses still occur, but the baseline rises as a positive-pressure breath is delivered (see Fig. 12.60B). These devices can be compared with time-cycled, pressure-limited ventilation when high-frequency pulsations are injected throughout the inspiratory phase. The resulting unit is called a HFPV.[62]

A ventilator that incorporates this principle is the Bird VDR-4 volumetric diffusive respirator (Percussionaire), which uses a sliding Venturi (Figs. 12.61 and 12.62). At the mouth

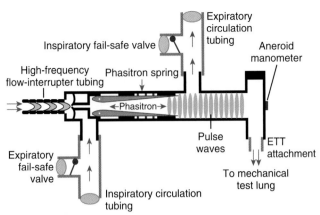

FIGURE 12.62 Schematic of the pulse generator (Phasitron), circulation tubing, and fail-safe valves. The open arrows denote airflow through the circuit. The bidirectional arrow denotes the sliding movement of the Phasitron component that creates the gas pulses. *ETT*, Endotracheal tube. (From Allen PF, Thurlby JR, Naworol GA, et al: Measurement of pulsatile tidal volume, pressure, amplitude, and gas flow during high frequency percussive ventilation, with and without partial cuff deflation. *Respir Care* 52:45, 2007.)

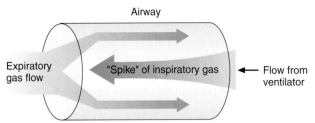

FIGURE 12.63 Effects of streaming in high-frequency jet ventilation (HFJV). Forward movement of the gas in the center, produced by pulsations from the jet, causes gas along the airway walls to be pushed backward.

of the Venturi is a jet orifice. Around the jet is a continuous bias flow of warm, humidified air. During inspiration a diaphragm connected to the Venturi fills with gas. This action slides the Venturi forward, toward the patient's airway, simultaneously blocking the expiratory port. During this time the jet is activated and begins delivering short pulses of gas. At the same time a large amount of air is entrained through the now open inspiratory ports, so that flow to the patient is high. The large gas flow is caused by the pressure gradient between the jet and the patient connector. As inspiration progresses and pressure builds in the patient's airway, this gradient is reduced, thereby reducing the flow. However, the jet pulsations continue throughout inspiration. When the set T_I is reached, inspiration ends. The diaphragm is no longer pressurized, and the Venturi slides back away from the patient, opening the expiratory port. During exhalation, a counterflow of gas is directed at the airway to maintain the set PEEP level.

Ventilation is controlled by the respiratory rate and peak airway pressure. Oxygenation is determined by the PEEP level, T_I, I:E ratio, and peak airway pressure. The high-frequency pressure oscillations also affect gas exchange, which makes clinical monitoring of these variables an important part of frequency adjustments.

The clinical benefits of HFPV may include facilitation of secretion removal.[62] HFPV has been used prophylactically in patients with thermal airway injury to help prevent pneumonia and atelectasis.[63-65]

Mechanisms of Action of High-Frequency Ventilation

The mechanisms of action of the various forms of HFV are not clearly understood; however, ventilation successfully occurs

even when the V_T is less than the patient's anatomical dead space volume (V_D). Alveoli located close to the airways are thought to be ventilated by convection, just as in conventional ventilation. Convection is the movement of air molecules associated with the pressures of ventilation.

The following additional mechanisms may be responsible:

- Pendelluft
- Gas streaming or helical diffusion
- Taylor dispersion
- Molecular diffusion
- Spike formation

Pendelluft is the movement of gases from one area of the lungs to another as a result of differences in the compliance and resistance of various lung regions; this is also called *out-of-phase ventilation*. This movement occurs through normal anatomical channels (e.g., alveolar ducts, the pores of Kohn, and the canals of Lambert). When lung tissue is oscillated, as occurs with HFV, this phenomenon may be enhanced.

Streaming or asymmetric velocity profiles occur when gas flows in both directions at once through a conductive airway. Inspired gas is believed to move into the lungs down the center of the airways in a parabolic fashion, whereas exhaled gas tends to move near the walls and out of the lungs (Fig. 12.63). This wall air movement may occur in a helical fashion and has been called *helical diffusion*.

Taylor dispersion is thought to occur in HFOV. It is the enhanced mixing of gases associated with the turbulent flow of high-velocity gases moving through small airways and their bifurcations. Taylor dispersion can occur where two gas streams meet. The erratic pattern of eddies and streams created is thought to enhance gas mixing and diffusion.

Simple molecular diffusion also occurs, at least at the terminal air spaces, and is another mechanism that adds to gas mixing. It is the result of the random thermal oscillation of molecules.

With regard to spike formation, one theory proposes that a spike (a parabolic-shaped front), a high-energy wave impulse of gas, travels rapidly through the center of the airway, much like a bullet. This gas movement may provide a larger area of gas mixing in the distal portions of the lungs.[66]

KEY POINTS

- Ventilators are electrically powered, pneumatically powered, or pneumatically powered and microprocessor (electrically) controlled. The gas flows from the source at the wall through output control valves to the patient's lungs down a pressure gradient.
- Contemporary ICU ventilators are primarily single-circuit ventilators. The source gas is the same as the gas that enters the patient's lungs.
- The flow-controlling valve currently used in most pneumatically powered ventilators is the proportional solenoid.
- Two key elements of fluidic devices are the Coanda effect and the flip-flop valve.
- The main parameter controlled by the ventilator is referred to as the *control variable*.
- The three variables the ventilator can control are volume, flow, and pressure. However, the ventilator can control only one of these variables at a time according to the equation of motion.
- Triggering begins a breath, and cycling ends a breath.
- A limiting variable limits the amount (value) a parameter (pressure, volume, flow) can reach during inspiration. However, the limit variable does not end the breath.
- The terminology used in the clinical setting to describe modes of ventilation has recently been revised to make mode nomenclature more understandable.
- A mode is defined by its control variable (VC or PC), breath sequence (CMV, IMV, and CSV), and targeting scheme.
- There are seven targeting schemes: set-point, dual, servo, adaptive, biovariable, optimal, and intelligent.

- All modes are variants of VC-CMV, PC-CMV, VC-IMV, PC-IMV, and CSV.
- PRVC (an adaptive target mode) is pressure-limited ventilation with a volume target.
- Volume support is PSV with a volume target.
- PAV (a servo-targeted mode) is a method of assisting spontaneous ventilation in which the practitioner adjusts the amount of WOB assumed by the ventilator based on the patient's elastance and resistance characteristics.
- ASV utilizes intelligent targeting, because the set-point is automatically adjusted by the ventilator to optimize the patient's WOB and prevent lung injury associated with ventilation.
- With NAVA (a servo-targeted mode), the ventilator begins inspiration as soon as diaphragmatic depolarization is detected. The depth and length of the breath are also established by the diaphragm's electrical activity. When diaphragmatic activity ends, inspiration ends.
- Smart Care, an intelligent targeted mode, is designed to promote weaning by automatically performing spontaneous breathing trials and recommending extubation.
- The two most frequently used forms of HFV are HFJV and HFOV.
- HFPV may improve oxygenation, support ventilation, and assist with secretion clearance.
- Five different mechanisms may be responsible for gas movement during HFV. They include pendelluft movement, gas streaming, Taylor dispersion, molecular diffusion, and spike formation.

ASSESSMENT QUESTIONS

See Appendix B for the answers.

1. All of the following are potential sources of power for a mechanical ventilator *except*:
   a. Compressed gas
   b. Electricity
   c. Compressed gas and electricity
   d. Fluidics

2. A ventilator measures a decrease in tidal volume (V_T) during pressure ventilation and automatically increases the pressure to return the volume to its original value. This is best described as:
   a. Pressure-controlled ventilation
   b. Adaptive targeting
   c. A closed-loop control system
   d. A pneumatically controlled ventilator

3. During operation of a ventilator, the respiratory therapist sets the V_T at 500 mL, the mandatory rate at 10 breaths/min, and an inspiratory flow of 50 L/min. These settings are associated with what type of ventilation?
   a. Pressure-targeted, flow-cycled ventilation
   b. Volume-targeted, flow-cycled ventilation
   c. Volume-targeted, time-cycled ventilation
   d. Volume-targeted, pressure-cycled ventilation

4. Which of the following are common phase variables for pressure-controlled continuous mandatory ventilation (PC-CMV)?
   1. Flow trigger
   2. Pressure limit
   3. Time cycle
   4. Flow limit
      a. 1 and 2 only
      b. 2, 3, and 4 only
      c. 1, 2, and 3 only
      d. 2 and 4 only

5. Which of the following is the most common flow control device on contemporary intensive care unit (ICU) ventilators?
   a. Rotary drive piston
   b. Proportional solenoid
   c. Bag-in-a-chamber
   d. Stepper motor with valve

6. A jet stream passes through an opening with a wall adjacent to its left side; the jet deflects toward the wall. What fluidic principle does this describe?
   a. Slip streaming
   b. Coanda effect

c. Flip-flop device

d. Separation bubble

7. Which of the following scalars would be used to describe volume-controlled continuous mandatory ventilation (VC-CMV)?

1. Square or rectangular flow
2. Linear pressure
3. Linear volume
4. Exponential flow

   a. 1 and 3 only
   b. 2 and 4 only
   c. 2, 3, and 4 only
   d. 1, 2, and 3 only

8. The following scalars are noted during ventilation of a patient: a descending flow pattern that returns to baseline before cycling into exhalation, and a square pressure scalar, in which the pressure decreases slightly below the baseline before the beginning of inspiration; volume delivery varies. This best describes what form of ventilation?

   a. Time-triggered, volume-variable ventilation
   b. Patient-triggered, pressure-limited, time-cycled ventilation
   c. Patient-triggered, volume-limited, flow-cycled ventilation
   d. Volume-triggered, pressure-limited, volume-cycled ventilation

9. A commonly used abbreviation for the mode described in question 8 is:

   a. PC-CMV
   b. PSV
   c. VC-CMV
   d. PRVC

10. What criteria must be met for a breath to be spontaneous?

1. The breath must be time triggered.
2. The breath must be pressure or time cycled.
3. The patient must trigger the breath.
4. The breath must be cycled by the patient's lung characteristics.

   a. 1 and 2 only
   b. 1 and 4 only
   c. 2 and 4 only
   d. 3 and 4 only

11. During patient ventilation the ventilator adjusts volume delivery to target the set V_T. This would be classified as:

   a. Adaptive
   b. Servo
   c. Set-point
   d. Biovariable

12. A pressure scalar indicates that the difference between the peak inspiratory pressure (PIP) and the plateau pressure (P_{plat}) is 5 cm H_2O. This value best describes:

   a. Static compliance
   b. Dynamic compliance
   c. Transairway pressure
   d. Airway resistance

13. An apneic patient is severely hypoxemic. The physician wants to use an appropriate mode with an elevated baseline pressure. What should the respiratory therapist recommend?

   a. Continuous spontaneous ventilation (CSV)
   b. Proportional assist ventilation (PAV)
   c. VC-CMV plus positive end-expiratory pressure (PEEP)
   d. Continuous positive airway pressure (CPAP)

14. A ventilator monitors end-tidal CO_2, the patient's spontaneous rate, and V_T. Then these data are used by the ventilator to recommend extubation. What targeting scheme is described?

   a. Set-point
   b. Adaptive
   c. Intelligent
   d. Optimal

15. A physician wants to use pressure ventilation that uses several seconds at a high CPAP that periodically drops to a lower CPAP. She wants to be sure that the lungs do not deflate during the periods of low CPAP. Which of the following modes of ventilation would the respiratory therapist recommend?

   a. Pressure-regulated volume control (PRVC)
   b. VC-CMV with set-point targeting
   c. PAV
   d. Airway pressure-release ventilation (APRV)

16. What high-frequency ventilation (HFV) technique provides an active inspiratory and expiratory phase?

   a. High-frequency positive-pressure ventilation (HFPPV)
   b. High-frequency flow interruption (HFFI)
   c. High-frequency jet ventilation (HFJV)
   d. High-frequency oscillatory ventilation (HFOV)

17. A patient is being ventilated by means of a Downs CPAP system set at 10 cm H_2O. The respiratory therapist notices that during spontaneous inspiration, the monitored inspiratory pressure is 5 cm H_2O and the expiratory pressure is 10 cm H_2O. To solve this problem, what should the therapist consider doing?

   a. Check the function of the one-way valve between the patient and the CPAP generator.
   b. Increase the flow to the system.
   c. Increase the pressure setting on the PEEP/CPAP valve.
   d. Check the system for leaks.

18. What lung mechanics are used by PAV to make adjustments in delivered pressure?

1. Compliance
2. Resistance
3. $P_{.01}$
4. Elastance

   a. 1 and 2 only
   b. 2 and 4 only
   c. 3 and 4 only
   d. 1, 2, 3, and 4

19. What information must the therapist enter into the ventilator to initiate automatic tube compensation (ATC)?
    1. Patient's height in cm
    2. Internal diameter of the artificial airway
    3. Patient's inspiratory flow
    4. Type of artificial airway
       a. 1 and 2 only
       b. 2 and 3 only
       c. 3 and 4 only
       d. 1, 2, and 4 only

20. A ventilator set for flow triggering has a base flow of 10 L/min and a flow trigger of 3 L/min. At what measured flow will the ventilator begin inspiration?
    a. When the expiratory flow drops from 10 L/min to 7 L/min
    b. When inspiratory sensitivity senses a rise in flow of 3 L/min
    c. When the expiratory flow increases from 10 to 13 L/min
    d. The answer cannot be determined from the information given.

21. While checking the ventilator graphics, the respiratory therapist notices no downward deflection of the pressure scalar before inspiratory flow begins. The inspiratory flow scalar is constant and has a fixed inspiratory time (T_I) of 1 second. What are the trigger and cycle variables, and is this breath-volume or pressure-targeted ventilation?
    a. Pressure-triggered, constant-flow, time-cycled ventilation
    b. Time-triggered, time-cycled, volume-targeted ventilation
    c. Time-triggered, constant-pressure, flow-cycled ventilation
    d. Patient-triggered, volume-limited, time-cycled ventilation

22. During ventilation the flow rises sharply to a peak of 100 L/min and progressively decreases. The pressure-time curve shows a sharp rise to plateau. The respiratory therapist notices that volume varies breath to breath. What type of ventilation is this?
    a. Volume-targeted ventilation
    b. Flow cycling
    c. PC-CMV
    d. APRV

23. During CSV (pressure-controlled CSV [PC-CSV]), what is the cycle variable?
    a. Time
    b. Flow
    c. Pressure
    d. Patient effort

24. Which of the following is the clinical name commonly applied to patient- or time-triggered, volume-targeted, and time-cycled ventilation?
    a. VC-CMV
    b. Controlled ventilation
    c. PCV
    d. Pressure augmentation

25. A breath begins as a decelerating-flow pressure-controlled breath, but the target V_T is not delivered in the set T_I, so the ventilator changes the breath to a volume-targeted breath to deliver the V_T. What target scheme does this describe?
    a. Set-point
    b. Adaptive
    c. Optimal
    d. Dual

26. Which of the following targeting schemes is defined by operator input of a patient's ideal body weight (IBW) and the use of a mathematical model by the ventilator to determine delivered parameters such as V_T and rate?
    a. Adaptive
    b. Set-point
    c. Intelligent
    d. Servo

27. What type of ventilation relies on detection of diaphragm depolarization?
    a. Neurally adjusted ventilatory assist (NAVA)
    b. PAV
    c. CSV
    d. HFV

28. During ventilation of a spontaneously breathing patient, the ventilator increases the respiratory rate so that the set minute volume is achieved. This best describes:
    a. Intermittent mandatory ventilation (IMV)
    b. CPAP
    c. NAVA
    d. Mandatory minute ventilation (MMV)

29. A ventilator has a breathing sequence in which there are mandatory pressure-controlled breaths, but the patient is able to breathe spontaneously between the mandatory breaths. This breathing sequence is called:
    a. CPAP
    b. PC-CMV
    c. Pressure-controlled intermittent mandatory ventilation (PC-IMV)
    d. PAV+

30. Which of the following breath sequences are described by Chatburn's classification system?
    1. Continuous mandatory ventilation (CMV)
    2. Synchronized intermittent mandatory ventilation (SIMV)
    3. Intermittent mandatory ventilation (IMV)
    4. CSV
       a. 1, 2, and 4 only
       b. 1, 2, and 3 only
       c. 1, 3, and 4 only
       d. 2, 3, and 4 only

REFERENCES

1. Cairo JM: *Pilbeam's mechanical ventilation: physiological and clinical applications,* ed 6, St. Louis, 2016, Elsevier.
2. Raniere VM: Optimization of patient-ventilator interactions: closed loop technology to turn the century [editorial]. *Intensive Care Med* 23:936, 1997.
3. Branson RD: Dual control modes, closed loop ventilation, handguns and tequila [editorial]. *Respir Care* 46:232-233, 2001.
4. Chatburn RL: *Fundamentals of mechanical ventilation,* Cleveland Heights, OH, 2003, Mandu Press.
5. Sanborn WG: Microprocessor-based mechanical ventilation. *Respir Care* 38(1):72-109, 1993.
6. Scanlan CL, Wilkins RL, Stoller JK: *Egan's fundamentals of respiratory therapy,* ed 7, St. Louis, 1999, Mosby.
7. Branson RD, Hess DR, Chatburn RL: *Respiratory care equipment,* ed 2, Philadelphia, 1999, Lippincott Williams & Wilkins.
8. Banner MJ: Expiratory positive pressure valves and work of breathing. *Respir Care* 32:431, 1987.
9. Mushin WW, Rendell-Baker L, Thompson PW, et al.: *Automatic ventilation of the lungs,* Philadelphia, 1980, FA Davis.
10. Chatburn RL: *Classification of mechanical ventilation,* Dallas, 1988, American Association for Respiratory Care.
11. Chatburn RL: A new system for understanding mechanical ventilators. *Respir Care* 36:1123-1155, 1991.
12. Branson RD, Hess DR, Chatburn RL: *Respiratory care equipment,* Philadelphia, 1995, JB Lippincott.
13. Chatburn RL, Primiano FP: A new system of understanding modes of mechanical ventilation. *Respir Care* 46(6):604-621, 2001.
14. Chatburn RL: Classification of ventilator modes: update and proposal for implementation. *Respir Care* 52:301-323, 2007.
15. Chatburn RL: Computer control of mechanical ventilation. *Respir Care* 49:507-517, 2004.
16. Chatburn RL, Volsko TA: Mechanical ventilators. In Wilkins RL, Stoller JK, Scanlan CL, editors: *Egan's fundamentals of respiratory care,* ed 8, St. Louis, 2003, Mosby/Elsevier.
17. Chatburn RL, Volsko TA, Hazy J, et al.: Determining the basis for a taxonomy of mechanical ventilation. *Respir Care* 57(4):514-524, 2012.
18. Chatburn RL, El-Khatib M, Miriles-Cabodevila E: A taxonomy for mechanical ventilation: ten fundamental maxims. *Respir Care* 59(11):1747-1763, 2014.
19. Hess DR, MacIntyre NR: *Respiratory care: principles and practice,* Philadelphia, 2002, WB Saunders.
20. MacIntyre N, Nishimura M: The Nagoya conference on system design and patient-ventilator interactions during pressure support ventilation. *Chest* 97:1463-1467, 1990.
21. Chatmongkolchart S, Williams P: Evaluation of inspiratory rise time and inspiratory termination criteria in new-generation mechanical ventilators: a lung model study. *Respir Care* 46:666-677, 2001.
22. Williams P, Mueluer M: Pressure support and pressure assist/control: are there differences?: an evaluation of the newest intensive care unit ventilators. *Respir Care* 45:1169-1181, 2000.
23. Unoki T, Serita A, Grap MJ: Automatic tube compensation during weaning from mechanical ventilation: evidence and clinical implications. *Crit Care Nurse* 28(4):34-42, 2008.
24. Stock MC, Downs JB: Airway pressure release ventilation: a new approach to ventilatory support during acute lung injury. *Respir Care* 32:517-521, 1987.
25. Foland JA, Martin J: Airway pressure release ventilation with a short release time in a child with acute respiratory distress syndrome. *Respir Care* 46:1019-1023, 2001.
26. Frawley PM, Habashi NM: Airway pressure release ventilation: theory and practice. *AACN Clin Issues* 12:234-246, 2001.
27. Myers TR, MacIntyre NR: Does airway pressure release ventilation offer important new advantages in mechanical ventilator support? *Respir Care* 52:452-458, 2007.
28. Rose L, Hawkins M: Airway pressure release ventilation and biphasic positive airway pressure: a systematic review of definitional criteria. *Intensive Care Med* 34:1766-1773, 2008.
29. Daoud EG, Farag HL, Chatburn RL: Airway pressure release ventilation: what do we know? *Respir Care* 57(2):282-292, 2012.
30. Branson RD, Chatburn RL: Should adaptive pressure control modes be utilized for virtually all patients receiving mechanical ventilation? *Respir Care* 52:478-485, 2007.
31. Bouadma L, Lellouche F, Cabello B, et al.: Use of an automated control system to adapt the level of pressure support and manage weaning. *Intensive Care Med* 28:s23, 2002.
32. Rose L, Presneill JJ, Johnston L, et al.: A randomized, controlled trial of conventional versus automated weaning from mechanical ventilation using SmartCare™/PS. *Intensive Care Med* 34:1788-1795, 2008.
33. Burns KEA, Lellouche F, Lessard MR: Automating the weaning process with advanced closed-loop systems. *Intensive Care Med* 34:1757-1765, 2008.
34. Hewlett AM, Platt AS: Mandatory minute volume: a new concept in weaning from mechanical ventilation. *Anaesthesia* 32:163-169, 1977.
35. Otis AB, Fenn WO, Rahn H: Mechanics of breathing in man. *J Appl Physiol* 2:592-607, 1950.
36. Chen C, Wu C, Dai Y, et al.: Effects of implementing adaptive support ventilation in a medical intensive care unit. *Respir Care* 56(7):976-983, 2011.
37. Hess DR: Mechanical ventilation strategies: what's new and what's worth keeping? *Respir Care* 47:1007-1017, 2002.
38. Branson R: Understanding and implementing advances in ventilator capabilities. *Curr Opin Crit Care* 10:23-32, 2004.
39. Yamada Y, Du HL: Effects of different pressure support termination on patient-ventilator synchrony. *Respir Care* 43:1048-1057, 1998.
40. Du HL, Ohtsuji M, Shigeta M, et al.: Expiratory asynchrony in proportional assist. *Am J Respir Crit Care Med* 165:972-977, 2002.
41. Sottiaux TM: Patient-ventilator interactions during volume-support ventilation: asynchrony and tidal volume instability—a report of three cases. *Respir Care* 46:255-262, 2001.
42. Keenan HT, Martin LD: Volume support ventilation in infants and children: analysis of a case series. *Respir Care* 42:281-287, 1997.
43. Grasso S, Ranieri VM: Proportional assist ventilation. *Respir Care Clin N Am* 7:465, 2001.
44. Kondili E, Xirouchaki N, Vaporidi K, et al.: Short-term cardiorespiratory effects of proportional assist and pressure-support ventilation in patients with acute lung

injury/acute respiratory distress syndrome. *Anesthesiology* 105:703-708, 2006.

45. Schulze A, Rieger-Fackeldey E, Gerhardt T, et al.: Randomized crossover comparison of proportional assist ventilation and patient-triggered ventilation in extremely low birth weight infants with evolving chronic lung disease. *Neonatology* 92:1-7, 2007.

46. Younes M: Proportional assist ventilation: a new approach to ventilatory support. I. Theory. *Am Rev Respir Dis* 145:114-120, 1992.

47. Younes M, Puddy A, Roberts D, et al.: Proportional assist ventilation: results of an initial clinical trial. *Am Rev Respir Dis* 145:121-129, 1992.

48. Schulze A, Schaller P: *Proportional assist ventilation: a new strategy for infant ventilation?* Boston, MA, Monograph series, 6:1-12, 1996, Tufts University.

49. Hart N, Hunt A, Polkey MI, et al.: Comparison of proportional assist ventilation and pressure support ventilation in chronic respiratory failure due to neuromuscular and chest wall deformity. *Thorax* 57:979-981, 2002.

50. Kondili E, Prinianakis G, Alexopoulou C, et al.: Respiratory load compensation during mechanical ventilation-proportional assist ventilation with load-adjustable gain factors versus pressure support. *Intensive Care Med* 32:692-699, 2006.

51. Leipälä JA, Iwasaki S, Lee S, et al.: Compliance and resistance levels and unloading in proportional assist ventilation. *Physiol Meas* 26:281-292, 2005.

52. Kacmarek RM: Proportional assist ventilation and neutrally adjusted ventilator assist. *Respir Care* 56(2):140-148, 2011.

53. Sinderby C, Beck J, Spahija J, et al.: Inspiratory muscle unloading by neurally adjusted ventilatory assist during maximal inspiratory efforts in healthy subjects. *Chest* 131:711-717, 2007.

54. Sinderby C, Navalesi P, Beck J, et al.: Neural control of mechanical ventilation in respiratory failure. *Nat Med* 5:1433-1436, 1999.

55. Sinderby C: Ventilatory assist driven by patient demand. *Am J Respir Crit Care Med* 168:729-730, 2003.

56. Fessler HE, Hess DR: Does high-frequency ventilation offer benefits over conventional ventilation in adult patients with respiratory distress syndrome? *Respir Care* 52:595-608, 2007.

57. Sjöstrand U: High-frequency positive pressure ventilation (HFPPV): a review. *Crit Care Med* 8:345-364, 1980.

58. Calkins JM: High-frequency jet ventilation: experimental evaluation. In Carlon CG, Howlan WS, editors: *High-frequency ventilation in intensive care and during surgery*, New York, 1985, Marcel Dekker.

59. English P, Mason SC: Neonatal mechanical ventilation. In Hess DR, MacIntyre NR, editors: *Respiratory care: principles and practice*, Philadelphia, 2002, WB Saunders.

60. Klain M, Smith RB: High-frequency percutaneous transtracheal jet ventilation. *Crit Care Med* 5:280-287, 1977.

61. Ferguson ND, Cook DJ, Guyatt GH, et al.: High frequency oscillation in early acute respiratory distress syndrome. *N Engl J Med* 368(9):795-805, 2013.

62. Toussaint M, De Win H, Steens M, et al.: Effect of intrapulmonary percussive ventilation on mucus clearance in Duchenne muscular dystrophy patients: a preliminary report. *Respir Care* 48:940-947, 2003.

63. Velmahos GC, Chan LS, Tatevossian R, et al.: High-frequency percussive ventilation improves oxygenation in patients with ARDS. *Chest* 116:440-446, 1999.

64. Reper P, Wibaux O, Van Laeke P, et al.: High frequency percussive ventilation and conventional ventilation after smoke inhalation: a randomized study. *Burns* 28:503-508, 2002.

65. Salim A, Martin M: High-frequency percussive ventilation. *Crit Care Med* 33:S241, 2005.

66. English P, Mason SC: Neonatal mechanical ventilation. In Hess DR, MacIntyre NR, editors: *Respiratory care: principles and practice*, Philadelphia, 2002, WB Saunders.

Mechanical Ventilators:
General Use Devices

Terry L. Forrette

OUTLINE

Note: Objectives and key terms are located at the beginning of each ventilator section.

This chapter provides detailed information about a variety of multipurpose ventilators that are primarily used to treat adult and pediatric patients in the intensive care unit (ICU). Each ventilator is presented in a separate section, with an outline, objectives, key terms, and references. The intent of this design is to allow the reader to examine all of the relevant material for one ventilator without having to move from one part of the text to another.

Every effort has been made to ensure that the information provided in this chapter is accurate and current. However, it is important for clinicians to consult the operating manuals and instructions from the manufacturers whenever using medical devices for patient care. Clinicians should also be aware that ventilator manufacturers release periodic software updates, as well as improvements and new features and functionality for their device. Staying abreast of these changes can be accomplished through a variety of resources, including manufacturer updates to customers and findings reported in the scientific literature.

COMMON FEATURES OF VENTILATORS

Common Internal Mechanisms

The internal mechanisms of many microprocessor-controlled machines have several similarities. Chapter 12 provides additional information on the internal drive mechanisms of ventilators, but Table 13.1 includes the ventilators discussed in this chapter and their associated drive mechanisms and power

TABLE 13.1 Common Ventilator Internal Mechanisms and Power Sources

Ventilator	Internal Drive Mechanism	Power Sources
CareFusion AVEA	A rigid accumulator	Pneumatic, electrical, internal battery
Dräger Evita Infinity V500/N500	Electromagnetic servo valves	Pneumatic, electrical, internal battery
Dräger EvitaXL	Electromagnetic servo valves	Pneumatic, electrical, internal battery
GE Carescape	Proportional solenoid valve	Pneumatic, electrical, internal battery
Hamilton-C3	Variable-orifice inspiratory valves	Pneumatic, electrical, internal battery
Hamilton-G5	Variable-orifice inspiratory valves	Pneumatic, electrical, internal battery
Medtronic Minimally Invasive Therapies Puritan Bennett 840/980	Proportional solenoid valve	Pneumatic, electrical, 12-V internal battery
Maquet Servo-i/ Servo-s/Servo-U	Proportional solenoid valve	Pneumatic, electrical, internal battery

sources. The drive mechanism is the mechanical device that produces gas flow to the patient. It is the mechanism used to convert the power source energy into a useful system to supply air to the patient. Ventilators are either electrically or pneumatically (pressured gas) powered, or they use a combination of each.

Historically, it was important for respiratory therapists (RTs) to understand specific details about the internal parts of ventilators to troubleshoot mechanical problems that could potentially arise. However, all of today's ventilators include onscreen troubleshooting and diagnostics to help users identify patient-ventilator problems that occur during mechanical ventilation. For this reason, much of the discussion of the internal function of ventilators in this chapter is presented in an abbreviated fashion.

Patient Parameters and Displays

Most ICU ventilators have light-emitting diode (LED) control panels, which show the operator the mode and parameters currently set and monitored, including graphic information. Some display screens or control panels are touch sensitive. Most control panels include a display window that can provide the operator with a written message, such as an alarm message.

Although Chapter 12 discusses general ventilator parameters, extended monitoring features for each ventilator are described with each ventilator covered in this chapter.

Modes of Ventilation

Chapter 12 describes a method of defining ventilator breaths and modes of ventilation. Unfortunately, manufacturers do not follow a consistent method for naming breath types and modes, which has resulted in a great deal of confusion. Each manufacturer may have a different name for the same mode and breathing pattern. This makes learning breath types and modes for each of the ventilators very difficult for the beginner. Table 13.2 attempts to clear up some of this difficulty by providing the manufacturer's name for the mode, breathing pattern, control type, and operational logic. It also provides a list of the ventilators presented in this chapter and the modes of ventilation for each device.

Alarms

Common alarms include high and low pressure, high and low oxygen percentage, high and low minute volume, high rate, and high and low positive end-expiratory pressure (PEEP)/continuous positive airway pressure (CPAP). Ventilators also have alarm-silencing buttons that usually silence audible alarms for 1 to 2 minutes. In many cases the type of alarm that is active is shown in a display window. Some ventilators illuminate the LEDs next to the violated alarms to indicate which alarms are being or have been activated. Some units scroll through the chronological order of the alarm events as the operator reads the display screen. Alarm information for each ventilator is covered in its section.

Understanding Individual Ventilators

Once clinicians have mastered the use of a newer, more sophisticated ventilator, they usually do not find it difficult to understand another brand. Manufacturers have tried to make their equipment user friendly and provide a variety of materials and services to explain their operation. Most ventilators have ventilator-based onscreen help menus with access to a variety of information and instruction. However, many companies still provide training DVDs, Web-based information, instruction and operation manuals, trained technicians and clinical application specialists, CD-ROM interactive programs, and product specialists via telephone or Internet. Users are encouraged to always refer to the operator's manual provided with each device.

Presentation of Specific Ventilators

It is assumed that readers have a basic understanding of the physical properties of ventilators as outlined in Chapter 12. The machines are presented in such a way as to help prepare readers to understand their standard and extended features such as monitoring displays, graphics, extended modes, and alarm function.

CAREFUSION AVEA (FORMERLY CARDINAL AVEA)[1,2]

OBJECTIVES

Upon completion of this section, you will be able to:
1. Identify the icons and waveforms on the main screen.
2. Describe visual and audible alarm signals.

TABLE 13.2 Comparison of Common Ventilator Modes

Ventilator	Assist/ Control CMV-Vol	PCV	VC-SIMV	PC-SIMV	PRVC	PRVC-SIMV	PSV/CPAP	APRV	Additional Mode(s) or Feature(s)
CareFusion AVEA	Volume A/C	Pressure A/C	Volume SIMV	Pressure SIMV	PRVC	PRVC SIMV	CPAP-PSV	APRV Biphasic	TCPL-A/C and TCPL-SIMV
Dräger Evita Infinity V500	CMV-Vol	CMV-Pres	SIMV (vol.) and PSV	SIMV (Press.)+ PSV	AutoFlow	AutoFlow with SIMV (volume)	CPAP with or without PSV	APRV	MMV, SmartCare PPS
Dräger EvitaXL	CMV	PCV+	SIMV (vol.) and PSV	SIMV (Press.)+ PSV	AutoFlow	AutoFlow with SIMV (volume)	PSV-CPAP	APRV	MMV & MMV + PS
GE CARESCAPE	CMV-Vol	CMV-Pres	SIMV (vol.) and PSV	SIMV (Press)+ and PSV	CMV-PRVC	SIMV— PRVC	PSV— CPAP	BiLevel	BiLevel-PRVC APRV VS NIV SBT
Hamilton-C3	N/A	PCV+	NA	SIMV+ With PSV	CMV-APV	SIMV-APV	Spont/PSV	DuoPAP	ASV
Hamilton-G5	CMV-VC	CMV-PC	SIMV-VC With PSV	SIMV-VC With PSV	CMV-APV	SIMV-APV	Spont/PSV	DuoPAP	INTELLiVENT-ASV
iMaquet Servo-i, Servo-s, and Servo-U	VC	PC	SIMV (Vol. Contr.)	SIMV (Press. Contr.)	PRVC	SIMV (PRVC)	PSV/CPAP	BiVent	VS, NAVA available on Servo-i/ Servo-U NIV
Medtronic Minimally Invasive Therapies PB 840 and 980	Assist/ control (volume)	Assist/ control (Press.)	SIMV (volume)	SIMV (pressure)	VC+	SIMV VC+	SPONT (PSV-CPAP)	Bilevel	PAV+ /VS

A/C, Assist/control; *APRV*, airway pressure-release ventilation; *APV*, adaptive pressure ventilation; *ASV*, adaptive support ventilation; *CMV*, continuous mandatory ventilation; *CPAP*, continuous positive airway pressure; *MMV*, mandatory minute ventilation; *NAVA*, neurally adjusted ventilatory assist; *NIV*, noninvasive positive-pressure ventilation; *PAP*, positive airway pressure; *PAV*, proportional assist ventilation; *PC-CMV*, pressure-controlled continuous mandatory ventilation; *PCV*, pressure-controlled ventilation; *PPS*, proportional pressure support; *PRVC*, pressure-regulated volume control; *PS*, pressure support; *PSV*, pressure-support ventilation; *SBT*, spontaneous breathing trial; *SIMV*, synchronized intermittent mandatory ventilation; *TCPL*, time cycled, pressure limited; *VS*, volume support.

3. Describe the purpose of each of the extended settings.
4. List differences between neonatal and adult modes of ventilation.

KEY TERMS (see Glossary)

Artificial airway compensation (AAC)
User interface module (UIM)
Variable-orifice (flow) pneumotachometer
Volume limit

The CareFusion AVEA ventilator originally was developed by VIASYS Healthcare, Critical Care Division (Fig. 13.1). In 2008 VIASYS was purchased by Cardinal Health's ventilator division, and the AVEA became part of Cardinal Health's critical care ventilator division. This purchase also included the acquisition of Bird, Bear, and SensorMedics ventilation products. CareFusion completed its spin-off from Cardinal Health in 2009. Becton, Dickinson and Company subsequently acquired CareFusion in 2015.

The AVEA is a servo-controlled, software-driven ventilator designed for neonatal, pediatric, and adult patients. Software upgrades can be uploaded to the ventilator when new product developments become available. The new software is electronically delivered to a laptop and then transferred to the ventilator; this process is performed by the company's technical support personnel.

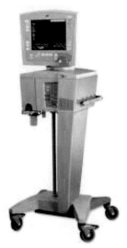

FIGURE 13.1 CareFusion AVEA ventilator. (Courtesy Care-Fusion, Inc., Yorba Linda, CA.)

OVERVIEW OF CONTROLS

The AVEA user interface is a full-color, active matrix, LCD touchscreen. Except for the on/off power switch, which is on the rear panel of the unit, all operator controls are on the front panel of the user interface. A data dial control is used to access and initiate the various control functions of the AVEA (Fig. 13.2).

Primary Breath Controls

Primary breath controls are rate, tidal volume, inspiratory pressure, peak flow, inspiratory pause, PEEP, pressure support, flow trigger, and F_iO_2 (fraction of inspired oxygen). These controls are displayed along the bottom of the touchscreen (see Fig. 13.2). Table 13.3 lists primary breath controls and their description.

MONITORING AND ALARMS

In addition to the display of standard data referenced in the introduction of this chapter (see Tables 13.1 and 13.2), the AVEA has both digital and graphic monitoring displays (Table 13.4). Extended monitoring features are available on the AVEA.

Alarms and Indicators

Alarms and indicators are used to alert clinicians when automatic and adjustable alarm limits are violated or when conditions affecting ventilator function are detected. All alarms have visual displays. Alarm messages appear in the ALARM INDICATOR at the upper right of the touchscreen. The highest priority alarm is always displayed in the top position.

Table 13.5 provides information on these ventilator alarms.

Extended Monitoring

The AVEA provides several extended monitoring options (Table 13.6). A complete description of these options can be found in the manufacturer's user's reference manual or on the manufacturer's website.

TABLE 13.3 Primary Breath Controls—CareFusion AVEA

Parameter	Range
RATE (bpbreaths/min)	1-120 breaths/min (adult), 1-150 breaths/min (pediatric/neonate)
V_T (mL)	100-2500 mL (adult), 25-500 mL (pediatric), 2-300 mL (neonate)
INSP PRESS (cm H_2O)	Inspiratory pressure: 0-90 cm H_2O (adult/pediatric), 0-80 cm H_2O (neonate)
INSPIRATORY RISE (This feature is referred to as PSV rise when PSV is used.)	A setting of 1 is the most rapid rise in pressure, and a setting of 9 is the slowest
PEAK FLOW (L/min)	3-150 L/min (adult), 1-75 L/min (pediatric), 0.4-30 L/min (neonate)
INSP TIME (s)	Inspiratory time: 0.2-5 s (adult/pediatric), 0.15-3 s (neonate)
FLOW CYCLE	0-45%
INSP HOLD (s)	0.0-3 s
PSV (cm H_2O)	Pressure-support ventilation: 0-90 cm H_2O (adult/pediatric), 0-80 cm H_2O (neonate)
PEEP (cm H_2O)	Positive end-expiratory pressure: 0-50 cm H_2O
FLOW TRIG (L/min)	Flow trigger sensitivity; 0.1-20 L/min
Pressure Trigger	Pressure triggering sensitivity 0.1 to 20 cm H_2O
WAVEFORMS	Square wave (constant flow) or a decelerating (descending) ramp
SIGH	1.5 times the set tidal volume every 100 breaths for adult and pediatric patients
% O_2	21-100%
PRES HIGH (cm H_2O)	High-pressure target in APRV: 0-90 cm H_2O (limited to total PIP of 90 cm H_2O)
TIME HIGH (s)	High-pres time in APRV: 0.2-30 s
TIME LOW (s)	Low-pres time in APRV: 0.2-30 s
PRES LOW (cm H_2O)	Low-pressure target in APRV: 0-45 cm H_2O

APRV, Airway pressure-release ventilation; *PIP,* peak inspiratory pressure; *PSV,* pressure-support ventilation.

STANDARD MODES OF VENTILATION

The AVEA offers a selection of modes and breath types. Box 13.1 lists the ventilation modes for adult, pediatric, and neonatal patients. Noninvasive ventilation for pediatric and adult patients and nasal CPAP for infants have been added since the original release. (*Note:* See Chapter 12 for a description of the basic function of each of these modes.)

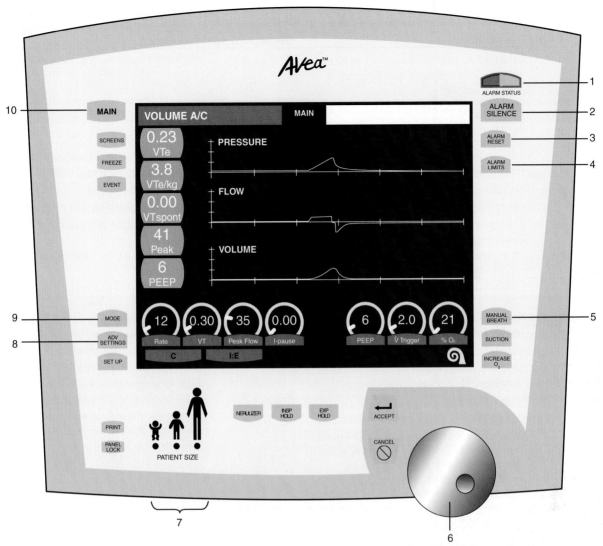

FIGURE 13.2 Front panel (user interface module) of the CareFusion AVEA ventilator, showing the membrane buttons, the light-emitting diodes (LEDs) and indicators, the DATA DIAL and the touchscreen displaying the normal operating screen. *(1)* This LED flashes for high- and medium-priority alarms and stays on continuously for low-priority alarms. *(2)* The alarm silence button silences an alarm for 2 minutes. *(3)* The alarm reset button cancels visual indicators of resolved alarms. *(4)* The alarm limits button opens and closes the alarm limits window. *(5)* The manual breath button delivers a single mandatory breath using current settings. *(6)* A data dial is used to change a highlighted field or control on the touchscreen. *(7)* Patient size LED indicators show the currently selected patient size. *(8)* The adv settings button opens and closes an advanced settings window for feature activation or parameter adjustment. *(9)* The mode button opens and closes the mode menu. *(10)* The main button returns to the main screen display from any screen. (Courtesy CareFusion, Inc., Yorba Linda, CA.)

EXTENDED MODES AND FEATURES

In addition to standard modes of ventilation, the AVEA provides extended modes. A complete description of these is found in Chapter 12 and on the manufacturer's website.

Machine Volume

Machine volume (MACH VOL) is another volume criterion that establishes a minimum volume delivery. It is active in pressure-targeted mandatory breaths, such as pressure A/C and pressure SIMV (synchronized intermittent mandatory ventilation).

PSV T$_{MAX}$

PSV T$_{MAX}$ sets the maximum length of inspiratory time allowed during a PSV (pressure-support ventilation) breath (range: 0.2 to 5 seconds [adult/pediatric patients] and 0.15 to 3 seconds [neonates]).

Independent Lung Ventilation

For clinicians who want to provide independent lung ventilation (ILV) to a patient through a double-lumen endotracheal tube, the AVEA can be synchronized with another AVEA. The

TABLE 13.4 **Standard Measured and Display Parameters—CareFusion AVEA**

Displayed Data	Description	Displayed Data	Description
V_{Te}	Exhaled tidal volume (mL)	f/V_T	Rapid, shallow breathing index (breaths/min/L); respiratory rate divided by tidal volume
V_{Te}/Kg	Milliliters of V_{Te} per kilogram adjusted for patient weight		
V_{Ti}	Inspired tidal volume (mL)	P_{PEAK}	Peak inspiratory pressure (cm H_2O)
Spon V_T	Spontaneous V_T (mL)	P_{MEAN}	Mean airway pressure (cm H_2O)
Spon V_T/Kg	Milliliters of Spon V_T per kilogram adjusted for patient weight	P_{PLAT}	Plateau pressure (cm H_2O), if available
		PEEP	Positive end-expiratory pressure (cm H_2O)
Mand V_T	Mandatory V_T (mL)	Auto-PEEP	Measurement of intrinsic PEEP
Mand V_T/Kg	Mandatory V_T per kilogram adjusted for patient weight	Air inlet	Air inlet pressure (psig)
		O_2 Inlet	Oxygen inlet pressure (psig)
Vdel	Volume of gas delivered by the ventilator	F_IO_2	Percent of oxygen displayed as a whole number
% Leak	Percent leakage; the difference between the inspiratory and expiratory volume in % difference	Cdyn	Dynamic compliance (characteristic) (mL/cm H_2O)
Ve	Calculated minute volume (L/min) based on set V_T and rate for volume breaths only	Cs (Cstat)	Static compliance (mL/cm H_2O); requires an inspiratory hold maneuver
Spon Ve/kg	Spontaneous minute volume adjusted for patient weight	Rrs	Respiratory system resistance (cm H_2O/L/sec); calculation is performed during an inspiratory hold maneuver
Rate	Respiratory rate (breaths/min)		
Spon Rate	Spontaneous rate (breaths/min)	PIFR	Peak inspiratory flow rate (L/min)
Mand rate	Mandatory rate (breaths/min)	PEFR	Peak expiratory flow rate (L/min)
Ti	Inspiratory time (sec)	Graphics	Graphic displays of breath delivery using pressure, volume, or flow scalars, or real-time displays of pressure-volume and flow-volume loops
Te	Expiratory time (sec)		
I:E	Calculated value for inspiratory to expiratory ratio, based on set rate, V_T, and peak flow for volume breaths, and rate, and inspiratory time for pressure, TCPL and PRVC breaths (range: 1:99.9 to 99.9:1)		

Additional monitored values are listed in the operator's manual.
PRVC, Pressure-regulated volume control; *TCPL,* time cycled pressure limited.

BOX 13.1 **Modes of Ventilation—CareFusion AVEA**

Adult/Pediatric Modes	Neonatal Modes
• Volume A/C	• Volume A/C
• Pressure A/C	• Pressure A/C
• PRVC A/C	• TCPL A/C
• Volume SIMV	• Volume SIMV
• Pressure SIMV	• Pressure SIMV
• PRVC SIMV	• TCPL SIMV
• APRV/BiPhasic	• Volume guarantee
• CPAP PSV	• CPAP PSV
• Apnea backup ventilation (ABV)	• Apnea backup ventilation (ABV)
• Noninvasive positive-pressure ventilation (NPPV or NIV)	• There is no NIV option in the neonatal mode for the AVEA

A/C, Assist/control; *APRV,* airway pressure-release ventilation; *CPAP,* continuous positive airway pressure; *PRVC,* pressure-regulated volume control; *PSV,* pressure-support ventilation; *SIMV,* synchronized intermittent mandatory ventilation; *TCPL,* time cycled, pressure limited.

ventilator provides an output (master) and an input (slave) for synchronization of the ventilators.

Heliox

Heliox delivery is available on the comprehensive AVEA package and as an option on the standard AVEA ventilator.

Neonatal Application

A neonatal application option is available with the AVEA. Either a hot wire or variable-orifice flow proximal airway flow sensor is recommended when the AVEA is used with infants who weigh less than 5 kg. In addition to standard modes of neonatal ventilation PC-SIMV, PRVC (pressure-regulated volume control), and PSV are available. Monitoring and alarm functions associated with these modes are very similar to the adult modes found on the AVEA. A complete description of the AVEA neonatal applications can be found on the manufacturer's website and operator's manual.

■ KEY POINTS

• The CareFusion AVEA can be used for conventional invasive or noninvasive positive-pressure ventilation and in neonatal, pediatric, and adult patients.

TABLE 13.5 Alarms—CareFusion AVEA

Alarm	Description
Vent Inop	Ventilator failure. The safety valve opens (SAFETY VALVE message appears). Spontaneously breathing patients can breathe room air.
Loss of Air	Wall or cylinder air below 18 psig. No compressor installed.
Loss of O_2	O_2 supply below 18 psig.
Loss of Gas Supply	All gas sources failed. Safety valve opens.
Low P_{PEAK}	Peak inspiratory pressure less than the set Low P_{PEAK} value.
High P_{PEAK}	Peak inspiratory pressure greater than the High P_{PEAK} value. Inspiration ends.
Ext High P_{PEAK}	High P_{PEAK} alarm has been active for longer than 5 seconds. Safety valve opens. No breaths are delivered.
Low PEEP	Baseline pressure drops below set Low PEEP level.
Low Minute Volume	Monitored exhaled $\dot{V}_E$ is less than set value for Low $\dot{V}_E$ alarm.
High Minute Volume	Monitored exhaled Ve is greater than set value for High $\dot{V}_E$ alarm.
High V_T	Monitored exhaled V_T is greater than set value for High V_T alarm.
Apnea	Ventilator does not detect a breath during set apnea interval.
High rate	Monitored total breath rate exceeds high rate value.
I-Time Limit	Inspiratory time exceeds set MAX I-time plus any set pause time (5 s [adult/pediatric patient], 3 s [neonate]).
I:E Limit	I:E ratio exceeds 4:1 for a mandatory breath; inspiration ends.
Low F_IO_2	Delivered O_2 falls below set F_IO_2 minus 6% or falls below 18%.
High F_IO_2	Delivered O_2 rises above set F_IO_2 plus 6%.

F_IO_2, Fraction of inspired oxygen; *I:E*, inspiratory time to expiratory time; V_T, tidal volume.

- Patient monitoring from the CareFusion AVEA includes esophageal, tracheal, and proximal airway pressure monitoring.
- The artificial airway compensation feature adjusts the pressure delivery from the CareFusion AVEA to compensate for the pressure drop across an artificial airway.
- NIV can be performed using any mode for pediatric and adult patients.
- Apnea backup ventilation is available in all modes in which spontaneous ventilation is available (SIMV, APRV [airway pressure-release ventilation]/BiPhasic, and CPAP/PSV modes).
- Machine volume (MACH VOL) establishes a minimum volume delivery when mandatory breaths are pressure targeted.

TABLE 13.6 Extended Monitoring—CareFusion AVEA

Feature	Description
Respiratory mechanics via esophageal catheter	Monitors and displays measurements of compliance and airway resistance
Volumetric capnography	Monitors end-tidal and mixed expired carbon dioxide values
Tracheal and esophageal pressure monitoring	Measures respiratory mechanics and auto-PEEP
Vsync	Changes volume breaths to pressure-limited, volume-targeted breaths

- Vsync changes volume breaths to pressure-limited, volume-targeted breaths.
- Respiratory mechanics that can be measured with the CareFusion AVEA include esophageal pressure measurement, MIP (maximum inspiratory pressure)/P_{100}, inflection point (Pflex), and autoPEEP.

REFERENCES

1. AVEA brochure RC 0105; AVEA 17 Comprehensive Spec Sheet RC 5860; AVEA nCPAP Spec Sheet; AVEA Neonatal Brochure Domestic RC 1198; AVEA Standard Spec Sheet, www.carefusion.com.
2. Cairo JM: *Pilbeam's mechanical ventilation: clinical and physiological application*, ed 6, St. Louis, 2016, Elsevier.

DRÄGER EVITAXL

OBJECTIVES

Upon completion of this section, you will be able to:

1. Identify the specific areas of the Dräger EvitaXL front control panel.
2. List the modes of ventilation available for the Dräger EvitaXL.
3. List differences between adult and neonatal modes of ventilation.

KEY TERMS (see Glossary)

Airway pressure-release ventilation (APRV)
Apnea ventilation
AutoFlow
Control panel
Expiratory hold
Mandatory minute ventilation (MMV)
NeoFlow
Occlusion pressure ($P_{0.1}$)
Pmax pressure limit

The Dräger EvitaXL is one of several ventilators in the Dräger Evita series. The two earlier versions, the Dräger E-4 and the

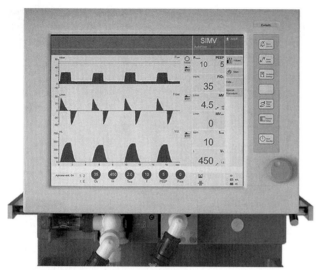

FIGURE 13.3 Front view of the Dräger EvitaXL. (© Drägerwerk AG & Co. KGaA, Lubeck, Germany.)

Evita 2 Dura, were developed after the original Evita ventilator. The EvitaXL is no longer sold in the United States but is available in Europe.

The E-4 and the Evita 2 Dura can be upgraded with the EvitaXL option to provide them with the options and features available with the EvitaXL. This section explains the features of the Dräger EvitaXL. The EvitaXL is designed to be used for ventilation of adults, children, and infants (minimum weight: 3 kg). To use the EvitaXL for infants, the NeoFlow option must be activated. The EvitaXL has a front control panel with touchpads, a dial (rotary) knob, and a computer screen (Figs. 13.3 and 13.4). The operating screen (control panel) contains the information and controls needed for ventilation.

OVERVIEW OF CONTROLS

A number of controls, monitors, and alarm settings are available on the Dräger EvitaXL. The EvitaXL uses a single rotary knob, several hard-touch keys on the side of the computer screen, and the touch-sensitive screen keys and screen knobs on the computer screen (see Fig. 13.4). The computer screen can display a variety of different pages, all of which display a similar layout (Fig. 13.5).

MONITORING AND ALARMS

In every mode of ventilation, the EvitaXL provides monitored parameters on the right side of the screen.

Standard Measured and Displayed Parameters

Table 13.7 lists the available ranges for primary breath control parameters. Many of the measured parameters on the EvitaXL are obtained with a hot wire pneumotachometer (see Chapter 8). In addition to the display of standard data referenced in the introduction of this chapter (see Tables 13.1 and 13.2), there are other basic parameters (Table 13.8), but the EvitaXL also can display extended monitoring (Table 13.9).

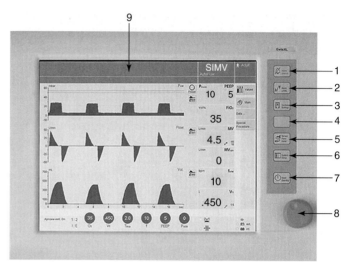

FIGURE 13.4 Details of the control panel on the EvitaXL. *(1)* Alarm silence key. *(2)* Alarm limits setting key. *(3)* Ventilator settings for ventilator modes and parameters. *(4)* Unassigned key for future use. *(5)* Sensor parameter key for calibrating sensors and activating and deactivating monitoring. *(6)* System setup key for configuring various ventilator functions. *(7)* Start/standby control. *(8)* Rotary dial knob for selecting and confirming settings. *(9)* Touch-sensitive screen for displaying various screen views. (© Drägerwerk AG & Co. KGaA, Lubeck, Germany.)

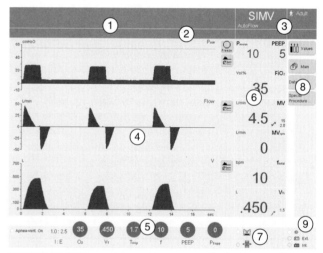

FIGURE 13.5 View of the typical screen display on the EvitaXL. *(1)* Space for display of alarm messages. *(2)* Space for display of operator prompts. *(3)* Mode of ventilation display, patient size selected (adult or child), and AutoFlow when selected. (AutoFlow is reviewed later.) *(4)* Graphic display of real-time waveforms, loops, and trends, depending on the page selected. *(5)* Digital display of set ventilation parameters. *(6)* Display of measured values. *(7)* Humidification type and status selected. *(8)* Touch-sensitive screen keys available for the currently selected page. *(9)* Power supply indicator. (© Drägerwerk AG & Co. KGaA, Lubeck, Germany.)

Extending Monitoring

The EvitaXL provides several extended monitoring options in addition to displaying standard measurements. Table 13.9 lists several of these options, and a complete description of these measurements can be found on the manufacturer's website.

TABLE 13.7 Primary Breath Controls—Dräger EvitaXL

Tidal Volume (Body Temperature and Pressure Saturated [BTPS] ± 10%)	
Adult	0.1-2 L
Pediatric	0.02-0.30 L
Neonate	0.03-0.10 L
Flow	
Adult	6-120 L/min (to 180 L/min with AutoFlow)
Pediatric	6-30 L/min (to 60 L/min with AutoFlow)
Neonate	0.25-30 L/min
Neonate continuous flow	6 L/min
Variable Ranges for All Patients	
Respiratory rate	0-100 breaths/min 0-150 breaths/min with NeoFlow
Inspiratory time	0.1-10 s
Inspiratory pressure (set) (Pinsp)	0-95 cm H$_2$O
Maximum inspiratory pressure limit (Pmax)	0-100 cm H$_2$O
Percent oxygen	21-100% (±5% of set)
PEEP	0-50 cm H$_2$O
Trigger sensitivity	0.3-15 L/min
Pressure support	0-95 cm H$_2$O
Rise time for PS	0-2 sec

PEEP, Positive end-expiratory pressure; *PS*, pressure support.

Alarms

Alarms can be set by pressing the ALARM LIMITS touchpad to the right of the display screen (see Figs. 13.4 and 13.5). Alarm parameters should always be set appropriately for the patient. Table 13.10 lists the ranges for the adjustable alarms.

STANDARD MODES OF VENTILATION

Box 13.2 lists the standard modes of operation available on the EvitaXL.

EXTENDED MODES AND FEATURES

The EvitaXL has several extended features to augment its standard modes of ventilation. They are described in general in Chapter 12 and in the owner's manual.

AutoFlow

AutoFlow is a dual control mode of ventilation (see Chapter 12). It can be activated when a volume-targeted mode of ventilation is selected, such as CMV (continuous mechanical ventilation), SIMV, or MMV (mandatory minute ventilation). AutoFlow provides pressure-limited breaths (pressure-controlled ventilation) that are volume targeted.

TABLE 13.8 Standard Measured and Displayed Parameters—Dräger EvitaXL

Parameter	Definition	Range
P$_{PEAK}$	Maximum airway pressure	0-120 cm H$_2$O
P$_{PLAT}$	Plateau pressure	0-99 cm H$_2$O
P$_{MEAN}$	Mean pressure	0-99 cm H$_2$O
PEEP	Positive end-expiratory pressure	0 to 50 cm H$_2$O
Auto-PEEP (intrinsic PEEP)	Pressure measured during an expiratory hold maneuver.	
P$_{MIN}$	Minimum airway pressure	20 to 99 cm H$_2$O
	Range	45 to 100 cm H$_2$O
	Resolution	1 cm H$_2$O
	Accuracy	4% (cm H$_2$O)
MV	Minute ventilation	0-100 L/min
MVspn	Spontaneous breathed minute volume	
	Range	0-120 L/min (BTPS)
	Resolution	0.1 L/min or values < 1 L/min: 0.01 L/min
	Accuracy	±8% of measured value
V$_{Te}$	Exhaled tidal volume	
	Range	0-6 L (BTPS)
	Resolution	1 mL
	Accuracy	±8% of measured value
f$_{tot}$	Breathing frequency	0-240 breaths/min
f$_{spn}$	Spontaneous frequency	
	Range	0-300 breaths/min
	Resolution	1 breath/min
	Accuracy	±1 breath/min
F$_I$O$_2$	Fractional inspired O$_2$ measured on inspiratory side	
	Range	15-100 vol.%
	Resolution	1 vol.%
	Accuracy	±3 vol.%
T	Breathing gas temperature	18°-51°C
R	Resistance	0-600 cm H$_2$O/L/s
C	Compliance	0-300 mL/cm H$_2$O
Waveforms	Pressure, volume, flow scalars	
Loops	Pressure-volume and flow-volume loops	

BTPS, Body temperature and pressure saturated.

TABLE 13.9   Extended Monitoring Features—Dräger EvitaXL

Feature	Description
Infrared carbon dioxide analyzer $P_{ET}CO_2$	Provides measurement of carbon dioxide production and dead space
Occlusion pressure at 100 ms ($P_{.01}$)	Evaluates neurological drive
Low-flow PV loop	Used to evaluate upper and lower inflection points

$P_{ET}CO_2$, Partial pressure of end-tidal carbon dioxide.

BOX 13.2   Modes of Ventilation—Dräger EvitaXL

- CMV—volume A/C
- PCV+ pressure A/C
- SIMV—volume or pressure with PS option
- CPAP—with or without PS
- APRV (airway pressure-release ventilation)
- ILV (independent lung ventilation)
- NIV (noninvasive mask ventilation)
- Apnea ventilation

A/C, Assist/control; *CMV,* continuous mandatory ventilation; *CPAP,* continuous positive airway pressure; *PCV,* pressure-controlled ventilation; *PS,* pressure support; *SIMV,* synchronized intermittent mandatory ventilation.

Mandatory Minute Ventilation

With MMV, the ventilator provides mandatory breathing only if the patient's spontaneous breathing is not adequate and drops below the preselected MMV setting. MMV is set by selecting that screen tab and then setting the MMV appropriate for the patient using the V_T (tidal volume), flow, f, and T_I (inspiratory time) settings. A pressure-support level should be set to ensure that the patient has adequate support for spontaneous breaths.

Neonatal Applications[1-3]

The EvitaXL, when configured using the NeoFlow proximal airway sensor, can be used for neonatal ventilation. With the exception of SmartCare, all invasive modes of ventilation available for adults are also available for neonatal patients. The neonatal modes of ventilation share many of the same monitoring and alarm functions used during adult ventilation. A complete description of neonatal options on the EvitaXL can be found on the manufacturer's website and in the operator's manual.

Automatic Leakage Compensation

During volume ventilation the EvitaXL can compensate for leakage. The unit has a leak compensation feature that can be turned off or on. When leak compensation is activated, the ventilator compares delivered flow with exhaled flow.

TABLE 13.10   Alarm Ranges—Dräger EvitaXL

Parameter	Range and/or Description
Expiratory Minute Ventilation	
Alarm at upper alarm limit	If MV has exceeded the upper limit MV 41-0.1 L/min
Alarm at lower alarm limit	If MV falls below the lower limit 0.01-40 L/min
Setting range for NIV	1-60 L/min
Volume	
Alarm at lower alarm limit	If the set V_T could not be applied (alarm limit is linked to set V_T)
Alarm at upper alarm limit	If applied V_T exceeds the alarm threshold, inspiration is interrupted and the exhalation valve opens
Setting range	21-4000 mL
High f_{spn}[a]	5-120 breaths/min; the rate is exceeded during spontaneous breathing
Airway Pressure (Paw)	
Alarm at upper alarm limit	If Paw high value is exceeded
Setting range	10-100 cm H_2O
Paw alarm at lower limit	If value of PEEP + 5 cm H_2O (linked to set PEEP value) is not exceeded for at least 96 ms in two consecutive ventilator breaths
Apnea Alarm Delay Time	If no breath is detected; range: 5-60 sec
End-Tidal CO₂ Alarm[b]	
High end-tidal CO₂ (ETCO₂)	If the upper limit has been exceeded
Range	0-98 mm Hg (1-15 vol.%)
Low ETCO₂	If the value drops below the lower alarm limit
Range	0-97 mm Hg (0-14.9 vol.%)
Inspired O₂% Alarm	
Alarm at upper alarm limit	If O₂% exceeds the upper alarm limit for at least 20 s
Alarm at lower alarm limit	If O₂% falls below the lower alarm limit for at least 20 s
Range	Both alarm limits are linked to the set value: Threshold for settings below 60 vol.%: ±4 vol.% Threshold for settings above 60 vol.%: ±6 vol.%

[a]No lower alarm limit available.
[b]Available only when CO_2 analyzer (capnograph) is added.
f_{spn}, Spontaneous frequency; *NIV,* noninvasive ventilation; *PEEP,* positive end-expiratory pressure; V_T, tidal volume.

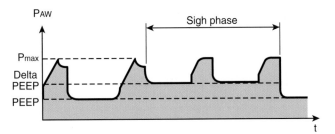

FIGURE 13.6 Example of the pressure-time waveform during the sigh mode with the EvitaXL. Pmax is maximum pressure, interim positive end-expiratory pressure (PEEP) is the PEEP applied during the sigh phase, and PEEP is the regular setting for PEEP before and after the sigh. (See text for additional information.) (© Drägerwerk AG & Co. KGaA, Lubeck, Germany.)

Sigh (Intermittent PEEP)

As with a normal sigh breath, the intended purpose of the sigh function on the EvitaXL is to open or keep open areas of the lung that are prone to collapsing (atelectasis). Sigh breaths are accomplished in the EvitaXL ventilator by intermittently increasing the PEEP level to the set sigh pressure value for two consecutive breaths in the CMV mode (Fig. 13.6). The range of baseline sigh pressure (PEEP) is 0 to 35 cm H_2O.

SmartCare

SmartCare/PS is a closed-loop form of ventilation designed to shorten weaning time for intubated or tracheostomy patients who are ready for ventilator discontinuation. The strategy of the software is to gradually reduce the level of assistance based on the patient's tolerance and comfort.

Automatic Tube Compensation

An automatic tube compensation (ATC) feature is available on the EvitaXL to compensate for the airway resistance associated with small artificial airways.

■ KEY POINTS

- The Dräger EvitaXL (version 7.0) is designed to be used for ventilation of adults, children, and infants (minimum weight: 3 kg).
- With the Dräger EvitaXL, the operator can choose invasive or noninvasive ventilation.
- Expiratory flow for the ventilator is measured with a hot wire pneumotachometer, and inspired oxygen concentrations are measured using a galvanic oxygen analyzer.
- As with the E-4, the EvitaXL can optimally include a mainstream carbon dioxide analyzer that provides information on end-tidal carbon dioxide, CO_2/time, and single-breath CO_2 (CO_2/volume).
- Available modes of ventilation include CMV, AutoFlow, SIMV, PCV+, MMV, CPAP, APRV, ILV, and apnea ventilation.
- AutoFlow is a dual-control mode that provides a pressure-limited, volume-targeted form of ventilation in which the ventilator adjusts the pressure to achieve the set volume.

- Special functions of the EvitaXL include compensation for patient circuit compliance, flow trigger, automatic leakage compensation, sigh (intermittent PEEP), and tubing compensation.
- Diagnostic functions available with the EvitaXL include measurement of intrinsic PEEP, occlusion pressure ($P_{0.1}$), low-flow PV loop, and negative inspiratory force, which requires the use of the expiratory hold function.
- SmartCare/PS, an option available with the EvitaXL, is a closed-loop form of ventilation designed to shorten weaning time for intubated or tracheostomy patients who are ready for ventilator discontinuation.

REFERENCES

1. Cairo JM: *Pilbeam's mechanical ventilation: physiological and clinical applications*, ed 6, St. Louis, 2016, Elsevier.
2. *The new generation of excellence in Dräger ventilation*, Marketing communications # 9051738, Lubeck, Germany, Drägerwerk AG & Co KGaA.
3. *Breathing support package, proportional pressure support PPS, tube compensation, ATC, supplement to the instructions for use of the Evita 4 as from software version 2.n 90 28 825-GA 5664.520 e*, ed 1, Telford, PA, 1996, and version 4.n, 2001, Dräger, Drägerwerk AG.

■ DRÄGER EVITA INFINITY V500 AND N500[1,2]

OBJECTIVES

Upon completion of this section, you will be able to:

1. Identify the specific areas of the Dräger Evita V500 and N500 control panels.
2. List the modes of ventilation available for the Evita V500 and Evita N500 ventilators.
3. List two extended monitoring features on the Evita V500 and Evita N500 ventilators.
4. Compare neonatal and adult ventilation on the Evita V500 and Evita N500.

KEY TERMS (see Glossary)

Automatic leakage compensation
Low-Flow PV Loop
SmartCare/PS
Smart Pulmonary View

The Dräger Evita Infinity Evita V500 (Evita V500) (Fig. 13.7) is the most recent addition to the Dräger Evita series manufactured by Drägerwerk in Lubeck, Germany. The Dräger EvitaXL ventilator is described in the previous section. The Evita Infinity N500 platform is very similar to that of the Evita V500 but is configured exclusively for neonatal ventilation.

OVERVIEW OF CONTROLS

The Evita V500 is an electrically powered, pneumatically driven, time-cycled, volume constant, pressure-controlled ventilator.

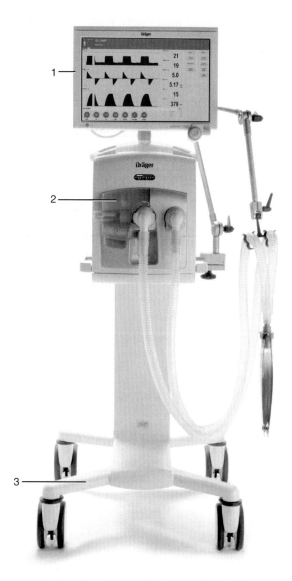

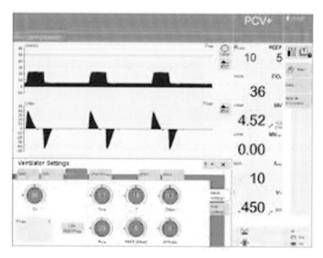

FIGURE 13.8 Medical cockpit of the Dräger Evita V500. (© Drägerwerk AG & Co. KGaA, Lubeck, Germany.)

FIGURE 13.7 Dräger Infinity Evita V500 Critical Care Unit. *(1)* Infinity C500 control and display unit. *(2)* Evita V500 ventilation unit. *(3)* Trolley 2, 90 cm. (© Drägerwerk AG & Co. KGaA, Lubeck, Germany.)

TABLE 13.11 Primary Breath Controls— Dräger Evita V500

Tidal Volume (Body Temperature and Pressure Saturated [BTPS] ± 10%)	
Adult	0.1-3 L
Pediatric	0.02-0.30 L
Neonate flow	0.002-0.10 L
Adult	2-120 L/min
Pediatric	2-30 L/min
Neonate	2-30 L/min
Neonate continuous flow	6 L/min
Variable Ranges for All Patients	
Respiratory rate	0-150 breaths/min
Inspiratory time	0.1-10 s
Inspiratory pressure (set) (Pinsp)	1-95 cm H_2O
Maximum inspiratory pressure limit (Pmax)	2-100 cm H_2O
Percent oxygen	21-100%
PEEP	0-50 cm H_2O
Trigger sensitivity	0.2-15 L/min
Pressure support	0-95 cm H_2O
Rise time for PS	0-2 s
Expiratory termination	1-80%

PEEP, Positive end-expiratory pressure; *PS,* pressure support.

The ventilator system comprises three major components: control system "Medical Cockpit," Evita ventilation unit, and power supply units (see Fig. 13.7).

Setting parameters is accomplished with the use of a rotary control found in the Medical Cockpit component. Likewise, patient-ventilator data are also displayed in this area (Fig. 13.8). In addition, the V500 offers the option to export logbooks, trends, and screen content to a USB stick and then print or email the data.

Table 13.11 lists the primary control features found on the Evita V500.

A number of controls, monitors, and alarm settings are available on the Dräger Evita V500. As does the Dräger EvitaXL, the Evita V500 uses a single rotary knob, several hard-touch keys on the side of the computer screen, and the touch-sensitive screen keys and screen knobs on the computer screen.

MONITORING AND ALARMS

In every mode of ventilation, the Evita V500 provides monitored parameters on the right side of the screen. The active mode appears in the top right corner. Graphics are centrally located. On the bottom is a row that displays the set parameters. Although these are the variables most commonly selected (Table 13.12), the displayed variables can be changed (see Fig. 13.8).

TABLE 13.12 Standard Measured and Displayed Parameters—Dräger Evita V500

Parameter	Definition	Range
P_{PEAK}	Maximum airway pressure	0-120 cm H_2O
P_{PLAT}	Plateau pressure	0-99 cm H_2O
P_{MEAN}	Mean pressure	0-99 cm H_2O
PEEP	Positive end-expiratory pressure	0-50 cm H_2O
Auto-PEEP (intrinsic PEEP)	Pressure measured during an expiratory hold maneuver.	
Pmin	Minimum airway pressure	−60 to 120 cm H_2O
MV	Minute ventilation	0-99 L/min
MVspn	Spontaneous breathed minute volume Range	0-99 L/min (BTPS)
V_{Te}	Exhaled tidal volume Range	0-5.5 L (BTPS)
f_{tot}	Breathing frequency	0-300 breaths/min
f_{spn}	Spontaneous frequency Range	0-300 breaths/min
F_IO_2	Fractional inspired O_2 measured on inspiratory side	
T	Breathing gas temperature	18°-51°C
R	Resistance	0-1000 cm H_2O/L/s
C	Compliance	0-650 mL/cm H_2O
Waveforms	Pressure, volume, flow scalars	
Loops	Pressure-volume and flow-volume loops	

BTPS, Body temperature and pressure saturated.

TABLE 13.13 Extended Monitoring Features—Dräger Evita V500

Feature	Description
Infrared carbon dioxide analyzer $P_{ET}CO_2$	Provides measurement of carbon dioxide production and dead space measurements
Occlusion pressure at 100 ms ($P_{.01}$)	Evaluates neurological drive
Low-flow PV loop	Used to evaluate upper and lower inflection points

$P_{ET}CO_2$, Partial pressure of end-tidal carbon dioxide.

TABLE 13.14 Alarms—Dräger Evita V500

Alarm	Value (Limits)
Expiratory minute volume	High/Low
Tidal volume	High/Low
Airway pressure	High/Low
F_IO_2	High/Low
Tachypnea	High/Low
Apnea	5-60 s
End-expiratory CO_2	High/Low

F_IO_2, Fraction of inspired oxygen.

BOX 13.3 Standard Modes of Ventilation—Dräger Evita V500

- CMV—volume A/C
- CMV—pressure A/C
- SIMV—volume or pressure with PS option
- CPAP—with or without PS
- APRV (airway pressure release ventilation)
- NIV—noninvasive mask ventilation with leak compensation
- Apnea ventilation

A/C, Assist/control; *CMV,* continuous mandatory ventilation; *CPAP,* continuous positive airway pressure; *PS,* pressure support; *SIMV,* synchronized intermittent mandatory ventilation.

Extended Monitoring

The V500 incorporates a feature called Smart Pulmonary View, which allows for real-time visualization of pulmonary function data. In addition to this information, the ventilator can show several extended displays of monitoring data. Table 13.13 lists some of these features.

Alarms

Many of the alarms on the Evita V500 can be set by pressing the ALARM LIMITS button on the main menu bar. Alarm parameters should always be set appropriately for the patient. Table 13.14 lists these alarms.

In addition to the user-adjustable alarm settings, the Evita V500 automatically has several alarm limits that cannot be set by the user. These are set based on the monitored values taken by the ventilator during start-up and throughout the course of ventilation. A complete description of these alarms can be found in the operator's manual.

STANDARD MODES OF VENTILATION

The Dräger Evita V500 has several manufacturer preset modes of ventilation, including assist control, SIMV, and spontaneous. In addition to these modes, volume- or pressure-control breath types are available. Box 13.3 lists the standard modes and breath types available on the Evita V500.

EXTENDED MODES AND FEATURES

The Dräger Evita V500 has several extended features to augment its standard modes of ventilation. These are described in Chapter 12 and also in the Evita V500 operator's manual.

AutoFlow

AutoFlow is a dual-control mode of ventilation (see Chapter 12). It can be activated when a volume-targeted mode of ventilation is selected, such as CMV, SIMV, or MMV. AutoFlow provides pressure-limited breaths (PCV) that are volume targeted.

Mandatory Minute Ventilation

With MMV the ventilator provides mandatory breathing only if the patient's spontaneous breathing is not adequate and drops below the preselected MMV setting. MMV is set by selecting that screen tab and then setting the MMV appropriate for the patient using the V_T, flow, f, and T_I settings. A pressure-support level should be set to ensure that the patient has adequate support for spontaneous breaths.

Automatic Leakage Compensation

During volume ventilation the Evita V500 can compensate for leakage. The unit has a leak-compensation feature that can be turned off or on. When leak compensation is activated, the ventilator compares delivered flow with exhaled flow.

Intermittent PEEP

As with a normal sigh breath, the intended purpose of the sigh function on the Dräger Evita V500 is to open up or keep open areas of the lung that are prone to collapsing (atelectatic). Sigh breaths are accomplished in the Evita V500 ventilator by intermittently increasing the PEEP level to the set sigh pressure value for two consecutive breaths in the CMV mode (see Fig. 13.6). The range of baseline sigh pressure (PEEP) is 0 to 35 cm H_2O.

Proportional Pressure Support

Proportional pressure support (PPS) is a spontaneous breathing mode in which pressure support (PS) is applied in proportion to the patient's breathing effort. Minimal breathing efforts are supported with a much lower level of support compared with stronger efforts that generate a higher level of PS from the ventilator. In PPS the ventilator can be programmed to provide support to overcome the elastance using volume assist and also flow assist to aid in overcoming airway resistance.

SmartCare

SmartCare/PS is a closed-loop form of ventilation designed to shorten weaning time for intubated or tracheotomized patients who are ready for ventilator discontinuation. The strategy of the software is to gradually reduce the level of assistance based on the patient's tolerance and comfort.

Automatic Tube Compensation

An ATC feature is available on the Evita V500 to compensate for the airway resistance associated with small artificial airways.

Neonatal Application

The Evita V500, when configured using the NeoFlow proximal airway sensor, can be used for neonatal ventilation. All invasive modes of ventilation, with the exception of SmartCare, are available during neonatal ventilation. Additionally, alarm and monitoring functions are very similar to those used with adult ventilation. A complete description of the neonatal options for the V500 and N500 can be found on the manufacturer's website and in the operator's manual.

KEY POINTS

- Control features, mode selection, and alarm functions are accessed in the cockpit area on the Dräger Evita V500.
- The Evita V500 offers the option to export logbooks, trends, and screen content to a USB stick and then print or email the data.
- The Evita V500 automatically sets several alarm limits that are based on the monitored values taken by the ventilator during start-up and throughout the course of ventilation.
- Smart Pulmonary View allows for real-time visualization of pulmonary function data.
- SmartCare/PS is a closed-loop form of ventilation designed to shorten weaning time for intubated or tracheotomized patients who are ready for ventilator discontinuation.

REFERENCES

1. Evita Infinity v500 SW 2 905260 en us; rsp evita V500 br 9066398 us en, Lubeck, Germany, 2013, Dräger, Drägerwerk AG & Co. KGaA.
2. *Instruction manual: Evita Infinity V500 Acute Care System—SW 2.n*, Lubeck, Germany, Drägerwerk AG & Co. KGaA.

GE HEALTHCARE CARESCAPE R860 (PREVIOUSLY KNOWN AS THE ENGSTRÖM CARESTATION[1])

OBJECTIVES

Upon completion of this section, you will be able to:
1. List the standard modes of ventilation found on the GE Carescape R860.
2. Describe the function of the ARC (airway resistance compensation) extended feature.
3. List measurements obtained with the gas modules.
4. Describe measurements obtained with the FRC INview module.
5. Describe options available for neonatal ventilation.

KEY TERMS (see Glossary)

FRC INview
Metabolic energy expenditure
Plug-and-play modules
SpiroDynamics

The GE Carescape R860 (Fig. 13.9) was released in 2015 with significant changes from the previous GE Engström CareStation. It delivers time- or flow-cycled breaths, depending on the breath type, using proportional flow control valves.

The ventilator can be set for adult, pediatric, or neonatal patients, depending on the software version used. A combination of a touch-sensitive screen and trim knob (Fig. 13.10) allow the user to select control variable, monitoring options, alarm settings, and modes.

OVERVIEW OF CONTROLS

Table 13.15 lists the primary breath controls for adult and pediatric patients. A complete listing of control variables may be found in the manufacturer's user's reference manual or at its website.

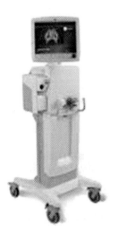

FIGURE 13.9 GE Healthcare Carescape. (Used with permission of GE Healthcare.)

MONITORING AND ALARMS

The Carescape R860 uses an expiratory flow transducer to measure exhaled parameters, which are updated on a breath-by-breath basis. Table 13.16 lists the standard measured parameters. Fig. 13.11 shows a screen display. A complete description of displayed parameters can be found in Chapter 12, and in the manufacturer's user's reference manual or website.

Extended Monitoring

The Carescape R860 provides the clinician with several patient monitoring options using its plug-and-play technology (Table 13.17). A complete description of these options is available in the manufacturer's user's reference manual and on its website.

Alarms

The Carescape R860 uses an escalating alarm feature with changes in tones if it is left unattended. Alarm settings may be manually selected or automatically set based on current values for each parameter. Table 13.18 lists the standard alarm ranges.

STANDARD MODES OF VENTILATION

A list of standard modes can be found in Box 13.4, and a complete general description of these modes may be found in Chapter 12. Additional information about the standard modes of ventilation is available in the manufacturer's user's reference manual and website.

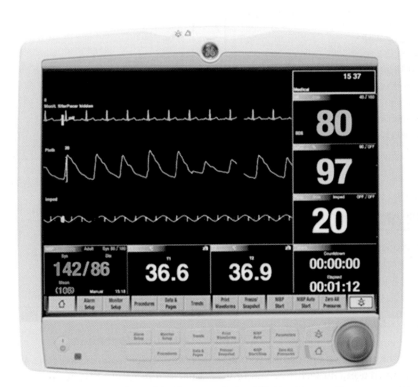

FIGURE 13.10 Display controls and indicators of the GE Healthcare Carescape. (Used with permission of GE Healthcare.)

TABLE 13.15 Primary Breath Controls (Adult and Pediatric)—GE Carescape R860

Parameter	Definition	Range
V max	Maximum peak flow	120 L
Flow	Flow	2-72 L/min pediatric 2-160 L/min adult
F_1O_2	Inspired oxygen	21-100%
Frequency	Respiratory rate	1-120 breaths/min (depending on mode and breath type)
I:E	Inspiratory to expiratory time	1:9 to 4:1 1:72 to 60:1 in BiLevel
T_1	Inspiratory time	0.25-15 s
T_E	Expiratory time	0.25-59.75 s
T_{high}	Time high during BiLevel	0.25-15 s
T_{low}	Time low during BiLevel	0.25-18 s
V_T	Tidal volume	20-2000 mL
PIP	Inspiratory pressure	1-98 cm H_2O
Phigh	High pressure during BiLevel	1-98 cm H_2O
Plow	Low pressure during BiLevel	1-50 cm H_2O
PEEP	Positive end-expiratory pressure	1-50 cm H_2O
PSV	Pressure support	0-60 cm H_2O
Rise Time	Rise to inspiratory pressure	0-500 ms
End Flow	Flow termination	5-80% of peak flow
Flow Trigger	Trigger effort	1 to 9 L/min
Pressure Trigger	Trigger effort	−10 to −0.25 cm H_2O
Bias Flow	Continuous in patient breathing circuit	2-10 L/min 8-20 L/min (NIV)

NIV, Noninvasive positive-pressure ventilation.

TABLE 13.16 Standard Measured and Displayed Parameters—GE Carescape R860

Parameter	Range
Tidal volume	5-2500 mL
Airway pressure	−20 to +120 cm H_2O
Patient flow	1-200 L/min
Minute volume	0-99.9 L/min
Rate	0-120 breaths/min
Inspired oxygen concentration	0-100%
Rapid shallow breathing index	0-9999 breaths/min/L
Waveforms	Scalars for pressure, volume, and flow
Spirometry loops	Display of PV, FV, or PF loops
Compliance	0.1-150 mL/cmH$_2$O
Resistance	1-500 cm H_2O/L/sec
PEEP	0-50 cm H_2O
Auto-PEEP	1-20 cm H_2O

FV, Flow volume loop; *PEEP,* positive end-expiratory pressure; *PF,* peak flow; *PV,* pressure volume curve.

TABLE 13.17 Extended Monitoring Features—GE Carescape R860

Feature	Description
Calculations View	Using monitored and collected data, the following parameters/indices can be calculated: P_AO_2, A-aDO$_2$, Pa/F$_1$O$_2$, CO, V$_d$/V$_T$
SpiroDynamics	Measurements of intrinsic PEEP using a tracheal catheter
FRC INview	Measurement of FRC based on nitrogen washout technique
Metabolic gas monitoring and nutritional assessment	Measurement of $\dot{V}O_2$ $\dot{V}CO_2$ are used to calculate respiratory quotient (RQ) and energy expenditure (EE)
Lung mechanics	$P_{0.1}$, NIF, vital capacity
SBT	Spontaneous breathing trial

A-aDO$_2$, Difference in alveolar-arterial oxygen gradient; *FRC,* functional residual capacity; *PEEP,* positive end-expiratory pressure; *NIF,* negative inspiratory force; *P$_{0.1}$,* occlusion pressure; *P$_A$O$_2$,* partial pressure of alveolar oxygen; *Pa/F$_1$O$_2$,* arterial oxygen pressure to inspired oxgyen ratio; *V$_d$/V$_T$,* deadspace to tidal volume ratio.

EXTENDED MODES AND FEATURES

In addition to standard modes of ventilation, the Carescape R860 provides several extended modes and features. A complete description of these can be found in the ventilator's operation manual.

BiLevel With Volume Guaranteed

With BiLevel with volume guaranteed, a patient is provided bilevel ventilation but with the additional option of a volume guarantee similar to the volume-guaranteed (VG) option available in CMV and SIMV.

Tube Compensation

Airway Resistance Compensation modifies the delivery pressure to correct for artificial airway resistance.

Leak Compensation

Leak Compensation allows the user to activate a leak compensation feature that automatically adjusts breath delivery to compensate for patient and system leaks.

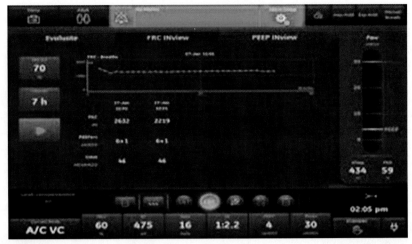

FIGURE 13.11 Monitoring screen view of the GE Healthcare Carescape. (Used with permission of GE Healthcare.)

TABLE 13.18 Standard Alarm Ranges—GE Carescape R860

Alarm	Value (limit)
Minute volume	Low: 0.01-40 L/min High: 0.02-99 L/min
Tidal volume	Low: 1-1950 mL High: 3-2000 mL
Respiratory rate	Low: 1-99/min High: 2-150/min
Inspired oxygen concentration	Low: 18-99% High: 24-100%
Airway pressure	High: 7-100 cm H_2O Low: 1-97 cm H_2O
PEEP	Low: 1-20 cm H_2O High: 5-50 cm H_2O
Auto-PEEP	1-20 cm H_2O
Apnea	5-60 s
Circuit leak	10-90%
End-tidal oxygen	Low: Off, 10-99% High: 11-100%
End-tidal carbon dioxide	Low: 0.1-14.9% or 0-114.5 mm Hg High: 0.2-15%, or 0.5-115 mm Hg

PEEP, Positive end-expiratory pressure.

BOX 13.4 Standard Modes of Ventilation—GE Healthcare Carescape

- CMV—Volume A/C
- CMV—Pressure A/C
- CMV—PCVG (pressure-controlled volume guaranteed)
- SIMV—Volume or pressure control with PS option
- SIMV—PCVG
- BiLevel/APRV—BiLevel with APRV capability
- CPAP with PSV
- NIV
- Apnea ventilation

A/C, Assist/control; *APRV,* airway pressure-release ventilation; *CMV,* continuous mandatory ventilation; *CPAP,* continuous positive airway pressure; *NIV,* noninvasive positive-pressure ventilation; *PS,* pressure support; *PSV,* pressure-support ventilation; *SIMV,* synchronized intermittent mandatory ventilation.

In addition to most of the standard and extended modes of ventilation, volume guarantee pressure support (VG-PS) is available with the neonatal option. A complete description of the neonatal option can be found on the manufacturer's website and in the operator's manual.

KEY POINTS

- The GE Healthcare Carescape R860 uses plug-and-play modules to provide a wide variety of displays and monitoring options.
- Extended monitoring features include nitrogen washout functional residual capacity (FRC) measurements and intrinsic PEEP measurements with an intratracheal catheter.
- Automatic compensation for artificial airways resistance is available using the ARC option.
- Measurements of oxygen consumption and carbon dioxide production are used to calculate respiratory quotient (RQ) and energy expenditure.

Trigger Compensation

Trigger Compensation allows the ventilator to automatically adjust the flow sensitivity for leaks in the patient breathing circuit and artificial airway.

Neonatal Applications

The neonatal option on the Carescape R860 provides ventilation for intubated neonatal patients weighing as little as 0.25 kg. A proximal flow sensor at the patient wye is used to monitor volumes. Monitoring and alarm function in the neonatal mode are similar to those available for adult and pediatric patients.

REFERENCE

1. *User's manual GE Healthcare Carescape R860*, Datax-Ohmeda, Inc., a General Electric Company, doing business as GE Healthcare, Finland.

HAMILTON-G5[1]

OBJECTIVES

Upon completion of this section, you will be able to:
1. Identify how control functions are accessed.
2. List the standard measured display of monitoring data.
3. Describe the use of the P/V tool.
4. List the standard modes of ventilation.
5. Describe the function of ASV.
6. Compare the differences between adult and neonatal ventilation.

KEY TERMS (see Glossary)

Adaptive support ventilation (ASV)
Auto alarm function
Dynamic Heart/Lung Panel
IntelliTrig

The Hamilton-G5 (G5) (Fig. 13.12) is an electronically controlled, pneumatically driven ventilator using variable-orifice inspiratory valves to deliver metered gas mixtures and flows. The ventilator can be used for adult, pediatric, or neonatal ventilation. Breath controls, alarm setting, and monitoring functions are accessed using a touchscreen and rotary knob control.

The Hamilton S1 ventilator, which is currently not available in the United States, includes many of the features found on the G5 model. The Hamilton S1 ventilator also offers a closed-loop feedback system, Adaptive Support Ventilation using exhaled carbon dioxide and SpO_2 (oxygen saturation as measured using pulse oximetry) measurements. (A version of ASV, INTELLiVENT-ASV is available in Europe)

OVERVIEW OF CONTROLS

Control functions on the Hamilton-G5 are accessed using a touchscreen (Figs. 13.13 and 13.14). Table 13.19 lists the primary breath controls.

MONITORING AND ALARMS

The G5 uses an airway sensor to measure flow, volume, and pressure at the patient's proximal airway. A complete description and operating characteristics of the airway sensor can be found in the G5 operator's manual, but Table 13.20 lists the standard measured displays and parameters. Fig. 13.15 shows the monitor display for the Hamilton-G5 ventilator.

The G5 provides a full array of alarm functions, which can be manually set or automatically set by the ventilator using

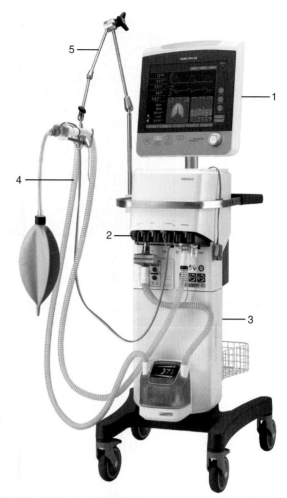

FIGURE 13.12 Hamilton-G5 with accessories. *(1)* Ventilation cockpit. *(2)* Breathing circuit connectors. *(3)* Trolley. *(4)* Breathing circuit. *(5)* Support arm. (Courtesy Hamilton Medical, Bonaduz, Switzerland.)

an Auto Alarm function. A complete description for setting and monitoring alarms (Table 13.21) can be found in the Hamilton-G5 user's manual.

Extended Monitoring

In addition to a display of standard measurements, the Hamilton-G5 has several extended monitoring features (Table 13.22). Many of these features are displayed using a Dynamic Heart/Lung Panel (Fig. 13.16). A description of these can be found in Chapter 12 and in the G5 user's manual.

STANDARD MODES OF VENTILATION

The Hamilton-G5 uses many of the standard modes of ventilation (Box 13.5) that previously described ventilators incorporate. A description of these modes can be found in Chapter 12 and in the G5 user's manual.

EXTENDED MODES AND FEATURES

In addition to the standard modes listed in Box 13.5, the G5 offers several "extended" modes of ventilation. A complete

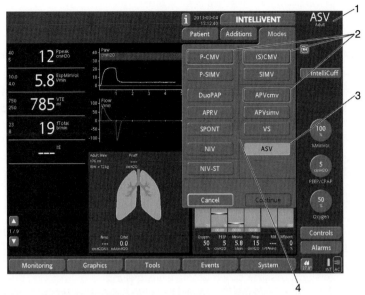

FIGURE 13.13 Hamilton-G5 Modes Window. *(1)* Active mode. *(2)* Backup mode for mode group. *(3)* New selected mode. *(4)* Box enclosed mode group. (Courtesy Hamilton Medical, Bonaduz, Switzerland.)

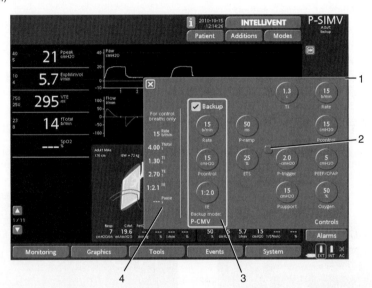

FIGURE 13.14 Hamilton-G5 Controls Window. *(1)* Control settings applicable to the mode. *(2)* Trigger-type selector (select and activate to select type). *(3)* Apnea backup ventilation enabled or disabled, and if enabled, backup mode and selected control settings for backup ventilation. *(4)* Timing parameters, based on the timing settings (if control breaths are permitted in the selected mode): • Rate and ratio of inspiratory time to expiratory time (I:E) • T_{total}: Total breath cycle time • T_I: Duration of inspiratory phase, including any pause • T_E: Duration of expiratory phase • Pause: Duration of pause or plateau • IRV (when applicable): Indicates that the insufflation + Pause time settings > 50% of total breath time • V_T/kg: Tidal volume per kg ideal body weight (Courtesy Hamilton Medical, Bonaduz, Switzerland.)

description of many of these can be found in Chapter 12 and also on the manufacturer's website.

Adaptive Pressure Ventilation

Adaptive pressure ventilation (APV) provides volume targeting during a pressure-controlled breath. The clinician sets a target tidal volume, and the ventilator adapts to changing lung mechanics by altering the delivery pressure. APV may be used with CMV- or SIMV-based ventilation.

Leak Compensation

Leak compensation is provided, using a proximal sensor to measure the difference between delivered and exhaled tidal volume. Using an IntelliTrig function, the ventilator automatically adjust leaks to improve synchrony.

Adaptive Support Ventilation

Adaptive support ventilation (ASV) is a form of closed-loop ventilation that provides for the delivery of minimum minute

TABLE 13.19 Primary Breath Controls—Hamilton-G5

Parameter	Definition	Range
Backup	Provides ventilation when apnea is detected	Enabled or disabled
ETS	Expiratory trigger sensitivity	5-70% of peak inspiratory flow
Flow pattern	Adjustable flow delivery	Sine, square, decelerating
Flow trigger	Effort from patient to initiate a breath	0.5-15 LMP
Gender	Setting used to compute IBW	Male, female
I:E	Inspiratory to expiratory time	1:9.0 to 4.0:1
% Minute volume	Used to set target MV in ASV	25-350%
F_IO_2	Delivered oxygen concentration	21-100%
P-ASV (see Fig. 13.15)	Maximum pressure set by ASV	PEEP 5-110 cm H_2O
Patient height	Setting used to calculate IBW	30-250 cm
Pause	Inspiratory pause	0-70% of cycle time
$P_{control}$	Pressure above PEEP during inspiratory phase for PCV breaths	5-100 cm H_2O
Peak flow	Maximum inspiratory flow	1-180 L/min
PEEP/CPAP	Baseline pressure	0-50 cm H_2O
P_{high} or P_{low}	Pressures applied with APRV or DuoPAP	0-50 cm H_2O
P-ramp	Rate of pressure rise	25-200 ms
Pressure support	Pressure above baseline during spontaneous breaths	0-100 cm H_2O
P-trigger	Effort from patient to initiate a breath above baseline pressure	0.1-10 cm H_2O
Rate	Mandatory breath rate	0.5-150 breaths/min
Sigh	Regularly delivered breaths at increased pressure or tidal volumes	Enabled or disabled
Thigh/Tlow	Duration of P_{high}/P_{low} setting	0.1-30 s
Ti	Time to deliver set V_T or $P_{control}$	0.1-10 s
%Ti	Time to deliver the required set V_T or $P_{control}$, as a percentage of the total breath cycle	10-80% to TCT
Tip	Inspiratory pause time	0-8 sec
TRC	Tube resistance compensation	10-100%
V_T	V_T delivered on mandatory breaths	20-2000 mL
V_{target}	Target V_T in APV modes	2-2000 mL

APRV, Airway pressure-release ventilation; *APV,* adaptive pressure ventilation; *ASV,* adaptive support ventilation; *CPAP,* continuous positive airway pressure; F_IO_2, fraction of inspired oxygen; *IBW,* ideal body weight; *PCV,* pressure-controlled ventilation; *PEEP,* positive end-expiratory pressure; *TCT,* total cycle time; V_T, tidal volume.

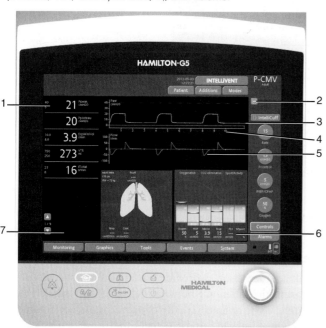

FIGURE 13.15 Monitor display. *(1)* Main monitoring parameters (MMPs) are freely configurable (selected during configuration). *(2)* Freeze button. *(3)* Waveforms. *(4)* Patient trigger indicator. *(5)* Ventilation cockpit panels. *(6)* Intelligent panels. *(7)* Secondary monitoring parameters (SMPs). (Courtesy Hamilton Medical, Bonaduz, Switzerland.)

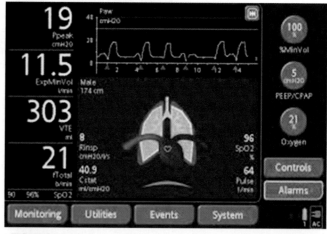

FIGURE 13.16 Dynamic Heart/Lung panel. (Courtesy Hamilton Medical, Bonaduz, Switzerland.)

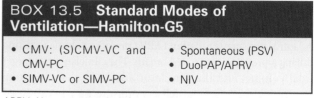

BOX 13.5 Standard Modes of Ventilation—Hamilton-G5

- CMV: (S)CMV-VC and CMV-PC
- SIMV-VC or SIMV-PC
- Spontaneous (PSV)
- DuoPAP/APRV
- NIV

APRV, Airway pressure-release ventilation; *CMV,* continuous mandatory ventilation; *NIV,* noninvasive positive-pressure ventilation; *PSV,* pressure-support ventilation; *SIMV,* synchronized intermittent mandatory ventilation.

TABLE 13.20　Standard Measured and Displayed Parameters—Hamilton-G5

Parameter	Range
Auto-PEEP	0-99 cm H_2O
Cstat—static compliance	0-200 mL/cm H_2O
Exp Flow—peak expiratory flow	0-999 L/min
Exp Min Vol	0.0-99.9 L/min
fSpont—spontaneous rate	0-999 breaths/min
fTotal—total breathing rate	0-999 breaths/min
I:E	1:99 to 99:1
Inspiratory Flow	0-999 L/min
Inspiratory Time	0.00-99.9 s
Expiratory Time	0.00-99.9 s
MV Spont	0.0-99.9 L/min
% Oxygen	18-100%
PEEP/CPAP	0-99 cm H_2O
P_{insp}	0-120 cm H_2O
$P_{minimum}$	–99-99 cm H_2O
$P_{mean/plateau}$	0-99 cm H_2O
R_{insp}/R_{exp}—resistance to inspiratory/respiratory flow	0-999 cm H_2O/L/s
RSB—rapid shallow breathing index	0-999 1/(L/min)
VLeak—leak volume	0-9999 mL
VTE—expiratory tidal volume	0-9999 mL
VTE_{spont}	0-9999 mL
Waveforms and Dynamic Loops	Scalars for pressure, volume, and flow; and dynamic loops for pressure-volume or flow-volume displays

CPAP, Continuous positive airway pressure; *I:E*, inspiratory time to expiratory time; *MV*, minute ventilation; *PEEP*, positive end-expiratory pressure.

TABLE 13.21　Standard Alarm Ranges—Hamilton-G5

Alarm	Range
Apnea Time	10-60 s
ExpMinVol (low and high)	Low: Off, 0.01-49 L/min High: Off, 0.03-50 L/min
Leak	Off, 5-80%
$P_{ET}CO_2$ (low and high)	Low: Off, 0-99 mm Hg High: Off, 1-100 mm Hg
Pressure (low and high)	Low: 2-119 cm H_2O High: 10-120 cm H_2O
Rate (low and high)	Low: 0-128 breaths/min High: 2-130 breaths/min
SpO$_2$ (low and high)	Low: 70-99% High: 71-100%
V_T (low and high)	Low: Off, 0-2950 mL High: Off, 1-3000 mL

$P_{ET}CO_2$, Partial pressure of end-tidal carbon dioxide; *SpO$_2$*, oxygen saturation as measured using pulse oximetry; *V_T*, tidal volume.

TABLE 13.22　Extended Monitoring Features—Hamilton-G5

Feature	Description
$F_{ET}CO_2$ and $P_{ET}CO_2$	Fractional/partial pressure of end-tidal CO_2 concentration used as an indirect assessment of $PaCO_2$
slopeCO$_2$ (%CO_2/L)	Slope of the alveolar plateau to evaluate inefficient ventilation
$\dot{V}CO_2$ (mL/min)	CO_2 elimination, which reflects metabolic rate
VDaw	Airway dead space
$\dot{V}$alv (mL/min)	Alveolar minute ventilation, which measures actual alveolar ventilation rather than Exp Min Vol
$P_{0.1}$ (cm H_2O)	Airway occlusion pressure during the first 100 ms of inspiration, which reflects respiratory drive
PTP (cm H_2O*s)	Inspiratory pressure time product, which is a reflection of work by the patient to trigger a breath
WOBimp (J/L)	Work of breathing imposed by the ventilator circuit and artificial airway
Integrated cuff pressure control	Regulates and maintains a predetermined artificial airway cuff pressure
P-V Tool	Generates a static pressure-volume curve to assess hysteresis during a lung recruitment maneuver
Transpulmonary pressure	Esophageal pressure monitoring to measure lung and chest wall compliance.

volume level through spontaneous or controlled breaths, or a combination of both breath types.

Neonatal Application

The Hamilton-G5 can be configured to provide neonatal ventilation using an infant flow sensor. The neonatal option has similar monitoring and alarm functions as adult ventilation. All infant/neonatal modes available in the G5 are pressure modes. ASV is not available with neonatal ventilation.

A complete description of the neonatal option can be found on the manufacturer's website and in the operator's manual.

■ KEY POINTS

- The Hamilton-G5 ventilator can be set for adult, pediatric, or neonatal ventilation.
- A sensor at the patient's proximal airway is used to measure flow, volume, and pressure.

- An Auto Alarm function allows for the automatic setting of alarm levels.
- A Dynamic Heart/Lung panel provides visual changes in lung mechanics.
- ASV, a form of closed-loop ventilation, provides for the delivery of a minimum minute volume with changing lung mechanics.

REFERENCE

1. *Operator's manual: Hamilton-G5*, Bonaduz, Switzerland, 2012, Hamilton Medical AG.

HAMILTON-C3[1]

OBJECTIVES

Upon completion of this section, you will be able to:
1. List the standard modes of ventilation.
2. Describe how APV differs from volume-controlled continuous mandatory ventilation (VC-CMV).
3. Describe how the Hamilton-C3 measures alveolar ventilation.
4. Compare the differences between adult and neonatal ventilation.

KEY TERMS (see Glossary)

Adaptive pressure ventilation (APV)
Adaptive support ventilation (ASV)
CO_2 elimination ($\dot{V}CO_2$)
Intelligent panels

The Hamilton-C3 (Fig. 13.17) is pneumatically powered and electronically controlled. The electrical systems control pneumatic gas delivery, monitor alarms, and distribute power. It is very similar in function to the Hamilton-G5, with the exception of providing pressure ventilation only in the form of PCV- and APV-type breaths. Additionally, there are some minor differences in control settings and displayed parameters (Tables 13.23 and 13.24). The C3 provides ventilation for adult, pediatric, and neonatal patients. (The C3 is an updated version of the Hamilton-C2, incorporating a larger user interface display.)

OVERVIEW OF CONTROLS

Table 13.23 provides a list of primary breath controls (adult and pediatric). A complete listing of control variables may be found in the manufacturer's user's reference manual or website. Control variables are accessed using a rotary knob and touch-screen (Fig. 13.18).

MONITORING AND ALARMS

The Hamilton-C3 measures flow, volume, and pressure using a proximal flow sensor. Table 13.24 lists the standard displays

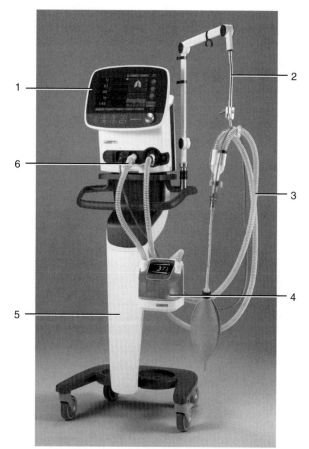

FIGURE 13.17 Hamilton-C3 with accessories. *(1)* Graphical user interface (GUI). *(2)* Support arm. *(3)* Breathing circuit. *(4)* HAMILTON-HC humidifier. *(5)* Trolley. *(6)* Breathing circuit connections. (Courtesy Hamilton Medical AG, Bonaduz, Switzerland.)

(Figs. 13.19 and 13.20). Monitored parameters are displayed using selective menus referred to as "Intelligent Panels."

Extended Monitoring

In addition to a display of standard measurements, the Hamilton-C3 has several extended monitoring features (Table 13.25). Many of these features are displayed using a Dynamic Heart/Lung Panel. A description of these may be found in Chapter 12 and in the C3 user's manual (see Fig. 13.16).

Alarms

The C3 provides a full array of alarm functions (Table 13.26), which can be manually set or automatically set by the ventilator using an Auto Alarm function. A complete description for setting and monitoring alarms can be found in the Hamilton C3 user's manual.

STANDARD MODES OF VENTILATION

The primary breath type delivered by the C3 is pressure-control ventilation with the option of providing adaptive pressure ventilation with a volume target. Box 13.6 lists the standard modes of ventilation. A description of adaptive

TABLE 13.23   Primary Breath Controls—Hamilton-C3

Parameter	Definition	Range
Backup	Provides ventilation when apnea is detected	Enabled or disabled
ETS	Expiratory trigger sensitivity	5-80% of peak inspiratory flow
Flow Pattern	Adjustable flow delivery	Sine, square, decelerating
Flow Trigger	Effort from patient to initiate a breath	1.0-15 LPM
Gender	Setting used to compute ideal body weight (IBW)	Male, female
I:E	Inspiratory to expiratory time	1:9.0-4.0:1
% Minute Volume	Used to set target MV in ASV	25-350%
F_IO_2	Delivered oxygen concentration	21-100%
P-ASV	Maximum pressure set by ASV	PEEP 5-60 cm H_2O
Patient height	Setting used to calculate IBW	30-250 cm
Pause	Inspiratory pause	0-70% of cycle time
$P_{control}$	Pressure above PEEP during inspiratory phase for PCV breaths	5-60 cm H_2O
Peak Flow	Maximum inspiratory flow	1-180 L/min
PEEP/CPAP	Baseline pressure	0-35 cm H_2O
P_{high} or P_{low}	Pressures applied with APRV or DuoPAP	0-60 cm H_2O
P-ramp	Rate of pressure rise	0-200 m/s
Pressure Support	Pressure above baseline during spontaneous breaths	0-60 cm H_2O
Rate	Mandatory breath rate	1-80 breaths/min
Sigh	Regularly delivered breaths at increased pressure or tidal volumes	Enabled or disabled
T_{high}/T_{low}	Duration of P_{high}/P_{low} setting	0.1-40 s
T_I	Time to deliver set V_T or $P_{control}$	0.1-12 s
TRC	Tube resistance compensation	0-100%
V_{target}	Target V_T in APV modes	20-2000 mL

APRV, Airway pressure-release ventilation; *APV,* adaptive pressure ventilation; *ASV,* adaptive support ventilation; *CPAP,* continuous positive airway pressure; *LPM,* liters per minute; *PCV,* pressure-controlled ventilation; *PEEP,* positive end-expiratory pressure; V_T, tidal volume.

TABLE 13.24   Standard Measured and Displayed Parameters—Hamilton-C3

Parameter	Range
Auto-PEEP	0-80 cm H_2O
Cstat—static compliance	0-200 mL/cm H_2O
Exp Flow—peak expiratory flow	0-210 L/min
Exp Min Vol	0.0-99.9 L/min
fSpont—spontaneous rate	0-999 breaths/min
fTotal—total breathing rate	0-999 breaths/min
I:E	1:99 to 99:1
Inspiratory Flow	0-210 L/min
Inspiratory Time	0.00-60 s
Expiratory Time	0.00-60 s
MV Spont	0.0-99.9 L/min
% Oxygen	18-105%
PEEP/CPAP	0-80 cm H_2O
P_{insp}	0-80 cm H_2O
$P_{mean/plateau}$	0-80 cm H_2O
R_{insp}—resistance to inspiratory	0-999 cm H_2O/L/s
RC_{exp}	0-99.9 s
RSB—rapid shallow breathing index	10-400 1/(L/min)
Leak	0-100%
V_{Te}—expiratory tidal volume	0-9000 mL
$V_{Te\ spont}$	0-9000 mL
Waveforms and Dynamic Loops	Scalars for pressure, volume, and flow; and dynamic loops for pressure-volume or flow-volume displays

CPAP, Continuous positive airway pressure; *I:E,* inspiratory time to expiratory time; *MV,* minute ventilation; *PEEP,* positive end-expiratory pressure.

TABLE 13.25   Extended Monitoring—Hamilton-C3

Feature	Description
$F_{ET}CO_2$ and $P_{ET}CO_2$	Fractional/partial pressure of end-tidal CO_2 concentration used as an indirect assessment of $PaCO_2$
slopeCO2 (%CO2/L)	Slope of the alveolar plateau to evaluate inefficient ventilation
$\dot{V}CO_2$ (mL/min)	CO_2 elimination, which reflects metabolic rate
VDaw	Airway dead space
$\dot{V}alv$ (mL/min)	Alveolar minute ventilation, which measures actual alveolar ventilation rather than Exp Min Vol
$P_{0.1}$ (cm H_2O)	Airway occlusion pressure during the first 100 ms of inspiration, which reflects respiratory drive
PTP (cm H_2O*s)	Inspiratory pressure time product, which is a reflection of work by the patient to trigger a breath

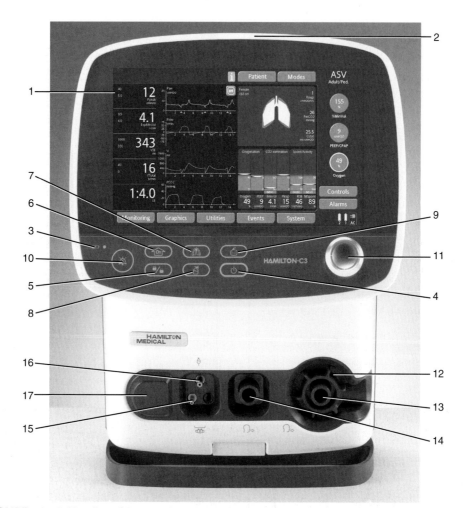

FIGURE 13.18 Hamilton-C3 control panel. *(1)* Touchscreen. *(2)* Alarm lamp. *(3)* Battery charge indicator. *(4)* Power/standby switch. Powers the ventilator on and off and accesses standby. *(5)* Screen lock/unlock key. *(6)* O₂ enrichment key. *(7)* Manual breath/inspiratory hold key. *(8)* Nebulizer on/off key. *(9)* Print screen key. *(10)* Alarm silence key. *(11)* Press-and-turn (P&T) knob. *(12)* Expiratory valve cover and membrane. *(13)* From patient port. *(14)* To patient port. *(15)* Flow sensor connection. *(16)* Pneumatic nebulizer output connector. *(17)* Oxygen cell with cover. (Courtesy Hamilton Medical, Bonaduz, Switzerland.)

TABLE 13.26 Adult Alarm Ranges—Hamilton-C3

Alarm	Range
Apnea Time	15-60 s
ExpMinVol (low and high)	Low: Off, 0.01-50 L/min High: Off, 0.03-50 L/min
$P_{ET}CO_2$ (low and high)	Low: Off, 0-99 mm Hg High: Off, 1-100 mm Hg
Pressure (low and high)	Low: 4-60 cm H₂O High: 15-70 cm H₂O
Rate (low and high)	Low: 0-99 breaths/min High: 0-99 to 130 breaths/min
V_T (low and high)	Low: Off, 10-3000 mL High: Off, 10-3000 mL

$P_{ET}CO_2$, Partial pressure of end-tidal carbon dioxide; V_T, tidal volume.

BOX 13.6 Standard Modes of Ventilation—Hamilton-C3

- (S)CMV+ (adaptive pressure ventilation[a])
- SIMV+ (adaptive pressure ventilation)
- PCV+
- PSIMV+
- Spontaneous/Pressure Support
- NIV
- DuoPAP/APRV

[a]Adaptive pressure ventilation allows volume targeting during a pressure-controlled breath.
APRV, Airway pressure-release ventilation; *NIV*, noninvasive positive-pressure ventilation; *PCV*, pressure-controlled ventilation; *PSIMV*, pressure-synchronized intermittent mandatory ventilation; *PC-IMV*, pressure controlled-intermittent mandatory ventilation; *PSV*, pressure-support ventilation; *(S)CMV*, PC-CMV; *SIMV*, synchronized intermittent mandatory ventilation.

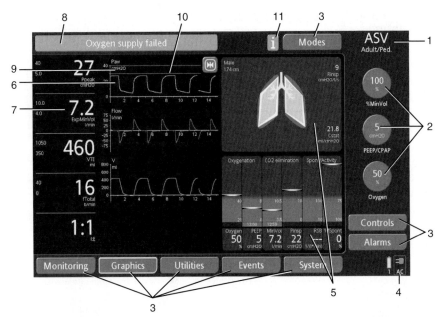

FIGURE 13.19 Default (basic screen). *(1)* Active mode and patient group. *(2)* Main controls. *(3)* Window buttons. *(4)* Input power. *(5)* Graphic display. *(6)* Trigger symbol. *(7)* Main monitoring parameters (MMPs). *(8)* Message bar. *(9)* Maximum pressure indication line. *(10)* Pressure limitation. *(11)* Inactive alarm indicator. (Courtesy Hamilton Medical, Bonaduz, Switzerland.)

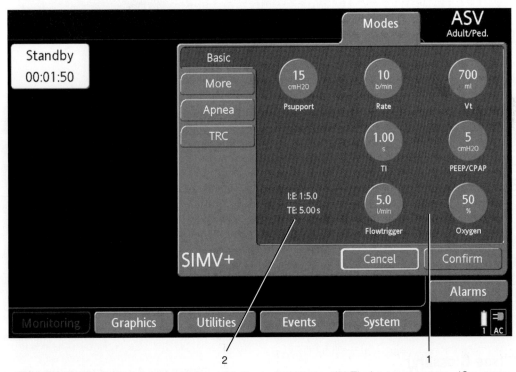

FIGURE 13.20 Basic control window. *(1)* Control settings. *(2)* Timing parameters. (Courtesy Hamilton Medical, Bonaduz, Switzerland.)

pressure ventilation and the other modes available on the C3 is provided in Chapter 12 and also in the manufacturer's user's manual.

EXTENDED MODES AND FEATURES

In addition to the standard modes listed in Box 13.6, the C3 offers several "extended" modes of ventilation. A complete description of many of these modes may be found in Chapter 12 and also on the manufacturer's website.

Leak Compensation

Leak compensation is provided using a proximal sensor to measure the difference between delivered and exhaled tidal volume. Using an IntelliTrig function, the ventilator automatically adjusts to leaks to improve synchrony.

Adaptive Support Ventilation

ASV is a form of closed-loop ventilation that provides for the delivery of minimum minute volume level through spontaneous or controlled breaths, or a combination of both breath types.

Neonatal Application

The Hamilton-C3 can be configured to provide neonatal ventilation using an infant flow sensor. The neonatal option has similar monitoring and alarm functions as adult ventilation. All neonatal modes available in the Hamilton C3 are pressure-controlled and pressure-regulated modes. ASV is not available with neonatal ventilation. A complete description of the neonatal option can be found on the manufacturer's website and in the operator's manual.

▎ KEY POINTS

- The Hamilton-C3 only provides for pressure breath types.
- An IntelliTrig functions automatically to compensate for leaks and improve synchrony.
- CO_2 elimination measurements provide for the calculation of alveolar dead space.

REFERENCE

1. *Operator's manual: Hamilton-C3*, Bonaduz, Switzerland, 2012, Hamilton Medical AG.

MEDTRONIC MINIMALLY INVASIVE THERAPIES PURITAN BENNETT 840 AND 980[1]

OBJECTIVES

Upon completion of this section, you will be able to:
1. Provide a definition of the parameter settings in the lower screen.
2. List the information contained in the upper screen.
3. Define the modes of ventilation available.
4. Define proportional assist ventilation plus (PAV+).
5. Compare the differences between adult and neonatal ventilation.

KEY TERMS (see Glossary)

Graphical user interface (GUI)
Proportional assist ventilation plus (PAV+)
Tube compensation (TC)
Volume control plus (VC+)

The Medtronic Minimally Invasive Therapies Puritan Bennett (PB) 840 ventilators (Fig. 13.21) are manufactured by Medtronic Minimally Invasive Therapies. In 2007 Covidien separated from Tyco Healthcare, the company that previously owned Puritan Bennett.

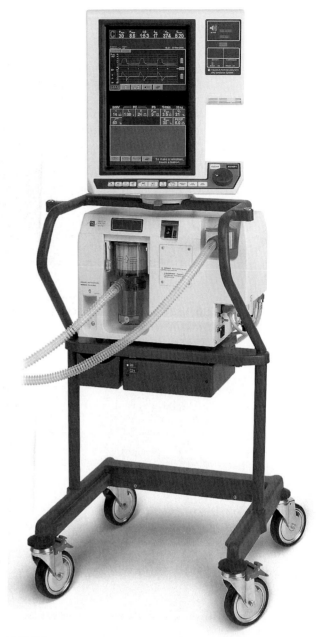

FIGURE 13.21 Medtronic Minimally Invasive Therapies PB 840 ventilator showing the graphical user interface and the breath delivery unit. (Copyright © 2013 Medtronic Minimally Invasive Therapies. All rights reserved. Reprinted with permission of Medtronic Minimally Invasive Therapies.)

The PB 840 was designed to ventilate neonatal, pediatric, and adult patients and is most commonly used in the acute care setting[2]. The ventilator includes a breath delivery unit (BDU) that controls ventilation and connects to the patient circuit. Above the BDU is a liquid crystal display (LCD), touch-sensitive interface screen. The screen, called the graphical user interface (GUI), displays monitored patient data and ventilator settings and information (Fig. 13.22).

The 980 ventilator system is the newest model of ventilator sold by Medtronic Minimally Invasive Therapies (Fig. 13.23A). It incorporates similar modes, alarms, monitoring,

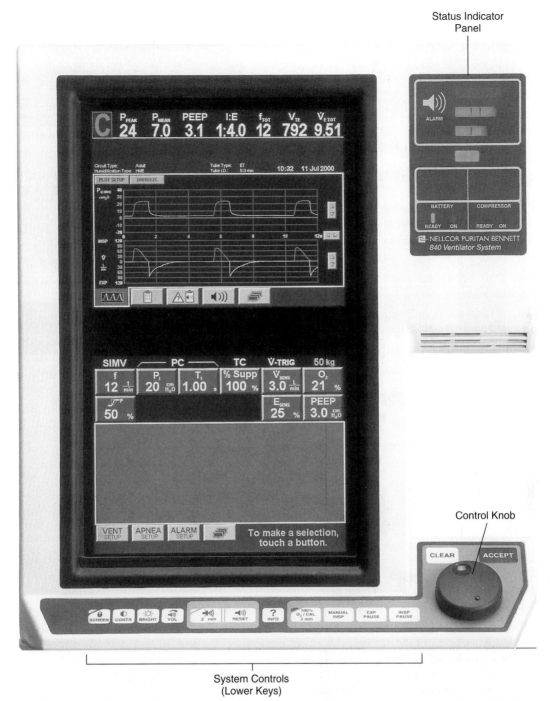

FIGURE 13.22 Medtronic Minimally Invasive Therapies PB 840 graphical user interface with the DualView screens, status indicator panel, lower row of system control keys, and the control knob. (Copyright © 2013 Medtronic Minimally Invasive Therapies. All rights reserved. Reprinted with permission of Medtronic Minimally Invasive Therapies.)

and extended features found on the 840 series ventilator. New for the 980 is a Ventilator Assurance feature that is automatically activated if the ventilator experiences unexpected changes in measured gas mixture or a fault in the gas delivery system. A complete description of Ventilator Assurance can be found in the 980 operator's manual. Additional updates include a touch, swipe, and pull-down screen, and a mixing chamber to improve metabolic (indirect calorimetry) measurements is available.

CONTROLS AND ALARMS

The controls and alarms are accessed through the GUI. Control features and alarm settings are managed with the use of a touchpad and a rotary control knob (see Fig. 13.23B).

Primary Breath Controls

Primary breath controls (Table 13.27) are accessed on the lower panel of the GUI. Changes are initiated by touching a

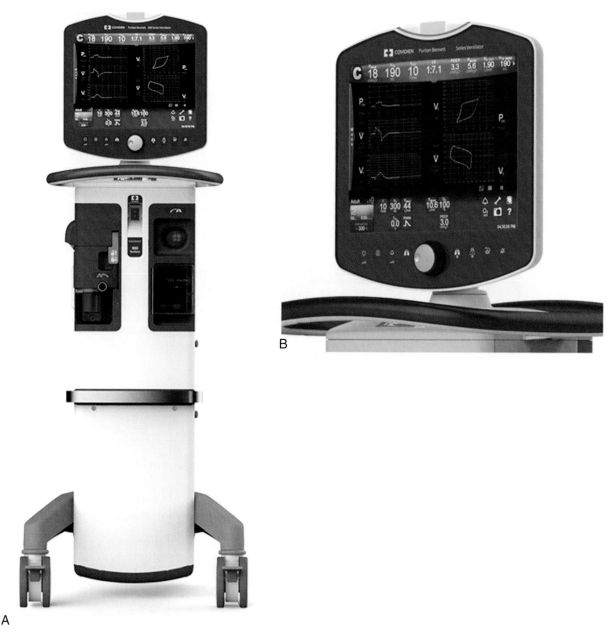

FIGURE 13.23 A, Medtronic Minimally Invasive Therapies PB 980. B, Graphical user interface with multiview screen, status indicator panel, system control keys, and the control knob. (Copyright 2015 Medtronic Minimally Invasive Therapies. All rights reserved, Reprinted with permission of Medtronic Minimally Invasive Therapies.)

control key, adjusting the setting with a rotary knob, and then pressing an accept key. A description of the various control features can be found in Chapter 12 and in the manufacturer's operation manual[1].

Monitoring and Parameters

Monitoring information is displayed on the top panel of the GUI. Displayed parameters are updated on a breath-by-breath basis (Table 13.28). A general description of standard measured parameters on the 840 can be found in Chapter 12 and the manufacturer's operation manual.

Extended Monitoring

In addition to displaying standard monitoring data, the PB 840/980 provides several extended monitoring features (Table 13.29). A description of these can be found on the manufacturer's website.

Alarms

The Medtronic Minimally Invasive Therapies PB 840/980 ventilators provide alarm functions (Table 13.30) during all modes of ventilation. Alarms are managed on the lower panel of the GUI

TABLE 13.27 Primary Breath Controls—Medtronic Minimally Invasive Therapies PB 840 and 980

Parameter	Definition	Range
Apnea Interval	Initiates back-up ventilation when no breath is detected	10-60 s
Constant During Rate Change	Determines which breath-timing variable is operator adjustable	TI, TE, or I:E
Dsens	Disconnect sensitivity	20-95%
Esens	Expiratory sensitivity	1-80%
T_E	Expiratory time	$\geq$0.2 s
Flow Pattern	Gas flow pattern for mandatory breaths (VC only)	Square or descending ramp
Vsens	Flow sensitivity	0.2-20 L/min
$T_{I\ Spont}$	High spontaneous inspiratory time during NIV	Based on set IBW
IBW	Ideal body weight	7.0-150 kg (adult)
I:E or T_H:T_L (BiLevel)	Inspiratory/expiratory time or time high to time low in BiLevel	1:299-4.00:1 1:299-149:1 (BiLevel)
P_I	Inspiratory pressure	5-90 cm H_2O
T_I or T_H in BiLevel	Inspiratory time/Time high	0.2-8.00 s/0.2-30 s
Mandatory Type	Sets mandatory breath type	VC, PC, or VC+
Mode	Sets ventilator mode	A/C, SIMV, Spont, CPAP, BiLevel
NIV	Noninvasive ventilation	NIV
O_2%	Inspired oxygen concentration	21-100%
Patient Circuit Type	Indicates type of patient circuit	Neonatal, pediatric, adult
V_{Max}	Peak inspiratory flow	3.0-150 L/min
PEEP	Positive end-expiratory pressure	0-45 cm H_2O
T_{PL}	Plateau time	0-2.0 s
Psens	Pressure sensitivity	0.1-20 cm H_2O
P_{Supp}	Pressure Support (PS)	0-70 cm H_2O
f	Sets mandatory breath respiratory rate	1.0-100/min
Rise Time Percent	Rate of rise to inspiratory pressure in PC or PS breaths	1-100%
Spontaneous Type	Sets spontaneous breath type	PS, TC, VS, PAV+
V_T	Tidal volume VC or VC+	25-2500 mL
Trigger Type	Flow or pressure trigger	See V_{Sens} and P_{Sens}
Tube Type/diameter	Characteristics of artificial airway	6.0-mm diameter; endotracheal or tracheostomy
Vent Type	Invasive or noninvasive ventilation	NA
Wave form	Determines flow pattern on VC breaths	Square or ramp
% Support	Level of support during PAV+	10-80%

A/C, Assist/control; *CPAP*, continuous positive airway pressure; *PAV+*, proportional assist ventilation plus; *SIMV*, synchronized intermittent mandatory ventilation; *TC*, tube compensation.

using the touch keys and rotary knob control. A general description of alarm functions can be found in Chapter 12 and in the manufacturer's operation manual.

STANDARD MODES OF VENTILATION

Box 13.7 lists the standard modes of ventilation. A description of these modes can be found in Chapter 12 and in the manufacturer's operation manual for the 840/980.

EXTENDED MODES AND FEATURES

In addition to the standard modes listed in Box 13.7, the 840/980 offers extended modes of ventilation. A complete

BOX 13.7 Standard Modes of Ventilation—Medtronic Minimally Invasive Therapies PB 840/980

- Assist Control (VC or VC+)
- SIMV (VC or VC+)
- BiLevel (APRV)
- Spontaneous
- Pressure support (PS)
- Proportional assist ventilation plus (PAV+)
- NIV
- Apnea ventilation

APRV, Airway pressure-release ventilation; *NIV*, noninvasive positive-pressure ventilation; *PS*, pressure support; *SIMV*, synchronized intermittent mandatory ventilation.

TABLE 13.28 Standard Measured and Displayed Parameters—Medtronic Minimally Invasive Therapies PB 840 and 980

Parameter	Range
Breath type	Control (C), Assist (A), or Spontaneous (S)
Delivered O_2 %	0-103%
End inspiratory pressure ($P_{I\ End}$)	–20-130 cm H_2O
Exhaled minute volume ($V_{E\ TOT}$)	0-99.9 L
Exhaled tidal volume (V_{TE})	0-6000 mL
I:E	1:5999 to 149:1
Intrinsic PEEP ($PEEP_I$)	–20-130 cm H_2O
Peak circuit/mean/plateau pressures ($P_{Peak}/P_{Mean}/P_{PL}$)	–20-130 cm H_2O
PEEP	–20-130 cm H_2O
Rapid shallow breathing index (f/V_T)	0-600 breaths/min/L
Spontaneous inspiratory time ($T_{I\ Spont}$)	0-10 s
Spontaneous minute volume ($V_{E\ Spont}$)	0-99.9 L
Spontaneous T_I/T_{TOT}	0-1
Static compliance (C_{STAT})	0-500 mL/cm H_2O
Static resistance (R_{STAT})	0-500 cm H_2O/L/s
Total PEEP ($PEEP_{TOT}$)	–20-130-cm H_2O
Total respiratory rate (f_{TOT})	0-200 min

I:E, Inspiratory time to expiratory time; *PEEP,* positive end-expiratory pressure; V_T, tidal volume.

TABLE 13.29 Extended Monitoring Features—Medtronic Minimally Invasive Therapies PB 840 and 980

Feature	Description
Leak	Leak flow and volume
Dynamic compliance and resistance	Breath-by-breath measurements of compliance and resistance
PSF	Peak spontaneous flow
WOB_{PI}/WOB_{TOT}	Work of breathing during PAV+
C_{PAV}/R_{PAV}	Compliance and resistance during PAV+
Breath timing bar	The breath timing bar shows the results of parameter setting changes on the I:E ratio.

I:E, Inspiratory time to expiratory time; *PAV,* proportional assist ventilation.

description of many of these may be found in Chapter 12 and also on the manufacturer's website.

Proportional Assist Ventilation

In proportional assist ventilation plus (PAV+) patient efforts and the ventilator combine to perform 100% of the work of

TABLE 13.30 Alarm Ranges—Medtronic Minimally Invasive Therapies PB 840 and 980

Alarm	Range
Apnea interval	10-60 s
High/low circuit pressure	1-100 cm H_2O
High/low exhaled minute volume	100-0.05 L/min or off
High/low exhaled tidal volume (mandatory)	3000-1 mL or off
High/low exhaled tidal volume (spontaneous)	2500-1 mL or off
High respiratory rate	Off to 110/min

breathing. The proportion assist (PA) breath targets a pressure based on the selected percentage of support (% SUPPORT) set by the operator and the flow and volume readings from the patient. As long as the patient is able to maintain a stable and adequate ventilatory pattern, PAV++ rhythmically unloads the respiratory muscles, allowing the patient to have a relatively normal breathing pattern.[3,4]

Tube Compensation

Tube compensation (TC) is a spontaneous breath type that is intended to reduce the work of breathing associated with an endotracheal (ET) or tracheostomy (trach) tube. The ventilator adjusts the delivered pressure in proportion to the inspiratory flow and the size of the artificial airway.

Volume Support

Volume support (VS) is pressure-support ventilation with a volume target. In VS, breaths are patient triggered (flow or pressure), pressure limited, and flow cycled. The ventilator automatically adjusts the pressure limit to achieve the set V_T.

Neonatal Application

Neonatal ventilation is available on the PB 840/980 using the Neomode software option. Monitoring and alarm function are very similar to those used for adult and pediatric ventilation. Pressure triggering is not available in the Neomode. Most of the adult modes of ventilation are available in the Neomode with the exception of PAV and tube compensation. A complete description of the Neomode option can be found on the manufacturer's website and in the operator's manual.

■ KEY POINTS

- The Medtronic Minimally Invasive Therapies PB 840/980 is designed to ventilate neonatal, pediatric, and adult patients. An ideal body weight (IBW) feature alerts the ventilator to the type of patient being ventilated.
- Control functions are accessed through a touch screen interface.
- Ventilator settings and alarm functions require a three-step process—touch, turn, and accept—to activate.
- PAV+ ventilation measures and targets a work of breathing level set by the operator.

REFERENCES

1. *Operator's and technical reference manual, Puritan Bennett 800 series ventilator system*, Boulder, CO, 2011, Covidien.
2. Cairo JM: *Pilbeam's mechanical ventilation: physiological and clinical applications*, ed 5, St. Louis, 2012, Elsevier.
3. Kondili E, Prinianakis G, Alexopoulou C, et al.: Respiratory load compensation during mechanical ventilation: proportional assist ventilation with load-adjustable gain factors versus pressure support. *Intensive Care Med* 32:692, 2006.
4. Puritan Bennett: PAV+ option addendum to the 840 ventilator operator's and technical reference manual, part no 10011698, Rev A, Boulder, CO, 2006, Puritan Bennett, a division of Covidien, Mansfield, MA.

MAQUET SERVO-i, SERVO-s, AND SERVO-U

OBJECTIVES

Upon completion of this section, you will be able to:
1. List the modes of ventilation available on the Maquet Servo-i, Servo-s, and Servo-U
2. Describe the alarms available with the Servo-i, Servo-s, and Servo-U.
3. Identify the extended monitoring features on the Servo-i, Servo-s, and Servo-U.
4. Describe the use of NAVA.
5. Compare the differences between adult and neonatal ventilation.

KEY TERMS (see Glossary)

Automode
Neurally adjusted ventilatory assist (NAVA)
Occlusion pressure ($P_{0.1}$)
Shallow breathing index (SBI)

The Maquet Servo-i ventilator system originally was released in the United States in 2002. The Servo-i and Maquet Servo-s ventilator (Fig. 13.24) can be used in acute care facilities and for transport in the hospital and also outside of the hospital. (It is approved for use in ambulances, fixed-wing aircraft, and helicopters.) The Servo-i and Servo-s are identical in functional design and user operation. The modes of ventilation available on the Servo-s are the same as those available on the Servo-i for both invasive and noninvasive ventilation. The primary differences are in the design of the carts, the location of the batteries, and the fact that the Servo-s cannot be used for neonatal ventilation. In addition, the Servo-s currently cannot be configured for use in a magnetic resonance imaging (MRI) suite.

Recently the Maquet Servo-U was released for sale in the United States (Fig. 13.25). It shares many of the same control features, modes and breath types, and alarm functions as the Servo-i and Servo-s. Additionally, the Servo-n was released, which is configured for neonatal application. New to the Servo-U and n models, a touch-and-hold feature, onboard

TABLE 13.31 Primary Breath Controls— Servo-i, Servo-s, and Servo-U[a]

Parameter	Range
Auto Mode	On/Off
Breathing Rate—SIMV	1-60/min
Breathing Rate—CMV	4-100
Edi Trigger (µV)	0.1-2.0
Flow trig sensitivity level	0-100%, 0-2.0 LPM[a]
I:E ratio	1:10-4:1
Inspiratory cycle-off (% of peak flow)	1-70
Inspiratory rise time (%)	0-20
Inspiratory rise time (s)	0-0.4
Leak compensation	On/Off[a]
Minute Volume (L/min)	0.5-60
NAVA level (cm H_2O/µV)	0.0-15.0
O_2 concentration (%)	21-100
PEEP (cm H_2O)	0-50
Phigh (cm H_2O)	2-50
Press trig sensitivity level (cm H_2O)	−20-0
Pressure level above PEEP (cm H_2O)	0-(120-PEEP)
PS above PEEP in Bivent (cm H_2O)	0-(120-PEEP)
PS above Phigh in Bivent (cm H_2O)	0-(120-PHigh)
Thigh (s)	0.2-10, 0.2-30 s[a]
Ti (s)	0.1-5
Tidal volume (mL)	100-2000, 100-4000[a]
Tpause (%)/(s)	0-30
Weight (kg)	10-250

[a]Updated parameter range for Servo-U.
CMV, Continuous mandatory ventilation; *I:E,* inspiratory time to expiratory time; *LPM,* liters per minute; *NAVA,* neurally adjusted ventilatory assist; *PEEP,* positive end-expiratory pressure; *PS,* pressure support; *SIMV,* synchronized intermittent mandatory ventilation.

tutorial feature, an enhanced touch-and-swipe user interface, and an improved expiratory gas cassette system are now available.

OVERVIEW OF CONTROLS

The user interface, or front panel, consists of a touchscreen and several knobs and touch keys for selecting and adjusting ventilator parameters. Fig. 13.26 shows the major components of the front panel. A complete description of the Servo-i and Servo-s primary breath controls (Table 13.31) can be found in the user's[1,2] manual or on the manufacturer's website.

MONITORING AND ALARMS

Measured values boxes are normally displayed numerically on the right side in the touchscreen (see Fig. 13.26). The values that appear can be customized by the operator (Table 13.32).

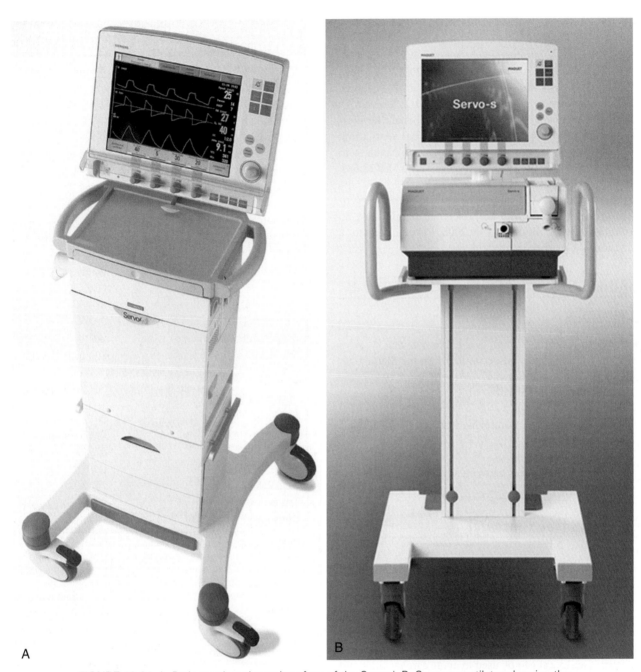

FIGURE 13.24 A, Patient unit and user interface of the Servo-i. B, Servo-s ventilator showing the user interface permanently mounted on the patient unit. (Courtesy Maquet, Inc., Bridgewater, NJ.)

Extended Monitoring Features

In addition to the standard display of monitoring data, the Servo-i and Servo-U can display an extended view of information (Table 13.33) depending on the mode or breath type that is selected. A complete general description of these features can be found in Chapter 12 or in the manufacturer's operation manual.[2]

Alarms

All alarms on the Servo-i and Servo-U are audible and visual (Table 13.34). The three alarm categories are high priority, medium priority, and low priority. Alarms may be manually set by using the control pads or through the use of an Autoset

function that uses measured values from patient data to determine alarm settings.

STANDARD MODES OF VENTILATION

The Servo-i and Servo-U provide several standard modes of ventilation (Box 13.8). A complete general description of these modes may be found in Chapter 12 and on the manufacturer's website.

EXTENDED MODES AND FEATURES

In addition to the standard modes of ventilation listed in Box 13.8, the Servo-i and Servo-U offer several extended modes

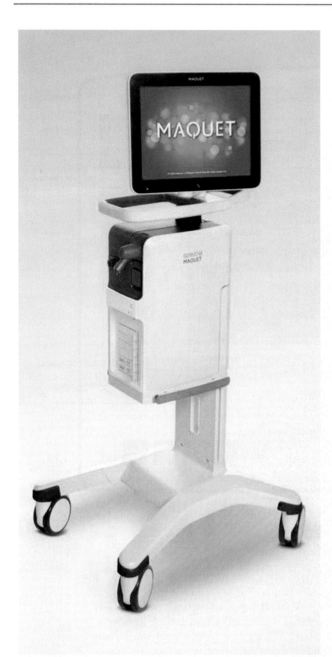

FIGURE 13.25 Servo-U ventilator. (Courtesy Maquet, Inc., Bridgewater, NJ.)

TABLE 13.32 Standard Measured and Displayed Parameters—Maquet Servo-i, Servo-s, and Servo-U

Parameter	Definition
P_{peak}	Maximum inspiratory pressure
P_{mean}	Mean airway pressure
PEEP	Total positive end-expiratory pressure
RR	Respiratory rate
Flowee	End-expiratory flow
I:E	Inspiratory-to-expiratory ratio (only during controlled ventilation)
T_I/T_{TOT}	Duty cycle or ratio of inspiration time to total breathing cycle time (only during spontaneous breathing)
O_2	Oxygen concentration in percentage
MV_e	Expiratory minute volume
VT_i	Inspiratory tidal volume
VT_e	Expiratory tidal volume
P_{plat}	Pressure during end-inspiratory pause
$PEEP_{tot}$	Intrinsic positive end-expiratory pressure
MV_i	Inspiratory minute volume
Cstatic	Static compliance, respiratory system
C dyn	Dynamic characteristics
SBI	Shallow breathing index

From Siemens Medical (Maquet Inc., Bridgewater, NJ).

TABLE 13.33 Extended Monitoring Features—Maquet Servo-i, Servo-s, and Servo-U

Feature	Description
Ri	Inspiratory resistance
Re	Expiratory resistance
WOBp	Work of breathing—patient
WOBv	Work of breathing—ventilator
Tc	Time constant
E	Elastance
$P_{0.1}$	Occlusion pressure during first 100 ms
Open lung tool (OLT)	Display of $P_{ET}CO_2$, $\dot{V}CO_2$, V_TCO_2
Edi peak and min	Peak and minimum electrical activity of the diaphragm
Wave Forms	Scalars for pressure, volume, and flow. Pressure-volume curve and flow volume loops

$P_{ET}CO_2$, Partial pressure of end-tidal carbon dioxide; $\dot{V}CO_2$, CO_2 minute elimination; $VTCO_2$, CO_2 tidal elimination; VT, tidal volume. From Siemens Medical (Maquet Inc., Bridgewater, NJ).[5]

BOX 13.8 Standard Modes of Ventilation—Maquet Servo-i, Servo-s, and Servo-U

- PC (PC-CMV)
- VC (VC-CMV)
- PRVC
- SIMV (VC) + PS
- SIMV (PC) + PS
- SIMV (PRVC) + PS
- Bi-Vent
- VS
- PS/CPAP
- NIV-PS and NIV-PC

CMV, Continuous mandatory ventilation; *CPAP,* continuous positive airway pressure; *NIV,* noninvasive positive-pressure ventilation; *PRVC,* pressure-regulated volume control; *PS,* pressure support; *PSV,* pressure-support ventilation; *SIMV,* synchronized intermittent mandatory ventilation; *VS,* volume support.

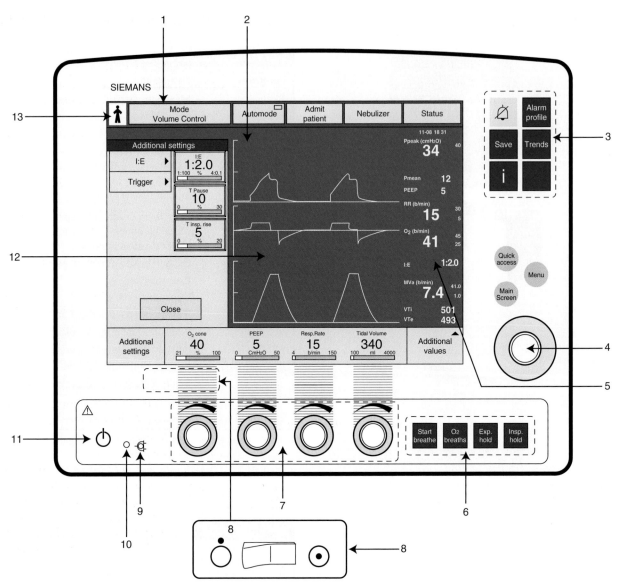

FIGURE 13.26 Control panel (user interface) of the Servo-i. *(1)* A menu touchpad area. *(2)* Text and alarm messages. *(3)* Fixed keys. *(4)* Main rotary dial. *(5)* Measured values boxes. *(6)* Special function keys. *(7)* Direct access knobs. *(8)* On/off switch (back panel of machine). *(9)* Service connector. *(10)* Main indicator (green). *(11)* Start ventilation/stop ventilation (standby). *(12)* Waveform area. *(13)* Patient category. (Courtesy Maquet, Inc., Bridgewater, NJ.)

of ventilation. A general description of these modes may be found on the manufacturer's website, in the operator's manual,[4] and in Chapter 12.

AutoMode

AutoMode allows the ventilator to automatically shift among controlled ventilation, supported ventilation, and spontaneous ventilation based on the effort sensed from the patient.

Neonatal Application

As previously mentioned, the Servo-s cannot be used for neonatal ventilation. Many of the monitoring features, alarm functions, and modes of ventilation available for adult ventilation on the Servo-i and Servo-U are also available for neonatal ventilation. A complete description of the neonatal option

can be found on the manufacturer's website and in the operator's manual.

MRI Capability

The Servo-i and Servo-U can be adapted for use in an MRI environment using up to a 3-Tesla magnet; this makes an ICU ventilator available in the MRI suite.

NAVA

NAVA is a mode of ventilation based on neural respiratory output[3]. NAVA relies on detection of the electrical activity of the diaphragm (EAdi) to control the timing and level of assistance delivered. NAVA requires the use of a special naso-gastric (NG) tube that is fitted with an array of miniaturized sensors.

TABLE 13.34 Alarm Ranges—Maquet Servo-i, Servo-s, and Servo-U

Alarms	Range
Airway pressure (upper)	16-120 cm H_2O
High continuous pressure	Set PEEP 15 cm H_2O exceeded for >15 sec
O_2 concentration	Set value ± 6% or ≤18%
Expired minute volume—high	0.5-60 L/min
Expired minute volume—low	0.5-40 L/min
Apnea	15-45 s
Gas supply	<2 kPa × 100 and >6.5 kPa × 100
Respiratory rate	1-160 breaths/min
High end-expiratory pressure (or CPAP)	0-55 cm H_2O
Low end-expiratory pressure (or CPAP)	0-47 cm H_2O (setting alarm to zero is alarm off position)

CPAP, Continuous positive airway pressure; *PEEP,* positive end-expiratory pressure;

KEY POINTS

- The Maquet Servo-s and Servo-i are identical in functional design and user operation.
- An optional available mode on the Maquet Servo-i, Servo-s, and Servo-U is BiVent, which is similar to airway pressure-release ventilation.
- The Servo-U is the latest model produced by Maquet.
- PRVC is a pressure-limited mode with a volume target.

ASSESSMENT QUESTIONS

See Appendix B for the answers.

1. Which of the following features are available for use with the CareFusion AVEA ventilator?
   1. Esophageal pressure monitoring
   2. Tracheal pressure monitoring
   3. Heliox gas delivery capability
   4. Nitric oxide gas delivery capability
      a. 1 and 2 only
      b. 3 and 4 only
      c. 1, 2, and 3 only
      d. 1, 2, 3, and 4
2. Measurements for volumetric capnography on the CareFusion AVEA ventilator are obtained with/by:
   a. Measuring end-tidal CO_2
   b. Performing a circuit leak test
   c. Requiring esophageal manometry
   d. Requiring the Vsynch software option
3. The PSV Tmax option on the CareFusion AVEA ventilator is used to:

- Volume support is patient triggered, pressure limited, and volume targeted.
- Automode facilitates weaning by allowing the patient to control his or her own breathing pattern (pressure support) as long as the individual is breathing spontaneously.
- The Open Lung Tool allows the operator to select any method of evaluating the pressure of overdistention and the pressure that occurs when the lung units collapse.
- Neurally adjusted ventilatory assist is a new option that uses the diaphragm's electrical activity to trigger and control spontaneous breaths. NAVA requires placement of a special monitoring NG tube.
- The Servo-s can be used for pediatric and adult patients but not for neonatal patients.
- The Servo-n can be used for neonates.
- Currently the Servo-s cannot be configured for use in a MRI suite.
- The modes of ventilation available on the Servo-s are the same as those available on the Servo-i for both invasive and noninvasive ventilation.

REFERENCES

1. Maquet: *User's manual, ventilator system ServoS V3.1 (US Version),* order no. 6664549, Solna, Sweden, 2012, Maquet.
2. Maquet: *User's manual (US Version), ventilator system Servo-I V3.1,* Maquet Critical Care, order no. 66-00-261, Solna, Sweden, 2012, Maquet.
3. Cairo JM: *Pilbeam's mechanical ventilation: physiological and clinical application,* ed 5, St. Louis, 2012, Elsevier.
4. Maquet: *Servo education, study guide,* Maquet Critical Care, order no. 66-72-817, Solna, Sweden, 2007, Maquet.
5. Maquet: *Lung recruitment: pocket guide,* Maquet Critical Care, order No. 66 61 271, Solna, Sweden, 2004, Maquet.

   a. Assess the patient's work of breathing
   b. Deliver independent lung ventilation (ILV)
   c. Terminate a spontaneous breath
   d. Generate an auto–positive end-expiratory pressure (auto-PEEP) measurement
4. Tracheal pressure measurements made with the CareFusion AVEA ventilator are used to:
   a. Assess a neonate's response to inhaled nitric oxide (INO)
   b. Measure auto-PEEP
   c. Determine the appropriate level of pressure when pressure-regulated volume control (PRVC) is used
   d. Activate a mandatory breath during continuous mechanical ventilation (CMV)
5. The internal drive mechanism on the AVEA ventilator is made of:
   a. A rigid accumulator
   b. A servo-controlled valve
   c. A Venturi fluidic block
   d. Variable-orifice inspiratory valves

6. A mode in which the operator sets P_{HIGH}, P_{LOW}, T_{HIGH}, and T_{LOW} is called:
   a. Airway pressure-release ventilation
   b. Pressure-regulated volume control ventilation
   c. Pressure-support ventilation
   d. Proportional assist ventilation

7. When comparing the Dräger EvitaXL with the Dräger Evita V500, the primary difference is:
   a. Available modes provided
   b. Main screen or user interface
   c. Internal gas delivery system
   d. Monitoring system

8. The purpose for using the low-flow pressure-volume loop feature with the Dräger EvitaXL is to:
   a. Determine the length of an apnea period in a patient with apneic episodes
   b. Deliver nebulized medications at a slower breath rate
   c. Evaluate for the upper and lower inflection points
   d. Measure the slow vital capacity of the patient

9. SmartCare is best defined as:
   a. Training of the respiratory care staff from the Dräger website
   b. Respiratory care personnel who have passed the Dräger EvitaXL examination
   c. Making appropriate ventilator adjustments while using pressure-support ventilation (PSV) for weaning
   d. A closed-loop form of ventilation designed to shorten weaning time

10. Which of the following are needed to use the Dräger EvitaXL for neonatal ventilation?
    a. Place a nitric oxide on the inspiratory limb of the ventilator circuit.
    b. Remove the expiratory flow transducer.
    c. Place a proximal sensor at the patient wye.
    d. Start the ventilator in the proportional pressure support (PPS) mode.

11. The function of NeoFlow on the Dräger Evita V500 is to provide flow triggering. True or false?
    a. True
    b. False

12. All of the following modes are available on the Dräger Evita N500 *except*:
    a. CMV
    b. Synchronized intermittent mandatory ventilation (SIMV)
    c. SmartCare
    d. PSV

13. To provide infant ventilation with the Dräger Evita V500, which of the following is required?
    a. Esophageal manometry
    b. SmartCare
    c. Proximal airway monitoring
    d. High-frequency oscillatory ventilation (HFOV) module

14. The primary difference between the Dräger Evita V500 and N500 is:

a. The Dräger Evita N500 is designed for neonatal ventilation only
b. Patient monitoring is accessed differently with the Dräger Evita V500 compared with the Dräger N500
c. The Dräger Evita N500 cannot provide pressure support ventilation (PSV)
d. The Dräger Evita V500 and Dräger Evita N500 use different power sources

15. The mode on the Dräger Evita V500 that provides mandatory breathing only if the patient's spontaneous breathing drops below the preselected setting is called:
    a. Mandatory minute ventilation (MMV)
    b. SIMV-PC
    c. PSV SmartCare
    d. Automatic tube compensation (ATC)

16. Which of the following controls sets the percentage of peak inspiratory flow that cycles the Maquet Servo-i/Servo-s ventilator out of inspiration during pressure support (PS) and volume support (VS)?
    a. Inspiratory cycle-off
    b. Inspiratory rise time
    c. Peak flow control
    d. Trigger timeout

17. On the Maquet Servo-i/Servo-s, neurally adjusted ventilatory assist (NAVA) is an extended mode that provides:
    a. Measurements of airways resistance
    b. Pressure–volume curves to set optimal PEEP
    c. Volume-targeting ventilation for spontaneous breaths
    d. Electrical signals from the diaphragm to trigger and cycle spontaneous breaths.

18. The Open Lung Tool on the Maquet Servo-i can trend which of the following parameters?
    1. Peak pressure
    2. PEEP
    3. Dynamic compliance
    4. Tidal volumes
       a. 3 only
       b. 1 and 2 only
       c. 3 and 4 only
       d. 1, 2, 3, and 4

19. The Maquet Servo-s has the following features in common with the Maquet Servo-i *except*:
    a. User interface
    b. Patient unit
    c. Magnetic resonance imaging (MRI) conditional cart
    d. Standard modes of ventilation

20. The Maquet Servo-s can be used for infant ventilation. True or false?
    a. True
    b. False

21. VC+ on the Medtronic Minimally Invasive Therapies PB 840 is similar to which mode on the CareFusion AVEA ventilator?
    a. PSV
    b. Pressure-controlled continuous mandatory ventilation (CMV-PC)
    c. Adaptive support ventilation (ASV)
    d. PRVC

22. Proportional assist ventilation plus (PAV+) is best described as a breath delivery method in which:
    a. The greater the patient effort, the higher the pressure delivered
    b. The pressure is set as a percentage of inspiratory effort
    c. The percent of support provided depends on the $P_{0.1}$ value of the patient
    d. Breaths are time or patient triggered

23. Which of the following best describes tube compensation on the Medtronic Minimally Invasive Therapies PB 840?
    a. An extended feature allowing the ventilator to adjust PSV to overcome the resistance of the artificial airway
    b. A mode similar to AutoFlow on the Dräger EvitaXL
    c. A method to terminate inspiration on a spontaneous breath
    d. A procedure performed during the short safety test (SST) to correct for circuit tubing compliance

24. BiLevel ventilation on the Medtronic Minimally Invasive Therapies PB 840 ventilator is similar to:
    a. PRVC
    b. Airway pressure-release ventilation (APRV)
    c. Rise time percent
    d. SmartCare

25. Which of the following is (are) *not* active with the Neomode on the Medtronic Minimally Invasive Therapies PB 840?
    1. VC+
    2. Rise time
    3. Pressure trigger
    4. SIMV
       a. 1 only
       b. 2 and 3 only
       c. 3 only
       d. 2 and 4 only

26. Standard modes of ventilation on the GE CareScape include all of the following *except:*
    a. CMV
    b. SIMV
    c. ASV
    d. Continuous positive airway pressure (CPAP)

27. Which feature on the GE Carescape allows the ventilator to automatically adjust the flow sensitivity for leaks in the patient breathing circuit and artificial airway?
    a. Leak compensation
    b. Pressure regulated volume guarantee (PRVG)
    c. FRC InView
    d. Trigger compensation

28. The InView Vent Calculations extended monitoring option on the GE Carescape provides which of the following?
    a. Measurements of oxygen consumption and carbon dioxide production
    b. Intrinsic PEEP
    c. Dead space
    d. Tracheal pressures

29. The tube resistance compensation (TRC) feature on the GE Carescape is used to:

a. Measure functional residual capacity (FRC) based on nitrogen
b. Compensate for artificial airway resistance
c. Determine total respiratory system compliance
d. Monitor inspiratory efforts when neonatal ventilation is selected

30. Lung mechanics measurements available on the GE Carescape include all of the following *except:*
    a. Work of breathing (WOB)
    b. Vital capacity
    c. Negative inspiratory force
    d. Occlusion pressure at 100 ms ($P_{0.1}$)

31. The primary difference between the Hamilton-G5 and Hamilton-C3 is:
    a. The Hamilton-G5 does not provide a neonatal option
    b. The Hamilton-C3 does not provide adaptive pressure ventilation (APV)
    c. The power source of the Hamilton-G5 is different from the Hamilton-C3
    d. Volume ventilation is not available with the Hamilton-C3

32. The IntelliTrig function on the Hamilton-C3 is used to:
    a. Compensate for leaks and improve synchrony
    b. Used to monitor proximal airway flows and volumes
    c. Calculate alveolar dead space measurements
    d. Measure negative inspiratory force (NIF) values during a spontaneous breathing trial (SBT)

33. An extended mode on the Hamilton-G5 that provides closed-loop ventilation for the delivery of a minimum minute volume is called:
    a. PAV
    b. ASV
    c. SmartCare
    d. PPS

34. Monitoring of airway pressures on the Hamilton-C3 and -G5 is accomplished with a(n):
    a. Active exhalation valve
    b. Esophageal catheter
    c. Proximal airway sensor
    d. Dynamic Heart/Lung monitor

35. The SlopeCO$_2$ feature on the G5 is used to:
    a. Calculate rise time to improve patient synchrony
    b. Detect and record apnea events
    c. Determine the WOB to trigger a breath via an esophageal catheter
    d. Measure the slope of the alveolar plateau to determine the efficiency of ventilation

36. Ventilators that incorporate proportional solenoid valves to control gas flow include:
    1. Maquet Servo-i
    2. Hamilton-G5
    3. Medtronic Minimally Invasive Therapies PB 840
    4. GE Carescape
       a. 1 only
       b. 2 and 3 only
       c. 1, 3, and 4 only
       d. 3 only

37. Which of the following ventilators provide(s) a battery backup power supply?
    1. GE CareScape
    2. Hamilton-C3
    3. Maquet Servo-s
    4. CareFusion AVEA
       a. 1 only
       b. 2, 3, and 4 only
       c. 4 only
       d. 1, 2, 3, and 4

38. NAVA, ASV, and PAV are all examples of:
    a. CMV ventilation modes
    b. Internal drive systems
    c. Methods to terminate spontaneous inspiration
    d. Closed-loop technologies

39. Ventilators that incorporate both a pneumatic and electrical power system include:
    1. CareFusion AVEA
    2. Medtronic Minimally Invasive Therapies PB 840
    3. GE Carescape
    4. Dräger Evita V500
       a. 1 only
       b. 2 and 3 only
       c. 1, 2, 3, and 4
       d. 3 and 4 only

40. When volume-targeted breaths are activated, triggering is based on which of the following?
    1. Time
    2. Flow
    3. Pressure
    4. Volume
       a. 1 only
       b. 2 and 3 only
       c. 1 and 3 only
       d. 1, 2, and 3 only

41. The maximum available inspiratory time to expiratory time (I:E) ratio for a mandatory breath is:
    a. 1:1
    b. 2:1
    c. 3:1
    d. 4:1

Infant and Pediatric Devices

OBJECTIVES

Upon completion of this chapter, you will be able to:

1. Systematically review continuous positive airway pressure (CPAP) delivery devices and ventilators used in the treatment of infant and pediatric patients.
2. List the various modes of ventilatory support provided by infant and pediatric ventilators.
3. Calculate the approximate tidal volume (V_T) delivered by a typical infant ventilator when given a particular flow and inspiratory time (T_I).
4. Describe the controls, monitors, alarm, and safety systems typically found on infant and pediatric ventilators.
5. Discuss precautions and key troubleshooting points for nasal CPAP devices and neonatal and pediatric ventilators.

OUTLINE

KEY TERMS

accumulator
amplitude
bias flow
circuit positive end-expiratory pressure (PEEP)
demand flow system
dump valve
electromagnetic
expiratory synchrony

hertz (Hz)
high-frequency jet ventilator
Hi-Lo jet tracheal tube
infrared sensor
jet solenoid
leak compensation
message log
oscillator subsystem

piston assembly
pneumatic safety valve
polarity voltage
proportioning valve
pulsation dampener
purge valve
square-wave driver
termination sensitivity

INFANT AND PEDIATRIC DEVICES IN THIS CHAPTER

Hudson RCI Infant Nasal Prong CPAP System
Nasopharyngeal CPAP
Mirage Kidsta Mask
CareFusion Infant Flow SiPAP
Fisher & Paykel Healthcare Bubble CPAP System
CareFusion V.I.P. Bird Infant Ventilator
Bird Partner IIi Monitor
CareFusion V.I.P. Bird Sterling and CareFusion Gold Infant/Pediatric Ventilators

Dräger Babylog 8000 Infant Ventilator
Dräger Babylog 8000 plus Infant Ventilator
Bunnell Life Pulse High Frequency Ventilator
Bunnell LifePort Endotracheal Tube Adaptor
CareFusion 3100A High Frequency Oscillatory Ventilator
CareFusion 3100B High Frequency Oscillatory Ventilator

Ventilatory support remains an essential component in the care of critically ill infants. Although the basic goal of mechanical ventilation, which is to ensure adequate ventilation and oxygenation, has remain unchanged, ventilatory strategies and the devices used to accomplish infant ventilation have significantly improved during the past 50 years.

The first published reports of the successful use of neonatal mechanical ventilation appeared in the 1960s. Historically, the majority of infants requiring mechanical ventilation have been treated using time-cycled, pressure-limited ventilation. Although there has been relatively limited scientific evidence to support that using this mode of ventilation is superior to volume-controlled ventilation, there was strong belief that the time-cycled, pressure-controlled ventilation reduced the risk for barotrauma in neonates.[1,2]

The introduction of positive end-expiratory pressure (PEEP) to restore functional residual capacity and prevent airway collapse resulted in the ability to use lower pressures during ventilation. By the 1970s, CPAP and intermittent mandatory ventilation (IMV) were common ventilatory modes, and neonatal ventilation had changed once again. High-frequency ventilation, surfactant replacement, *extracorporeal membrane oxygenation* (ECMO), and the introduction of microprocessor-based mechanical ventilators have led to improved outcomes for infants requiring ventilatory support.

Advances in ventilator technology have also allowed for more precise patient monitoring and have enabled implementation of additional modes that were previously associated with only adult and pediatric patients. Manufacturers have introduced ventilators with a wide range of modes, including both volume-targeted and pressure-targeted modes and modes that allow an element of patient control of the ventilator. These include initiation and termination of inspiration, as well as control of flow. Some modes are even hybrids, combining the best features of both the pressure-targeted and volume-targeted modes.

Various modes for ventilation are available on current-generation mechanical ventilators along with improved monitoring capabilities. Neonatal ventilation is no longer solely concerned with providing adequate gas exchange and oxygenation; ventilator management strategies have evolved during the past decade, which allow clinicians to reduce lung injury by optimizing mechanical ventilation.

This chapter provides an overview of various devices that are used for invasive and noninvasive mechanical ventilation of neonates and pediatric patients. It is divided into three sections: (1) CPAP devices; (2) infant ventilators; and (3) high-frequency jet and oscillatory ventilators. Additional information about neonatal and pediatric features of the general-use ventilators can be found in Chapter 13. Although every attempt has been made to ensure that the information within this chapter was accurate at the time of publication, ventilator manufacturers update their devices, and the reader is advised to refer to manufacturers' user manuals, review safety precautions, and remain alert to device updates.

CONTINUOUS POSITIVE AIRWAY PRESSURE SYSTEMS

Continuous positive airway pressure (CPAP) has been used for many years in the treatment of hypoxemia in infants and children. Historically, CPAP has been administered by using a constant flow of a gas mixture adjusted to provide a single pressure level at the airway. One method to accomplish this is for an infant ventilator to serve as the driver for the system. Today, however, freestanding systems are available with interfaces that alter flow characteristics between inspiration and expiration. For example, a freestanding system may be able to provide either constant expiratory pressure or biphasic pressure (i.e., pressure on inspiration and expiration). "Bubble CPAP," which provides a single pressure and flow, has been used in the past and is experiencing a reemergence in popularity.

In recent years a popular practice has been to fit infant ventilator circuits with noninvasive CPAP interfaces such as nasal prongs. This fitting is accomplished by adding one of the many available interfaces designed for infant nasal CPAP. An example interface is the Argyle CPAP nasal cannula (Medtronic Minimally Invasive Therapies), which connects directly to a standard infant ventilator circuit (Fig. 14.1). Some interfaces, such as the Hudson RCI Infant Nasal Prong CPAP System (Teleflex), provide both the integrated ventilator circuit and the nasal-prong interface (Fig. 14.2).

Nasopharyngeal CPAP provides an alternative to noninvasive interfaces, such as nasal prongs. Nasopharyngeal CPAP is provided by trimming endotracheal tubes (ETTs) to fit the

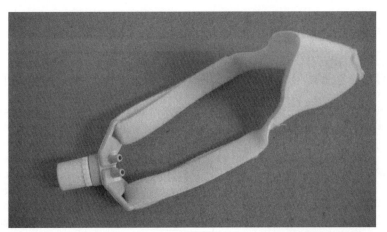

FIGURE 14.1 Kendall Health Argyle continuous positive airway pressure (CPAP) nasal prongs and headgear.

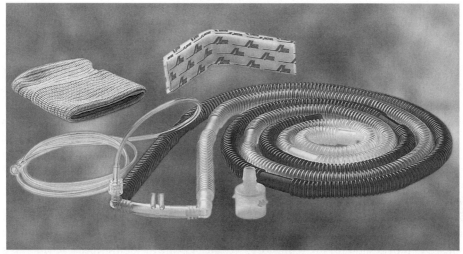

FIGURE 14.2 Hudson RCI Infant Nasal Prong CPAP circuit and patient interface. (Courtesy Teleflex, Morrisville, NC.)

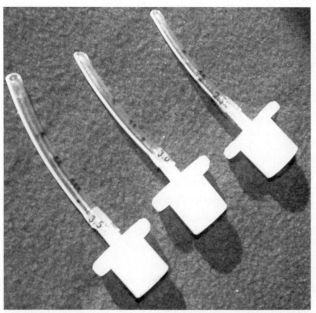

FIGURE 14.3 Nasopharyngeal continuous positive airway pressure (CPAP).

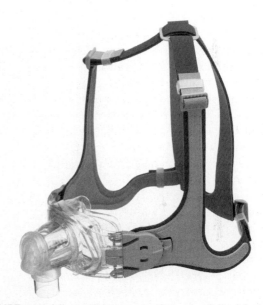

FIGURE 14.4 Mirage Kidsta mask. (Courtesy © ResMed 2009. Used with permission.)

infant's upper airway (Fig. 14.3).[2] Nasopharyngeal CPAP may be used in situations in which nasal appliances and headgear cannot be used because of potential aggravation of a surgical site or skin condition. In addition, nasopharyngeal CPAP may be better tolerated by some patients, or its use may simply be the preference of clinicians.[3]

Even though many clinicians lean toward one type of CPAP system and interface over another, no clinical research data are available at this time that conclusively show the superiority of one system or interface type. Moreover, because CPAP is used in the management of several clinical situations, it cannot yet be stated that one type of system or interface is more effective for a certain clinical circumstance than another. Convenience, economics, and staff experience often dictate the type of CPAP system and interface a facility chooses to use.

It is not uncommon for clinicians to use nasal-prong or nasopharyngeal CPAP interfaces in children up to the age of 6 months. For older children, nasal masks are the preferred device because most available prong sizes are too small. Also, masks and accompanying headgear seem to stay in position better in the older, more active child.

Today, many brands of masks are available for small children. An example, the ResMed Mirage Kidsta mask (ResMed, Inc.), is shown in Fig. 14.4. Nasal masks are preferred over full-face designs. Although it is known that older children are not obligate nose breathers, most "settle in" to breathing through these masks after becoming accustomed to them. If the patient does not tolerate a nasal mask, it is often because the nasal passages are not fully patent. It is usually a good practice to take measures to clear the nose, if possible, and offer the patient a trial with a nasal mask to evaluate its effectiveness before resorting to a full-face mask.

Although not all clinicians agree, the use of conventional adult CPAP drivers, whether they are ventilators or standalone devices, is generally appropriate for providing nasal CPAP to children older than 6 months of age.

This section of the chapter reviews a few examples of CPAP application devices, including the CareFusion Infant Flow synchronized inspiratory positive airway pressure (SiPAP) and the Fisher & Paykel Healthcare Bubble CPAP System.

CAREFUSION INFANT FLOW SiPAP SYSTEM

The CareFusion Infant Flow SiPAP system (Becton, Dickinson and Company) is designed to provide noninvasive ventilatory support for infants and pediatric patients (Fig. 14.5).[4] The SiPAP system provides a means by which patients can be

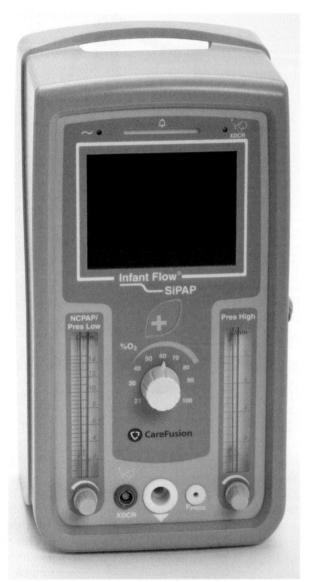

FIGURE 14.5 The Infant Flow SiPAP. (Courtesy Becton, Dickinson, and Company [CareFusion], Franklin Lakes, NJ.)

transitioned from intubation to successful extubation while more support is provided than with traditional noninvasive CPAP. SiPAP may provide support efficiently enough that some patients can avoid intubation.

Many infants are placed on noninvasive CPAP systems in an effort to reduce the frequency of apneic periods, such as those seen in apnea of prematurity. With the availability of a bilevel airway pressure device for small infants, it is possible that the problem of spontaneous apnea can be better managed. Moreover, an immediate response and resolution to apneic episodes are possible with this capability of providing manual breaths and backup apnea ventilation.

Available Configurations

The Infant Flow SiPAP system is available in two configurations: the Plus and the Comprehensive. The Plus configuration offers nasal CPAP (nCPAP) and time-triggered biphasic ventilation with breath-rate monitoring. The Comprehensive configuration offers these same features plus patient-triggered biphasic ventilation (called "BiPhasic tr") with backup breath-rate monitoring in the case of apnea. Both configurations deliver blended gas mixtures and incorporate a graphics screen for monitoring and displaying settings, touchscreen technology, patient monitoring, alarm systems, and backup battery power.

In the Comprehensive model, in addition to the patient circuit, an abdominal transducer known as a *Grasby* capsule is part of the design. This capsule is necessary to the detection of apnea when the "BiPhasic tr" mode is being used.

Power Source

The Infant Flow SiPAP system connects to 100 AC to 230 AC power and 50-psi (pounds per square inch) O_2 and compressed air power sources. An internal battery can provide up to 2 hours of operating time if the AC power source is lost. The battery requires 16 hours to become fully charged from a discharged state.

When the Infant Flow SiPAP system is powered on, it automatically performs internal electrical and pneumatic checks. Once the setup screen is visible, the user must calibrate the oxygen sensor and perform the patient circuit leak test and alarms test (see the operator's manual).[5]

Once the preuse tests are completed, the clinician can select the desired mode and settings (Box 14.1). As the unit begins operation, monitoring data are displayed on the driver screen. Box 14.2 lists monitored parameters, and Table 14.1 lists the ranges for monitored parameters.

Mechanism of Operation

The Infant Flow SiPAP system consists of a driver, a standard ventilator humidifier, and the patient circuit. The pneumatic components of the Infant Flow SiPAP driver consist of two separate flowmeters labeled the "NCPAP/Pres Low" flowmeter and the "Pres High" flowmeter. The other components are an oxygen/air blending system and a monitoring/alarms system.

A proprietary Infant Flow Generator, which is capable of alternating between two levels of flow and pressure, is incorporated into the patient circuit near the nasal interface. The

BOX 14.1 Main Mode Controls on the Infant Flow SiPAP System

- Nasal continuous positive airway pressure (nCPAP)
- nCPAP with breath-rate monitoring and low breath-rate alarm
- BiPhasic (time triggered)
- BiPhasic (time triggered) with breath-rate monitoring and low breath-rate alarm
- BiPhasic tr (time triggered) with breath-rate monitoring, low breath-rate alarm, and apnea
- Backup (Comprehensive models only)

SiPAP, Synchronized inspiratory positive airway pressure.

BOX 14.2 Parameters Monitored by the Infant Flow SiPAP System

- PEEP
- CPAP
- Mean airway pressure ($P_{\overline{aw}}$)
- Peak inspiratory pressure (PIP)
- O_2%
- I:E ratio (ratio of inspiratory time to expiratory time)
- Spontaneous rate (Rsp)
- Battery charge level

CPAP, Continuous positive airway pressure; *PEEP,* positive end-expiratory pressure; *SiPAP,* synchronized inspiratory positive airway pressure.

TABLE 14.1 Monitored Parameter Ranges on the SiPAP

Parameter	Range
Inspiratory time (T_I)	0.1-3.0 s
Rate (R)	1-150 breaths/min (non-US configuration parameters) 1-54 breaths/min (US configuration parameters)
Apnea interval (T_{apnea})	10-30 s, 5-s intervals (non-US configuration parameters)
Apnea interval (TLBR)	10-30 s, 5-s intervals (US configuration parameters)
nCPAP/Pres Low flowmeter	0-5 L/min; accuracy ±15% of selected output
Pres High flowmeter	0-15 L/min; accuracy ±15% of selected output
Manual breath	×1
O_2%	21-100%

nCPAP, Nasal continuous positive airway pressure; *SiPAP,* synchronized inspiratory positive airway pressure.

Infant Flow SiPAP system delivers a humidified flow of gas to produce a targeted level of pressure. It is worth mentioning that the Infant Flow SiPAP unit is capable of alternating between two targeted pressures.

Fig. 14.6 shows the relationship of flow and pressure. The low pressure is produced by the "NCPAP/Pres Low" flowmeter from the driver. Flow to the Infant Flow Generator from the

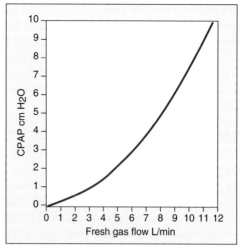

FIGURE 14.6 A graph flow-pressure nomogram for the Infant Flow SiPAP unit showing the continuous positive airway pressure (CPAP) on the *y* axis (cm H_2O) and fresh gas flow (L/min) on the *x* axis. Note the exponential rise in fresh gas as the CPAP increases. (Redrawn from information provided by Becton, Dickinson, and Company, Franklin Lakes, NJ.)

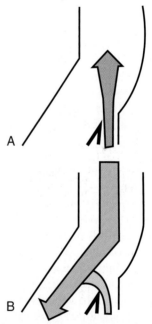

FIGURE 14.7 Twin injector nozzles of the Infant Flow Generator for the SiPAP driver. A, When the patient makes an inspiratory effort, the flow generator converts the kinetic energy of flow to pressure, to stabilize pressure delivery at the patient interface. B, As the patient exhales, the pressure from the exhaled gas causes the flow from the driver to flip around toward the expiratory limb. When expiratory flow stops, the flow from the driver instantly flips back to the inspiratory position (A).

"NCPAP/Pres Low" flowmeter is directed toward its expiratory limb (Fig. 14.7). This creates an expiratory pressure equal to the targeted CPAP.

When the patient takes a breath, the inspiratory effort diverts gas flow away from the expiratory limb to mix with an existing inspiratory flow (see Fig. 14.7). The inspiratory flow is produced by the "Pres High" flowmeter. The sum of the two flows, which is larger than the expiratory flow alone, creates the targeted inspiratory PAP (IPAP). After inspiration, pressure from the patient's expiratory flow diverts gas to the expiratory limb to return to the expiratory baseline flow and expiratory PAP (EPAP). The inspiratory-to-expiratory function uses fluidics.

Patient Interface and Humidification

A variety of patient interfaces are available, including nasal prongs and nasal masks. The circuit/interface is fitted to the patient by using a fabric bonnet, also available in different sizes. A complete guide accompanies the Infant Flow SiPAP system to enable the practitioner to select and fit the appropriately sized nasal cannula, nasal mask, and bonnet. It is important to use the sizing templates provided to ensure a good fit. The best performance from the system greatly depends on how well the interface fits the patient.

Once the interface is fitted and the unit is operational, the clinician must periodically check the interface for patency and general condition. (*Note:* Any patient interface can become obstructed, misaligned, or dislodged.) In addition, interfaces can cause skin damage if they are not properly sized or positioned.

The manufacturer does not recommend the use of a specific humidifier. However, the humidifier selected for use must be capable of providing inspired gas temperatures between 36°C (96.8°F) and 37°C (98.6°F). A continuous-feed water source for the humidifier chamber is strongly recommended to maintain stable circuit compliance.

Control Settings

Once the Infant Flow SiPAP is powered on, the default parameter settings are displayed. The front panel of the Infant Flow SiPAP driver is shown in Fig. 14.5. All parameter controls on the Infant Flow SiPAP driver are accessed through its touch-screen design. Box 14.1 lists the main controls.

When a parameter is touched, it becomes highlighted and *increase* and *decrease* buttons appear. After the parameter is selected and changed, the button is touched once again to confirm the new setting. If the setting is not confirmed within 15 seconds, the highlighted parameter will return automatically to its last keystroke and the screen will return to its prior configuration.

If no control is touched for 120 seconds, the screen panel automatically locks to prevent inadvertent changes. The "screen lock" button must be touched to unlock the controls. However, if a high-priority alarm is activated, the screen immediately unlocks to allow parameter changes.

If a setting is changed that is incompatible with other parameters, the driver software will automatically adjust other settings to bring them back into compatibility. If the clinician returns the adjusted parameter back to its original setting within 15 seconds, the automatically adjusted parameter(s) will return to their original settings.

One of the parameters available is time triggering. Timed triggering from EPAP to IPAP can be controlled by selecting an inspiratory time (T_I) on the touch screen. In addition, breath frequency can be set. This is a backup setting, however, and is operational only when the patient does not actively cycle respirations. (*Note:* In the Comprehensive configuration, an apnea backup rate, time interval, and apnea alarm can be set.)

By using the two flowmeters, the clinician can set both an inspiratory and an expiratory pressure. If only CPAP is desired, only the "NCPAP/Pres Low" flowmeter is set to deliver flow. The "Pres High" flowmeter is turned off unless it is desirable to deliver a manual breath, in which case the "Pres High" flowmeter is set. (*Note:* When operating the system in the NCPAP mode and the "Pres High" flowmeter is set, "biphasic" manual breaths can be delivered by pressing the manual breath button.)

The actual pressure for a given flow (as shown in Fig. 14.6) can fall outside of the predicted value by as much as 10%. The predicted flow-to-pressure relationship increases to more than 10% when flows are decreased to achieve low pressures (e.g., 2 cm H_2O). For this reason, it is recommended that the Infant Flow SiPAP system not be used to deliver pressures of 2 cm H_2O or less.

Alarms

The driver automatically sets some alarm limits based on the parameter settings that have been selected. Other alarms are preset. Table 14.2 lists alarms and conditions that trigger alarms. By pressing the alarm mute/reset button, the clinician can silence alarm conditions for 30 seconds. If the button is pressed and held for 3 seconds, alarms are reset.

TABLE 14.2 **Alarms and Conditions That Trigger Alarms on the SiPAP**	
Alarm	**Trigger**
Supply gases failure	Activates with a ±20-psi pressure change in either gas line
High airway pressure	Activates with a pressure rise 3 cm H_2O over set pressure
Airway overpressure limit	Activates at 11 cm H_2O in nCPAP and BiPhasic
	Activates at 15 cm H_2O in "BiPhasic tr" mode
Low airway pressure	Activates if pressure falls 2 cm H_2O below set pressure
High and low %	Activates if measured oxygen concentration is greater than ±5% of set value
Low battery charge	Activates if battery charge falls below 40%
Low battery voltage	Activates if battery voltage falls below 10 V

nCPAP, Nasal continuous positive airway pressure; *SiPAP,* synchronized inspiratory positive airway pressure.

Modes of Ventilation

Box 14.1 lists the available modes for the SiPAP. The Infant Flow SiPAP system provides two basic modes: CPAP and BiPhasic. The other mode choices are simply additional features for these two basic modes.

Summary: Infant Flow SiPAP

Noninvasive bilevel airway pressure has been an effective tool in adult and pediatric patients for many years. As is the case with mechanical ventilators, a practical device to provide the same type of support to the smallest of infants has been a technical challenge. In the meantime, a gap between CPAP and mechanical ventilation has persisted in neonatal critical care settings. This gap has led to many extubation failures and untold additional ventilator days for patients. The Infant Flow SiPAP System is the first practical infant bilevel application that may effectively bridge that gap and provide a real alternative to more invasive care.

FISHER & PAYKEL HEALTHCARE BUBBLE CPAP SYSTEM

The Fisher & Paykel Healthcare Bubble CPAP System (Fisher & Paykel Healthcare) was introduced to provide clinicians with a commercially available freestanding CPAP delivery device that takes advantage of the "high-frequency," or "bubbling," effect that is reported to be unique to this system. The application of bubble CPAP has been associated with reduced incidence of chronic lung disease in premature infants.[5] However, no randomized trials have been published that compare this method with the more conventional forms of CPAP delivery.

The Fisher & Paykel Healthcare Bubble CPAP System consists of two components: a delivery system and a patient interface. These components can be used together as a single system or can be used separately as parts of clinician-designed hybrid systems.

Delivery System

A schematic of the Fisher & Paykel Healthcare Bubble CPAP System is shown in Fig. 14.8. The manufacturer recommends the use of a Fisher & Paykel Healthcare MR290 humidifier chamber (Fig. 14.9), which is designed to operate with either the MR850 or the MR730 humidifier unit. If the MR850 is used, it is set to the "invasive" mode. If the MR730 is used, the temperature control is initially set at 40°C (104°F) and the chamber control at −3. Fine adjustments to these settings may be necessary once the system is in use. A continuous-feed

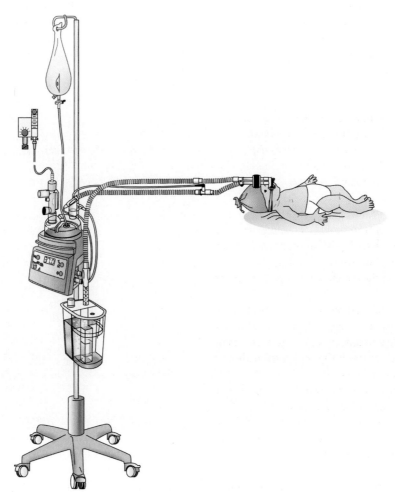

FIGURE 14.8 Fisher & Paykel Healthcare Bubble CPAP System.

sterile water system keeps a constant water level within the chamber.

The system also depends on a standard air/oxygen blender, a 0 L/min to 15 L/min flowmeter, and standard oxygen tubing to deliver inspiratory gas flow to the unit. Flow enters the system by way of a plastic manifold (Fig. 14.10), which is connected to the inlet of the humidifier chamber. This manifold system incorporates a safety pressure vent, as well as optional ports, to place an oxygen analyzer sensor and a pressure-monitoring device or alarm.

The hot-wire inspiratory limb of the patient circuit is connected to the humidifier outlet. Two temperature probes in the circuit provide servo feedback to the humidifier unit. Humidified gas with a minimum of condensation flows to the patient interface, which is described later in this section. Gas exiting the patient interface flows to the CPAP generator (Fig. 14.11).

The generator, which is usually mounted on the same stand as the humidifier, consists of a clear plastic container made up of two compartments. With the plastic funnel provided, the clinician fills the main compartment of the humidifier with either sterile water or a weak acetic acid solution. The main compartment is filled until it begins to overflow into the other compartment. The desired CPAP level is set by adjusting the CPAP probe, which is a tube with numbers exactly embedded at 1-cm increments in the plastic. The number that is positioned directly above the lid is the CPAP setting. A CPAP range from 3 cm H_2O to 10 cm H_2O is available.

The manufacturer recommends a system test for leaks; instructions for this test are included with the circuit packaging. The manufacturer packages the manifold, humidifier chamber, and circuit limbs together as a convenience.

Patient Interface

The patient interface consists of a choice of 3 lengths of nasal tubing, 4 sizes of head bonnets, 3 sizes of head straps (called *headgear*), 11 sizes of nasal prongs, and 4 sizes of chin straps.

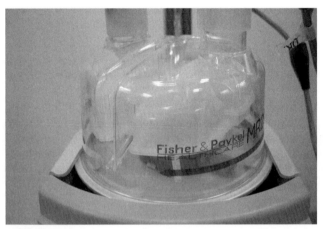

FIGURE 14.9 Fisher & Paykel Healthcare MR290 humidifier for the Bubble CPAP System.

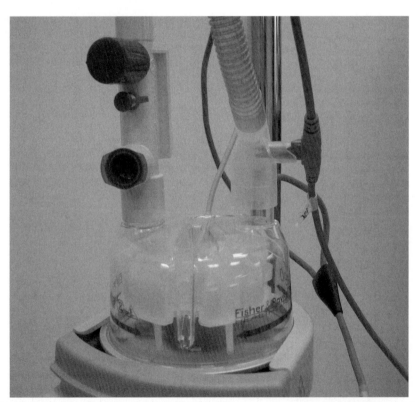

FIGURE 14.10 The attachment of an oxygen line (*top center*) to the humidifier manifold system for the Fisher & Paykel Healthcare Bubble CPAP System. This manifold integrates a safety pressure vent, as well as optional ports to place an oxygen analyzer sensor and a pressure-monitoring device or alarm. Two temperature probes in the circuit provide servo feedback to the humidifier unit (*right side*).

In part because of so many different component sizes, the Fisher & Paykel Healthcare patient interface system is one of the most complex of all CPAP application devices on the market today. Appropriate sizes of prongs, head straps or bonnets, and nasal tubing have to be chosen. The clinician must be skilled at fitting and adjusting the various mounting straps. If proper emphasis is not given to both sizing and proper fitting, CPAP delivery may be ineffective, and patient stress caused by discomfort may be excessive.

The method by which the interface is applied is to first measure the patient's head circumference and choose the head strap or bonnet whose range corresponds to the measurement. Bonnets are usually chosen for premature infants because they offer more stability and provide some aid in preserving core temperature.

The next step is to select the proper size of nasal prongs (Fig. 14.12). To assist with this, the manufacturer recommends its sizing guide, which consists of templates used to match nares opening sizes and septum gap. Generally, it is recommended that the clinician choose the largest prong size that occupies the entire nares opening, but that does not stretch the skin. The prong set that meets those criteria, but with the narrowest septum gap, should be tried. However, the clinician often must move up or down one size after a brief trial period with the system.

Once prongs are sized, the nasal tubing must be selected. From the three available sizes, the clinician selects the size in which the clear tubing extends from the patient's nares to just before the top of the head. The clinician should also see that the accompanying foam block allows the tubing to lie parallel to the patient's face. Foam strips can be peeled away one at a time to adjust the foam block. Fig. 14.13 shows the prongs, nasal tubing, and foam strips.

With the nasal tubing selected and sized, the nasal-prong set is then attached to its end. The patient circuit is then attached, and a flow of 6 L/min to 8 L/min is set. The prongs can then be inserted into the nares and the nasal tubing secured by using the Velcro strap at the patient's forehead. Finally, the glider clips are secured in such a way that a slight bend is seen. Box 14.3 describes the key steps in setting up the Bubble CPAP device (Clinical Scenario 14.1).

Some clinicians have used the Fisher & Paykel Healthcare patient interface with other CPAP systems and with ventilators that provide CPAP. Also, the Fisher & Paykel Healthcare CPAP delivery system has found its way into other types of applications, such as in the delivery of high-flow oxygen by nasal cannula and in helium/oxygen mixtures.

The Fisher & Paykel Healthcare Bubble CPAP System offers the clinician a convenient and inexpensive means of providing noninvasive ventilatory support to infants, especially those who are premature or who cannot tolerate conventional face masks.

THE INFANT VENTILATOR

As previously mentioned, infants have been ventilated primarily in the time-cycled, pressure-limited (TCPL) mode. The

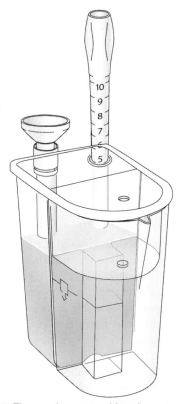

FIGURE 14.11 The continuous positive airway pressure (CPAP) probe for the Fisher & Paykel Healthcare Bubble CPAP System. The desired CPAP level is set by adjusting the CPAP probe. The number that is positioned directly above the lid is the CPAP setting (3 to 10 cm H$_2$O).

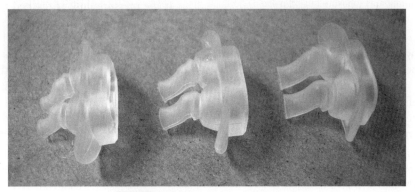

FIGURE 14.12 Infant nasal prongs.

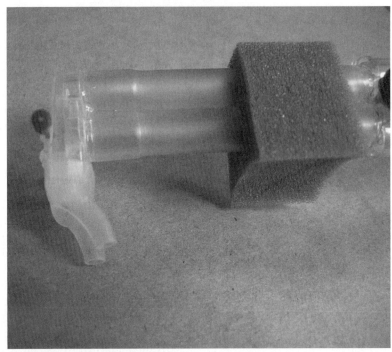

FIGURE 14.13 The prongs, nasal tubing, and foam strips *(left side)* with the nasal prong attached to the far-left end. The patient circuit is then attached *(right side)*. The prongs can then be inserted into the nares and the nasal tubing secured by using the Velcro strap at the patient's forehead. (See text for additional information.)

CLINICAL SCENARIO 14.1

Following a cesarean delivery at 41 weeks' gestational age, a 4.1-kg newborn has a respiratory rate of 50 to 70 breaths/min and is in respiratory distress. After admission to a level III neonatal intensive care unit, she is placed on a Fisher & Paykel Healthcare Bubble CPAP system. CPAP is set at 6 cm H_2O, flow at 8 L/min and F_IO_2 at 0.60.

Approximately 45 minutes after CPAP has been initiated, the infant continues to breathe at a respiratory rate of 50 to 70 breaths/min with mild retractions. A F_IO_2 of 0.70 is required to maintain the patient's SpO_2 at 93% to 95%. The infant also shows periods of irritability and frequently cries and moves her head in a side-to-side motion. What should be the respiratory therapist's concerns at this time? What should the respiratory therapist evaluate?

See Appendix A for answers.

CPAP, Continuous positive airway pressure; *F_IO_2,* fractional inspired oxygen; *SpO_2,* oxygen saturation as measured using pulse oximetry.

reason for this probably relates to the historical evolution of infant ventilators. Advocates for the use of TCPL believed that this mode reduced the risk for barotrauma and was superior to volume control in infants.[1] As a result, until recently, infant ventilators were designed to provide TCPL and CPAP exclusively. These devices were simple in design and incorporated many similar features.

Today, however, more-precise monitoring and patient sensing have made it possible to apply additional modes of ventilation in infants. These modes were associated only with adult and pediatric patients. Manufacturers have introduced more-sophisticated models with unique features. Although these infant ventilators have retained the basic design that enables them to provide TCPL and CPAP, many now offer additional options. For example, volume-controlled ventilation and pressure support are available on many models.

Most infant ventilators have been designed to provide a continuous flow of an air/oxygen mixture into the ventilator circuit (Fig. 14.14A).[6] In this design a positive-pressure breath results when the machine's exhalation valve closes, permitting the gas mixture to flow to the patient (see Fig. 14.14B). During the inspiratory phase, when a preset pressure limit is reached, pressure is maintained until the ventilator time-cycles into expiration (see Fig. 14.14C). When the exhalation valve opens, the expiratory phase begins. As long as the exhalation valve remains open, a constant flow of the gas mixture passes through the patient's airway and is available for spontaneous breaths.

If the pressure limit is reached in this type of ventilator, tidal volume will depend on flow, pressure limit, and inspiratory time (see calculation, Box 14.4). However, alterations in the patient's compliance and airway resistance can affect the tidal volume. For example, consider the patient whose compliance improves over a few hours. If the ventilator settings are not modified, the patient's lungs will accommodate flow from the ventilator over a longer period during the inspiratory phase. Peak pressure will be reached later in the inspiratory phase. Therefore a larger-than-desired tidal volume may be delivered by the ventilator. Inspiratory time and flow are set and digitally displayed on most infant ventilators. The calculation shown in Box 14.4 can be used to estimate the available

BOX 14.3 Bubble CPAP: Key Steps to Setup and Use

- Attach oxygen tubing to flowmeter and connect to humidifier inlet. Adjust flow to 5 to 10 L/min. This flow will provide sufficient CPAP.
- Verify system tightness by observing bubbling of water in CPAP generator. Look for a gentle, continuous bubbling. Vigorous bubbling is not recommended.
- Set required F_IO_2 on air/oxygen blender.
- Fill bubble chamber with sterile water (or weak acetic acid solution) up to fill mark, and set CPAP tubing to desired level. Depth of the tubing under the water controls the amount of positive pressure in system.
- Choose appropriately sized nasal tubing.
- Choose the appropriately sized nasal prongs by using the size guide included in the nasal tubing packaging. Prongs should fit the nares snugly without pinching the nasal septum. If prongs are too small, there will be an increase in airway pressure and gas will leak from the system, making it difficult to maintain the desired positive pressure.
- Patient's mouth, nose, and pharynx should be thoroughly suctioned before the nasal prongs are inserted.
- Prongs can be moistened with saline, sterile water, or small amounts of water-soluble lubricant before they are placed curve-side down into the infant's nose. Long-term use of prongs may necessitate use of a hydrocolloid dressing to protect nasal openings.
- Nasal prongs should fill nasal openings completely without stretching the skin or putting undue pressure on the nares. Blanching around the rim of nostrils suggests that prongs are too large.
- Correct positioning reduces the risk for trauma and ensures effective delivery of CPAP.
- If the infant's mouth is open, this can cause a significant decrease in airway pressure. This situation should be prevented or corrected by placing a pacifier in the infant's mouth. Mouth breathing will usually stop once the infant adjusts to the system. Chin straps, although available, are not recommended and should be used only as a last resort.

CPAP, Continuous positive airway pressure; F_IO_2, fractional inspired oxygen.

BOX 14.4 Calculation of Maximum Available Tidal Volume for Time-Triggered, Pressure-Limited, Time-Cycled Ventilation (TPTV)

$$V_T = \frac{\text{Inspiratory time (seconds)} \times \text{Flow (L/min)}}{60}$$

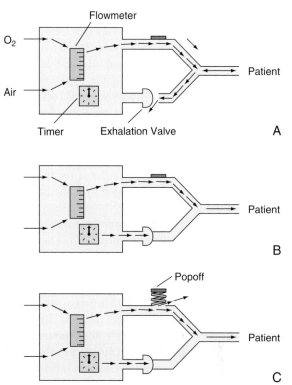

FIGURE 14.14 The typical continuous-flow ventilator circuit designed for time-triggered, pressure-limited, time-cycled ventilation. A, Spontaneous phase; B, inspiratory phase; C, pressure-limiting phase. (From Koff PB, Eitzman D, Neu J: *Neonatal and pediatric respiratory care*, ed 2, St. Louis, 1993, Mosby-Elsevier.)

inspiratory flow. The ventilator matches the patient's inspiratory flow. Demand flow is believed by some clinicians to be advantageous to operator-selected continuous-flow systems, because continuous-flow systems tend to produce resistance to expiration at the airway, commonly known as **circuit positive end-expiratory pressure (PEEP)**. For patients whose ventilatory needs include high inspiratory flows but low end-expiratory pressure, the demand system eliminates the need to set a high continuous flow. Some patients may present with highly variable ventilatory patterns. The use of a demand system may ensure sufficient flow to meet transiently high inspiratory flow needs.

In a typical demand system, a minimal preset continuous flow is delivered by the ventilator. On spontaneous inspiration, this flow will increase to maintain the baseline pressure. When the ventilator delivers a mandatory breath, the flow increases to the value set with the flow control knob.

With the development of improved flow-sensing capability, current ventilator models can now enable the clinician to distinguish between the patient's inspiratory flow and machine-generated flow, even in very tiny patients. This allows the clinician to select the TCPL mode and adjust the ventilator to deliver patient-triggered mandatory breaths. This type of continuous-flow IMV is possible even with small ETT leaks. Flow-sensing capability has led to other advances, many of which are unique to a specific ventilator model. The ways in

tidal volume if the pressure limit is reached. However, if the pressure limit is reached early in the inspiratory phase, tidal volume could be substantially less than calculated.

Some ventilators use a demand flow system to provide inspiratory gas for spontaneous breaths. This type of system delivers flow at a variable rate proportional to patient

which flow-sensing applications have been developed are discussed with each ventilator that uses this technology.

The same flow-sensing technology that provides better ventilator–patient synchrony has enabled clinicians to return to volume modes of ventilation in infants. By closely monitoring inspired and expired tidal volume, ventilatory pressures, and waveforms, clinicians can better adjust ventilator settings according to physiological changes. Compliance and airway resistance measurements are now possible. Providing the appropriate level of support, responding to physiological changes more quickly, and weaning infants from the ventilator more effectively are greatly facilitated by some of the latest developments in infant ventilators.

As pressure-limited, volume-targeted modes of ventilation (e.g., pressure-regulated volume control [PRVC]) increasingly have been used in adults, their application in infants and pediatric patients has been growing as well. (See Chapter 12 for more information on these modes.) Clinicians working with adults have long recognized that pressure control and pressure support modes are desirable in many clinical situations, primarily because of their decelerating waveforms. With the addition of a volume-targeting capability to these modes, a patient receives a more consistent tidal volume in spite of compliance or airway resistance changes. In infants, rapid and sometimes dramatic changes are often seen in compliance after surfactant replacement therapy.[7] In many pediatric patients, marked compliance or airway resistance changes can occur very rapidly because of the progression of a disease process or after an intervention. Therefore a ventilator that is capable of delivering consistent tidal volumes with pressure ventilation (e.g., PRVC and volume support) while providing decelerating flow can be very useful in both the neonatal and the pediatric settings.

In small infants, such as those weighing less than 1000 g, use of pressure-limited, volume-targeted breath delivery has not yet gained widespread acceptance. The tried and proven TCPL mode, with its simplicity and safety, continues to be the most widely used in premature and very low-birth-weight infants.

With infants, some clinicians continue to prefer to use mechanical ventilators that were designed exclusively for infants and small children. This section provides information on ventilators specifically designed for infants and children. However, manufacturers are beginning to design models that are suitable for any size patient. (See Chapter 13 for details on general use ventilators.) Features such as flow triggering and flow cycling, short response times, volume monitoring, and low internal compressible volume are being incorporated into most new ventilator designs.

It is important to mentioned that although some hospitals have chosen a single ventilator model that can be used with adult, pediatric, and neonatal patients, extra care must be used when these ventilators are used in very small patients, especially with uncuffed artificial airways. It is good practice to monitor tidal volume at the infant s airway when using these ventilators; this measure will enable a more precise determination of ventilator function. The use of calculations to correct for compressible volume does not take artificial airway leak into account. Moreover, in situations in which compliance is markedly low or airway resistance is markedly high, volume loss in the patient/circuit system can be greater than that calculated.

This following section reviews several ventilators that have been specifically designed for the ventilation of infants and children.

CAREFUSION V.I.P. BIRD INFANT/PEDIATRIC VENTILATOR

The V.I.P. Bird ventilator (CareFusion) mechanically supports neonatal, infant, and pediatric patients with the most common ventilator modes (Fig. 14.15). It is electrically powered with 110-V AC and pneumatically powered by external compressed air and oxygen at 40 psig to 75 psig. DC power operation from an external power source is possible.

The V.I.P. Bird is microprocessor-controlled by three processors. Flow triggering and flow cycling can be accomplished by using the Bird Partner IIi Volume Monitor and infant flow sensor. An oxygen blender auxiliary output flowmeter (0 to 15 L/min) is located on the side of the ventilator for use with a nebulizer or handheld resuscitator.[8]

Noteworthy Internal Functions

The microblender mixes the two gases according to the set oxygen percentage. The blended gas then enters the 1.1-L accumulator. The accumulator reserves pressurized gas during the expiratory phase to meet high inspiratory flow demands of the patient with maximum flow capabilities up

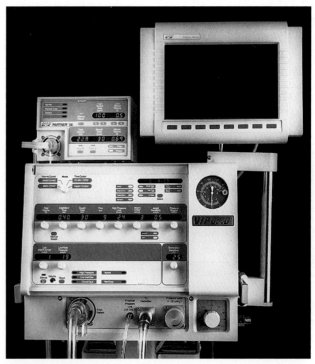

FIGURE 14.15 The V.I.P. Bird Ventilator. (Courtesy CareFusion, Inc., Yorba Linda, CA.)

BOX 14.5 Function of the High-Pressure Control

The high-pressure limit controls the set peak inspiratory pressure in the time-cycled, pressure-limited (TCPL) modes. Its function in the volume-cycled (VC) modes is a high-pressure limit.

TABLE 14.3 Specifications for the V.I.P. Bird Infant/Pediatric Ventilator

Tidal volume	20-995 mL
Inspiratory time	0.1-3.0 s
Rate	0-150 breaths/min
Flow (TC modes)	3-40 L/min
Flow (VC modes)	3-120 L/min
Peak inspiratory pressure	0-80 cm H_2O
TC Modes	
High-pressure limit	0-120 cm H_2O
VC Modes	
PEEP/CPAP	0-24 cm H_2O
Assist sensitivity	Off, 0.1-5.0 L/min
TC Modes	
Assist sensitivity	Off, 1-20 cm H_2O
VC Modes	
Pressure support	0-50 cm H_2O
Trigger mechanism	Pressure (VC)/flow (TC)
Alarms	Low PEEP/CPAP, low peak pressure, high pressure, low inlet pressure, circuit fault, apnea, ventilator inoperative

CPAP, Continuous positive airway pressure; *PEEP*, positive end-expiratory pressure; *TC*, time-cycled; *VC*, volume-cycled.

to 120 L/min. The gas exits the accumulator and enters a pneumatic regulator that adjusts the flow-control valve, driving pressure to 25 psig. A pulsation dampener is located between the regulator and the flow-control valve and is used to stabilize pressure and maintain driving pressure to the flow-control valve.

Gas flow is delivered to the patient by means of an electromechanical proportioning valve and an electromagnetic exhalation valve. Delivered flow rates are determined by the system driving pressure and the diameter of the valve opening. Flow rates are unaffected by downstream patient circuit pressures of up to 350 cm H_2O with a system pressure of 25 psig.

Because of the possibility of inadvertent PEEP developing from the continuous flow present in the expiratory limb of the patient circuit during TCPL ventilation, a jet Venturi is incorporated into the exhalation manifold. The jet solenoid controls the driving pressure to the exhalation valve jet Venturi and is controlled by the microprocessor. It is active when the flow rate control is set at 5 L/min or greater with a PEEP of 0 cm H_2O to 5 cm H_2O or when PEEP is set at 0 and flow at any setting.

A pneumatically driven safety valve is activated when a ventilator-inoperative event or electrical power failure occurs. This allows the spontaneously breathing patient to breathe room air.

If a pressure difference of 20 psig occurs between the air and oxygen sources, the gas source with the highest pressure will be used by the ventilator. This will result in a delivered oxygen concentration of either 21% or 100%.

Control and Alarm Panel

Fig. 14.16 is a diagram of the control and alarm panel. The mode selector knob is located on the front top-left panel and has two groups of modes. The volume-cycled (VC) modes are assist/control (A/C) and synchronized intermittent mandatory ventilation (SIMV)/CPAP. The time-cycled (TC) modes are A/C and (S)IMV/CPAP.

The front-panel control settings are tidal volume, inspiratory time, rate, flow, high pressure (Box 14.5), PEEP/CPAP, assist sensitivity, and pressure support. Table 14.3 lists parameter specifications and their available ranges for the V.I.P. Bird infant/pediatric ventilator. The manual breath-control button is located on the control panel and is a single, operator-initiated controlled breath that is available in all modes.

Illumination of displays highlights the controls that are functional for that specific mode. Dimmed displays are controls that are not functional in a certain mode. For example, tidal volume will have a dimmed display when the ventilator is operating in a TCPL mode. During CPAP the inspiratory time

and peak inspiratory pressure (PIP) displays remain illuminated and are functional during manual ventilation.

Directly below the control section is the alarm section, which includes the following knobs: low PEEP/CPAP (−9 to 24 cm H_2O), low peak pressure (off, 3 to 120 cm H_2O), high pressure, low inlet gas, circuit fault, apnea (inactive with continuous flow), vent inop (inoperative), alarm silence (60 seconds), and reset. An additional safety feature is the mechanical pressure-relief knob, which is located next to the oxygen concentration dial and can be adjusted between 0 cm H_2O and 130 cm H_2O in all modes. Turning the pressure-relief knob clockwise increases the value, and turning it counterclockwise decreases the value. The high-pressure limit is normally set below the overpressure relief valve setting for the high-pressure limit to be activated (see Box 14.5).

When the power switch located on the rear top-left panel is turned off, the ventilator inoperable alarm can be silenced by depressing the alarm silence button. The alarm silence button is located on the front bottom-left panel. It will silence the alarm for 60 seconds, unless the reset button located on the right is depressed.

Table 14.4 lists the front-panel digital displays. There are some additional displays worth mentioning. The patient effort light-emitting diode (LED) will flash when the patient's inspiratory effort exceeds the assist sensitivity setting. The demand LED will flash when the demand flow system is triggered by spontaneous efforts decreasing airway pressure 1 cm H_2O below the baseline pressure during TC IMV. Airway pressures

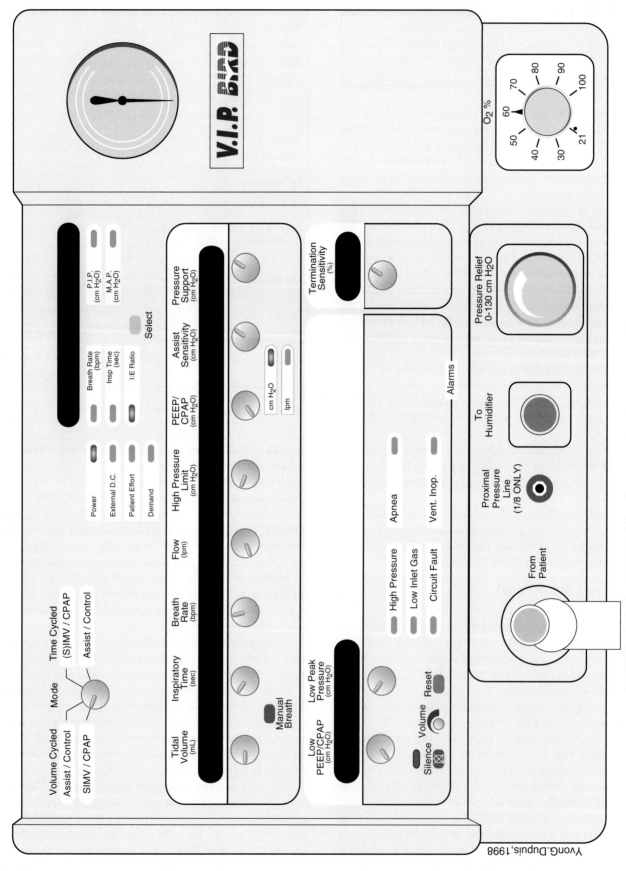

FIGURE 14.16 The V.I.P. Bird Ventilator control and alarm panel. (Courtesy Yvon Dupuis.)

TABLE 14.4 Digital Displays on the V.I.P. Bird Ventilator

Parameter	Range
Breath rate	0-250 breaths/min
Inspiratory time	0.05-60 s
I:E ratio	1:0.1 to 1:60
PIP	0-130 cm H_2O
MAP	0-120 cm H_2O
Power	Illuminates when power is on
External DC	Illuminates when external DC power source is being used
Patient effort	Illuminates when assist sensitivity is met
Demand	Illuminates when demand system is triggered

DC, Direct current; *I:E ratio,* ratio of inspiratory time to expiratory time; *MAP,* mean airway pressure; *PIP,* peak inspiratory pressure.

BOX 14.6 Breath Termination Ranges According to Tidal Volume

- For delivered tidal volume (V_T) of 0 mL to 50 mL, the flow-cycle value is 5% of peak flow.
- For delivered V_T 50 mL to 200 mL, the flow-cycle value is a range of 5% to 25% of peak flow.
- For delivered V_T > 200 mL, the flow-cycle value is 25% of peak flow.

are displayed on a pressure gauge. In the IMV mode, only the mandatory breaths are shown in the breath-rate display. The inspiratory time-to-expiratory time (I:E) ratio LED flashes when an inverse I:E ratio is present.

Modes of Ventilation

Two basic types of breath delivery or modes are provided by the V.I.P. Bird: VC and TC.

Volume-Cycled Modes

In the A/C VC mode, inspiration is time triggered or pressure triggered, volume targeted, flow limited, and volume cycled. Inspiration can be pressure cycled if the airway pressure reaches the set high-pressure alarm setting. The operator sets the following parameters: tidal volume, breath rate, flow, high-pressure limit, PEEP/CPAP, and assist sensitivity.

In the SIMV/CPAP VC mode, mandatory breaths are time triggered or pressure triggered, volume targeted, flow limited, and volume cycled. Inspiration can be pressure cycled if the airway pressure reaches the set high-pressure alarm setting. Spontaneous respiratory efforts between mandatory breaths are pressure triggered, pressure targeted, and time cycled. Pressure support can be added to spontaneous efforts and are pressure triggered, pressure limited, and flow cycled. (*Note:* The maximum demand flow available is 120 L/min for spontaneous and pressure-supported breaths.) The operator sets the following parameters: tidal volume, inspiratory time (pressure support time limit), breath rate, flow, high-pressure limit, PEEP/CPAP, assist sensitivity, and pressure support (if desired).

Pressure support termination criteria are set up differently with the V.I.P. Bird ventilator because of the varied patient population that can be ventilated with this device. For example, if the unit fails to flow cycle at 25% of peak flow because of an air leak around the artificial airway, this may result in excessive inspiratory times (some units will time cycle at 2 to 3 seconds). The termination criteria for the V.I.P. Bird are

based on delivered tidal volume ranges (Box 14.6). The pressure-support display will flash when the breath is time cycled.

Time-Cycled Modes

In the IMV time-cycled mode, mandatory breaths are time triggered, pressure targeted, and time cycled. In IMV the operator sets the following parameters: breath rate, inspiratory time, flow, high-pressure limit (PIP desired), and PEEP/CPAP. The continuous-flow and demand-flow systems support spontaneous efforts. Continuous flow is determined by the flow knob setting (range: 0 to 15 L/min). Demand flow is available when spontaneous inspiration decreases the airway pressure 1 cm H_2O below the baseline pressure. The maximum level of demand flow is 120 L/min. Sensitivity is set at 1 cm H_2O below baseline pressure in the IMV/CPAP mode. CPAP is activated when the breath-rate setting is 0.

In (S)IMV/CPAP (with the Bird Partner IIi Volume Monitor and infant flow sensor), the mandatory breath is flow triggered or time triggered, pressure targeted, and time cycled. CPAP is activated when the breath-rate setting is 0. In SIMV the operator sets the following parameters: breath rate, inspiratory time, flow, high-pressure limit, PEEP/CPAP, and assist sensitivity (L/min).

In the A/C mode, inspiration is flow triggered or time triggered, pressure targeted, and flow cycled or time cycled. The patient receives the set pressure with every spontaneous respiratory effort. The breath-rate setting acts as a backup rate in the event of decreased respiratory effort. The operator sets the following parameters: breath rate, inspiratory time, flow, high-pressure limit, PEEP/CPAP, assist sensitivity (L/min), and termination sensitivity.

The termination sensitivity control is an additional feature that adjusts the flow termination point of the breath, preventing air trapping and an inverse I:E ratio, thus providing expiratory synchrony. It is used only in the A/C TC mode. Termination sensitivity ranges are off, and they are 5% to 25% of peak flow. For example, a setting of 25% means that the breath will be terminated when the inspiratory flow (measured at the proximal airway) decreases to 25% of measured peak inspiratory flow. If the flow fails to decrease to the percentage set, which might occur with a low percentage setting and the presence of an air leak around the artificial airway, the breath is time cycled. The termination percentage setting will flash to indicate that the breath is time cycled. Airway graphics are helpful in evaluating patient–ventilator synchrony, and their use is strongly recommended with this mode of ventilation (Box 14.7).

The assist sensitivity control is adjustable from 0.2 L/min to 5 L/min with the use of the infant flow sensor. By pressing the continuous flow button on the Bird Partner IIi monitor, the operator can evaluate the real-time flow signal by observing the continuous flow readout at end exhalation. If the digital readout returns to 0, the operator should set the assist sensitivity value at 0.2 L/min to provide optimal patient-triggering capabilities. If there is a leak (flow readout does not return to 0), the assist sensitivity should be adjusted to 0.2 L/min above the digital readout. Adjusting the sensitivity to a level above the leak helps prevent autocycling and requires the patient to generate only the flow difference between the leak and the assist sensitivity setting.

Graphics Displays

Airway graphics are an invaluable tool that allows the clinician to monitor and adjust ventilatory strategies for each patient. Graphical analysis also provides real-time and trend assessment of ventilator parameters and of patient–ventilator interactions. The Bird Graphics Monitor is designed for use with the V.I.P. Bird and Bird 8400STi ventilators. It requires use of the Bird Partner or Bird Partner IIi monitor (see the following subsection on the Partner IIi monitor). The graphics monitor is easily moved between ventilators. A communication port is available for connection to a printer. Compatible printers include the HP (Hewlett-Packard Company) ThinkJet and Epson FX-850 (Epson America, Inc.).

The graphics monitor displays real-time scalar waveforms for pressure, flow, and volume (vertical axis) plotted over time (horizontal axis). The waveform-select screen allows the clinician to select two waveforms at a time. Positive values (above 0 on the vertical axis) relate to the inspiratory phase, and negative values to the expiratory phase of ventilation.

Pressure/volume and flow/volume loops are also available, along with reference loop storage. The pressure/volume graphic loop displays tidal volume on the vertical axis and airway pressure on the horizontal axis. The flow/volume graphic loop displays flow on the vertical axis and tidal volume on the horizontal axis. The freeze screen provides movable target and reference cursors that allow the clinician to hold and evaluate significant events. The trend feature has 10 selectable parameters and can be set for 15 minutes or 1-, 2-, 4-, 8-, or 24-hour windows.[9]

Special Features of the V.I.P. Ventilator

One of the notable special features with the V.I.P. Bird is leak compensation. Leak compensation is used to stabilize baseline pressure, prevent autocycling, and optimize assist sensitivity in the presence of leaks. It is recommended for use only with leaks around artificial airways. It is not recommended for those patients with minimal respiratory effort and no leak, because some patients are unable to trigger appropriately with leak compensation active. Leak compensation is functional only in the VC modes.

When pressure decreases 0.25 cm H_2O below baseline pressure, the leak-compensation feature introduces small amounts of flow into the circuit, an attempt to reestablish baseline pressure. The amount of leak compensation needed is learned by the exhalation valve pressure transducer so that the flow-control valve returns to the determined value after each breath. The amount of flow is reevaluated every 8 milliseconds. The maximum amount of flow available is either 5 L/min with assist sensitivity set at −1 cm H_2O or 10 L/min with assist sensitivity set at −2 cm H_2O to −5 cm H_2O. The default setting after any power-up is "leak compensation on." The leak compensation is turned on or off by pressing the select button until the desired feature is displayed in the digital window (top-left digital display).

Bird Partner IIi Monitor

The Bird Partner IIi monitor (CareFusion, Inc.) is a microprocessor-controlled volume monitor with a variable-orifice, differential-pressure, flow-measuring device that is placed in the patient circuit near the upper airway. (See Chapter 8 for a description of the variable orifice differential pressure transducer.) The flow-measuring device does the following:

- Measures effective inspiratory and expiratory volumes
- Displays digital measured values (tidal volume, breath rate, minute ventilation, and the real-time flow signal—only with infant sensor)
- Displays digital alarm parameters (high rate, low minute ventilation)
- Provides an adjustable apnea alarm (10 to 60 seconds in 5-second increments)

Alarm limits can be set by using the monitor s touchpad controls. The apnea button (red) is located on the rear panel of the monitor. The clinician can visualize the current apnea setting by depressing the red button and observing the displayed value in the tidal volume window. Repeated depression of the button will allow the clinician to adjust the apnea setting.

The monitor can be used with the infant sensor or the pediatric sensor. The infant sensor is placed at the proximal airway and circuit Y-connector. It can be used only with artificial airways having an internal diameter (ID) of 4.5 mm or less (Fig. 14.17). The sensor (B) is placed with the arrow pointing toward the patient (A) and the monitoring tubes (C) facing upward to prevent condensation or secretion accumulation within the lines. Box 14.8 contains important information about cleaning the infant sensor.

The gas inlet on the back of the ventilator connects to a 50-psig source and is used to inject 12 mL/min of gas through the pressure line to prevent obstructions within the line and to prevent water from entering the differential pressure transducer. The gas flow is synchronized with the expiratory phase so no additional volume is delivered to the patient during inspiration. The tidal volume readout is the effective tidal

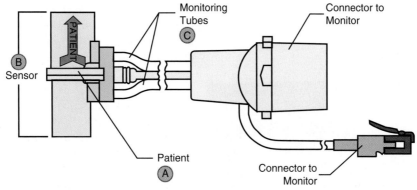

FIGURE 14.17 Infant sensor used with the Partner IIi monitor and the V.I.P. Bird. (See text for explanation.) (Courtesy CareFusion, Inc., Yorba Linda, CA.)

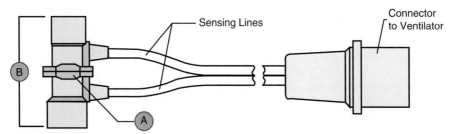

FIGURE 14.18 Pediatric sensor used with Partner IIi monitor and V.I.P. Bird. (Courtesy Care-Fusion, Inc., Yorba Linda, CA.)

BOX 14.8   Clinical Note: Flow Sensor

The infant flow sensor should be cleaned every 24 hours to maintain accurate tidal volume measurements and flow-triggering capabilities. The sensor can be sterilized in a cold solution or gas sterilized. Steam autoclave or pasteurization cannot be used because the high temperatures will damage the flow element.

BOX 14.9   Use of a Capnograph With an Inline Sensor

When performing capnographic monitoring, place the end-tidal CO_2 sensor between the infant sensor and the patient circuit Y-sensor to provide optimal flow-triggering capabilities. There are special connectors available to facilitate the additional monitoring. The infant sensor has less than 1 mm of dead space.

volume, because the sensor placement is at the patient s airway. Box 14.9 explains the use of a capnograph with an infant flow sensor.

If a continuous artificial airway leak is present, the "CONT V" function can be used to determine the liter flow of the leak. By pressing and holding the "CONT V" on the touchpad, a real-time flow through the infant sensor is displayed. The clinician can use the baseline leak or the flow displayed between breaths to determine the best trigger sensitivity setting and to prevent autotriggering. Generally, trigger sensitivity is set

0.2 L/min to 0.4 L/min above the baseline leak flow. Measurement of artificial airway leak is possible only with use of the infant sensor.

The pediatric sensor (*B* in Fig. 14.18) is placed just before the expiratory valve with the arrow pointing toward the direction of gas flow. The tidal volume readout includes compressible volume and effective tidal volume. Tidal volume measurements are derived from the measurement of flow. As flow passes through the sensor and past the variable-orifice flow element (*A*), which is located between two chambers, the flow element bends in the direction of flow, creating a small pressure difference between the two chambers. The differential pressure transducer measures the pressure differences between the two chambers, then sends an analog signal that is read by the microprocessor, which compares the signal with a calibration curve and translates the value to a volume.[9,10]

CAREFUSION V.I.P. BIRD STERLING AND GOLD INFANT/PEDIATRIC VENTILATORS

The V.I.P. Sterling and Gold infant/pediatric ventilators are improved models of the original V.I.P. (see Fig. 14.15 and compare with Fig. 14.19). The internal design and most of the controls, alarms, and specifications are identical to the original. Therefore only the changes and new features will be presented here.

The most noteworthy differences are in two areas. First, both ventilators use redesigned flow sensors called the *Infant "Smart" Flow Sensor* and the *Pediatric "Smart" Flow Sensor*. The other major change is the incorporation of the functions

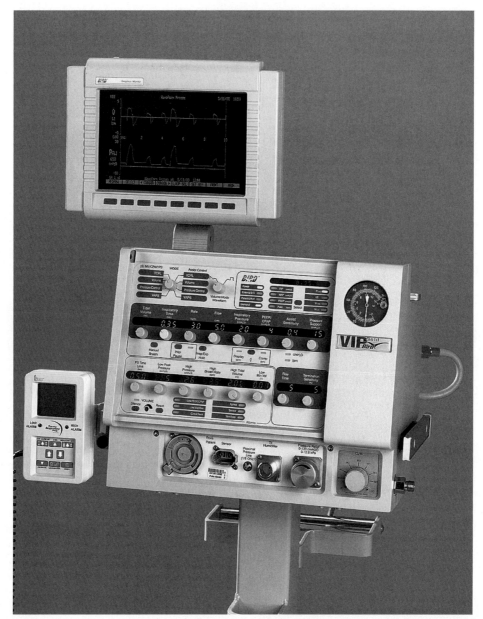

FIGURE 14.19 The V.I.P. Bird Gold infant ventilator. (Courtesy CareFusion, Inc., Yorba Linda, CA.)

of the Partner IIi monitor into the main ventilator housing. Some expanded setting limits and some new features have also been added. Volume-assured pressure support (VAPS), a dual-control mode, is a key addition on the V.I.P. Gold. It is described later in this section.

The heart of the redesigned flow sensors for both the Sterling and the Gold is a stainless steel flap that replaces the former plastic design. A variable-orifice differential pressure transducer, similar to that in the original sensors, is used to measure flow. With the new design the Infant "Smart" Flow Sensor can be used with artificial airway sizes up to 5.5-mm ID. For larger ETTs, the Pediatric "Smart" Flow Sensor is necessary. This sensor is placed at the exhalation valve rather than at the artificial airway.[10]

The ventilator's microprocessor is able to determine which flow sensor is in use. When the Infant "Smart" Flow Sensor

is in use, a bias flow of 3 L/min is present unless the ventilator is operating in the TCPL mode. In the TCPL mode, flow is set by the operator. When the Pediatric "Smart" Flow Sensor is in use, bias flow can be turned on or off by pressing the bias flow control. Bias flow operates at a fixed 5 L/min with the pediatric sensor when turned on.

Changes in Controls/Alarms

Although many of the controls, indicators, and alarms on the Sterling and Gold models are identical to those of the original V.I.P., some additions and changes have been made. The front panel of the V.I.P. Bird Gold is shown in Fig. 14.20. The layout of controls and indicators is very similar to that of the original. As in the original model, push buttons are used to activate functions, visualize certain parameter settings, or turn functions on or off. A single selector switch is used

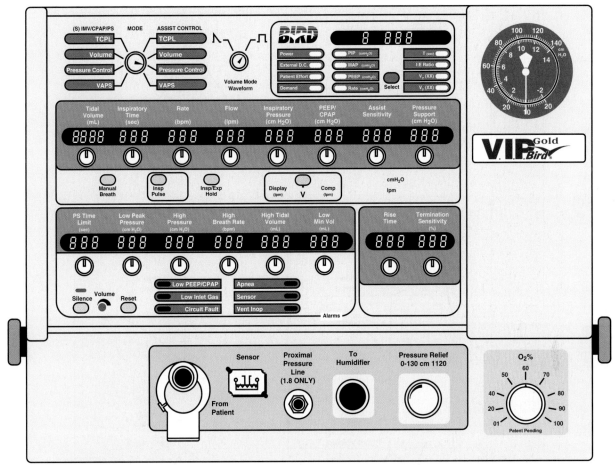

FIGURE 14.20 The operating panel of the V.I.P. Bird Gold infant ventilator. (Courtesy CareFusion, Inc., Yorba Linda, CA.)

to change modes. Dials are used to adjust parameters and alarm limits.

Ventilator Modes and the Mode Select Switch

The mode select switch, located in the upper-left portion of the front control panel, is a multiposition dial. The position of the switch sets either the mode or the breath type. As is the case in the original V.I.P., some controls are deactivated when certain modes are selected. Displays for deactivated controls remain illuminated but dimmed.

The A/C modes for both the Sterling and Gold models are grouped in a mode category column to the right of the control dial. The TCPL mode and the volume-limited mode are the only A/C modes available on the Sterling in this mode category. Two additional A/C modes are available on the Gold model: pressure control and VAPS (described later). The left column of both models lists the (S)IMV/CPAP/PS (pressure support) modes. On the Sterling, only TCPL and volume modes are available in this mode category. CPAP can be provided in either of these modes, and pressure support can be added to nonmandatory breaths. In addition to the two (S)IMV/CPAP/PS modes that are included on the Sterling, the Gold also provides pressure control and VAPS in this mode category. When adding PS to spontaneous breaths, the level can be adjusted with a separate control, allowing separate inspiratory pressures for mandatory and pressure-supported, spontaneous breaths.

The VAPS mode is available only on the V.I.P. Bird Gold model. It is a dual-control mode that guarantees that a pressure-controlled breath, a pressure-supported breath, or a TCPL breath will reach a preset volume. During a VAPS breath, V_T may be augmented by extending the inspiratory phase at the set flow for a segment of time beyond the point that flow would otherwise terminate. An example of how the ventilator augments a breath is represented by waveforms in Fig. 14.21. Breath A is a pressure-supported breath that terminates at a set flow. In this breath the desired V_T is reached within the set inspiratory time. In contrast, Breath B represents a breath in which delivery of the set V_T is not achieved during the allotted inspiratory time. When the ventilator determines that the delivered volume is too low, it allows flow to decelerate to its minimum set-point. However, rather than terminating, the set flow continues over a slightly lengthened inspiratory time, causing the PIP to rise. The breath is therefore augmented to the desired V_T. An augmented breath essentially transitions from a pressure-controlled or TCPL breath to a volume-controlled breath. With VAPS, electronic extension of the inspiratory phase occurs only if the microprocessor determines that the pressure settings alone cannot deliver the preset tidal volume (Clinical Scenario 14.2).

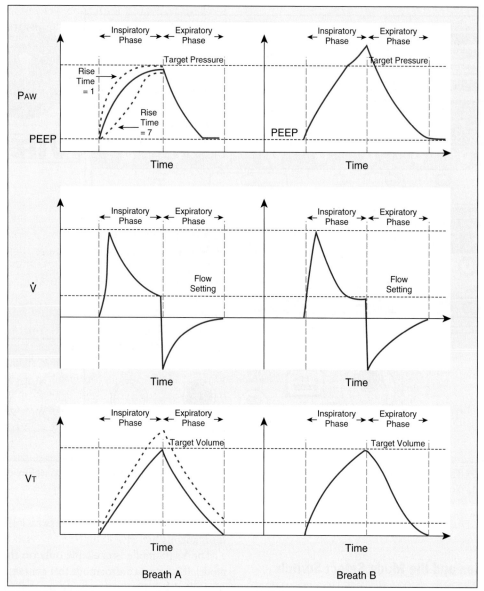

FIGURE 14.21 Volume-assured pressure support (VAPS) breath delivery with V.I.P. Bird Sterling and Gold infant ventilators. Breath A *(left column)* depicts breaths that flow cycle at the set flow after the minimum tidal volume has been delivered. (*Note:* The target pressure is delivered. Flow decelerates to the flow setting. Tidal volume [V_T] has met or exceeded the set V_T. The breath cycles out of inspiration at the set flow.) Breath B *(right column)* shows a transition from a pressure-supported breath to a volume-assured breath. Transition occurs when flow drops to the set peak flow and the set V_T has not been delivered. (*Note:* The target pressure is delivered. Flow decelerates to the flow setting. V_T has not met the set V_T. Flow remains constant at the set peak flow until the set V_T is achieved. Peak pressure continues to rise and T_I increases until V_T is delivered.) *PAW,* Airway pressure; *PEEP,* positive end-expiratory pressure; $\dot{V}$, flow. (Courtesy CareFusion, Inc., Yorba Linda, CA.)

VAPS can be selected from either the (S)IMV/CPAP/PS column or the A/C column of the mode select switch. When selected from the (S)IMV/CPAP/PS column, mandatory pressure-controlled breaths are delivered at a guaranteed volume. The clinician must set V_T, inspiratory pressure, rate, and flow. Nonmandatory breaths in this form of VAPS will be unsupported if no pressure support level is present.

When the clinician sets a PS level and a PS/VAPS time limit, both pressure support breaths and mandatory pressure-controlled breaths will be delivered at a guaranteed volume. The PS level and the PS/VAPS time limit controls must be set by the clinician.

When VAPS is selected from the A/C column, breaths delivered to the patient are either patient-triggered or

PEEP, Positive end-expiratory pressure; *VAPS,* volume-assured pressure support; V_T, tidal volume.

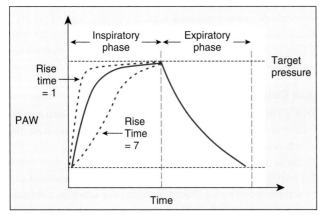

FIGURE 14.22 The rise time control available on the Gold model tapers pressure delivery at the beginning of inspiration. (See text for a description.) *PAW,* Airway pressure. (Courtesy CareFusion, Inc., Yorba Linda, CA.)

mandatory TCPL breaths. In this version of VAPS, the clinician sets inspiratory pressure as well as V_T, flow, PS/VAPS time limit, and rate.

Pressure Support/VAPS Time Limit Control

This control is active only in the PS mode on both the Sterling and Gold, and in the VAPS mode on the Gold. It is automatically activated when these modes are selected. This control sets a time limit for the inspiratory phase in case of a leak or any other condition in which inspiratory flow does not drop to the termination level. Adjustable from 0.1 second to 3.0 seconds, the PS/VAPS Time Limit is displayed in a window above the control.

Rise Time Control

Available on the Gold model only, the rise time control allows the inspiratory pressure rise time to be adjusted. This control is active only in the pressure control, VAPS, and PS modes. The control is adjustable from a setting of 1 to 7. At a setting of 1, the fastest rise time, the set PIP is reached quickly and is held for the duration of the set inspiratory time (Fig. 14.22). At the slowest setting, 7, inspiratory flow is decreased to allow a gradual rise to set PIP. The selected setting is displayed in a

window above the control knob. The inspiratory time and the breath cycle are not affected by this control.

Tidal Volume Control

Tidal volume for both the Sterling and Gold models is set and adjusted in the same way as for the original V.I.P. However, the V_T limit has been increased to 1200 mL. On the Gold model in the VAPS mode, the V_T control setting establishes a target volume. This volume is not necessarily delivered if the set V_T, measured on exhalation, is achieved by the effects of inspiratory pressure settings alone.

Volume Mode Waveform Switch

The two-position volume mode waveform switch is active only when volume-controlled breaths are delivered. The left position sets a decelerating (descending) flow waveform during the inspiratory phase. The right position sets a square (constant) waveform.

Apnea Indicator and Apnea Interval Switch

A period of apnea equal to the set apnea interval will trigger an audible alarm and a flashing visual indicator. The audible alarm can be silenced with the alarm silence button, or it will silence itself once the alarm condition is corrected. The visual indicator will continue to flash until the reset button is pressed.

The apnea interval is set by the operator and is adjustable from 10 seconds to 60 seconds. The current apnea interval can be determined by pressing and holding the select button for 2 seconds. The interval will appear in the monitor display window. The apnea interval is also displayed when the apnea interval switch is pressed. This switch is a push button located on the rear panel of the ventilator. Upon pressing the button one time, the current apnea interval is displayed in the monitor display window for 3 seconds. Each push of the button after the first time will increase the apnea interval by 5-second increments up to a maximum of 60 seconds. After the operator toggles to the 60-second maximum, pressing the button again returns the interval to 10 seconds.

Bias Flow, Assist Sensitivity, and Triggering

The purpose of bias flow within the patient circuit is to provide a reference flow for the sensors to put flow triggering into operation. When the infant sensor is in use, the bias flow is automatically on and delivering 3 L/min. With the infant sensor the bias flow status will not appear in the monitor display window. When the pediatric sensor is used, the bias flow level runs at a preset 5 L/min. However, with the pediatric sensor, the bias flow status can be viewed in the monitor display window by using the select button. Repeatedly pressing the select button enables you to scroll through all monitored parameters. After the final parameter is scanned, the message "BF ON" or "BF OFF" will be displayed. At this point the operator can turn the bias flow on or off by pressing and holding the select button for 2 seconds. When no flow sensor is used, no bias flow is delivered.

Both the V.I.P. Bird Sterling and Gold ventilators provide either flow triggering or pressure triggering in all modes. The assist sensitivity control sets either the flow or pressure necessary to trigger the ventilator into inspiration, depending on the type of triggering that is active. An indicator for each type of triggering illuminates when active. Triggering can be locked out completely by turning the assist sensitivity control to the off position. When using the infant flow sensor, only flow triggering is active and is adjustable from 0.1 L/min to 3.0 L/min through the assist sensitivity control. When the pediatric flow sensor is in use and bias flow is turned on, flow triggering is active and is adjustable from 2.2 L/min to 5.0 L/min. When the bias flow is turned on, pressure triggering is active with the pediatric sensor and is adjustable from 1 cm H_2O to 20 cm H_2O. If no flow sensor is used, both models automatically default to pressure triggering in all modes.

Flow Display/Compensation

The "Flow Display Comp" button on both the Sterling and Gold models replaces the "CONT V" button on the original Partner IIi monitor. This control serves the same function as the CONT V button when the infant flow sensor is in use. When the Flow Display Comp button is pressed, the display indicator to the left will illuminate. Flow values will then be displayed in the ventilator s monitor display window. The operator can then use the select button to toggle between inspiratory and expiratory real-time flows. This function is particularly useful in determining the amount of baseline leak at the artificial airway and adjusting the assist sensitivity to eliminate autotriggering. The clinician can toggle to the inspiratory flow, note the amount of baseline leak, and set the assist sensitivity control at least 0.2 L/min above the detected leak.

With the use of the pediatric flow sensor, the Flow Display Comp button serves another function. With this sensor, pressing the button establishes a zero point for the volume monitor based on the set level of continuous flow. This function is called *flow compensation*. To accurately monitor volumes, flow compensation is activated each time the flow setting is changed. When the Flow Display Comp button with the pediatric sensor connected is pressed, the "Comp" indicator to the right will illuminate for 3 seconds, and the level of flow compensation will appear in the monitor display window. To disable flow compensation, the Flow Display Comp function must be pressed and held for 2 seconds. The Flow Display Comp function is not available when the ventilator is operated without either of the flow sensors.

Inspiratory/Expiratory Hold

An inspiratory/expiratory hold function is available on the V.I.P. Bird Gold model only. When the "Insp/Exp Hold" button is pressed once, an "I/E Hold" prompt will appear in the monitor display window. If the Select button is pressed once while this message is displayed, it will toggle to the "I Hold" message. To attain an inspiratory hold for up to 3 seconds, the Insp/Exp Hold button is pressed and held. When the button is released, the inspiratory plateau pressure appears in the monitor display window.

An expiratory hold can be performed by first pressing the Insp/Exp Hold button to bring up the I/E Hold prompt in the monitor display window. The select button is then pressed twice to display the "E Hold" message. To attain an expiratory hold for up to 3 seconds, the Insp/Exp Hold button is pressed and held. When the button is released, the expiratory plateau pressure appears in the monitor display window.

Inspiratory Pause

An inspiratory pause control is available only on the V.I.P. Bird Gold. This control allows an inspiratory pause time to be set when operating the ventilator in either volume-targeted or VAPS modes. When the "Insp Pause" button is pressed once, the current setting, if any has been selected, is shown in the display monitor window. The window will first show IP followed by the current pause setting. While the pause time is being displayed, the value can be changed by pressing the select button. Each time the select button is pressed, the inspiratory pause time will increase by 0.1 second up to a maximum of 2 seconds. If the clinician holds the button, this action will also allow the pause time to increase. To reset the pause time to 0 (zero), the clinician must press the reset button.

Leak Compensation Control

Leak compensation has been changed on the Sterling and Gold models. This function is no longer available with the infant flow sensor. It can be activated only when using the pediatric sensor with the bias flow turned off or when using the ventilator without a flow sensor. Leak compensation can be activated on the V.I.P. Bird Sterling only when in a volume mode or on the V.I.P. Bird Gold when in a volume mode or in pressure control or VAPS.

Leak compensation can be activated by scrolling through the displayed parameters using the select button until the current leak compensation message appears in the monitor display window. This message will be either "LK ON" or "LK OFF." Pressing and holding the select button will enable you to toggle between the "LK ON" and "LK OFF" settings.

Leak compensation is used when artificial airway leak prevents the ventilator from otherwise maintaining the PEEP level. Small increments of flow are introduced into the circuit to provide back pressure compensation for the leak. When you use leak compensation, you must be aware that the patient's ability to trigger may be diminished. Careful attention to the assist sensitivity setting is necessary. In some cases, removal of the source of the leak is preferable to the use of the leak compensation function (Clinical Scenario 14.3).

Table 14.5 lists the specifications for the V.I.P. Bird Gold and Sterling ventilators.

📌 CLINICAL SCENARIO 14.3

A respiratory therapist is assessing a patient being ventilated with the V.I.P. Bird Gold ventilator. The therapist notices the patient using accessory muscles to inspire. The patient's efforts do not trigger a ventilator breath even though the trigger sensitivity seems to be at an appropriate setting. What is a possible cause of the problem?

See Appendix A for the answer.

TABLE 14.5	Specifications for V.I.P. Bird Gold and Sterling Ventilators		
Controls	**Available Settings and Ranges**	**Controls**	**Available Settings and Ranges**
Mode Select		Apnea switch	10-60 s
Waveform select	Square wave/decelerating flow	Alarm intensity	Minimum 66 dB
Tidal volume	10-1200 mL	O_2 concentration	21-100%
Inspiratory time	0.10-3.0 s		
Breath rate	0-150 breaths/min	**Monitors and Indicators**	**Available Settings and Ranges**
Flow	3-120 L/min—volume modes and VAPS (Gold only)	Peak inspiratory pressure	0-130 cm H_2O
	3-40 L/min—TCPL, inspiratory flow	Airway pressure manometer	–20 to 140 cm H_2O
	3-15 L/min—TCPL, expiratory bias flow	Inspiratory time	0.05-60 s
		Mean airway pressure	0-120 cm H_2O
Inspiratory pressure	3-80 cm H_2O	I:E ratio	1:0.1 to 1:60
PEEP/CPAP	0-24 cm H_2O	Minute volume	0.0-99.9 L (with flow sensor)
Assist sensitivity	Pressure-triggered: 1-29 cm H_2O	PEEP	0-24 cm H_2O
	Flow-triggered—Infant "Smart" Flow Sensor: 0.02-3 L/min	Tidal volume	0-9999 mL (with flow sensor)
	Flow-triggered—Pediatric "Smart" Flow Sensor: 1-5 L/min	Respiratory rate	0-250 breaths/min
Pressure support	1-50 cm H_2O	Alarms	Low peak pressure
Termination sensitivity	5%, 10%, 15%, 20%, and 25% of peak flow		High pressure
			Low PEEP/CPAP
Rise time	1-7 (1, fastest; 7, slowest)		Pressure-support/VAPS time limit
Manual breath	0-2 s		High tidal volume
Inspiratory pause			Low minute volume
Inspiratory/expiratory hold	3 s (maximum)		High breath rate
Flow Display Comp			High/prolonged pressure
Alarm silence			Low inlet gas pressure
Alarm reset			Blender input gas
Monitor display select			Circuit fault
			Apnea
			Sensor
			Ventilator inoperative

CPAP, Continuous positive airway pressure; *I:E ratio,* ratio of inspiratory time to expiratory time; *PEEP,* positive end-expiratory pressure; *TCPL,* time-cycled, pressure-limited; *VAPS,* volume-assured pressure support.

DRÄGER BABYLOG 8000 INFANT VENTILATOR

The Dräger Babylog 8000 plus Infant Ventilator (Drägerwerk AG & Co. KGaA) (Fig. 14.23) is used to mechanically ventilate premature babies and infants. The weight limit use for the ventilator is 20 kg. It is electrically and pneumatically powered, and microprocessor and pneumatically controlled. A proximal flow sensor, which is a hot wire anemometer, is placed at the patient's Y-connector. It allows the Babylog to monitor flow and detect patient effort at the ETT level, thereby providing improved patient–ventilator synchrony[11] (Clinical Scenario 14.4).

Noteworthy Internal Functions

The compressed air and oxygen sources pass through a filter and nonreturn valve before entering the pressure regulators. The two gas sources then enter the solenoid valves and flow adjusters, which blend and control the gas flowing through the inspiratory limb of the patient circuit. In the event of a gas supply or electrical failure, the patient can spontaneously breathe room air through a filter and nonreturn valve.

> ### 📌 CLINICAL SCENARIO 14.4
>
> An infant is being ventilated on the Dräger Babylog 8000 in the synchronized intermittent mandatory ventilation (SIMV) mode with volume guarantee. A proximal flow sensor alarm activates, and the airway pressure increases to 30 cm H_2O, although average pressures for breath delivery have been 19 cm H_2O. The infant appears to be breathing out of synchrony with the ventilator. A nurse silences the alarm and notifies the respiratory therapist. What might have caused the pressure to rise to 30 cm H_2O in this situation?
> See Appendix A for the answer.

Expiratory gas flow from the patient circuit is regulated by a pneumatic exhalation valve. The pneumatic safety valve directs excessive pressure buildup within the ventilator system through the exhalation valve.

Control and Alarm Panel

Fig. 14.24 provides an illustration of the control and alarm panel of the Babylog 8000 plus, which is almost identical to

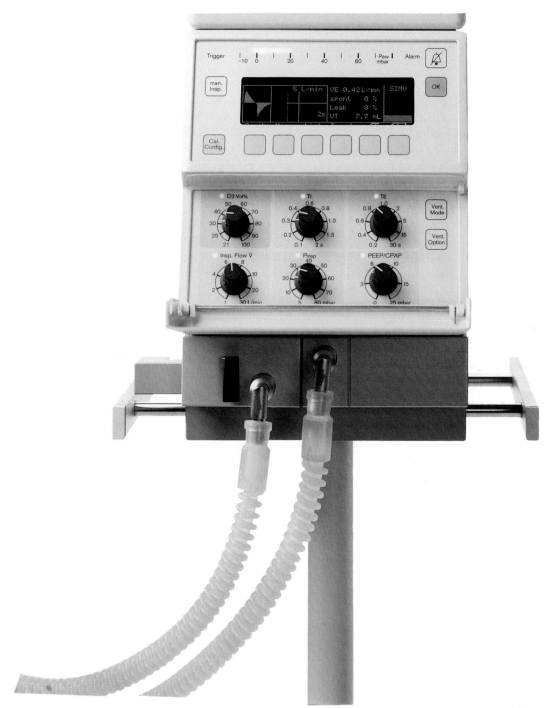

FIGURE 14.23 The Dräger Babylog 8000 plus Infant Ventilator. (Courtesy Drägerwerk AG & Co. KGaA, Lübeck, Germany.)

the 8000 (see following section on the 8000 plus). In the 8000 plus the continuous mandatory ventilation (CMV) soft-key pad of the 8000 is replaced with "Vent. Options." The CPAP pad of the 8000 is replaced with the vent mode.

The panel contains a rotary dial panel and a display/soft-key panel. The dial panel contains buttons for the operating modes (CPAP and intermittent positive-pressure ventilation [IPPV]) and rotary dials for ventilator parameters. Activated modes are indicated by an illuminated LED located within

the button. The button must be depressed until the green LED is continuously illuminated for the mode to be activated. This is a safety feature that is in place to prevent accidental mode changes. Illuminated green LEDs indicate mandatory parameters to be set for that particular mode of ventilation. If a parameter has been internally limited or needs attention, the green LED will flash.

The rotary dial panel contains six dials: "OXYGEN CONCENTRATION %," "INSPIRATORY TIME," "EXPIRATORY

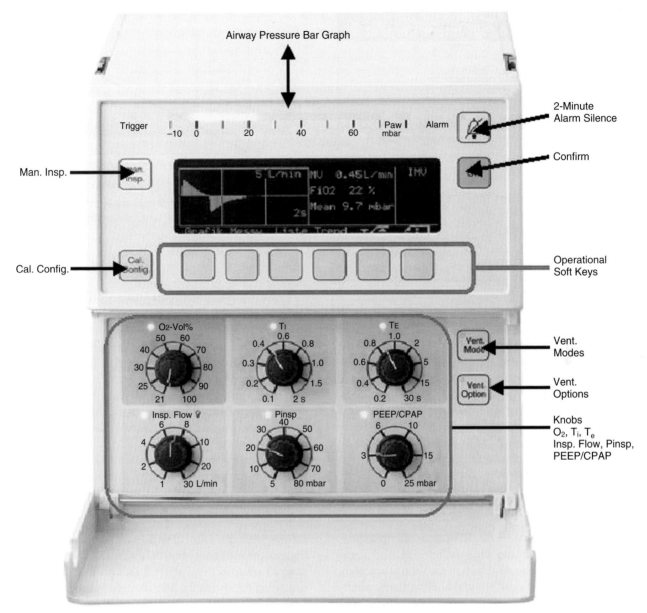

Airway Pressure Bar Graph

Trigger | −10 0 | 20 | 40 | 60 | Paw | Alarm
mbar

2-Minute Alarm Silence

Confirm

Man. Insp.

Cal. Config.

Operational Soft Keys

O2-Vol% | Ti | TE

Vent. Modes

Vent. Options

Insp. Flow | Pinsp | PEEP/CPAP

Knobs
O₂, Tᵢ, Tₑ
Insp. Flow, Pinsp,
PEEP/CPAP

FIGURE 14.24 The control and alarm panel of the Babylog 8000 plus Infant Ventilator. (See text for further information.) (Courtesy Drägerwerk AG & Co. KGaA, Lübeck, Germany.)

TIME," "INSPIRATORY FLOW," "INSPIRATORY PRESSURE LIMIT," and PEEP/CPAP. Table 14.6 provides parameter specifications for the Dräger Babylog 8000 plus Ventilator.

The screen and soft-key panel that are located on the top of the ventilator serve various functions. The waveform display window displays either pressure or flow scalar waveforms over time. The measured values window digitally displays minute ventilation, oxygen concentration, PIP, mean airway pressure ($P_{\overline{aw}}$), and PEEP. The current mode of ventilation and other pertinent information are displayed on the far right in the status window.

The soft keys are used to select ventilation modes and ventilator functions, as well as to access other windows. The menu keys are located on the bottom of the screen. The screen functions are selected from the monitoring and functions menu with their respective submenus. Green LED illuminating lights will indicate whether monitoring or functions has been selected. The manual soft key is located above the monitoring LED and activates a manual breath or an *extension* of an existing breath in progress. The maximum inspiratory time available is 5 seconds. Text messages are displayed as pop-up windows at the top of any current screen.

The alarm silence and reset/check soft keys are located on the top-right panel. The alarm silence button silences the alarm for 2 minutes, whereas the reset/check button allows the clinician to recognize those messages and clear them from the screen. A red alarm light will flash when a warning or caution message is displayed on the screen.

Inspiratory and expiratory pressure sensors calculate the airway pressure, which is then displayed as real-time airway

TABLE 14.6 **Specifications for the Dräger Babylog 8000 Plus Infant Ventilator**	
Inspiratory time	0.1-2.0 s
Expiratory time	0.2-30 s
Inspiratory flow	1-30 L/min
Expiratory flow	1-30 L/min
Peak inspiratory pressure	10-80 cm H_2O
PEEP/CPAP	0-15 cm H_2O
O_2 concentration	21-100%
Rate	2-150 breaths/min
Trigger mechanism	Flow/volume trigger
Alarms	Loss of PEEP/CPAP, high pressure, high minute ventilation, low minute ventilation, minute ventilation delay, and apnea

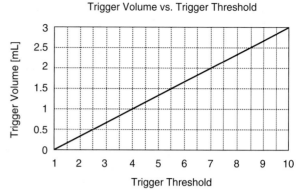

FIGURE 14.25 The trigger sensitivity setting on the Babylog 8000 Infant Ventilator. (See text for further information.)

pressure measurements on an illuminating bar graph located on the top of the monitor. The yellow LED is illuminated when inspiration is triggered.

The oxygen concentration alarm limits are set internally at ±4%. The alarm limits for PEEP and P_{insp} are also set internally by the microprocessor. The loss of PEEP/CPAP limit is −4 cm H_2O, with a minimum of −2 cm H_2O. The high-pressure alarm is automatically set to P_{insp} +10 cm H_2O or PEEP/CPAP +4 cm H_2O. In the event of excessive pressure buildup within the circuit, the exhalation valve opens, allowing exhalation. Adjustable alarm limits include high minute ventilation, low minute ventilation, minute ventilation delay (0 to 30 seconds), and apnea (5 to 20 seconds).

The ventilator alarms are arranged in order of importance. The alarms are grouped into advisory, warning, and alarm messages that are digitally displayed on the ventilator screen, eliminating the guesswork of troubleshooting alarm conditions. Incidents such as obstructed ETT, kinked circuit, and apnea are clearly identified on the ventilator screen. Each alarm level has a distinctive audible tone that indicates its level of importance. Every message is recorded in the message log, which is capable of storing the 100 most recent entries. The log records the time of occurrence, displayed text, and information on the response.

Modes of Ventilation

The mandatory breaths in A/C and SIMV are time triggered or patient triggered, pressure targeted, and time cycled. The operator sets the following parameters: inspiratory time, expiratory time, inspiratory flow, inspiratory pressure, PEEP, and trigger sensitivity. Mandatory breaths are volume triggered when a patient's spontaneous inspiratory volume is equal to or greater than the set trigger volume (set value of 2 or greater); otherwise the mandatory breath is time triggered.

Continuous flow supports spontaneous respiratory efforts between the mandatory breaths in the CPAP mode. The amount of continuous flow available is determined by either the inspiratory flow control or the VIVE (variable inspiratory, variable expiratory) flow option.

The VIVE operating mode allows the clinician to adjust the flow during the expiratory phase to match the patient's needs during mandatory and spontaneous breaths. The inspiratory flow rate is displayed on the left bar graph, and adjustments can be made with the rotary dial. The expiratory flow rate is displayed on the right bar graph and can be adjusted with the up and down menu buttons.

Trigger sensitivity is set by accessing the main menu function and selecting the trigger button. The trigger sensitivity range is 1 to 10, with 1 (minimum) representing increased trigger sensitivity and 10 (maximum) representing the least-sensitive trigger. The trigger threshold of 1 to 10 corresponds with a volume of 0 mL to 3 mL. The recommended setting is minimum; a yellow trigger LED is illuminated with each triggered breath. A setting of 1 indicates that when the Babylog measures a flow change of 0.25 L/min (straight flow-trigger), the mandatory breath is then synchronized with the patient's effort. Settings above 1 indicate that the Babylog is evaluating the system for flow changes, but it is waiting until a particular volume moves across the flow sensor, and then it will synchronize the breath with the patient's negative effort (Fig. 14.25).

The IMV breath is time triggered, pressure targeted, pressure limited or flow limited, and time cycled or pressure cycled. The operator sets the following parameters: oxygen concentration, inspiratory time, expiratory time, inspiratory flow, inspiratory pressure, and PEEP. The mandatory rate is calculated by adding the inspiratory time and expiratory time that are set and dividing the sum into 60 seconds. The mandatory breath is time triggered based on the rate calculation.

Nasal CPAP can be used, but the flow measurement has to be disabled by disconnecting the connector from the proximal flow sensor and pressing the reset/check button. The operator sets the following parameters: oxygen concentration, inspiratory flow, and PEEP.

Graphics Displays

Real-time pressure and flow scalar waveforms are displayed on the monitoring screen. The waveforms are accessed through the monitoring main menu; one must select the graph submenu then press either the "P–aw" or flow button. The waveform scale is automatically set by the ventilator. The displayed flow scalar waveform indicates the inspiratory flow pattern above the baseline and expiratory flow below. Freeze and trend options are also available if desired. The trend feature stores a 24-hour window.

Special Features

The ventilator performs an automatic calibration of the oxygen analyzer every 24 hours. Calibration can also be done manually under the function menu and the "cal sub-menu" (calibration submenu). The calibration takes approximately 5 minutes to complete. The flow sensor calibration is accessed through the function menu and calibration submenu. To calibrate the flow sensor, the operator simply follows the instructions given on the screen. The monitoring of minute ventilation and apnea is made possible only with a calibrated flow sensor. It is recommended that calibration of the flow sensor be performed every time the ventilator is turned on, after sensor assembly, and after sensor replacement.

DRÄGER BABYLOG 8000 PLUS INFANT VENTILATOR

The Dräger Babylog 8000 has had several upgrades. Software version 4 is the original. The next two upgrades were versions 5 and 6. The company then added "plus" to the unit's name, a term that is probably best defined as indicative of (1) extra monitoring, (2) pressure support, and (3) the addition of a volume guarantee. (*Note:* Some individuals do not consider pressure support to be part of the "plus" package.)

The Dräger Babylog 8000 plus is an updated version of the original 8000 model. In this newer model, additional monitoring parameters have been added. A pressure support ventilation mode and volume guarantee are available as options. A high-frequency feature capable of rates from 5 Hz to 20 Hz is another option with this model, but this feature is not available in the United States.

Additional monitoring includes measurement of lung mechanics. These parameters are accessible from the monitoring menu and include airway resistance, dynamic compliance, time constant, C20/C, and *r*, which is the correlation coefficient of linear regression. A low tidal volume alarm is also available.

The pressure support ventilation mode is provided as a spontaneous-only mode. It cannot be combined with other modes or used with mandatory breaths. However, if apnea is detected, the ventilator will begin delivering mandatory breaths according to the set pressure and inspiratory and expiratory times. Pressure support breaths are flow triggered and either flow cycled or time cycled. When inspiratory flow drops to a fixed 15% of peak flow, inspiration terminates. Flow termination is not adjustable. Time cycling will occur if the set T_I is reached.

Volume guarantee is a dual-mode feature that can be used in all patient-triggered modes. As its name implies, a tidal volume can be set by the clinician. However, the ventilator will continue to provide characteristic waveforms of pressure-targeted ventilation. In other words, volume guarantee is pressure-limited ventilation with a volume target. The clinician continues to have control over the delivered peak pressure, but he or she also can select a V_T target. The volume guarantee feature can be used only when the airway flow sensor is in use.

When volume guarantee is activated, the ventilator software continuously measures and compares inspired and expired tidal volume. Each following breath uses the comparisons from the previous breath to make adjustments to the PIP so that a V_T as close as possible to the preset value can be delivered. The lowest inspiratory pressure that can result in delivery of the target V_T is then administered.

When activating the volume guarantee, the clinician sets the maximum PIP. This setting becomes an inspiratory pressure limit. Over the next six to eight breaths, the ventilator determines the appropriate inspiratory pressure and begins to achieve and maintain the target V_T. If the patient's inspiratory effort adds to the V_T, the ventilator PIP will immediately decrease. If the total inspiratory V_T exceeds the set target volume by 130%, the expiratory valve will open and no additional ventilator-driven gas will be delivered to the patient.

The clinician needs to exercise care when using the volume guarantee and closely monitor patient–ventilator interaction. Because the patient is breathing spontaneously, an increase in metabolic demand or change in pulmonary compliance can dramatically affect the patient's ventilatory pattern. An appropriate target tidal volume must be selected based on the patient's weight. A clinically safe PIP must be set as must an appropriate value for the low V_T alarm. Frequent patient assessment and careful monitoring are essential. The volume guarantee is potentially hazardous in the face of significant continuous or positional ETT leak. Its use is discouraged under these conditions.

HIGH-FREQUENCY VENTILATORS

High-frequency ventilation (HFV) is an alternative method of ventilation in infants, children, and adults. The two HFV instruments currently used are high-frequency jet ventilation (HFJV) and high-frequency oscillation (HFO) devices. These have been used most frequently in infants, but one oscillator, the CareFusion Model 3100B, is available for use in the adult population. These high-frequency devices will be reviewed. The theory behind how HFV achieves gas exchange is described elsewhere.[2]

BUNNELL LIFE PULSE HIGH FREQUENCY VENTILATOR

The Bunnell Life Pulse High Frequency Ventilator (Bunnell Incorporated,) is indicated for patients with severe respiratory distress syndrome complicated by pulmonary air leak that has been untreatable with conventional mechanical ventilation strategies (Fig. 14.26). The Bunnell HFJV system is a

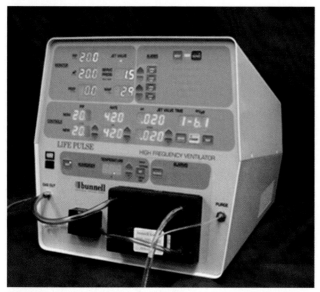

FIGURE 14.26 The Bunnell Life Pulse High Frequency Ventilator. (Courtesy Bunnell Incorporated, Salt Lake City, UT.)

microprocessor-controlled, pressure-limited, time-cycled, constant-flow, high-frequency jet ventilator that works in conjunction with a conventional ventilator. The conventional ventilator provides background conventional ventilation (if desired), supplies entrained gas, and regulates the PEEP level.[12]

Control and Alarm Panel

The on/off switch is located midway on the front left panel. If you press the button once, this powers the ventilator on (displays green light); pressing the button again turns the ventilator off (no light). Fig. 14.27 provides a diagram of the seven components of the ventilator.

Monitoring Display

The ventilator monitoring displays provide pertinent information on the patient and on ventilator performance and are located on the front top-left panel of the control panel. These displays are PIP, ΔP (PIP-PEEP), PEEP, servo pressure, and $P_{\overline{aw}}$. The four patient pressures are sensed at the distal end of the Hi-Lo jet tube (if used) and measured by the transducer in the patient box. The displays are averages calculated over a short period and are not reflective of alveolar pressures. Mean airway pressure can be increased by increasing PIP, increasing PEEP, and increasing the rate and tidal volume of the sigh breaths. The PEEP level is controlled by the conventional ventilator even though it is displayed on the Bunnell's control panel.

The servo pressure measurement (0 to 20 psig) is the amount of internal pressure required to generate the PIP displayed in the NOW (current requirement) display and is a clinical indicator of improved lung status or acute changes (e.g., tension pneumothorax, ETT leak, atelectasis). For example, a decrease in lung compliance may result in a decrease in servo pressure, because less gas is required to meet the set PIP. Increases in lung compliance or the development of a

pneumothorax may result in elevated servo pressures (Clinical Scenario 14.5).

The pinch valve on/off lights located on the front top-left panel (monitor panel, Fig. 14.27) indicate the communication between the ventilator and pinch valve (located on patient box, see Fig. 14.27). The illuminated on light indicates the valve is signaled to open for inspiration. The illuminated off light indicates the valve is signaled to close for expiration. The light will alternate rapidly between the on and off displays.

Alarm Display

The ventilator alarm displays are located on the front top-right panel and consist of the following: a servo pressure button (+1 cm H_2O present value), a mean airway pressure ($P_{\overline{aw}}$) button (+1.5 cm H_2O), a high PIP button (i.e., >5 cm H_2O PIP for 2 seconds or >10 cm H_2O for 30 seconds), and loss of PIP button (i.e., < 25% PIP). The $P_{\overline{aw}}$ and servo pressure upper and lower limits can be adjusted manually.

The high PIP, jet valve fault, ventilator fault, low gas pressure, cannot meet PIP, and loss of PIP alarms are backlit displays. The jet valve fault alarm alerts the clinician that the pinch valve in the patient box is not functioning appropriately. The microprocessor is continuously monitoring the pinch valve and activates the alarm when malfunctions are detected. The Life Pulse continues to operate even if the pinch valve is not cycling. The ventilator fault alarm alerts the clinician that a problem is present within the Life Pulse's electronics or valves. A numeric code will be displayed in the jet valve on/off time window to indicate the type of failure.

The low gas pressure alarm alerts the clinician that the gas supply is less than 30 psig. The "cannot meet PIP" alarm warns the clinician that the ventilator is unable to deliver the pressures within a set range although the servo pressure has increased to the maximum level available. The alarm can be a result of a leak in the humidifier cartridge/patient circuit; incomplete connection of the circuit to the jet tube; a defective or damaged jet tube (e.g., a kinked tube, improper positioning, occlusion, or leak); the present settings being insufficient to ventilate larger patient; a patient fighting the Life Pulse; or the pinch valve opening action is not effective, resulting in higher servo pressures being necessary to meet current settings.

The reset, ready light, and alarm silence (60 seconds) buttons are located above the ventilator alarm displays. The reset button has the machine recalculate automatic upper and lower limits for the servo pressure, PIP, and $P_{\overline{aw}}$ parameters. It is recommended for use when changes are made on the

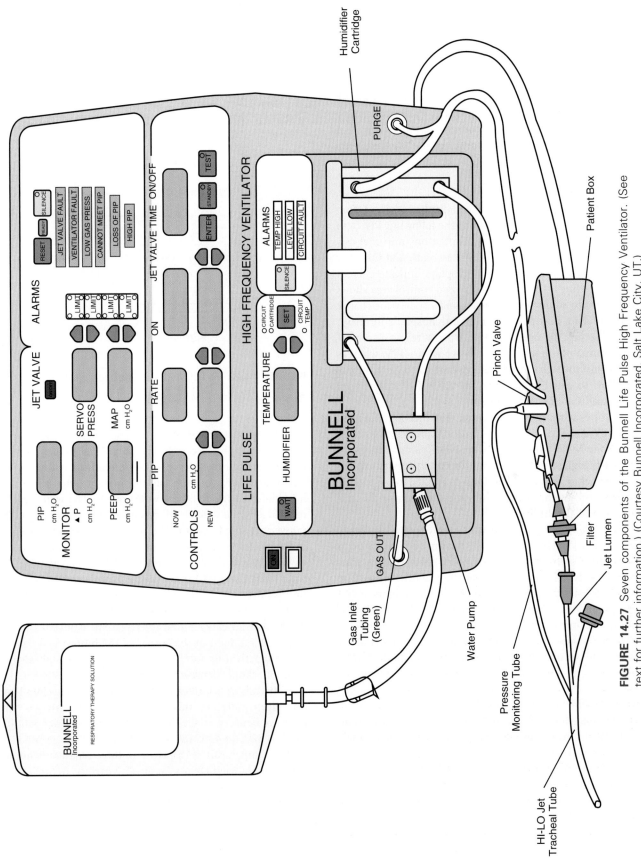

FIGURE 14.27 Seven components of the Bunnell Life Pulse High Frequency Ventilator. (See text for further information.) (Courtesy Bunnell Incorporated, Salt Lake City, UT.)

conventional side of ventilation and manual adjustments are not made. When the reset button is pressed, the ready light turns off and alarm indicators are inactive. The Life Pulse calculates new alarm limits; after this is accomplished, the ready light will illuminate and all alarms are reactivated. The ready light indicates that the machine is ready for operation and has stabilized after start-up or reset, calculated alarm limits, and is ready for operation. The silence button will silence audible alarms for 60 seconds. The alarm will resume after this period of time if the condition has not resolved. A red light will illuminate in the corner of the silence button when the silence function is in effect.

Control Parameters

The ventilator control parameters and displays are located on the front middle panel and consist of the following: PIP (8 to 50 cm H_2O), RATE (240 to 660 insufflations/min), jet ON time (inspiratory time; 0.02 to 0.034 second), and ON/OFF ratio (1:1.2 to 1:12). The NOW displays indicate current operating settings. The NEW display and control area allows the operator to adjust set parameters and visualize the change before entering new parameters. Some hospitals interrupt HFJV by setting the sigh breath peak pressure (on a conventional ventilator) higher than it is set with HFJV, whereas others adjust the sigh breath peak pressure (on a conventional ventilator) to equal or less than the HFJV PIP setting (i.e., HFJV breaths are not interrupted).

The operating mode selection buttons are ENTER, STANDBY, and TEST. If the enter button is pressed, this action changes the NOW parameters to the NEW parameters. Inappropriately high servo pressure may occur if the enter button is pressed before the patient circuit is connected to the patient, possibly resulting in high pressures and the delivery of excessively high tidal volumes.

The standby mode is used when the operator wants to interrupt HFJV temporarily (i.e., during suctioning or to monitor the effectiveness of conventional ventilation). Alarms are inactive while the system is in the standby mode. The functioning standby mode is indicated by red lights, and a 5-second audible alarm and is automatically set up with ventilator power-up.

The test mode is an automatic test that checks the ventilator systems and circuitry for proper function and should ***not*** be performed with a patient connected to the jet ventilator.

Humidification

The disposable humidifier cartridge/patient breathing circuit is a closed system that provides humidity, heating, and monitoring of the gas exiting the ventilator (Fig. 14.28). The humidifier cartridge heats and humidifies the gas before patient delivery. The cartridge receptacle holds the humidifier cartridge in place by securing the latch in place. The water in the cartridge is warmed by the anodized aluminum heater plate.

The "gas-out" and "purge pneumatic" connectors located on the front panel are of different sizes to prevent improper connections. The short, green gas-inlet tube connects the gas flow from the ventilator to the cartridge. The clear water-inlet

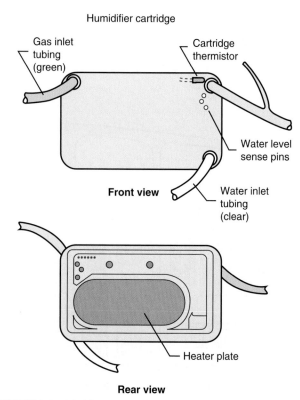

FIGURE 14.28 The humidifier cartridge/patient breathing circuit of the Bunnell Life Pulse High Frequency Ventilator.

tube transfers water from the pump when the water-level sensors detect a decrease in the water level, thus filling the humidifier cartridge. Water is transferred from a nonpressurized source (i.e., solution bag or bottle) to the pressurized humidifier cartridge by the water pump. The water level is regulated by the water-level sensor pins in the cartridge. The purge port supplies gas to the purge valve, which is located in the patient box. The gas is used to provide a moisture-free environment in the monitoring line of the Hi-Lo jet tube. The small, clear, second lumen of the patient circuit connects to this port.

The "humidifier wait" button turns off the heater and water pump, allowing easy removal and replacement of the cartridge/circuit. A red light in the corner of the button will flash to indicate activation of the wait feature. To resume normal function, simply depress the button again.

A thermistor is located at the patient breathing circuit and cartridge connection; this device ensures adequate gas temperature delivery to the patient. The available temperature range is 32°C to 42°C (89.6°F to 107.6°F).

The temperature is displayed in three separate windows, which are labeled *circuit (desired)*, *cartridge (desired)*, and *circuit temperature (actual temperature)*. The set button allows the clinician to select the temperature setting/measurement to be displayed. The window display will automatically return to the circuit temperature display reading. The humidifier system has a separate "silence" button (separate from the ventilator's alarm silence button) and various backlit alarm messages. The messages warn the clinician of any

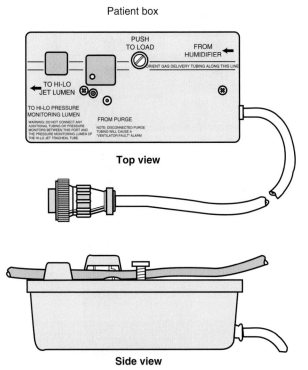

FIGURE 14.29 The patient box on the Bunnell Life Pulse High Frequency Ventilator.

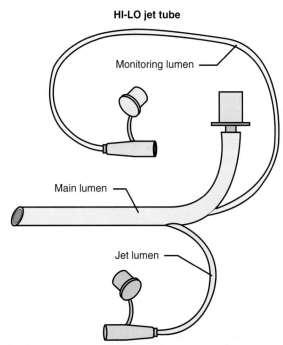

FIGURE 14.30 Triple-lumen Hi-Lo jet tracheal tubes for use in high-frequency jet ventilation. (Courtesy Medtronic Minimally Invasive Therapies, Yorba Linda, CA.)

temperature/water level changes and electrical problems within the cartridge/circuit.

Patient Box and Pinch Valve

The patient box is a satellite component that contains the pinch valve, purge valve, and pressure transducer (Fig. 14.29). It is designed for placement near the patient's head to ensure accurate pressure monitoring and delivery of jet bursts.

The patient box electrical cable connects to the rear panel of the ventilator. An electromagnetic solenoid activates the pinch valve. The pinch valve breaks the flow of pressurized gas into small bursts with the pinch-and-release action on the silicone tube of the patient breathing circuit. The "push to load" button opens the valve to allow for correct placement of the silicone tube within the patient box and to facilitate repositioning of the silicone tube. The silicone tube should be moved 2 mm every 8 hours to prevent areas of wear and to prevent tearing.

A bacterial filter is present downstream from the pinch valve to provide particle filtration. A millimeter measuring guide is printed on the patient box for visual use. The purge valve maintains a moisture-free, pressure-monitoring line of the ETT by allowing pressurized gas from the ventilator to pass through the line. A 10-millisecond burst of gas is introduced through the monitoring line. The pressure transducer measures tracheal pressure and sends the information to the microprocessor.

Rear Panel

The rear panel contains the mixed-gas input connection, oxygen sensor connection, hour meter, circuit breaker, alarm volume control, patient box connector, analog output, and dump valve outlet. The gas-input fitting connects the ventilator to an oxygen blender to provide varied oxygen concentrations. A 30-psig to 100-psig supply source is required. The oxygen sensor connection allows continuous monitoring of fractional inspired oxygen (F_IO_2). The dump valve is a safety valve that releases internal pressure.

Special Features

Two special-function devices worth noting are the Hi-Lo jet ETT and the LifePort Endotracheal Tube Adapter.

Hi-Lo Jet Endotracheal Tube

The triple-lumen Hi-Lo jet tracheal tubes (Fig. 14.30) are uncuffed and range in size from 2.5-mm to 6.0-mm ID in 0.5-mm increments. The external diameter is approximately equal to the external diameter of a standard ETT that is a half-size larger. For example, a 3.0-mm ID Hi-Lo jet tube has an external diameter that is approximately equal to a 3.5-mm ID standard ETT.[13]

The three lumens of the Hi-Lo jet tube serve various functions. The main lumen contains a 15-mm connector that provides the connection point for the conventional ventilator circuit Y-connector. The jet lumen provides the connection to the patient breathing circuit from the patient box. The jet bursts are delivered through this lumen. The monitoring lumen is used to monitor pressures at the distal end of the Hi-Lo jet tube. This lumen is connected to the "To Hi-Lo Pressure Monitoring Lumen" connection on the patient box.

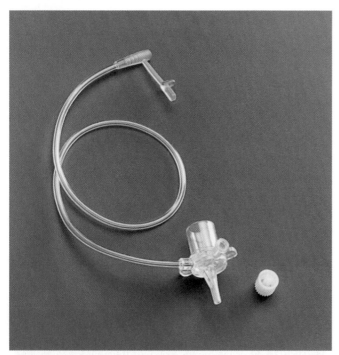

FIGURE 14.31 Bunnell LifePort Endotracheal Tube Adapter for use in high-frequency jet ventilation. (Courtesy Bunnell Incorporated, Salt Lake City, UT.)

LifePort Endotracheal Tube Adapter

The development of the LifePort Endotracheal Tube Adapter (Fig. 14.31) has nullified the requirement of intubating/reintubating patients with the specialized jet tube before the initiation of HFJV. With the use of the double-port ETT adapter and a conventional single-lumen ETT, HFJV can be implemented easily and quickly. The adapters are available with ID sizes of 2.5 mm, 3.5 mm, and 4.5 mm. To initiate HFJV, the operator simply replaces the 15-mm standard ETT adapter with the 15-mm connection of the jet tube adapter. The jet port facilitates the entry of gas from the jet ventilator. The inspired gas is redirected through a nozzle, which increases the gas's velocity. The momentum of the gas is converted to pressure as the gas exits from the nozzle.

Bunnell Incorporated suggests that, when using the 2.5-mm ID LifePort adapter, the HFJV PIP must be adjusted to equal that of the conventional PIP. When the larger adapters are used, the clinician should set up the initial HFJV PIP at 90% of the conventional PIP.

CAREFUSION 3100A HIGH FREQUENCY OSCILLATORY VENTILATOR

The BD CareFusion (formerly SensorMedics[a]) model 3100 high-frequency oscillator was the first of two high-frequency oscillators for use with neonates, originally introduced by

---

[a]SensorMedics Corporation was purchased by Viasys Healthcare. Then, in June 2008, Viasys Healthcare was subsequently purchased by CareFusion, which is now part of Becton, Dickinson and Company.

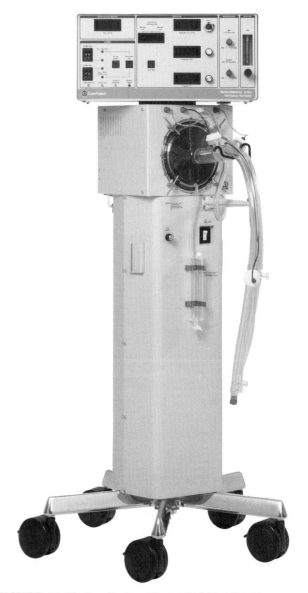

FIGURE 14.32 CareFusion Model 3100A High-Frequency Oscillatory Ventilator by CareFusion. (Courtesy CareFusion, Inc., McGaw Park, IL.)

the SensorMedics Corporation of Yorba Linda, California. An improved model, the 3100A (Fig. 14.32), replaced the 3100. Both of these models have been used extensively in the treatment of acute respiratory failure in infants. The 3100A has also been used in older pediatric patients and adult patients.

Noteworthy Internal Functions

The heart of the CareFusion models is the oscillator subsystem, or the piston assembly (Fig. 14.33). The system incorporates an electronic control circuit, or square-wave driver, which powers a linear-drive motor. The motor consists of an electrical coil within a magnet, which is similar to the configuration of a permanent magnet speaker. When positive polarity is applied to the square-wave driver, the coil is driven

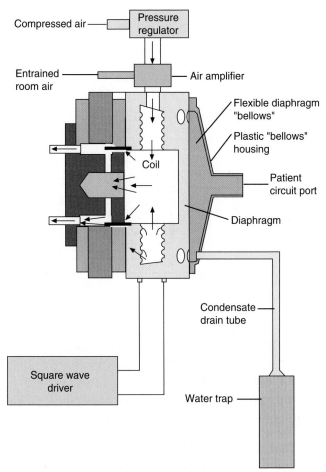

FIGURE 14.33 The piston assembly of the CareFusion Model 3100A High-Frequency Oscillatory Ventilator. (Courtesy Becton, Dickinson, and Company [CareFusion], Franklin Lakes, NJ.)

forward. The coil is attached to a rubber bellows, or diaphragm, to create a piston. When the coil moves forward, the piston moves toward the patient airway, creating the inspiratory phase. When the polarity changes to negative, the electrical coil and the attached piston are driven away from the patient, creating an active expiration.[13]

The amount of polarity voltage applied to the electrical coil determines the distance that the piston will be driven toward or away from the patient airway. Therefore, increasing the polarity voltage increases piston movement, or amplitude. Piston excursion is limited, however, by resistance from the pressure within the patient circuit. The oscillator subsystem also limits the piston stroke to 365 mL. The total time for a piston stroke is a few milliseconds.

When oscillations are at low frequencies, the piston has sufficient time to travel the available excursion length during either the inspiratory or expiratory phase and remain at maximum position until it begins its movement in the opposite direction. Conversely, as oscillating frequency is increased, the excursion time of the piston becomes a larger percentage of the breath phase. The percentage of time the piston remains completely forward or backward decreases. At very high frequencies, the polarity to the coil changes so rapidly that the piston does not have time for a complete excursion and arrival to its maximum position. In fact, it may travel only a fraction of its potential distance before changing direction. Therefore volume delivered by the piston is decreased as oscillatory frequency is increased.

Although the piston subsystem is designed to produce as little friction as possible, the rapid movement of the piston generates some heat. Therefore a Venturi-type air amplifier is used on the 3100A to introduce cooling air around the electrical coil. A separate compressed air source of at least 30 psig serves this system, which consists of a regulator and Venturi. The regulator reduces airflow to 15 L/min, and the Venturi entrains 45 L/min of room air. This provides 60 L/min of cooling air for the subsystem.

Circuit Design

Fig. 14.34 shows the basic circuit of the 3100A. After exiting the back panel of the ventilator and passing through a humidifier, blended gas enters the patient circuit at the bias flow inlet. Flow is set by using the bias flow control on the front panel. The gas mixture fills the space in front of the piston, then flows past the limit valve and on toward the ETT connection. Gas then passes the dump valve and exits through either the control valve or a small restricted orifice next to the control valve housing. The oscillating piston moves the circuit gas in a forward and backward direction toward the airway. The rate of bias flow, the pressure maintained at the airway, and the speed and excursion of the piston are all set by the clinician.

Any standard humidifier can be used with the 3100 and 3100A. Circuits are designed to accommodate heater sensors to provide servo-controlled temperature at the airway. Hot wire circuits are available to reduce water condensation. All circuits incorporate a water outlet, tubing, and water trap that permit water condensate to drain away from the piston.

Controls
On/Off Switch

The ventilator's on/off switch is located on the front of the unit below the piston and to the right (see Fig. 14.32). If power to the unit is turned off or electrical power is interrupted while the ventilator is in operation, an audible alarm will sound and the red "power failure" LED on the front control panel will be illuminated. This alarm can be silenced only by depressing the reset button on the front panel. With any interruption in ventilator operation, pressurization of the circuit's three mushroom valves stops immediately, allowing the circuit to vent to the atmosphere. This venting allows the patient to breathe room air. The proximity of the vented dump valve close to the airway enables the spontaneously breathing patient to breathe room air with minimal resistance from the ventilator circuit.

Piston Centering

The forward and backward excursions of the piston are limited by two mechanical stops. If time and amplitude allow the piston to encounter one of the stops, it will remain stationary for the duration of the inspiratory or expiratory time and

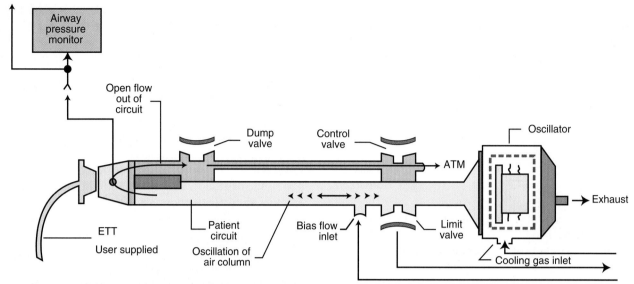

FIGURE 14.34 The basic breathing circuit of the CareFusion Model 3100A High-Frequency Oscillatory Ventilator. *ATM,* Atmospheric pressure; *ETT,* endotracheal tube. (Courtesy Becton, Dickinson, and Company, Franklin Lakes, NJ.)

then change direction. An infrared sensor is used to track the movement of the piston between the mechanical stops. Piston movement is displayed by a bar graph on the control panel. The left end of the bar graph is labeled *MIN INSP LIMIT* and the right, *MAX INSP LIMIT*. The dot represents the piston's center position.

The piston centering control knob adjusts an electrical counterforce to the piston. This counterforce acts in opposition to the $P_{\overline{aw}}$ on the front side of the piston. The result of this opposing counterforce is a centering effect on the piston. At a constant $P_{\overline{aw}}$, as the piston centering control knob is turned clockwise, the piston will move toward the "MAX INSP LIMIT," one of the mechanical stops. The oscillator should not be operated so that the piston is driven against a mechanical stop for an extended period of time. The piston needs to be maintained in the center of the bar graph to maintain piston efficiency and to maximize the life of the oscillator mechanism.

Adjusting other controls, such as the mean pressure adjust control or the power control, will change the piston position. The clinician should regularly check and adjust piston centering after making changes in other settings.

Bias Flow

The bias flow control sets the rate of continuous flow through the patient circuit. Adjusting this control counterclockwise increases flow to an internal limit of 40 L/min. Gas flow is indicated by a ball float that is located within a glass tube. The tube is graduated in 5-L/min increments.

F_IO_2

A standard air/oxygen blender is used to provide blended gas to the ventilator. A minimum pressure of 30 psig is required. The gas mixture should be adjusted to the desired F_IO_2 before it enters the ventilator.

Mean Pressure Adjust

The mean pressure adjust control knob adjusts the $P_{\overline{aw}}$. This control varies the resistance placed on the control valve, the mushroom valve in the patient circuit at the end of the expiratory limb. $P_{\overline{aw}}$ is digitally displayed in the mean pressure monitor window. Although the mean pressure adjust control is the primary determinant of $P_{\overline{aw}}$, other controls will also affect it. For example, increasing bias flow will increase $P_{\overline{aw}}$. Changes to the power, frequency, inspiratory time, and piston centering controls will also change the $P_{\overline{aw}}$. Therefore, if a change in $P_{\overline{aw}}$ occurs because another control has been adjusted, the mean pressure adjust control knob should be used to return the $P_{\overline{aw}}$ to the desired level.

Mean Pressure Limit

The mean pressure limit control knob is normally used to set a limit above which the $P_{\overline{aw}}$ cannot be exceeded. Adjustable to a maximum of 45 cm H_2O, this control can be used to protect the patient from an inadvertent rise in $P_{\overline{aw}}$. This control sets a pressure in the limit valve, a mushroom valve located close to the bias flow inlet of the patient circuit. If the pressure within the circuit were to exceed this pressure, the limit valve would open to permit excess pressure to be vented to the atmosphere.

An alternative use of the mean pressure limit control is to set it above the $P_{\overline{aw}}$ that would otherwise exist when the clinician uses only the mean pressure adjust control. Using the control in this way assures the clinician that $P_{\overline{aw}}$ will not exceed that prescribed, regardless of changes made in bias flow, percentage of inspiratory time, or frequency. However, the clinician should be aware that changes made to controls that result in an uncentered piston can still change $P_{\overline{aw}}$, regardless of where the mean pressure limit control is set. Increasing the power, or amplitude, also can increase $P_{\overline{aw}}$.

Power/ΔP

The power control determines the amount of polarity voltage applied to the oscillator's subsystem electrical coil. Adjusting this control clockwise increases the forward and backward displacement of the piston, thereby increasing oscillatory pressure (ΔP), which is also called *amplitude,* and delivered volume. Pressure is adjustable from approximately 7 cm H_2O to 90 cm H_2O.

The extent to which the ΔP increases depends on the resistance to forward movement the piston encounters. For example, when the oscillator is used with a patient with extremely low pulmonary or chest wall compliance, the piston will meet a high resistance in the inspiratory phase. Increasing the power setting will increase ΔP, but not in the same proportion as the amount of resistance the piston encounters from the $P_{\overline{aw}}$. Therefore, if a low level of $P_{\overline{aw}}$ is present, ΔP adjustments for the same change in power will be greater than if a high level of $P_{\overline{aw}}$ is present.

Percentage of Inspiratory Time

The fraction of time that the piston is in the inspiratory position is determined by the "% Inspiratory Time" control. For example, if the control is set at 33%, the piston will spend 33% of the breath cycle in the inspiratory position and the remaining 67% in the expiratory position. The control is adjustable from 30% to 50%. The setting is digitally displayed in the window to the left of the control knob.

Changing the inspiratory time affects the symmetry of the oscillator waveform. If, for example, the clinician decreases the % inspiratory time control from 50% to 33%, the amount of time for the piston to travel during the inspiratory phase may be limited. This is especially true at high frequencies. Therefore the ΔP and $P_{\overline{aw}}$ can be affected by changes in the percentage of inspiratory time.

Frequency

The frequency control sets the oscillatory frequency, or breaths per minute, in hertz (Hz); 1 Hz is equal to 60 cycles, or 60 breaths, per minute. The control is adjustable from 3 Hz to 15 Hz, and the setting is digitally displayed in the window to the left of the control.

As frequency is increased, excursion of the piston will be limited by the time allotted for each breath cycle. Changes in the frequency will affect $P_{\overline{aw}}$ and ΔP (Boxes 14.10 and 14.11).

Start/Stop

The start/stop control button either enables or disables oscillator operation. Pressing this start/stop button will light the green LED labeled *OSCILLATOR STOPPED* if the ventilator's microprocessor determines that the unit is safe to operate. This control allows the oscillator to begin operation only if the startup procedure was properly performed.

Reset

The reset button sets or resets the unit's safety alarms and the power failure alarm. Conditions triggering an alarm must be corrected before resetting can occur. This button does not

---

BOX 14.10 Clinical Example of Changing Frequency With the 3100A

A patient is on the CareFusion 3100A at a frequency of 15 Hz. The clinician decides to lower the frequency to 10 Hz. Doing so allows the piston more travel time. This results in greater piston displacement, or more delivered volume to the patient. The exact amount of the volume increase is unknown. In some patients an inadvertent (and unknown) increase in tidal volume may contribute to volutrauma. Therefore the clinician should always use caution when lowering the oscillatory frequency.

BOX 14.11 Effect of Control Changes on Mean Airway Pressure

Many of the controls on the 3100 affect more than one parameter. For example, when adjusting the amplitude with the power control, the alteration in piston thrust will change the level of mean airway pressure. When the frequency is adjusted, changes in amplitude, piston position, and mean airway pressure will occur. Therefore the clinician should use caution when making a setting change and carefully readjust other settings that might also change.

---

function unless the ventilator has been activated with the start/stop button.

Certain alarm conditions, such as the "PAW <20% SET MAX PAW" alarm, cause the circuit dump valve to immediately deflate. When the clinician depresses the reset button, the dump valve will reinflate. It is necessary to press the reset button until the airway pressure exceeds 20% of that on the "SET MAX PAW" thumbwheel. Otherwise, reset may not occur.

The reset button also is used to silence the ventilator's battery-powered audible power failure alarm if the unit is turned off or if electrical power is interrupted.

Alarms
45-Second Silence

For most alarm conditions, the audible portion can be silenced for 45 seconds by pressing the "45-SEC SILENCE" button. When activated, the button's yellow LED will light until the silence period lapses.

When the oscillator is turned off at the power switch or the oscillator stops because of a power interruption, the audible alarm can be silenced only by pressing the reset button.

Set Maximum and Minimum $P_{\overline{aw}}$

The "SET MAX PAW" and "SET MIN PAW" thumbwheel switches enable the clinician to set maximum and minimum limits for $P_{\overline{aw}}$. Because some drifting of $P_{\overline{aw}}$ may be attributable to ETT leaks or spontaneous breathing, a safety range needs to be set. When either limit is reached, a red LED next to the corresponding thumbwheel will light and an audible alarm will sound. The ventilator continues to operate, but the alarm condition will persist until the mean pressure adjust control is readjusted or new alarm limits are set.

PAW <20% SET MAX PAW

Conditions causing a sharp drop in $P_{\overline{aw}}$ to a level less than 20% of the value set on the "SET MAX PAW" thumbwheel will result in an alarm condition. The thumbwheel will trigger a "PAW <20% SET MAX PAW" alarm. When this alarm is triggered, the oscillator stops, the red LED lights to indicate this alarm condition, and the audible alarm sounds. Bias flow will continue to be delivered to permit spontaneous ventilation.

PAW >50 cm H₂O

The "PAW >50 cm H_2O" alarm is activated if $P_{\overline{aw}}$ rises above 50 cm H_2O for any reason. When this alarm is activated, the dump valve opens, causing the oscillator to stop. The red LED lights up to indicate this alarm condition, and an audible alarm sounds. Although the audible alarm can be silenced with the "45-SEC SILENCE" button, the oscillator will not resume operating until the reset button is pressed and held until $P_{\overline{aw}}$ exceeds 20% of that set with the "SET MAX PAW" thumbwheel.

Power Failure

The battery-powered power failure alarm is activated if the power switch to the ventilator is turned off or if electrical power is interrupted. If the unit's main circuit breaker is tripped or the main power supply fails, this alarm condition also occurs. The power failure LED lights up, and the audible alarm sounds. Both can be extinguished by pressing the reset button.

When power is restored to the ventilator, the circuit must be occluded and the reset button pressed and held until $P_{\overline{aw}}$ exceeds 20% of that set with the "SET MAX PAW" thumbwheel. Only then will oscillations resume (Box 14.12).

Battery Low

The yellow "battery low" LED lights up when the battery serving the power failure alarm is low. No audible alarm is activated.

Source Gas Low

The yellow "source gas low" LED lights up whenever gas pressure from the blender falls below 30 psig. This LED also lights up if the pressure drops below 30 psig in the separate compressed-air source for cooling the piston subsystem. The most common cause of this alarm condition is obstruction of the inlet filter cartridge with dirt. If this problem is not corrected, the piston subsystem is likely to overheat, resulting in piston failure.

Oscillator Overheated

The yellow "OSCILLATOR OVERHEATED" LED lights when the oscillator coil temperature reaches 175°C (347°F). No audible alarm sounds. If this problem is not corrected, piston failure can result.

Troubleshooting

The array of visual and audible alarms assists the clinician in troubleshooting specific problems with the CareFusion oscillator. The instruction manual also provides a troubleshooting guide.

Circuit leaks are most likely to occur at the many connection points. For example, the pressure line going from the airway Y-connector to the front of the unit may be loose. Lines going from the front to each of the mushroom valves can be the source of leaks. All of these lines have Luer-Lok connections that need to be tight. Although it occurs only rarely, any of the mushroom valves can rupture, which will cause the unit to stop oscillating and will activate the alarm.

When a circuit not equipped with heater wires is used, pooling of water can occur at any low point in the circuit. If the patient is positioned lower than the circuit, excessive condensate can run into the patient's airway. Therefore care must be taken to keep water drained from the circuit.

If the CareFusion 3100A is operated for long periods of time at very low frequencies, the piston can begin to fail. If the piston housing is not connected to a compressed-air source or if the unit is operated without sufficient piston centering, the piston will wear out more rapidly than normal. Piston failure is usually indicated by a knocking sound and by drifting in the $P_{\overline{aw}}$ and amplitude levels.

Every clinician who uses CareFusion 3100A oscillators needs to be capable of performing a system calibration and check. An outline of this procedure is printed on the left side and top of the unit. If a clinician notes problems in maintaining the desired settings, the patient must be removed from the ventilator and provided with another means of ventilation support. Then the clinician should perform a system calibration and check. Doing so often reveals the source of the problem.

CAREFUSION 3100B HIGH FREQUENCY OSCILLATORY VENTILATOR

The CareFusion 3100B High Frequency Oscillatory Ventilator, a different version of the model 3100A, is intended to be used with adult patients. Appropriate for the patient with a weight more than 35 kg, the model 3100B (Fig. 14.35A) is designed with greater power, flow, and pressure capabilities than the 3100A. Because the design and controls of the two models are very similar, only the differences between the two are discussed here.

BOX 14.12 **Returning the Oscillator to Operation After Disconnect**

When alarm conditions occur, especially those that shut down the oscillator, the clinician should immediately remove the patient from the circuit and provide manual ventilation. After the cause of the alarm condition is corrected, the airway connector should be plugged and oscillations restarted by using the reset button. Plugging the circuit and restarting oscillations are necessary to confirm safe operation. When that is done, the plug is then removed and the connection is immediately occluded by hand. Next, the circuit is quickly reconnected to the patient's airway.

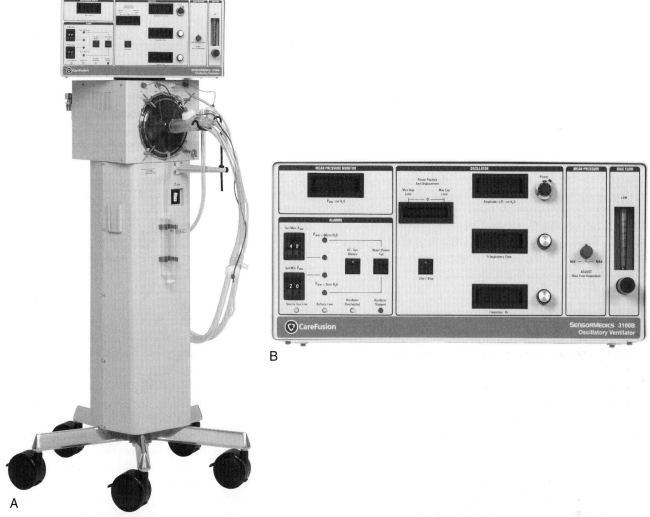

FIGURE 14.35 A, The CareFusion Model 3100B High-Frequency Oscillatory Ventilator. B, Control panel of the 3100B. (Courtesy Becton, Dickinson, and Company [CareFusion], Franklin Lakes, NJ.)

Differences Between 3100A and 3100B Models

Power and $P_{\overline{aw}}$ controls for the 3100B are identical to those for the 3100A. Although the power control remains a graduated 10-turn locking dial, the ΔP is adjustable to greater than 90 cm H_2O of the maximum amplitude of the proximal airway pressure. Mean airway pressure is adjustable to approximately 55 cm H_2O. Piston-centering is performed automatically by updated electronic sensors. Therefore the center piston control has been eliminated from this model.[14]

The mean pressure limit control has also been eliminated. The "SET MAX PAW" is the only adjustable control that prevents inadvertent increases in P_{aw}. The limit controls are discussed next.

The bias flow capability of the 3100B has been expanded to an internal limit of 60 L/min. The rotameter glass tube, which indicates flow, is graduated from 0 L/min to 60 L/min in 5-L/min increments (see Fig. 14.35B).

The frequency control and digital display, which operate identically to the same controls on the 3100A, permit the

operator to adjust the frequency from 3 Hz to 15 Hz. These are the same limits that are used on the 3100A. The inspiratory time control is also identical, with limits from 30% to 50%.

The alarm panel on the model 3100B is arranged identically to that on the 3100A. However, there are several differences in alarm limits and function. A major difference is in the set maximum $P_{\overline{aw}}$ control. The maximum setting for this control is 59 cm H_2O. When the ventilator is operating and the set pressure limit is reached or exceeded by the proximal pressure, the unit no longer shuts down entirely. The audible and visual alarm will activate, but instead of shutting down, the ventilator will depressurize the limit valve seat until the $P_{\overline{aw}}$ falls to a level of 12 cm H_2O (±3 cm H_2O) below the set mean. After the pressure drops to this point, the limit valve will allow the circuit to repressurize and rise again and the audible and visual alarms will be deactivated. If the proximal pressure rises again to meet or exceed the limit setting, the same cycle of events will repeat until the alarm condition is resolved.

The "PAW >60 cm H_2O" red LED and audible alarm operate the same as the "PAW >50 cm H_2O" LED on the 3100A, with the only difference being the higher pressure required to trigger the alarm condition. The "PAW <5 cm H_2O" red LED and alarm operate identically to the "PAW <20% OF SET MAX PAW" button, except that a $P_{\overline{aw}}$ less than 5 cm H_2O will trigger the alarm.

CHAPTER SUMMARY

The ventilators discussed in this chapter represent those that are widely used in the infant and pediatric settings. In many clinical settings, mechanical ventilation is provided to patients of all ages and sizes by staff members who also work with this wide range of patients. In such settings, a ventilator that is easily adapted to fit any need presents a cost savings and time savings in terms of staff technical training. General-purpose ventilators that were originally designed to be used with adults have been found to be easily adapted to pediatric applications and, in some cases, to neonatal applications.

Infant and pediatric ventilators will continue to be developed, particularly to provide better monitoring capabilities. Additional developments in specialized applications unique to the neonatal/pediatric population are certain, including ventilatory support to spontaneously breathing patients and high-frequency technology. In addition, some clinicians have shown interest in ventilators capable of delivering subambient oxygen concentrations. Others have envisioned systems capable of providing specialty gases, such as nitric oxide and heliox. In the planning stages for years, prototype closed-loop systems that monitor arterial blood and expired gases and adjust their own ventilator settings are now being tested.

As with all technology, necessity drives the scope and the direction of advancement. As clinical problems present themselves, technical innovation will provide more-sophisticated solutions. Factors such as medical advances, economics, demographics, and even ideology will continue to affect the infant/pediatric ventilator market.

KEY POINTS

- The CareFusion Infant Flow generator consists of two fluidic jets, which on inspiration direct flow through the nasal prongs; on expiration, pressure from the expiratory gas flow "flips" the direction of flow away from the prongs and through an expiratory port.
- When using the CareFusion Infant Flow SiPAP, the clinician can set both an inspiratory and an expiratory pressure by adjusting the two flowmeters.
- Bubble CPAP, such as the Fisher & Paykel Healthcare Bubble CPAP System, provides a single pressure and flow, but with minute oscillations around the set pressure level, and has been associated with reduced incidence of chronic lung disease in premature infants.
- With the CareFusion V.I.P. Bird, flow triggering and flow cycling are accomplished by using the Bird Partner IIi Volume Monitor and the Infant "Smart" Flow Sensor.
- The termination sensitivity control on the V.I.P. Bird allows adjustment of the flow-termination point of the breath and is used only in the A/C time-cycled mode.
- Leak compensation available with volume-cycled modes on the V.I.P. Bird is recommended for use only with leaks around artificial airways and is not for use with patients who have minimal inspiratory effort and no leakage.
- In the V.I.P. Bird Sterling and Gold ventilators, the functions of the Partner IIi Volume Monitor have been directly incorporated into the main ventilator housing.
- VAPS, available on the V.I.P. Bird Gold, is a dual-control mode that begins as a pressure-targeted breath (descending flow) but switches to constant-flow delivery with a volume-target, if the *set* volume has not been achieved during the breath.
- With the Dräger Babylog 8000, the high-pressure alarm is automatically set to a pressure of 10 cm H_2O or a PEEP/CPAP of 4 cm H_2O. In the event of excessive pressure buildup within the circuit, the exhalation valve opens, allowing exhalation.

- During IMV with the Dräger Babylog 8000, the mandatory breath is time triggered based on the rate calculation.
- The application of nasal CPAP with the Dräger Babylog 8000 requires disabling of the flow measurement by disconnecting the attachment from the proximal flow sensor and pressing the reset/check button.
- The volume guarantee feature on the Dräger Babylog 8000 plus provides pressure-limited ventilation with a volume target (a dual-control mode) and can be used only when the airway flow sensor is in use.
- The Bunnell Life Pulse High Frequency Ventilator is a microprocessor-controlled, pressure-limited, TC, constant-flow, high-frequency jet ventilator that works in conjunction with a conventional ventilator.
- On the Bunnell High Frequency Ventilator, an electromagnetic solenoid activates the pinch valve, which interrupts the flow of pressurized gas and gives small bursts of air to the patient's airway.
- The Bunnell HFJV system is indicated for patients with severe respiratory distress syndrome complicated by pulmonary air leak that has been untreatable with conventional mechanical ventilation strategies.
- With the CareFusion HFO system, volume delivered by the piston is decreased as oscillatory frequency is increased.
- Any interruption of ventilator operation on the CareFusion HFO system pressurization of the circuit's three mushroom valves stops immediately, allowing the circuit to open to the atmosphere.
- When using the CareFusion HFO system, the mean pressure adjust control is the primary determinant of $P_{\overline{aw}}$, although increasing bias flow will increase $P_{\overline{aw}}$ and changes to the power, frequency, inspiratory time, and piston-centering controls will also alter the $P_{\overline{aw}}$.
- When the CareFusion HFO system is turned off at the power switch or the oscillator stops because of a power interruption, the audible alarm can be silenced only by pressing the reset button.

ASSESSMENT QUESTIONS

See Appendix B for the answers.

1. One of the most common modes of ventilation used in infants for more than 30 years is:
   a. Volume ventilation
   b. Synchronized intermittent mandatory ventilation (SIMV) with pressure support
   c. Time-triggered, pressure-limited, time-cycled ventilation
   d. Volume-assured pressure support (VAPS)

2. Better ventilator-to-patient synchrony has been developed in infant ventilation because of the technological advancement of which of the following devices?
   a. Floating expiratory valves
   b. Flow-sensing devices
   c. Volume-measuring devices
   d. Rapid-response pressure monitors

3. In children up to the age of 6 months, the interface most often used to provide nasal continuous positive airway pressure (CPAP) is the:
   a. Nasal prong
   b. Nasopharyngeal CPAP interface
   c. Nasal mask
   d. Nasal trumpet

4. When the patient takes a breath from the CareFusion SiPAP, the inspiratory effort results in which of the following?
   a. Gas flow is diverted away from the expiratory limb to mix with existing inspiratory flow.
   b. The inspiratory flow is produced by the "Pres Low" flowmeter.
   c. The targeted inspiratory positive airway pressure (IPAP) is the "Pres High" flowmeter alone.
   d. Pressure from the patient's inspiratory flow draws gas from the expiratory limb.

5. The Fisher & Paykel Healthcare Bubble CPAP System requires which of the following components?
   1. A humidifier chamber with a continuous-feed sterile water system
   2. A standard air/oxygen blender with standard oxygen tubing
   3. A hot wire inspiratory limb of the patient circuit
   4. A CPAP generator
      a. 4 only
      b. 2 and 4 only
      c. 1, 2, and 3 only
      d. 1, 2, 3, and 4

6. When the Bubble CPAP System is in use, the desired CPAP level is set by:
   a. Increasing the flow from the gas source
   b. Adjusting the position of the CPAP probe
   c. Increasing the generator's pressure
   d. Increasing the CPAP setting

7. When the Fisher & Paykel Healthcare MR730 humidifier is used with the Bubble CPAP System, what should the temperature control and chamber control be set for?
   a. Temperature control at 37°C and chamber control at −1
   b. Temperature control at 39°C and chamber control at +3
   c. Temperature control at 42°C and chamber control at −2
   d. Temperature control at 40°C and chamber control at −3

8. Termination sensitivity is an added feature on the V.I.P. Bird ventilator that:
   a. Allows the clinician to adjust the flow-termination point of the breath
   b. Operates in all modes
   c. Can be adjusted from 0% to 55% in increments of 10%
   d. Sets the breath trigger sensitivity to patient effort

9. On the V.I.P. Bird the termination sensitivity setting flashes when the:
   a. Breath is terminated at the set value
   b. Breath is time cycled (TC)
   c. Breath is both flow triggered and flow cycled
   d. Expiratory time is deemed too short by the ventilator's microprocessor

10. On the V.I.P. Bird, leak compensation is:
    1. Available in all modes
    2. Available only in volume-cycled (VC) modes
    3. Used to stabilize baseline pressure in the presence of leaks
    4. Available in pressure control and pressure support (PS)
       a. 1 only
       b. 2 only
       c. 4 only
       d. 1 and 3 only

11. The flow sensor in the Sterling and Gold versions of the V.I.P. Bird differs from the original because it:
    a. Incorporates a hot wire anemometer
    b. Contains a stainless steel flap in the variable-orifice differential pressure transducer
    c. Uses an ultrasonic wave–detection monitor
    d. Incorporates a laser beam splitter

12. In the Dräger Babylog 8000 infant ventilator, all of the following are automatically set by the microprocessor *except:*
    a. Oxygen concentration alarms
    b. Positive end-expiratory pressure (PEEP) alarm limits
    c. Low tidal volume (V_T) alarm
    d. Inspiratory pressure alarm

13. When the V.I.P. Gold ventilator rise time control is set at 1:
    a. A rapid rise to set pressure occurs
    b. Only volume breaths are affected
    c. The inspiratory time increases
    d. The respiratory rate increases

14. When the V.I.P. Bird mode switch is set at TC SIMV, what are the breath variables for mandatory breaths?
    1. Time triggering or patient triggering
    2. Volume-targeted breaths
    3. Pressure-targeted breaths
    4. TC
       a. 3 only
       b. 1 and 2 only
       c. 1, 3, and 4 only
       d. 1, 2, and 4 only

15. The Bunnell Life Pulse High Frequency Ventilator:
    1. Operates in tandem with a conventional ventilator
    2. Requires the use of the Hi-Lo jet tube
    3. Delivers rates of 240 insufflations/min to 660 insufflations/min
    4. Operates independently with the use of another device
       a. 1 and 2 only
       b. 2 and 4 only
       c. 1 and 3 only
       d. 3 and 4 only

16. The triple-lumen Hi-Lo jet tube:
    a. Is the only type of endotracheal tube (ETT) that can be used with the Bunnell Life Pulse High Frequency Ventilator
    b. Ranges in size from 2.5-mm internal diameter (ID) to 6.0-mm ID
    c. Must be replaced with a standard ETT when the patient is switched to conventional ventilation
    d. All of the above

17. The Dräger Babylog 8000 infant ventilator:
    a. Is used to ventilate premature and term infants
    b. Has a weight limit of 10 kg
    c. Has a built-in battery
    d. All of the above

18. Which of the following statements is (are) true regarding the use of the activated volume guarantee feature of the Dräger Babylog 8000 plus?
    1. The proximal flow sensor must be attached when this feature is used.
    2. The clinician sets the maximum peak inspiratory pressure.
    3. The maximum peak inspiratory pressure becomes an inspiratory pressure limit.
    4. Over six to eight breaths, the ventilator determines the appropriate inspiratory pressure and begins to achieve and maintain the target tidal volume.
       a. 1 only
       b. 3 only
       c. 1 and 2 only
       d. 1, 2, 3, and 4

19. During volume guarantee on the Dräger Babylog 8000 plus, the volume is set at 5 mL, but the patient's inspiratory effort results in a 7-mL volume demand. How will the ventilator respond?
    a. The ventilator's peak inspiratory pressure (PIP) will immediately decrease.
    b. If the total inspiratory tidal volume exceeds the set target volume by 200%, the expiratory valve will open and no additional ventilator-driven gas will be delivered to the patient.
    c. The 7-mL volume will be given and displayed without a ventilator response.
    d. A high tidal volume alarm will activate.

20. The power control on the CareFusion 3100A is primarily used to change the:
    a. Mean airway pressure
    b. Frequency
    c. Bias flow
    d. Amplitude

21. If the frequency on the CareFusion 3100A is increased from 10 Hz to 15 Hz and no other settings are changed, which of the following will occur?
    a. Inspiratory time will increase.
    b. Volume delivered by the piston will decrease.
    c. Amplitude will increase.
    d. None of the above

22. Mean airway pressure in the CareFusion 3100A high-frequency oscillator can be affected by which of the following?
    1. Bias flow
    2. Frequency setting
    3. Percentage of inspiratory time (% T_I)
    4. Piston centering
    5. Mean airway adjustment control
       a. 5 only
       b. 1 and 3 only
       c. 2, 4, and 5 only
       d. 1, 2, 3, 4, and 5

23. A new feature of the CareFusion 3100B oscillator compared with the 3100A is the:
    a. Frequency control
    b. Inspiratory time control
    c. Automatic piston centering
    d. Mean airway pressure control

REFERENCES

1. Chatburn RL: Principles and practices of neonatal and pediatric ventilation. *Respir Care* 36:573, 1991.
2. Watson K: Neonatal and pediatric mechanical ventilation. In Pilbeam SP, Cairo JM: *Mechanical ventilation—physiological and clinical application*, St. Louis, 2006, Elsevier.
3. Watson K: Infant and pediatric devices. In Cairo JM: *Mosby's respiratory care equipment*, ed 9, St. Louis, 2014, Elsevier.
4. CareFusion: *Operator's manual*, Infant Flow SiPAP 675-101-101.
5. de Klerk AM, de Klerk RK: Use of continuous positive airway pressure in preterm infants: comments and experience from New Zealand. *Pediatrics* 108:761-763, 2001.
6. Betit P, Thompson JE, Benjamin PK: Mechanical ventilation. In Koff PB, Eitzman D, Neu J, editors: *Neonatal and pediatric respiratory care*, ed 2, St. Louis, 1993, Mosby.
7. Thompson MA: Early nasal CPAP and prophylactic surfactant for neonates at risk of RDS: the IFDAS trial, presented at the European Society for Paediatric Research, annual meeting, Helsinki, Finland, August 2001.
8. *Instruction manual: V.I.P. Bird Infant-Pediatric Ventilator*, Palm Springs, CA, 1991, Viasys Healthcare Systems, Critical Care Division.
9. *Instruction manual: V.I.P. graphics instruction manual*, Palm Springs, CA, 1991, Viasys Healthcare Systems, Critical Care Division.
10. *Operator's manual: V.I.P. Bird Gold and Sterling Ventilator Systems*, Palm Springs, CA, 2000, Viasys Healthcare Systems, Critical Care Division.
11. Dräger Medical AG & Co: *Operator's manual: Dräger Babylog 8000*, 1st U.S. edition, Lübeck, Germany, 1993, Dräger Inc.
12. Bunnell Incorporated: *Operator's manual: Life Pulse High-Frequency Jet Ventilator*, Salt Lake City, UT, 1991, Bunnell Incorporated.
13. *Operator's manual: 3100A High-Frequency Oscillatory Ventilator*, form P/N 767124, Palm Springs, CA, 1991, (CareFusion) Viasys Healthcare Systems, Critical Care Division.
14. *Operator's manual: 3100B High-Frequency Oscillatory Ventilator*, form P/N 767164, rev. J, Palm Springs, CA, 2001, (CareFusion) Viasys Healthcare Systems, Critical Care Division.

Transport, Home Care, and Noninvasive Ventilatory Devices

OBJECTIVES

Upon completion of this chapter, you will be able to:

1. Give the value in liters per minute of the logical flow for the patient-disconnect feature when the pNeuton model A ventilator is in use.
2. Determine the length of time that elapses between a low-battery event and a ventilator-inoperative event with the Crossvent ventilator when there is a power loss.
3. State the value for the gas supply pressure that will result in a low source-pressure alarm when the Crossvent 4+ is in use.
4. Describe the operating features, alarms, and parameter ranges of the following ventilators: Bio-Med Crossvent, Bio-Med MVP-10, Zoll 731 Series EMV+, CareFusion LTV 1200, Newport HT70, and the CareFusion ReVel.
5. Describe the effect of the oxygen flow on oxygen delivery in the Oxylog 3000 Plus.
6. Review the function of the low-pressure "eyeball" alarm in the Smiths Medical Pneupac ventiPAC ventilator.
7. Discuss the ability of the Newport HT50 to provide enriched oxygen delivery.
8. Describe the adjustment of the positive end-expiratory pressure/continuous positive airway pressure (PEEP/CPAP) control on the HT50 ventilator.
9. Estimate the amount of time the Newport HT70 secondary backup battery maintains operation without interruption when the main Power Pac battery is depleted.
10. Name the two operator-adjustable alarms on the Respironics BiPAP Focus.
11. Discuss the optional AVAPS (average volume-assured pressure support) mode with the Respironics V60 ventilator.
12. Give the patient size limit for the Respironics Synchrony ventilator.
13. List the alarms available on the Puritan Bennett GoodKnight 425.
14. List the adjustable level of PEEP available with the ResMed Stellar 100.

OUTLINE

KEY TERMS

accumulator/silencer
expiratory positive airway pressure (EPAP)
pressure-relief valve

General-use ventilators utilized in the intensive care unit (ICU) were described in Chapters 12 and 13. This chapter provides a review of ventilators that are primarily used in patient transport and home care. As such, this chapter presents information about devices, such as portable ventilators, bilevel airway pressure equipment and continuous positive airway pressure (CPAP) machines, noninvasive positive-pressure ventilators, and noninvasive negative-pressure ventilators.

I. TRANSPORT VENTILATORS

There are few procedures that require greater care and skill than the transportation of critically ill patients. The movement of a patient from one location to another should never be considered routine. It is important to recognize that transport of a critically ill patient is not without the risk for complications.[1] Loss of an intravenous line; changes in body temperature; hyperventilation or hypoventilation, which can perpetuate cardiac arrhythmias; along with equipment malfunction are potential problems associated with the transport of a ventilator-dependent patient. Additionally, providing manual ventilation to ventilator-dependent patients during transport has been reported to be associated with episodic hypotension, hyperventilation, and ventilation asynchrony.[2,3] Indeed, every attempt should be made to ensure that monitoring, ventilation, oxygenation, and patient care are adequately maintained during transport of critically ill patients to ensure patient safety. Institutional protocols should guide the decision to transport critically ill patients and serve as a checklist for the transport team. Preparation and communication are vital components of a successful transport.

The attributes commonly shared among transport ventilators are compact size, light weight, and a reliable power source. The power source must allow the ventilator to operate from an internal battery or a gas source to permit mobility. Durability and ease of operation are additional features that are desired when selecting a good transport ventilator. The incorporation of microprocessors and the miniaturization of components have increased the capabilities and functionality of modern transport ventilators, including improvements in monitoring and available alarms. Current transport ventilators have features that were once associated only with costly intensive care ventilators (e.g., flow triggering, pressure support [PS], and high-frequency ventilation).[4,5] The current generation of transport ventilators can also provide a variety of alarms and modes of ventilation similar to those found on ICU ventilators.

Respiratory therapists must understand the capabilities and limitations of ventilators used during the transport process. Although the use of a transport ventilator can reduce the risks associated with manual ventilation, it is also important to recognize that a knowledgeable, well-qualified operator is essential to ensuring the proper application of the equipment.

Transport ventilators must be able to function properly in extreme conditions, including temperature extremes, vibrations, and altitude changes. These devices should also contain sufficient shielding to protect the ventilator's internal mechanisms from electromagnetic interference.

In addition to durability, transport ventilators should be easy to operate. This does not imply that the machine should be basic in operation; it only suggests that the user controls should be readily accessible and easy to adjust. The volume, rate, and pressure controls should be large and easy to find, and all displays should be clearly visible in both daytime and nighttime lighting to reduce the chance of mistakes caused by missed or misread information.

The American Association for Respiratory Care (AARC) has developed a clinical practice guideline specifically addressing the purpose, indications, methods of providing, and complications associated with transporting mechanically ventilated patients, which is a valuable resource to practitioners interested in transport ventilation (Clinical Practice Guideline 15.1).[3,4] It is important for all clinicians involved in the transport of critically ill patients to understand that although many transport ventilators have functional capabilities comparable to contemporary ICU ventilators, ensuring patient safety must always be the clinician's first priority.

AIRON pNEUTON

The pNeuton (Airon Corporation) is designed to provide invasive and noninvasive ventilation for pediatric and adult patients who weigh 23 kg (50.7 lb) or more (Fig. 15.1).[5] It is pneumatically powered and controlled. The modes of operation offered are continuous mandatory ventilation (CMV), intermittent mandatory ventilation (IMV), and CPAP, and this unit also includes a pressure-limiting feature. It measures 4 in in height (H) by 8 in in width (W) by 6 in in depth (D) and weighs 2.7 kg (6.0 lb), and it is magnetic resonance imaging (MRI) compatible up to a 3-T static field. Table 15.1 provides a summary of some of the specifications of the pNeuton transport ventilator.

Power Source

The pNeuton is a pneumatically powered ventilator and requires a 55-pounds per square inch (psi) (±15 psi) gas source to operate. It has no battery backup or alternating current (AC) power option. Two models of the pNeuton are available: an A model and an S model. The internal system of the A model with the patient-disconnect alarm requires 4 L/min of

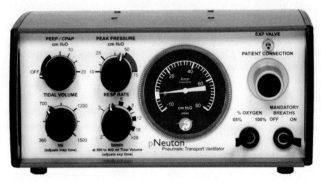

FIGURE 15.1 Airon pNeuton transport ventilator. (Courtesy Airon Corporation, Melbourne, FL.)

CLINICAL PRACTICE GUIDELINE 15.1
In-Hospital Transport of the Mechanically Ventilated Patient

Definition/Description
Transportation of mechanically ventilated patients for diagnostic or therapeutic procedures is always associated with a degree of risk. Every attempt should be made to ensure monitoring, ventilation, oxygenation, and patient care remain constant during movement. Patient transport includes preparation and movement to and from and time spent at the destination.

Indications
Transportation of mechanically ventilated patients should be undertaken only after a careful evaluation of the risk-to-benefit ratio.

Contraindications
Contraindications include the inability to do the following: maintain an airway, provide adequate oxygenation and ventilation, maintain acceptable hemodynamic performance, and adequately monitor cardiopulmonary signs during transport.

Precautions and Complications
The potential hazards and complications of transport include the following:

- Hyperventilation during manual ventilation, resulting in respiratory alkalosis, cardiac dysrhythmias, and hypotension
- Loss of positive end-expiratory pressure/continuous positive airway pressure (PEEP/CPAP), resulting in hypoxemia
- Position changes that result in hypotension, hypercarbia, and hypoxemia
- Dysrhythmias
- Equipment failure, which causes inaccurate data or loss of monitoring capabilities
- Inadvertent disconnection of intravenous pharmacological agents, which results in hemodynamic instability
- Accidental extubation
- Accidental removal of vascular access
- Loss of oxygen supply, resulting in hypoxemia

Limitations
The literature suggests that nearly two-thirds of all transports for diagnostic studies fail to yield results that affect patient care.

Monitoring
Monitoring provided during transport should be maintained at the level of stationary care.

For complete guidelines, see Chang DW, American Association for Respiratory Care: Clinical practice guideline: in-hospital transport of the mechanically ventilated patient—2002 revision & update. *Resp Care* 47:721-723, 2002.

TABLE 15.1 Specifications for pNeuton Ventilator

Control Settings	Range
Modes	Nonsynchronized IMV, CPAP
Power source	Pneumatic powered
Rate	3-50 breaths/min
Noninvasive ventilation mode	Yes
Peak pressure range	15-75 cm H_2O
Tidal volume	360-1500 mL
Inspiratory time	Auto set
PEEP/CPAP	0-20 cm H_2O
Oxygen percent	65% or 100% oxygen
Pressure support	N/A
Monitors/displays	Analog pressure gauge range: 0-120 cm H_2O
Dimensions	4 in × 8 in × 6 in, weighs 2.7 kg (6 lb)
Gas consumption	4 L/min
Alarms	Low oxygen inlet pressure alarm; patient disconnect alarm
Battery duration	N/A

CPAP, Continuous positive airway pressure; *IMV*, intermittent mandatory ventilation; *PEEP*, positive end-expiratory pressure.

up to an altitude of 15,000 ft. Note that altitude will not affect pressure settings. However, tidal volume (V_T) will increase and respiratory rate will decrease with increases in altitude. This is because the ventilator's internal calibration is set for sea level. The accuracy of V_T delivery at higher altitudes should be checked with an external respirometer.

Controls and Alarms

The pNeuton contains several front-panel controls for setting ventilator parameters and for monitoring patient data and alarms.

PEEP/CPAP

Positive end-expiratory pressure/continuous positive airway pressure (PEEP/CPAP) is adjustable between 0 cm H_2O and 20 cm H_2O. The trigger sensitivity does not need to be readjusted with increases in PEEP/CPAP, because this is done automatically by the ventilator.

Peak Pressure

Peak pressure control of mandatory breaths is adjustable from 10 cm H_2O to 75 cm H_2O, and pressure is displayed on an analog pressure manometer. When peak pressures are set higher than 50 cm H_2O, the control pointer will be in the red bar area, indicating that the set pressure is high.

Tidal Volume and Respiratory Rate

The V_T is set using a knob in the lower left-hand corner. The available V_T range is 360 to 1500 mL. For ease of use there are V_T markings at 360, 700, 1100, and 1500 mL. The respiratory

source gas for operation. The model S without the disconnect alarm uses 3 L/min of source gas for operation of the internal logical system.

The pNeuton typically operates from a 55-psi oxygen source. The operator can select either the 100% or the 65% oxygen setting, with the lower setting entraining room air to lower the oxygen concentration. The pNeuton can operate normally

rate is set with a control knob located next to the V_T knob on the control panel. It is adjustable from 2 breaths/min to 50 breaths/min in the CMV/IMV mode (i.e., mandatory breath is turned on).

It is important to mention that the V_T and respiratory rate controls determine the mandatory breath inspiratory and expiratory times. The pNeuton provides a fixed flow (i.e., 36 L/min or 600 mL/s) during mandatory breaths. Therefore the inspiratory time will reflect the range of V_Ts available (i.e., 360 to 1500 mL). The ventilator V_T output does not change with increasing patient circuit pressure, but the actual V_T delivered to the patient changes due to compression of gas in the ventilator circuit.

The respiratory rate control is calibrated for set V_Ts between 500 and 900 mL.[5] The calibrated respiratory rate range optimizes the interdependence between the expiratory and inspiratory time.[5] Consequently, V_Ts set below 500 mL will result in higher rates than marked on the Respiratory Rate control. Conversely, V_Ts set above 900 mL will result in lower rates than marked on the Respiratory Rate control.

It is suggested that independent validation of V_T and rate be performed using external spirometers and timing devices.[5]

Percentage Oxygen

The F_IO_2 (fraction of inspired oxygen) is controlled by a two-position switch located in the upper right-hand corner of the control panel. As previously mentioned, the available options are 100% and 65% O_2.

Mandatory Breaths Control

This function is controlled by a two-position (on/off) switch located in the upper right-hand corner of the control panel next to the percentage oxygen switch. This control determines whether the pNeuton is operating in CMV/IMV or CPAP mode and thus represents the mode control for the ventilator.

Pressure Gauge

The pNeuton has an analog pressure gauge located in the center of the control panel. It displays delivered peak pressures and PEEP/CPAP levels in a range from 0 cm H_2O to 80 cm H_2O.

Alarms

The pNeuton has a totally pneumatically powered alarm system. A low oxygen inlet pressure alarm will activate when the source pressure falls below 30 psi. The low-pressure alarm will continue to sound until all pressure has been lost in the system or pressure is reestablished to at least 35 psi.[5]

The pNeuton also provides a high-pressure release. The patient circuit peak pressure, which is adjustable using the Peak Pressure control, can be set from 10 to 75 cm H_2O. The factory preset value is 50 cm H_2O. (*Note*: In addition to the Peak Pressure control, the pNeuton has an internal safety pressure release valve. This valve automatically limits circuit pressure to approximately 80 cm H_2O.)[5]

The pNeuton has an internal Anti-Suffocation System, which allows the patient to breathe on his or her own if the ventilator malfunctions. When the ventilator senses a *negative* pressure of approximately 2 cm H_2O, an internal valve opens, allowing unimpeded ambient air to enter the patient circuit to the patient, regardless of the ventilator control settings, including PEEP/CPAP.[5]

Modes of Operation

The pNeuton offers volume-controlled (VC)-CMV, pressure-controlled (PC)-CMV, VC-IMV, PC-IMV, and CPAP modes. These modes can be easily used as noninvasive modes, if desired, when an appropriate face mask or other interface is used.

The ventilator's CPAP demand flow system provides gas for spontaneous breathing at adjustable CPAP pressure up to 20 cm H_2O. During PEEP/CPAP the pneumatic system provides a continuous flow of gas through the circuit of approximately 10 L/min to meet the inspiratory demand during spontaneous breaths. If the patient's inspiratory flow demand exceeds the continuous flow of gas, additional flow will be needed to meet patient demand. The flow sensitivity is preset and not adjustable. The CPAP system will meet patient needs greater than 100 L/min by attempting to maintain a balance between the flow and pressure at the expiratory valve.[5]

BIO-MED CROSSVENT

The Crossvent ventilator (Bio-Med Devices, Inc,) is a compact ventilator that can be used for transport or in the ICU. It is an electronically controlled, pneumatically powered ventilator. It can be time triggered or patient triggered, volume targeted or pressure targeted, and time cycled.[6]

Crossvent ventilators come in several models; Table 15.2 provides a comparison of model features. The Crossvent 4+ ventilator is capable of ventilating newborns through adult-sized patients, depending on which model is selected. The following discussion focuses on the Crossvent 4+ model (Fig. 15.2).

The Crossvent 4+ is designed to provide CMV, IMV, CPAP, and pressure-support ventilation (PSV). (*Note*: The Crossvent ventilator control panel utilizes synchronized intermittent mandatory ventilation [SIMV] to designate IMV). The Crossvent 4+ weighs 4.8 kg (10.5 lb) and is 10 in H × 11 in W × 5.5 in D. Table 15.3 outlines specific features.

Electrical Power Source

As mentioned, the Crossvent is electrically controlled and therefore requires an electrical power source to function properly. It can use either a standard AC electrical outlet or its internal direct current (DC) battery power. When the Crossvent is connected to an AC power outlet, it will automatically default to the AC power source. When AC power is not available, the Crossvent switches to its internal DC battery. The battery operational time is approximately 6 hours when fully charged. The Crossvent's source of operational power is displayed on the liquid crystal display (LCD) screen in the lower left-hand corner. When the battery is within approximately 20 minutes of remaining power, the alarm menu will

TABLE 15.2 Available Features of the Crossvent Models CV-4+, VC-3+, CV-2+, and CV-2i+

	CV-4+	CV-3+	CV-2+	CV-2i+
Display				
C = Color Display; M = Monochrome Display	M	C	C	C
Modes				
Adult	✓	✓		
Pediatric	✓	✓	✓	
Neonatal	✓		✓	✓
Assist/control	✓	✓	✓	✓
SIMV	✓	✓	✓	✓
CPAP	✓	✓	✓	✓
PEEP	✓	✓	✓	✓
SIGH	✓	✓		
Pressure support	✓	✓	✓	✓
Pressure limit	✓	✓	✓	✓
Monitors/Alarms				
Pressure	✓	✓	✓	✓
Rate	✓	✓	✓	✓
Oxygen %	✓	✓	✓	✓
Temperature	✓			
Mean pressure	✓	✓	✓	✓
PEEP	✓	✓	✓	✓
Exhale tidal volume	✓	✓	✓	✓
Exhale minute volume	✓	✓	✓	✓
PWI (pressure wave index)	✓			
Low battery	✓	✓	✓	✓
Low supply pressure	✓	✓	✓	
Apnea	✓	a	a	a

[a]May be alerted to apneic condition by use of other alarms in the alarm menus.
CPAP, Continuous positive airway pressure; *PEEP*, positive end-expiratory pressure; *SIMV*, synchronized intermittent mandatory ventilation.

flash "Low Battery, Connect External Power" on the LCD screen and sound an alarm. The ventilator should be connected to AC power as soon as possible to prevent power loss when the battery charge is depleted. When AC power is detected, the Crossvent will then switch to AC power as its primary source and the internal battery will begin to recharge.

Internal Mechanism/Oxygen Source

The Crossvent requires a compressed-gas source of 31 psi to 75 psi to ensure adequate gas flow to a patient. If the supply pressure falls below the minimum 31 psi, a low source pressure alarm will activate.

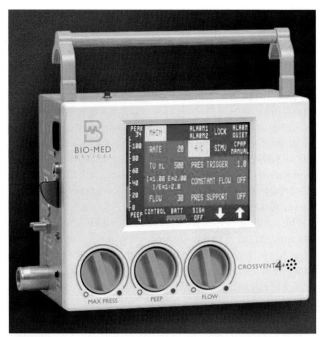

FIGURE 15.2 Bio-Med Crossvent 4+ Ventilator. (Courtesy Bio-Med Devices, Inc., Guilford, Ct.)

An air/oxygen blender can be used to deliver a precise F_IO_2. The output of the blender is connected to the Crossvent's supply inlet connection. For optimum performance the gas sources to the blender should provide 45 to 75 psi of pressure. The Crossvent delivers the oxygen concentration set on the blender. An optional air entrainment module can be used instead of a blender. The air entrainment module offers the ability to deliver 50% oxygen or 100% oxygen to the patient.

Controls and Alarms

The main controls for the Crossvent are located on the front LCD panel of the ventilator (see Fig. 15.2). The operator can either use the touchscreen LCD controls or the three control knobs located below the LCD screen.

Flow Control

The flow-control knob is located on the lower right side of the Crossvent 4+. The inspiratory gas flow ranges from 1 L/min to 120 L/min. The set value is displayed on the ventilator's LCD screen.

PEEP Control

The PEEP control is located to the left of the flow control. The Crossvent can deliver a PEEP/CPAP range of 0 cm H_2O to 35 cm H_2O. Adjusting the PEEP control sets the amount of PEEP or CPAP applied to the exhalation valve. The PEEP level is internally controlled in the Crossvent, which can deliver a PEEP range of 0 cm H_2O to 35 cm H_2O. The sensitivity control automatically compensates for the set level of PEEP, so sensitivity does not have to be readjusted when the PEEP/CPAP level is changed. (*Note*: If the Crossvent is connected to an active gas source and not in use, the PEEP control

TABLE 15.3 Specifications for Bio-Med Crossvent 4+

Control Settings	Range
Modes	CMV, SIMV, Pressure Support, CPAP
Power source	AC power; internal DC battery
Rate	CMV mode 5-150 breaths/min; SIMV mode 0.6-50 breaths/min
Noninvasive ventilation mode	N/A
Flow rate	1-120 L/min
Pressure trigger	−0.2 to −10 cm H_2O
Peak pressure	0-120 cm H_2O
Tidal volume	2-2500 mL
Inspiratory time	0.1-3.0 s
I:E ratio	3:1 to 1:99
PEEP/CPAP	0-35 cm H_2O
Oxygen percent	21-100% oxygen
Pressure support	0-50 cm H_2O
Monitors/displays	LCD screen
Dimensions	10 in H × 11 in W × 5.5 in D, weighs 4.8 kg (10.5 lb)
Gas consumption	4 L/min
Alarms	Peak pressure, high respiratory rate, exhaled tidal volume, PEEP/CPAP, high and low mean airway pressure, high and low oxygen percentage, low battery alarm
Battery duration	6 h when fully charged

CMV, Continuous mandatory ventilation; *CPAP,* continuous positive airway pressure; *D,* deep; *H,* high; *I:E,* inspiratory time to expiratory time; *LCD,* liquid crystal display; *PEEP,* positive end-expiratory pressure; *SIMV,* synchronized intermittent mandatory ventilation; *W,* wide.

should be turned fully counterclockwise to conserve gas supply [Clinical Scenario 15.1]).

Maximum Pressure

The maximum pressure control is located to the left of the PEEP control. Adjusting this knob sets the pressure applied to the exhalation valve and to an internal adjustable pressure-relief valve. The set pressure determines the maximum amount of pressure delivered during patient-triggered or time-triggered mandatory breaths. The maximum pressure control value is adjustable from 0 cm H_2O to 120 cm H_2O. (*Note:* The maximum pressure control value should always be set higher than the set PEEP level to ensure that the correct PEEP level is delivered.)

Display Interface and Menus

Several menus are available and are listed in Box 15.1. A menu item or parameter is selected by touching the desired variable or parameter on the LCD screen. Once the parameter is selected, it is highlighted in yellow for 30 seconds. If no change is made,

CLINICAL SCENARIO 15.1 Using a Crossvent + for Patient Transport

A respiratory therapist uses the Crossvent+ to transport a patient to radiology. Once in radiology the patient is switched to another ventilator, and the Crossvent is placed in the hallway for the return transport back to the ICU.

One hour later the therapist returns to transport the patient but finds the oxygen cylinder that was originally used is completely empty. What is one possible cause for this problem? See Appendix A for the answer.

ICU, Intensive care unit.

BOX 15.1 Crossvent Menus Available on the LCD Screen

- Main menu
- Functions menu
- Primary Alarms menu
- Secondary Alarms menu
- Set Up menu

LCD, Liquid crystal display.

the highlighted area deactivates. Changes in parameters are accomplished by touching the up (↑) and down (↓) arrows located on the lower right-hand side of the screen. It is not necessary to use onscreen arrows to select a menu or mode. These can also be adjusted by simply pressing the desired key (e.g., the SIMV mode key).

The value for flow is displayed in the flow key itself, but it can be adjusted only by using the flow-control knob. The I:E ratio (the ratio of inspiratory time to expiratory time) is a displayed value only. The I:E is calculated from the set rate, V_T, and flow.

On the left side of the screen is a digital display of delivered airway pressures. The top and bottom keys are always available for use unless the setup screen is activated. As shown in Fig. 15.2, the top row of touchscreen keys allows the user to move between menus, as well as silence the alarm and lock the touchscreen. The bottom row provides information on the type of breath that is delivered (i.e., mandatory or spontaneous); operating power source; application of sigh breaths; and the setup screen key.

The LCD has a backlit screen. The default setting ensures that this backlight is always on, but it can be turned off to save battery life. (*Note:* When the backlight is not active, the LCD screen is not viewable.)

Alarms

The Crossvent has three alarm menu screens; alarm menus 1 and 2 are accessed by pressing the corresponding top row of keys located on the LCD screen (see Fig. 15.2). The third alarm menu screen appears only during a specific alarm situation, such as a low battery alarm or a ventilator failure alarm. Available alarms include exhaled V_T, peak inspiratory pressure (PIP), PEEP, mean pressure, low supply pressure, rate, oxygen concentration, and low battery. Table 15.4 provides an alarm overview with ranges and set limits.

TABLE 15.4 Crossvent 4+ Alarm Parameter Ranges and Alarm Limits

Parameter Range	Display Range	SET LIMITS Low	SET LIMITS High
Peak pressure (cm H_2O)	0-125	3-124	4-125
Rate (breaths/min)	0-199	4-159	5-160
Exh. tidal volume (mL)	50-4000	50-3199	51-3200
Exh. minute volume (L)	0-200	0-99	1-100
PEEP/CPAP (cm H_2O)	0-99	0-99	0-100
Mean airway pressure (cm H_2O)	0-125	0-124	1-125
Oxygen (%)	0-100	18-100	19-100

CPAP, Continuous positive airway pressure; *PEEP,* positive end-expiratory pressure.

BOX 15.2 Crossvent Modes of Operation

- Continuous mandatory ventilation (CMV)
- Intermittent Mandatory Ventilation (IMV)
- Continuous Positive Airway Pressure (CPAP)/Manual Ventilation
- Pressure Support Ventilation (PSV)

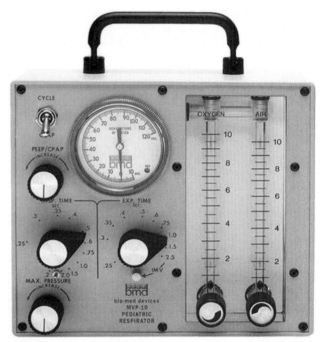

FIGURE 15.3 Bio-Med MVP-10. (Courtesy Bio-Med Devices, Inc., Guilford, CT.)

Modes

The Crossvent provides a variety of ventilatory modes: control, assist CMV, IMV, CPAP, manual ventilation, and PSV (Box 15.2).

Continuous Mandatory Ventilation

The CMV mode provides either patient-triggered or time-triggered mandatory breaths. (*Note:* Crossvent ventilators utilize the term assist/control (A/C) ventilation to designate this mode of ventilation.) The operator can set breaths to be either volume targeted or pressure targeted. The set respiratory rate range in the CMV mode is from 5 breaths/min to 150 breaths/min.

Intermittent Mandatory Ventilation

As is the case with the CMV mode, mandatory breaths during the IMV mode can be patient triggered or time triggered, and volume targeted or pressure targeted as desired. Notice that with IMV, only the set mandatory breaths are delivered at set parameters, whereas the patient's spontaneous effort between mandatory breaths is met by a fresh supply of gas. The set rate range in the IMV mode is 0.6 breaths/min to 50 breaths/min. The sigh breath option is available in the volume-targeted IMV mode and operates as described in the following section.

Sigh Breaths

A sigh breath option is available in the VC-CMV and VC-IMV modes. Once the sigh key is activated through the LCD screen, beginning with the next breath, one sigh breath is provided every 100 breaths or one every 7 minutes, whichever occurs first. The V_T delivered during the sigh breath is equal to 1.5 times the normal set V_T. This is accomplished by increasing the inspiratory time for that breath. The maximum V_T is 2500 mL and an inspiratory time limit of 3 seconds for these sigh breaths. The expiratory time for a sigh breath is also increased to maintain the same I:E ratio for a set ventilator breath.

CPAP/Manual Mode

Gas flow during the CPAP/manual mode is provided for spontaneous breaths at the set PEEP/CPAP level or atmospheric pressure when PEEP/CPAP is set at 0. The manual breath key will initiate one mandatory breath each time the key is pressed, delivering the set V_T and inspiratory time set on the backup rate control. This mode also offers an apnea backup rate. If the patient has a significant apnea episode, the ventilator will switch to a selected rate, V_T, inspiratory time, and F_IO_2.

Pressure Support

The Crossvent 4+ also can provide PS in the IMV and CPAP modes (range: 0 to 50 cm H_2O). When PS is selected, the Crossvent provides the set PS level for the spontaneous breaths.

BIO-MED MVP-10

The Bio-Med MVP-10 (Bio-Med Devices, Inc.) is a gas-powered ventilator that is controlled by a fluidic logic circuit. Breath delivery is time cycled and pressure limited. The MVP-10 was designed for respiratory support of neonatal and pediatric patients, both during transport and in the hospital.[7] It is designed for all applications, ranging up to a 400-mL V_T. It is a continuous-flow ventilator that can operate in IMV or CPAP mode or provide continuous-flow oxygen. The MVP-10 is portable and lightweight. It weighs 2.3 kg (5 lb 2 oz) and measures 8 in H × 9 in W × 3 in D (Fig. 15.3). The MVP-10

TABLE 15.5 Specifications for Bio-Med MVP-10

Control Settings	Range
Modes	IMV, CPAP, or continuous flow oxygen
Power source	Completely pneumatically powered
Rate	0-120 breaths/min
Noninvasive ventilation mode	N/A
Peak pressure range	0-120 cm H_2O
Tidal volume	up to 400 mL
Inspiratory time	0.2-2.0 s
PEEP/CPAP	0-18 cm H_2O
Oxygen percent	21-100%
Pressure support	N/A
Monitors/displays	Analog pressure gauge
Dimensions	8 in × 9 in × 3 in, 2.3 kg (5 lb 2 oz)
Gas consumption	4 L/min
Alarms	N/A
Battery duration	N/A

CPAP, Continuous positive airway pressure; *IMV*, intermittent mandatory ventilation; *PEEP*, positive end-expiratory pressure.

is also available in an MRI-compatible version. Table 15.5 lists important specifications of the MVP-10.

Power Source

The MVP-10 requires medical-grade oxygen and compressed air at 50 psi (±5 psi). The gas sources may be a cylinder or a wall outlet with a Diameter Index Safety System (DISS) connector. The fluidic logic circuits are normally powered by oxygen. If only one source gas is used, it must be connected to the oxygen power line connector in order for the fluidic logic circuits to receive pressurized gas. If compressed air is used in the oxygen power line, the set time intervals are approximately 10% less than if powered by 100% oxygen because of the difference in gas density. A blender may be connected to the oxygen power line. If oxygen and air from a blender are used, a biomedical device (BMD) Y-adapter would be needed.

The fluidic logic consumes approximately 4 L/min of gas supply and needs to be included in gas-supply calculations. Clinical Scenario 15.2 illustrates some examples of calculating oxygen cylinder duration. As seen with other uncompensated transport ventilators, such as the Bio-Med IC-2A, the set inspiratory and expiratory time may also be affected during air transport because of the changes in barometric pressure that occur at different altitudes.

Controls and Alarms

Fig. 15.3 shows the front panel of the MVP-10 and its controls. The primary controls are the mode switch, PEEP/CPAP dial, inspiratory time control, expiratory time control, maximum

 CLINICAL SCENARIO 15.2
Calculation of Cylinder Duration for the Bio-Med MVP-10

You are transporting a infant of 34 weeks' gestation on the MVP-10. You are on 60% F_iO_2, IMV rate of 30, peak pressure 25 cm H_2O, and PEEP 5 cm H_2O. To obtain the desired peak pressure and 60% F_iO_2, you require 2 L/min of oxygen and 2 L/min of air (see Fig. 15.4). You know that the MVP-10 requires 4 L/min of oxygen for logical flow to operate and needs an additional 2 L/min of oxygen for the delivered F_iO_2 for a total oxygen consumption rate of 6 L/min. For the estimated cylinder duration for the MVP-10 in the IMV mode, use the following formula:

Pressure of gas supply = tank pressure × conversion factor

For example:
2200 psig = tank pressure
0.28 = conversion factor for an E cylinder
Volume of gas supply = (2200 psig) (0.28) = 616 L
You can now calculate cylinder duration one of two ways. First you can calculate minutes of duration simply by dividing the needed 6 L/min into the 616 L in the E cylinder Dividing 6 L/min into 616 L, 616/6 = approximately 103 min. To calculate hourly duration, multiply the 6 L/min consumption × 60 min for an hourly consumption of 360 L.

How long will it take for the tank to be completely empty?

616 L/360 L/h = 1.71 h

What if you were now on 100% and required 4 L/min of oxygen to provide the desired peak pressure and F_iO_2? The E cylinder has 1800 psi remaining. How long will the cylinder last?
See Appendix A for the answer.

F_iO_2, Fraction of inspired oxygen; *IMV*, intermittent mandatory ventilation; *PEEP*, positive end-expiratory pressure.

 CLINICAL SCENARIO 15.3 MVP-10

You are transporting a term newborn on the MVP-10 by air with settings of 60% F_iO_2, IMV rate of 30, Peak Pressure of 25 cm H_2O, and PEEP of 5 cm H_2O. The transporter is loaded in the aircraft.

While securing yourself in the aircraft, you note the ventilator is now not cycling. However, the PEEP is being maintained at a level of 5 cm H_2O. The flowmeters show gas flow from both oxygen and compressed air sources. What is a likely cause of the malfunction?
See Appendix A for the answer.

F_iO_2, Fraction of inspired oxygen; *IMV*, intermittent mandatory ventilation; *PEEP*, positive end-expiratory pressure.

pressure dial, and the built-in air/oxygen blender. The MVP-10 has no built-in alarms.

Mode Switch

The cycle/CPAP switch is a two-position switch that enables the selection of either a time-cycled mode or the CPAP position. The ventilator allows a noncycling flow of gas with or without a continuous PEEP. Clinical Scenario 15.3 presents a scenario based on this control.

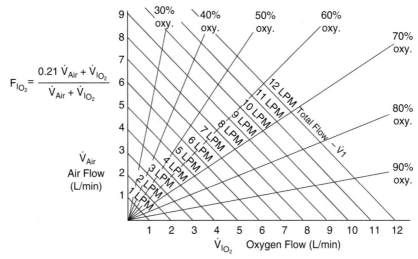

FIGURE 15.4 Bio-Med MVP-10 air–oxygen mixing ratio chart. *LPM,* L/min. (Information from Bio-Med Devices, Inc., Guilford, CT.)

PEEP/CPAP

In adjusting the PEEP/CPAP dial, a positive pressure will be maintained in the patient's ventilator circuit during expiration in either the time-cycled IMV mode or in the CPAP mode. Adjustment of this control places a controlled pressure on the expiration valve while maintaining the set pressure in the patient's circuit during exhalation. The PEEP/CPAP range is variable up to 16 cm H_2O (±4 cm H_2O) at a flow of 6 L/min. The levels of PEEP/CPAP are affected by flow. When flow to the built-in blender is increased, the set pressures may increase somewhat. These changes can be noted on the pressure gauge and readjusted accordingly.

Inspiratory and Expiratory Time Controls

The IMV rate on the MVP-10 is set using the inspiratory and expiratory time controls. The inspiratory time control is adjustable from 0.2 second to 2.0 seconds, whereas the expiratory time control is adjustable from 0.25 second to 2.5 seconds. The inspiratory and expiratory time controls determine the respiratory rate (variable from 0 to 120 breaths/min). The pneumatic logic circuit controls the opening and closing of the expiratory valve, cycling the ventilator into inspiration and expiration. Adjustment of the inspiratory and expiratory time controls determines how quickly the gas pressure builds in the pneumatic logic controller and switches from inspiration to expiration and back to inspiration.

Maximum Pressure Control and Pressure Gauge

The maximum pressure control is used to set the maximum peak pressure to be delivered in the patient circuit during inspiration. This control is located on the back panel of the MVP-10. The maximum pressure that can be set is adjustable up to 70 cm H_2O (±10 cm H_2O), allowing the establishment of a pressure-limited breath mode.

The delivered peak and set PEEP pressures can be observed on the analog pressure gauge, which is designed to show pressure in the patient circuit of −10 cm H_2O to +120 cm H_2O. The MVP-10 is typically used as a pressure-control ventilator. If the set inspiratory flow and inspiratory time are not sufficient

for the set peak pressure to be delivered, the MVP-10 becomes a flow controller.

Oxygen and Air Flowmeters

The MVP-10 has two built-in Thorpe tube flowmeters. Each flowmeter can be adjusted to deliver 0 L/min to 10 L/min of gas. The air and oxygen flowmeters control the level of continuous flow through the patient circuit, in addition to the oxygen concentration. Manipulation of the air and oxygen flowmeters together delivers an approximate F_IO_2. Fig. 15.4 shows a chart (and formula) that can be used to estimate the F_IO_2 delivered based on the set air and oxygen flow rates. For example, a ratio of 1:1 (air-to-oxygen) provides an F_IO_2 of approximately 0.6. (The F_IO_2 can also be estimated using the method for calculating air entrainment ratios described in Fig. 4.20.) It is recommended that the operator carefully measure the F_IO_2 of delivered gas using an external oxygen analyzer because the MVP-10 does not have a built-in oxygen analyzer.

Modes

The MVP-10 has two optional modes of ventilation. The first is IMV, in which the ventilator will time-trigger a pressure-targeted mandatory breath based on the set inspiratory time and rate. For this mode to be activated, the mode switch must be in the cycle position.

The second operational mode is the CPAP mode, in which a continuous supply of gas is provided through the patient circuit at the set level of CPAP.

DRÄGER OXYLOG 3000 PLUS

The Dräger Oxylog 3000 Plus (Drägerwerk Medical AG & Co. KGaA) (Fig. 15.5) is an updated version of the Oxylog 3000 model. The Oxylog 3000 Plus is a time-triggered or patient-triggered, volume-controlled or pressure-controlled, time-cycled ventilator for patients requiring V_T of 50 mL to 2000 mL. The ventilator (excluding the handle) is 11.4 in H × 7.24 in W × 6.89 in D. It weighs 5.8 kg (12.7 lb), including the internal

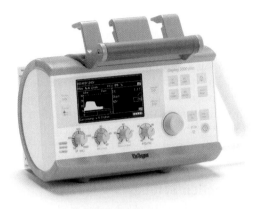

FIGURE 15.5 The Dräger Oxylog 3000 Plus ventilator. (© Drägerwerk AG & Co. KGaA, Lubeck, Germany.)

TABLE 15.6 Specifications of the Dräger Oxylog 3000 Plus

Control Settings	Range
Modes	CMV, SIMV/PS, CPAP/PS, PCV/PS, BiPAP
Power source	AC power, external; 10-32-V power source, internal rechargeable lithium battery
Rate	2-60 breaths/min
Noninvasive ventilation mode	Yes
Peak pressure range	20-100 cm H_2O
Tidal volume	50-2000 mL
Pressure control	3-55 cm H_2O
Inspiratory time	0.2-10 s
PEEP/CPAP	0-20 cm H_2O
Oxygen percent	40-100% oxygen
Pressure support	0-35 cm H_2O
Monitors/displays	Electroluminescence screen
Dimensions	11.4 in × 7.24 in × 6.89 in; 5.8 kg (12.7 lb)
Gas consumption	0.1-0.5 L/min
Alarms	Low Supply Pressure; High Peak Airway Pressure; Low Airway Pressure; Leakage; Apnea; High Frequency
Battery duration	3 h with nickel metal-hydride battery; 4 h with lithium ion battery

BiPAP, Bilevel positive airway pressure; *CMV,* continuous mandatory ventilation; *CPAP,* continuous positive airway pressure; *PCV,* pressure-controlled ventilation; *PEEP,* positive end-expiratory pressure; *PS,* pressure support; *SIMV,* synchronized intermittent mandatory ventilation.

battery.[8] Table 15.6 provides some of the available parameters and features of the Oxylog 3000 Plus.

The Oxylog 3000 Plus has additional optional features not available on the Oxylog 3000. The optional features on the 3000 Plus include the Autoflow mode, integrated end-tidal CO_2 monitoring, data export, and a side handle.

The Autoflow (AF) mode delivers the set V_T using a decelerating flow pattern to achieve the lowest peak airway pressure possible. The Oxylog 3000 Plus determines the pressure required to deliver the set V_T based on lung characteristics (i.e., resistance and compliance relationships) and the patient's spontaneous breathing demand. If the set V_T cannot be achieved and the maximum inspiratory pressure is reached, the alarm V_T *low, pressure limit* is generated. If the V_T is reached (inspiratory flow = 0), before the inspiratory time (T_I) has fully elapsed, the Oxylog 3000 Plus ensures that the patient can draw inspiratory flow during the remaining inspiratory time.

A second additional feature available with the Oxylog 3000 Plus is downloadable data communication though the MEDIBUS protocol only. Measured values available for transfer through these features are graphic recordings, alarms, alarms settings, user settings, and data (trigger) to enable the ventilator graphics monitoring. Finally, the Oxylog 3000 Plus has the additional feature of incorporated end-tidal carbon dioxide monitoring. Additional information about this feature is available by request from Dräger Medical. The Oxylog 3000 Plus also automatically compensates for changes in altitude.

Power Source

The Dräger Oxylog 3000 Plus requires both an electrical power source and a pneumatic power source to properly function. The electronic control system can use three separate electrical power sources:

1. An AC/DC power supply (100 to 240 volts AC (VAC) / (50 to 60 Hz
2. An external 12/24/28 volts DC (VDC) power source via an optional DC/DC converter
3. An internal rechargeable lithium ion battery

When the ventilator is connected to one of the two external power sources, the green "power connected" status light goes on and the rechargeable internal battery pack starts charging regardless of whether the ventilator is on or off. This internal battery is essential for the operation of the machine. The internal battery can provide power for "typical ventilation" for approximately 7.5 hours with the lithium ion battery when fully charged. The internal lithium ion battery requires approximately 4 hours to recharge. (*Note:* The battery pack can be "hot-swapped," which means that it can be replaced by a charged battery within a few seconds without having to restart the ventilator.)

The pneumatic power source requires a high-pressure medical-grade gas (oxygen or air) supplied in a range of 39 psi to 87 psi. The source gas can be derived from a cylinder, wall outlet, or oxygen/air blender with a DISS connector.

Internal Mechanism

High-pressure oxygen enters through the inlet port located on the right side of the Oxylog, and it is immediately filtered and reduced to a constant working pressure by a regulator. The source gas then passes into an electronically controlled pressure regulator, which governs the rate and pattern of flow of the gas. After it passes through the electronically controlled pressure regulator, the gas enters the pneumatic connection block, which internally controls PEEP during exhalation, and with the ventilation accessories provides the interface with the patient. The incoming oxygen supply is also routed to the metering block, which entrains room air through a patented Venturi component, blending it to the desired F_IO_2 (range: 0.4 to 1.0).

Oxygen Supply

The metering block controls the F_IO_2 delivered to the patient. An oxygen concentration of 40% to 100% can be delivered using flows from 9 to 35 L/min. If the flows are less than 9 L/min or greater than 35 L/min, the minimum concentration of 40% can no longer be guaranteed. The internal pneumatic components of the ventilator consume only 0.1 L/min to 0.5 L/min of gas to support their functions, so the bulk of oxygen used is for patient ventilation.

Controls

Start/Standby Key and LED Indicators

The start/standby soft key is located in the lower right-hand corner of the control panel. Pressing this soft key will power up the Oxylog 3000 Plus. To the immediate left of the start/standby soft key are two light-emitting diode (LED) indicators. The Ext Power indicator will illuminate if the ventilator is operating on external power—either AC or external DC power. Just above the Ext Power LED is the charge indicator, which is illuminated in orange when the battery is charging and in green when the battery is fully charged.

Inspiratory Hold

The inspiratory hold soft key is located directly above the start/standby soft key. Depressing the inspiratory hold key will either extend the momentary ventilation breath or start a new inspiratory breath and hold it for a maximum of 15 seconds.

O_2 Inhalation

A 100% O_2 support function is available to help reduce the risk for hypoxia during bronchial suctioning. The O_2 inhalation soft key is located to the left of the inspiratory hold soft key. Depressing this soft key will increase the F_IO_2 to 100% for 3 minutes regardless of the preset F_IO_2. A green LED on the soft key is illuminated when this feature is active. The set F_IO_2 will be automatically restored after the 3-minute period or if the 100% O_2 key is depressed again. (*Note:* If medical air is used as the drive gas, the 100% O_2 function will not deliver pure oxygen.) This feature is designed to help oxygenate before suctioning or intubation in noninvasive positive-pressure ventilation (NIV).

Alarms: Reset and Silence

The alarm reset soft key is located just above the inspiratory hold soft key. Depressing this key will reset all alarms to their set limits and clear the display of any alarm messages.

The alarm silence soft key is located directly above the alarm reset key. Depressing this soft key will silence the alarm condition for 2 minutes. Once the alarm silence key is active, an LED is illuminated on the soft key. If the alarm condition has not been remedied, the alarm will sound again.

Mode Keys

The Oxylog 3000 Plus has four mode soft keys located just above the control dial. Available modes include VC-CMV, VC-SIMV/PS, Spontaneous-CPAP/PS (SPN-CPAP/PS), and PC-SIMV+. The desired default ventilation mode can be set in the "user configuration" menu so that the Oxylog 3000 Plus will begin ventilation in the mode of choice. Activating the soft key for any of the modes of ventilation enables that mode to become operational. The modes are reviewed later in this section.

Rotary Selection/Settings

A rotary control dial is located below the mode soft keys. Used in conjunction with the settings and alarm soft keys, the operator can select desired operating parameters using a process of "select-change-confirm." The operator can select any function or value displayed in the settings or alarm menu by rotating the button until the desired value is highlighted; then by pushing the button to select the desired value; by rotating the button to change the value or function; and, finally, by pushing the button to confirm the new setting. Requiring an active confirmation of a new setting helps support patient safety.

Additional Controls

The O_2% control dial is located to the left of the rotary selection dial. This dial allows adjustment of F_IO_2 from 0.4 to 1.0. As previously mentioned, the Oxylog 3000 Plus blends room air through the Venturi system to achieve the selected F_IO_2, which is displayed on the screen.

The P_{max} control is located to the left of the oxygen control. It allows the operator to set a maximum pressure limit (adjustable range: 20 to 100 cm H_2O).

The frequency control is adjustable from 2 breaths/min to 60 breaths/min. It is color coded to assist the operator in setting a respiratory rate appropriate for the patient's size (Table 15.7). The green range is for infants who weigh from 10 to 20 kg (22 to 44.1 lb) (respiratory rate range: 30 to 40 breaths/min). The blue range is for children 20 to 40 kg (44.1 to 88.2 lb) (respiratory rate range: 20 to 30 breaths/min). The brown range is for adults who weigh more than 40 kg (88.2 lb) (respiratory rate range: 5 to 20 breaths/min).

TABLE 15.7 Oxylog 3000 Plus Color-Coded Settings for Patient Size, Minute Ventilation, and Rate

Color Patient Size Range (kg)	Minute Ventilation	Ventilator Rate
Green (infants) 10-20 kg	0.1-0.3 L	30-40 breaths/min
Blue (children) 20-40 kg	0.3-0.8 L	20-30 breaths/min
Brown (adults) more than 40 kg	0.8-1.5 L	5-20 breaths/min

© Drägerwerk AG & Co. KGaA, Lubeck, Germany.

The V_T control is also color coded in a manner similar to the frequency control. The V_T is adjustable from 50 mL to 2000 mL.

The Oxylog 3000 Plus measures V_T at body temperature and pressure saturated (BTPS) conditions. The Oxylog 3000 Plus can automatically compensate for V_T delivery when altitude changes.

Curves/Volumes (Ventilator Graphics)

The soft keys for generating ventilator graphics are located to the left of the electroluminescence display screen. These soft keys allow the operator to change displayed waveforms to either flow/time or pressure/time. These soft keys also allow for changes in displayed volumes, including the following: minute volume, set frequency, exhaled V_T, PEEP, peak pressure, mean airway pressure, plateau pressure, spontaneous minute volume, spontaneous respiratory rate, and oxygen percentage.

Alarms

The Oxylog 3000 Plus has multiple built-in alarms and has three distinct levels of alarm conditions. Each alarm condition has its own display and audible alert. Box 15.3 provides additional details about the alarm conditions.

The Oxylog 3000 Plus has an auto alarm function to help support quick startup of the ventilator. After ventilation has been initiated, the auto alarm function can be activated in the settings menu. The function "auto alarm limits" sets the alarm limits on the ventilator based on the actual measured values at the time of activation:

- Minute ventilation high alarm (MVhigh) = measured minute ventilation + 2 L/min
- Minute ventilation low alarm (MVlow) = measured minute ventilation − 2 L/min
- Spontaneous frequency alarm (fspn) = measured spontaneous frequency + 5 breaths/min

Supply Pressure Low

This alarm is activated when the supply pressure of the source gas is below 39 psi. Audible and visual alarm indicators are active with this condition.

High Peak Airway Pressure

This alarm is activated when the delivered peak airway pressure exceeds the operator-set limit. The peak airway pressure is adjustable from 20 cm H_2O to 100 cm H_2O and is set with the P_{max} control dial, which was described earlier in this chapter. Audible and visual alarm indicators are active with this condition.

Low Airway Pressure

This alarm is activated when the pressure difference between the delivered peak airway pressure and the expiratory pressure is less than 5 cm H_2O or when the set peak airway pressure is not attained. Audible and visual alarm indicators are active with this condition.

Apnea Alarm

An apnea alarm condition is activated when no respiratory activity is detected. This alarm response time is adjustable from 15 seconds to 60 seconds. Audible and visual alarm indicators are active with this condition.

Leakage

A volume leakage alarm activates when the measured expired V_T is approximately 60% lower than the measured inspired V_T. This alarm is not available in the NIV mode.

High Frequency

The high-frequency alarm is activated when the total respiratory rate exceeds the high respiratory rate limit set by the operator. The adjustable range of the high-frequency alarm is from 2 breaths/min to 60 breaths/min.

Modes of Ventilation

Box 15.4 lists the modes of ventilation available on the Oxylog 3000 Plus. An apnea backup rate is available on the Oxylog 3000 Plus with an adjustable apnea delay activation time from 15 seconds to 60 seconds. When the apnea ventilation activation time (T_{apnea}) is selected, the Dräger 3000 Plus will ask the operator to select a desired apnea rate and V_T to be applied during an apneic event. This means that once set, apnea ventilation will remain unchanged until the values (rate and volume) are changed in the menu.

BOX 15.3   Dräger Oxylog 3000 Plus Alarm Conditions

In the event of an alarm, the red or yellow alarm LED flashes. The alarm message appears on the right of the top line on the screen.

Oxylog 3000 assigns corresponding priority to the alarm message, highlights the text with the appropriate number of exclamation marks, and generates different tone sequences for the respective alarms:

!!! = Warning
!! = Caution
! = Advisory

Warning

A warning is an alarm with top priority. The red alarm LED flashes. Warnings are highlighted by three exclamation marks and displayed in inverted form. The Oxylog 3000 generates a sequence of five tones that sound twice and repeat every 7.5 s.

Caution

A caution is an alarm of medium priority. The yellow alarm LED flashes. Caution messages are highlighted by two exclamation marks. Oxylog 3000 generates a three-tone sequence that is repeated every 20 s.

Advisory

An advisory is a low-priority alarm. The yellow alarm LED lights up. Advisory messages are identified by one exclamation mark. The Oxylog 3000 generates a two-tone alarm sequence that sounds only once.

LED, Light-emitting diode.

BOX 15.4 Oxylog 3000 Plus Modes of Operation

- VC-CMV
- VC-SIMV/PS
- SPN-CPAP/PS
- PC-BIPAP

BIPAP, Bilevel positive airway pressure; *CMV,* continuous mandatory ventilation; *CPAP,* continuous positive airway pressure; *PC,* pressure controlled; *PS,* pressure support; *SIMV,* synchronized intermittent mandatory ventilation; *SPN,* spontaneous; *VC,* volume controlled.

 ## CLINICAL SCENARIO 15.4
Oxylog 3000 Plus

You are asked to transport a 63-year-old male patient from the cardiac catheterization laboratory post stent placement with the Oxylog 3000 Plus. The patient is on an F_IO_2 of 45%, SIMV rate of 14, V_T of 800 mL, and PEEP of 12 cm H_2O. As you enter the patient's settings in the Oxylog 3000 and connect the patient to the Oxylog 3000, an alarm sounds and a message appears in the display window: "PEEP >10 mbar?" What must you do to clear this alarm message?

See Appendix A for the answer.

F_IO_2, Fraction of inspired oxygen; *PEEP,* positive end-expiratory pressure; *SIMV,* synchronized intermittent mandatory ventilation; *V_T,* tidal volume.

VC-CMV (VC-AC)

The VC-CMV mode provides breaths that are patient or time triggered, volume targeted, and time cycled. The controls for respiratory rate (range: 5 to 60 breaths/min) and V_T (range: 50 to 2000 mL) establish a baseline minute ventilation. All breaths deliver the set V_T.

VC-AC is used for patients who can generate some spontaneous effort. Adjustment of the trigger sensitivity is necessary to synchronize with the patient's breathing efforts. Trigger sensitivity is accessed through the settings menu.

VC-SIMV

The VC-SIMV mode provides a maximum number of mandatory breaths and allows the patient to breathe spontaneously between the mandatory breaths. Mandatory breaths can be either time triggered or patient triggered, volume targeted or pressure targeted, and time cycled. Spontaneous breaths can be supplemented with PS. PS breaths are patient triggered, pressure limited, and flow cycled.

Selecting the VC-SIMV mode soft key allows the operator to set an IMV rate ranging from 2 breaths/min to 60 breaths/min and a V_T of 50 mL to 2000 mL. PS is available in this mode from 0 cm H_2O to 35 cm H_2O above baseline (set PEEP). Both PEEP and PS levels can be changed through accessing the settings menu on the display screen. PEEP levels greater than 10 cm H_2O have to be confirmed with an additional step for patient safety (Clinical Scenario 15.4).

PC-BIPAP

PC-BIPAP (bilevel positive airway pressure) is a mode in which the patient can breathe spontaneously at any time, even during the inspiratory inflation cycle. Mandatory breaths are time triggered or patient triggered, pressure targeted, and time cycled. This mode is similar to that found in a high-flow CPAP device because of the presence of an open expiratory valve system.

In the PC-BIPAP mode the operator sets the minimum respiratory rate, inspiratory pressure above PEEP, and the flow trigger. The patient's spontaneous breaths independent of the set mandatory breaths can be assisted with PS. The delivered V_T and minute ventilation may vary, so the operator needs to carefully set minute ventilation alarm limits.

Activating the PC-BIPAP soft key allows the operator to set a rate from 2 breaths/min to 60 breaths/min with an adjustable set inspiratory control pressure value ranging from PEEP 3 cm H_2O to 55 cm H_2O.

SPN-CPAP

The SPN-CPAP mode is used for spontaneously breathing patients who may require only a set level of PEEP to restore their functional residual capacity and possibly reduce work of breathing. The operator sets the desired PEEP level and F_IO_2. PS can also be added.

The apnea backup function is operational in this mode and should be set to provide adequate ventilation if apnea should occur.

Touching the SPN-CPAP soft key allows the operator to set a CPAP level from 0 cm H_2O to 20 cm H_2O. The maximum inspiratory flow for spontaneous breaths is 100 L/min, which includes leakage. The PS level is adjustable, as described earlier, from 0 cm H_2O to 35 cm H_2O relative to the set PEEP level.

ZOLL 731 SERIES EMV+

The Zoll 731 Series EMV+ (Zoll Medical Corporation) is a microprocessor-controlled volume- and pressure-targeted, time- or flow-cycled ventilator. The EMV+ (Fig. 15.6) is indicated for use in the management of infant through adult patients weighing 5 kg (11 lb) or more with acute or chronic respiratory failure. It is appropriate for use in hospitals, aeromedical and ground transport, as well as mass casualty situations. The EMV+ dimensions are 8.0 in W × 12.5 in H × 4.5 in D; it weighs 4.4 kg (9.7 lb).[9] The EMV+ can provide assist/control (A/C), SIMV, and CPAP with and without pressure support. The EMV+ utilizes an internal compressor to help generate gas flow to the patient. Table 15.8 summarizes important features of the EMV+.[9]

Power Source

The 731 EMV+ requires an electric power supply to operate properly. The electronic system can use one of the following three sources to power the microprocessor and its electrical components:

- An internal DC battery
- A 120-V AC outlet (with a converter)
- An external 12- or 24-V DC battery

The EMV+ is designed to use external power when available rather than its internal battery pack. When an acceptable external power source is present, the internal battery pack is

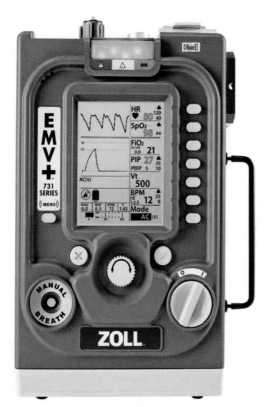

FIGURE 15.6 The Zoll EMV+ 731 Series ventilator. (Courtesy Zoll Medical Corporation, Chelmsford, MA.)

TABLE 15.8 Specifications for the Zoll EMV+ 731 Series Ventilator

Control Settings	Range
Modes	CMV (A/C), SIMV, CPAP with and without Pressure Support and with and without Noninvasive Positive-Pressure Ventilation (NIV)
Breath target	Volume and pressure
Power source	Pneumatic and electric power internal DC battery, external DC battery or 120-V AC outlet (with a converter)
Rate	1-60 breaths/min
Noninvasive ventilation mode	Yes
Peak pressure	80 cm H_2O
Tidal volume	50-1500 mL
Inspiratory time	0.3-3 s
PEEP/CPAP	0-25 cm H_2O external valve
Oxygen percent	21-100%
Pressure support	0-60 (cm H_2O)
Monitors/displays	Alphanumeric display and digital bar graph
Dimensions	12.5 in × 8 in × 4.5 in, weighs approximately 4.4 kg (9.7 lb)
Logic gas consumption	N/A
Alarms	High and Low Tidal, Volume, PEEP not met, Apnea, Low Battery, High and Low Peak Pressure

A/C, Assist/control; *CMV,* continuous mandatory ventilation; *CPAP,* continuous positive airway pressure; *PEEP,* positive end-expiratory pressure; *SIMV,* synchronized intermittent mandatory ventilation.

automatically charged while the unit operates. When an external power failure occurs, the EMV+ automatically switches to its internal battery pack for operating power and activates the EXTERNAL POWER FAILURE alarm; there is no interruption in operation and/or loss of any alarms. When external power returns, operating power automatically switches from internal power to the external source. The internal battery is rated for 10 hours of use.

Internal Mechanism

High-pressure O_2 and/or ambient air enter the device via their respective inlets. A proportional solenoid (PSOL) controls the output flow and timing of O_2 into the manifold. Compressed ambient air is discharged into the manifold via the integrated radial compressor. A microprocessor controls the output of the components to deliver either a volume- or pressure-targeted breath. Pneumotachometers monitor the PSOL and compressor output, providing feedback on the output flow and timing, while a transducer monitors the pressure delivered to the patient's airway.

During inspiration the flow from the PSOL and compressor are proportioned to provide the desired F_1O_2 while achieving the volume or pressure target. Gas from the manifold flows into the patient circuit, causing a pressure rise that displaces the diaphragm in the exhalation valve, which channels the gas flow into the patient. At the end of inspiration, either flow or pressure cycled, the pressure in the diaphragm is released, allowing gas from the patient to exhaust through the exhalation valve. PEEP is maintained by allowing pressure from the

circuit to displace the exhalation valve diaphragm at the end of exhalation to maintain the desired baseline pressure.

Oxygen Source

Oxygen delivery on the EMV+ has a dual means of increasing delivered oxygen percentage via either a high-pressure or low-pressure oxygen source. When a 55-psi high-pressure O_2 source is connected to the high-pressure oxygen inlet, the internal blender allows the F_1O_2 to be set from 21% to 100%.

When the F_1O_2 is set to 21%, the operator may connect a low-flow O_2 source at the Fresh Gas/Emergency Air Intake using the reservoir bag. The EMV+ can use O_2 from low-flow sources, O_2 flow meters, and O_2 concentrators to provide supplemental O_2 to patients. To do this, O_2 is entrained through the Fresh Gas/Emergency Air Intake when the internal compressor of the EMV+ cycles to deliver a breath. To ensure efficient O_2 delivery, the manufacturer recommends that the operator use the Oxygen Reservoir Bag Assembly. This assembly performs a number of functions:

1. It acts a reservoir collecting O_2 during the expiratory phase of ventilation.

2. It provides interface to the ventilator and the attachment of the low-flow O_2 supply hose.

3. It provides an inlet for air in the event the low-flow O_2 supply fails or the V_T is greater than the supplied O_2. O_2 Reservoir mode is indicated on the display with a plus (+) sign next to the F_IO_2 value.

Controls and Displays

The control panel of the EMV++ (see Fig. 15.6) incorporates all controls and the LCD display. The EMV+ controls and indicators facilitate ease of use and visibility in a variety of operating environments. An LCD provides continuous display of control settings, operating conditions, power, and alarm status information (Fig. 15.7). Special designated parameter buttons can be used to control most EMV+ functions. Pressing the PARAMETER button highlights the primary parameter. When the parameter the operator wishes to change is highlighted, the operator turns the Rotary Encoder dial clockwise or counterclockwise to adjust the parameter to the desired value and confirms the new value by pressing the CONFIRM/SELECT button. After this is done, the highlight goes away and the unit begins operation using the new parameter. Details for each control are described in the following sections of the text.

Power On/Off

The power switch is located on the front lower right-hand side of the EMV+. Turning the POWER OFF/ON to the right will apply power. The EMV+ automatically performs a self-check that includes a check for preexisting alarm conditions. The ventilator circuit must be open to ambient atmospheric conditions (not connected to the patient) during start-up. Ventilator operation begins immediately following the self-check. Alarm conditions are checked continuously following the initial start-up. The ventilator will operate on the internal battery with a rated life of 10 hours of continuous use. The battery is capable of achieving 90% recharge in 2 hours.

Heart Rate (HR)

Pressing the HR button highlights the High Heart Rate alarm limit and enables its value to be changed. Pressing the HR button a second time will highlight the current value of the Low Heart Rate Alarm Limit and enable its value to be changed. (*Note*: The HR parameters are functional only when the pulse oximeter is connected.) Both limits are adjustable in 1 beat/min increments. The default value at start-up for the high alarm limit is 120 beats/min; the low alarm limit is 40 beats/min.

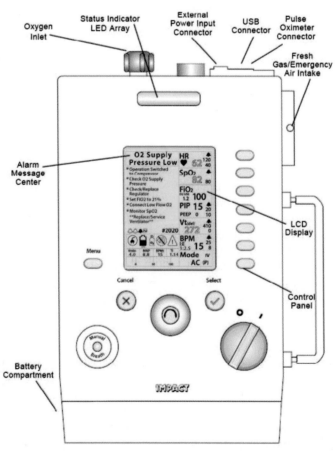

FIGURE 15.7 The EMV+ 731 Series ventilator control panel. *LCD*, Liquid crystal display; *LED*, light-emitting diode. (Courtesy Zoll Medical Corporation, Chelmsford, MA.)

SpO₂

The EMV+ contains a built-in pulse oximeter with alarms. Pressing the SpO₂ (oxygen saturation as measured using pulse oximetry) button highlights the Low SpO₂ Alarm Limit and enables its value to be changed. The SpO₂ display is active only when the pulse oximeter is connected. If the probe is not attached to the patient during start-up or the operator places the pulse oximeter in standby, "stby" will be displayed in the parameter window. The default low SpO₂ value at start-up is 94%.

F₁O₂

Pressing the F₁O₂ button displays the current value and enables this parameter to be changed. There are no adjustable secondary parameters. The default value at start-up is 21% whether O₂ is present or not. If a high-pressure O₂ source is present and an F₁O₂ value greater than 21% is saved for Power Up settings, the unit will start up with that saved F₁O₂ value. If high-pressure O₂ is not present, the unit will start up with F₁O₂ = 21% and O₂ SUPPLY PRESSURE LOW alarm will not be activated. The secondary display in the parameter window is O₂ Use. This is the flow (L/min) of high-pressure O₂ used by the unit to support the patient at the current settings. O₂ Reservoir mode is indicated on the display with a plus "+" sign next to the F₁O₂ value. (The "O₂ Use" value does not include O₂ use in the O₂ Reservoir.)

Peak Inspiratory Pressure (PIP)

In volume-targeted modes the primary field shows the delivered PIP because that value will change dependent on the patient's pulmonary resistance and compliance values. In pressure target modes the PIP target is displayed and can be adjusted. The PIP High Limit, PIP Low Limit, and PEEP are also available as secondary parameters. The High Peak Inspiratory Pressure is adjustable between 10 and 80 (cm H_2O).

Pressure Support

This is the amount of pressure applied for spontaneous pressure-supported breaths, which are available in SIMV and CPAP. The level of set PS can range from 0 to 60 (cm H_2O).

Tidal Volume (V$_T$)

In volume-targeted modes the primary field shows the set V$_T$. The set V$_T$ can be adjusted from 50 to 1500 mL. In pressure-target modes the delivered V$_T$ is shown as outlined text and is based on the patient's pulmonary mechanics. The V$_T$ High and Low Limits are also available as secondary parameters.

Breath Rate (BPM)

Pressing the BPM button highlights the current value and enables it to be changed. The breaths per minute value can be set between 1 and 60 breaths/min.

Secondary parameters include high breath rate, low breath rate, and I:E ratio, which can be adjusted by pressing the CONTROL PARAMETER button the appropriate number of times. By selecting the desired parameter with the Control Parameter selection process, the operator can select which parameter is dependent or independent.

- *Selecting I:E*—results in the ventilator maintaining the I:E ratio while the inspiratory time (T$_I$) varies when the breathing rate is changed.
- *Selecting T$_I$*—maintains a constant inspiratory time while the I:E ratio varies when the rate is changed.

When the EMV+ is operating in CPAP, the patient's actual breathing rate is displayed as the BPM.

Rise time. The EMV+ allows the operator to adjust the time it takes to reach the full inspiratory flow and peak inspiratory pressure during pressure-targeted breathing and when PS is being used. The range is 1 to 10, where 1 is the shortest rise time and 10 is the longest rise time. When the unit is turned on, either the default Rise Time (3) or a User Setting Rise Time will be used. Using the pressure-time waveform as reference will assist the operator in setting the rise time. The rise time settings should be reassessed and adjusted after the patient is placed on the ventilator and initially stabilized. To minimize patient's work of breathing and potential for pressure overshoots, operators must take the following into consideration when setting the rise time:
- Patient's respiratory pattern
- Patient's comfort
- Patient's flow demand
- Resistance (mechanical/physiological)
- Compliance characteristics

The rise time for a passive lung is determined primarily by airway resistance and is fairly independent of compliance. The rise time can be determined by utilizing Table 15.9. An adult patient with high resistance may benefit from a rise time setting of 3 to 4 for optimal breath delivery. Rise times of 8 to 10 are optimized for infants and are flow limited. (The infant circuit is not intended for flows >60 L/min.)

MODE

Pressing the MODE button will highlight the current ventilation mode. Pressing the PARAMETER button again will allow for the selection of volume or pressure targeting, which are shown as either "(V)" for volume or "(P)" for pressure. Selecting volume ensures that a constant volume is delivered to the patient in the inspiratory time using a constant flow. Pressure-targeted ventilation provides a constant airway pressure for the duration of the inspiratory time using a decelerating flow pattern. Turning the Rotary Encoder will toggle between the pressure control mode (P) and the volume control mode (V). Pressing the CONFIRM/SELECT button will lock the type of breath desired. Once the operator selects either a pressure or volume mode, the operator can select from the following

TABLE 15.9 **EMV+ 731 Series Rise Time Determinants**	
Resistance	**Rise Time**
5	1
20	3
50	5
200	10

modes: A/C (i.e., CMV), SIMV with or without pressure support, and CPAP—noninvasive mask CPAP with or without pressure support with automatic leak compensation.

Again, once the mode of ventilation is highlighted, rotating the Rotary Encoder dial will toggle through the options of ventilation offered by the EMV+ Once the correct mode is highlighted, pressing the CONFIRM/SELECT button will lock in that mode of ventilation.

CONFIRM/SELECT

Once a parameter has been adjusted to the desired level, pressing the CONFIRM/SELECT button will confirm the new control setting. This control may also be utilized to select additional parameters from a secondary menu or setting option. The CONFIRM/SELECT button switch is labeled with a green check mark "√."

MANUAL BREATH

Pressing the MANUAL BREATH button delivers one control breath based on the V_T or PIP settings. If the MANUAL BREATH is pressed during inspiration or before baseline is reached in the expiratory period, a manual breath will not be triggered. If there is incomplete exhalation, it will not be possible to trigger a manual breath. This is to prevent accidental breath stacking. When operating in CPAP, a breath is delivered using the PIP value from the Apnea Backup settings.

ROTARY ENCODER

Turning the Rotary Encoder knob will allow the operator to change the value of a selected parameter or highlight a particular menu option such as ventilator rate or PEEP setting.

MUTE/CANCEL

Pressing the MUTE/CANCEL button allows the operator to mute most medium priority alarms, to cancel/acknowledge low priority alarms, or to cancel an action that is no longer desired (e.g., a parameter value change).

Pressing the MUTE/CANCEL button can also be used to cancel any current operation and return to the normal operating screen. The MUTE/CANCEL button switch is labeled with a red "X."

MENU

Pressing the MENU control button provides access to user menus and special functions. The operator uses the rotary encoder to scroll to the desired menu option and presses the CONFIRM/SELECT button to access the menu control. Pressing CONFIRM/SELECT then accesses the parameter variable that is changed by turning the Rotary Encoder to the desired value. To accept the new parameter value, the operator presses the CONFIRM/SELECT (the highlight moves from the parameter variable back to the parameter label). For parameters with multiple options, pressing CONFIRM/SELECT opens a submenu where the various parameters, such as screen contrast and trigger level, are selected using the Rotary Encoder and changed using the process described earlier. At any point the operator can cancel an operation, return to the previous MENU level, or exit the MENU control by pressing the MUTE/CANCEL button.

Alarms

The EMV+ provides a comprehensive set of alarms to alert the operator and guide the operator's actions to resolve the alarm condition and ensure patient safety. At the onset of an alarm, the screen displays the alarm name and then a series of context-sensitive help messages. When multiple alarms occur, they are prioritized and displayed based on the risk to the patient. The number of active alarms is indicated at the bottom of the Alarms Message Center (AMC) as a series of ALARM BELL icons with each bell indicating an active alarm.

Alarms are prioritized based on the risk to the patient. The alarm with the greatest risk to the patient is always presented first. All messages are context based and suggest what is causing the condition and/or how it can be resolved.

Alarm Priorities

Alarm priorities define the operational state of the ventilator regarding its ability to provide mechanical ventilation. The level of the alarm priority is indicated by a three-color LED display, similar to a traffic light (red, yellow, and green), on the top face of the ventilator.

The level of alarm determines what effect pressing the MUTE/CANCEL button has. High and medium priority alarms are highlighted by a red LED indicator located on the top face of the ventilator.

There are three priorities:

1. *High Priority:* Mechanical ventilation under operator control is no longer possible. This alarm category requires immediate intervention by the operator. This includes system failure alarms where the CPU has failed and a backup has taken over to sound the audible and visual alarms. It also includes the situation in which the device is turned on and there is no internal or external power source. Pressing the MUTE/CANCEL button has no effect on the high-priority alarm. The alarm can only be silenced by turning off the ventilator.

2. *Medium Priority:* Mechanical ventilation is active or is possible (maybe for a finite period of time), but there is a failure/fault with the patient, ventilator circuit, a pneumatic subsystem, or pulse oximeter. This alarm category requires immediate intervention by the operator. Pressing the MUTE/CANCEL button mutes medium-priority alarms for 30 seconds. If after 30 seconds the alarm-causing condition still exists, the audible alarm will recur until it is muted again for another 30-second period or resolves.

3. *Low Priority (Advisory):* Safe mechanical ventilation is active, but there is a fault that the operator must be aware of to ensure safe management of the patient and/or ventilator. Low-priority alarms present with both an audible and yellow LED alarm signal alerting the user to the condition. Pressing the MUTE/CANCEL button cancels the audible signal. If the alarm is not resolved, the yellow LED remains illuminated to remind the operator of the fault or failure.

Modes of Ventilation

As previously mentioned, the EMV+ offers a range of modes using both pressure and volume targeting that can be selected to optimally manage mechanical ventilation of the patient. The EMV+ offers CMV, IMV (which can be supported with pressure support), and CPAP. Spontaneous breaths can be either unsupported or supported using pressure support.

In the CMV mode the patient receives either controlled or assisted breaths. When the patient triggers an assisted breath, he or she receives a breath based on either the volume or pressure target. The CMV mode lets the patient initiate mandatory breaths and ultimately controls the total rate of the ventilator. The breaths may be either volume targeted or pressure targeted as set by the operator. The CMV mode breaths are patient triggered or time triggered, volume targeted, and time cycled.

In the IMV mode mandatory breaths are patient triggered or time triggered and volume targeted or pressure targeted as desired. However, with IMV, only the set mandatory breaths are delivered at set parameters, whereas the patient's spontaneous effort between mandatory breaths is met by a fresh supply of gas.

In the CPAP/manual mode, gas flow is provided for spontaneous breaths at the set PEEP/CPAP level or atmospheric pressure when PEEP/CPAP is set at 0.

The MANUAL BREATH button key will initiate one controlled breath each time the key is pressed, delivering the set V_T and inspiratory time set on the backup rate control.

CAREFUSION LTV 1000

The CareFusion LTV (laptop ventilator; CareFusion) is currently available in five models: the LTV 1200, 1000, 950, 900, and 800.[10,11] The LTV 1200 and 1000 ventilators are primarily used in the transport and hospital settings, whereas the 950, 900, and 800 are mainly used in the home care setting. Box 15.5 lists the basic differences among the 1000, 950, 900, and 800. The LTV 950, 900, and 800 are discussed in the home care section of this chapter. The 1200 is also reviewed later. Table 15.10 lists important features of the LTV 1000 and 1200. However, this section's discussion is restricted to the LTV 1000.

BOX 15.5 The Basic Differences in the LTV 1000, 950, 900, and 800 Ventilators

- The 1000 has a built-in oxygen blender and can provide PCV.
- The 950 does not have a built-in blender but does provide PCV.
- The 900 has flow triggering, volume ventilation, and pressure support, but neither the blender nor PCV.
- The LTV 800 and 900 models have volume-targeted mandatory breaths only.
- The 800 is strictly a pressure-trigger, volume-controlled ventilator without PSV.
- "Low Pressure O₂ Source" button is on the LTV 1200 and 1000 but not available with the 800, 900, or 950 models.

PCV, Pressure-controlled ventilation.

The LTV 1000 (Fig. 15.8) is an electrically powered unit that uses an internal rotary compressor to generate gas flow to the patient. On the left side of the unit are the connecting ports for the ventilator (Fig. 15.9). These consist of a power cord connector (*1*), a patient assist call cable or a remote alarm port (*2*), a communications port (*3*), and an oxygen hose connector (*4*). On the same side are two vents. The ventilator uses room air and oxygen to provide gas flow to the patient. The room air enters the ventilator through a large opening covered by a filter (*5*). This opening must not be blocked, or flow to the patient will be restricted. The second, smaller opening allows air to be drawn in to cool the internal components of the unit (*6*). It also must be kept unblocked. The oxygen-connecting port can be attached to either a high-pressure or a low-pressure oxygen source. An example of a high-pressure source is wall oxygen (40 to 70 psig). For low-pressure oxygen sources such as an oxygen concentrator, a female DISS oxygen adapter is available that allows connection

TABLE 15.10 Specifications for CareFusion LTV 1000 and 1200

Control Settings	Range
Modes	CMV (A/C), SIMV, CPAP, NIV, Apnea Backup
Power source	AC power, internal DC power, external DC power
Rate	1-80 breaths/min
Noninvasive ventilation mode	Yes
Peak pressure	120 cm H₂O
Tidal volume	50-2000 mL
Inspiratory time	0.3-9.9 s
PEEP/CPAP	0-20 cm H₂O
Oxygen percent	21-100%
Pressure support	1-60 cm H₂O
Monitors/displays	Digital Airway Pressure Gauge, LED display window
Dimensions	10 in × 12 in × 3 in, 6.1 kg (13.4 lb)
Logic gas consumption	None
Alarms[a]	Apnea Interval, High Respiratory Rate, High PEEP, Low PEEP, High Pressure Limit, High/Low Oxygen Pressure, Low Minute Ventilation, Low Pressure Alarm
Battery duration	Approximately 6 h with external DC battery; 2 h internal battery

[a]Additional alarms detailed in LTV 1200 manual and in the section on the LTV 1000. (*LTV® 1200 Ventilator/MR Conditional LTV® 1200 System operator's manual,* P/N 18247-001, rev. G, Minneapolis, MN, 2009, Pulmonetic Systems.)
A/C, Assist/control; *CMV,* continuous mandatory ventilation; *CPAP,* continuous positive airway pressure; *LED,* light-emitting diode; *NIV,* noninvasive positive-pressure ventilation; *PEEP,* positive end-expiratory pressure; *SIMV,* synchronized intermittent mandatory ventilation.

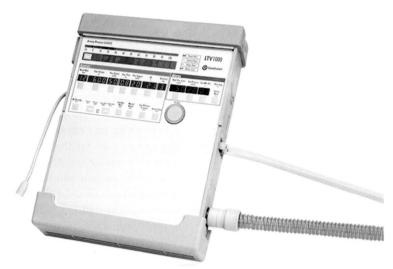

FIGURE 15.8 CareFusion LTV 1000 ventilator. (Courtesy CareFusion, Inc., Yorba Linda, CA.)

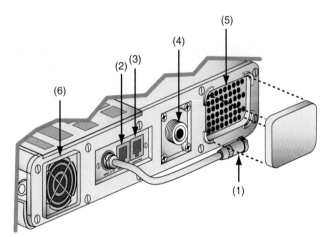

FIGURE 15.9 Left side of CareFusion LTV 1000 ventilator. (Courtesy CareFusion, Inc., Yorba Linda, CA.)

TABLE 15.11 Internal Battery— AC Power Not Connected—LTV Series

When the internal battery is operational, the battery level indicator illuminates. The color code provides information about available charge time remaining.

LED Color	Battery Time[a]	Approximate Internal Battery Level
Green	Acceptable	60 min
Yellow	Low	30 min
Red	Critically low	7 min

[a]Approximate value. Available time depends on currently active ventilator settings. To conserve power, the other screen displays go blank. Only the pressure manometer remains illuminated. *LED,* Light-emitting diode.

to regular oxygen tubing. Other low-pressure O_2 sources might include an O_2 flowmeter attached to a wall outlet or an O_2 cylinder with a regulator and flowmeter attached. (*Note:* The internal oxygen blender is available only on the LTV 1000 and 1200.) Oxygen enters the ventilator and blends with room air in the mixing chamber, which is called an **accumulator/ silencer**. This chamber both blends the gas and acts as an acoustic silencer to reduce compressor noise.

Power Source

The LTV series units are designed to run on AC or DC (12-V) power. Although the unit normally uses an AC power cord adapter, more recently released LTV models have a 6-in pigtail adapter located on the left side of the ventilator (see Fig. 15.9). When connected to an AC power outlet, the internal battery is continuously charged.

For DC power the LTV can use either its own internal battery or one of two available external DC batteries. The internal battery can last approximately 60 minutes when fully charged (Table 15.11). The fully charged large external battery can provide up to approximately 8 hours of power; the smaller

battery, approximately 3 to 4 hours. It takes up to 8 hours to recharge the large external battery when it is completely depleted. (*Note:* An optional auto lighter adapter is also available for LTV use while in a car.)

Patient Circuit

On the right side of the ventilator are the connections for the patient circuit and a small opening for the alarm sound (Fig. 15.10, *[1]*). This alarm opening should not be covered, or the alarm volume will be reduced. There is a 22-mm connector for the main inspiratory flow line (see Fig. 15.10 *[2]*) and a small connector for the exhalation valve line (see Fig. 15.10, *[3]*) that powers the external exhalation valve.

There are also two flow transducer connectors located on the right side (see Fig. 15.10, *[4]*). Two small-gauge gas lines are attached to these connectors and to the two connectors located on the patient Y-adapter. The transducer located by the patient Y-connector is used for flow, volume, and pressure monitoring. A pulse of gas is sent through these lines with each breath during the first minute of ventilation and then once a minute thereafter. This helps keep the lines clear of moisture.

In addition to closing the patient circuit during inspiration, the exhalation valve of the LTV also controls the PEEP levels. This is done by pushing the PEEP valve lock with one hand and rotating the valve with the other to increase and decrease PEEP levels (Fig. 15.11, *detail A*).

Controls and Alarms

The commonly used controls are located on the front panel of the LTV. As with many of the newer ventilators that use built-in microprocessors, some controls are menu driven and are not located on the panel itself but are pulled up on the display window when needed.

Front-Panel Controls

The front panel (Fig. 15.12) contains controls, alarm, and monitoring displays. The controls are divided into two rows.

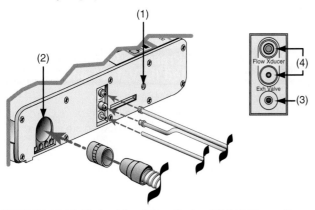

FIGURE 15.10 Right side of CareFusion LTV 1000 ventilator. (Courtesy CareFusion, Inc., Yorba Linda, CA.)

The bottom row contains main function buttons or touchpads, and the upper row contains parameter-setting buttons.

Above the row of parameter controls is a display window that has two main functions. It displays current ventilator data and provides access to additional control functions. To the right of the controls, alarm-setting keys are located. Just below the alarm keys is a set value knob.

The ON/STANDBY button turns the ventilator on and illuminates the LED above it (Box 15.6). The ventilator automatically begins to ventilate the patient by using the last settings. To place the ventilator into standby, the operator presses and holds the button for 3 seconds. As long as the unit is plugged into an AC outlet and placed in standby, the internal battery will be charged.

The SELECT (VOLUME/PRESSURE) button allows the operator to choose either volume-targeted or pressure-targeted breaths. Pressing the button toggles between the two choices. The currently active breath type is continuously illuminated. Pressing the button causes the new selection to flash. A change in breath type is confirmed by pressing the button again. If the button is not pressed to confirm the change, the ventilator simply remains in the current breath type. (*Note:* The LTV 800 and 900 models have only volume-targeted mandatory breaths.)

BOX 15.6 The LTV 1000 Warm-up Period

When the ventilator is first turned on, the transducers need 60 s to warm up to ensure normal function. During this period the message "WARMUP XX" appears in the display window. This message is removed after the warm-up period. The leak test and calibration should not be run during this period.

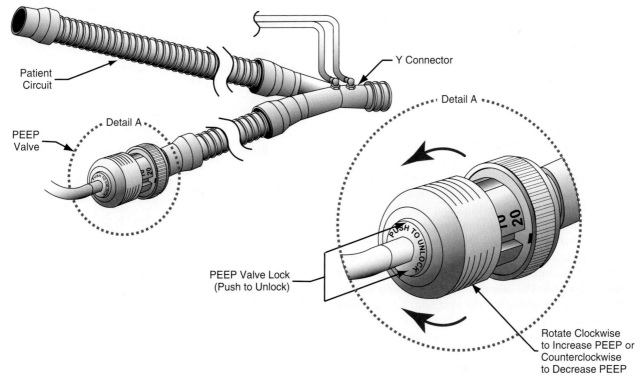

FIGURE 15.11 CareFusion LTV 1000 ventilator's patient circuit. *PEEP,* Positive end-expiratory pressure. (Courtesy CareFusion, Inc., Yorba Linda, CA.)

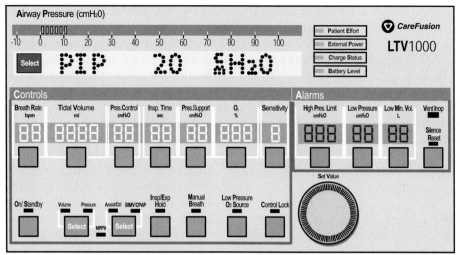

FIGURE 15.12 CareFusion LTV 1000 ventilator's control panel. (Courtesy CareFusion, Inc., Yorba Linda, CA.)

Between the BREATH-TYPE button and the MODE button is an indicator labeled NIV, for noninvasive positive-pressure ventilation. This illuminates when the NIV mode has been selected from the extended features menu. A noninvasive interface, such as a mask, can be used to connect a patient to the LTV during any mode of ventilation. However, when NIV is enabled, some of the alarms are deactivated (see the section "Modes of Ventilation").

The mode-control select provides the options of A/C or SIMV/CPAP. To select a mode, the operator presses the SELECT button. The flashing LED indicates that the mode that is selected will become active if the select key is pressed again.

The INSP/EXP HOLD (inspiratory/expiratory hold) button allows the operator to perform either of these two functions. The operator presses the button and reads the display window (monitoring screen), which will show one of the following: INSP HOLD or EXP HOLD. Pressing the INSP/EXP HOLD button scrolls through the choices on the screen. Following the screen prompts will guide the operator through the desired procedure.

The next control is the MANUAL BREATH button. When this button is pressed, a manual breath based on current volume or pressure settings is delivered to the patient. In addition, a bolus of air purges the flow sensor line.

The low-pressure O_2 source is a feature available only for the LTV 1200 and LTV 1000. Certain changes in alarm features occur when oxygen is supplied from a low-pressure/low-flow O_2 source and the low-pressure O_2 feature is activated (Box 15.7). When the low-pressure/O_2 source is NOT on, a high-pressure oxygen source is expected and gas-blending is done within the ventilator. The delivered O_2 concentration is determined by the O_2% setting on the ventilator's front panel. (*Note:* The ventilator does not have a built-in O_2 analyzer.)

The CONTROL LOCK button allows the screen to be locked so that the settings cannot be accidentally changed. Pushing once turns the lock on. The LED above the CONTROL LOCK illuminates (which means the panel is locked). If the operator tries to change a setting when the panel is locked,

---

BOX 15.7   Low-Pressure O2 Source—Not Installed or Installed (LTV 1000 and 1200)

O_2 Blending Option NOT Installed

Oxygen may still be provided from a low-pressure O_2 source through the low flow inlet, but the following are inactive:

- LOW PRESSURE O_2 SOURCE button
- O_2% control
- Oxygen Inlet Pressure alarms (high and low)

O_2 Blending Option Installed

The LOW PRESSURE O_2 SOURCE button is active only when the oxygen blending option is installed. To activate this option, the operator pushes the LOW PRESSURE O_2 SOURCE button until it is on and its LED illuminated. While it is on:

- The O_2 inlet pressure low alarm is NOT active
- The O_2 pressure high alarm activates when the O_2 source is more than 10 psi
- The % O_2 display shows only dimmed dash lines and the % O_2 cannot be set
- The O_2 inlet flow must be set to obtain the desired O_2%
- O_2% delivery varies with the input O_2 flow (L/min) and the minute volume (V_E) based on the figure below.

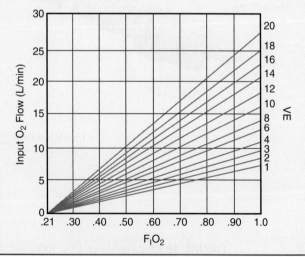

F_IO_2, Fraction of inspired oxygen; *LED*, light-emitting diode.

the display window reads "LOCKED" and the LED flashes. Pressing the "CONTROL LOCK" button again unlocks the screen.

The **HARD** method of locking should be used when children or others may have access to the ventilator, such as in the patient's home. The operator selects "CTRL UNLOCK" from the extended features menu (reviewed later in this section). If **HARD** lock has been selected in this menu, the operator must press the "CONTROL LOCK" button for 3 seconds to unlock the control panel.

The upper row of controls contains the parameter settings such as rate and V_T. The procedure for changing the variables in this row, and in the alarms, is basically the same. The PARAMETER button is touched to make a change. This action brightly illuminates the set value for the parameter and dulls the displays for all other parameters. The "set value" knob is rotated until the desired value appears in the display above the PARAMETER button. The change is immediately active if the set value knob is pressed again or after 5 seconds.

The number in the window above each parameter represents the value set for that parameter. Numbers appear bright when the parameter is active in the current mode and breath type. They appear dim when they are not. A parameter's digital display will also brighten if it is selected for changing. All others then dim. Three parameters—sensitivity, PS, and respiratory rate—can be turned off. The respective display for any of those three parameters will be blank ("- -") when it is turned off.

When the LTV is being powered by the internal battery, after 60 seconds all the digital displays turn off, if no button has been pushed or any controls changed. The displays can be reilluminated by pushing any button or turning the set value knob. Flashing displays will also occur (Box 15.8).

The breath rate control sets the minimum mandatory breath rate (breaths/min). It can be turned off ("- -"). The rate range is 1 to 80 breaths/min. The V_T button controls volume delivery during volume-targeted ventilation (range: 50 to 2000 mL). The T_I button sets the length of inspiration for volume-targeted and pressure-targeted breaths (range: 0.3 to 9.9 seconds). Inspiration cannot be shorter than 300 milliseconds. When V_T or T_I is being adjusted, the calculated flow ($\dot{V}$ calc) is shown in the display window. The peak flow is based on the setting of T_I and V_T (Box 15.9).

PCV (pressure-controlled ventilation) is a feature available in the LTV 1200, 1000, and 950 models. The "PRESS. CONTROL" button establishes the inspiratory pressure for pressure-targeted breaths. The operator pushes the PRESS. CONTROL button and uses the set value knob to change to the desired inspiratory pressure (range: 1 to 99 cm H_2O). This pressure is not added to the baseline PEEP. PEEP/CPAP is set mechanically by using the expiratory/PEEP valve.

The PRESS. SUPPORT button establishes the target pressure above 0 baseline for pressure-supported spontaneous breaths (range: off ["- -"], or 1 to 60 cm H_2O). PS is available for spontaneous breaths with SIMV in either pressure- or volume-targeted ventilation and for CPAP breaths (see the section "Modes of Ventilation").

The $O_2\%$ button establishes the percent O_2 delivery when it is on and a high-pressure oxygen source is available. (*Note:* The low-pressure O_2 button must be in the off position.)

The SENSITIVITY button is used to set the flow-trigger sensitivity level for assisted or spontaneous breaths. The range is off ("- -") and 1 to 9 L/min. The most sensitive setting is 1 L/min. The base flow is preset at 10 L/min and requires no setting by the operator. When a trigger is detected, the patient effort LED illuminates.

There are only a few clinical circumstances in which turning off the sensitivity might be appropriate. For example, if a patient has a large air leak through a bronchopleural fistula (BPF); for example, if the leak resulting from the BPF is more than 15 L/min, even with the sensitivity at 9 L/min (least sensitivity) and leak compensation available (newer models compensate at 6 L/min leak), air may still leak from the system. Large air leaks can prolong inspiration and also result in accidental early triggering of a breath during exhalation (auto-triggering). The leak is falsely seen as a patient effort. In this case it may be appropriate to set a mandatory breath rate and turn the sensitivity off.

In addition to flow triggering, there is a backup pressure-sensing trigger that will pressure trigger a breath in the following circumstances:
- Sensitivity is set between 1 L/min and 9 L/min.
- The ventilator is in exhalation.
- A minimum expiratory time has elapsed (300 milliseconds).
- The airway pressure drops below −3 cm H_2O.

BOX 15.8 Conditions When Displays Will Flash With the LTV 1000

1. When the limit has been reached for a value as the operator is adjusting that value, the display will flash. For example, when setting V_T, if the V_T is set too high for the available peak flow based on the set T_I, the V_T display will flash.
2. A flashing display results when alarm conditions are occurring or an alarm has just occurred.
3. If a control display flashes, a special condition has occurred. For example, PS breaths are normally flow cycled. If a time-cycled PS breath occurs, the PS indicator will flash.
4. The message "Locked" will flash in the display window if someone has tried to change the controls when the panel is locked. It will flash for 3 s.

T_I, Inspiratory time; V_T, tidal volume.

BOX 15.9 Flow Pattern and Peak Flow in the LTV

The flow pattern is automatically set as a descending ramp for all volume-targeted breaths. The peak flow at the beginning of inspiration is calculated by the ventilator such that the tidal volume can be delivered during the set T_I, and inspiration ends when flow drops to 50% of the peak or 10 L/min, whichever is highest. The range of available flow is 10 to 100 L/min for a mandatory breath.

T_I, Inspiratory time.

The leak-compensation feature in newer versions is constantly measuring for leaks and adjusting the baseline of the ventilator to compensate for leaks (up to 6 L/min). For example, if the operator sets the flow sensitivity to 2 L, the ventilator would normally trigger a breath when a 2-L change in baseline (bias flow) was detected during expiration. Suppose a 4-L/min leak exists with a 2-L/min sensitivity setting. The ventilator identifies the 4-L/min leak and adjusts the baseline flow so that the required patient effort is still only 2 L/min to trigger a breath and autotriggering is prevented.

In earlier versions of the LTV 1000, which do not have leak compensation, the sensitivity is usually set higher than the leak measurement. The operator can check the current leak measurement by going into the "RT XDCR DATA" menu and selecting the "LEAK" measurement displayed. For example, if the leak is measured at 2.38 L/min, an appropriate sensitivity setting would be 3 L/min. The difference would represent the trigger (3 − 2.38 = 0.62). An effort of 0.62 L/min would have to be inhaled by the patient from the bias flow to trigger the next breath.

Alarms

The alarm controls and settings are to the right of the parameter controls. The first alarm is the "High Press. Limit" (cm H_2O). This control establishes the maximum pressure allowed in the patient circuit. If the set value is reached, an audible alarm sounds, the display window reads "HIGH PRES," inspiration ends, and the exhalation valve opens. If a high-pressure condition continues for more than 3 seconds, the internal turbine stops rotating and circuit pressure empties to the atmosphere. The audible alarm automatically stops when the pressure drops to the high-pressure limit −5 cm H_2O or drops to a circuit pressure of 25 cm H_2O, whichever is less. To set the high-pressure limit, the operator presses the button and rotates the set value knob to the desired value (range: 5 to 100 cm H_2O).

To set the low-pressure alarm value (cm H_2O), the operator pushes the LOW-PRESSURE button and rotates the set value knob. The actual value appears in the display window. The knob is rotated until the desired value is seen (range: 1 to 60 cm H_2O). The low-pressure alarm has two possible functions. The LTV can apply the low-pressure alarm to all breaths, both spontaneous and mandatory ("ALL BREATHS" selection) or to mandatory breaths only ("VC/PC ONLY" selection). The mandatory breaths can be pressure targeted or volume targeted.

The operator accesses the extended menu functions (discussed later in this section) to set the low-pressure alarm for either all breaths or for mandatory breaths only (Box 15.10). When the LPPS (low peak pressure *spontaneous*) alarm is turned off, the message "LPPS OFF" appears in the display window. Spontaneous breaths have no low-pressure alarm. This is an informational message only. (*Note:* The operator can remove the LPPS Off message from the screen by activating the scroll feature of the display window [Box 15.11].)

The "Low Min. Vol." (LMV) alarm sets the minimum expected exhaled $\dot{V}_E$ (range: Off ["- -"] or 0.1 to 99 L). If $\dot{V}_E$

BOX 15.10   **Low Pressure Alarm Settings: All Breaths Versus Mandatory Breaths**

Assume the ventilator is set with the inspiratory pressure at 25 cm H_2O in SIMV pressure-targeted ventilation with a pressure support of 15 cm H_2O.

If ALL breaths are monitored for low pressure, the operator would set the low pressure alarm to a value lower than the PS level. In this case it might be approximately 10 cm H_2O. If the circuit pressure does not rise to 10 cm H_2O for any breath, the alarm will sound.

If only mandatory breaths were monitored, the operator might set the low pressure alarm at approximately 20 cm H_2O. The alarm would occur only if a mandatory breath's pressure dropped below 20 cm H_2O. The alarm would not be active for spontaneous breaths.

PS, Pressure support; *SIMV,* synchronized intermittent mandatory ventilation.

BOX 15.11   **The Scroll Feature for the LTV**

Double clicking (pressing twice) on the SELECT button adjacent to the display window results in a scrolling of ventilator parameters in the window. For example, peak airway pressure, PEEP, respiratory rate, and other ventilator parameters appear consecutively in the window. Each parameter remains in the window with the current measured value for 2 s, and then the next parameter appears.

When scrolling is active, the "LPPS off" message appears for 2 s as well, notifying the operator that LPPS (low peak pressure spontaneous) is off.

If the operator wants to stop the scrolling to freeze a particular parameter in the window, the operator presses the SELECT button once when the desired parameter is in the window. This allows continuous monitoring of a specific parameter such as respiratory rate.

To reactivate scrolling, simply press the SELECT button twice.

When scrolling is active and the low minute volume alarm is off, the "LMV Alarm off" message appears in the message window in the sequence of ventilator parameters.

PEEP, Positive end-expiratory pressure.

---

drops below the set value, an audible alarm sounds and the message "LOW MIN VOL" appears in the message window. If the low $\dot{V}_E$ alarm is turned to the off ("- -") position, a message will appear saying "LMV-off alarm off" in the display window after 60 seconds. It is an informational message only. The operator can resume scrolling of parameters by pressing the SELECT button twice (see Box 15.11). (*Note:* The LMV alarm is not active in the NIV mode.)

The message "LMV LPPS OFF" appears in the window when both the low $\dot{V}_E$ and low peak pressure for spontaneous breath alarms are off (Clinical Scenario 15.5). The message appears in the window after the disabling of the alarm(s) as a safety feature and at all times, unless scrolling is active. If

CPAP, Continuous positive airway pressure; *LMV,* Low Min. Vol; *LPPS,* low peak pressure spontaneous.

scrolling is active, the message becomes one of the scrolled parameters.

The "Vent Inop" indicator just right of the alarm controls is illuminated only when the ventilator is in the inoperative state. This occurs under the following conditions:

1. The ventilator has been put into standby (i.e., the ON/ STANDBY button is held for 3 seconds).
2. The power sources, either internal or external, are insufficient to operate the ventilator.
3. The ventilator has been turned off.
4. A condition exists that renders the ventilator unable to provide patient ventilation and is unsafe.

When a ventilator inoperative alarm occurs, the inspiratory flow stops; the exhalation valve opens, allowing the patient to breathe spontaneously from room air; the oxygen blender solenoids close; the "INOP" LED is red; and an audible alarm sounds continuously. Another mode of ventilating must be provided for the patient immediately.

The SILENCE/RESET button is used to silence an alarm for 60 seconds. This button can also be used to start a 60-second alarm silence period—for example, before disconnecting the patient for some procedure or when the ventilator is placed in standby. After an alarm condition has been resolved, this button can also be used to clear the visual alarm displays. The SILENCE/RESET button also silences the Vent Inop audible alarm, but the Vent Inop LED will remain lit for at least 5 minutes.

In addition to the alarms described, additional alarm conditions may occur and present an alarm message in the display window.

Set Value Knob

This knob allows adjustment of the numerical values of the ventilator parameters and alarms, and it scrolls through menu items that appear in the display window.

Airway Pressure Bar Graph and Display Window

At the very top of the operating panel is the airway pressure display. This horizontal bar graph displays the pressure in the patient circuit (range: −10 to +108 cm H_2O).

The display window shows monitored data, alarm messages, and the extended features menu. During normal operation the monitored data are presented sequentially. Table 15.12 provides a list of monitored data tand how the values are calculated. Each item is displayed for 3 seconds.

TABLE 15.12 LTV 1000 (and 1200) Monitored Data

Parameter	Description
PIP	Peak inspiratory pressure (cm H_2O). Greatest pressure measured during inspiration and the first 300 ms of exhalation.
MAP	Mean airway pressure (cm H_2O). Calculation of mean airway pressure for the last 60 s, displayed in 10-s intervals.
PEEP	Positive end-expiratory pressure (cm H_2O). The measured pressure at the end of exhalation.
f	Total respiratory rate per minute based on the last 8 breaths. Updated every 20 s. Includes all breath types.
Vte	Measured exhaled tidal volume. Measured and displayed at the end of each exhalation.
V_E	Minute volume monitor displays the exhaled tidal volume for the last 60 s as calculated from the last 8 breaths. Recalculated and displayed every 20 s or the completion of every exhalation, whichever occurs first.
I:E	Displays the calculated ratio of inspiration to expiration with the smaller of the two reduced to a value of 1. Displays regular and inverse ratios.
$\dot{V}$calc	The calculated peak flow, which occurs at the beginning of the breath for a volume-targeted breath (not included with pressure ventilation). The calculation is based on set V_T, T_I, and a predetermined minimum flow at the end of inspiration. Flow normally drops in a descending ramp fashion to 50% of the calculated peak or 10 L/min, whichever is greater.

T_I, Inspiratory time; V_T, tidal volume.

Select Button—Display Screen

The SELECT button to the left of the display screen has several functions. It is used to stop the normal scrolling of monitored ventilator parameters. Pushing the button once while the normal data scan is active halts the screen with the current parameter data showing. Each time the button is pushed after that, the next data item in the list is displayed. Scanning can be resumed by pressing the button twice within 3 seconds.

The extended features menu is selected by pushing the SELECT button for 3 seconds. The first menu item is displayed in the window (see the section "Extended Features," which follows the next section).

Front-Panel Indicators

To the right of the pressure manometer are four indicators. The patient effort indicator illuminates when the ventilator detects a patient's inspiratory effort based on the sensitivity setting. The external power illuminates when the unit is

TABLE 15.13 Battery Charge Status and LED Color Indicators (Charge Status LED)— LTV Series

LED Color	Charge Status
Flashing yellow	The ventilator is performing precharge qualification testing of the internal battery before beginning the charging procedure. Occurs when the external power is first applied to the unit. Takes from a few seconds to an hour on a very depleted battery
Green	Internal battery fully charged
Yellow	Internal battery is being charged but has not reached a full charge level
Red	The internal battery cannot be charged. The ventilator has detected a charge fault or internal battery fault. Remove from service, and contact a certified service technician

LED, Light-emitting diode.

CLINICAL SCENARIO 15.6

You are transporting a patient with the LTV 1200 with an SIMV/PS rate of 8 breaths/min; the peak flow measured by the ventilator is 35 L/min. The flow termination is set at 10%. At what flow will inspiratory flow end?
  See Appendix A for the answer.

PS, Pressure support; *SIMV*, synchronized intermittent mandatory ventilation.

operating from an external power source. This can be an AC power source or an external battery. The adjacent LED is green when power is adequate and yellow when external power is low. Table 15.11 and Table 15.13 provide information on the battery-charging status and related indicator colors.

Extended Features

Other than the alarms available on the operating panel, the extended features menu accesses additional alarm controls. Several other functions are available through this menu, including oxygen cylinder duration calculation. The extended features menu can be accessed by pushing the SELECT button for 3 seconds. The first menu item is displayed in the window. While scrolling through the features menu, the operator will come to a useful tool for transport operation. The LTV 1200 and 1000 have built-in oxygen cylinder duration calculators. The operator only needs to select the cylinder size and pressure in the cylinder in pounds per square inch (psi), and the cylinder duration will be calculated with the current settings. Users are advised to follow the ventilator maintenance procedures outlined in the operator's manual provided by the manufacturer for viewing the following: transducer autozero, real-time transducer data, event trace, and ventilator maintenance.

Breath Types

As with other ventilators, the LTV series distinguishes between breath type and mode. For example, breaths can be volume targeted or pressure targeted. Each of these breath types is available in the A/C mode or SIMV mode.

There are four breath types in the LTV unit: volume control, pressure control, PS, and spontaneous. To select volume or pressure breaths, the operator toggles the SELECT—VOLUME (or) PRESSURE button to establish breath type (bottom row of controls).

Volume-controlled breaths are patient triggered (flow or pressure), time triggered, or manually triggered. The limiting

value is the set V_T. Flow is delivered in a descending ramp waveform. The cycling method is T_I. The operator can also set breath rate, O_2%, and sensitivity.

Pressure-controlled breaths are also patient triggered, time triggered, or manually triggered. (*Note:* The LTV 900 and 800 do not have pressure control.) The target inspiratory pressure is set with the "PRESS. CONTROL" button (cm H_2O). The target pressure is the maximum pressure delivered by the ventilator during inspiration and is NOT additive to PEEP.

PEEP is set by the mechanical PEEP valve located on the expiratory valve. For example, if the pressure control is set to 25 cm H_2O and the PEEP is at 5 cm H_2O, the normal pressure reached during inspiration will be 25 cm H_2O. Baseline pressure will be 5 cm H_2O. The usual cycle mechanism for a pressure-controlled breath is time. Breath rate, T_I, O_2%, and sensitivity are also set.

If desired, the operator can select flow cycling for pressure-controlled breaths rather than time cycling by activating the flow-termination percent feature through the extended features menu. Flow-cycling percent can be adjusted from 10% to 40% of peak flow. The default setting is 25%. For example, if the peak flow during inspiration is 50 L/min and the flow-cycling setting is 25%, inspiratory flow ends when the flow drops to 12.5 L/min (25% of 50 L/min). A pressure-controlled breath will time cycle unless the flow-termination setting occurs before the set inspiratory time elapses. If a long T_I is set, such as 1.5 seconds, it is more likely that the flow will drop to the set flow-termination point before 1.5 seconds have elapsed.

A rise-time profile can also be set with pressure control to taper pressure and flow delivery at the beginning of inspiration. This is also selected by using the extended features menu. The default setting for rise time is profile no. 4. (*Note:* The fastest rise-time setting is no. 1, and the slowest is no. 9.)

PS breaths are patient triggered, pressure limited, and flow cycled. As with pressure-controlled breaths, PS assumes a 0 baseline, so the set value is not added to the PEEP pressure as in most other ventilators. Flow cycling can be adjusted by using the flow-termination feature described earlier. A default of 3 L/min is preset so that inspiratory flow cannot drop lower than 3 L/min (Clinical Scenario 15.6).

PS breaths are time cycled if T_I exceeds the time termination limit (range: 0.3 to 3 seconds), which is set through the extended features menu. PS breaths will also time cycle if T_I exceeds the length of two breath periods. The "PRESS. SUPPORT" display will flash briefly when a breath is time cycled. As with pressure control, the rise-time profile may be selected from the extended features menu for PSV.

CLINICAL SCENARIO 15.7

A physician wants his patient weaned from mandatory breaths and orders a pressure support of 12 cm H_2O plus a PEEP of 3 cm H_2O for a total inspiratory pressure of 15 cm H_2O. How would the therapist adjust these values on the LTV 1000? See Appendix A for the answer.

PEEP, Positive end-expiratory pressure.

BOX 15.12 Alarms Available During NIV With the LTV[a]

- High pressure
- Internal battery low
- Apnea alarm and Apnea backup
- Internal battery empty ventilation
- Sense line disconnected
- Vent Inop
- External power low
- Defaults

[a]All other alarms are disabled. The displays for low minute volume and low peak pressure are set to dimmed dashes, showing they are not active.
NIV, Noninvasive positive-pressure ventilation.

Spontaneous breaths are designed to meet patient demand and maintain the circuit pressure at the measured PEEP value from the previous breath. The breath is cycled when the flow drops below 10% of the maximum flow measured during inspiration or 2 L/min, whichever occurs first. Spontaneous breaths will also time cycle if the breath time exceeds two breath periods.

Modes of Ventilation

The LTV series ventilator provides the following modes of ventilation: CMV, IMV, CPAP, apnea backup ventilation, and NIV.

CMV is available when the "ASSIST/CTRL" LED is illuminated near the mode SELECT button. The manufacturer considers control to be active when the sensitivity is set to off ("−"). However, there is seldom a good reason to make a ventilator insensitive to the patient (see previous discussion on sensitivity setting).

Assist/control is considered active when a value greater than 0 sensitivity is set. The breath type is established by the BREATH-TYPE SELECT button (volume targeted or pressure targeted). The minimum rate is set by the breath rate control. The patient can trigger additional mandatory breaths.

The IMV mode is active when the "IMV/CPAP" LED is illuminated near the MODE-SELECT button. The breath rate (1 to 80 breaths/min) establishes the maximum mandatory breath rate. Patients can spontaneously breathe between mandatory breaths. Spontaneous breaths can be from the set baseline pressure (0 or PEEP) and can also be supported with PS.

CPAP is considered the active mode if the "IMV/CPAP" LED is illuminated and the Breath Rate is off ("−"). In CPAP, spontaneous breaths can be from the baseline pressure and can also be given PS (Clinical Scenario 15.7).

Apnea backup ventilation is available should the patient become apneic. The apnea interval can be set using the extended features menu. The ventilator begins apnea backup ventilation in the A/C mode based on the current settings. The active controls are displayed at full intensity, and others are dimmed. If the set breath rate is greater than or equal to 12 breaths/min, the apnea breath rate is the set breath rate. If the set breath rate is less than 12 breaths/min and the breath rate is not limited by other control settings, the apnea breath rate is 12 breaths/min. If the set breath rate is limited to less than 12 breaths/min, because of V_T, flow, and T_I settings, the apnea breath rate is the highest allowed rate. Normal ventilation resumes when two consecutive patient-triggered breaths occur or when the operator resets the apnea alarm using the silence/reset control.

NIV is provided as a secondary mode that may be selected in addition to the primary ventilation mode. NIV is selected through the extended features menu, and specific alarms are available (Box 15.12). When activated, ventilation is delivered according to the selected mode and breath type that are currently active. The NIV LED is lit when it is on. The number of alarms in NIV is limited when it is active.

Special Features

One of the optional features of the LTV series is a monitor screen that provides several display windows, including scalars, loops, and data. Fig. 15.13 shows the waveform screen with scalars for pressure-time, flow-time, and volume-time displayed. The screen can be frozen to view an event or scaled to size the waveforms. Another screen provides pressure-volume and flow-volume loops.

The data screen displays information normally scrolled in the display window of the operating panel. The data include PIP, PEEP, Vte (exhaled tidal volume), mean airway pressure (P_{aw}), f (respiratory rate), $\dot{V}_E$, I:E, $\dot{V}$ calc, and peak flow. The right side of the data screen lists information on current parameter and alarm settings and also settings of the items available in the special features menu such as flow termination and rise time. The advantage of having a monitoring screen is the easy and immediate access to information, including trends.

Troubleshooting

To prevent difficulties in ventilator operation, it is appropriate to run the ventilator checkout tests before the LTV is used on a new patient and following a circuit change. Before running the checkout tests, the patient circuit and all related components should be attached. The patient should be disconnected from the unit during any testing.

General Troubleshooting

The exhalation valve is cleaned during regular maintenance. This valve is delicate and needs to be handled carefully. If apparent leak problems occur and the circuit does not pass the leak test, the operator should be sure the exhalation valve diaphragm is correctly seated.

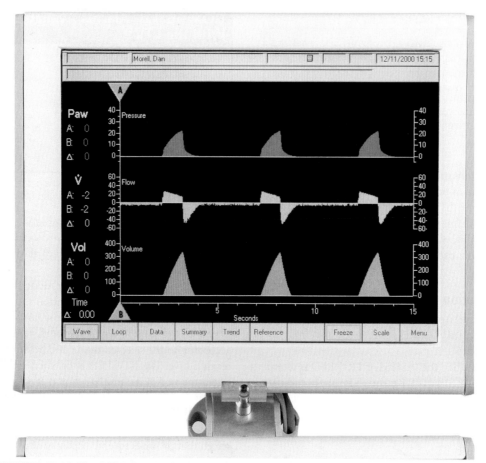

FIGURE 15.13 The LTM Graphics Monitor. The "communications port" on the LTV series ventilators (900, 950 and the 1000) allows for attachment to this monitor. (Courtesy CareFusion, Inc., Yorba Linda, CA.)

The operator's manual contains a section on troubleshooting that is symptom based. For example, suppose a control does not operate. The manual explains that the control may not be active in the current mode or breath type. Or the controls could be locked. Or perhaps the control has not been "selected" by pushing the associated button. The user is advised to review the suggestions listed in the troubleshooting section of the operator's manual for more detail.

CAREFUSION LTV 1200

The LTV 1200 (CareFusion) is similar to the LTV 1000 ventilator. It also features an electromechanical pneumatic turbine system under the control of a microprocessor, which delivers patient ventilation. The turbine technology allows the ventilator to operate without a compressed-gas source. This section focuses on the LTV 1200 and will illustrate differences between it and the LTV 1000.

The LTV 1200 ventilator (Fig. 15.14) is designed for use on adults and pediatric patients who weigh a minimum of 5 kg (11 lb) and who need either invasive or noninvasive ventilation. The dimensions of the LTV 1200 are 10 in × 12 in × 3 in, and it weighs 6.1 kg (13.4 lb).[11]

The internal mechanisms, operating controls, modes, alarms, and features are similar to those found on the LTV 1000

ventilator. Currently the LTV 1200 has a method to present ventilator settings for rapid patient setup that is not available on other models of the LTV. (See also the operations section that follows shortly.)

Power Source

Like the LTV 1000, the LTV 1200 ventilator is designed to run on a 110-V or 220-V AC power source, or an 11-V to 15-V DC power source. This may be an external battery or a DC power system. When connected to an AC power outlet, the internal battery is continuously charged.

For DC power the LTV can use either its own internal battery or one of many available external DC batteries. The internal battery can last approximately 60 minutes when fully charged. An external lithium ion battery is available for transport and hospital that lasts 3 hours each and the UPS (universal power supply) that lasts 4 hours fully charged. There is also an optional auto lighter adapter that enables the use of the LTV unit while in a car.

Internal Mechanism

The internal mechanism of operation is similar to that of the LTV 1000. Room air is drawn into the LTV unit from a flexible foam inlet filter on the side of the LTV unit. Once past the filter, the air then enters an accumulator/

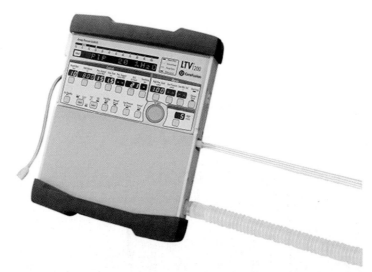

FIGURE 15.14 CareFusion LTV 1200 ventilator. (Courtesy CareFusion, Inc., Yorba Linda, CA.)

silencer, where it mixes with oxygen supplied from the oxygen blender.

The gas flow then enters a rotary compressor, where the gas is pressurized to deliver the correct flow rate and pressure needed to meet the set parameters. Unlike the case with the LTV 1000, the PEEP control is internal in the LTV 1200. A PEEP transducer is used in conjunction with the airway pressure transducer and monitored by the LTV's software to deliver the set PEEP level. The PEEP on the LTV 1200 is adjusted on the front panel of the unit.

Oxygen Source

Both the LTV 1200 and 1000 have a dual means of increasing delivered oxygen percentage via either a high-pressure or a low-pressure oxygen source.

In the LTV 1200, oxygen blending requires a high-pressure source and is active only when the low-pressure O_2 source is not selected. The high-pressure system is controlled by the O_2% (O_2 flush) button. (The O_2 flush control is described later in this section.)

When the low-pressure O_2 source is selected, the oxygen percentage display window will display dimmed dashes (–) and cannot be adjusted. The low-pressure oxygen source allows oxygen to be supplied from a low-pressure source such as a flowmeter or an oxygen concentrator. The percentage of oxygen delivered is not regulated by the ventilator but is instead dependent on the oxygen inlet flow and the total minute ventilation set on the ventilator. See Box 15.7 for a description and illustration of the approximate delivered F_IO_2 based on the set minute ventilation and the oxygen flow. As with any bleed-in system, it is recommended that a calibrated oxygen analyzer be used to determine the exact delivered F_IO_2.

Operations

To turn on the LTV 1200, the operator presses the ON/STANDBY button. The front panel (Fig. 15.15) will illuminate, and an audible alarm will activate for 1 second. If the "patient query" function is active, the message "SAME PATIENT" is

displayed in the LED window. If this is the same patient, a press of the SELECT button will begin ventilation with the settings used during the last power-down.

If this is a new patient, the operator should turn the set value knob until "NEW PATIENT" is displayed, then press the SELECT button. A new query will then be displayed in the LED window, asking the operator if this patient is an adult, pediatric, or infant patient. The operator should then turn the set value knob until the desired patient type is displayed. Pressing the SELECT button again will cause the ventilator to begin ventilating with appropriate preset settings for the selected patient type. If the patient query function is turned off, the ventilator will begin to immediately ventilate the patient with the settings set during the last power-down.

Controls and Alarms

The commonly used controls are located on the front panel of the LTV. As with many of the newer ventilators that use built-in microprocessors, some controls are menu driven and are not located on the panel itself but are pulled up on the display window when needed.

Front-Panel Controls

The front-panel diagram (see Fig. 15.15) shows how the controls and displays are arranged. The controls are divided into two rows. The bottom row contains main function buttons or touch pads, and the upper row contains parameter-setting buttons.

Above the row of parameter controls is a display window, which has two main functions. It displays current ventilator data and provides access to additional control functions. Alarm setting keys are located to the right of the controls. Just below the alarm keys is a set value knob. Table 15.14 lists the five types of controls available with the LTV 1200 ventilator.

Select (Volume/Pressure) Button

As in the LTV 1000, this control allows the operator to choose either volume-targeted or pressure-targeted breaths. (See the

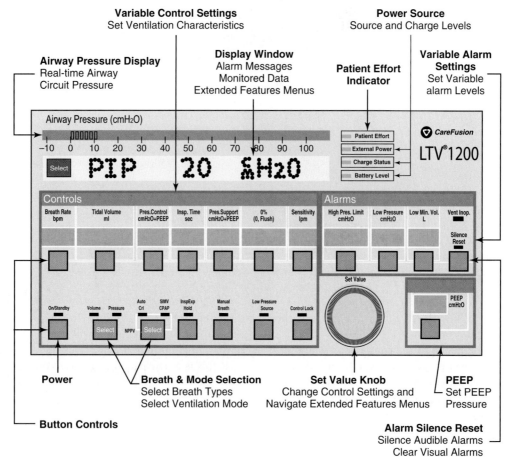

FIGURE 15.15 CareFusion LTV 1200 ventilator's control panel. *PEEP,* Positive end-expiratory pressure. (Courtesy CareFusion, Inc., Yorba Linda, CA.)

TABLE 15.14 Five Types of Controls on the LTV 1200 Ventilator	
Types of Controls	**Description**
Variable controls	Controls and alarms that have front-panel displays
Buttons	Push buttons that select an option or perform a function
Set value knob	Used to set control values and navigate extended features menus
Extended features	Ventilation options that do not have front-panel controls but are available through a special menu
Mechanical cords	Controls, such as Over Pressure Relief, that are hardware regulated and not operator adjustable

section "Front-Panel Controls" in the LTV 1000 section for more information on this control.)

Select Mode Control

The mode control select provides the options of A/C or IMV/CPAP and NIV. It is similar in function to the same control on the LTV 1000 with the following differences. Each press of the button advances or confirms your selection as follows:

- One press selects the first mode in the series (A/C) and the associated LED flashes. A second press confirms the selection, and the associated LED lights solid green.
- If you press the button again, the IMV/CPAP LED flashes. Pressing again confirms and causes the IMV/CPAP LED to solid light green.
- Press once more to select NIV mode, and the NIV LED flashes. To confirm NIV mode, you must press the button again, but be aware that the NIV LED will continue to flash until the inspiratory positive airway pressure (IPAP) and expiratory positive airway pressure (EPAP) values have been set.
- *Note:* The LTV 1000 toggles only between A/C and IMV. NIV is selected from the menu function.

Inspiratory/Expiratory Hold Button

The INSPIRATORY/EXPIRATORY HOLD button allows the operator to perform either of these two functions. The operator presses the button and reads the display window (monitoring screen), which will show one of the following: "INSP HOLD" or "EXP HOLD." If the operator presses the INSP/

EXP HOLD button, to the operator can scroll through the choices on the screen.

Manual Breath Button

When the MANUAL BREATH button is pressed, a manual breath with volume and pressure based on current settings is delivered to the patient. In addition, a bolus of air purges the flow sensor line.

Low-Pressure O₂ Source Button

When selected, this option allows oxygen to be supplied from a low-pressure/low-flow oxygen source, such as an oxygen concentrator or a line-mounted flowmeter. Oxygen from the low-pressure source is mixed with air inside the ventilator. The O_2 percentage delivered to the patient is determined by the O_2 inlet flow and the total minute volume and is not regulated by the ventilator.

When the low-pressure O_2 source option is selected and a high O_2 pressure source is attached to the ventilator, an automatic high O_2 switchover safety response generates a "HIGH O_2 PRES" alarm, switches the ventilator to high-pressure O_2 source mode, and sets the percentage of oxygen to be delivered in the gas flow to 21%. When the low-pressure O_2 source option is not selected, a high-pressure oxygen source is expected, and oxygen blending is done within the ventilator. The ventilator expects an oxygen source with a pressure of 40 psi to 80 psi. The O_2 percent delivered to the patient is determined by the O_2% setting on the ventilator's front panel.

Selecting the low-pressure O_2 source. To select this option, the operator pushes and holds the LOW-PRESSURE O_2 SOURCE button for 3 seconds. As the low-pressure O_2 source is being selected, the associated LED will be flashing. Once the low-pressure O_2 source has been selected, the associated LED will remain on continually.

While the low-pressure O_2 source is on, the O_2 inlet pressure low alarm is inactive, but the O_2 pressure high alarm is set to activate at more than 10 psi. The O_2% (O_2 flush) display will display dimmed dashes, and O_2% cannot be set. To set the desired oxygen percentage, the flow of oxygen inlet must be adjusted.

O₂% (O₂ Flush) Button

The O_2% (O_2 FLUSH) button is a dual-function control (O_2% **and** O_2 FLUSH). When the button is being used to set the percentage of oxygen delivered by the ventilator through the oxygen-blending system (O_2%), the operator pushes and releases the O_2% (O_2 FLUSH) button, and changes the setting with the set value knob. When the button is being used to elevate the F_1O_2 to 100% for a preset period of time (O_2 flush), the operator pushes and holds the O_2% (O_2 FLUSH) button for 3 seconds.

The O_2% control establishes the percentage of oxygen to be delivered through the oxygen-blending system.

PEEP Control

Adjustment of the PEEP on the LTV 1200 is different from adjustment of the externally mounted PEEP valve on the LTV

1000. On the LTV 1200 the operator pushes the PEEP control button, which highlights the PEEP LED window. The PEEP level can be adjusted by turning the set value knob to the desired level and then confirming by pressing the PEEP control button. The adjustable range of PEEP is 0 cm H_2O to 20 cm H_2O. The LTV 1200 has PEEP-compensated PS and pressure control.

Upper-Row Parameters

The upper row of controls contains the parameter settings such as rate and V_T. The procedure for changing the variables in this row, and in the alarms, is basically the same as for the lower row. The PARAMETER button is touched to make a change. This action brightly illuminates the set value for the parameter and dulls the displays for all other parameters. The set value knob is rotated until the value desired appears in the display above the PARAMETER button. The change is immediately active when the desired PARAMETER button is pressed again or after 5 seconds.

The number in the window above each parameter represents the value set for that parameter. Numbers appear bright when the parameter is active in the current mode and breath type. They appear dim when they are not. A parameter's digital display will also brighten if it is selected for changing. All others then dim.

Three parameters—sensitivity, PS, and respiratory rate—can be turned off. The respective display for any of those three parameters will be blank ("- -") when it is turned off.

When the LTV is being powered by the internal battery, after 60 seconds all the digital displays turn off if no button has been pushed or any control changed. The displays can be reilluminated by pushing any button or turning the set value knob. Flashing displays will also occur.

Breath rate. The breath rate control sets the minimum mandatory breath rate (in breaths/min). It can be turned off, so that the breaths LED display will show dashes ("- -"). The rate range is 1 to 80 breaths/min. The process for selecting the desired rate is similar to that described with the PEEP control on the LTV 1200. Pressing the BREATH RATE button will brighten the breaths LED. The operator turns the select value knob to the desired rate, then confirms by pressing the BREATH RATE button again.

Tidal volume. The TIDAL VOLUME button controls volume delivery during volume-targeted ventilation. The adjustable V_T range is from 50 mL to 2000 mL. Pressing the TIDAL VOLUME button will brighten the V_T display LED. The operator turns the select value knob until the desired V_T is displayed, then confirms by pressing the TIDAL VOLUME button again.

Pressure control button. The PRESS. CONTROL button establishes the inspiratory pressure for pressure-targeted breaths. The operator pushes the PRESS. CONTROL button and uses the set value knob to change to the desired inspiratory pressure (range: 1 to 99 cm H_2O). With the LTV 1000 this pressure is not added to the baseline PEEP. PEEP/CPAP is set mechanically by using the expiratory/PEEP valve. However, in the LTV 1200, pressure is automatically set above the PEEP level.

Inspiratory time. The "Insp Time" control sets the length of inspiration for volume-targeted and pressure-targeted breaths (range: 0.3 to 9.9 seconds). Inspiration cannot be shorter than 300 milliseconds. When V_T or T_I is being adjusted, the calculated flow ($\dot{V}calc$) is shown in the display window. The peak flow is based on the setting of T_I and V_T.

Pressure support. The PRESS. SUPPORT button control establishes the target pressure above baseline for pressure-supported spontaneous breaths (range: off ["- -"] or 1 to 60 cm H_2O). For the LTV 1000 unit the baseline will always be 0, whereas for the LTV 1200 the PS level will be above PEEP level. PS is available for spontaneous breaths with SIMV in either pressure-targeted or volume-targeted ventilation and for CPAP breaths (see the section "Modes of Ventilation").

O_2% button. The O_2% button establishes the percentage of O_2 delivery when it is on and a high-pressure oxygen source is available. If the operator presses the O_2 button, this will highlight the LED window; the operator must then rotate the set value knob to the desired percentage. Pressing the O_2 button again will confirm the new setting. The LED display will return to the normal intensity as will all other active parameters. (*Note:* The low-pressure O_2 button must be in the off position.)

Sensitivity

The SENSITIVITY button is used to set the flow-trigger sensitivity level for assisted or spontaneous breaths. The range goes from off ("- -") up to 1 L/min to 9 L/min. The most sensitive setting is 1 L/min. The base flow is preset at 10 L/min and requires no setting by the operator. When a trigger is detected, the patient effort LED illuminates. (See the section on the LTV 1000 for additional information on sensitivity.)

Leak compensation. The leak-compensation feature enables constant monitoring for leaks and adjustment of the baseline of the ventilator to compensate for leaks (up to 6 L/min). (See earlier discussion.)

Alarms. The alarm controls and settings are to the right of the parameter controls. These alarms are similar to those described with the LTV 1000 ventilator in the preceding section.

Airway pressure bar graph and display window. At the very top of the operating panel is the airway pressure display. This horizontal bar graph displays the pressure in the patient circuit (range: −10 to +108 cm H_2O).

The display window displays monitored data, alarm messages, and the extended features menu. During normal operation the monitored data are presented sequentially. Each item is displayed for 3 seconds. See Table 15.12 for a complete list of displayed items.

Select Button—Display Screen

As is the case with the LTV 1000, the SELECT button to the left of the display screen has several functions. It is used to stop the normal scrolling of monitored ventilator parameters. If the button is pushed once while the normal data scan is active, this halts the screen with the current parameter data showing. Each time the button is pushed after that, the next

data item in the list is displayed. Scanning can be resumed by pressing the button twice within 3 seconds.

Breath Types and Modes of Ventilation

As with the LTV 1000, the LTV 1200 has specific breath types and modes. The reader is directed to the preceding section on the LTV 1000 to learn about these two features. Only the differences are reviewed here.

If desired, the operator can select flow cycling for pressure-controlled (PC) breaths rather than time cycling by activating the flow termination percent feature using the extended features menu. The flow-cycling percent can be adjusted from 10% to 40% of peak flow. With the LTV 1200, the default setting is made in terms of the patient type selected (i.e., adult, pediatric, or infant) when the machine is powered on, or it can be adjusted in the extended features menu.

The LTV series ventilator provides the following modes of ventilation: CMV, IMV, CPAP, apnea backup ventilation, and NIV. These modes are described in the preceding section on the LTV 1000 ventilator.

On the LTV 1200 unit, NIV can be easily set up on the front panel as discussed earlier with the LTV 1000. With NIV used in the LTV 1000 and 1200, masks must be *nonvented* to operate correctly and not consume excess gas supply.

Additional Features

Two additional features are accessed through the extended features mode. The extended features menu is selected by pushing the SELECT button for 3 seconds. The first menu item is displayed in the window. Scrolling through the features menu, the operator will find a useful tool for transport operation. The LTV 1200 and 1000 have built-in oxygen cylinder duration calculators. The operator needs to select only the cylinder size and pressure in psi and the cylinder duration will be calculated with the current settings. As is the case with any procedure, readers are directed to consult the manufacturer's manual for the particular ventilator they are using.

With the LTV 1200 an additional feature found in the extended menu is a spontaneous breathing trial (SBT) mode. With the SBT option the operator can temporarily minimize ventilatory support and perform clinical assessments of a patient's dependence on, or ability to be removed from, positive-pressure ventilation (PPV). The SBT mode should be used only when a respiratory therapist or other properly trained and qualified personnel are present.

CAREFUSION REVEL

The CareFusion ReVel (CareFusion) is the Palm Top Ventilator (PTV) based on the LTV series ventilators. The ReVel is electrically powered and incorporates an ActivCore blower technology to power the ventilator (Fig. 15.16). It is designed for critical care transport for pediatric patients ($\geq$5 kg [11 lb]) to adult patients. The ReVel's dimensions are 11.3 in high × 7.1 in wide × 3.3 in deep, and it weighs 4.5 kg (9.9 lb).[12] The ReVel offers CMV, IMV, CPAP plus Pressure Support, NIV, and Apnea Backup. The operator interface is based on the LTV

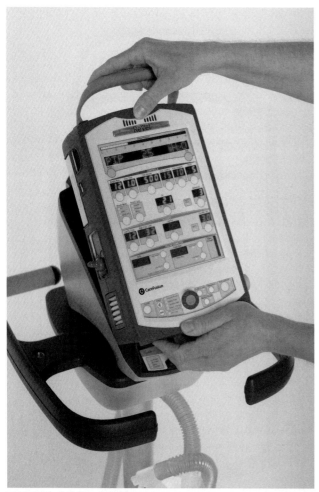

FIGURE 15.16 CareFusion ReVel ventilator. (Courtesy Care-Fusion, Inc., Yorba Linda, CA.)

TABLE 15.15 Specifications for CareFusion ReVel

Control Settings	Range
Modes	Volume Control, Pressure Control, PRVC (Pressure-Regulated Volume Control), PRVS (Pressure-Regulated Volume Support), Pressure Support, Spontaneous
Power source	AC power, internal DC power, external DC power
Rate	1-80 breaths/min
Noninvasive ventilation mode	Yes
Peak pressure	120 cm H_2O
Tidal volume	50-2000 mL
Inspiratory time	0.3-9.9 s
PEEP/CPAP	0-20 cm H_2O
Oxygen percent	21-100%
Pressure support	1-60 cm H_2O
Monitors/displays	Digital Airway Pressure Gauge, LED display window
Dimensions	11.3 in high × 7.1 in wide × 3.3 in deep, 4.5 kg (9.9 lb)
Logic gas consumption	None
Alarms	Apnea, High Pressure, High Frequency, High PEEP, High Pulse, High SpO_2, Low F_IO_2, Low Minute Volume, Low Peak Pressure, Low PEEP, Low Pulse, Low SpO_2
Battery duration	4-h internal battery (hot swappable)

F_IO_2, Fraction of inspired oxygen; *LED*, light-emitting diode; *PEEP*, positive end-expiratory pressure; *SpO_2*, oxygen saturation as measured using pulse oximetry.

Series Ventilator platform. Table 15.15 lists modes, ventilator parameters, and other features of the CareFusion ReVel specifications.

Power Source

The ReVel series ventilators are designed to run on AC or DC (12-V) power. When connected to an AC power outlet, the internal battery is continuously charged. The ventilator normally operates from external DC power. There is an external power port on the side of the ventilator enabling direct connection to a number of approved external DC power sources. The ReVel also has an optional portable docking station to recharge the ventilator. A removable DC battery pack powers the unit.

The design of the battery pack allows the operator to easily pull and hot swap the battery from its bay and replace it with another charged battery without interruption of ventilation. While the removable battery pack is being changed, the internal transition battery provides power to the ventilator for up to 1 minute. Both the removable battery pack and the transition battery are charged when an approved external DC power source is connected to the ventilator. (*Note*: An optional auto

lighter adapter is also available for using the ReVel ventilator while in a car.)

Internal Mechanism

The ReVel ventilator is powered by the ActivCore blower technology. The ActivCore blower draws room air into the accumulator/filter, where it is mixed with oxygen from the O_2 blender module. Room air from the ActivCore blower is delivered through a filter and bias valve to the inspiratory limb of the patient circuit in a flow pattern to achieve the set patient settings.

A flow transducer downstream of the pneumatic system provides flow feedback to the pneumatic system processor. The exhalation control module closes the exhalation valve during inspiration to direct the air to the patient.

During exhalation the pneumatic system delivers bias flow and the exhalation valve is servo controlled to achieve the desired amount of PEEP. During exhalation, flow is monitored through the patient flow transducer to detect patient triggering. With leak compensation enabled, the pneumatic system ensures minimal work of breathing by delivering bias flow at the intended level above leak flow, thereby maintaining PEEP and patient triggering sensitivity, even in the presence of large patient leaks. Patient flows are sensed by monitoring the differential pressure across a patient flow transducer. The patient flow transducer design is a fixed orifice integrated into the patient. This design achieves sensitive breath detection and minimal dead space while adding robustness. It also reduces the costs of replacing/cleaning the flow sensor. Differential pressure from the patient flow transducer is returned to the ventilator via the sense lines, where the pressure transducer module determines both the airway pressure and the patient flow. The transducers on the pressure transducer module are regularly auto-zeroed to ensure accurate performance throughout changing environmental conditions, such as patient transport.

A safety valve is incorporated into the inspiratory port to ensure that the patient does not receive excessive pressure in the event that the expiratory limb gets blocked, and to allow the patient to inspire spontaneously if the ventilator is inoperative.

Oxygen Source

The oxygen connecting port can be attached to either a high-pressure or a low-pressure oxygen source. An example of a high-pressure source is wall oxygen (40 to 70 psig). For low-pressure oxygen sources, such as an oxygen concentrator, a female DISS oxygen adapter is available that allows connection to regular oxygen tubing. When the O_2% control is set to LPS (low pressure source), oxygen can be supplied from a low-pressure/low-flow oxygen source of less than 10 psi (<69 BAR, <69 kPa) such as a flowmeter. The blended gas delivery can be monitored with an external F_IO_2 sensor and the values displayed on the user interface. When high-pressure oxygen is attached to the O_2 inlet port, the ventilator is able to drive a nebulizer to deliver aerosolized drugs to the patient while at the same time compensating for the added gas delivery.

Operations

To activate the ReVel the operator must push the ON/OFF button located on the lower left-hand side of the front face of the ventilator (Fig. 15.17). The LED on this control button will then illuminate. The ventilator will then go through its diagnostics before setting the patient's ventilator settings

To initiate mechanical ventilation on the ReVel, the operator has two options similar to the LTV 1200. Normal ventilation can be initiated using either the patient ventilation settings that were in effect the last time the ventilator was powered down (SAME PATIENT), or ventilation controls and alarm configurations/limits automatically set to initial values clinically appropriate for a new patient (NEW PATIENT). To adjust any ventilator parameter, the operator need only follow the same Select-Adjust-Confirm found on the LTV control panel (see the LTV 1200 section earlier).

- *To turn the ventilator off:* Push and hold the ON/OFF button for 3 seconds. A Vent Inoperative alarm occurs and the Vent Inop LED is illuminated. To silence the alarm and

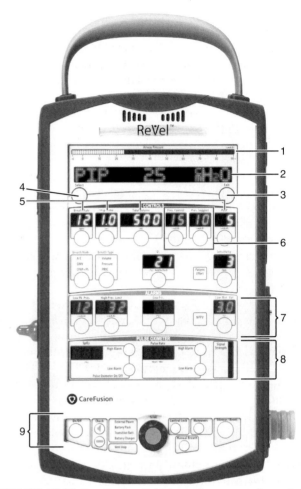

FIGURE 15.17 CareFusion ReVel ventilator control panel. *(1)* Airway pressure display. *(2)* Display window. *(3)* Exit button for extended features. *(4)* "Select" button for patient setup, extended features, and manual scrolling. *(5)* Highlighted controls are active. *(6)* Dimmed controls are *not* active. *(7)* Alarm displays for low peak, high pressure, low fraction of inspired oxygen (F_IO_2), low exhaled minimum volume (Ve). *(8)* Optional pulse oximeter. *(9)* Power, scroll knob, power status, control lock, maneuvers, manual breath, and alarm silence/reset. (Courtesy CareFusion, Inc., Yorba Linda, CA.)

extinguish the Vent Inop LED, the operator needs to push the SILENCE/RESET button.

Controls and Alarms

The commonly used controls are located on the front panel of the ReVel. As with many of the newer ventilators that use built-in microprocessors, some controls are menu driven and are not located on the panel itself but are pulled up on the display window when needed. There are three main types of ventilation and alarm controls on the ReVel front and lower interface panels: adjustable controls, push buttons, and scroll knob.

The face of the ReVel can be broken down to into two sections: the lower interface panel and upper front panel, which contain the airway pressure manometer, display window, control panel, alarms panel, and pulse oximeter panel.

Front-Panel Controls

The front-panel diagram (see Fig. 15.17) shows how the controls and displays are arranged on the ReVel ventilator. The controls are divided into two rows. The bottom row contains main function buttons or touchpads, and the upper row contains parameter display/setting LEDs.

Above the row of parameter controls is a display window, which has two main functions. It displays current ventilator data and provides access to additional control functions similar to the LTV series ventilators.

Located just above the display window is the alphanumeric, dot matrix LED display airway pressure manometer bar, which shows developed ventilator pressures during operation. The range of the airway pressure manometer is -6 cm H_2O to $90+$ cm H_2O.

Each illuminated LED represents a pressure increment of 2 cm H_2O, except for $90+$, which represents air pressure of 90 cm H_2O or higher.

Display window. The display window near the top of the front panel is an alphanumeric LED array that displays multiple types of information in a prioritized (highest to lowest) order, including Alarm Messages, Alert Messages Battery/Power Check Information, Test Results, Startup/Extended Features Menus, and Monitored Data, which can be displayed as automatically scrolling or paused on a selected parameter.

Below and to the left of the Display Window is the SELECT button. The SELECT button has several functions. It is used to stop the normal scrolling of monitored ventilator parameters. If the button is pushed once while the normal data scan is active, this halts the screen with the current parameter data showing. Each time the button is pushed after that, the next data item in the list is displayed. Scanning can be resumed by pressing the button twice within 3 seconds.

Below and to the right of the Display window is the EXIT button. The EXIT button is used to restart automatic scrolling of monitored data on the LED display window, exit Standby mode, and exit Startup and Extended Features menus or configuration settings displayed (without changing the setting).

Control panel. Most of the ventilator's front panel adjustable ventilation and alarm limit controls use a simple three-step method of "Select, Change, and Confirm" to set configuration values similar to the LTV ventilator series. The number in the window above each parameter represents the value set for that parameter. Numbers appear bright when the parameter is active in the current mode and breath type. They appear dim when they are not. A parameter's digital display will also brighten if it is selected for changing.

Three parameters—sensitivity, PS, and respiratory rate—can be turned off. The respective display for any of those three parameters will be blank ("- -") when it is turned off.

Selecting the desired parameter needing to be changed, such as breath rate, entails the following process. The operator presses the soft key below the desire parameter. The selected parameter LED will remain bright while the remaining parameter LEDs will be dimmed.

Rotating the Scroll knob located at the bottom of the ReVel will change the value of the desired parameter. Once the desired value is attained, the operator will then press the soft key below that selected parameter to confirm the new value. At this point all other LED parameter indicators will be brighten to normal levels.

Table 15.16 shows the parameters that can be adjusted on the ReVel ventilator.

Control panel parameters. There are eight adjustable parameters and three indicator controls contained in the control panel. All are adjustable except for the Patient Effort indicator. The Patient Effort LED indicator is illuminated (green) briefly each time a patient triggers a breath.

Breath rate. The breath rate control sets the minimum mandatory breath rate (in breaths/min). It can be turned off, so that the breaths LED display will show dashes ("- -"). The rate range is 1 breath/min to a maximum of 80 breaths/min. The process for selecting the desired rate is described earlier using the select-change-confirm process.

Pressing the BREATH RATE button will brighten the breaths LED. The operator turns the scroll knob to the desired rate, then confirms by pressing the BREATH RATE button again.

Inspiratory time. The "Insp Time" control sets the length of inspiration for VC-CMV, PC-CMV, and PRVC (pressure-regulated volume control) breaths with an adjustable range of 0.3 to 9.9 seconds. When V_T or T_I is being adjusted, the calculated flow ($\dot{V}$calc) is shown in the display window. The peak flow is calculated based on the settings of T_I and V_T. Inspiration cannot be shorter than 300 milliseconds.

Tidal volume. The TIDAL VOLUME button controls volume delivery during volume-targeted ventilation. The adjustable V_T range is from 50 mL to 2000 mL. Pressing the TIDAL VOLUME button will brighten the V_T display LED. The operator turns the scroll knob until the desired V_T is displayed, then confirms by pressing the TIDAL VOLUME button again.

Pressure control. The PRESS. CONTROL button establishes the inspiratory pressure for pressure-targeted breaths. The operator pushes the PRESS. CONTROL button and uses the set value knob to change to the desired inspiratory pressure (range: 1 to 99 cm H_2O). With the ReVel, pressure control setting is automatically set above the PEEP level.

Pressure support. The PRESS. SUPPORT button control establishes the target pressure above baseline for pressure-supported spontaneous breaths (range: off ("- -") or 1 to 60 cm H_2O). For the ReVel the PS level will be above PEEP level. PS is available for spontaneous breaths with SIMV in either pressure-targeted or volume-targeted ventilation and for CPAP breaths. The Pressure Support control is inactive in CPAP+PS (PRVC) mode. Support breaths are delivered as PRVS (pressure-regulated volume support) breaths.

PEEP control. On the ReVel the operator pushes the PEEP control button, which highlights the PEEP LED window. Adjustment of the PEEP level is accomplished by turning the Scroll knob to the desired level and then confirming by pressing the PEEP control button. The adjustable range of PEEP is 0 to 20 cm H_2O. The ReVel has PEEP-compensated PS and pressure control.

O_2% and flush control. The O_2 control is a dual-function control, because it is also used for the O_2 flush procedure

TABLE 15.16   Adjustable Parameters for the CareFusion ReVel Ventilator

Controls	BREATH MODE AND TYPE										
	Intubated Patient Interface									Noninvasive Patient Interface (NPPV)	
	A/C + Volume	A/C + Pressure	A/C + PRVC	SIMV + Volume	SIMV + Pressure	SIMV + PRVC	CPAP + PS + Volume	CPAP + PS + Pressure	CPAP + PS + PRVC	A/C + Pressure	CPAP + PS Pressure
Bias Flow[a]	X	X	X	X	X	X	X	X	X	X	X
Breath Rate	X	X	X	X	X	X	X		X	X	
Flow Term[a]		X[b]	X[b]	X	X	X	X	X	X	X[b]	X
Insp. Time	X	X	X	X	X	X	X	X	X	X	
Leak Comp[a]	X	X	X	X	X	X	X	X	X	X	X
O₂	X	X	X	X	X	X	X	X	X	X	X
PC Flow Term[a]		X	X		X	X				X	
PEEP	X	X	X	X	X	X	X	X	X	X	X
Pres. Trigger[a]	X	X	X	X	X	X	X	X	X	X	X
Pres. Control		X			X					X	
Pres. Support				X	X	X	X	X	X		X
Rise Time[a]		X	X	X	X	X	X	X	X	X	X
Sensitivity	X	X	X	X	X	X	X	X	X	X	X
Tidal Volume	X		X	X		X			X		
Time Term[a]				X	X	X	X	X			X

[a]Control accessed while in normal ventilation modes through the Extended Features menus.
[b]Available when Pressure Control Flow Termination (PC Flow Term) is on.
A/C, Assist/control; *CPAP*, continuous positive airway pressure; *NPPV*, noninvasive positive-pressure ventilation; *PEEP*, positive end-expiratory pressure; *PRVC*, pressure-regulated volume control; *PS*, pressure support; *SIMV*, synchronized intermittent mandatory ventilation.
Information from CareFusion, Inc., Yorba Linda, CA.

described later. The O₂% control button establishes the percentage of O_2 delivery when it is on and a high-pressure oxygen source is available. If the operator presses the O_2 button, this will highlight the LED window; the operator must then rotate the Scroll knob to the desired percentage. Pressing the O_2 button again will confirm the new setting.

The LED display will return to the normal intensity, as will all other active parameters. When an O_2 flush procedure is started, displayed monitored values will stop scrolling in the front panel display window, and the percentage of O_2 increased and the remaining time for the procedure (beginning at the set duration of time and reducing every second and minute until no time is left) is displayed.

Additionally, the total percentage of oxygen being delivered to the patient will be flashed in the O_2 control display window while the procedure is being performed.

Sensitivity control. The Sensitivity control is used to set the flow-trigger sensitivity level for assisted or spontaneous breaths. The range goes from off ("- -") up to 1 to 9 L/min. The most sensitive setting is 1 L/min, and 9 L/min is the least sensitive for flow triggering.

The ReVel may also be set to enable pressure triggering by the patient. A P in the display window indicates that pressure triggering is enabled and flow triggers are disabled. The base flow is preset at 10 L/min and requires no setting by the operator. When a trigger is detected, the patient effort LED illuminates.

Breath mode. The Breath Mode control is used to select between the following ventilation breath modes: CMV, IMV, and CPAP+PS. Selecting the breath mode entails pressing the soft key and turning the scroll knob until the LED next to the desired mode is highlighted. Pressing the soft key will then activate that mode.

Breath type. The Breath Type control is used to select between the following ventilation breath types: Volume, Pressure, or PRVC. Selection of the desired breath type follows the process noted earlier with the Breath Mode selection process (see Table 15.16).

Front-Panel Alarms

The ReVel ventilator generates several unique types of audible alarm and signal notification sound patterns. The volume at which these are generated depends upon on the type of sound and the set audible volume level. Table 15.17 shows the different levels and sounds of alarms provided by the ReVel ventilator. There are four adjustable alarms and one mode indicator found on the ReVel front panel. They are adjusted and set with the previously described select-adjust-confirm process.

Low peak pressure. The Low Pk. Pres. (Low Peak Pressure) control is used to set the low peak pressure alarm limit value. The adjustable range of this alarm is 1 to 60 cm H_2O in increments of 1, or "- -" (off).

High airway pressure limit. The High Pres. Limit (High Airway Pressure Limit) control is used to set the high airway pressure limit alarm value. The range of this alarm is 5 to 100 cm H_2O in increments of 1 cm H_2O.

TABLE 15.17 ReVel Alarm Levels and Signs

Alarm/Signal Sound Type	Sound Pattern	Audible Volume Level
Vent Inop alarm	A continuously repeated group of 8 pulsed tones	Sounds at fixed volume of 80 ± 5 dBA
High Priority alarm	Continuously repeated groups of 10 pulsed tones (3-2-3-2)	Sounds between >45 dBa and 80 ± 5 dBA, and is automatically adjusted to a higher audible volume level than that of Low Priority alarms
Medium Priority alarm	A continuously repeated group of 3 pulsed tones	
Low Priority alarm	A continuously repeated group of 2 pulsed tones	Sounds between >45 dBa and <80 ± 5 dBA, and is automatically adjusted to a lower audible volume level than that of High and Medium Priority alarms
Accessory Attach signal	A group of 2, ascending-pitch, pulsed tones	
Key Click signal	A single medium-frequency note	
Battery Use alarm	A periodic audible tone, once per minute	Sounds at set Battery Use Tone volume
SpO₂ Pulse Tone signal	A single audible tone, repeated for each pulse detected	Sounds at set Pulse Tone volume

SpO₂, Oxygen saturation as measured using pulse oximetry. Information from CareFusion, Inc., Yorba Linda, CA.

Low F_lO_2. The Low F_lO_2 control is used to set the low F_lO_2 alarm limit value. The range of this alarm is 18 to 95% in increments of 1, or "- -" (off).

Low exhaled minimum volume. The Low Min. Vol. (Low Minimum Volume) control is used to set the low exhaled minimum volume alarm limit value. The adjustable range of this alarm is 0.1 to 99 L, or "- -" (off).

NIV LED indicator. The NIV LED indicator is illuminated (red) when an NIV ventilation mode is active.

Breath Types and Modes of Ventilation

The ReVel has several breath types and modes available. The ReVel ventilator provides the following breath types: Pressure Control, Pressure Regulated Volume Control (PRVC), Pressure Support, Spontaneous, Volume Control, and Volume Targeted Pressure Support. The reader is directed to the preceding section on the LTV 1000 to learn about these features.

If desired, the operator can select flow cycling for PC breaths rather than time cycling by activating the flow-termination percentage feature using the extended features menu. The flow-cycling percentage can be adjusted from 10% to 40% of peak flow. With either the LTV 1000 or the LTV 1200, the default setting is made in terms of the patient type selected (i.e., adult, pediatric, or infant) when the machine is powered on, or it can be adjusted in the extended features menu.

The ReVel ventilator also provides an Apnea Backup mode of ventilation. When the set Apnea Interval (Apnea Int) (maximum time allowed between the beginning of one breath and the beginning of the next breath) is exceeded, the Apnea alarm is generated and the ventilator will enter Apnea Backup ventilation mode based on current ventilator settings.

NIV is a secondary, supplementary mode that may be selected with the primary ventilation mode. NIV can be applied in the A/C or CPAP+PS modes, when these modes are selected. The ventilator is capable of performing NIV with a standard dual-limb circuit. Adjust sensitivity to accommodate patient effort without autocycling. Activating leak compensation or increasing the level of bias flow may help overcome leaks and optimize the sensitivity setting. Set the alarms to avoid unnecessary alerts while maintaining adequate monitoring. As with the LTV 1200 ventilator, a nonvented mask should be used.

Additional features are accessed through the extended features mode. The extended features menu is selected by pushing the select button for 3 seconds. The first menu item is displayed in the window. Scrolling through the features menu, the operator will find a useful tool for transport operation. The ReVel, LTV 1200, and LTV 1000 have built-in oxygen cylinder duration calculators. The operator needs to select only the cylinder size and pressure in psi and the cylinder duration will be calculated with the current settings. As is the case with any procedure, readers are directed to consult the manufacturer's manual for the particular ventilator they are using.

As with the LTV 1200, an additional feature found in the extended menu is an SBT mode. With the SBT option you can temporarily minimize ventilatory support and perform clinical assessments of a patient's dependence on, or ability to be removed from, positive-pressure ventilation.

The SBT mode should be used only when a respiratory therapist or other properly trained and qualified personnel are present. Finally, the ReVel ventilator offers three optional additional features, including a nebulizer option, Pulse Oximetry (SpO_2), and F_1O_2 Sensor.

Next to the ON/OFF button is the DISPLAY/ALARM CHECK button, and directly below it is the BATTERY/POWER CHECK button. The BATTERY/POWER CHECK button is used to check the status of the battery and power system without interfering with the ventilator's operation. If you push and hold the BATTERY/POWER CHECK button, the ventilator displays a message in the Display Window for each of the four possible sources of power available to the ReVel ventilator indicating their detection and current status. The DISPLAY/ALARM CHECK button is used to check the displays, indicators, and audible alarm system without interfering with the ventilator's operation.

If you push and hold the DISPLAY/ALARM CHECK button, the ventilator illuminates all front panel and lower interface panel window displays and indicator LEDs in the colors as indicated later and sounds two audible tones of similar volume, followed by the High Priority Alarm Signal at the set volume. To the right of these control buttons are a series of five LED indicators, four indicating the current power source of the ReVel and a Vent Inop LED.

The Scroll knob is the next control on the lower interface panel. It is a rotary encoder knob used to change the settings of selected adjustable controls or to scroll through various configuration menus displayed in the front panel display window.

To the right of the Scroll knob are three soft keys, the CONTROL LOCK, MANUAL BREATH, and MANEUVERS buttons. The CONTROL LOCK button is activated to prevent accidental changes to ventilation controls and alarm limits settings. To turn Control Lock on, push the CONTROL LOCK button. The Control Lock LED is illuminated whenever the front-panel controls are locked. The MANUAL BREATH button will deliver one machine breath. The machine breath is defined by the current Breath Type settings.

The Manual Breath LED is illuminated during the Manual Breath inspiration. When in CPAP+PS breath mode, the ventilator will deliver one breath based on the A/C setting for the current breath type.

The MANUAL BREATH button is enabled only during exhalation. The MANEUVERS button is used to initiate Inspiratory or Expiratory Hold maneuvers. To begin an Inspiratory Hold, the operator must press and release the MANEUVERS button located on the lower interface panel. I-Hold is then displayed in the front panel display window, and the Maneuvers LED does not illuminate at this point. To perform an Expiratory Hold, rotate the Scroll knob until E-Hold appears in the display window, then proceed as follows. When the name of the desired maneuver is displayed, push and release the MANEUVERS button again.

The Maneuvers LED begins flashing to indicate that the displayed/selected maneuver is armed and ready to run. Maneuver arming automatically terminates if 60 seconds elapse in the same phase of a maneuver without a button press. To activate the maneuver, push and hold the MANEUVERS button. The Maneuvers LED illuminates continuously, and on the next appropriate breath the ventilator will initiate the "Hold." The maneuver will occur while the MANEUVERS button is held for a maximum of 6 seconds. If the button is released before the 6 seconds has expired, the maneuver will be terminated. In either case, the ventilator returns to normal ventilation immediately following termination of the maneuver. During an Inspiratory Hold maneuver, the inspiratory phase of a breath is held for a period of time sufficient to determine and display Delta Pressure (Δ Pres xx), Plateau Pressure (P Plat xx), and Static Lung Compliance (C Static xx). The obtained scrolling maneuver data will then appear over the Display Screen until the operator pushes the EXIT button on the front panel.

The final soft key on the lower interface panel is the SILENCE/RESET button. The SILENCE/RESET button is used to temporarily silence active audible alarms, remove visible alarm messages in the display window, and reset alarms. If pushed once during an active alarm condition (alarm

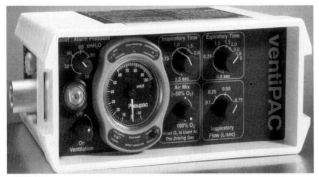

FIGURE 15.18 Smiths Medical ventiPAC. (Courtesy Smiths Medical, Inc., Waukesha, WI.)

sounding, alarm message flashing in the display window), the audible alarm is silenced for 60 seconds and the Silence/Reset LED is illuminated. If alarm conditions are resolved during the 60-second silence period, the audible alarm will not be reactivated.

SMITHS MEDICAL PNEUPAC VENTIPAC

The ventiPAC (Smiths Medical) is a portable, time-cycled, volume ventilator that is designed for adults and for children who weigh more than 5 kg (11 lb). It is totally pneumatically operated and is MRI compatible. The ventiPAC's dimensions are 3.7 in × 8.7 in × 6.4 in, and it weighs 3 kg (6.6 lb) without integrated alarms (3.1 kg [6.8 lb] with integrated alarms) (Fig. 15.18). Table 15.18 lists modes, ventilator parameters, and other features of the Smiths Medical Pneupac ventiPAC.[13]

Power Source

The ventiPAC unit is totally pneumatically powered with medical-grade oxygen at 45 to 70 psi. The ventiPAC unit has no battery backup or AC power option.

Internal Mechanism

A compressed-gas source enters the ventiPAC through a DISS connection in the rear of the unit. The gas source is then filtered and directed to the internal flow-control mechanism. The ventiPAC does not incorporate an internal PEEP control. A disposable PEEP valve must be added to the circuit and adjusted as indicated.

Oxygen Source

The ventiPAC has two options for supplied F_IO_2 to the patient. Either 50% or 100% oxygen may be selected by adjusting the air mix selector. (Air mix is discussed in greater detail later in this chapter.)

Controls

The ventiPAC has six individual controls to select the desired settings required by the patient. Fig. 15.18 shows the controls on the front of the unit. The ON VENTILATION/OFF VENTILATION switch is in the lower left-hand corner. The ventiPAC has an analog pressure gauge to display delivered pressures to

TABLE 15.18 Specifications for Smiths Medical ventiPAC

Control Settings	Range
Modes	Synchronized Minimum Mandatory Ventilation (SMMV) Demand/CPAP
Power source	Pneumatic
Rate	7-60 breaths/min
Noninvasive ventilation mode	Yes
Peak pressure	80 cm H₂O
Tidal volume	50-1500 mL
Inspiratory time	0.5-2.0 s
PEEP/CPAP	Optional 0-20 cm H₂O
Oxygen percent	50% or 100%
Pressure support	N/A
Monitors/displays	Analog Airway Pressure Gauge, Low Pressure Display
Dimensions	3.7 in × 8.7 in × 6.4 in
Logic gas consumption	Not specified
Alarms	High Pressure, Low Pressure Disconnect, Low Gas Supply
Battery duration	N/A

CPAP, Continuous positive airway pressure; *PEEP*, positive end-expiratory pressure.

the patient as measured at the ventilator outlet. The range of this gauge is −10 to +100 cm H_2O.

The ventiPAC does not have an internal PEEP mechanism. PEEP is generated via an external PEEP valve incorporated into the patient circuit. The adjustable range of this valve is from 0 cm H_2O to 20 cm H_2O. The PEEP pressure value (in cm H_2O) will be displayed only if the optional PEEP valve is attached to the ventilator circuit. The external PEEP valve is MRI compliant.

Respiratory Rate

Respiratory rate (RR) is set by manipulation of the inspiratory and expiratory time control knobs located on the upper right side of the control panel. Inspiratory time is adjustable from 0.5 second to 2 seconds. Expiratory time is adjustable from 0.6 second to 6 seconds. The deliverable respiratory rate is from 7 breaths/min to 60 breaths/min.

Tidal Volume

Deliverable V_T is a product of the set T_I and the inspiratory flow, which is adjustable from 6 L/min to 60 L/min. The V_T range of the ventiPAC is 50 to 1500 mL. V_T is calculated by multiplying the inspiratory flow in liters per second by the set inspiratory time in seconds (T_I). The following formula illustrates this concept:

$$\text{Inspiratory flow (L/sec)} \times T_I \text{ (seconds)} = V_T \text{ (L)}$$

(See Clinical Scenario 15.8.)

CLINICAL SCENARIO 15.8
Smiths Medical ventiPAC

A respiratory therapist is asked to transport a 60-year-old male patient who recently suffered a cardiac arrest. Upon arrival at the local referral facility, the therapist finds the patient is on the ventiPAC ventilator using a 100% oxygen cylinder. The T_I is set at 1 s and the T_E is set at 4 s. The inspiratory flow is set at 0.5 L/s. What is the set respiratory rate and V_T delivery?

See Appendix A for the answer.

T_E, Expiratory time; T_I, inspiratory time, V_T, tidal volume.

Air Mix Control

The position control is a two-position rotary switch—AIR MIX or 100% O_2. When in the Air Mix position, ambient air mixes with the drive gas to a ratio of 2:1 via a Venturi system. This will result in 45% O_2 being delivered to the patient when 100% oxygen is used as the drive gas. The Air Mix position is more efficient, providing an approximate 70% savings in drive-gas consumption when it is selected.

When the AIR MIX switch is in the 100% O_2 position, the supply gas will be delivered to the patient. This could be 21% or 100% oxygen, depending on whether air or an oxygen source is being used.

Pressure Relief

This control is located in the upper left-hand corner of the control panel and is adjustable from 20 cm H_2O to 80 cm H_2O. This rotary control knob allows continuous adjustment of the maximum patient inflation pressure through the setting of the spring-loaded relief valve. An audible alarm sounds when the set limit is reached.

Alarms

The ventiPAC has incorporated visual and audible alarms into a display ring surrounding the pressure gauge. The alarms consist of a high-pressure alarm, low pressure/disconnect, and other safety features. A visual eyeball type of indicator is used to warn the user of a low gas supply, and an audible and visual alarm is used to warn of low battery level. The battery provides power to the alarms.

High-Pressure Alarm

The high-pressure alarm is a pneumatically operated alarm with an electronically generated audible and visual indicator on the alarm monitor. The high-pressure alarm activates after the set high-pressure alarm has been maintained for a period of 1 second.

Low Inflation Pressure (Disconnect) Alarm

An audible and visual alarm warns the operator if the inflation pressure does not rise above the set level of 10 cm H_2O at least once in a 10-second period. This is not affected by PEEP applications.

Breathing Detector

The breathing detector illuminates when a spontaneous breathing effort has been detected and the low inflation pressure is reset.

Low Battery Alarm

A yellow visual indicator illuminates when the internal battery is at a reduced voltage. The rate at which the yellow indicator flashes gives the user an idea of how low the voltage level is. When the flash rate increases to twice a second, an audible alarm will sound for the remainder of the battery life.

Low Gas Supply Indicator

Directly below the relief/alarm pressure control is a visual indicator relaying to the operator when the operating gas supply is nearly exhausted. When the supply gas pressure is adequate, the gas-supply indicator will show white. When the supply pressure is low enough to not allow the ventilator to operate properly, the indicator will turn red. At 45 psi the indicator will begin to change color from white to red. Any visible red in the indicator means that the gas supply is inadequate. In most cases the display will oscillate between white and red as the supply pressure falls. This visual indication will be accompanied by an electronically generated medium-priority audible alarm. If this alarm is ignored for more than 60 seconds, the alarm will shut itself off to conserve battery power.

Synchronized Minimum Mandatory Ventilation/Demand

This control has two positions. First is the ventilation off (demand), in which only the internal demand valve is powered by the gas supply. Any spontaneous breathing effort by the patient is met by flow from the demand valve. This position allows the operator to provide 100% oxygen therapy.

In the ventilation on position, the ventiPAC offers a mode of ventilation called synchronized minimum mandatory ventilation (SMMV). SMMV allows the patient to breathe spontaneously without the risk for stacking mandatory breaths on top of spontaneous breaths.

If an adult patient has an adequate ventilation level, mandatory cycling by the ventiPAC will not occur. This is true as long as the minute ventilation is maintained. If the spontaneous rate becomes inadequate, the set rate and V_T will be delivered. This SMMV feature applies only to V_T of more than 400 mL.

For a spontaneous V_T between 150 mL and 400 mL during SMMV, the mandatory breath is inhibited until spontaneous exhalation is completed and the expiratory time is proportionally extended, as long as the set minute ventilation is maintained.

With a spontaneous V_T of less than 150 mL, the ventilator will deliver a mandatory breath.

SUMMARY OF TRANSPORT VENTILATORS

The ideal transport ventilator is small, lightweight, and able to withstand the rigors of transport in a variety of environmental extremes, while providing adequate, safe ventilation to the patient at all times. For this reason, facilities looking to purchase a ventilator for transport should first determine the conditions in which they will be used.

When transporting patients, particular care must be taken to ensure optimal monitoring of patient status, ventilation, oxygenation, and patient safety.[2,14] Choosing and using the right equipment are part of the respiratory therapist's responsibilities.

Operating features available with a particular ventilator may be changed frequently by the manufacturers. For example, a new range for trigger sensitivity may be added or a new alarm added to a ventilator. For this and patient safety reasons, the user should always refer to the operating manual and information from the manufacturer when operating a ventilator.

Transport ventilators are becoming increasingly popular, not only for their intended purpose of transporting patients, but for use as ventilators in response to both natural and human-made disasters. Many states are now purchasing transport ventilators to help meet any potential catastrophic event.

II. HOME CARE VENTILATORS

Home care in the United States began more than 100 years ago.[1] Individuals discharged from the hospital who required routine follow-up care were the primary candidates for this emerging sector of medicine. Today it is one of the fastest-growing areas of health care. With the continued rise in the cost of caring for patients in the acute or extended care environment, home care is a realistic alternative for individuals battling primarily chronic diseases. Conditions that might meet the indications for home ventilatory support are not limited to the following: ventilatory muscle disorders, alveolar hypoventilation syndrome, primary respiratory disorders, obstructive lung diseases, restrictive lung diseases, and cardiac disorders, including congenital anomalies. The goals of home invasive mechanical ventilation are as follows[15,16]:

- To sustain and extend life
- To enhance the quality of life
- To reduce morbidity
- To improve or sustain physical and psychological function of all patients needing ventilator assistance and to enhance growth and development in the pediatric patients who need ventilator assistance
- To provide cost-effective care

The following section focuses on the technical aspects of the equipment available for home care ventilation. The supportive measures include primarily positive-pressure ventilators, which are the most commonly used, and noninvasive positive-pressure ventilators.[17,18]

NEWPORT HT50

The Newport HT50 (formerly manufactured by Newport Medical Instruments, now a company of Medtronic Minimally Invasive Therapies) is a portable ventilator designed for home care, subacute care, transport use, and hospital use (Fig. 15.19).

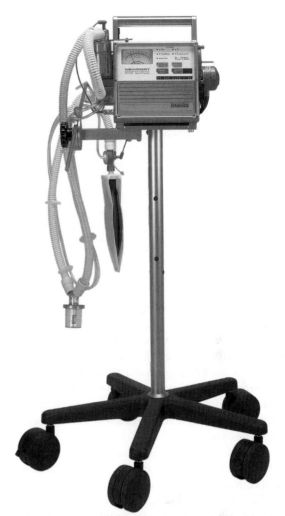

FIGURE 15.19 Newport HT50 ventilator. (Copyright © 2013 Medtronic Minimally Invasive Therapies. All rights reserved. Reprinted with permission of Medtronic Minimally Invasive Therapies.)

It is a microprocessor-controlled ventilator that may be used for adult or pediatric patients (who weigh ≥10 kg [22 lb]).[19]

The device functions in three modes: CMV, IMV, and spontaneous ventilation (spont). It is lightweight (6.8 kg [15 lb] without a humidifier) and compact (10.6 in × 7.87 in × 10.24 in).

Power Source

The HT50 is electrically powered and requires no gas sources to properly perform all of its operations. Oxygen enrichment is available through a 50-psi entrainment (0 bleed) mixer or a low-flow blending bag kit. The electronic system can use three possible power sources:

1. A standard AC outlet (100 to 240 V)
2. An external DC battery (12 to 30 V)
3. An internal DC battery

Indicators on the top right section of the front provide information about the current power source (Ext. Power/Charging Int. Battery, Int. Battery [Push to Test]).

The internal battery can sustain ventilator operation for up to 10 hours and requires 8 hours to fully recharge from any AC or DC power source, even while the ventilation is in operation. Newport recommends charging the battery for a minimum of 5 hours after the battery has been completely depleted (approximately 80% of a full charge).

The HT50 has a universal power entry module. This module allows the clinician to use the same port for connecting the plug for AC as it does for an external DC. To use external DC the source must be capable of delivering a minimum of 12 V and a maximum of 30 V to be compatible with the ventilator. The auto DC power connector allows for powering the HT50 from the cigarette lighter in an automobile.

The HT50 is equipped with several battery indicators and alarms that monitor the status of the power supply to the ventilator. The indicators are located in the upper right section of the front panel. The button labeled "INT BATTERY (PUSH TO TEST)", allows the operator to read the battery charge level in the pressure gauge window when operating from the internal battery. When the LED adjacent to this control is amber, the internal battery is partially to fully charged. When red, the battery is low.

The message display window in the center of the front panel will provide written messages of battery conditions. They include the following: battery low alarm, battery empty alarm, and "No ext. power" (a power switchover alarm).

When the "battery low" message appears in the message display window, an audible, intermittent three-pulse cautionary beep sounds and a visible alert (i.e., the LED blinks red adjacent to "Int. Battery") is activated. This alarm indicates that the internal battery is in use and less than 1 hour of battery charge remains. Pressing the SILENCE/RESET button can silence the audible alarm, but the visual alarm will remain illuminated until the ventilator is plugged into an AC outlet or an external battery is connected.

The battery empty message is activated when less than 30 minutes of power remains in the internal battery. It is accompanied by an audible, intermittent three-pulse cautionary alarm and a visible alert (LED blinks red adjacent to "Int. Battery").

The power switchover alarm notifies the clinician that the external power source has failed and the internal battery is now in use. It occurs when a switch from an external battery to the internal battery has occurred because of disconnection from the power cord or a power interruption. The message "No Ext. Power" appears in the message window, the LED next to the "Int Battery" blinks red, and the red LED next to the "Ext. Power/Charging Int. Battery" message is constantly lit. This alarm can be silenced by pressing the SILENCE/RESET button or by plugging the ventilator into a working outlet.

The internal pneumatic circuit does not require external compressed air but does require a medical-grade high-pressure oxygen gas source capable of delivering 35 to 90 psi of low-flow oxygen. The 35- to 90-psi oxygen source may be a cylinder or wall outlet. The low-flow source may be a flowmeter from a cylinder, wall outlet, liquid system, or concentrator.

Internal Mechanism

All gas enters the HT50 through an opening in the filter cover located on the right side of the machine. If neither oxygen accessory is connected, the ventilator delivers room air to the patient. For oxygen enrichment, either the air-oxygen entrainment mixer or oxygen-blending bag kit is inserted into the opening (see the following section, "Oxygen Source"). This ventilator uses a dual-micropiston delivery system that allows the ventilator to operate without an external air compressor.

The respiratory rate, trigger sensitivity, pressure control or V_T, PEEP, and PS set by the clinician determine the stroke rate and stroke speed of the pistons.

Oxygen Source

The HT50 comes with two oxygen-delivery options: (a) an optional air-oxygen entrainment mixer and (b) an oxygen-blending bag kit. The air-oxygen entrainment mixer attaches to the fresh gas intake valve on the right side of the ventilator and allows for the attachment of a high-pressure oxygen gas source. This device allows the clinician to control the oxygen percentage delivered to the patient from 21% to 100% oxygen with a knob located on the blender itself. It is a unique high-pressure ambient mixing system that uses no bleed.

The oxygen-blending bag kit also attaches to the fresh gas intake valve on the right side of the ventilator and allows for the attachment of a low-flow oxygen gas source. This device allows the clinician to control the oxygen percentage delivered to the patient by varying the flow set on a flowmeter attached to the blending bag kit. Two charts (one for use with PEEP and one for use without PEEP) assist the clinician in setting proper flow rates to achieve a given F_IO_2.

Humidifier

The HT50 offers a humidifier option. When the humidifier is attached (left side of machine), it is functional only if the ventilator is powered by an external AC power source.

The humidifier is activated by a button located on the front right of the control panel, which allows the operator to activate the humidifier and set a temperature ranging from 19°C to 39°C. The operator presses the HUMIDIFIER button to adjust the temperature and uses the up and down arrows in the center of the front panel to increase and decrease the temperature setting. During ventilation the displayed temperature is measured at the patient connector. The displayed temperature is measured at the humidifier bottle outlet. To turn off the humidifier, the operator presses and holds the button for 3 seconds.

If the message "Check Humidifier" appears in the message display window and the LED adjacent to the humidifier control blinks red, a malfunction has been detected. The humidifier shuts down. One of five possible messages is displayed. The user is advised to see the operating manual for instructions.

Patient Circuit

The connections for the patient circuit are located on the left side of the ventilator. They include a temperature plug when the humidifier is attached, a proximal pressure line with filter, a drive line for the externally mounted exhalation valve, and the main inspiratory line.

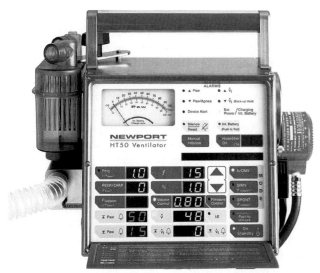

FIGURE 15.20 The Newport HT50 ventilator's control panel (see text for further description). (Copyright © 2013 Medtronic Minimally Invasive Therapies. All rights reserved. Reprinted with permission of Medtronic Minimally Invasive Therapies.)

Control Panel and Alarms

The front panel of the HT50 contains several controls for setting parameters and monitoring patient data and alarms, as well as for powering up the ventilator (Fig. 15.20). The ON/STANDBY selector is located at the bottom right of the front panel. It allows the user to select one of three operating conditions by pressing the ON/STANDBY button.

In the first condition, the ventilator is in the off/standby mode. Standby means that the ventilator is plugged into an external power supply and the internal battery is charging.

The second condition (button pressed once) is the settings feature. The settings feature allows the clinician to program the ventilator settings before turning the machine on and connecting it to a patient. It is also the condition during which an exhalation valve calibration is performed (Box 15.13). This simple procedure (occlude the circuit and press the MANUAL INFLATION button twice) performs a leak check on the breathing circuit and also provides a linearization curve for the ventilator pressure management in conjunction with the exhalation valve in use. When operating in settings, the parameter values that are entered (e.g., V_T, respiratory rate) do not have to be confirmed by pressing the key a second time, as they do during normal operation (Box 15.14).

To begin ventilation, the third condition, the ON/STANDBY button, is pressed again. Two safety features help prevent any accidental changes in the set parameters from occurring. The first is a panel cover, which blocks the control settings from view and must be opened to gain front-panel access. The second is the panel lock feature located at the bottom right of the ventilator, just above the ON/STANDBY selector. When activated, it locks all settings on the ventilator and prevents someone from inadvertently changing the parameters.

Control Parameters

The front panel is divided into roughly three sections: the top section of monitored data and alarm indicators, the central

panel containing parameter controls and modes, and the bottom section of alarms (see Fig. 15.20).

As a general rule, when changing parameter values, the operator first presses the desired parameter button, uses the up or down arrow to change the displayed setting, and then presses the parameter button again to confirm and activate the change. Alarms are set in the same way. A setting limitation message will appear in the message display window when the operator adjusts a parameter to its limits. Table 15.19 lists setting limitation messages.

The first control parameter displayed is trigger sensitivity (P_{TRIG}; 0 to −9.9 cm H_2O). The sensitivity is automatically PEEP compensated. For example, if PEEP is 5 cm H_2O and the sensitivity is −0.5 cm H_2O, the breath triggers when an inspiratory effort drops the airway pressure to 4.5 cm H_2O. The P_{TRIG} LED indicator light illuminates every time a spontaneous breath is detected, allowing the clinician to track the patient's breathing pattern.

The PEEP/CPAP (0 to 30 cm H_2O) control governs the baseline pressure. PEEP/CPAP cannot be set higher than the pressure-control target setting of −5 cm H_2O. This is to ensure that the ventilator is able to deliver a breath during pressure ventilation, even if it is just 5 cm H_2O (i.e., the difference between set pressure target and PEEP).

PS has an available range of 0 to 60 cm H_2O. The ventilator will not allow the combined value of PEEP/CPAP plus PS to be greater than 60 cm H_2O.

The available mandatory respiratory rate (f) range is 1 to 99 breaths/min. T_I is adjustable from 0.1 second to 3.0 seconds. The next control is the volume control (100 to 2200 mL)/pressure control (5 to 60 cm H_2O). This control allows the operator to select either volume-targeted or pressure-targeted

TABLE 15.19 Setting Limitation Messages on the Newport

Messages	Meaning
Reached max $\dot{V}$	Maximum flow setting reached
Reached min $\dot{V}$	Minimum flow setting reached
Inverse I:E	An inverse I:E ratio has been set
Reached max I:E	The maximum inverse ratio of 3:1 has been reached
$\dot{V}$ unavailable	Flow value cannot be displayed during pressure ventilation
PEEP + PS too high	Maximum limit of PEEP + PS is 60 cm H_2O
PC—PEEP too low	PC/PEEP is <5 cm H_2O
↑ PEEP too low	High P_{limit}—PEEP is <5 cm H_2O
Reminder Messages	
Panel lock	Operator has tried to change a parameter with the panel lock activated
Press again	Pressing the same button is required to confirm and activate the parameter change requested

PC, Pressure control; *PEEP,* positive end-expiratory pressure; *PS,* pressure support.

breaths and set the desired parameter value—that is, volume in liters or pressure in cm H_2O.

Mode controls include CMV, SIMV, and SPONT (see the section "Modes of Ventilation"). To activate the mode the operator presses the desired mode once and then a second time to activate it. However, before confirming a mode, all the appropriate parameter settings for that mode should be set and checked.

The lower section of the panel includes the high- and low-pressure alarm controls (airway pressure [Paw]), inspiratory flow display, and I:E ratio display, minute volume display, and the high and low minute volume alarm controls ($\dot{V}_I$). (The alarms are reviewed later in this section.)

The inspiratory flow ($\dot{V}$) and I:E ratio LCD displays allow the clinician to select viewing either one or the other in the adjacent display window by touching the desired parameter control. To the left is the flow display.

When operating in volume-controlled ventilation, the flow delivered to the patient is determined by the inspiratory time and the V_T setting:

$$V_T \text{ (L)} = T_I \text{ (seconds)} \times \text{Flow (L/sec)}$$

The calculated flow value is displayed in an LCD panel in the bottom middle of the front panel as $\dot{V}$. (*Note:* If the T_I allows the flow to reach a maximum- or minimum-range level [range is 6 to 100 L/min], adjustment of T_I stops and a beep sounds. A setting limitation message appears in the message display window.) The flow display is not available during pressure control or spontaneous ventilation.

The I:E ratio is determined by the frequency and the inspiratory time settings (range: 1:99 up to 3:1). When the entered parameters generate an inverse I:E ratio, the ventilator briefly alarms, making the clinician aware of the changes, but continues with ventilation. The I:E ratio cannot exceed 3:1.

The upper portion of the control panel contains a pressure gauge (−10 to 100 cm H_2O or mBar) that monitors real-time airway pressure. This section of the front panel also includes a manual inflation control (3 seconds maximum) and the humidifier control described previously.

The manual inflation feature is active only in the A/CMV and SIMV modes. It allows the clinician to control the amount of the V_T for the manual breath by controlling the T_I. The flow is determined by the variables of V_T and T_I set in volume-targeted A/CMV and SIMV. In pressure control the set pressure is delivered. A manual breath is terminated under three conditions:

1. The clinician stops pressing the control.
2. The set high-pressure alarm limit is reached.
3. Three seconds have elapsed.

A backup safety feature will not allow the clinician to deliver a manual breath while the patient is in inspiration or if the airway pressure is greater than 5 cm H_2O above PEEP.

Just below the manual inflation control is the message display window discussed previously. When the display is blank, the operator can view monitored parameters by using the up and down arrows on the front panel. Monitored values that appear include V_T, $\dot{V}_I$, f, or Paw (peak, mean, and base). These are updated every 10 seconds or at the end of each breath, allowing the operator to record current values.

Airway Pressure and Minute Ventilation Alarms

The high airway pressure alarm control is located on the lower left portion of the control panel and has an adjustable range of 4 to 99 cm H_2O. When the set high-pressure level is reached, audiovisual alarms are activated and the machine cycles into exhalation.

The visual indicator is in the top section of the front panel. The high peak pressure alarm cannot be set below the PEEP setting.

The low airway pressure alarm control is below the high airway pressure alarm control. Its operating range is 3 to 98 cm H_2O. The low airway pressure alarm is active only during mandatory breaths in the CMV and IMV modes. It activates when the rise in pressure does not exceed the alarm setting during the inspiratory phase for two consecutive patient-triggered or time-triggered mandatory breaths. The visual indicator is in the top section of the front panel.

The high and low minute ventilation alarm controls are also located on the lower panel. The high $\dot{V}_I$ (high inspiratory minute volume) alarm has a setting range of 1.1 to 50 L. The low $\dot{V}_I$ (low inspiratory minute volume) has a setting range of 0.3 to 49 L. If the measured minute volume falls outside of the set limits, the appropriate alarm becomes active, producing both an audible and a visible alert. The visual indicator is in the upper section of the front panel. (*Note:* The alarm measures the volume delivered from the ventilator and not what is exhaled by the patient.) If at any time the minute ventilation falls below the "low minute ventilation" alarm value, the backup ventilation (BUV) feature is activated and the $\dot{V}_I$ ("Back-up Vent.") indicator illuminates. This feature is active in all modes and is described in the section on modes of ventilation.

Additional Alarms

Additional alarms that are monitored and have messages that appear in the message display window include the following: High Baseline Pressure, Occlusion, Low Baseline Pressure, Check Proximal Line, Apnea, PC cannot be reached, and device alerts.

High baseline pressure alarm. The High Baseline Pressure alarm occurs when the baseline pressure is greater than the low airway pressure alarm setting at the beginning of a time-triggered mandatory breath. The alarm message will display "HIGH Pbase." The alarm will reset when airway pressure drops to within 5 cm H_2O of the PEEP/CPAP level.

Occlusion alarm. The Occlusion alarm activates when the airway pressure remains +15 cm H_2O above the PEEP setting for 3 seconds after exhalation has begun or at the end of exhalation, whichever comes first. It is corrected if airway pressure falls to within 5 cm H_2O of baseline.

If this alarm occurs, no additional mandatory breaths are delivered until it is corrected. The device alert indicator blinks, and the ventilator attempts to release pressure through the redundant safety system. The safety system allows the patient to draw ambient air into the breathing circuit through an emergency intake valve when no other flow is available. The patient effort required to open this valve is approximately 2 cm H_2O.

Low baseline pressure alarm. The Low Baseline Pressure alarm ("LOW Pbase") indicates an unstable baseline. For example, this could occur with a large leak in the patient circuit (pressure $\geq$ 2 cm H_2O below baseline for 3 seconds). In addition to the message displayed, the low Paw indicator blinks. The alarm resets when the baseline pressure difference is less than 2 cm H_2O (Clinical Scenario 15.9).

Check proximal line alarm. The Check Proximal Line ("CHECK PROX LINE") alarm occurs during inspiration when the proximal pressure measured is significantly different from the internal backup pressure sensor measurement taken inside the ventilator. In addition to the message, the low Paw/Apnea indicator blinks red. Causes include disconnections, kinking of the circuit, and a water-filled proximal sensor line. Ventilation continues during this condition by using the pressure monitored by the internal pressure transducer.

⚑ CLINICAL SCENARIO 15.9 Low Pressure Alarm on a Newport HT50

You are called to an intermediate care area to troubleshoot a reported alarm by nursing. You arrive to find the following message on the ventilator's message window: ("LOW Pbase"). What is the meaning of the alarm message?

See Appendix A for answer.

Apnea alarm. When a patient breath goes undetected for 30 seconds, an Apnea alarm occurs ("APNEA").

PCV not reached alarm. "PCV not reached" signals to the operator that the maximum inspiratory pressure measured is less than 50% of the set pressure during PCV. The operator should check the patient to be sure the patient is being adequately ventilated and then check the circuit for leaks.

Device alert. When the device alert LED illuminates, a steady red and an internal beep occur. This indicates that the ventilator has detected one of four message conditions:

1. OCCL Shutdown
2. Motor Fault
3. 10 V SHUTDOWN
4. SYSTEM ERROR

With the exception of an occlusion alert, in all these conditions the ventilator will stop ventilating. Another method must be found to ventilate the patient, and the HT50 should be taken out of service and not used on patients until it is checked by a qualified technician.

Alarm/silence-reset. The ALARM/SILENCE-RESET button is in the upper alarm indicator section on the control panel. When it is activated, this control silences the alarm for 60 seconds. It is also used to clear "latched" alarms that are no longer active, including alarm messages in the message window.

Modes of Ventilation

The mode settings located on the right front panel of the HT50 are A/CMV, SIMV and "Spont.," or spontaneous. When selecting a mode after the ventilator has been turned on, the operator must press the button twice to confirm the selection. If the button is not pressed a second time within 5 seconds, the selection is canceled.

When operating in the CMV or IMV mode, the ventilator can be programmed for either VC or PC ventilation for the mandatory breaths. This control was described previously. When VC ventilation is chosen, the LED display allows the clinician to determine the V_T delivered.

If PC is the desired option, then the LED display allows the clinician to determine the pressure target delivered to the patient.

In A/CMV VC mode, the clinician sets the V_T, frequency (minimum respiratory rate), T_I, and trigger sensitivity. PEEP can also be set. All breaths have the same V_T delivered, regardless of whether they are patient triggered or time triggered.

The SIMV VC mode lets the patient breath spontaneously between mandatory breaths without receiving the set V_T. The operator sets V_T, breath rate, T_I, PS for spontaneous breaths, PEEP, and trigger sensitivity.

For PC mandatory breaths, the operator selects the PC option and adjusts the pressure to the desired target value. Mandatory breaths in either CMV or IMV then become pressure targeted rather than volume targeted.

When the spontaneous mode is used to ventilate, all breaths become patient triggered and pressure targeted. PS may be used in addition to PEEP/CPAP to aid the spontaneous breaths. When a patient circuit is disconnected during PC or PS, flow may increase through the circuit to compensate for the low pressure. After reconnecting the patient circuit, the operator should press the PC or PS button twice to quickly readjust the flow to a lower level.

BUV is a safety feature that becomes active, as noted, when the low $\dot{V}_I$ alarm is activated It is available in all modes. During BUV the message "Low $\dot{V}_I$ (BUV)" is displayed. When the HT50 is operating in the spontaneous mode and BUV becomes active, the ventilator delivers a pressure-targeted breath. The pressure delivered to the patient is 15 cm H_2O above the PEEP setting, and it is maintained for 1 second at a respiratory rate of 15 breaths/min.

The BUV feature is deactivated if there is a recorded rise in minute ventilation to 10% above the set low $\dot{V}_I$ alarm value. It is important to note that the "low minute ventilation" alarm responds to the volume delivered from the ventilator, not the volume exhaled from the patient. If there is a leak or the circuit becomes disconnected, the alarm will not sound and BUV will not be activated. A high minute volume is usually the indicator of an increase in leak or disconnection.

NEWPORT HT70

The Newport HT70 series (Medtronic Minimally Invasive Therapies) are microprocessor-controlled ventilators designed to provide continuous or intermittent positive-pressure mechanical ventilatory support for the care of individuals who require mechanical ventilation through invasive or non-invasive interfaces.

The Newport HT70 (Fig. 15.21) is applicable for infant, pediatric, and adult patients who weigh 5 kg (11 lb) or more. The Newport HT70 series of ventilators are designed to be utilized in such settings as hospitals, subacute, emergency

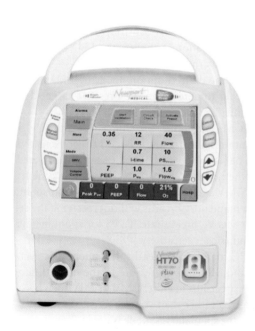

room, and home care environments, as well as for transport and emergency response applications. The HT70 is 10.25 in high × 9.75 in wide × 11 in deep and weighs 7 kg (15.4 lb).[20] The device functions in multiple modes, including: A/C mode ventilation (A/CMV), SIMV, spontaneous ventilation (spont), NIV, PS, PC, VC, and Backup Ventilation.

Power Source

The HT70 may be operated from a variety of AC (100 to 240 V AC at 50/60 Hz) or DC (12 to 24 V DC) external power sources, or from the internal dual battery system. The optional DC auto lighter power adapter accessory enables connection to an automobile-type DC outlet. Anytime the ventilator is connected to external power, both batteries in the internal dual battery system are charged, even while the ventilator is in use. The internal dual battery system can provide up to 10 hours of operation when new and fully charged (under standard conditions).

The HT70 has a dual-battery configuration to supply power for operation consisting of two independent, but coordinated, lithium ion batteries; the integrated, hot swappable primary Power Pac battery, and the secondary backup battery. The backup battery will provide a minimum of 30 minutes of emergency backup power.

Newer style Power Pac batteries have an LED on the bottom edge to show the charge condition. Pushing the status button will display the charge level of the battery with green indicating approximately 90% or higher charge level; amber indicating charge not completed; and red indicating battery depleted.

Internal Mechanism

The HT70 utilizes a micropistons pump to deliver a variable flow, enabling the HT70 to provide a full range of operating modes and breath types with a servo-controlled, leak-compensated PEEP. This dual-micropiston delivery system allows the HT70 to operate without an external air compressor. The respiratory rate, trigger sensitivity, pressure control, V_T, PEEP, and PS set by the clinician determine the stroke rate and stroke speed of the pistons.

All gas enters the HT70 through an opening in the filter cover located on the right side of the machine. The ventilator would deliver room air to the patient. For oxygen enrichment, either the air-oxygen entrainment mixer or low flow oxygen reservoir oxygen-blending bag kit is inserted into the opening, similar to the HT50.

Oxygen Source

The HT70 has a dual means of providing supplemental oxygen to the patient. The first is a high-pressure source connected to an air/oxygen entrainment mixer used to blend atmospheric air with high-pressure medical-grade oxygen at a precise ratio. A control knob on this mixer allows for incremental oxygen adjustment from 21% to 100%. The mixer attaches to the fresh gas intake port on the filter cover, located on the right side of the ventilator. It is imperative to ensure that the medical-grade 100% oxygen source gas is on when the mixer is attached during ventilator operation.

The second method of oxygen enrichment is accomplished by utilizing a low-flow oxygen reservoir to blend atmospheric air with a low-flow (0 to 10 L/min) medical-grade oxygen source. The low-flow oxygen reservoir threads into the fresh gas intake port, located on the right side of the ventilator. This system allows the user to ventilate patients with oxygen-enriched gas from 21% up to 100%, depending on patient settings. Oxygen delivery is affected by use of the bias flow, PEEP, delivered minute volume, and F_IO_2 of source gas. Use a calibrated oxygen monitor to verify the level of oxygen enrichment. Refer to the oxygen supply flow graphs that are included with the low-flow oxygen reservoir instructions for use and also located below (with PEEP) (Fig. 15.22).

Control Panel

The HT70 front panel (Fig. 15.23) consists of easy-access membrane buttons, LED indicators, and the patient connection manifold. The center touchscreen panel provides access to alarm and parameter settings. The ON/OFF momentary-type power switch is located on the left side rear of the ventilator along the bottom edge. The operator presses the power switch once and waits for the startup screen to appear. The ventilator will initially be in standby mode, where the operator can make setting changes and perform the circuit check before ventilation. To start ventilation the operator touches the START VENTILATION button at the top of the screen.

Most parameters are changed with a simple touch-adjust-accept method seen with many newer microprocessor interactive screen ventilators. The operator must first activate the desired control by touching it (button will appear highlighted on the screen). The operator utilizes the UP/DOWN button (located on the right side of the front panel just below the ACCEPT and CANCEL buttons) to adjust the settings. Once the desired settings of the parameter are adjusted, the operator need only press the ACCEPT button to accept the change. The operator can make several parameter adjustments before accepting the changes. When satisfied with all of the changes, the operator can accept them by pressing the ACCEPT button once.

If the operator would like to go back to the previous ventilator settings, simply pressing the CANCEL button will revert back to the previous settings. Fig. 15.23 shows the HT70's controls and indicators. The adjustable parameters on the touchscreen of the HT70 can also be viewed in Fig. 15.23.

Alarms

The Newport HT70 ventilator has an extensive alarm package to accurately monitor patients, whether they are being supported invasively or noninvasively. Some alarms are automatic, whereas others are adjustable and require the operator to enter a desired value to an alarm setting. Table 15.20 lists the adjustable alarms.

To access the alarm parameters, the operator need only touch the ALARMS button on the upper left corner of the touchscreen of the HT70. The alarm controls are changed just like the parameter controls, with the simple touch-adjust-accept method described earlier. It is possible to make several alarm adjustments before accepting the all the alarm parameter changes. Pressing the ACCEPT button once will confirm all alarm parameter changes.

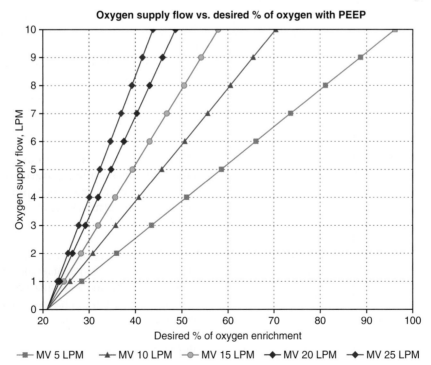

FIGURE 15.22 Newport HT70 oxygen supply flow graphs. *LPM*, L/min; *MV*, minute volume; *PEEP*, positive end-expiratory pressure. (Copyright © 2013 Medtronic Minimally Invasive Therapies. All rights reserved. Reprinted with permission of Medtronic Minimally Invasive Therapies.)

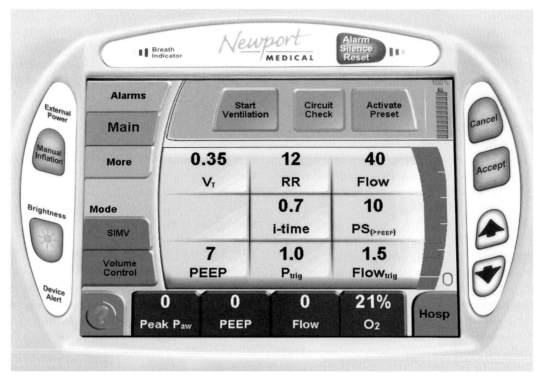

FIGURE 15.23 Newport HT70 ventilator's main screen. (Copyright © 2013 Medtronic Minimally Invasive Therapies. All rights reserved. Reprinted with permission of Medtronic Minimally Invasive Therapies.)

TABLE 15.20	**Newport HT70 Alarms**
Condition	**Alarm**
High Pressure	Min Vol (High Inspiratory Minute Volume)
Low Pressure	Min Vol (Low Inspiratory Minute Volume)
RR (High Respiratory Rate)	F_IO_2 (optional) (High Oxygen Concentration)
Apnea (time adjust)	F_IO_2 (optional) (Low Oxygen Concentration

F_IO_2, Fraction of inspired oxygen.

The HT70 is capable of automatically setting the alarm limits by the operator pressing the ALARM QUICK SET button on the touchscreen and confirming this action by pressing the ACCEPT button. The HT70 will monitor ventilation for 30 seconds and then set the appropriate alarm limits. During this 30-second period the touchscreen will not respond unless an alarm occurs or the CANCEL button is pressed. If an alarm occurs during the monitoring period, the Quick Set procedure is canceled.

When an alarm limit is violated, the message area in the touchscreen changes color according to alarm priority, and an alarm message is displayed. The HT70 also has three methods of notification during alarm conditions. First the alarm LEDs in the handle of the HT70 will flash, followed by the ALARM parameter button on the alarms screen (if it is an adjustable alarm) being highlighted. Finally, an audible alarm sounds. When the alarm violation is no longer in effect, the alarm

message remains steadily visible until it is reset by pressing the ALARM SILENCE/RESET button.

The ALARM SILENCE/RESET button is located on the top right corner of the ventilator control interface. Pressing the ALARM SILENCE/RESET button will silence the audible alarm for 1 minute (60 seconds). Located next to ALARM SILENCE/RESET button, the LED remains lit during the 1-minute alarm silence period. Once an alarm condition has been corrected, pressing this button will clear (reset) the alarm message. If there are multiple alarm messages present, the operator may press repeatedly to clear all the alarm messages or hold down the button for 3 seconds to clear all messages at once.

Not all alarms on the HT70 are adjustable by the operator. Table 15.21 lists the automatic alarm parameters monitored by the ventilator. All automatic alarms are displayed similarly to the adjustable alarms discussed earlier.

Domains

A three-tiered management domain system makes it very easy for critical caregivers to manage all controls while providing quick access to the more essential elements in transport situations and significantly enhanced safety and simplicity in the home care environment.

Modes

The mode settings located on the left portion of the touchscreen of the HT70 are A/CMV, SIMV, and "Spont.," or spontaneous. When selecting a mode after the ventilator has been turned on, the operator must press the ACCEPT button.

TABLE 15.21 Newport HT70 Nonadjustable Alarms

Condition	Alarm
High Baseline Pressure	Alarm Pressure Control Setting Not Reached alarm
Low Baseline Pressure	Alarm Backup Battery Low Charge alarm
Occlusion alarm	No External Power alarm
Sustained Occlusion alarm	Shut Down Alert alarm
Check Circuit alarm	Backup Battery Low
Device Alert alarm	Backup Battery Shutdown Imminent
Power Pac Battery Pack Low	Internal Temperature alarm
Switching to Backup Battery	Backup Battery Temperature alarm
Running on Backup Battery Power Pac	Temperature alarm
Motor Fault	Backup Battery Failure

BOX 15.15 Back-up Ventilation in Spontaneous Mode

The factory default setting for Back-up Ventilation in the SPONT mode will implement these changes:
- SPONT = SIMV mode
- Rate = 15 breaths/min
- Pressure Control breath type: 15 cm H_2O above set PEEP
- I-Time—1.0 s

I-Time, Inspiratory time; *PEEP,* positive end-expiratory pressure; *SIMV,* synchronized intermittent mandatory ventilation.

When operating in the CMV or IMV mode, the ventilator can be programmed for either VC or PC ventilation for the mandatory breaths. When VC ventilation is chosen, the screen display allows the clinician to determine the V_T delivered. If PC is the desired option, then the screen display allows the clinician to determine the pressure target delivered to the patient.

In VC-CMV mode, the clinician sets the V_T, frequency (minimum respiratory rate), T_I (or flow), and trigger sensitivity. PEEP can also be set. All breaths have the same V_T delivered, regardless of whether they are patient triggered or time triggered.

The VC-IMV mode lets the patient breathe spontaneously with or without PS between mandatory breaths without receiving the set V_T. The operator sets V_T, breath rate, inspiratory time, PS for spontaneous breaths, PEEP, and trigger sensitivity.

For PC mandatory breaths the operator selects the PC option and adjusts the pressure to the desired target value. Mandatory breaths in either CMV or IMV then become pressure targeted rather than volume targeted.

When the spontaneous mode is used to ventilate the patient, all breaths will become patient triggered and pressure targeted. PS may be used in addition to PEEP/CPAP to aid the spontaneous breaths.

Back-up Ventilation

Back-up Ventilation activates when the currently linked alarm occurs. This function can be linked with the Low Minute Volume (MVI) alarm, the Apnea alarm, or both alarms. During Back-up Ventilation, the linked alarm(s) will sound and the message window will indicate that Back-up Ventilation is in use. There are default Back-up Ventilation parameters, but the user may adjust these in the Advanced Screen. Back-up Ventilation is functional in all modes.

Back-up Ventilation is not active for 60 seconds after the user adjusts ventilator controls, changes modes, or starts ventilation from the Setting condition. During Back-up Ventilation the ALARM SILENCE/RESET button can be pressed to silence the audible alarm. This will not cancel Back-up Ventilation. When linked with the Low Minute Volume alarm, Back-up Ventilation is based on the delivered inspiratory minute volume. The inspiratory minute volume may be different from the expiratory minute volume in some conditions, such as in the case of a patient breathing circuit or airway leak or circuit disconnect.

Back-up Ventilation in A/CMV and SIMV Modes

The factory default setting for Back-up Ventilation in these two modes will increase the respiratory rate by 1.5 times the set rate, up to a maximum of 99 breaths/min. The minimum breath rate delivered is 15 breaths/min. The respiratory rate (RR) will increase only up to a rate that produces a 1:1 I:E ratio, even if the calculated Back-up Ventilation rate is higher.

Back-up Ventilation in Spontaneous Mode

The factory default setting for Back-up Ventilation in the SPONT mode will implement the changes identified in Box 15.15.

Cancellation of Back-up Ventilation

User canceled. If during Back-up Ventilation the user adjusts any ventilation parameter, Back-up Ventilation is suspended for 1 minute and all user-selected ventilation parameters are employed. Sixty seconds must pass after parameter adjustments before a linked alarm violation will result in Back-up Ventilation.

Patient canceled. If linked to low minute volume, Back-up Ventilation is canceled when delivered inspiratory minute volume exceeds the Low MVI alarm setting by 10%. If linked to Apnea alarm, Back-up Ventilation is canceled after 2 minutes. At that time the audible alarm stops, the alarm indicator latches, and the HT70 resumes ventilation at the user-selected parameters. Press the ALARM SILENCE/RESET button to cancel the latched alarm indicator and alarm message in the message display window.

NEWPORT HT70 PLUS

The Newport HT70 Plus model adds an on-airway flow sensor with onscreen graphics, exhaled tidal and minute volume monitoring/alarms, and flow trigger. The Plus model is also compatible with an optional plug-and-play oximeter.

CAREFUSION LTV 800

The LTV 800 ventilator (CareFusion) (Fig. 15.24) is the base model of the LTV series and is designed for use in the home or skilled nursing facility for patients who require ventilatory support. The LTV 800 is designed to ventilate adult through pediatric patients who weigh (5 kg [11 lb]) or more.[21] Its dimensions are 12 in × 10 in × 3 in, and it weighs 5.4 kg (12 lb). In general, the 800, 900, and 950 are used in home care and skilled nursing facilities. A previous section in this chapter focused on the LTV 1000 and 1200. This section focuses on the LTV 800 and points out some differences among the 800, the 900, and the 950. For a detailed comparison of these models, the reader is directed to the CareFusion website.

Power Source

The LTV series ventilators are designed to run on AC or DC (12-V) power. Although the unit normally uses an AC power cord adapter, when connected to an AC power outlet, the internal battery is continuously charged via a pigtail adapter. For DC power the LTV 800 can use either its own internal battery or one of two available external DC batteries. The internal battery can last approximately 60 minutes when fully charged. The fully charged large external battery can provide up to 8 hours of power, whereas the smaller battery, approximately 3 to 4 hours. It takes up to 8 hours to recharge the large external battery when it is completely depleted. (*Note:* An optional auto lighter adapter is also available for use of the LTV unit while in a car.)

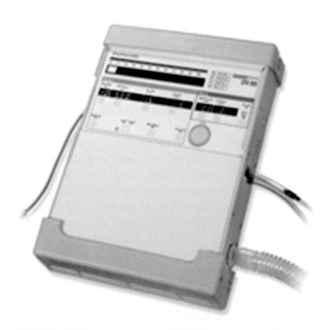

FIGURE 15.24 CareFusion LTV 800 ventilator. (Courtesy CareFusion, Inc., Yorba Linda, CA.)

Internal Mechanism

The LTV 800 ventilator is electrically powered with an internal rotary compressor to generate gas flow to the patient. Air is entrained into the LTV through the air inlet port on the left side of the ventilator. The microprocessor then controls the inspiratory flow to deliver the desired V_T and respiratory rate.

The LTV 800 is strictly a pressure-triggered, volume-controlled ventilator. Low-pressure oxygen enters the ventilator from a flowmeter, oxygen cylinder, or concentrator and blends with room air in the mixing chamber, which is called an *accumulator/silencer*. This chamber both blends the gas and acts as an acoustic silencer to reduce compressor noise. The 800, 900, and 950 have no internal blender and require a low-pressure oxygen source to enrich the delivered gas supply to the patient. The use of the oxygen analyzer is recommended to determine the exact F_IO_2.

Controls/Displays

The most commonly used controls are located on the front panel of the LTV 800. As with many of the newer ventilators that use built-in microprocessors, some controls are menu driven and are not located on the panel itself but are pulled up on the display window when needed. The front panel of the LTV 800 (Fig. 15.25) contains controls, alarm, and monitoring displays. The controls are divided into two rows. The bottom row contains main function buttons or touchpads, and the upper row contains parameter-setting buttons.

Above the row of parameter controls is a display window, which has two main functions. It displays current ventilator data and provides access to additional control functions. Alarm-setting keys are located to the right of the controls. Just below the alarm keys is a set value knob.

On/Standby

The ON/STANDBY button turns the ventilator on and illuminates the LED above it. The ventilator automatically begins to ventilate the patient by using the last settings. To place the ventilator into standby, the operator presses and holds the button for 3 seconds.

Mode-Selection Key

This button allows the operator to choose the desired delivery mode. The operator may choose CMV, IMV/CPAP, or non-invasive modes. Pushing the MODE-SELECTION button will cause the desired mode LED to flash for 5 seconds. Once the desired mode has been highlighted, the operator must press the MODE button a second time to confirm the mode selected. The ventilator will now begin to operate in the selected mode.

Control Lock

The CONTROL LOCK button allows the screen to be locked so that the settings cannot be accidentally changed. Pushing once turns the lock on. The LED above the control lock illuminates (i.e., the panel is locked). If the operator tries to change a setting when the panel is locked, the display window reads "LOCKED" and the LED flashes. Pressing the CONTROL LOCK button again unlocks the screen.

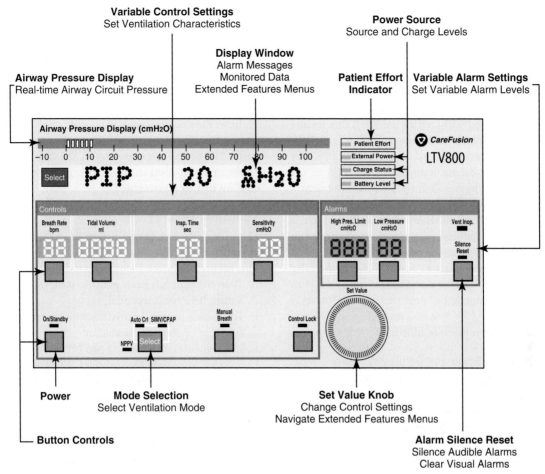

FIGURE 15.25 CareFusion LTV 800 ventilator's control panel. (Courtesy CareFusion, Inc., Yorba Linda, CA.)

Set Value

The SET VALUE knob is located to the right of the control lock soft key. This knob allows adjustment of the numerical values of the ventilator parameters and alarms, and it scrolls through menu items that appear in the display window.

Parameter Controls

The upper row of controls contains the parameter settings such as rate and V_T. The procedure for changing the variables in this row, and in the alarms, is basically the same. The parameter button is touched to make a change. This action brightly illuminates the set value for the parameter and dulls the displays for all other parameters. The Set Value knob is rotated until the value desired appears in the display above the parameter button. The change is immediately active when the parameter button is pressed again or after 5 seconds.

The number in the window above each parameter represents the value set for that parameter. Numbers appear bright when the parameter is active in the current mode and breath type. They appear dim when they are not. A parameter's digital display will also brighten if it is selected for changing. All others then dim. Three parameters—sensitivity, PS, and respiratory rate—can be turned off. The corresponding display for

each of those three parameters will be blank ("- -") when it is turned off.

Respiratory rate. The breath rate control sets the minimum mandatory breath rate (breaths/min). It can be turned off ("- -"). The adjustable rate range is 0 to 80 breaths/min. Pressing the button below the respiratory rate LED display will highlight that parameter. The operator turns the Set Value control to attain the desired value on the respiratory rate LED. Pressing the RATE button again will activate the new setting.

Tidal volume. The V_T soft key controls volume delivery during volume-targeted ventilation. The adjustable V_T range is 50 to 2000 mL. Pressing the soft key below the V_T LED display will highlight that parameter. With the Set Value knob the operator can attain the desired value on the V_T LED. Pressing the TIDAL VOLUME button will activate the new setting.

Inspiratory time. T_I sets the length of inspiration for volume-targeted and pressure-targeted breaths (range: 0.3 to 9.9 seconds). Inspiration cannot be shorter than 300 milliseconds. When V_T or T_I is being adjusted, the calculated flow ($\dot{V}calc$) is shown in the display window. The peak flow is based on the setting of T_I and V_T. The procedure for setting the T_I is the same as that described earlier for setting the respiratory rate and V_T.

Sensitivity. The Sensitivity soft key is used to set the pressure trigger sensitivity level for assisted or spontaneous breaths. The range is from off ("- -") up to −2 to +20 cm H_2O. When a trigger is detected, the patient effort LED illuminates. The LTV 950 has flow triggering with an adjustable range of 1 to 9 L/min.

Leak compensation. A leak-compensation feature is available on both the 900 and 950 (not in the 800); this feature constantly measures for leaks and adjusts the baseline of the ventilator to compensate for leaks of up to 6 L/min. In earlier models of the LTV that do not have leak compensation, the sensitivity is usually set higher than the leak measurement.

PEEP/CPAP. In the LTV 800, 900, 950, and 1000 ventilators, PEEP is not internally controlled. An external PEEP valve is required as part of the ventilator circuit and is illustrated in Fig. 15.11 *(detail A)*. The adjustable range for PEEP/CPAP is 0 to 20 cm H_2O. The operator can adjust PEEP by pushing the PEEP valve lock with one hand and rotating the valve with the other hand. It is important to note that the PEEP level is not compensated on the LTV 800, 900, and 950, so sensitivity must be readjusted when PEEP is added.

Airway Pressure Bar Graph and Display Window

At the very top of the operating panel is the airway pressure display. This horizontal bar graph displays the pressure in the patient circuit (range: −10 to +108 cm H_2O). The display window shows monitored data, alarm messages, and the extended features menu. During normal operation, the monitored data are presented sequentially. Each item is displayed for 3 seconds.

Select Button—Display Screen

The SELECT button to the left of the display screen has several functions. It is used to stop the normal scrolling of monitored ventilator parameters. Pushing the button once while the normal data scan is active halts the screen with the current parameter data showing. Each time the button is pushed after that, the next data item in the list is displayed. Scanning can be resumed by pressing the button twice within 3 seconds.

Front-Panel Indicators

To the right of the pressure manometer are four indicators. The patient effort indicator illuminates when the ventilator detects a patient's inspiratory effort based on the sensitivity setting. The external power illuminates when the unit is operating from an external power source. This can be an AC power source or an external battery. The adjacent LED is green when power is adequate and yellow when external power is low.

Alarms

The alarm controls and settings are to the right of the parameter controls. The first alarm is the "High Pressure Limit" alarm (in cm H_2O). This control establishes the maximum pressure allowed in the patient circuit. If the set value is reached, an audible alarm sounds, the display window reads "HIGH PRES," inspiration ends, and the exhalation valve opens. If a high-pressure condition continues for more than

3 seconds, the internal turbine stops rotating and circuit pressure empties to the atmosphere. The audible alarm automatically stops when the pressure drops to the high-pressure limit of −5 cm H_2O or drops to a circuit pressure of 25 cm H_2O, whichever is less. To set the high-pressure limit, the soft key is pressed and the Set Value knob is rotated to the desired value (range: 5 to 100 cm H_2O).

To set the low-pressure alarm value (cm H_2O), the operator pushes the Low Pressure soft key and rotates the Set Value knob. The actual value appears in the display window. The knob is rotated until the desired value is seen (range: from OFF up to 1 to 60 cm H_2O).

Vent-Inop Display

The VENT INOP indicator just right of the alarm controls is illuminated only when the ventilator is in the inoperative state. This occurs under the following conditions:

1. The ventilator has been put into standby (ON/STANDBY button held for 3 seconds).
2. The power sources, either internal or external, are insufficient to operate the ventilator.
3. The ventilator has been turned off.
4. A condition exists that renders the ventilator unable to provide patient ventilation and unsafe to use.

When a ventilator inoperative alarm occurs, the inspiratory flow stops; the exhalation valve opens, allowing the patient to breathe spontaneously from room air; the oxygen blender solenoids close; the VENT INOP LED is red; and an audible alarm sounds continuously. The patient needs to be removed from the ventilator, and another mode of ventilating must be provided for the patient immediately.

Alarm Silence

The SILENCE/RESET button is located to the right of the pressure alarm LED display and is used to silence an alarm for 60 seconds. This button can also be used to start a 60-second alarm-silence period, for example, before disconnecting the patient for some procedure or when the ventilator is placed in standby. After an alarm condition has been resolved, this button can also be used to clear the visual alarm displays. The SILENCE/RESET button also silences the audible ventilator inoperative alarm, but the VENT INOP LED will remain lit for at least 5 minutes.

Modes of Ventilation

The LTV 800 series ventilator provides the following modes of ventilation: control, A/C, SIMV, CPAP, Apnea BUV, and NIV. The LTV 800 and 900 provide only volume-controlled ventilation breaths, whereas the LTV 950 can provide both volume-controlled and pressure-controlled breaths.

Control and Assist/Control

Control and A/C are available when the "ASSIST/CTRL" LED is illuminated near the mode select button. Control is considered active, by the manufacturer, when the sensitivity is set to off ("- -"). If using the control mode, the operator must consider the patient's effort to breathe over the set rate, because this could be very uncomfortable for the patient and lead to patient–ventilator dyssynchrony.

Assist/Control

A/C is considered active when a value greater than zero sensitivity is set. The breath type is established by the BREATH-TYPE SELECT button (volume-targeted or pressure-targeted, in the 950 unit only). The rate is set by the breath rate control. In the A/C mode the set rate can be the minimum rate setting. The patient can trigger additional mandatory breaths as desired.

SIMV

The SIMV mode is active when the SIMV/CPAP LED is illuminated near the MODE SELECT button. The breath rate (1 to 80 breaths/min) establishes the minimum mandatory breath rate. Patients can spontaneously breathe between mandatory breaths. Spontaneous breaths can be from the set baseline pressure (0 or PEEP) and can also be supported with PS with the LTV 950.

CPAP

The CPAP mode is considered the active mode if the SIMV/CPAP LED is illuminated and the breath rate is off ("- -"). In CPAP, spontaneous breaths can be from the baseline pressure and can also be pressure supported with the LTV 900 and 950.

Pressure Support

The LTV 800 does not offer a PS mode, but the LTV 900 and 950 both offer PS. The adjustable range goes from off up to 1 to 60 cm H_2O.

Apnea Backup

Apnea backup ventilation is available should the patient become apneic. The apnea interval is set by using the extended features menu. The ventilator begins Apnea BUV in the A/C mode based on the current settings.

The active controls are displayed at full intensity, and others are dimmed. If the set breath rate is ≥12 breaths/min, the apnea breath rate is the set breath rate. If the set breath rate is <12 breaths/min and the breath rate is not limited by other control settings, the apnea breath rate is 12 breaths/min. If the set breath rate is limited to <12 breaths/min, because of V_T, flow, and T_I settings, the apnea breath rate is the highest allowed rate. Normal ventilation resumes when two consecutive patient-triggered breaths occur or when the operator resets the apnea alarm using the SILENCE/RESET control.

NIV

NIV is provided as a secondary mode that may be selected in addition to the primary ventilation mode. NIV is selected by using the extended features menu. When activated, ventilation is delivered according to the selected mode and breath type that are currently active by way of a full mask or other noninvasive interface. The NIV LED is lit when it is on. The number of alarms in NIV is limited when it is active and is similar to those on the LTV 1000 (see Box 15.12). Again, the operator must remember that the LTV 800 and 900 can support

only volume-targeted ventilation and the LTV 950 can supply both volume and pressure ventilation.

SUMMARY OF THE LTV 800, 900, 950, 1000, AND 1200

The LTV 800, 900, and 950 ventilators are primarily designed for home care and skilled nursing facilities. The LTV 1000 and 1200 are primarily designed for transport and acute care.

PURITAN BENNETT 540

The Medtronic Minimally Invasive Therapies Puritan Bennett 540 (PB 540) ventilator (Medtronic Minimally Invasive Therapies) (Fig. 15.26) is indicated for the continuous or intermittent mechanical ventilatory support of patients weighing at least (5 kg [11 lb]) who require mechanical ventilation. The ventilator is suitable for use in institutional, home, and portable settings. It is not intended for use as an emergency transport ventilator. Specifically, the ventilator is applicable for adult and pediatric patients who may require invasive or noninvasive ventilation with both pressure-targeted and volume-targeted modes The PB 540's dimensions are 9.25 in wide × 12.40 in deep × 6.0 in high, and it weighs 4.5 kg (9.9 lb).[22] Table 15.22 lists the specifications of the PB 540.

Power Source

The PB 540 may operate on any of four power sources: AC power, 12- to 30-V DC power, internal battery power, or auxiliary DC car adapter (cigarette lighter) can be used to power the ventilator. But when AC power is available, the ventilator will automatically select AC power as its primary operating power source. The internal lithium battery may provide up to 11 hours (depending on ventilator settings and other factors) of battery life.

Internal Mechanism

The operation of the PB 540 is based on a self-adapting, closed-loop drive system. The speed of the flow generator

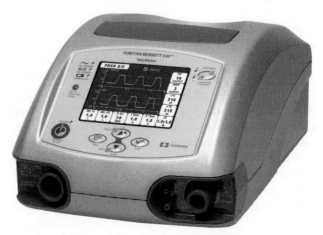

FIGURE 15.26 Puritan Bennett 540 ventilator. (Copyright © 2013 Medtronic Minimally Invasive Therapies. All rights reserved. Reprinted with permission of Medtronic Minimally Invasive Therapies.)

TABLE 15.22 Puritan Bennett 540 Ventilator Specifications	
Modes	Assisted Controlled Volume, Assisted Controlled Pressure, Synchronous Intermittent Mandatory Ventilation Volume, Synchronous Intermittent Mandatory Ventilation Pressure, CPAP, PSV
Power source	AC power, internal DC power, external DC power
Rate	1-80 breaths/min
Noninvasive ventilation mode	Yes
Peak pressure	120 cm H_2O
Tidal volume	50-2000 mL
Inspiratory time	0.3-6 s
PEEP/CPAP	0-20 cm H_2O
Oxygen percent	21-100%
Pressure support	5-55 cm H_2O
Monitors/displays	Digital Airway Pressure Gauge, LED display window
Dimensions	6 in × 12.4 in × 9.25 in, 4.5 kg (9.9 lb)
Alarms[a]	Apnea Interval, High Respiratory Rate, High PEEP, Low PEEP, High Pressure Limit, High/Low Oxygen Pressure, Low Minute Ventilation, Low Pressure Alarm
Battery duration	Approximately 11 h with fully charged internal battery at setting of PIP 10 cm H_2O, V_T 200 mL, rate 20 breaths/min

[a]A full list of alarms for the PB 540 can be found in the PB 540 User manual available from your Puritan Bennett representative. *CPAP*, Continuous positive airway pressure; *PEEP*, positive end-expiratory pressure; *PIP*, peak inspiratory pressure; *PSV*, pressure-support ventilation; *V_T*, tidal volume.

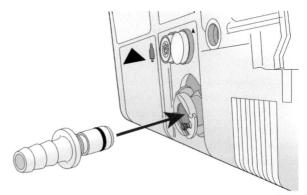

FIGURE 15.27 Medtronic Minimally Invasive Therapies PB 540 ventilator's oxygen connector. (Copyright © 2013 Medtronic Minimally Invasive Therapies. All rights reserved. Reprinted with the permission of Medtronic Minimally Invasive Therapies.)

can also be used to determine the end of the inspiration phase in certain ventilation modes. The flow measurement is automatically corrected as a function of the atmospheric pressure measured inside the ventilator with the Altitude Compensation feature. The flow and volume are in BTPS conditions.

Oxygen Source

Oxygen administered to the patient is introduced from an external source into the machine through the oxygen connector at the rear of the ventilator. It is essential that you also use the special factory coupler supplied with the ventilator to attach the external low-pressure oxygen source to the connector. The connector is also fitted with a nonreturn airtight valve system. The nonreturn airtight valve system includes a stud and a locking tab (Fig. 15.27). The specific oxygen flow to the patient depends on the physiological characteristics of the patient and the ventilator settings. The operator must ensure that the oxygen supply pressure to the machine never exceeds 7.25 psi or a flow of 15 L/min. F_IO_2 enrichment up to 50% can be attained with the PB 540. Because the PB 540 does not include an internal oxygen analyzer, it is recommended to always measure the delivered oxygen with a calibrated oxygen analyzer that features a high and low concentration alarm so as to ensure that the prescribed oxygen concentration is delivered to the patient.

Operation of the Ventilator

Operation of the 540 ventilator begins by moving the protective cover over the ON/OFF (I/O) rocker-type switch. The 540 has power applied when the switch is in the I position and switched off in the O position. Once the power has been applied to the 540 ventilator, the ventilator will go through several diagnostic steps. First a *Power On Self-Test* (POST) is initiated when the ventilator is plugged into an AC power source.

The second event that occurs is that all the front-panel indicators flash except for the indicator that displays the type of power supply being utilized and the audible alarms will briefly sound. The ventilator's display backlight will illuminate, and the PURITAN BENNETT logo will be briefly displayed.

The blue VENT STDBY indicator to the right of the VENTILATION ON/OFF key illuminates, indicating the device is

(turbine) is servo-controlled according to the patient pressure signal or the inspired flow signal. The turbine speed control algorithms themselves are based on equations that vary according to the ventilation modes, settings, and the respiratory cycle phases. Thus fixing the pressure rise time or flow pattern has an influence on the level of turbine acceleration at the start of the inspiration phase. The transition between the inspiration phase and expiration phase is controlled by a deceleration or braking algorithm proportional to the pressure difference between the two phases. The expiratory solenoid valve (three-way valve) is fully closed during the inspiratory phase and is proportionally controlled during the expiratory phase to obtain the bias flow.

The speed of the turbine adapts to the expiratory pressure threshold during the entire expiratory phase to maintain the operator-set PEEP. The flow measurement completes the system by enabling detection of patient inspiratory effort and the triggering of inspiration phases. The flow measurement

now in the standby mode. The display panel will then produce a Welcome Menu screen for approximately 5 seconds. The data provided includes the hours of operation of the ventilator, as well as the number of hours and minutes the patient has been utilizing the ventilator.

It is possible to skip the Welcome Screen and directly begin ventilation by pressing the VENTILATION ON/OFF key to start ventilation immediately. The Ventilation menu is then displayed, along with a visual prompt to press the VENTILATION ON/OFF key to start ventilation, as shown in Fig. 15.26. The starting ventilation mode that follows the Welcome menu is by default the last ventilation mode and settings last utilized. If the ventilator's memory of the last utilized settings is faulty, a CHECK SETTINGS alarm is activated. If this alarm occurs, the operator should reenter the desired parameters and resave them; otherwise the ventilator will operate on default parameter values.

Initiating Ventilation

With the ventilator on and in standby, a message will appear on the right-hand side of the screen that prompts the ventilator operator to press the VENTILATION ON/OFF key to start ventilation. Pressing and then releasing the VENTILATION ON/OFF key will cause the blue Ventilator Standby light indicator to extinguish, and the ventilator will sound a beep. Ventilation will then commence with the values of the monitored ventilator parameters displayed in the right-hand window. The manufacturer recommends that the operator allow the ventilator to complete one full breath cycle before connecting the ventilator to the patient.

To stop ventilation the operator must press and hold down the VENTILATION ON/OFF key for approximately 3 seconds. A message will appear in the screen prompting the user to release the VENTILATION ON/OFF key to stop ventilation.

The ventilator will sound two beeps, at which point the operator can release the key and mechanical ventilation will stop. The blue LED located to the upper right of the VENTILATION ON/OFF key will again illuminate to indicate ventilation is on Standby. To totally power down the ventilator, move the I/O rocker switch in the rear of the ventilator to the O position. The blue LED Standby light and the ventilator screen will turn off. When the ventilator is completely stopped, but while it is still connected to the AC power source (the green AC POWER indicator is illuminated), the internal battery will continue charging.

Operational Controls

The PB 540 ventilator uses a microturbine and the patient circuit with integral exhalation valve to provide ventilatory support to patients. The 540 ventilator is capable of providing both invasive and noninvasive support. Clinicians may use a variety of interfaces to connect patients to the ventilator: nasal or full face masks; endotracheal or tracheotomy tubes.

All operational controls are accessed through the control panel (see Fig. 15.26) located on the top of the ventilator. The control panel features the controls for setting up and operating the ventilator as well as LEDs to indicate the ventilator's power source, ventilation On/Off status, and alarm priority level. Control functions include turning the ventilation on and off, configuring ventilation modes, silencing and canceling alarms, and setting device and alarm parameters. The display screen displays current modes, ventilation settings, patient data and waveforms, and configuration of the ventilator, as well as alarm management.

To access the setting controls, the operator needs to press the MENU key. Fig. 15.26 illustrates the ventilator parameter selection screen. Each adjustable parameter has a small open square next to it on the left side of the screen. A white-filled cursor square will be noted next to the ventilator parameter that may be adjusted. Utilizing the Up or Down arrows on the control panel, the operator may select any parameter needing adjustment. Pressing the MENU screen again will change the display to the alarm settings screen or the graphics screen with the mode and ventilator settings displayed along the bottom and right side of the screen.

Alarms

The alarms or faults generated by the PB 540 ventilator are classified into two categories:
- Ventilation (or utilization) alarms
- Technical faults

Some of the PB 540's ventilator alarms are adjustable, depending on ventilation modes. Other alarms are automatic and nonadjustable to create safe patient ventilation. Alarms that are activated indicate events likely to affect the patient's ventilation in the short term and necessitate rapid correction of the alarm parameter. Alarms on the 540 are classified into three levels of priority. The alarm hierarchy for signaling the level of alarm criticality is listed below.
- *Very High Priority (VHP): Immediate critical situation; ventilation is impossible:* Continuous sound signaling/with or without continuous red LED illumination/with or without message/with or without display lighting (it is possible for an alarm condition to occur that may not have **both** a message and lighting).
- *High Priority (HP): Critical situation in the short term; ventilation is potentially compromised:* High-frequency sound signaling/flashing red LED illumination/with message/with display lighting
- *Medium Priority (MP): Critical situation in the long term; ventilation is not affected in the short term:* Medium-frequency sound signaling/flashing yellow LED illumination/with message/with display lighting
- *Note:* There are currently no Low-Priority (LP) Alarms.

During operation, when an alarm is activated, one of the red or yellow alarm indicators to the left of the ALARM CONTROL key will illuminate and flash, and an alarm tone sounds. A message is displayed and flashes in reverse video at the lower right-hand portion of the Ventilation Menu or Alarm Menu screen. In the event several alarms are activated at the same time, the highest priority audible and visual alarm is highlighted; however, all active messages are displayed, in the sequence in which they occurred. All alarms are recorded in the internal memory of the ventilator at the time they are activated.

The Alarm Logs menu is used to display the last eight alarms activated, along with their date and time of activation. The operator accesses the Alarm Log menu by pressing the MENU key to access the alarm setting menu (if this is not the menu currently displayed). Then the operator presses the DOWN key until the cursor is on the "Alarm Logs" line at the bottom of the page. Pressing the ENTER key will then display the Alarm Logs screen.

The audible portion of alarms may be silenced for 60 seconds at a time. Pressing the ALARM CONTROL key results in canceling the audible portion of all activated alarms. The visual portions (light indicator and message) of activated alarms will remain visible until the alarm situation is resolved and the alarm is reset. For a list of alarms available on the 540 ventilator, readers are referred to the ventilator's operating manual.

Modes of Ventilation

The PB 540 ventilator offers A/C, SIMV, and CPAP modes of ventilation. The types of breaths can be classified into Volume Control, Pressure Control, and Pressure Support categories. When set to an A/C mode, machine-initiated breaths are delivered at a clinician-set volume or pressure, inspiratory time, and rate. If the patient triggers a spontaneous breath between machine breaths, the ventilator will deliver a breath based on the volume or pressure settings and inspiratory time. Whether initiated by the patient or the ventilator, all breaths are delivered at the same preset volume or pressure and inspiratory time.

The names of the A/C modes are:
- VOL A/C, if the breaths are based on a volume setting
- PRES A/C, if the breaths are based on a pressure setting

When set to a SIMV Mode, machine-initiated breaths are delivered at a clinician-set volume or pressure, inspiratory time, and rate. These mandatory breaths are synchronized with patient effort. If the patient triggers a spontaneous breath between machine breaths, the ventilator will deliver a spontaneous breath, which is pressure supported. CPAP spontaneous breaths are not available in SIMV modes.

The names of the SIMV modes are:
- V SIMV, if mandatory breaths are based on a volume setting
- P SIMV, if mandatory breaths are based on a pressure setting

In CPAP the ventilator maintains a constant level of positive pressure in the patient's airway. The level of CPAP is adjustable from 0 to 20 cm H_2O.

Like CPAP mode, PSV/CPAP mode maintains a constant level of pressure in the patient's airway. In addition, the ventilator applies a clinician-set PS adjustable to 5 to 55 cm H_2O on each of the patient's breaths. This has the same benefits as CPAP, with the additional benefit of assisting the patient in decreasing work of breathing.

III. NONINVASIVE VENTILATION

The first successful use of NIV was recorded in the mid-18th century. During the course of the following 200 years, advances

in the equipment technology enabled clinicians to test this mode of ventilation as a possible form of treatment for patients requiring mechanical ventilatory support. Dräger, one of the earliest supporters of NIV, used a face mask and a compressed gas source to manage the airway of drowning victims as early as 1911.[23] The experiments with NIV continued in the late 1930s, when Barach and colleagues used intermittent positive-pressure ventilation (IPPV) to treat patients with pulmonary edema, and in the 1950s, with Motely and colleagues for the treatment of acute respiratory failure.[23] It is worth mentioning, however, that the mainstay of ventilatory support in the United States until the 1960s was the iron lung, with intermittent positive-pressure breathing (IPPB) being relegated mainly to the administration of aerosolized medication.

During the 1960s and 1970s, invasive ventilation by way of endotracheal tubes progressively became more popular than NIV by iron lung. Cuffed endotracheal tubes provided better protection to the airway, and PPV provided superior ventilatory support. These two factors significantly decreased interest in NIV for a number of years.

In the 1980s, improved patient interfaces (masks) and success with the treatment of obstructive sleep apnea (OSA) through mask ventilation led to the revival of NIV as an alternative mode to traditional invasive mechanical ventilation.[24] Since then NIV has gained widespread approval for use in the acute care and home care environments. This increased interest can be attributed to several factors (Box 15.16), including the advent of portable and safe ventilators, user-friendly interfaces, and a better understanding of respiratory muscle function.[1,25] The use of NIV in conjunction with appropriate medical therapies is now considered the standard of care for a select population of patients with acute respiratory failure caused by severe exacerbations of chronic obstructive pulmonary disease. Indeed, clinicians have chosen to use NIV for a variety of disease states that were previously managed with conventional mechanical ventilation.[26-28]

Clinical trials evaluating the effectiveness of NIV for patients with neuromuscular disease, chronic obstructive pulmonary disease necessitating nighttime respiratory muscle rest, and acute respiratory failure, as well as for postoperative support and the facilitation of weaning, have provided valuable information on the effectiveness of NIV. Randomized, controlled

---

BOX 15.16   Factors Contributing to NIV Interest[28,41]

- Success in obstructive sleep apnea[2]
- Improved patient interfaces[2]
- Does not inhibit natural pulmonary defense mechanisms
- Allows the patient to eat, drink, and verbalize
- Allows the patient to expectorate secretions
- Less costly than conventional mechanical ventilation
- Possibility of use in acute and chronic ventilatory failure
- Avoidance of complications of intubation and tracheostomy[2]
- Ability to be used when patients refuse intubation[2]

NIV, Noninvasive positive-pressure ventilation.

trials indicate that NIV is associated with lower rates of endotracheal intubation, lower intensive care and hospital mortality rates, and a decreased number of admission days in the ICU and hospital.[28,29]

The following information focuses on the various patient interfaces used to provide NIV along with a description of examples of noninvasive positive-pressure ventilators.

THE PATIENT INTERFACE

Effective application of NIV requires the use a properly fitting mask that combines minimal air leakage with maximum comfort.[26] Lack of comfort leads to poor compliance, resulting in less use and a deterioration of the patient's medical condition. The interfaces typically used include nasal mask, nasal pillows, oronasal mask, total face mask, and mouthpiece.

The nasal mask is the most commonly used mask and often the most difficult to properly apply to the patient (Fig. 15.28). Selecting the correct mask size, particularly nasal mask size, can be a challenging task for the respiratory therapist. The most common mistake associated with these devices involves using a larger-than-necessary mask. It is important to recognize that the patient's nose, not the face, needs to be covered. The top of the mask should lie at the junction of the nasal bone

and the frontal bone and be fitted to cover the nares snugly. The sizes most frequently used for adult patients are small and medium. Most nasal mask manufacturers provide a gauging device that the clinician can use to estimate the proper size mask for a patient. (*Note*: Gauging devices are manufactured specifically for the home ventilator or CPAP device in use and should not be used with other equipment.)

Nasal pillows are a second form of nasal NIV and are often used as an alternative to the nasal mask (Fig. 15.29). The interface consists of two cushions that are inserted into the nares of the patient that allow for ventilation. Pressure is not applied to the bridge of the nose as with the nasal mask, thereby reducing the risk for pressure sores. It is not uncommon to alternate between the nasal mask and nasal pillow interfaces to reduce the risk for developing pressure sores.

The oronasal mask is slightly larger than the nasal mask (Fig. 15.30). Fitting the mask begins with placement above the junction of the nasal bone and frontal bone and includes the mouth and the nose. The bottom of the mask should rest just under the bottom lip. When first fitting the mask, it is not unusual to have large air leaks around the mouth. A period of adjustment is usually required that allows the patient to acclimate to the oronasal mask. This adjustment generally results in a reduction in the amount of leakage. Nonetheless, leaks are inevitable. It is important to mention that using a mask that is too tightly fitted for the patient may cause the

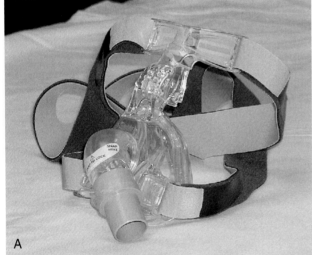

A

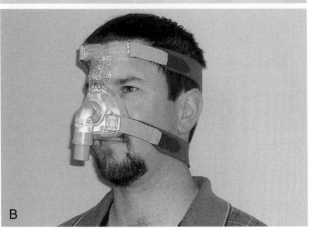

B

FIGURE 15.28 Example of nasal mask.

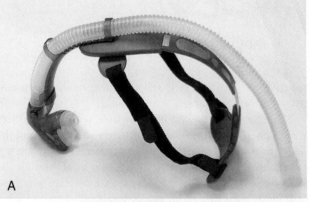

A

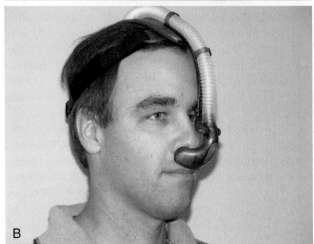

B

FIGURE 15.29 Example of nasal pillows.

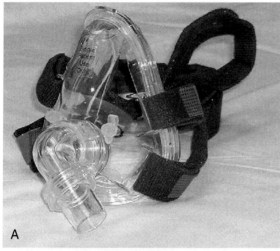

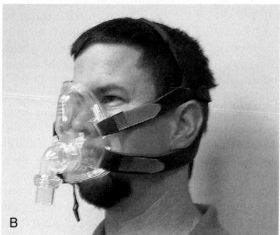

FIGURE 15.30 Example of oronasal mask.

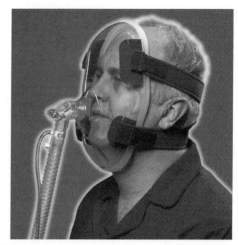

FIGURE 15.31 Full face mask. (Courtesy Philips Respironics, Murrysville, PA.)

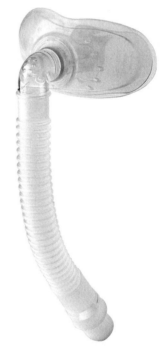

FIGURE 15.32 Oral continuous positive airway pressure (CPAP) device.

patient to be uncomfortable and place the person at increased risk for pressure necrosis.

NIV machines that are typically used with these devices are designed to compensate for relatively small leaks and the subsequent loss of volume. Large, uncontrolled leaks are not acceptable. A chin strap may be effective at alleviating the problem if an excessive leak persists. Chin straps are most commonly used with nasal masks or pillows.

Another alternative for patients who experience claustrophobia or who cannot tolerate nasal or oronasal masks is the full-face mask. The total face mask is a clear, lightweight plastic faceplate surrounded by a soft, inflatable cushion that seals the perimeter of the face (Fig. 15.31). Full-face masks reduce the tendency for pressure sores because these devices seal the entire face.

The final type of interface that can be used for NIV is the oral mask. An oral mask allows IPPV when patients have trouble tolerating or achieving a seal with other conventional mask options. The Oracle Mask (Fig. 15.32), which was designed and manufactured by Fisher & Paykel Healthcare in 2000, was the first oral mask available for CPAP/bilevel therapy. This device uses a soft silicone oblong design that seals through the interaction of two silicone flanges that fit against the inside and outside of the patient's mouth. The chief benefit of the

mouth seal is that it rarely contributes to the development of pressure sores. It is also easy to use.

The equipment used to attach the masks to the client is often overlooked. Securing the various interfaces is just as important as selecting the appropriate size. The apparatus most commonly used consists of cloth straps and Velcro headgear (see Fig. 15.30). It is customary to have three points of attachment (prongs or slots) on the oronasal and nasal mask that allow the straps to fasten to the headgear. These prongs or slots for straps are often found on the outer edge of the mask and allow the clinician to evenly distribute the pressure on the face, thereby reducing leaks. The slots for the Velcro straps or the plastic prongs are positioned to evenly distribute the mask on the face of the user. It is easiest if the

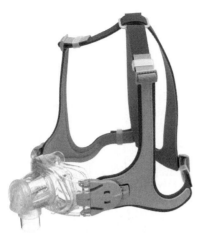

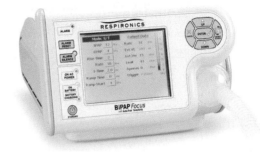

FIGURE 15.35 Respironics BiPAP Focus. (Courtesy Respironics, Inc., Murrysville, PA.)

FIGURE 15.33 Mirage Kidsta. (©ResMed 2013. San Diego, CA.)

> **BOX 15.17 BiPAP Focus Contraindications**
>
> - Lack of spontaneous respiratory drive
> - Inability to maintain a patent airway or adequately clear secretions
> - At risk for aspiration of gastric contents
> - Acute sinusitis or otitis media
> - Hypotension

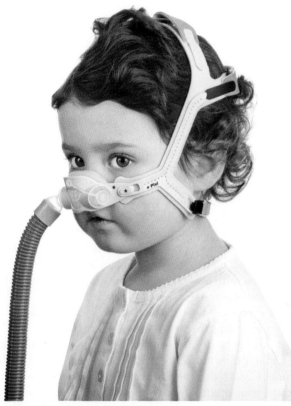

FIGURE 15.34 Pixi. (©ResMed 2013. San Diego, CA.)

clinician makes all strap attachments before placing the mask on the client.

Figs. 15.33 and 15.34 provides examples of noninvasive interfaces that can be used for pediatric patients.

VENTILATORS

Home care NIV ventilators and other support devices may have any of the following features:
- The ability to provide full ventilatory support
- The ability to ventilate at night only

- Bilevel support or CPAP
- High-pressure, low-pressure, and apnea alarms

Controls that are common to noninvasive positive-pressure ventilators include the following: A/C, SIMV, PSV, bilevel pressure ventilation modes, volume ventilation, respiratory rate, T_I, PEEP, F_IO_2, and humidification. Following is information about several NIV modes that are commonly used today.

Respironics BiPAP Focus

The BiPAP Focus noninvasive ventilator (Philips Respironics, Inc.) provides noninvasive breathing support for adult patients who weigh 30 kg (66.1 lb) or more, and is used for the treatment of respiratory insufficiency, respiratory distress, and OSA (Fig. 15.35).[30] The Focus is microprocessor controlled and offers two modes of support. The BiPAP Focus features CPAP and spontaneous/timed (S/T) modes to provide needed noninvasive support. The unit weighs 4.5 kg (10 lb), and its dimensions are 5.5 in × 11.4 in × 14 in. The BiPAP Focus is contraindicated for the conditions listed in Box 15.17.

Power Source

The BiPAP Focus is designed to operate on 100-V AC/230-V AC and 50/60 Hz via a DC power converter. The unit also has an internal battery as a backup power source. This internal battery is designed to operate the unit for 45 minutes. The internal battery will be charged when the unit is connected to the AC power and the ON/OFF switch in the back of the unit is in the On position, which is denoted by an illuminated charging LED. The battery charge time is typically less than 5 hours, but it can be longer because of environmental conditions, such as lower temperatures. The battery is intended only as a backup power source and for use during transport

TABLE 15.23 **BiPAP Focus Internal Battery Life Expectancy**	
CPAP or IPAP Setting	**Approximate Battery Life**
10 cm H$_2$O	60 minutes
15 cm H$_2$O	50 minutes
20 cm H$_2$O	40 minutes
25 cm H$_2$O	30 minutes
30 cm H$_2$O	20 minutes

Warning: When running on battery, the high flows that occur during a patient disconnect will cause the battery to deplete in as little as 2 min. Connect to AC power immediately as soon as the battery depletion alarm sounds to avoid total loss of power. *CPAP,* Continuous positive airway pressure; *IPAP,* inspiratory positive airway pressure.

within the hospital. The manufacturer warns that the BiPAP Focus will not operate without a functioning battery installed in the unit. Estimated internal battery life is illustrated in Table 15.23.

Internal Mechanism

The ventilator uses a blower-driven, sleeve valve–controlled system that is able to deliver and maintain pressures from 0 cm H$_2$O to 35 cm H$_2$O at one constant level (CPAP) or at two levels (IPAP and EPAP) or bilevel ventilation. The delivery of a breath begins with room air that is entrained through an inlet filter at the rear of the ventilator and then pressurized by the internal blower. The entrained air moves from the blower to the pressure valve assembly (PVA), which regulates the desired inspiratory, expiratory, or continuous pressures that are selected for the patient.

In line after the PVA, and just before the machine outlet, is the airflow module. This device monitors total gas flow and patient pressures. This information is sent to the main control system of the Focus, where it is processed and used to maintain set pressure levels and trigger and cycle thresholds.

Oxygen Source

The BiPAP Focus is designed to provide noninvasive support, primarily at room air concentrations. Supplemental oxygen may be added by placing a Respironics oxygen-enrichment adapter and an oxygen safety valve in line with the patient circuit immediately after the bacteria filter on the breathing circuit connector on the front of the unit. The potential range of supplemental oxygen concentration is dependent on factors such as given V$_T$, pressures used, and flow of supplemental oxygen into the enrichment adapter. The use of a calibrated oxygen analyzer is recommended, and oxygen flow into the enrichment adapter should not exceed 15 L/min.

Leak Compensation

Leaks are inherent to user interfaces and patient circuits in NIV machines. These leaks can affect the device's ability to trigger and cycle a breath effectively. In addition, the estimation of a leak is important for proper analysis of the signal to ensure patient–ventilator synchrony. Therefore monitoring and

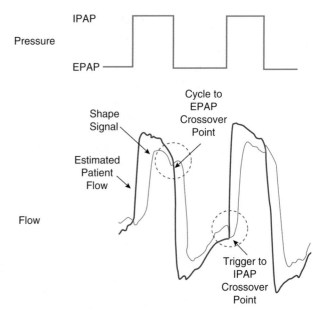

FIGURE 15.36 Respironics BiPAP Focus shape signal. *EPAP,* Expiratory positive airway pressure; *IPAP,* inspiratory positive airway pressure. (Courtesy Philips Respironics, Inc., Murrysville, PA.)

compensating for changes in leaks are critical for maintaining the appropriate trigger and cycle levels for the ventilator.

The BiPAP Focus uses a digital trigger-sensitivity system called Digital Auto-Trak sensitivity that features a combination of different mechanisms to identify and modify baseline values in response to leaks. It also automatically adjusts its variable trigger and cycle threshold to maintain performance in the presence of leaks.

The built-in microprocessor governs the digital signal process. It does this by modeling the patient's flow patterns. In this process it analyzes and estimates leak rates to provide triggering sensitivity. The ventilator works to synchronize the transition between inhalation and exhalation.

The expiratory flow rate adjustment primarily works to make course adjustments in baseline values. When the ventilator is initially turned on, it measures the total flow through the circuit before it is connected to the patient. This includes the intentional leak created by the exhalation port. The BiPAP Focus is then attached to the patient, and the expiratory flow through the circuit is measured after the machine has cycled into expiration. Through measurement and calculation, the ventilator is able to determine the intentional and unintentional leak of the system. This allows the ventilator to establish and monitor the baseline pressure, which allows the trigger and cycle values to be set.

Triggering to inspiration (IPAP) occurs by two methods. The first is by volume triggering. When 6 mL of volume from patient effort is inhaled from the circuit, the ventilator volume triggers to IPAP.

The second method for triggering to IPAP is the shape signal. The shape signal is actually a shadow image of the patient's actual flow/time waveform that is "redrawn" by the microprocessor to overlap the actual signal (Fig. 15.36).

The shape signal is part of the Digital Auto-Trak sensitivity. When the patient flow intersects the shadow flow from the shape signal, the ventilator triggers to IPAP.

Cycling to exhalation (EPAP) occurs when the patient's flow intersects the shape signal flow. A second method of cycling to EPAP occurs when the microprocessor's electronic signal rises in proportion to the inspiratory flow waveform.

Sometimes a patient's mouth will open at the end of inspiration during BiPAP ventilation. This results in a rise in flow from the ventilator to maintain the set IPAP pressure. The sudden rush of flow through the upper airway and sinuses can rouse the patient and adversely affect cycling. When this occurs with the Focus, the Digital Auto-Trak system recognizes the rapid increase in flow at end inspiration as a result of a leak and immediately cycles to EPAP to maintain patient–ventilator synchrony.

Tidal Volume Estimation

Although the BiPAP Focus does not directly measure volume, it is able to estimate inspiratory and expiratory V_Ts based on the patient flow and the time spent in inspiration and expiration. Differences that occur between the inspiratory and expiratory V_Ts are then assumed to be the result of a change in the amount of intentional leak and are accounted for by an adjustment in baseline for the next breath. This feature allows the ventilator to adjust the baseline on a breath-to-breath basis, thereby reducing large corrections.

Controls and Displays

The BiPAP Focus is powered up by pressing the ON/OFF switch located on the back of the unit, followed by pressing the STANDBY button on the front of the unit in the lower left-hand corner. It is recommended that a preoperational check be completed before the unit is connected to the patient.

The front panel of the BiPAP Focus consists of three sections. On the left-hand side of the unit, you will find a STANDBY key, a battery charging/on battery indicator, AC power indicators, an ALARM SILENCE key, ALARM RESET, and an alarm indicator.

The second section consists of the navigation LCD screen, which provides three different screen options for the operator to view. The option screen allows the operator to view or change mode and settings. This screen can also display real-time patient data (Fig. 15.37). The patient data screen will display the total respiratory rate, estimated V_T, estimated minute volume, percent leak, number of apneic events, and trigger, whether patient initiated or time triggered by the ventilator. A pressure bar graph is located on the right side of the patient data screen.

The second screen option is the alarm settings screen. In this screen the operator can view or adjust needed alarms, and these are detailed in the following section, "Alarms." The third screen option allows the operator to change the unit's audio and visual settings such as alarm volume, contrast, brightness, and display units. In any of the three option screens, real-time patient data are displayed.

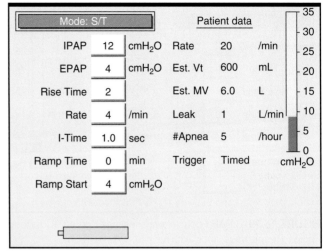

FIGURE 15.37 BiPAP Focus patient data screen. (Courtesy Philips Respironics, Inc., Murrysville, PA.)

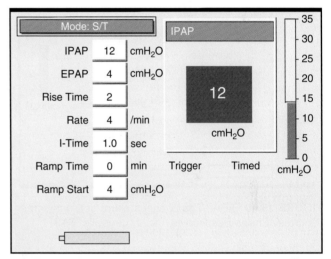

FIGURE 15.38 BiPAP Focus pop-up window. (Courtesy Philips Respironics, Inc., Murrysville, PA.)

Accessing the LCD screen is accomplished through an adjustable control. For the purpose of this discussion, this control is referred to as the mode and operations selector switch (MOSS).

To change modes or settings, the operator need only use the arrow keys to highlight the desired parameter on the LCD screen and press the enter key. A popup window for the setting will then appear (Fig. 15.38). Using the UP or DOWN arrow keys, the operator can apply a new setting. Pressing the ENTER key again confirms the new setting; pressing the CANCEL key allows the user to exit the popup screen without changing the setting.

Parameters that can be adjusted in the CPAP mode screen include the CPAP level, ramp time, and ramp pressure initiation level. Adjustable parameters in the S/T mode screen include IPAP, EPAP, rise time, respiratory rate, inspiratory time, ramp time, and ramp pressure start.

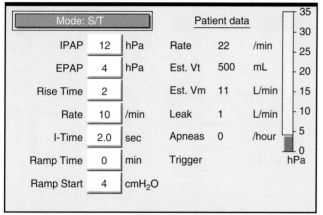

FIGURE 15.39 BiPAP Focus alarm message screen. (Courtesy Philips Respironics, Inc., Murrysville, PA.)

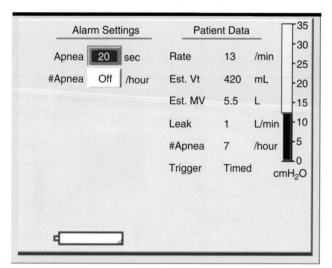

FIGURE 15.40 BiPAP Focus apnea alarm settings screen. (Courtesy Philips Respironics, Inc., Murrysville, PA.)

Alarms

The BiPAP Focus alarm system has two types of alarms: autoresettable and nonresettable. Autoresettable alarms automatically reset after an alarm situation occurs and is corrected. Nonresettable alarms must be manually reset.

When an alarm is activated, the alarm indicator flashes, an alarm message is displayed in the lower right-hand corner on the LCD screen (Fig. 15.39), and the Focus sounds a repeated sequence of beeps. Most of the alarms found on the BiPAP Focus are preset from the manufacturer; only the apnea detection time and number of apnea events in an hour are adjustable by the operator and are illustrated in Fig. 15.40. The apnea period is defined by the Focus as the amount of time with no spontaneous patient breathing effort. The number of apnea events is the second programmable alarm on the BiPAP Focus. This alarm will count the number of apnea events lasting 10 seconds or more in the previous hour of operation. The operator must note that in the first hour of operation, this value is only estimated. Major preset alarms include high- or low-pressure alarm, apnea, patient disconnect, low power, and loss of main power.

TABLE 15.24 The Adjustable Parameters for the BiPAP Focus in the S/T Mode[a]

Parameter	Range
Rate	1-30 breaths/min
IPAP	4-30 cm H_2O
EPAP	4-25 cm H_2O
Inspiratory time	0.5-3 s
Rise time	1-6, where 1 = 0.1 s and 6 = 0.6 s
Ramp time	0-45 min
Ramp pressure initiation level	4 cm H_2O EPAP

[a]In the CPAP mode the adjustable parameters are CPAP level, ramp time, and ramp start (with a default level of 4 cm H_2O). *CPAP*, Continuous positive airway pressure; *EPAP*, expiratory positive airway pressure; *IPAP*, inspiratory positive airway pressure; *S/T*, spontaneous/timed.

Modes of Ventilation

The BiPAP Focus system has two modes available: CPAP and spontaneous timed (S/T) modes. In the CPAP mode the adjustable parameters are CPAP level, ramp time, and ramp start, which has a default level of 4 cm H_2O.

Table 15.24 lists the S/T mode's adjustable settings. The S/T breaths may be flow triggered by the patient or time triggered dependent on the set rate. In the S/T mode the rate control does not guarantee a set number of mandatory breaths. Instead, it gives a set number of breaths regardless of whether they are patient triggered or time triggered by the machine.

Respironics V60

The Respironics V60 ventilator (Philips Healthcare HRC) is a microprocessor-controlled, pneumatic, BiPAP ventilatory assist system that provides NIV and invasive ventilatory support for spontaneously breathing adult and pediatric patients (Fig. 15.41). The ventilator is intended to support pediatric patients weighing 20 kg (44.1 lb) or greater to adult patients.[31]

Power Source

Standard 120-volt AC power supplies the main operation of the V60 ventilator. Should there be AC power failure, an optional internal backup battery can power the ventilator for up to 6 hours if fully charged. When the V60 ventilator is powered by the battery, a battery symbol will appear in the display screen that shows the approximate battery time remaining in hours and minutes, and it shows the capacity graphically. Should the V60 not have the optional battery installed, an icon will highlight the lack of a backup power source. If AC power is lost as a result of depletion or lack of a backup battery, an audible alarm annunciates for at least 2 minutes.

Internal Mechanism

The ventilator uses ambient air and a high-pressure oxygen source. Room air enters through an inlet filter. Oxygen enters though a high-pressure inlet, and a proportioning valve provides the operator-set concentration. The system mixes the

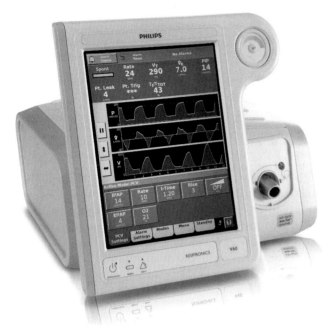

FIGURE 15.41 Respironics V60 ventilator. (Philips Healthcare HRC, Carlsbad, CA.)

air and oxygen, pressurizes it in the blower, and then regulates it to the user-set pressure. To do this, the ventilator compares the proximal airway pressure with the ventilator (internal system) pressure, and adjusts the machine pressure to compensate for the pressure drop across the inspiratory filter, patient circuit, and humidifier. This helps ensure accurate and responsive pressure delivery and leak compensation. The ventilator delivers gas to the patient through a main flow (inspiratory) bacteria filter, a single-limb patient breathing circuit, a humidification device (optional) and a patient interface, such as a mask or endotracheal tube (ETT). A pressure tap proximal to the patient is used to monitor patient pressure. The exhalation port continually exhausts gas from the single-limb circuit during inspiration and exhalation to minimize rebreathing and ensure CO_2 removal.

Oxygen Source

The V60 ventilator allows the clinician to deliver an enriched oxygen mixture (F_IO_2 range: 0.21 to 1.0) to the patient by attaching a high-pressure gas source to the oxygen module found on the rear of the machine. The F_IO_2 setting found in the graphical user interface allows the clinician to regulate the amount of oxygen delivered to the patient. For patient transport, oxygen cylinders may be utilized as an oxygen source. (*Note:* To provide a continuous and adequate supply of oxygen during transport, ensure that all cylinders are full (13,790 kPa/2000 psig or more), and only one cylinder should be opened. Devices such as cylinder/regulators that limit flow should not be used.)

Leak Compensation

Leaks are inherent to patient interfaces and circuits in NIV machines. Therefore monitoring and compensating for leaks

associated with NIV is critical for maintaining the appropriate trigger and cycle levels for the ventilator. The V60 continuously calculates and compensates for the total leak rate, which is a sum of known or *intentional* leak and unintentional leak (patient leak). The clinician enters the known intentional leakage value specific to the mask/patient interface and the circuit's exhalation port so that the ventilator can accurately calculate and display the patient leak. This is critical to assessing mask seal efficacy and preventing overtightening of the mask that may result in pressure sores. If intentional leaks are unknown, the ventilator displays the total leak value. The V60 uses a system called Auto-Trak Sensitivity, which employs a combination of two mechanisms to identify and modify baseline values in response to leaks. These are expiratory flow rate and V_T adjustments. The shape signal created by Auto-Trak is actually a shadow image of the patient's actual flow/time waveform that is "redrawn" by the microprocessor to overlap the actual signal. The shape signal is part of the digital Auto-Trak sensitivity. When the patient flow intersects the shadow flow from the shape signal, the ventilator triggers to IPAP. Cycling to exhalation (EPAP) occurs when the patient's flow intersects the shape signal flow. A second method of cycling to EPAP occurs when the microprocessor's electronic signal rises in proportion to the inspiratory flow waveform.

The expiratory flow rate adjustment primarily works to make course adjustments in baseline values. At the end of expiration, total flow should equal the total leak rate. This total flow is compared to an originally established value of baseline leak. If the two are not equal, the unit will adjust its calculation of the baseline leak. This, in turn, allows the trigger and cycle thresholds to be maintained in the presence of changing leak.

The V_T adjustment is used for fine-tuning the baseline flow on a breath-to-breath basis. Although the V60 does not directly measure volume, it is able to estimate inspiratory and expiratory V_Ts based on the patient flow and the time spent in inspiration and expiration. Differences that occur between the inspiratory and expiratory V_Ts are then assumed to be the result of a change in the amount of leak and are accounted for by an adjustment in baseline for the next breath. This feature allows the ventilator to adjust the baseline on a breath-to-breath basis, thereby reducing the need for large corrections.

The V60 also has an optional feature called Auto-Trak+. The Auto-Trak+ option for the Respironics V60 ventilator lets the operator further adjust thresholds of the Auto-Trak algorithm that manage trigger and cycling, the level of Auto-Trak Sensitivity, a feature that recognizes and compensates for intentional and unintentional leaks. When Auto-Trak+ settings are adjusted, these multiple trigger and/or cycle thresholds are adjusted simultaneously, retaining all the autoadaptive features of Auto-Trak Sensitivity in the face of changing leak. The base Auto-Trak algorithm or the "normal" settings on Auto-Trak+ work well for most patients. Pediatric patients, however, may benefit from more-sensitive trigger settings, and some adult patients may benefit from more- or less-sensitive cycle settings.

Controls and Displays

The Respironics V60 is powered up by pressing the ON/SHUTDOWN key located on the lower left-hand side of the device. The operator will hear tones from both the backup alarm (high pitch) and the primary alarm (lower pitch). The V60 will display the last settings applied before shutdown. It is recommended that the operator always complete a preoperational check before connecting to the patient. The operator must be familiar with using the touchscreen or navigation ring to select, adjust, activate, and confirm parameters.

All interactions, such as ventilator settings, patient data, and alarms, with the V60 are conducted through the graphical user interface. During V60 operation the upper screen displays alarms and patient data. The middle screen displays real-time graphic waveforms and alarm and informational messages. The lower screen lets the operator access modes and other ventilator settings, display help information, and see the power status.

The front panel of the V60 consists of touchscreen tab controls shown in the lower portion of the screen in Fig. 15.41. The use of these touch tabs is the primary method of selecting adjustments to the V60. Touching any of the control tabs will open another interactive screen for the parameters chosen. Table 15.25 lists the touchscreen tabs and the functions accessed by their activation.

For example, to change mode the operator presses the MODES tab on the graphical user interface. A second popup menu will appear with the available modes offered by the V60. To change modes or settings, the operator need only touch the screen, pressing the desired mode. Once the mode has been confirmed, a second popup screen will appear with adjustable settings for the selected mode. Fig. 15.42 shows this window where the IPAP setting is displayed for adjustment. To increase or decrease the selected setting, the operator may use the arrows located on either side of the selected parameter, which is highlighted. A second option to make a parameter adjustment is to slide your finger around the navigation ring. Sliding your finger around the navigation ring clockwise or counterclockwise will increase or decrease the selected parameter value, respectively. To confirm the new value the operator can press either the green check mark in the center of the navigation ring or press the ACCEPT tab on the parameter display. This process can be followed to change any parameter or alarm.

Alarms

The Respironics V60 ventilator has an extensive alarm package to accurately monitor patients, whether they are being supported invasively or noninvasively. System alarms are automatically set, whereas others are adjustable and require the operator to enter a desired value to an alarm setting. The adjustable alarms include High Peak Airway Pressure, Low Inspiratory Pressure, High Respiratory Rate, Low Respiratory Rate, High Tidal Volume, Low Tidal Volume, Low Minute Ventilation, and Low Inspiratory Pressure Delay Time Alarm.

The V60 has two levels of alarms, and each has its own visual and auditory characteristic. A low-priority alarm will result in an intermittent tone at an interval of approximately 20 seconds, and a yellow alert bar will appear at the top of

TABLE 15.25	**Touchscreen Tabs and Functions Accessed With the V60**
Standby	Standby lets the operator safely suspend ventilation to temporarily disconnect the patient from the ventilator or to set up the ventilator before connecting the patient. Alarms are disabled during standby
Menu	Screen Brightness, Alarm Volume, Mask/Port Interface, Ventilator Information, Auto Trak+ (if enabled as an option)
Modes	CPAP, Batch ST, PCV, AVAPS, and PPV (optional)
Alarm Settings	High Respiratory Rate, Low Respiratory Rate, High Tidal Volume, Low Tidal Volume, High Pressure, Low Pressure, Low Minute Ventilation, Low Inspiratory Pressure Delay time
CPAP Settings	Allows operator to enter CPAP settings

AVAPS, Average volume-assured pressure support; *CPAP,* continuous positive airway pressure; *PCV,* pressure-controlled ventilation; *PPV,* positive-pressure ventilation; *S/T,* spontaneous/timed.

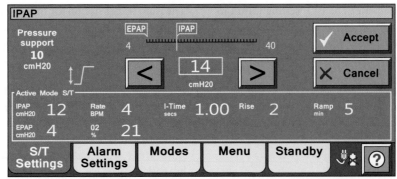

FIGURE 15.42 Respironics V60 ventilator pop-up window. (Philips Healthcare HRC, Carlsbad, CA.)

the graphical user interface. A high-priority alarm will result in a repeating sequence of five tones and an alternating red and black message bar, again located on the upper portion of the graphical user interface.

The operator can silence alarms by simply touching the graphical user interface in the upper left-hand corner. Once activated, the alarm will be silenced for 2 minutes and the alarm silence bar will display a 2-minute countdown until the alarm is once again active. To reset a resolved alarm, the operator need only touch the alarm reset tab on the graphical user interface immediately to the right of the alarm silence tab. Resetting the alarm also clears any displayed alarm messages.

High peak airway pressure alarm. The High Peak Airway Pressure alarm is adjustable from 5 to 50 cm H_2O. When this alarm is triggered, both an audible and a visual alarm become active, with a specific high-pressure alarm message displayed in the graphical user interface display.

Low inspiratory pressure alarm. The Low Inspiratory Pressure alarm can be adjusted from OFF to 40 cm H_2O. When this alarm is triggered, both an audible and a visual alarm become active, with a specific high-pressure alarm message displayed on the graphical user interface display.

Tidal volume alarms. The high V_T alarm limits are from 200 to 3500 mL, whereas the low V_T alarm range is OFF to 1500 mL. When either alarm is triggered, both an audible and a visual alarm are activated, with a specific alarm message displayed on the graphical user interface display.

High rate alarm. The High Respiratory Rate (high-frequency) alarm is adjustable from 5 to 90 breaths/min. As with all adjustable alarms, it is signaled by both an audible alarm and a visual message in the alarm window portion on the graphical user interface display.

Low rate alarm. The Low Respiratory Rate alarm is adjustable from 1 to 89 breaths/min. As with all adjustable alarms, it is signaled by both an audible alarm and a visual message in the alarm window portion on the graphical user interface display.

Lo V_E (low minute ventilation alarm). The Low Minute Volume alarm is adjustable from OFF to 99.0 L/min. As with all adjustable alarms, it is signaled by both an audible alarm and a visual message in the alarm window portion on the graphical user interface display.

LIP T (low inspiratory pressure delay time). Low Inspiratory Pressure Delay Time alarm is adjustable from 5 to 60 seconds. As with all adjustable alarms, it is signaled by both an audible alarm and a visual message in the alarm window portion on the graphical user interface display.

Setting Definitions

- IPAP setting represents the inspiratory positive airway pressure; this pressure is expressed as PIP on the patient parameters in the display.
- EPAP represents the expiratory positive airway pressure, otherwise known as PEEP in conventional invasive ventilation.
- PS is the difference between IPAP and EPAP values.

- Rise time sets the initial inspiratory flow rate and thus defines the time in which the IPAP is achieved, where the lower the setting number the faster the rise to IPAP.

Modes

The Respironics V60 ventilator offers a range of conventional pressure modes, CPAP, PCV, S/T, and PPV. The volume-targeted AVAPS mode combines the attributes of pressure-controlled and volume-targeted ventilation.

CPAP. CPAP is used for spontaneously breathing patients who may require only a set level of PEEP/CPAP to decrease work of breathing, to increase their functional residual capacity, or to treat problems such as OSA. The adjustable range of CPAP is 4 to 25 cm H_2O. This mode is truly a spontaneous mode, relying entirely on the patient to maintain the patient's own minute ventilation.

The optional C-Flex setting available with the V60 enhances traditional CPAP by reducing the pressure at the beginning of exhalation—a time when patients may be uncomfortable with CPAP—and returning it to the set CPAP level before the end of exhalation.

PCV. The PCV mode delivers pressure-controlled mandatory breaths, triggered by the ventilator (Timed) or the patient (Spont). Triggering of spontaneous patient breaths are triggered based on the ventilator's Auto-Trak Sensitivity algorithms, which include volume trigger or Shape Signal. Box 15.18 shows the control settings active in the PCV mode. The IPAP setting defines the applied pressure for all breaths, and I-Time (inspiratory time) defines the breath timing for all breaths whether spontaneous or machine triggered.

The S/T mode guarantees breath delivery at the operator-set rate. It delivers pressure-controlled, time-cycled mandatory and pressure-supported spontaneous breaths, all at the IPAP pressure level. If the patient fails to trigger a breath within the interval determined by the rate setting, the ventilator triggers a mandatory breath with the set I-Time. It is not necessary to set patient triggering or cycling sensitivities: the patient triggers and cycles based on the ventilator's Auto-Trak Sensitivity algorithms. The trigger algorithms include Volume trigger and Shape Signal. The cycling of spontaneously triggered breaths are cycled by any of the following four thresholds: SET (spontaneous expiratory threshold, a flow base criteria), Shape Signal, Flow reversal, and Maximum I time (3.0 seconds). The control settings active in the S/T mode are the same as in the PCV mode and are shown in Box 15.18.

BOX 15.18 **V60 Control Settings Active in the PCV Mode**

• IPAP	• Rise
• Rate	• EPAP
• F_IO_2	• I-Time
• Ramp Time	• S/T mode

EPAP, Expiratory positive airway pressure; *FIO2*, fraction of inspired oxygen; *IPAP*, inspiratory positive airway pressure; *I-Time*, inspiratory time; *PCV*, pressure-controlled ventilation; *S/T*, spontaneous/timed.

AVAPS mode. Unlike most pressure modes, the AVAPS mode allows for the delivery of a target V_T. It achieves the target volume by regulating the pressure applied following an initial pressure ramp-up. The AVAPS mode delivers time-cycled mandatory breaths and pressure-supported spontaneous breaths. If the patient fails to trigger a breath within the interval determined by the rate control, the ventilator triggers a mandatory breath with the set I-Time. Mandatory and spontaneous breaths are delivered at a pressure that is continually adjusted over a period of time to achieve the volume target (i.e., V_T). Min P and Max P define the range of pressures that can be used to achieve that target V_T. The pressure titration occurs slowly because the pressure change is limited to a 1- to 2.5-cm H_2O change per minute. The operator sets no patient triggering or cycling sensitivities: the patient triggers and cycles are based on the ventilator's Auto-Trak Sensitivity algorithms.

PPV mode (optional). The PPV mode provides patient-triggered breaths that deliver pressure in proportion to patient effort. Additionally, a user-settable backup rate activates machine-triggered, pressure-limited, and time-cycled breaths in the case of apnea. In the PPV mode, patient effort determines the pressure, flow, and V_T delivered by the ventilator. The ventilator responds to patient effort, allowing the patient to determine when to start and end a breath and how flow and pressure change as the patient inspires. The end result is that the level of PS is controlled by the inspiratory effort of the patient. Because the patient completely controls ventilatory output, PPV may significantly improve patient–ventilator synchrony and ultimately, patient comfort.

IV. HOME BILEVEL DEVICES

The ever-increasing understanding of sleep medicine and the ability to have smaller bilevel airway pressure units designed for home and institutional use have led to an expanding portion of noninvasive support for patients with OSA or treatment of respiratory insufficiency. There are many devices on the market today to help treat these patients. This section looks at a few models of these kinds of devices. The theory of operation in these models is similar to that used in all units.

RESPIRONICS SYNCHRONY

The BiPAP Synchrony (Fig. 15.43) is designed to provide noninvasive ventilatory assistance to adult patients (those who weigh 30 kg [66.1 lb] or more) for the treatment of respiratory insufficiency or OSA. The Synchrony is designed for use with nasal masks and full masks, as recommended by the manufacturer (Respironics, Inc.). The Synchrony is 12 in × 7 in × 6 in and weighs approximately 2.7 kg (6 lb).[32]

Power Source

The BiPAP Synchrony has two power options available for operation. The primary power source is 100-V to 240-V AC power or 12-V DC.

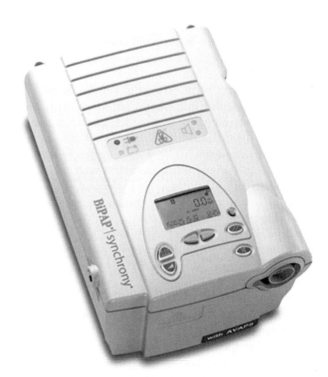

FIGURE 15.43 Respironics BiPAP Synchrony. (Courtesy Philips Respironics, Inc., Murrysville, PA.)

Internal Mechanism

Air is drawn into the Synchrony unit through the air inlet located in the back of the unit. The air is then directed to the microprocessor-controlled blower, where the set IPAP, EPAP, and rate control are located.

Oxygen Source

The BiPAP Synchrony is designed to operate primarily with room air, but it can be supplemented with an oxygen source. To provide enriched oxygen the BiPAP Synchrony must be equipped with an optional oxygen valve, which would be located on the right side of the unit. The oxygen source cannot exceed 15 L/min in flow or more than 50 psi.

Supplemental oxygen can also be added to the mask port of the patient's interface. As with any blended system, it is recommended that the delivered gas be periodically analyzed with an oxygen analyzer.

Operations/Controls

The control panel for the BiPAP Synchrony, illustrated in Fig. 15.44, is located on the top of the unit. Once the Synchrony is connected to a power source, the operator needs to press the STANDBY button. The Synchrony will sound two beeps and briefly illuminate the alarm indicators and display the startup screen, followed by the self-test screen. The available controls are listed in Box 15.19.

Display Screen

The display screen has two different windows–the Control screen and the Monitoring screen. The activity indicator (•)

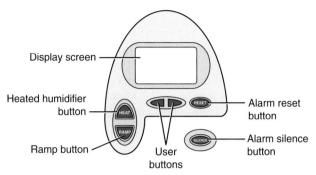

FIGURE 15.44 Respironics Synchrony BiPAP control panel. (Courtesy Philips Respironics, Inc., Murrysville, PA.)

BOX 15.19 BiPAP Synchrony Controls

The following controls are available:

- *AC power indicator:* A green LED is lit when AC power is present to operate the unit.
- *DC power indicator:* A green LED is lit when DC power is present to operate the unit.
- *STANDBY key:* The STANDBY key starts and stops the Focus unit.
- Control keys (UP, DOWN, ENTER): These keys allow the operator to change menu screens and adjust modes of operation and set parameters.
- *RAMP/ALARM SILENCE key:* The RAMP/ALARM SILENCE key is a dual-function key. In a nonalarm situation, pressing this key will activate the ramp feature, in which the Focus unit begins pressure at the EPAP level and gradually increases the IPAP level slowly at each breath until the set IPAP level is achieved.
- *Yellow alarm indicator:* When the yellow indicator light is flashing, this indicates the presence of a medium-priority alarm. If the yellow indicator light is continuously illuminated, this denotes a silenced medium alarm condition or a low-priority alarm.
- *Red alarm indicator:* When the red indicator light is flashing, this indicates the presence of a high-priority alarm. If the red indicator light is continuously illuminated, this denotes a loss of power or silenced alarm condition.

EPAP, Expiratory positive airway pressure; *IPAP,* inspiratory positive airway pressure; *LED,* light-emitting diode.

TABLE 15.26 Alarm Levels of the BiPAP Synchrony

High (Red Flashing)	Medium (Yellow Flashing)	Low (Yellow/Constant)
Apnea	Battery Voltage Too High	Battery in Use
Low Pressure Support	Low Battery	Call for Service
High Pressure		Momentary Loss of Power
Low Minute Ventilation		Power Failure (Battery in Use)
Invalid Prescription		
Low Pressure		
Patient Disconnect		
Ventilator Failure		
Battery Failure		

---

is shown next to the IPAP icon and alternates between the IPAP icon and the EPAP icon as the unit cycles the breath. The activity indicator is also present when an alarm is activated, alerting the operator to the alarm message. The selection symbol (▸) indicates a parameter that can be adjusted. The navigation symbol (◆) (shown here as up and down arrows) illustrates a parameter or screen that can be changed.

Alarms

The Synchrony has three levels of alarms, each with a distinct audio tone and an illuminating LED on the ALARM soft key located on the right side of the unit. To silence or reset the alarm, the operator need only press the RAMP/SILENCE key located on the bottom-middle portion of the control panel.

The first level of alarms is the high-priority level, which is announced by a flashing red LED on the alarm display and a series of three beeps followed by a series of two beeps. An alarm message also appears in the display window. This level of alarm requires immediate attention to correct the situation. Depending on the nature of the high-priority alarm, the Synchrony unit might not continue to operate, hence the need for immediate attention. There is one priority alarm condition that will result in a constant red LED display on the ALARM key, and that occurs with a total loss of power.

The second level of alarm is the medium-priority alarm, which is signaled by a flashing yellow LED in the ALARM key, followed by a series of three beeps sounds and display of an alarm message. Second-level alarms require a prompt response to assess the nature of the problem.

Low-priority alarms are announced by a steady yellow LED light on the ALARM key, followed by a series of two beeps sounds and the display of an alarm message or error code on the screen. The Synchrony unit will continue to function during medium- and low-level alarms. Table 15.26 shows the alarm levels and their associated alarm conditions.

Modes of Ventilation

The BiPAP Synchrony has four modes of operation: CPAP, spontaneous, S/T (upgrade), timed (upgrade), and pressure-controlled (upgrade). The modes listed with an upgrade symbol (upgrade) are optional modes.

CPAP

During CPAP the unit maintains the pressure set at the EPAP set level throughout inspiration and expiration. There is no apnea backup rate available.

Spontaneous Ventilation

Spontaneous ventilation is a bilevel mode that responds to the patient's inspiration and expiration by increasing pressure during inhalation and decreasing the delivered pressure during exhalation. There is no mandatory rate in this mode.

Spontaneous/Timed

S/T is an optional bilevel mode that responds to both the patient's inspiration and expiration effort by increasing the delivered pressure during inhalation and decreasing the delivered pressure when exhalation is detected. If the patient does not initiate a breath within a set time period, the Synchrony will initiate a breath. During these timed breaths the Synchrony controls the time of inhalation and decreases the delivered pressure for exhalation within a set time period.

Timed Mode

The timed (T) mode of ventilation is also an optional bilevel mode in which the Synchrony controls both the inspiration and exhalation components (time, pressure) of the delivered breath independent of the patient's spontaneous effort.

Pressure-Controlled

PC is a bilevel mode that responds to the patient's inspiratory effort by increasing the delivered pressure. The length of the inspiration is controlled by the Synchrony. As in the S/T mode, if the patient does not initiate a breath within a set time period, the Synchrony will automatically initiate a breath.

PURITAN BENNETT GOODKNIGHT 425

The Puritan Bennett GoodKnight 425 is a bilevel positive airway pressure device designed for use in treating OSA in spontaneously breathing patients who weigh more than 30 kg (66.1 lb) (Fig. 15.45). The GoodKnight 425 can be used in the home or hospital setting. It is not intended for invasive ventilation. The GoodKnight's dimensions are 5.6 in × 2.9 in × 7.7 in, and it weighs 0.7 kg (1.5 lb) without the power supply.[33]

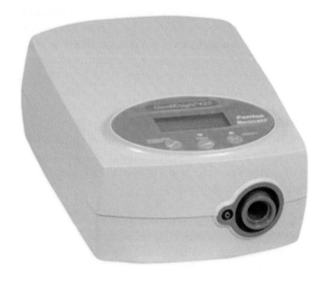

FIGURE 15.45 Puritan Bennett GoodKnight 425. (Copyright © 2013 Medtronic Minimally Invasive Therapies. All rights reserved. Reprinted with permission of Medtronic Minimally Invasive Therapies.)

Power Supply

The GoodKnight 425 is primarily powered by a 100-V or 240-V AC power source and can also be powered by an optional 12-V automotive battery. DC operation is possible without a DC/AC inverter by using an optional cable and adapter. An additional adapter may be needed to plug the unit into a wall outlet if the user is outside the United States.

Oxygen

The GoodKnight delivers room air under normal conditions but can be supplemented with oxygen by using an oxygen adapter placed just distal to the unit's patient circuit outlet connector. The supplemental oxygen may also be added to the mask port of the patient's interface. The maximum recommended supplemental bleed is 10 L/min. The F_IO_2 delivered to the patient will depend on factors such as pressure settings, patient breathing pattern, interface selection, leak rate, and flow of the oxygen source. It is recommended that the oxygen concentration from the unit be periodically analyzed.

Internal Mechanism

The GoodKnight 425 is powered by a microprocessor blower that entrains room air through the air inlet located in the rear of the unit. The microprocessor-controlled blower then develops the set IPAP, EPAP, and rate set by the operator.

Operations/Controls

The main controls of the GoodKnight unit are located on the top panel. To power up the unit, the operator need only push the ON/OFF soft key located in the lower right-hand corner of the control panel. To access all settings the operator must press and hold the "hidden button" located under the word *GoodKnight* and simultaneously press the INFORMATION-ACCESS button located in the lower left-hand corner of the control panel.

Alarms

The GoodKnight 425 has no built-in alarms.

Modes of Ventilation

The GoodKnight 425 has two modes of operation: CPAP and spontaneous bilevel positive airway pressure ventilation. There is no apnea backup rate on the GoodKnight 425. However, the GoodKnight 425 S/T model does have an apnea backup rate option.

CPAP

The CPAP mode delivers CPAP to the patient circuit and requires that the patient trigger each breath. The range of CPAP available on the GoodKnight 425 is 4 to 25 cm H_2O.

Spontaneous Mode

This bilevel mode is not a timed mode but rather a strictly spontaneous mode. The pressure settings available on the GoodKnight 425 are an IPAP of 4 to 25 cm H_2O and an EPAP setting of 4 to 25 cm H_2O. If apneic events are a significant issue, the patient should be placed on the 425 S/T to ensure adequate ventilation.

RESMED STELLAR 100

The ResMed Stellar 100 (Fig. 15.46) is a bilevel positive airway pressure device that is intended to provide ventilation for nondependent, spontaneously breathing adult and pediatric patients (weighing 13.6 kg [30 lb] and above) with respiratory insufficiency or respiratory failure, with or without OSA. The device is for noninvasive use, or invasive use with an uncuffed or deflated tracheostomy tube. The ResMed Stellar 100's dimensions are 9 in long × 6.7 in wide × 4.7 in high, and it weighs 2.1 kg (4.6 lb).[34]

The ResMed Stellar 100 offers both bilevel and CPAP modes of operation.

Power Supply

The ResMed Stellar 100 is primarily powered by a 100-V or 240-V AC power source or on its internal lithium-ion battery. The estimated battery life is 2 hours at EPAP 5, IPAP 15, and 20 breaths/min. The unit can be powered by an optional power device such as the ResMed Power Station II or any external power supply unit or other DC power supply that meets the required 24-V/3-A DC voltage and current specifications.

Oxygen Supply

The ResMed Stellar 100 delivers room air under normal conditions but can be supplemented with oxygen added by using a factory-designed oxygen adapter line placed in the back of the unit. The maximum recommended supplemental bleed is 30 L/min at maximum oxygen pressure of 0.73 psi (50 mbar). The F_IO_2 delivered to the patient will depend on factors such as pressure settings, patient breathing pattern, interface selection, leak rate, and flow of the oxygen source. It is

recommended that the oxygen concentration from the unit be periodically analyzed.

Internal Mechanism

The ResMed Stellar 100 is powered by a microprocessor-controlled blower that entrains room air through the air inlet located in the rear of the unit. The microprocessor-controlled blower then develops the set IPAP, EPAP, and rate set by the operator.

Operations/Controls

The main controls of the unit are located on the top panel of the unit. Press the power switch at the back of the device once to turn on the device. Check that the alarm sounds a test beep and the LEDs for the ALARM SIGNAL and the ALARM MUTE buttons flash. The device is ready for use when the treatment screen is displayed.

To access all settings the operator must press the MENU button located on the right side of the LCD screen. The MENU button lets the operator access therapy and alarm settings of the Stellar 100. Once the menu screen appears, the operator utilizes the PUSH DIAL located directly below the LCD screen. The PUSH DIAL acts as an enter/select button in changing between settings: Rotating the PUSH DIAL moves the selected parameter, which is marked dark blue. Once a selected parameter is located, the operator needs to press the PUSH DIAL. Pressing the PUSH DIAL will then display the parameter in orange. Rotating the PUSH DIAL either clockwise or counterclockwise will increase, decrease, or change the parameter. To confirm the setting change, the operator is required to press the PUSH DIAL within 3 seconds or the setting change times out.

Alarms

The ResMed Stellar 100 has both adjustable and nonadjustable alarms. Adjustable alarms are set using the same procedure as changing modes or parameter settings described previously. Adjustable alarms are listed in Box 15.20, and nonadjustable alarms are listed in Box 15.21. As always, readers are

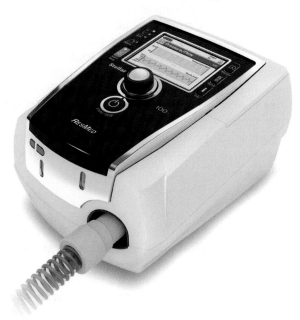

FIGURE 15.46 Stellar 150. (©ResMed 2013. San Diego, CA.)

BOX 15.20 Stellar 100 Adjustable Alarms

- High Leak
- High Pressure
- Low Minute Ventilation
- Low Pressure
- High Respiratory Rate
- Low Respiratory Rate
- Apnea
- Non-vented mask
- High F_IO_2
- Low F_IO_2
- Low SpO_2

F_IO_2, Fraction of inspired oxygen; SpO_2, oxygen saturation as measured using pulse oximetry.

BOX 15.21 Stellar 100 Nonadjustable Alarms

- Circuit disconnected
- Over pressure
- Blocked tube
- Internal battery empty

encouraged to contact their local representative for complete alarm parameters.

Modes of Ventilation

The ResMed Stellar 100 has five available modes: S/T, PAC (Pressure-Assisted Control), CPAP, S (Spontaneous), and T (Timed).

Spontaneous/Timed

S/T is an optional bilevel mode that responds to both the patient's inspiration and expiration effort by increasing the delivered pressure during inhalation and decreasing the delivered pressure when exhalation is detected. If the patient does not initiate a breath within a set time period, the ResMed Stellar 100 will initiate a breath. During these timed breaths, ResMed Stellar 100 controls the time of inhalation and decreases the delivered pressure for exhalation within a set time period. The adjustable parameters are an IPAP of 2 to 40 cm H_2O; EPAP of 2 to 25 cm H_2O; Respiratory Rate of 5 to 60 breaths/min; and Inspiratory Time range of 0.1 to 4 seconds.

PAC

PAC is a bilevel mode that responds to the patient's inspiratory effort by increasing the delivered pressure. The length of the inspiration is controlled by the ResMed Stellar 100. As in the S/T mode, if the patient does not initiate a breath within a set time period, the ResMed Stellar 100 will automatically initiate a breath.

CPAP

The CPAP mode delivers CPAP to the patient circuit and requires that the patient trigger each breath. The range of CPAP available on the ResMed Stellar 100 is 2 to 25 cm H_2O.

Spontaneous Mode

This bilevel mode is not a timed mode but rather a strictly spontaneous (S) mode. The pressure settings available on the ResMed Stellar 100 are similar to the ST mode with an IPAP of 2 to 40 cm H_2O and an EPAP setting of 2 to 25 cm H_2O. If apneic events are a significant issue, the patient should be placed on the S/T mode to ensure adequate ventilation.

Timed Mode

The timed (T) mode of ventilation is also a bilevel mode in which the ResMed Stellar 100 controls both the inspiration and exhalation components (time, pressure) of the delivered breath independent of the patient's spontaneous effort. Adjustable parameters are similar to the S/T mode described earlier.

SUMMARY OF HOME CARE EQUIPMENT

With increasing life expectancy of the adult population in America and our ability to support diseases once thought to be untreatable, home care has become a viable alternative to hospital care for the ventilator-dependent patient. In addition, there are a growing number of children who also require continuous mechanical respiratory support for chronic conditions. Home care provides an option for these children as well.[35,36]

In addition to the diagnosis of chronic pulmonary disease, there has been a shift in diagnoses to neurogenic respiratory insufficiency. This shift has resulted in implications for both hospital and community-based providers in extending services to the home setting.[37-40]

A study by Luján et al.[37] compared the effectiveness and efficiency of an initiation protocol for *noninvasive home mechanical ventilation* (NIHMV) carried out at a pulmonary outpatient clinic with the standard in-hospital model. The NIHMV model reduced costs by 50%. Indihar did a cost-based study comparing five different sites of chronic ventilator care.[38] In a comparison of the step-down unit in a hospital with home care supported by the family, it was found that the costs were reduced by approximately one-third. Cost is not the only reason for home care ventilation, but it is a major reason why home mechanical ventilation is so aggressively pursued.

The estimate of health-related quality of life (HRQOL) needs to be included in the assessment of costs and benefits of modern treatment modalities such as home mechanical ventilation. The level of HRQOL is dependent on the type of disease process involved.[39,40] When choosing among positive-pressure ventilators, invasive or noninvasive techniques, negative-pressure ventilators, or supportive aids, it is important that the patient and family are educated about the operation of the equipment. They should be aware of the potential problems that might arise and how to identify them. When looking at supportive devices for the home, the clinician should choose one that is simple and operator friendly, with clear alarms to alert the user of any malfunctions. It is important to remember that the primary operators of home care devices are nonmedical personnel. Operators should refer to the manufacturer's instructions to accomplish correct operation of any life support device.

■ KEY POINTS

- The pNeuton transport ventilator has no battery backup or AC power option and operates strictly from pneumatic power.
- With the Crossvent ventilator the alarm menu will flash "Low Battery, Connect External Power" on the LCD screen and sound an alarm when operating from the internal battery with only 20 minutes of remaining power. At this point the ventilator must be connected to AC power to continue operation.
- When the Crossvent is connected to an active gas source and not in use, the PEEP control should be turned fully counterclockwise to conserve gas supply.
- The Bio-Med MVP-10 has no alarms, so it should not be left to operate unattended.

- In the Oxylog 3000 Plus, the F_IO_2 delivery is controlled by the metering block. In flow ranges of 9 to 35 L/min, an oxygen concentration of 40% to 100% can be delivered.
- The Model 731 EMV+ is indicated for use in the management of infant through adult patients weighing 5 kg (11 lb) or more with acute or chronic respiratory failure.
- The hard method of locking the LTV 1000 ventilator should be used when children or others may have access to the ventilator, such as in the patient's home.
- The flow pattern for the LTV 1200 ventilator is automatically set as a descending ramp for all volume-targeted breaths and occurs naturally in all pressure-targeted breaths.
- The select button on the LTV 1200 is used to stop the normal scrolling of monitored ventilator parameters.
- The extended features menu of the LTV 1000 and 1200 ventilators is selected by pressing the select button for 3 seconds.

- A visual indication on the Smiths Medical Pneupac ventiPAC ventilator will begin to turn red and sound an audible alarm when the gas supply source is losing pressure. If this alarm is ignored for more than 60 seconds, the alarm will shut itself off to conserve battery power.
- The Newport HT50 has a universal power entry module that allows the same port to be used for connecting to an AC or external DC power source.
- The Newport HT70 is applicable for infant, pediatric, and adult patients weighing 5 kg (11 lb) or more.
- The BiPAP Focus will not operate without a functioning battery installed in the unit.
- To provide enriched oxygen the BiPAP Synchrony must be equipped with an optional oxygen valve.
- The GoodKnight 425 CPAP device has two modes of operation: CPAP and spontaneous bilevel, and includes no built-in alarms.

ASSESSMENT QUESTIONS

See Appendix B for the answers.

1. How many liters per minute is the logical flow for the Airon pNeuton model S for the patient without the disconnect feature?
   a. 3 L/min
   b. 4 L/min
   c. 6 L/min
   d. 10 L/min

2. When the sigh parameter is active on the Bio-Med Crossvent ventilator, how often will the sigh maneuver be completed?
   a. Sigh breath is provided every 100 breaths or 1 every 7 minutes, whichever occurs first
   b. Sigh breath is provided every 50 breaths or 1 every 10 minutes, whichever occurs first
   c. Sigh breath is provided every 120 breaths or 1 every 20 minutes, whichever occurs first
   d. Sigh breath is provided every 80 breaths or 1 every 15 minutes, whichever occurs first

3. Which alarm parameter cannot be disabled on the Crossvent alarm screen?
   a. Mean airway pressure
   b. Exhaled minute volume
   c. High respiratory rate
   d. Oxygen alarm

4. If compressed air is used to power the Bio-Med MVP-10, the set time intervals are approximately how much less than if powered by 100% oxygen because of the difference in gas density?
   a. 5%
   b. 10%
   c. 15%
   d. 20%

5. The Bio-Med MVP-10 can be magnetic resonance imaging (MRI) compatible. True or false?
   a. True
   b. False

6. What is the maximum gas logic consumption rate on the Dräger Oxylog 3000 Plus?
   a. 0.1 L/min
   b. 0.3 L/min
   c. 0.5 L/min
   d. 1.0 L/min

7. What is the minimum patient weight recommended for the Zoll 731 Series EMV+?
   a. 2.5 kg (5.5 lb)
   b. 5 kg (11 lb)
   c. 10 kg (22 lb)
   d. 15 kg (33.1 lb)

8. Pressing the MUTE/CANCEL button on the EMV+ during a high-priority alarm will cancel the alarm for how much time?
   a. 15 seconds
   b. 30 seconds
   c. 45 seconds
   d. 0 seconds

9. When the CareFusion LTV 1000 internal battery is operational and the battery level indicator illuminates red, how long will the ventilator possibly still operate?
   a. 1 minute
   b. 3 minutes
   c. 5 minutes
   d. 7 minutes

10. The CareFusion LTV 1200 offers which of the following features?
    1. Noninvasive ventilation mode
    2. External positive end-expiratory pressure (PEEP) valve
    3. Cylinder duration calculator
    4. High-frequency ventilation
    a. 2 and 3 only
    b. 1 and 4 only
    c. 3 and 4 only
    d. 1 and 3 only

11. What type of mask needs to be utilized for the CareFusion LTV 1000 and LTV 1200 to operate correctly in the non-invasive mode?
    a. Vented masks
    b. Partial vented mask
    c. Nonvented masks
    d. All of the above

12. The CareFusion ReVel internal transition battery provides power to the ventilator for up to how many minutes?
    a. 1 minute
    b. 2 minutes
    c. 5 minutes
    d. 10 minutes

13. Noninvasive positive-pressure ventilation (NIV) can be activated with the CareFusion ReVel in which modes?
    1. Assist/Control
    2. Synchronized intermittent mandatory ventilation (SIMV)
    3. Continuous positive airway pressure (CPAP)
       a. 1 only
       b. 1 and 2 only
       c. 2 and 3 only
       d. 1 and 3 only

14. At what psi will the Smiths Medical ventiPAC low-pressure "eyeball" alarm begin to change from white to red, indicating a low gas supply pressure?
    a. 40 psi
    b. 25 psi
    c. 45 psi
    d. 30 psi

15. The Newport HT50 can provide an enriched oxygen delivery by which of the following methods?
    1. An optional oxygen blender through a high-pressure oxygen gas source
    2. An oxygen-blending bag for providing additional oxygen for spontaneous breaths
    3. By using the two high-pressure gas sources required for powering the device
    4. By bleeding oxygen into the patient circuit
       a. 3 only
       b. 4 only
       c. 1 and 2 only
       d. 1 and 4 only

16. A respiratory therapist is increasing the PEEP/CPAP control on the Newport HT50 from 5 to 10 cm H_2O. The patient's pressure setting is 10 cm H_2O. The ventilator does not allow the increase in PEEP. The most likely reason is:
    a. The therapist must toggle past a safety switch to increase PEEP above 9 cm H_2O.
    b. The high-pressure alarm is set at 20 cm H_2O, and the settings would cause this alarm to activate.
    c. The PEEP/CPAP level cannot be set higher than the pressure setting −5 cm H_2O.
    d. The low-pressure alarm must be readjusted before the change in PEEP can occur.

17. Which of the following alarms on the Newport HT70 is not adjustable?
    a. High Pressure
    b. Apnea
    c. Low Baseline Pressure
    d. High Inspiratory Minute Volume

18. After pressing the QUICK SET ALARM key on the control panel of the Newport HT70, how long will it be until the ventilator has set the alarm limits?
    a. 10 seconds
    b. 15 seconds
    c. 20 seconds
    d. 30 seconds

19. The internal ventilator battery on the CareFusion LTV 800 is rated for how long?
    a. 45 minutes
    b. 120 minutes
    c. 60 minutes
    d. 30 minutes

20. The leak compensation on the CareFusion LTV 900 and LTV 950 can compensate for leaks up to:
    a. 6 L/min
    b. 3 L/min
    c. 1 L/min
    d. 8 L/min

21. What fraction of inspired oxygen (F_IO_2) enrichment percentage may be attained with the Puritan Bennett 540 with a maximal bleed in flow of 15 L/min?
    a. 40%
    b. 50%
    c. 60%
    d. 100%

22. What is the minimum weight of a patient who can be set up on the Puritan Bennett 540 ventilator?
    a. 5 kg (11 lb)
    b. 7.5 kg (16.5 lb)
    c. 10 kg (22 lb)
    d. 12 kg (26.5 lb)

23. The Respironics BiPAP Focus has two operator-adjustable alarms in which combination?
    a. High pressure and apnea detection time
    b. High respiratory rate and low pressure
    c. Apnea detection time and number of apnea events in 1 hour
    d. Number of apnea events in 1 hour and low tidal volume (V_T)

24. The Respironics Synchrony is designed to be used on patients whose weight is greater than or equal to:
    a. 20 kg (30.1 lb)
    b. 30 kg (66.1 lb)
    c. 20 kg (44.1 lb)
    d. 35 kg (77.2 lb)

25. The Puritan Bennett GoodKnight 425 alarms include:
    a. High pressure
    b. Apnea alarm
    c. Low pressure
    d. No alarm

REFERENCES

1. Pierson JD: Noninvasive positive pressure ventilation: history and terminology. *Respir Care* 42(4):370, 1996.
2. Chipman DW, Caramez MP, Miyoshi E, et al.: Performance comparison of 15 transports ventilators. *Respir Care* 52(6):740-751, 2007.
3. American Association for Respiratory Care: Clinical practice guideline: transport of the mechanically ventilated patient. *Respir Care* 47:721-723, 2002.
4. Austin NP, Johannignan AJ: Transport of the mechanically ventilated patient. *Respir Care Clin N Am* 8:1, 2002.
5. pNeuton transport ventilator operators manual, CD-S-005 Rev I, Melbourne, FL, 2015, Airon Corporation.
6. Crossvent 4+ operators manual, Guilford, CT, 2005, Bio-Med Devices, Inc.
7. Bio-Med MVP-10 operators manual, Guilford, CT, 2003, Bio-Med Devices.
8. Oxylog 3000 Plus operators manual, Telford, PA, 2010, Drager Medical Inc.
9. Zoll portable critical care ventilator operator's manual (REF 906-0731-01 Rev F), Chelmsford, MA, 2015, Zoll Medical Corporation.
10. LTV Series ventilator operator's manual, part no. 10664 revision T, Minneapolis, MN, 2005, Pulmonetics Systems, Inc., Division of Viasys Health Care.
11. LTV 1200 Operators Manual, part no. 18247-001, Rev G, Minneapolis, MN, 2009, Pulmonetics Systems, Inc., Division of Viasys Health Care.
12. CareFusion ReVel ventilator, operator's manual, P/N 12432-001 Rev. A, San Diego, CA, 2011, CareFusion Corporation.
13. VentiPAC: Operators Manual, Waukesha, WI, 2005, Smith Medical, Inc.
14. Day D: Keeping patients safe during intrahospital transport. *Crit Care Nurse* 30:18-32, 2010.
15. American Association for Respiratory Care: Clinical practice guideline: long-term invasive mechanical ventilation in the home. *Respir Care* 52:1056-1062, 2007.
16. McKim DA, Road J, Avendano M, et al.: Home mechanical ventilation: a Canadian Thoracic Society clinical practice guideline. *Can Respir J* 18(4):197-215, 2011.
17. Dunne PJ, McInturff SL: *Respiratory home care: the essentials*, Philadelphia, 1998, FA Davis.
18. Lewarski JS, Gay PC: Current issues in home mechanical ventilation. *Chest* 132(2):671-676, 2007.
19. Newport HT50 operator's manual, Newport Beach, Calif, 2008, Newport Medical Instruments.
20. Newport HT70 ventilator operating manual, OPRHT70 Rev. F, Costa Mesa, CA, 2011, Newport Medical Instruments, Inc.
21. LTV 800 operators manual, Minneapolis, MN, 2008, Viasys Healthcare Systems, Inc.
22. Puritan Bennett 540 ventilator user's manual, Boulder, CO, 2009, Nellcor Puritan Bennett LLC.
23. Dominique R, Barry M: Part 1. Noninvasive ventilation: from the past to the present. In Elliot M, Nava S, editors: *Noninvasive ventilation and weaning principles*, London, UK, 2010, Edward Arnold Publishers Ltd.
24. Sullivan CE, Berthon-Jones M, Issa FG: Reversal of obstructive sleep apnea by continuous positive airway pressure applied through the nose. *Lancet* 1:862, 1981.
25. Cairo JM: Basic concepts of noninvasive positive pressure ventilation. In *Pilbeam's mechanical ventilation—physiological and clinical application*, ed 5, St. Louis, 2016, Mosby/Elsevier.
26. Barreiro TJ, Gemmel DJ: Noninvasive ventilation. *Crit Care Clin* 23(2):201-222, 2007.
27. Sinuff T, Kahnamoui K, Cook DJ, et al.: Practice guidelines as multipurpose tools: a qualitative study of noninvasive ventilation. *Crit Care Med* 35:776-782, 2007.
28. Hostetler MA: Use of noninvasive positive pressure ventilation in the emergency department. *Emerg Med Clin North Am* 26:929-939, 2008.
29. Epstein LJ, Kristo D, Strollo PJ Jr, et al.: Clinical guideline for the evaluation, management and long-term care of obstructive sleep apnea in adults. *J Clin Sleep Med* 5:263-276, 2009.
30. Respironics BiPAP Focus clinical manual, Murrysville, PA, 2006, Respironics, Inc.
31. Respironics V60 ventilator user manual, 1047358 Rev F, Carlsbad, CA, 2009, Respironics California, Inc.
32. Respironics Synchrony operating manual, Pittsburgh, PA, 2006, Respironics, Inc.
33. Puritan Bennett GoodKnight 425 operators manual, Pleasanton, CA, 2005, Puritan Bennett Inc.
34. ResMed Stellar 100 operators manual, San Diego, CA, 2011, ResMed Corp.
35. Gramlich T: Long-term ventilation. In Cairo JM: *Pilbeam's mechanical ventilation—physiological and clinical applications*, St. Louis, 2012, Mosby/Elsevier.
36. Graham RJ, Fleeger EW, Robinson WM: Chronic ventilator need in the community: a 2005 pediatric census of Massachusetts. *Pediatrics* 119(6):e1280-e1287, 2007.
37. Lujan M, Moreno A, Veigas C, et al.: Non-invasive home mechanical ventilation: effectiveness and efficiency of an outpatient initiation protocol compared with the standard in-hospital model. *Respir Med* 101:1177-1182, 2007.
38. Indihar SF: Cost of comparison care for chronic ventilator patients. *Chest* 99:260, 1991.
39. Windisch W, Criee CP: Quality of life in patients with home mechanical ventilation. *Pneumologie* 60:539-546, 2006.
40. Windisch W: Impact of home mechanical ventilation on health-related quality of life. *Eur Respir J* 32(5):1328-1336, 2008.
41. Yeow ME, Santanilla JI: Noninvasive positive pressure ventilation in the emergency department. *Emerg Med Clin North Am* 26(3):835-847, 2008.

Suggested Answer Key for Clinical Scenarios

AUTHORS' NOTE

Decisions made in the clinical setting vary considerably among individuals and hospitals. There is usually more than one acceptable solution to a problem in patient care. The answers provided here represent only one or two possible choices of treatment. Readers are encouraged to talk these cases over with instructors, mentors, and colleagues.

CHAPTER 1 BASIC PHYSICS FOR THE RESPIRATORY THERAPIST

Clinical Scenario 1-1

You can calculate the volume of gas in his lungs as he descends the pond by applying Boyle's law. We know that at sea level, where pressure surrounding the diver equals 1 atm (atmospheric pressure), the volume in his lungs equals 3000 mL. As the diver descends, the pressure surrounding him increases by 1 atm for every 33 feet. Thus, at 33 feet, the pressure exerted on the diver equals 2 atm. We can calculate the volume of gas in his lungs using the following variation of Boyle's law:

- $V_2 = V_1 P_1 / P_2$
- $V_2 = (3000 \text{ mL}) (1 \text{ atm})/(2 \text{ atm})$
- $V_2 = 1500 \text{ mL}$

At a depth of 66 feet, the pressure exerted on the diver equals 3 atm and his volume is calculated as

- $V_2 = V_1 P_1 / P_2$
- $V_2 = (3000 \text{ mL}) (1 \text{ atm})/(3 \text{ atm})$
- $V_2 = 1000 \text{ mL}$

Thus, at 33 feet below the surface of the pond, the pressure to which the diver is exposed equals 2 atm, causing the diver's lung volume to decrease to one-half (1500 mL) of the original volume at 33 feet and one-third (1000 mL) of the original volume at 66 feet.

Clinical Scenario 1-2

According to Gay-Lussac's law, the pressure of a gas within a cylinder is directly related to the temperature at which the cylinder is exposed. Consequently, increasing this temperature causes a proportional increase in the pressure of the gas within the cylinder. Thus, in this example, if the fire is not controlled and the temperature in the basement rises, the pressure within the cylinders can increase, creating an explosion hazard. Moving the cylinders removes the hazardous condition.

Clinical Scenario 1-3

In this problem, $P_1 = 760$ mm Hg; $V_1 = 6$ L; $T_1 = 273$ K; $T_2 = 37°C$ (310 K); $P_2 = 3$ atm or 2280 mm Hg; $V_2 =$ unknown. Thus,

- $P_1 V_1 / T_1 = P_2 V_2 / T_2 V_2 = P_1 V_1 T_2 / P_2 T_1$
- $V_2 = [(760 \text{ mm Hg})(6 \text{ L})(310 \text{ K})]/[(2280 \text{ mm Hg})(273 \text{ K})]$
- $V_2 = 2.27$ L

Clinical Scenario 1-4

Various conditions can cause a reduction in the rate of oxygen diffusion across the alveolar-capillary membrane. Decreasing the surface area of the membrane (e.g., resection of a lobe of the lung), increasing the thickness of the alveolar-capillary membrane (e.g., pulmonary fibrosis or the presence of pulmonary edema), and reducing the partial pressure gradient for oxygen between the alveoli and the blood flowing through the pulmonary capillary (e.g., reducing the partial pressure of inspired oxygen, such as when one ascends to high altitude) will reduce the rate at which oxygen crosses the alveolar-capillary membrane.

CHAPTER 2 PRINCIPLES OF INFECTION CONTROL

Clinical Scenario 2-1

The clinical manifestations described point to a diagnosis of pneumonia. The laboratory findings suggest a bacterial pneumonia; *Streptococcus pneumoniae* is most commonly associated with bacterial pneumonia.

Clinical Scenario 2-2

- *Pseudomonas aeruginosa* is a highly motile, Gram-negative bacillus found in the human gastrointestinal tract. It is a contaminant in many aqueous solutions (vehicle route).
- Human immunodeficiency virus (HIV) is transmitted through the exchange of body fluids (e.g., sexual contact) with an HIV-infected individual.
- Tuberculosis is a chronic bacterial infection that is almost exclusively transmitted within aerosol droplets produced by the coughing or sneezing of an individual with active tuberculosis.
- Malaria is a parasitic infection that is transmitted by mosquitoes (vector).

Clinical Scenario 2-3

First, determine whether the device is contaminated. Microbiological identification requires that the hospital's clinical laboratory staff work with the staff of the respiratory care department to determine whether infectious organisms are in the devices in question. The clinical microbiologist can provide information about nosocomial infections from direct smears and stains, cultures, serological tests, and antibiotic susceptibility testing.

Ongoing surveillance is required to ensure that an infection control program is adequately protecting patients and health care providers. Surveillance typically consists of the following: equipment processing quality control, routine sampling of in-use equipment, and microbiological identification. Equipment processing is monitored with chemical and biological indicators. Routine sampling of in-use equipment can be done with sterile cotton swabs, liquid broth, and aerosol impaction. Aerosol impaction is an effective method for sampling the particulate output of nebulizers.

Clinical Scenario 2-4

Most major burn wounds become infected during the first 48 to 72 hours after the incident. Care should therefore be directed to minimizing situations in which wound colonization can occur. For this reason, the most effective strategy is to use strict contact isolation procedures.

CHAPTER 3 MANUFACTURE, STORAGE, AND TRANSPORT OF MEDICAL GASES

Clinical Scenario 3-1

(1) Frozen carbon dioxide (dry ice); (2) heliox; (3) oxygen; (4) nitric oxide.

Clinical Scenario 3-2

There is an apparent leak at the connection. The valve stem should first be closed, then the connection between the cylinder outlet and the regulator tightened.

Clinical Scenario 3-3

Turn off the zone valve that controls oxygen flow from the main oxygen supply to the affected area (in this case, the fifth floor of the north wing). Call for assistance to provide E cylinders of oxygen for patients requiring oxygen therapy.

CHAPTER 4 ADMINISTERING MEDICAL GASES: REGULATORS, FLOWMETERS, AND CONTROLLING DEVICES

Clinical Scenario 4-1

The flow rate of oxygen is 6 L/min or 100 mL/s (6000 mL/60 s). If the expired gas is exhaled in the first 1.5 seconds of expiration, then 0.5 second is available for filling the anatomical reservoir, which is approximately 50 mL for this patient. The anatomical reservoir includes the nose, nasopharynx, and oropharynx, which is approximately one-third of the patient's dead space, or 150 mL (1 mL for every pound is a good estimate of the amount of dead space in a normal patient). The patient's inspiration lasts 1 second, so he will inspire 100 mL of 100% oxygen. Therefore the anatomical reservoir and the inspiratory flow deliver 150 mL of 100% oxygen to the patient. The remaining 350 mL of tidal volume will be entrained room air, which has an F_IO_2 of approximately 0.20. This 350 mL of room air contains 70 mL of 100% oxygen (350 mL × 0.20 = 70 mL).

The delivered F_IO_2 can now be estimated:
- 50 mL of 100% oxygen from the anatomical reservoir
- 100 mL of 100% oxygen (O_2 flow = 100 mL/s)
- 350 mL of 21% oxygen (350 mL × 0.20 = 70 mL)
- 220 mL of 100% oxygen/500 mL tidal volume
- Estimated delivered $F_IO_2 = 0.44$

Clinical Scenario 4-2

These are common complaints of patients who use nasal cannulas for long-term oxygen therapy. You could suggest that he consider using a transtracheal oxygen (TTO) device. These devices are more comfortable for patients requiring long-term oxygen therapy and are generally well tolerated by patients. Just as important, they are cosmetically more pleasing to most patients than are nasal cannulas. If the patient agrees to try the TTO device, you must teach him how to properly care for it. Adequate education is an essential part of ensuring patient compliance with any type of long-term oxygen therapy device.

Clinical Scenario 4-3

The actual flow of gas being administered to the patient receiving an 80%:20% heliox gas mixture through an O_2 flowmeter at 10 L/min as the driving gas for nebulizing the β_2-bronchodilator is 18 L/min = (1.8 × liter flow).

Clinical Scenario 4-4

You should remove the helium–oxygen mixture, switch the patient to 100% oxygen (i.e., nonrebreathing mask), and immediately notify the physician of the patient's condition. You should recheck the concentration of oxygen delivered from the cylinder. It is possible that the contents of the cylinder were "unmixed," and thus the F_IO_2 delivered to the patient was actually much less than expected.

CHAPTER 5 AIRWAY MANAGEMENT DEVICES AND ADVANCED CARDIAC LIFE SUPPORT

Clinical Scenario 5-1

The greatest priorities are the establishment of the ABCs—airway, breathing, and circulation (in that order). If the patient has a patent airway, one should then begin to establish breathing mask ventilation. If a patient is lying on the ground, the laryngoscopist will need to lower himself or herself to the ground, supporting his or her weight with the right hand. This frees up the left hand and arm for laryngoscopy.

Clinical Scenario 5-2

There are several possibilities. The tube could be in the esophagus, the patient's cardiac output could be low, or there could be no perfusion of blood through the lungs, as might occur as a result of a massive pulmonary embolus.

Clinical Scenario 5-3

Two devices that can be used in this emergency situation are laryngeal mask airways (LMAs) and the Combitube. Others include the Fastrach LMA, fiberoptic scope, and a surgical airway.

CHAPTER 6 HUMIDITY AND AEROSOL THERAPY

Clinical Scenario 6-1

The problem is that the device is unable to meet the inspiratory flow needs of the patient. As a consequence, he must entrain room air, which reduces the F_IO_2 that is being delivered. You can correct the situation by choosing a high-flow aerosol generator, such as a Misty Ox device. Alternatively, you can connect two low-flow aerosol nebulizers together with a Briggs adapter to increase flow. The key point is to choose an aerosol delivery device that can provide an inspiratory flow that will exceed the patient's inspiratory flow needs.

Clinical Scenario 6-2

- *Patient A:* No humidification required for the 60-year-old patient with emphysema who is receiving oxygen via a nasal cannula at 3 L/min.
- *Patient B:* No humidification required for the 48-year-old patient with chronic bronchitis who is receiving 35% oxygen (that is, the flow rate is <4 L/min.
- *Patient C:* Heat and moisture exchange required for the 28-year-old postoperative patient with an endotracheal tube that will not be in place for more than 24 hours.
- *Patient D:* A heated humidifier is required for the 72-year-old patient with chronic obstructive pulmonary disease (COPD) and thick secretions requiring mechanical ventilation.

Clinical Scenario 6-3

Spacers and holding chambers, small-volume nebulizers, and vibrating mesh nebulizers are all clinically appropriate forms of aerosol generators used to administer medications to the lung of a 6-year-old child with asthma since the age of 1 year.

Clinical Scenario 6-4

The following steps should be taken:
- *Step 1:* Check that the driving pressure supplied to the nebulizer is adequate, and adjust upward for adequate output.
- *Step 2:* Check that the flow rate is adequate, and if not, adjust to 6 to 10 L/min until adequate output is achieved.
- *Step 3:* Check that the nebulizer matches the compressor according to the data supplied by the manufacturer, and obtain correct nebulizer if not correct.

- *Step 4:* Check whether the plastic device's venture orifice is clogged and there is build-up of electrostatic charge in the device. If present, clean the device and dry thoroughly.

Clinical Scenario 6-5

The proper protective measure that should be taken to ensure safe delivery of pentamidine in a private room is the administration of the drug in a room equipped for negative-pressure ventilation with adequate air exchange (at least six per hour). HEPA (high-efficiency particulate air) filters should be used to filter the room air or vent exhaust, or the aerosol should be scavenged to the outside. In areas where more than one patient is being treated: booths or stations (such as the Aerostar aerosol protection cart [Respiratory Safety Systems]) should be used for sputum induction and aerosolized medication treatments. The area should be designed to provide adequate airflow to draw aerosol and droplet nuclei from the patient into an appropriate filtration system or an exhaust system directly to the outside. Booths and stations should be adequately cleaned between patients. Filters should be treated as hazardous waste. Goggles, gowns, and gloves should be worn. Continuous ongoing safety education should be performed.

CHAPTER 7 LUNG EXPANSION THERAPY AND AIRWAY CLEARANCE DEVICES

Clinical Scenario 7-1

This is a fairly common problem encountered by respiratory therapists. Most patients who have undergone abdominal surgical procedures avoid taking deep breaths because of the intense pain that occurs when the diaphragm pushes on the abdominal contents. This patient should be started on an aggressive plan that includes bronchial hygiene and lung expansion therapy to prevent postoperative atelectasis and pneumonia. The plan could include incentive spirometry, cough training (with instructions on splinting), aerosol therapy, and possibly chest physiotherapy and postural drainage.

Clinical Scenario 7-2

Although the patient is a candidate for antibiotic therapy as a medical treatment, respiratory care is needed to help clear secretions and reexpand lung bases that seem to be secretion filled and/or atelectatic. Because the patient is unable to cooperate to perform therapies such as incentive spirometry and/or coughing and deep breathing, intermittent positive-pressure breathing (IPPB) is an appropriate form of therapy in this case. This therapy might be accompanied by a β-adrenergic agent and a mucolytic to help mobilize secretions so that they can be cleared with suctioning. Postural draining and percussion might also be beneficial, particularly because this patient is not mobile.

Clinical Scenario 7-3

This is a primary indication for using intrapulmonary percussive ventilation (IPV). Although it is a relatively new lung expansion technique, early studies indicate that IPV can be a useful bronchial hygiene technique for treating cystic fibrosis patients. Because of the acute nature of the patient's present illness, it is reasonable to give an initial IPV treatment and then reassess the patient in 1 to 2 hours. If the treatment improves gas exchange, as evidenced by physical assessment and pulse oximetry, further treatments would be indicated, thus preventing impending respiratory failure, which would require endotracheal intubation and mechanical ventilation. Other therapeutic modalities that might be considered would include aerosol therapy, chest physiotherapy and postural drainage, and positive expiratory pressure (PEP) therapy.

CHAPTER 8 ASSESSMENT OF PULMONARY FUNCTION

Clinical Scenario 8-1

There are several things that could interfere with the operation of the device: (1) The mouthpiece is connected to the wrong side of the device, and thus the exhaled gas cannot be measured; (2) the patient did not perform the test properly because either the technique was not clearly explained to him or he did not give a good effort; (3) the device was not plugged into the electrical outlet; or (4) the patient's exhaled gas is leaking around the mouthpiece.

Clinical Scenario 8-2

The forced vital capacity (FVC), forced expiratory volume in 1 second (FEV_1), and forced expiratory flow from 25% to 75% of the vital capacity ($FEF_{25-75\%}$) are considerably reduced. The FEV_1/VC is also reduced. The residual volume (RV) and functional residual capacity (FRC) are elevated, indicating the presence of air trapping. These findings are consistent with an individual with moderate to severe chronic obstructive pulmonary disease (COPD).

Clinical Scenario 8-3

One possible explanation for this type of problem is that there is a leak in the sampling line. This problem can also occur when moisture builds up in the sampling line.

Clinical Scenario 8-4

Phase II represents the transition between airway and alveolar gas exchange and as phase II decreases with increased positive end-expiratory pressure (PEEP), dead space increases and less CO_2 is exhaled per breath.

Clinical Scenario 8-5

The erratic changes seen in the $\dot{V}O_2$ can be related to fluctuations in the F_1O_2, separation of the patient's inspired and expired gases from the continuous gas flow from the ventilator, or from the presence of excessive amounts of water vapor. Problems associated with fluctuations in F_1O_2 can be alleviated to some extent by using an air/oxygen blender or premixed gases. The problem is particularly difficult to alleviate when the patient is breathing $F_1O_2 > 0.5$ because of the Haldane transformation. Inspired and expired gases can be separated using isolation valves supplied by the manufacturer of the metabolic monitor. Water vapor is nearly always difficult to address when continuous measurements are being obtained from ventilator-dependent patients, particularly when a cascade humidifier is being used. Replacing the humidifier with an artificial nose may help to minimize the problem.

CHAPTER 9 ASSESSMENT OF CARDIOVASCULAR FUNCTION

Clinical Scenario 9-1

The ventricular rate is 187 beats/min. The rate can be calculated by using the formula: effective ventricular rate = 1500 ÷ (R-R interval); thus 1500 ÷ 8 = 187 beats/min.

Clinical Scenario 9-2

This electrocardiogram demonstrates elevated P waves in lead II (2.5 mm), suggesting right atrial enlargement. There are QS complexes throughout the precordial leads, suggesting the presence of a transmural infarction. The presence of peaked T waves also suggests this diagnosis. Note the presence of a prominent Q wave in lead I and aVL, suggesting an anterior lateral myocardial infarction (MI). The prominent Q waves seen in the inferior leads (II, III, and aVF) and the T-wave changes seen in these leads also suggest an inferior infarct.

Clinical Scenario 9-3

(1) Measurements obtained from hypovolemic patients ventilated with positive end-expiratory pressure (PEEP) will typically show exaggerated variations in pressure. This is particularly evident in patients ventilated with high inspiratory pressures, such as those patients with asthma or acute respiratory distress syndrome (ARDS). (2) This problem can occur if the catheter is too proximal or if the balloon ruptures. (3) Excessive noise on the pressure tracing is usually associated with catheter whip or the catheter tip being located too close to the pulmonary valve.

Clinical Scenario 9-4

The cardiac output can be calculated using the Fick equation, or
$$\dot{V}O_2 = \dot{Q} \times (CaO_2 - C\overline{v}O_2)$$
The steps for making this calculation follow:
$$CaO_2 = (Hb \times 1.34) SaO_2 + (PaO_2 \times 0.003)$$
$$CaO_2 = (12 \text{ gm\%} \times 1.34) 0.92 + (60 \text{ mm Hg} \times 0.003)$$
$$CaO_2 = 14.97 \text{ vol\%}$$
$$C\overline{v}O_2 = (Hb \times 1.34) S\overline{v}O_2 + (P\overline{v}O_2 \times 0.003)$$
$$C\overline{v}O_2 = (12 \text{ gm\%} \times 1.34) 0.60 + (30 \text{ mm Hg} \times 0.003)$$
$$C\overline{v}O_2 = 9.74 \text{ vol\%}$$
$$\dot{Q} = \dot{V}O_2 \div (CaO_2 \times C\overline{v}O_2) 10$$
$$\dot{Q} = 200 \text{ mL/min} \div (14.97 \text{ mL/100 mL} - 9.74 \text{ mL/100 mL}) 10$$
$$\dot{Q} = 3.82 \text{ L/min}$$

CHAPTER 10 BLOOD GAS MONITORING

Clinical Scenario 10-1

The presence of an air bubble will cause the PCO_2 (partial pressure of carbon dioxide) to be lower than normal and the

PO$_2$ (partial pressure of oxygen) to be higher than normal. The reason for this discrepancy is that room air has a PCO$_2$ of approximately 0.3 mm Hg and a PO$_2$ of approximately 150 mm Hg. (See Chapter 3 for a full discussion of partial pressures of gases in room air.)

Clinical Scenario 10-2

The interpretation of respiratory alkalosis is probably correct. The PO$_2$ (partial pressure of oxygen) results, however, need to be evaluated by another method because capillary PO$_2$ does not always correlate well with PaO$_2$ (partial pressure of arterial oxygen).

Clinical Scenario 10-3

Neither the SpO$_2$ (oxygen saturation as measured using pulse oximetry) nor the calculated SaO$_2$ (arterial oxygen saturation) accurately reflects the true oxygen saturation when CO poisoning is suspected. SpO$_2$ can be falsely high. SaO$_2$ is calculated by the arterial blood gas (ABG) analyzer's microprocessor; PaO$_2$ (partial pressure of arterial oxygen) is a measure of dissolved (not bound) O$_2$. The patient's blood sample should be run on a CO-oximeter, which directly measures the oxyhemoglobin saturation and carboxyhemoglobin levels. For example, suppose that the CO-oximeter measured the following: O$_2$Hb = 83%; COHb = 15%; and thus HHb = 2%. Assume that the total hemoglobin equals 15 gm%. Then 83% of 15 gm% of Hb = 12.45 gm%; 15% of 15 gm% = 2.25 gm%; 2% of 15 gm% = 0.3 gm%. Notice that the pulse oximeter detects only the levels of O$_2$Hb and HHb. That is, the pulse oximeter reading suggests that only 2% of the hemoglobin is unsaturated and that 98% is saturated with oxygen. So 98% of the 15 gm% of Hb represents 14.7 gm% O$_2$Hb. Therefore the pulse oximeter overestimates the true level of oxyhemoglobin by approximately 2.25 gm%.

CHAPTER 11 SLEEP DIAGNOSTICS

Clinical Scenario 11-1

Several important facts suggest that Mr. H. may have a sleep-related disorder: He has been referred to the laboratory after an automobile accident when he "fell asleep at the wheel." He also reports excessive daytime sleepiness, and his wife says that he snores and that his sleeping pattern has become increasingly restless during the last 6 months. It is also mentioned that he has a long history of smoking cigarettes (possibly indicating the presence of some chronic respiratory problem, such as small airway disease) and that alcohol seems to exacerbate his snoring episodes. All of these findings suggest that Mr. H might have obstructive sleep apnea.

An effective strategy here would be to schedule this patient for an overnight sleep study involving polysomnography. This information, coupled with a complete history and physical examination, should allow for a diagnosis of sleep apnea, if that is the case. Furthermore, the results of these studies will provide valuable information on the severity of the disorder, thus helping you to devise an appropriate treatment plan.

Clinical Scenario 11-2

This is a typical polysomnographic recording of a patient with mixed sleep apnea. Notice that an initial central apnea is followed by an obstructive apnea that usually produces significant oxygen desaturation.

CHAPTER 12 INTRODUCTION TO VENTILATORS

Clinical Scenario 12-1

Part I: An open-loop system. The ventilator was told to deliver 650 mL and it did, but it did not make any adjustments when the exhaled volume was less than the set volume.

Part II: A closed-loop system. The ventilator has compared the exhaled volume with the set volume and progressively increased the peak pressure to achieve the set tidal volume.

Clinical Scenario 12-2

Problem 1: It seems that inspiratory flow is inadequate because pressures are dropping so low during inspiration. The patient may be opening the safety pop-in valve. Check the gas source to be sure it is on and connected and that the flow is adequate.

Problem 2: There is probably a leak in the system, and pressure in the system cannot be maintained.

Clinical Scenario 12-3

The pressure must drop from +10 cm H$_2$O minus the sensitivity setting (i.e., 10 − 1 = +9 cm H$_2$O). In other words, inspiration starts when the pressure drops to +9 cm H$_2$O or 1 cm H$_2$O below baseline pressure of 10 cm H$_2$O. This answer assumes that the ventilator is positive end-expiratory pressure (PEEP) compensated, which most are.

Clinical Scenario 12-4

Base flow = 6 L/min − trigger flow. Measured flow must drop to 4 L/min.

Clinical Scenario 12-5

The trigger variable is pressure, the control variable is pressure, the limit variable is pressure, and the cycling variable is time. In this example the control variable and the limit variable are the same.

Clinical Scenario 12-6

Technically, referring to the variable as "volume cycled" is incorrect, if volume cycling is defined as the measurement of volume and the ending of inspiratory flow when the volume was achieved. A classic example of this cycling mechanism is the historic MA-1. In the MA-1 the rising of the bellows and the contact of a switch near the top of the bellows ended inspiration (i.e., until the volume left the bellows [a volume device], inspiration did not end). The MA-1 ventilator provides an example of true volume cycling.

One could argue, however, that the measurement of flow over time is a volume measurement because volume = flow/time. Current ICU ventilators have flow-controlling valves that are very accurate in their flow delivery. Should we split hairs over this issue? What is most important in the clinical setting? We are interested in volume ventilation or delivery of a tidal volume. We would want to know that the volume left the ventilator at the end of inspiratory flow. This is the case.

Both are correct. One is technically correct by very strict standards and definition. The other is correct based on common clinical usage and an acceptance that flow/T_I = volume.

Clinical Scenario 12-7

Pressure is being limited to a certain value, as is volume. Without knowing the mechanism by which the breath is delivered, one cannot precisely determine the limit variable. For example, if this is a bag-in-a-box design, the volume could be limited to the volume within the bag. This would also limit pressure delivery. Or it could be a linear drive piston with a pop-off valve designed to limit the pressure in the circuit during the excursion of the piston. However, it can be determined that the breath is time cycled. None of the variables went into exhalation until a specific time had elapsed. This is illustrated by the flow-time curve, which went from a constant flow to a zero flow baseline before exhalation occurred.

Clinical Scenario 12-8

Part I:
- C_T = volume/PIP, C_T = 90 mL/45 cm H_2O = 2 mL/cm H_2O
- Volume lost = PIP × C_T = 20 cm H_2O × 2 mL/cm H_2O = 40 mL

Set tidal volume was 300 mL minus 40 mL lost to the circuit. The patient will receive 260 mL.
Part II:
- 3 mL/cm H_2O × 28 cm H_2O = 84 mL will be lost to the circuit; 640 mL − 84 mL = 556 mL will reach the patient.

Clinical Scenario 12-9

No, the ventilator will measure a minute ventilation of 7.5 L/min (25 breaths/min × V_T of 0.3 = 7.5 L/min), which is well above the set minimum of 4.0 L/min. The patient has an increased work of breathing. Unless the high-rate alarm is set correctly, the operator will be unaware of the patient's problem.

Clinical Scenario 12-10

The transairway pressure will be peak inspiratory pressure (PIP) − $P_{plateau}$ or 24 − 18 cm H_2O, or 6 cm H_2O. This might be a safe starting point to set pressure support (PS) to overcome the resistance of the ventilator system and airway.

For an 80-kg patient, using a tidal volume target of 5 to 6 mL/kg, an exhaled V_T of between 400 and 480 mL would be appropriate.

Clinical Scenario 12-11

We know that pressure-support ventilation (PSV) is patient triggered and that patients determine their own tidal volume based on their lung characteristics and their inspiratory effort, as well as by the set pressure. The ventilator algorithm that ends the breath does so when a predetermined flow that is a percentage of peak flow is reached. It can be argued that the programmer designed the algorithm so that the ventilator knows the patient's inspiration is ending (i.e., flow is declining). Therefore the programming is based on what the patient's breath is doing. So you could argue that it really is the patient's breathing pattern that determines all phases of a pressure-supported breath.

CHAPTER 13 MECHANICAL VENTILATORS: GENERAL USE DEVICES

None

CHAPTER 14 INFANT AND PEDIATRIC DEVICES

Clinical Scenario 14-1

Usually after a short time, an infant with this kind of history will "settle in" to continuous positive airway pressure (CPAP) and begin to breathe more slowly and comfortably. Oxygen requirement should be decreasing, not increasing. For the infant who is not improving, the first thing that the respiratory therapist needs to check is the fit of the prongs. Often with an infant this large, the prongs are too small. They need to fit snugly into the nares, but without "stretching out" or blanching the nostrils. It is not so important that the prongs intrude into the nares, but that they have a snug fit. It is also important to check the connections of the system to ensure that there are no leaks. Comfort measures may also be considered, including bundling, oral pacifier, and positioning.

Clinical Scenario 14-2

This is an example in which the patient is probably actively inspiring because the set tidal volume (V_T) is less than the delivered V_T. The breath is not volume cycled. Because flow drops to zero before the end of inspiration, the breath is not flow cycled.

Clinical Scenario 14-3

The therapist should check to see whether the leak compensation is turned on. If it is turned on, the sensitivity control may need to be readjusted. In some cases, efforts to remove leaks are preferable to using the leak compensation feature. The therapist should also check to be sure no auto–positive end-expiratory pressure (auto-PEEP) is present, which can make triggering the ventilator difficult.

Clinical Scenario 14-4

This clinical round is presented to provide some important information on the use of the proximal flow sensor with the Dräger Babylog. If the proximal sensor becomes clogged with mucus or moisture, the Babylog will not be able to detect the infant's inspiratory efforts. For safety reasons the ventilator will use a back up breathing pattern. If the ventilator is set in the synchronized intermittent mandatory ventilation (SIMV) mode with VG (volume guarantee), the ventilator reverts to intermittent mandatory ventilation (IMV) at the set peak inspiratory pressure (PIP). If the ventilator is operating in SIMV only, it reverts to IMV at the current ventilator settings. It would have been more appropriate for the respiratory therapist to set a lower back up pressure to avoid exposing the infant to the higher level of pressure in the event that the sensor no longer functioned. Periodic inspection of the proximal sensor might help to avoid the problem, especially when the infant is known to have excess secretions. The Dräger Babylog will revert back to the operating mode of pressure-support ventilation (PSV) with VG if it again detects patient efforts without the clinician having to respond to the event.

Clinical Scenario 14-5

With improvement in blood gas levels and breath sounds, the increase in servo pressure may indicate an improvement in compliance.

CHAPTER 15 TRANSPORT, HOME CARE, AND NONINVASIVE VENTILATORY DEVICES

Clinical Scenario 15-1

The therapist may have forgotten to turn the positive end-expiratory pressure (PEEP)/continuous positive airway pressure (CPAP) control to the off position (fully counterclockwise) once the transport was completed, resulting in gas being used from the transport oxygen cylinder. Unless this control is turned to the off position, the ventilator will continue to use supply gas to maintain the PEEP/CPAP valve.

Clinical Scenario 15-2

- $1800 \text{ psi} \times 0.28 = 504 \text{ L oxygen}$
- $4 \text{ L/min logical} + 4 \text{ L/min} = 8 \text{ L/min}$
- $504 \text{ L} \div 8 \text{ L/min} = 63 \text{ min}$

Clinical Scenario 15-3

The likely cause is that the CYCLE/continuous positive airway pressure (CPAP) switch is in the CPAP position and may have been inadvertently moved during the loading process.

Clinical Scenario 15-4

To apply a positive end-expiratory pressure (PEEP) level greater than 10 mbar, the operator must confirm this PEEP level by depressing the rotary dial located in the front of the control panel.

Clinical Scenario 15-5

This message indicates that both the low minute volume and low peak pressure for spontaneous breath alarms are turned off. The therapist should activate the LMV alarm and note that the LPP alarm is off and consider turning it to "all breaths." It is important, particularly with a spontaneously breathing patient, that a minimum safe minute ventilation is monitored. With CPAP being used, it is also appropriate to have a low peak pressure monitored for spontaneous breaths.

Clinical Scenario 15-6

The flow termination point is 3.5 L/min (10% of 35 L/min). The preset default flow in the LTV is 2 L/min.

Clinical Scenario 15-7

The therapist should change the breath type to Pressure, the mode to synchronized intermittent mandatory ventilation/continuous positive airway pressure (SIMV/CPAP), the breath rate to "—," the sensitivity to a level appropriate for the patient, and the pressure support to 15 cm H_2O. Remember that on the LTV the pressure setting for pressure support (PS) is not added to the positive end-expiratory pressure (PEEP) value. The PEEP valve/expiratory valve is manually adjusted to a PEEP of 3 cm H_2O. The pressure graph displays the value for the PEEP setting. The exhaled measured tidal volume should also be checked to see whether it is appropriate for the patient.

Clinical Scenario 15-8

The rate will be 60 seconds divided by the sum of inspiratory time (T_I) and expiratory time (T_E): $60/(1+4) = 60/5 = 12$ breaths/min.

The tidal volume (V_T) will be the flow (L/s) $\times T_I = 0.5 \text{ L/s} \times 1 \text{ s} = 0.5 \text{ L}$ (500 mL).

Clinical Scenario 15-9

The low baseline pressure alarm ("LOW Pbase") indicates an unstable baseline. For example, this could occur with a large leak in the patient circuit (pressure ≥ 2 cm H_2O below baseline for 3 seconds). You find the volume on the cuff of the patient's tracheostomy tube is low and causing a large intermittent leak, in turn causing the alarm. You adjust the cuff to minimal seal, and the alarm situation resolves.

CHAPTER 1 BASIC PHYSICS FOR THE RESPIRATORY THERAPIST

1. (a) 38.89°C; (b) 77°F; (c) 310 K; (d) 310 K
2. (a) 2.94 kPa; (b) 759.77 mm Hg; (c) 14.71 mm Hg; (d) 29.4 lb/in² (PSI)
3. (a) 160 mm Hg; (b) 593 mm Hg; (c) 0.228 mm Hg
4. (c) 750 mm Hg
5. 793.15 mm Hg
6. 3.12 L
7. The density of oxygen = 32/22.4 = 1.43 g/L. The density of carbon dioxide = 1.96 g/L.
8. (a) Length of the tube and viscosity of the gas
9. (a) Increasing the surface area of the membrane and increasing the partial pressure gradient of the gas across the membrane
10. (d) Increased density of the gas, increased radius of the conducting tube, and decreased viscosity of the gas
11. 2 A
12. (1) Ensuring that all devices attached to patients are electrically grounded; (2) ensuring that equipment circuit interrupters are functioning; (3) ensuring that all electrical devices used with a microshock-sensitive patient are well insulated and connected to outlets with a common, low-resistance ground
13. A 1000-watt air compressor used for 24 hours would require 24 kilowatt-hours of energy (1000 W × 24 h = 24,000 W/24 h or 24 kilowatts/24 h). If the cost of 1 kilowatt-hour is $0.10, then the total cost to operate the air compressor for 24 hours would be $2.40 (24 h × 0.10 = $2.40).
14. (d) 1 A
15. (b) 132 mm Hg

CHAPTER 2 PRINCIPLES OF INFECTION CONTROL

1. (a) *Pseudomonas aeruginosa*
2. (c) Acid-fast bacteria
3. (d) HIV
4. The Centers for Disease Control and Prevention updated its recommendations for hand-washing technique in 2009. See the CDC website for more information.
5. (c) Glutaraldehyde
6. (a) Semicritical; (b) critical; (c) noncritical; (d) semicritical; (e) semicritical
7. (b) Pertussis
8. (d) High-level disinfection with ortho-phthaladehyde
9. (b) Steam autoclave
10. (c) Hepatitis
11. (d) Foley catheters, intravenous catheters, endotracheal tubes, and burns all have the potential to cause skin and mucosal barrier disruption.
12. (d) Spore-producing bacterium
13. (1) A source of pathogens; (2) a mode of transmission of the infectious agent; (3) a susceptible host
14. (1) Monitoring equipment processing; (2) sampling in-use equipment routinely; (3) microbiologically identifying suspected pathogens
15. (d) The patient should have a private room; articles contaminated with secretion must be disinfected or discarded; and masks must be worn by all individuals who will be in close contact with the patient.
16. Standard precautions: Hands should be washed between tasks and procedures on the same patient to prevent cross-contamination of different body sites. Gloves, masks, protective eyewear, and gowns should be worn when there is a chance of contacting blood. Needles and other sharp objects should be handled with care to prevent injuries. Needles should be recapped after use. Used needles and other sharps should be disposed of in specially marked containers.
17. (1) e; (2) a; (3) c; (4) d; (5) b
18. (a) Hepatitis A, venereal disease, HIV, *Staphylococcus* spp. enteric bacteria; (b) salmonellosis, hepatitis A; (c) tuberculosis, diphtheria; (d) bubonic plague

CHAPTER 3 MANUFACTURE, STORAGE, AND TRANSPORT OF MEDICAL GASES

1. (b) Carbon dioxide
2. (d) Gray
3. (c) The pin positions of the regulator are not the same as those on the cylinder
4. (d) 10 feet
5. (d) 43 hours
6. (c) 15 hours, 42 minutes
7. (a) 50 psi

8. (b) An average day's supply
9. (b) 40%
10. (b) The rate of gas flow and the age of the sieve beds
11. (a) The frangible disk ruptures from the increased pressure, allowing gas to escape from the cylinder.
12. (b) The time between the test dates shown exceeds recommendations.
13. (c) This action clears the debris from the connector.
14. (a) NFPA
15. False. The compressor will draw air in from the local environment and therefore will contain pollutants that may contaminate the local environment.

CHAPTER 4 ADMINISTERING MEDICAL GASES: REGULATORS, FLOWMETERS, AND CONTROLLING DEVICES

1. The easiest way to determine the number of stages in a regulator is to count the number of pressure-relief valves. Each chamber should have its own pressure-relief valve.
2. (c) Air entrainment mask
3. (d) Gas flow from these flowmeters stops if resistance creates a back pressure that exceeds the source gas pressure.
4. (c) They require lower oxygen flow to achieve a given F_IO_2 than do standard nasal cannulas, and they are less obtrusive (i.e., more cosmetically pleasing) than nasal cannulas.
5. (d) 3:1
6. (c) 50%
7. (b) 300 mm Hg
8. (a) Air embolism and carbon monoxide poisoning
9. (d) Managing postextubation stridor in pediatric trauma patients; providing ventilator support for patients with severe airway obstruction resulting from chronic bronchitis and emphysema; administering anesthetic gases to patients with small-diameter endotracheal tubes; and delivering oxygen therapy to asthmatic children
10. (d) Nonrebreathing mask
11. (c) It has been used successfully to treat persistent pulmonary hypertension of the newborn; it can be used as an adjunct to the treatment of congenital cardiac defects
12. (c) 16 L/min
13. (d) Pulse, blood pressure, respirations, and mental status
14. (c) Nitrogen dioxide and nitric oxide are toxic if inhaled, and the therapeutic dose of nitric oxide is 5 to 80 parts per million (ppm).
15. (d) Hypertension, bounding pulse, $PaCO_2$ >70 mm Hg, and multiple premature ventricular contractions

CHAPTER 5 AIRWAY MANAGEMENT DEVICES AND ADVANCED CARDIAC LIFE SUPPORT

1. (a) Establishing a patent airway
2. (c) Prominent incisors

3. (c) Bypasses upper airway obstructions
4. (d) Prevents pressure injuries and damage to pharyngeal tissues
5. (b) Breath sounds over the epigastrium
6. (b) Oral intubation with a cuffed tube
7. (b) The lung is not protected from aspiration
8. (a) The airway catching on the back of the tongue
9. (d) Subcutaneous emphysema
10. (a) Failure to recognize esophageal intubation
11. (d) All of the above
12. (a) 10 French (Fr)
13. Possible answers: mouth opening, dental examination, Mallampati classification, thyromental distance, cervical range of motion
14. (c) #3
15. (d) Hypoxia, hemorrhage, nerve injury, and gas dissection of the tissues surrounding the tracheotomy site
16. (d) Tracheal ulcers, cartilage loss, malacia, and rupture
17. (b) 3-mm ID
18. (c) Request placement of a TT
19. (c) Double-lumen endotracheal tube (DLT)
20. (c) 0.85 with an oxygen flow of 15 L/min
21. (b) Manual resuscitators must be able to operate at a relative humidity of 40% to 96%, and adult resuscitators must deliver a tidal volume of at least 600 mL into a test lung set at a compliance of 0.02 L/cm H_2O

CHAPTER 6 HUMIDITY AND AEROSOL THERAPY

1. (d) 43.9 mg/L of water vapor
2. (b) Absolute humidity increases
3. (c) 30 mg/L
4. (c) 43%
5. (b) 31°C to 35°C (87.8°F to 95°F)
6. (d) Atelectasis, destruction of the airway epithelium, inspissation of secretions, and mucociliary dysfunction
7. (a) Minute volume >10 L/min
8. (d) Heat and moisture exchanger
9. (1) Simple HMEs; (2) heat and moisture exchanging filters; (3) hygroscopic condenser humidifiers; (4) hygroscopic condenser humidifiers with filters
10. (b) Slow inspiratory flow rate
11. (b) 1 to 5 μm
12. (b) 6 to 8 L/min
13. (b) Inspiratory flow rate
14. (a) Less than 1%
15. (1) Nebulizer design, (2) gas pressure, (3) gas density, (4) temperature, (5) humidity, and (6) medication characteristics

CHAPTER 7 LUNG EXPANSION THERAPY AND AIRWAY CLEARANCE DEVICES

1. (a) To prevent atelectasis
2. (1) Upper abdominal surgery; (2) thoracic surgery; (3) presence of a restrictive lung defect associated with

quadriplegia or a dysfunctional diaphragm; (4) to prevent atelectasis in patients with COPD who are scheduled for surgery

3. The most common problem encountered involves a leak in the system caused by a crack in the device, defective tubing, or failure of the patient to maintain a tight seal around the mouthpiece.

4. (b) Inspiratory capacity

5. This patient is a good candidate for incentive spirometry; he is alert and cooperative. Although he does experience some pain when he takes deep breaths, he should be able to take deep breaths (vital capacity >10 mL/kg).

6. (d) Active hemoptysis, nausea, intracranial pressure >15 mm Hg, and recent esophageal surgery

7. (d) Forced vital capacity (FVC) = 50% predicted and vital capacity (VC) = 15 mL/kg

8. (c) Peak inspiratory pressure

9. (c) 40 L/min

10. (b) 25 to 40 cm H_2O

11. (1) Underwater seals, (2) weighted ball resistors, (3) spring-loaded valve resistors, and (4) magnetic valve resistors

12. (d) Increased sputum production, resolution of hypoxemia, and diminished breath sounds become adventitious sounds that can be auscultated over the larger airways

13. (d) All of the above

14. (c) Oscillate the chest wall to promote secretion clearance

15. (b) Duchenne muscular dystrophy

CHAPTER 8 ASSESSMENT OF PULMONARY FUNCTION

1. (a) Wright respirometers and hot wire respirometers

2. (c) The linearity and frequency response of the device, the device's sensitivity to environmental conditions, and the frequency of calibration

3. (c) 0.5 to 8 L ± 3% of the reading, or 50 mL, whichever is greater

4. (b) Exhaled nitrogen concentration is less than 1.5%

5. (b) Upper airway obstruction

6. (b) Residual volume (RV) and total lung capacity (TLC)

7. (c) −60 to −100 cm H_2O

8. (b) Peak expiratory flow (PEF)

9. (c) $\dot{V}/\dot{Q}$ imbalances, such as occur with patients with emphysema or chronic bronchitis

10. (d) 1500 to 3000

11. (a) Inert gas techniques measure communicating lung volumes; body plethysmographs measure thoracic gas volumes (including gas trapped behind closed airways). For patients with air trapping, the N_2 washout techniques underestimate the true FRC by the amount of trapped air present.

12. (c) Chemiluminescence analyzer and electrochemical analyzer

13. (c) The patient appears agitated, the measurement is performed immediately after the patient receives a physical therapy treatment, and the fractional inspired oxygen (F_1O_2) is 0.8.

14. (d) 1

15. (b) Fever

CHAPTER 9 ASSESSMENT OF CARDIOVASCULAR FUNCTION

1. (a) $Na^+ > K^+$

2. (d) The slope of phase 4 of the sinoatrial (SA) node is greater than that of the ventricular myocyte.

3. (d) Left leg

4. (c) 100 beats/min

5. (c) Lead V_4

6. (d) Epicardial surface of the base of the left ventricle

7. (b) The R-R interval is constant.

8. (d) Greater than 100 beats/min

9. (c) Lead aVF

10. (c) Wolff-Parkinson-White (WPW) syndrome

11. (c) Second-degree (Mobitz II) AV block

12. (c) The threshold potential for this type of tissue is more negative than the threshold potentials for a nodal myocyte.

13. (b) The dicrotic notch of the aortic pressure tracing is associated with closure of the aortic and pulmonary valves, and the pressure in the left ventricle is higher than aortic pressure during the period of maximum ejection.

14. (b) Right ventricular end-diastolic pressure (RVEDP)

15. (d) 6 L/min

CHAPTER 10 BLOOD GAS MONITORING

1. (a) Gloves and protective eyewear (goggles)

2. (b) A patent ulnar artery

3. (c) Radial artery

4. (c) Acute respiratory alkalosis with mild hypoxemia

5. (a) Barbiturate intoxication

6. (a) Poor perfusion state

7. (d) Low perfusion states, such as hypovolemic shock; dark blue nail polish; and methemoglobinemia

8. (a) Hypercarbia and acute acidosis

9. (b) Saturated potassium chloride

10. (b) Protein buildup on the electrode

11. (d) Organic calcium

12. (a) Daily

13. *Quality control* may be defined as a system that includes analyzing control samples (with known values of pH, PCO_2, and PO_2), assessing the results of these measurements against defined limits, identifying problems, and specifying corrective actions.
Quality assurance involves proficiency testing, which provides a dynamic process of identification, evaluation, and resolution of problems that affect blood gas measurements.

14. (a) 70 mm Hg

15. (a) Thermal injury

16. (c) A $PtcO_2/F_1O_2$ <200 is an indication of hypoperfusion and should prompt the clinician for further evaluation and possible intervention.

17. (c) CO-oximetry

CHAPTER 11 SLEEP DIAGNOSTICS

1. (c) Sleep spindles and K-complexes are seen on an electroencephalogram (EEG); slow, pendulous, and disconjugate movements of the eyes; and a relatively low threshold for arousal from sleep

2. Neonates do not follow the pattern of sleep that is typically found in adult sleepers. For example, adults enter sleep through NREM and progress over a period of 90 minutes through NREM stages 1 to 4 to REM sleep. Neonates enter sleep through an active sleep state, which is comparable with REM sleep in the adult. Furthermore, as any parent can attest, neonates awaken on a more regular basis, such as every 2 to 3 hours.

3. As the sleeper passes through the various stages of non-REM sleep, there is a progressive reduction in chemosensitivity and respiratory drive. The reduction in respiratory drive that occurs during the early stages of non-REM sleep (stages 1 and 2) predisposes the person to periods of apnea (i.e., Cheyne-Stokes respiration) as he or she fluctuates between being awake and being asleep. With the establishment of non-REM slow-wave sleep (stages 3 and 4), nonrespiratory inputs become minimized, and minute ventilation is regulated by metabolic control.

Minute ventilation decreases by 1 to 2 L/min when compared with wakefulness. As a consequence, $PaCO_2$ rises by 2 to 8 mm Hg, and PaO_2 decreases by 5 to 10 mm Hg. As the sleeper enters REM sleep, breathing becomes irregular as the ventilatory response to chemical and mechanical respiratory stimuli is further reduced and even transiently abolished. There is decreased skeletal muscle activity, including inhibition of the upper airway muscles and the intercostal and accessory muscles of respiration. Inhibition of the upper airway muscles leads to an increase in upper airway resistance, and inhibition of the intercostal and accessory muscles is associated with diminished thoracoabdominal coupling and short periods of central apnea (10 to 20 seconds in duration). $PaCO_2$ and PaO_2 levels are variable but are generally similar to those during the latter stages of non-REM sleep.

4. (b) Blood pressure decreases by as much as 25 mm Hg during REM sleep.

5. True

6. (b) 5

7. (1) Oxygen saturation; (2) nasal-oral airflow; (3) respiratory effort

8. (d) Chronic loud snoring, excessive daytime sleepiness, personality changes, and obesity

9.

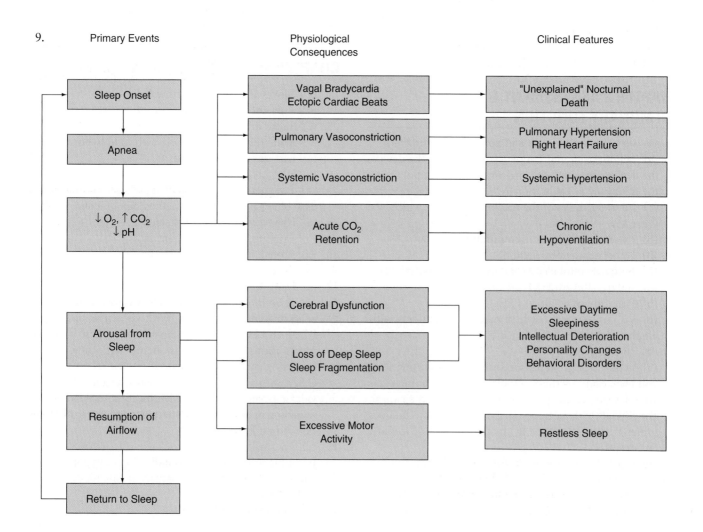

| Primary Events | Physiological Consequences | Clinical Features |

10. (c) Alveolar hypoventilation, myasthenia gravis, and stroke
11. (d) Pulmonary hypertension
12. (c) Phasic oxygen desaturation, hypercarbia, and intermittent paradoxical respiratory efforts
13. (c) These patients rarely report insomnia, or gasping for air upon awakening after an apneic event, and depression is a common finding in these patients.
14. The AI is the number of apneic periods observed divided by the total number of hours of sleep; the AHI includes both apneic and hypopneic episodes for the total number of hours of sleep. Normative data for asymptomatic individuals from Guilleminault and Dement suggest that males average about seven apneic episodes per 8 hours of sleep and females average about two episodes per 8 hours of sleep.
15. (c) Ethanol, sedatives, and hypnotics

CHAPTER 12 INTRODUCTION TO VENTILATORS

1. (d) Fluidics
2. (c) A closed-loop control system
3. (c) Volume-targeted, time-cycled ventilation
4. (c) Flow trigger, pressure limit, and time cycle
5. (b) Proportional solenoid
6. (b) Coanda effect
7. (d) Square or rectangular flow, linear pressure, and linear volume
8. (b) Patient-triggered, pressure-limited, time-cycled ventilation
9. (a) PC-CMV
10. (d) The patient must trigger the breath, and the breath must be cycled by the patient's lung characteristics.
11. (a) Adaptive
12. (c) Transairway pressure
13. (c) VC-CMV plus positive end-expiratory pressure (PEEP)
14. (c) Intelligent
15. (d) Airway pressure-release ventilation (APRV)
16. (d) High-frequency oscillatory ventilation (HFOV)
17. (b) Increase the flow to the system
18. (b) Resistance and elastance
19. (b) Internal diameter of the artificial airway and patient's inspiratory flow
20. (b) When inspiratory sensitivity senses a rise in flow of 3 L/min
21. (b) Time-triggered, time-cycled, volume-targeted ventilation
22. (c) PC-CMV
23. (b) Flow
24. (a) VC-CMV
25. (d) Dual
26. (a) Adaptive
27. (a) Neurally adjusted ventilatory assist (NAVA)
28. (d) Mandatory minute ventilation (MMV)
29. (c) Pressure-controlled intermittent mandatory ventilation (PC-IMV)
30. (c) Continuous mandatory ventilation (CMV), intermittent mandatory ventilation (IMV), and continuous spontaneous ventilation (CSV)

CHAPTER 13 MECHANICAL VENTILATORS: GENERAL USE DEVICES

1. (c) Esophageal pressure monitoring, tracheal pressure monitoring, and heliox gas delivery capability
2. (a) Measuring end-tidal CO_2
3. (c) Terminate a spontaneous breath
4. (b) Measure auto-PEEP
5. (a) A rigid accumulator
6. (a) Airway pressure-release ventilation
7. (b) Main screen or user interface
8. (c) Evaluate for the upper and lower inflection points
9. (d) A closed-loop form of ventilation designed to shorten weaning time
10. (c) Place a proximal sensor at the patient wye
11. (b) False
12. (c) SmartCare
13. (c) Proximal airway monitoring
14. (a) The Dräger N500 is designed for neonatal ventilation only
15. (a) Mandatory minute ventilation (MMV)
16. (a) Inspiratory cycle-off
17. (d) Electrical signals from the diaphragm to trigger and cycle spontaneous breaths
18. (d) Peak pressure, PEEP, dynamic compliance, and tidal volumes
19. (c) Magnetic resonance imaging (MRI) conditional cart
20. (b) False
21. (d) PRVC
22. (a) The greater the patient effort, the higher the pressure delivered
23. (a) An extended feature allowing the ventilator to adjust PSV to overcome the resistance of the artificial airway
24. (b) Airway pressure-release ventilation (APRV)
25. (c) Pressure trigger
26. (c) ASV
27. (d) Trigger compensation
28. (c) Dead space
29. (b) Compensate for artificial airway resistance
30. (a) Work of breathing (WOB)
31. (d) Volume ventilation is not available with the Hamilton-C3
32. (a) Compensate for leaks and improve synchrony
33. (b) ASV
34. (c) Proximal airway sensor
35. (d) Measure the slope of the alveolar plateau to determine the efficiency of ventilation
36. (c) Maquet Servo-i, Medtronic Minimally Invasive Therapies PB 840, and GE Carescape
37. (d) GE Carescape, Hamilton-C3, Maquet Servo-s, and CareFusion AVEA
38. (d) Closed-loop technologies

39. (c) CareFusion AVEA, Medtronic Minimally Invasive Therapies PB 840, GE Carescape, and Dräger V500
40. (d) Time, flow, and pressure
41. (d) 4:1

CHAPTER 14 INFANT AND PEDIATRIC DEVICES

1. (c) Time-triggered, pressure-limited, time-cycled ventilation
2. (b) Flow-sensing devices
3. (a) Nasal prong
4. (a) Gas flow is diverted away from the expiratory limb to mix with existing inspiratory flow.
5. (d) A humidifier chamber with a continuous-feed sterile water system; a standard air/oxygen blender with standard oxygen tubing; a hot wire inspiratory limb of the patient circuit; and a CPAP generator
6. (b) Adjusting the position of the CPAP probe
7. (d) Temperature control at 40°C and chamber control at −3
8. (a) Allows the clinician to adjust the flow-termination point of the breath
9. (b) Breath is time cycled (TC)
10. (d) Only available in all modes and used to stabilize baseline pressure in the presence of leaks
11. (b) Contains a stainless steel flap in the variable-orifice differential pressure transducer
12. (c) Low tidal volume (V_T) alarm
13. (a) A rapid rise to set pressure occurs
14. (c) Time triggering or patient triggering, pressure-targeted breaths, and TC
15. (c) Operates in tandem with a conventional ventilator and delivers rates of 240 insufflations/min to 660 insufflations/min
16. (b) Ranges in size from 2.5-mm internal diameter (ID) to 6.0-mm ID
17. (a) Is used to ventilate premature and term infants
18. (d) The proximal flow sensor must be attached when this feature is used; the clinician sets the maximum peak inspiratory pressure; the maximum peak inspiratory pressure becomes an inspiratory pressure limit; and over six to eight breaths, the ventilator determines the appropriate inspiratory pressure and begins to achieve and maintain the target tidal volume.

19. (a) The ventilator's peak inspiratory pressure (PIP) will immediately decrease.
20. (d) Amplitude
21. (b) Volume delivered by the piston will decrease.
22. (d) Bias flow, frequency setting, percentage of inspiratory time (%T_I), piston centering; and mean airway adjustment control
23. (c) Automatic piston centering

CHAPTER 15 TRANSPORT, HOME CARE, AND NONINVASIVE VENTILATORY DEVICES

1. (a) 3 L/min
2. (a) Sigh breath is provided every 100 breaths or 1 every 7 minutes, whichever occurs first
3. (c) High respiratory rate
4. (b) 10%
5. (a) True
6. (c) 0.5 L/min
7. (b) 5 kg (11 lb)
8. (d) 0 seconds
9. (d) 7 minutes
10. (d) Noninvasive ventilation mode and cylinder duration calculator
11. (c) Nonvented masks
12. (b) 2 minutes
13. (d) Assist/control and continuous positive airway pressure (CPAP)
14. (c) 45 psi
15. (c) An optional oxygen blender through a high-pressure oxygen gas source and an oxygen-blending bag for providing additional oxygen for spontaneous breaths
16. (c) The PEEP/CPAP level cannot be set higher than the pressure setting minus 5 cm H_2O
17. (c) Low Baseline Pressure
18. (d) 30 seconds
19. (b) 120 minutes
20. (a) 6 L/min
21. (b) 50%
22. (a) 5 kg (11 lb)
23. (c) Apnea detection time and number of apnea events in 1 hour
24. (b) 30 kg (66.1 lb)
25. (d) No alarm

Normal Reference Ranges

Adult Complete Blood Count: Serum RBCs, WBCs, Platelets

CBC Component Conventional Units (SI Units)	Reference Ranges
WBC count × 10³/µL (×10⁹/L)	4.5-11.5
RBC count × 10⁶/µL (×10¹²/L)	M: 4.60-6.00 F: 4.00-5.40
Hemoglobin g/dL (g/L)	M: 14.0-18.0 (140-180) F: 12.0-15.0 (120-150)
Hematocrit % (L/L)	M: 40-54 (0.40-0.54) F: 35-49 (0.35-0.49)
Segmented neutrophils	40-75%
Bands	0-6%
Eosinophils	0-6%
Basophils	0-1%
Lymphocytes	20-45%
Monocytes	2-10%
Platelet count	150,000-400,000/mm³

Blood Gases

Normal Arterial Blood Gas Values for Children, Adolescents, and Adults

pH (range)	7.40 (7.35-7.45)
$PaCO_2$ (range)	40 (35-45) torr
PaO_2 (range)	95 (85-100) torr
SaO_2	≥97%
HCO_3^- (range)	24 (22-26) mEq/L
BE (range)	0 (−2 to +2) mEq/L

Other Blood Gas Values

SpO_2	≥97%
SvO_2	75%

Normal Neonatal Arterial Blood Gas Values

	Normal Preterm (at 1-5 h)	Normal Term (at 5 h)	Normal Preterm (at 5 days)
pH (range)	7.33 (7.29-7.37)	7.34 (7.31-7.37)	7.38 (7.34-7.42)
$PaCO_2$ (range) torr	47 (39-56)	35 (32-39)	36 (32-41)
PaO_2 (range) torr	60 (52-68)	74 (62-86)	76 (62-92)
SaO_2	90%	95%	95%
HCO_3^- (range) mEq/L	19 (18-20)	21 (20-22)	21 (20-22)
BE (range) mEq/L	−4 (−5 to −2)	−3 (−6 to −2)	−3 (−6 to −2)

Other Blood Gas Values

	Normal Preterm (at 1-5 h)	Normal Term (at 5 h)	Normal Preterm (at 5 days)
SpO_2	90%	95%	95%

BE, Base excess; *torr*, Torricelli (1 torr = 1 mm Hg pressure).

Cardiovascular

Normal Values for ECG Interpretation With Common Alterations

Variable	Normal Range	Common Alterations
Arterial blood pressure	90-140 mm Hg 60-90 mm Hg	>140/90 mm Hg (hypertension) <90/60 mm Hg (hypotension)
Heart rate	60-100 bpm	>100 bpm (tachycardia) <60 bpm (bradycardia)
PR interval	0.12-0.20/s	>0.20 s (tachycardia; bradycardia; first-, second-, and third-degree heart block; premature ventricular complexes; atrial contractions; atrial fibrillation; atrial flutter; elevated ST segment; inverted T wave; ventricular tachycardia; fibrillation; asystole)
QRS interval	<0.10/s	>0.10 s (ectopic foci)
ST segment	Isoelectric	Elevated or depressed; myocardial ischemia
T wave	Upright, round, and asymmetrical	Inverted with ischemia; tall and peaked with electrolyte imbalances
Cardiac output	4-8 L/min	>8 L/min (elevated): stress, septic shock, fever, hypervolemia drugs <4 L/min (decreased): left ventricular failure, myocardial infarction, pulmonary embolus, PPV, PEEP, pneumothorax, blood loss, hypovolemia
Cardiac index	2.5-4.0 L/min per m^2	>4 L/min per m^2 (fluid overload, right ventricular failure, pulmonary hypertension, valvular stenosis, pulmonary embolus, cardiac tamponade, pneumothorax, positive pressure ventilation, PEEP, left ventricular failure) <2.5 L/min per m^2 (hypovolemia, blood loss, shock, peripheral vasodilation, cardiovascular collapse)
Central venous pressure	2-6 mm Hg	>6 mm Hg (fluid overload, right ventricular failure, pulmonary hypertension, valvular stenosis, pulmonary embolus, cardiac tamponade, pneumothorax, positive pressure ventilation, PEEP, left ventricular failure) <2 mm Hg (hypovolemia, blood loss, shock, peripheral vasodilation, cardiovascular collapse)
Pulmonary artery pressure	20-35 mm Hg 5-15 mm Hg	>35/15 mm Hg (pulmonary hypertension, left ventricular failure, fluid overload) <20/5 mm Hg (pulmonary hypotension, hypovolemia, cardiovascular collapse)
Mean pulmonary artery pressure	10-20 mm Hg	>20 mm Hg (pulmonary hypertension, left ventricular failure, fluid overload) <10 mm Hg (pulmonary hypotension, hypovolemia, cardiovascular collapse)
Pulmonary capillary wedge pressure	5-10 mm Hg (<18 mm Hg)	>18 mm Hg (left ventricular failure, fluid overload) >20 mm Hg (interstitial edema) >25 mm Hg (alveolar filling) >30 mm Hg (frank pulmonary edema) <5 mm Hg (hypovolemia, shock, cardiovascular collapse)
Systemic vascular resistance	11.25-17.5 mm Hg/L/min 900-1400 dynes-sec/cm^3	>1400 dynes-sec/cm^3 (vasoconstrictors, hypovolemia, late septic shock) <900 dynes-sec/cm^3 (vasodilators, early septic shock)
Pulmonary vascular resistance	1.38-3.13 mm Hg/L/min 110-250 dynes-sec/cm^3	>250 dynes-sec/cm^3 (hypoxemia, decreased pH, PaCO$_2$, vasopressors, emboli, emphysema, interstitial fibrosis, pneumothorax) <110 dynes-sec/cm^3 (pulmonary vasodilators, nitric oxide, O$_2$, calcium blockers)

Coagulation Test Values

	Partial Thromboplastin Time (PTT) (s)	Prothrombin Time (PT) (s)
Infant, 1 day old	37.1-48.7	11.6-14.4
Infant, 5 days old	34-51.2	10.9-15.3
Adult	25-39	12-15

Chemistry Panel: Serum Electrolytes and Glucose

Common Chemistry Panels With Sample Test Reference Ranges

Panel and Analytes Measured	Common Reference Ranges
Albumin	2.9-5.5 mg/dL
Blood urea nitrogen (BUN)	8-23 mg/dL
Calcium (Ca)	8.6-10.5 mmol/dL
Ionized calcium (Ca^{++})	2.25-2.75 mEq/L
CO_2	22-29 mmol/L
Chloride (Cl$^-$)	98-107 mEq/L
Creatinine (Cr)	0.7-1.3 mg/dL
Glucose	<100 mg/dL
Magnesium (Mg^{++})	1.7-2.4 mg/dL
Potassium (K$^+$)	3.5-5.0 mEq/L
Sodium (Na$^+$)	135-145 mEq/L

Pulmonary Function Testing (PFT)

Common Parameters Used for Ventilatory Assessment[a]

Parameter	Common Reference Range	Critical Value
Tidal volume (V_T)	5-8 mL/kg PBW	<4-5 mL/kg or <300 mL
Frequency (f)	12-20 breaths/min	>30-35 breaths/min
Rapid shallow breathing index (RSBI)		>105 without PS or CPAP
Dead space-to-tidal volume ratio (V_D/V_T)	0.25-0.40	>0.60
Minute volume (V_E)	5-6 L/min	>10 L/min
Vital capacity (VC)	65-75 mL/kg	<10-15 mL/kg
Maximum inspiratory pressure (MIP)	−80 to −100 cm H_2O	0 to −20 cm H_2O

[a]These values do not apply to neonatal or young pediatric patients. *CPAP*, Continuous positive airway pressure; *PBW*, predicted body weight; *PS*, pressure support.

Vital Signs: Normal Respiratory and Heart Rates and Blood Pressure

Age	Resting Pulse (beats/min)	Respiratory Rate (breaths/min)	Heart Rate (beats/min)	Blood Pressure (mm Hg)
Infants (<1 yr)	90-170	30-60	90-120	80/50 (1-6 mo) 90/65 (6-12 mo)
Toddler (1 to 3 yr)	80-160	24-40	80-100	95/65 (1-2 yr)
Preschooler (4 to 5 yr)	80-120	22-34	70-90	100/60 (2-6 yr)
School age (6 to 12 yr)	70-110	18-30	70-90	110/60
Adolescent (13 to18 yr)	70-110	16-22	60-80	110/65 (12-16 yr)
Adult	60-100	12-20	60-100	<120/80

Frequently Used Formulae and Values

GAS LAWS

Definitions of Standard Conditions

	Temperature (°C)	Pressure (mm Hg)	Water Vapor
STPD		760	Zero
ATPD		Atmospheric	Zero
ATPS		Atmospheric	Saturated
BTPS		Atmospheric	47 mm Hg

Gas Cylinders

Oxygen cylinder factors for common cylinder sizes:

D Cylinder	0.16
E Cylinder	0.28
G Cylinder	2.41
H Cylinder	3.14
K Cylinder	3.14

$$\text{Cylinder factor} = \frac{\text{cubic feet in full cylinder} \times factor}{\text{pressure of full cylinder}}$$

Duration of gas (min)
= (Amount of gas in cylinder [L])/(Flow [L/min])

Amount of gas in cylinder

$$= \frac{\text{Liquid O}_2 \text{ weight (lb)} \times 860}{2} .5\,\text{lb/L}$$

FLOW RATES, AND MIXING AIR AND OXYGEN

Air-to-Oxygen Ratios and Total Flows of Several Common Venturi Devices

%	Oxygen Flow Rate (L/min)	Air/Oxygen Ratio	Total Flow (L/min)
24	4	25.3:1	105
28	4	10.3:1	45
31	6	6.9:1	47
35	8	4.3:1	42
40	8	3:	32
50	12	1.7:1	32
60	24	1:	48
70	24	0.6:1	38

FORMULAE USED WITH GAS LAWS

Boyle's law (solving for pressure): $P_2 = \dfrac{P_1 \times V_1}{V_2}$

Boyle's law (solving for volume): $V_2 = \dfrac{P_1 \times V_1}{P_2}$

Charles' law (solving for volume): $V_2 = \dfrac{P_1 \times T_2}{T_1}$

Gay-Lussac's law (solving for pressure): $P_2 = \dfrac{P_1 \times T_2}{T_1}$

Combined-gas law (solving for volume): $V_2 = \dfrac{V_1 \times P_1 \times T_2}{P_2 \times T_1}$

Combined-gas law (solving for pressure): $P_2 = \dfrac{V_1 \times P_1 \times T_2}{V_2 \times T_1}$

Combined-gas law (solving for temperature):
$$T_2 = \frac{P_2 \times V_2 \times T_1}{P_1 \times V_1}$$

Density:
$$d = \frac{m}{V}$$

Notes: Where d is the density, m is the object's mass, and V is the volume the mass occupies. In clinical practice, weight is used for the mass which provides a weight density d_w and for gases, mass is measured by gmw, and the volume is expressed in liters.

or

$$d_w = \frac{\text{weight}}{\text{volume}}$$

Notes: Where d_w is the weight density.

FORMULA USED WHEN MIXING AIR AND OXYGEN

$$\%O_2 = \frac{(\text{air flow rate} \times 21) + (O_2 \text{ flow rate } 100\%)}{\text{total flow rate}}$$

FORMULAE USED WHEN CALCULATING HUMIDITY

$$\text{(relative) } \%RH = \frac{\text{Content (Absolute humidity)}}{\text{Saturated Capacity}} \times 100$$

(absolute) AH

$$= \frac{\text{water output}\left(\dfrac{\text{millimeters}}{\text{minute}}\right) \times 1000 \text{ mg/mL}}{\text{gas flow in } \dfrac{\text{liters}}{\text{min}}}$$

$$\text{(body) } \%BH = \left(\frac{AH}{43}.8\right) \times 100$$

FORMULAE USED WITH MECHANICAL VENTILATION

Ideal Body Weight:

Men: IBW (lb) = 106 + 6[height (in) − 60]

Women: IBW (lb) = 105 + 5[height (in) − 60]

Spontaneous Tidal Volume:

Spontaneous tidal volume

$$= \frac{\text{spontaneous minute ventilation}}{\text{spontaneous breath rate}}$$

Tidal Volume:

$$V_T = \dot{V}_E \div f$$

V_T (Lost Because of Compressed Gas):

Volume lost = Tubing compliance
$\times$ (Peak pressure − PEEP)

$$V_T \text{ (delivered)} = V_T \text{ (set)} - V_T \text{ (lost)}$$

$$\text{I:E ratio} = \frac{T_E}{T_I}$$

FORMULAE USED WITH COMPLIANCE AND RESISTANCE

Compliance:

$$\text{Compliance} = \frac{V_T}{\text{plateau pressure} - \text{PEEP}}$$

Dynamic Compliance:

$$\frac{V_T}{\text{PIP} - \text{PEEP}}$$

Flow Resistance:

$$R = \frac{(P_1 - P_2)}{\dot{V}}$$

Lung Compliance:

$$C_L = \frac{\Delta V \text{ (liters)}}{\Delta P_{plat} \text{ (cm H}_2\text{O)}}$$

Notes: Where C_L is the compliance (L/cm H$_2$O) for the lung. ΔV (L) is the change in volume from the beginning to the end of inspiration. ΔP_{plat} (cm H$_2$O) is the change in pressure from the beginning to the end of inspiration.

Airway Resistance:

$$R_{aw} = \frac{\text{PIP} - P_{plat}}{\text{Flow}}$$

Notes: Where R_{aw} (cm H$_2$O/L/s) is the airway resistance, PIP is the peak inspiratory pressure (cm H$_2$O), P_{plat} is the plateau pressure (cm H$_2$O). The presence of an artificial airway changes the airway resistance. This measurement is easily assessed on patients receiving ventilator support. A constant flow pattern (square) should be used for this measurement. Remember that ventilators normally report the flow rate in L/min, and this value needs to be converted to L/s.

Inspiratory Resistance:

$$R_{aw} = \Delta P / \Delta F = \frac{(P_{peak} - P_{plat})}{\text{flow}}$$

Static Compliance:

$$\text{Static compliance} = \frac{V_T}{P_{plat} - \text{PEEP}}$$

FORMULAE USED WHEN CALCULATING DEAD SPACE

Dead Space to Tidal Volume Ratio:

$$\frac{V_D}{V_T} = \frac{\text{PaCO}_2 - \text{P}_{\bar{E}}\text{CO}_2}{\text{PaCO}_2}$$

Notes: Where $\bar{V}_T$ is the dead space to tidal volume ratio (%), PaCO$_2$ is the partial pressure of arterial carbon dioxide (mm Hg), and P$_{\bar{E}}$CO$_2$ is the partial pressure of mixed expired carbon dioxide (mm Hg). The measurement for P$_{\bar{E}}$CO$_2$ is a mixed expired carbon dioxide value. This value can be measured by collecting expired gas in a large reservoir such as a Douglas bag. Newer capnometers use microprocessors to calculate the average (mixed) carbon dioxide value from individual breaths.

Dead Space Ventilation:

$$\dot{V}_D = V_D \times f$$

Notes: Where $\dot{V}_D$ is dead space ventilation (L/min), V_D is dead space volume (L), and f is frequency (breaths/min).

GLOSSARY

absolute humidity The actual mass or content of water in a measured volume of air. It is usually expressed in grams per cubic meter or pounds. (Chs 1, 6)

absorbance sensor An apparatus designed to react to physical stimuli from light or other radiant energy. (Ch 10)

accumulator A device that allows a volume of gas to be held for a period of time and then releases the gas at a preset rate. Used as a timing or limiting mechanism. Also referred to as *silencer* (Chs 14, 15)

accuracy The state or quality of being precise or exact. (Ch 8)

acid-fast bacteria Of, or pertaining to, certain bacteria (especially *Mycobacterium* spp.) that retain red dyes after an acid wash. (Ch 2)

acid-fast stain (Also called *Ziehl-Neelsen stain.*) Used to identify bacteria that belong to the genus *Mycobacterium*. (Ch 2)

acoustics The science of sounds.

actual bicarbonate The concentration of HCO_3^- that is present in the plasma of anaerobically drawn blood. It is derived from measurements of pH and partial pressure of arterial carbon dioxide ($PaCO_2$) with the Henderson-Hasselbalch equation. (Ch 10)

adaptive pressure ventilation (APV) A closed-loop (servo-controlled) mode of ventilation available on the Hamilton-G5 ventilator that provides pressure-targeted ventilation with a volume guarantee. (Ch 13)

adaptive support ventilation (ASV) A closed-loop mode of ventilation available on the Hamilton-G5 that uses pressure-targeted ventilation to ensure a certain minute volume. The ventilator enables prediction of tidal volume and respiratory rate based on the patient information entered by the operator, constantly monitors patient and ventilator parameters, and adjusts breath delivery to establish the least amount of work possible for the patient. (Chs 12, 13)

adaptive targeting A closed-loop ventilator control scheme in which automatic adjustments of one set-point are made to maintain a different selected set-point. (Ch 12)

adhesive forces Attractive forces between two different kinds of molecules. (Ch 1)

adiabatic A process occurring without exchange of heat of a system with its environment. (Ch 6)

adjustable, multiple-orifice flow restrictors Uses a series of calibrated openings in a disk that can be adjusted to deliver different flows. As with the fixed-orifice flow restrictor, the operating pressure is crucial to the accuracy of the device. (Ch 4)

adjustable reducing valve See *adjustable regulator.*

adjustable regulator A valve that allows the user to determine (adjust) pressure limits. (Ch 4)

aerobe A microorganism that lives and grows in the presence of free oxygen. (Ch 2)

aerosol A suspension of solid or liquid particles in a gas. (Ch 6)

airborne Carried in the air via aerosol droplets, droplet nuclei, or dust particles. (Ch 2)

airborne precautions Safeguards designed to reduce the risk for airborne transmission of infectious agents. (Ch 2)

airway pressure Pressure achieved in the patient airway. (Ch 12)

airway pressure-release ventilation (APRV) A mode of ventilation during which the patient breathes spontaneously at an elevated baseline, but the airway is periodically "released" to allow expiration. (Ch 13)

airway resistance (R_{aw}) A measure of the impedance to ventilation caused by gas movement through the airways. It is computed as the change in pressure along a tube, divided by the gas flow through the tube. (Ch 8)

Allen test A test for the patency of the ulnar or radial artery. The patient's hand is formed into a fist while the therapist compresses the radial and ulnar arteries. Compression continues while the fist is flexed. If blood perfusion through the ulnar artery is adequate, the hand should flush and resume normal (pink) coloration when the ulnar artery compression is released. (Ch 10)

alternating supply system A gas supply system that has two supplies of compressed gas (primary and secondary). The secondary system is used when the primary system fails. (Ch 3)

alveolar ventilation The volume of air that ventilates all the perfused alveoli, measured as minute volume in liters per minute. This figure is also the difference between total ventilation and dead space ventilation. The normal average is from 4 to 5 L/min. (Ch 8)

American Standards Association (ASA) indexing A type of safety system for high-pressure gas connections. ASA connections are noninterchangeable to prevent the interchange of regulator equipment among gases. ASA indexing has separate systems for large and small cylinders. (Ch 3)

ammeter An instrument for measuring the strength of an electric current in terms of amperes. (Ch 1)

ammonia A chemical compound composed of nitrogen and hydrogen (NH_3). It is found in trace quantities in the atmosphere and is produced from the breakdown of nitrogenous organic matter. (Ch 8)

amorphous solids A solid, such as glass or margarine, in which the constituent atoms and molecules are arranged in a fashion that is not rigid. In contrast, the constituent particles of crystalline solids are more rigidly arranged. (Ch 1)

ampere The standard unit of measurement of electrical current. (Ch 1)

amperometric Refers to measuring an electrical current at a single applied potential. (Ch 10)

amplitude The height of a waveform; usually indicative of intensity. (Ch 14)

anaerobe A microorganism that grows and lives in the absence of oxygen. (Ch 2)

anemometer A gauge for determining the force or speed and sometimes the direction of the wind or air. (Ch 8)

aneroid barometer See *aneroid manometer.*

aneroid manometer A pressure-measuring device that compares a reference pressure with an observed pressure (by using one of several methods). (Ch 8)

apnea ventilation Emergency back-up ventilation triggered when no patient breath is detected for a certain period of time. (Ch 13)

Archimedes principle States that when an object is submerged in a fluid, it will be buoyed up by a force equal to the weight of the fluid that is displaced by the object. (Ch 1)

arousal threshold Ease of awakening. Can be monitored by an increase in the tension developed by the skeletal muscles. (Ch 11)

artificial airway compensation (AAC) A feature on the AVEA ventilator that adjusts the pressure delivery to compensate for the pressure drop across an artificial airway. (Ch 13)

assisted breath Breath in which the patient begins inspiration, but the ventilator controls the inspiratory phase and ends inspiration. (Ch 12)

atom The smallest division of an element that exhibits all the properties and characteristics of that element, including neutrons, electrons, and protons. The number of protons in the nucleus of every atom of a given element is the same and is called its *atomic number.* (Ch 1)

atomic theory The concept that all matter is composed of submicroscopic atoms that are, in turn, composed of protons, electrons, and neutrons. A chemical element is identified by the number of protons in its atoms. (Ch 1)

atomizer A device that produces an aerosol suspension of liquid particles without using baffles to control particle size. (Ch 6)

atrial fibrillation A cardiac rhythm characterized by disorganized electrical activity in the atria accompanied by an irregular ventricular response that is usually rapid. (Ch 9)

atrial flutter A type of atrial tachycardia with rates greater than 230 beats/min. The atria lose their ability to contract normally and typically appear to quiver. (Ch 9)

atrial premature depolarization An atrial beat that occurs earlier than expected. Also known as *premature atrial beat.* (Ch 9)

auto alarm function A feature on the Hamilton-G5 and Hamilton-C3 models that allows for automatic adjustment of alarm levels. (Ch 13)

autoclave An apparatus that uses steam under pressure to sterilize articles and equipment. (Ch 2)

autoflow A dual mode of ventilation that provides pressure-targeted breaths with volume guarantee whenever *volume ventilation* (continuous mandatory ventilation [CMV], synchronized intermittent mandatory ventilation [SIMV], or mandatory minute ventilation [MMV]) is simultaneously selected in the Dräger Evita Infinity V500 ventilator. It also alters the function of the inspiratory and expiratory valves, allowing patients to receive whatever inspiratory flow they demand—up to 180 L/min in any volume mode—regardless of the volume settings. (Chs 12, 13)

automaticity The property of the heart to initiate an action potential in the absence of external stimuli. (Ch 9)

automatic leakage compensation See *automatic tube compensation*. (Ch 13)

automode A ventilator feature (available on the Servo-i and Servo-U) designed to switch from a control to a support mode of ventilation if the patient triggers two consecutive breaths. The ventilator remains in the support mode as long as the patient keeps triggering breaths. (Ch 13)

auto-PEEP (positive end-expiratory pressure) Abnormal and usually undetected residual pressure above atmospheric pressure remaining in the alveoli at end-exhalation caused by dynamic air trapping. Also called *intrinsic PEEP*. (Chs 8, 12)

autotroph Organisms that require simple inorganic nutrients to sustain themselves. (Ch 2)

Avogadro's number The number of particles (i.e., atoms or molecules) in one mole of a particular substance. It has been determined to be approximately 6.02×10^{23} molecules. (Ch 1)

B

bacilli Aerobic or facultatively aerobic, spore-bearing, rod-shaped microorganisms of *Bacillaceae* spp. (Ch 2)

bactericide Any drug or other agent that kills bacteria. (Ch 2)

baffle Any obstruction in an aerosol's path that breaks the aerosol into smaller particles. (Ch 6)

base excess/deficit The number of millimoles of strong acid or base required to titrate a blood sample to a pH of 7.4, a partial pressure of carbon dioxide (PCO_2) of 40 mm Hg, and a temperature of 37°C. (Ch 10)

baseline pressure The pressure level at which inspiration begins and ends. (Ch 12)

beam deflection The change in the direction of a beam or jet of gas when it is hit with another jet of gas moving through a fluid device. (Ch 12)

Bell factor In a water-sealed spirometer, the number of milliliters of gas that must be displaced to cause a kymographic pen to move 1 mm. (Ch 8)

bias flow Flow in the circuit during the expiratory phase of mechanical ventilation that makes fresh gas immediately available when the patient inhales. Bias flow also reduces the ventilator's response time for triggering a breath. (Ch 14)

bilevel positive airway pressure (BiPAP) A spontaneous breath mode of ventilatory support that allows separate regulation of the inspiratory and expiratory pressures. Also called *bilevel ventilation, bilevel pressure assist, bilevel pressure support*. (Chs 12, 13)

BiPAP Abbreviation for bilevel positive airway pressure.

body plethysmography A method of studying alveolar pressures, lung volumes, and airway resistance. The patient sits or reclines in an airtight compartment and breathes normally. The pressure changes in the alveoli are reciprocated in the compartment and recorded automatically by the body plethysmograph. (Ch 8)

boiling point The temperature at which a liquid begins to turn to a gas. For water at 1 atm: 100°C, 212°F, or 373 K absolute. (Ch 1)

Boltzmann Universal Gas Constant A fundamental physics constant named for Ludwig Boltzmann, who determined its value as being equivalent to the ratio of the universal gas constant to Avogadro's number. It has a value of 1.380662×10^{-23} joules per kelvin. (Ch 1)

Boothby-Lovelace-Bulbulian (BLB) mask An apparatus for administering oxygen; consists of a mask fitted with an inspiratory-expiratory valve and a rebreathing bag. (Ch 4)

Bourdon flowmeter A flowmeter that incorporates a Bourdon gauge. (Ch 4)

breath-actuated nebulizer Generates aerosol only during inspiration. This feature eliminates waste of aerosol during exhalation and increases the delivered dose threefold or more over continuous and breath-enhanced nebulizers. (Ch 6)

breath-enhanced nebulizer Generates aerosol continuously, using an inspiratory vent that allows the patient to draw in air through the nebulization chamber containing aerosolized drug. (Ch 6)

Brownian motion The random movement of molecules/particles caused by the molecules being struck by other molecules/particles. (Ch 6)

BTPS Abbreviation for body temperature and pressure saturated (with water vapor). (Ch 6)

bubble humidifier A device that increases the water content of a gas by passing it through a volume of water. (Ch 6)

buffer base The total blood buffer capable of binding hydrogen ions. Normal buffer base (NBB) ranges from 44 to 48 mmol/L. (Ch 10)

buoyancy When an object is immersed in a fluid, it appears to weigh less than it does in air. (Ch 1)

C

capillary blood gases (CBGs) Gases dissolved in the blood that are obtained from a capillary sample. Results include pH, PCO_2, and partial pressure of oxygen (PO_2) values, which may differ from arterial blood gas values. (Ch 10)

capnogram A tracing that shows the proportion of carbon dioxide in exhaled air. (Ch 8)

capnograph A device that measures and provides a graphic representation of the amount of carbon dioxide in a gas sample. A mainstream capnograph analyzes gas at the airway. With a sidestream capnograph, however, the gas to be analyzed is aspirated from the airway through a narrow-bore polyethylene tube and transferred to a sample chamber. (Ch 8)

carbogen Carbon dioxide–oxygen mixtures. (Ch 4)

cardiac cycle The pressure, volume, and flow events that occur in the heart and great vessels during a typical heartbeat. (Ch 9)

cardiac work The product of pressure and volume measurements that accompany ventricular contraction. (Ch 9)

cardiopulmonary resuscitation (CPR) A basic emergency procedure for life support involving artificial respiration and manual external cardiac massage. (Ch 5)

Celsius (C) Temperature scale in which 0° is the freezing point of water and 100° is the boiling point of water at sea level. (Ch 1)

center body The metallic divider in the midportion of the Bird Mark series that was a site for gas channels and control devices. (Ch 11)

central processing unit (CPU) The component of a computer that controls the encoding and execution of instructions. Mainly consists of an arithmetic unit, which performs arithmetic functions, and an internal memory, which controls the sequencing of operations. Also called a *processor*. (Ch 10)

check valve A device usually consisting of a one-way valve that prevents back or retrograde gas flow. (Ch 3)

chemical sterilant Any chemical agent that destroys all living organisms, including viruses, in a material. (Ch 2)

chemiluminescence monitoring A type of nitrogen oxide monitoring system routinely used during nitric oxide administration. It involves the quantification of gas-specific photoemission. See also *electrochemical monitoring*. (Ch 8)

chest cuirass The shell-like part of a negative-pressure ventilator. (Ch 12)

chlorofluorocarbons (CFCs) CFCs, such as Freon, were the propellants used in pressurized metered-dose inhaler (pMDIs) since their introduction in 1956. (Ch 6)

Clark electrode The electrode most commonly used to measure the partial pressure of oxygen. (Ch 10)

cleaning The removal of all foreign material, especially organic matter (e.g., blood, serum, pus, and fecal matter), from objects by using hot water, soaps, detergents, and enzymatic products. (Ch 2)

Clinical Laboratory Improvement Amendments of 1988 (CLIA-88) The amendments require routine calibrations of instruments, as well as programs to assess quality control (QC) and quality assurance (QA). (Ch 10)

closed-circuit calorimeter

closed-circuit method The patient breathes into and out of a container prefilled with oxygen. Oxygen consumption is determined by measuring the oxygen volume used by the patient. (Ch 8)

closed-loop system A hardware–software combination that controls a mechanical or electronic process without user input. (Ch 12)

clutch plate In the Bird Mark series, the steel plates that are connected by a wire shaft and suspended between two magnets. The clutch plates act as on/off switches for gas flow.

CO_2 elimination ($\dot{V}CO_2$) The amount of carbon dioxide (in mL or L) exhaled per unit of time. It is most often reported in units of milliliters (mL) per minute or liters (L) per minute. (Ch 13)

Coanda effect A term in fluidics that refers to the sidewall attachment phenomenon of gas streams. (Ch 12)

cocci Bacteria that are round, spherical, or oval, such as gonococci, pneumococci, staphylococci, and streptococci. (Ch 2)

cohesive forces Attractive forces between like kinds of molecules. (Ch 1)

Combitube A double-lumen device designed to provide a patent upper airway when inserted blindly after failed intubation or in a comatose patient with airway difficulties. (Ch 5)

compound A substance composed of two or more elements, chemically combined in definite proportions, that cannot be separated by physical means. (Ch 1)

condensation Change of state from gas to liquid, such as with water vapor condensation. (Chs 1, 6)

conductivity The property of cardiac muscle to propagate an impulse throughout the heart. (Ch 9)

constant positive airway pressure See *continuous positive airway pressure (CPAP)*.

contact precautions Safeguards designed to reduce the risk for transmission of epidemiologically important microorganisms by direct or indirect contact. (Ch 2)

continuous mandatory ventilation (CMV) A mode of ventilation that provides control or assist/control ventilation. Breaths are time triggered or patient triggered, volume targeted or pressure targeted, and volume cycled or time cycled. (Ch 12)

continuous positive airway pressure (CPAP) A method of providing positive pressure without mechanical assistance (i.e., mandatory breath delivery) for spontaneously breathing patients. A technique for increasing functional residual capacity and arterial oxygenation. (Ch 12)

continuous spontaneous ventilation A method of delivering ventilatory support in which the patient determines when a breath is initiated and when it is terminated. (Ch 12)

continuous supply system A mechanism that delivers a gas or an aerosol throughout the ventilatory cycle. (Ch 3)

control panel The user interface, with the controls for the operator to set desired parameters. (Chs 12, 13)

control variable Four elements of breath delivery: flow, volume, pressure, and time. The elements are controlled or limited by the ventilator. The operator sets the numeric values for each element on the front panel of the ventilator. (Ch 12)

critical point The critical temperature and the critical pressure of a substance. (Ch 1)

critical pressure The pressure above which a material cannot exist as a gas. (Ch 1)

critical temperature The temperature below which a material cannot exist as a gas. (Ch 1)

cryogenic Producing extremely low temperatures. (Ch 3)

cycle variable The phase variable that is measured and used to end inspiration; the element of breath delivery that determines the end of inspiration. See also *control variable*. (Ch 12)

D

dead space ventilation Ventilation characterized by respired gas volume that does not participate in gas exchange. Alveolar dead space is characterized by alveoli that are ventilated but not perfused. (Ch 8)

decontamination The process whereby contaminants are removed from objects, usually by simple physical means (e.g., washing). (Ch 2)

demand flow system An automatic device that provides additional flow to the patient in response to patient effort. (Ch 14)

density An expression of the amount of mass per unit of volume a substance possesses.

deposition The process in which aerosol particles are deposited within the respiratory system during inspiration as a result of gravity, impaction, Brownian motion, or turbulence. (Ch 6)

Diameter Index Safety System (DISS) A safety system for compressed-gas fittings. The DISS is used in respiratory care when equipment is connected to a low-pressure gas source (≤200 psi). (Ch 3)

diaphragm compressor A gas-delivery system that operates to reduce gas volume by increasing pressure via movement of a flexible diaphragm. (Ch 3)

diaphragm valves Comparatively thin, flat valves that have many applications in respiratory care. They may separate high- and low-pressure areas as one-way valves or as backflow-prevention devices. (Ch 3)

diastasis A longer period of reduced filling that typically follows the rapid filling period during the beginning third of ventricular filling.

diffusion The physical process whereby atoms or molecules tend to move from an area of higher concentration or pressure to an area of lower concentration or pressure. (Chs 1, 6)

diluter regulator A mechanism that controls the entrained air in an oxygen diluter system. (Ch 7)

diplobacilli Bacilli that occur in pairs. (Ch 2)

diplococcus A member of the *Eubacteriales* family that occurs in pairs because of incomplete cell division. Diplococci are often found as parasites of saprophytes. Also used to describe bacteria of the *Coccaceae* family that occur as pairs of cocci. (Ch 2)

dipole–dipole interaction The interaction of equal and opposite electrical charges. (Ch 1)

direct-acting valve A device that provides volume or flow by direct action from a control knob or device, such as the valve connected to a water faucet. As the faucet is turned, the valve opens or closes. (Ch 3)

direct contact Mutual touching of two individuals or organisms. Many communicable diseases may be spread by direct contact between infected and healthy persons. (Ch 2)

direct-drive piston A piston whose movement is governed by linear (straight line) movement of a shaft that is connected to the piston head. Also called a *linear-drive piston*. (Ch 12)

disconjugate Refers to eye movements seen during non–rapid eye movement (NREM) sleep, in which the eyes do not move in the same direction (i.e., eye movements are not paired). (Ch 11)

disinfection The process of destroying at least the vegetative phase of pathogenic microorganisms by physical or chemical means. (Ch 2)

DISS See *Diameter Index Safety System*.

Doppler effect The apparent change in frequency of sound or light waves emitted by a source as it moves away from or toward an observer. The frequency increases as the source moves toward the observer and decreases as it moves away (e.g., the rising pitch of an approaching train and the falling pitch of a departing train). The Doppler effect is also observed in electromagnetic radiation (e.g., light and radio waves). (Ch 8)

double-lumen endotracheal tube (DLT) A specialized endotracheal tube that allows the right and left lungs to be ventilated separately (i.e., independent lung ventilation). (Ch 5)

driving pressure The amount of pressure required to move a fluid through a tube. To maintain a given level of fluid flow through a tube, the driving pressure will increase in proportion to the resistance offered by the tube. (Ch 4)

droplet precautions Safeguards designed to reduce the risk for transmitting infectious agents by droplet. (Ch 2)

dry powder inhaler A type of metered-dose inhaler that delivers a drug as a powder rather than as a liquid aerosol. (Ch 6)

dry rolling seal spirometer A type of device measuring volume changes in the airway opening. Consists of a canister containing a piston sealed to it with a rolling diaphragmlike seal. (Ch 8)

Dual set-point (dual) targeting Mode of ventilation in which the control variable (pressure, volume, flow) switches during a breath. (Ch 12)

duckbill/diaphragm/fishmouth valves Valves made of elastic materials that have a slit in the middle; the slit opens when pressurized to allow gas flow. (Ch 5)

dump valve A ventilator circuit mechanism that allows expired gas to exit the ventilator. (Ch 14)

Dynamic Heart/Lung Panel A type of graphic display on the Hamilton-G5 that includes the Dynamic Lung, Vent Status, ASV target graphics window, and ASV monitored data window panels. (**Ch 13**)

E

electrical impedance The total opposition offered by an electric circuit to the flow of an alternating current of electrons. Impedance is a combination of the effects of electrical resistance and reactance. (**Ch 8**)

electrically powered Energy supplied by the activity of electrons or other subatomic particles in motion. Also said of a mechanical device or ventilator requiring electricity to operate. (**Ch 12**)

electricity A form of energy expressed by the activity of electrons and other subatomic particles in motion—as in dynamic electricity—or at rest, as in static electricity. Electricity can be produced by heat; generated by a voltaic cell; or produced by induction, rubbing on nonconductors with dry materials, or chemical activity. (**Ch 1**)

electrochemical monitoring A type of monitoring system routinely used when oxygen or nitric oxide is administered. Gases diffusing across a semipermeable membrane react with an electrolyte solution, generating a current flow between two polarized electrodes as electrons are liberated or consumed. See also *chemiluminescence monitoring*. (**Ch 8**)

electrochemical sensor An apparatus designed to react to physical stimuli that accompany chemical activity produced by electrical influence. (**Ch 10**)

electrode A contact for the induction or detection of electrical activity. Also a medium for conducting an electrical current from the body to physiological monitoring equipment. (**Ch 10**)

electromagnetic Relating to the electromagnetic force, which is one of the four fundamental forces of nature. It is concerned with the magnetic field that is produced by an electrical current. (**Ch 14**)

electromotive force (EMF) The electrical potential, or the ability of electric energy to perform work. Usually measured in joules per coulomb or volts. Any device, such as a storage battery, that converts some form of energy into electricity is a source of EMF. (**Ch 1**)

element One of more than 100 primary, simple substances that cannot be broken down into any other substance by chemical means. Each atom of any element contains a specific number of protons in the nucleus and an equal number of electrons outside the nucleus. The nucleus contains a variable number of neutrons. An element with a disproportionate number of neutrons may be unstable, in which case the nucleus undergoes radioactive decay into a more stable elemental form. (**Ch 1**)

emitted dose The mass of drug leaving the mouthpiece of a nebulizer or inhaler as aerosol. (**Ch 6**)

end-expiratory pause See *expiratory hold*. (**Ch 12**)

endospores Intermediate bacterial forms that develop in response to adverse condition. (**Ch 2**)

endotracheal tube A type of artificial airway inserted through the mouth or nose and the larynx into the trachea. (**Ch 5**)

energy expenditure The metabolic cost (in calories or kilojoules) of various forms of physical activity. (**Ch 8**)

epoch A standard 30-second duration of the sleep recording that is assigned a sleep stage designation; for special purposes, occasionally longer or shorter epochs are scored. (**Ch 11**)

eukaryotic Of or pertaining to cells with true nuclei bounded by a nuclear membrane and capable of mitosis. (**Ch 2**)

evaporation The process by which liquids change into the vapor state. This occurs because of changes in temperature, pressure, and vapor pressure gradients. (**Chs 1, 6**)

excitability The ability of the heart to respond to a stimulus by producing an action potential. (**Ch 9**)

exhalation valve A one-way valve system through which exhaled gases exit the ventilator and its circuit. (**Ch 7**)

expiratory flow cartridge In the Bird Mark series, an accumulator cartridge that used an adjustable and controlled leak to vary expiratory time.

expiratory hold A mechanical ventilator control that delays mandatory breath delivery when it is pressed during the end of exhalation, used for measuring auto-PEEP. (**Chs 12, 13**)

expiratory pause See *expiratory hold*.

expiratory positive airway pressure (EPAP) The pressure measured in a patient circuit during exhalation. A parameter that can be set during BiPAP ventilation that governs pressure delivery during exhalation. (**Chs 12, 15**)

expiratory synchrony Ideal matching between the end of a patient's inspiratory effort and the termination of ventilator flow (ventilator cycling). (**Ch 14**)

expiratory time accumulator See *expiratory flow cartridge*.

expiratory time control See *expiratory flow cartridge*.

expiratory timer See *expiratory flow cartridge*.

external circuit The portion of the pneumatic circuit consisting of tubing from a ventilator to a patient. Also called a *patient circuit* or a *ventilator circuit*. (**Ch 12**)

external positive end-expiratory pressure (PEEP) valve A threshold or flow resistor added to the exhalation valve assembly of a ventilator or breathing device (e.g., resuscitation valve) to provide positive pressure during exhalation. (**Ch 15**)

extreme extension See *sniffing position*.

F

face mask ventilation (FMV) Bag-mask-valve ventilation. (**Ch 5**)

facultative Not obligatory; having the ability to adapt to more than one condition (e.g., a facultative anaerobe that can live with or without oxygen). (**Ch 2**)

Fahrenheit (F) A temperature scale in which the boiling point of water is 212°F and the freezing point of water is 32°F at sea level. (**Ch 1**)

Fastrach Consists of a laryngeal mask airway (LMA) cuff mounted on a curved, hollow metal shaft, preformed to fit into an average-sized airway. (**Ch 5**)

feedback channel In pneumatic or fluid devices, a mechanism that provides a signal or flow to a control device.

feedback line See *feedback channel*.

fetal hemoglobin (HbF) A hemoglobin variant that has a greater affinity for oxygen than adult hemoglobin. HbF is gradually replaced over the first year of life by HbA (adult hemoglobin). (**Ch 10**)

fiberoptic bronchoscope Considered the gold standard for intubation of a patient known to have a difficult airway or an unstable neck; allows endotracheal tube insertion under laryngeal visualization using the scope as a guide for the endotracheal tube. (**Ch 5**)

fine-particle fraction (FP) The percentage of the aerosol small enough to have a good chance of depositing in lung (1 to 5 μm). (**Ch 6**)

fishmouth valve See *duckbill/diaphragm/fishmouth valves*.

fixed orifice A hole in a device that has a specific, unchanging size. (**Ch 4**)

fixed-performance oxygen-delivery system Oxygen therapy equipment that supplies inspired gases at a consistent preset oxygen concentration. Also called a *high-flow system*. (**Ch 4**)

Fleisch pneumotachometer A device that operates on the principle that the flow of gas through the device is proportional to the pressure drop that occurs as the gas flows across a known resistance (a bundle of brass capillary tubes arranged in parallel). (**Ch 8**)

flip-flop component A fluidic element that contains two outlets and two control ports. The main flow switches flow from one outlet to the other when a signal gas pulse acts on the main flow. (**Ch 12**)

floating electrode Electrocardiographic (ECG) electrodes, which consist of a silver–silver chloride electrode that is encased within a plastic housing. The surface of the electrode is covered with a conductive gel or paste. The entire electrode assembly can be attached to the skin with a double-sided ring, which adheres to the patient's skin and to the plastic housing of the electrode. These electrodes are referred to as "floating" electrodes because the only conductive path between the electrode and the patient's skin is the electrolyte gel or paste. (**Ch 9**)

flow control See *flow-control valve*.

flow-control valve A device that controls and adjusts inspiratory flow on a ventilator, thus affecting respiratory rate and volume. (**Ch 12**)

flow-dependent incentive spirometer A device that encourages a patient to take slow, deep breaths. The patient is encouraged to achieve a specific airflow during inspiration by using a visual cue that indicates airflow. (**Ch 7**)

flow rate control See *flow-control valve.*

flow resistance Difference in pressure between the two points along a tube, divided by the actual flow. **(Ch 12)**

flow resistor See *flow restrictor.*

flow restrictor A device that reduces the flow of a fluid/gas out of a system by providing an in-stream obstruction, usually in the form of an orifice of reduced size, thus causing back pressure in the system. Increases or decreases in gas flow result in increases or decreases in the back pressure created by the restrictor. **(Ch 4)**

flow restrictor/regulator See *flow restrictor.*

flow triggering When the ventilator detects a drop in gas flow, then inspiration is set to occur. **(Ch 12)**

fluid logic A method for delivering gas flow that uses fluidic elements that do not require moving parts. See also *fluidic.*

fluidic Referring to hydrodynamic principles used to direct gas flow through circuits, resulting in switching of flow directions and signal amplification. Also used in pressure sensing and flow sensing. **(Ch 1)**

fluidic drive A type of pneumatically powered ventilator or device that uses fluidic principles (elements). A mechanism to provide the primary power source for gas delivery with fluidics.

fluidic ventilators One type of pneumatically powered ventilator. **(Ch 12)**

fluorescent sensor An optical blood gas sensor that uses dyes that fluoresce when struck by light in the ultraviolet or near-ultraviolet visible range. The pH, PCO_2, or PO_2 of arterial blood can be determined by using these devices. **(Ch 10)**

flutter valve A mucus clearance device that consists of a pipe-shaped apparatus with a steel ball in a bowl covered with a perforated cap. The flutter valve uses the principles associated with positive expiratory pressure and high-frequency airway oscillations. **(Ch 7)**

fomite Nonliving material, such as bed linens or equipment, that may transmit pathogenic organisms. **(Ch 2)**

fractional distillation of liquid air A method of reducing air to its component gases using pressure and temperature changes. **(Ch 3)**

fractional hemoglobin saturation The amount of oxyhemoglobin measured divided by the amount of all four types of hemoglobin (Hb) present, written as follows:

Fractional O_2Hb
$= O_2Hb \div (HHb + O_2Hb + COHb + MetHb).$

(Ch 10)

FRC See *functional residual capacity.*

FRC INview Module on the GE Carescape that allows for measurement of FRC using a technique based on the nitrogen washout method. **(Ch 13)**

freezing point The temperature at which a liquid becomes a solid. **(Ch 1)**

French scale A measurement scale commonly used to delineate the external diameter of catheters; 1 French unit equals approximately 0.33 mm. **(Ch 4)**

French sizes See *French scale.* **(Ch 5)**

functional hemoglobin saturation The oxyhemoglobin concentration divided by the concentration of hemoglobin capable of carrying oxygen, written as follows:

Functional $O_2Hb = O_2Hb \div (HHb + O_2Hb).$

(Ch 10)

functional residual capacity (FRC) The total amount of gas left in the lungs after a normal, quiet exhalation. **(Ch 8)**

fungicide An agent that is destructive to fungi. **(Ch 2)**

fusible plug A type of pressure-relief mechanism made of a metal alloy that melts when the temperature of the gas in the tank exceeds a predetermined temperature. Fusible plugs operate on the principle that as the pressure in a tank increases, the temperature of the gas increases, which causes the plug to melt. The melting of the plug releases excess pressure. **(Ch 3)**

G

galvanic analyzer An electric analyzer that determines gas concentrations by measuring the change in resistance of electric current in both reference and sampling circuits. **(Ch 8)**

geometric standard deviation (GSD) A measure of the variability of particle diameters within an aerosol. The higher the GSD, the wider the range of particle sizes. **(Ch 6)**

germicide A drug that kills pathogenic microorganisms. **(Ch 2)**

glucose oxidase An enzyme used to coat electrodes when measuring glucose. **(Ch 10)**

Gram-negative Having the pink color of the counterstain used in the Gram method of staining microorganisms. This property is a primary method of characterizing organisms in microbiology. **(Ch 2)**

Gram-positive Retaining the violet color of the stain used in the Gram method of staining microorganisms. This property is a primary method of characterizing organisms in microbiology. **(Ch 2)**

Gram stain The method of staining microorganisms by using a violet stain and an iodine solution; decolorizing with an alcohol or acetone solution; and counterstaining with safranin. The retention of either the violet color of the stain or the pink color of the counterstain is a primary means for the identification and classification of bacteria. Also called the *Gram method.* **(Ch 2)**

graphical user interface (GUI) A graphic control panel is located on the front of most ventilators. It contains the controls by which the operator can adjust input variables, such as the mandatory rate, tidal volume, PEEP, and inspiratory time. **(Ch 13)**

graphics A visual representation of monitored parameters, such as pressure, volume, and flow per unit time. See also *scalars.* **(Ch 12)**

gravitational potential energy The potential energy an object can gain by falling, as a result of gravity. **(Ch 1)**

Guedel airway An upper airway device (oropharyngeal airway) used to provide air passage distal to an obstructing tongue. **(Ch 5)**

H

Haldane transformation Mathematical formula used in the open-circuit indirect calorimetry technique to calculate oxygen consumption by multiplying the inspired oxygen concentration by the ratio of expired-to-inspired nitrogen concentration. The calculation is based on the assumption that because nitrogen is inert, the inspired and expired nitrogen concentrations are equivalent. **(Ch 8)**

half-cells One of two cells connected by a potassium chloride (KCl) bridge in the standard pH electrode. **(Ch 10)**

health care–associated infections (HAIs) See *nosocomial.* **(Ch 2)**

heart blocks A group of arrhythmias in which impulses fail to propagate in a normal manner because of an increased refractoriness of one or more conductive paths in the heart (e.g., atrioventricular blocks). **(Ch 9)**

heat and moisture exchanger (HME) A passive, disposable device that humidifies and warms incoming gases in patients receiving mechanical ventilation by using the principles of condensation and evaporation. Also called an *artificial nose.* **(Ch 6)**

heliox A low-density therapeutic mixture of helium with at least 20% oxygen; used in some institutions as part of large airway obstruction treatment. **(Ch 4)**

Henderson-Hasselbalch equation The chemical formula relating pH, pKa, and the ratio of the conjugate base (bicarbonate) to the weak acid (carbonic acid). **(Ch 10)**

hertz (Hz) Cycles per second. **(Ch 14)**

heterodisperse Containing particles of many different sizes. **(Ch 6)**

heterotrophs Bacteria that require complex organic nutrients. **(Ch 2)**

HFJV See *high-frequency jet ventilation.*

HFO See *high-frequency oscillation.*

HFV See *high-frequency ventilation.*

high-frequency jet ventilation (HFJV) A type of high-frequency ventilation that provides a jet gas pulse to the airway via a small-lumen catheter within the endotracheal tube at rates of approximately 100 to 200 pulses/min. **(Chs 12, 14)**

high-frequency oscillation (HFO) A type of high-frequency ventilation that cycles at rates of 60 to 3000 times per minute. **(Ch 12)**

high-frequency oscillatory ventilation (HFOV) See *high-frequency oscillation.* **(Ch 12)**

high-frequency percussive breaths Part of intrapulmonary percussive ventilation. **(Ch 7)**

high-frequency ventilation (HFV) A method of ventilation at rates of more than 100 breaths per minute. See also *high-frequency jet ventilation* and *high-frequency oscillation.* **(Ch 12)**

high-level disinfection The use of chemical sterilants at reduced exposure times (less than 45 minutes) to kill bacteria, fungi, and viruses. High-level disinfection does not kill a high level of bacterial spores. Compare intermediate-level disinfection and low-level disinfection. (**Ch 2**)

horsepower   Common term for power; measure of the rate at which work is being performed (P = W/t). (**Ch 1**)

hot film anemometer   A flow-sensing device used in some ventilators that works by measuring the temperature of the gas flow. Similar to hot-wire flow transducers.

humidifier   A device that adds invisible molecular water to gas. (**Ch 6**)

humidity   The amount of water vapor in a system expressed as weight/volume (e.g., g/L). Also water in the molecular form. (**Ch 6**)

humidity deficit   A condition in which the available humidity is less than the potential humidity; that is, the percentage relative humidity is less than 100 (e.g., the humidity deficit at a body temperature of 37°C is compared with its capacity of 44 mg/L). (**Ch 6**)

hydrofluoroalkane   A pMDI propellant. (**Ch 6**)

hydrogen bonding   The attractive force of compounds in which a hydrogen atom covalently linked to an electronegative element (e.g., oxygen, nitrogen, fluorine) has a large degree of positive character relative to the electronegative atom, thereby causing the compound to have a large dipole. (**Ch 1**)

hydrometer   A device that determines the specific gravity or density of a liquid by comparing its weight with that of an equal volume of water. A calibrated, hollow, glass device is placed in the liquid being examined, and the depth to which the device settles in the liquid is noted. (**Ch 1**)

hydrophobic   The property of repelling water molecules. (**Ch 6**)

hygrometer   Used to measure humidity. (**Ch 6**)

hygroscopic   The property of attracting and binding water molecules. (**Ch 6**)

hyperbilirubinemia   Above-average amounts of the bile pigment bilirubin in the blood; often characterized by jaundice, anorexia, and malaise. (**Ch 10**)

I

impedance cardiography   A noninvasive technique for measuring cardiac output based on the principle of impedance plethysmography. In this technique, two sets of electrodes are placed on the thorax to measure electrical impedance. (**Ch 9**)

impedance plethysmography   A technique for detecting blood vessel occlusion that determines volumetric changes in an area of the body (e.g., limb blood flow) by measuring changes in its girth as indicated in the electrical impedance of mercury-containing polymeric silicone (Silastic) tubes in a pressure cuff. (**Ch 9**)

IMV (pressurized breaths)   See *intermittent mandatory ventilation*.

incisura   A notch or indentation that appears on the aortic pressure tracing. It is thought to be associated with retrograde flow of blood from the aorta back toward the left ventricle at the end of ventricular systole. (**Ch 9**)

indirect contact   Contacting a susceptible host with a contaminated intermediate object (usually inanimate) in the patient's environment. (**Chs 2**)

inert gas techniques   Includes techniques such as nitrogen washout and helium dilution. (**Ch 8**)

inertial impaction   The deposition of particles by collision with a surface; the primary mechanism for pulmonary deposition of larger particles (usually more than 5 μm in diameter). Large particles tend to travel in a straight line and collide with surfaces in their pathway (e.g., airway branches, baffles). (**Ch 6**)

infection surveillance   The procedures of a hospital or other health facility to minimize the risk for spreading of nosocomial or community-acquired infections to patients or staff members. (**Ch 2**)

inflating port   An orifice through which ventilating gas flows.

infrared sensor   An electronic device that measures infrared radiation emanating from an object. This technology is often used in the measurement of exhaled CO_2 (capnography). (**Ch 14**)

inhaled mass   The amount of drug inhaled; represents only a portion of the emitted dose. (**Ch 6**)

inhaler   Generates medical aerosols. (**Ch 6**)

injector   A device that adds a quantity of liquid or gas to a main flow source. See also *jet*.

inspiratory hold (plateau)   A ventilatory maneuver in which delivered volume is held in the lungs before exhalation. Inspiratory gas flow stops, and the expiratory valve is maintained briefly in the closed position, thus keeping the delivered volume (and pressure) in the lungs. Commonly used to measure plateau pressure for the calculation of static compliance. (**Ch 12**)

inspiratory pause   See *inspiratory hold*. (**Ch 12**)

inspiratory positive airway pressure (IPAP)   The pressure measured in a patient circuit during inspiration. A parameter that can be set during bilevel positive airway pressure (BiPAP) ventilation and governs pressure delivery during inspiration. (**Ch 12**)

inspiratory pressure calibration control   Allows the inspiratory pressure limit to be set.

inspiratory pressure level   The maximum amount of pressure allowed during mechanical ventilation.

inspiratory pressure-relief control   A device that sets the "pop-off" pressure on a mechanical ventilator.

inspissated   Dried, heavy, or intense. (**Ch 6**)

insulator   A nonconducting substance that is a barrier to heat or electricity passage. (**Ch 1**)

intelligent panels   Graphic display on the Hamilton-C3 ventilator used to show measured parameters (e.g., tidal volume, inspiratory flow). (**Ch 13**)

intelligent targeting   Ventilator modes in which targets (e.g., pressure, volume) are automatically adjusted according to a rule-based expert system. (**Ch 12**)

IntelliTrig   A function on the Hamilton-C3 ventilator that automatically adjusts to circuit leaks to improve synchrony using a proximal sensor to measure the difference between delivered and exhaled tidal volume. (**Ch 13**)

intermediate-level disinfection   Removing vegetative bacteria, tubercle bacteria, viruses, and fungi, but not necessarily killing spores. Compare high-level disinfection and low-level disinfection. (**Ch 2**)

intermittent mandatory ventilation (IMV) (pressurized breaths)   A time-triggered ventilatory mode that permits spontaneous ventilation and intersperses required pressurized breaths at predetermined intervals. See also *synchronized intermittent mandatory ventilation*. (**Ch 12**)

internal circuit   A series of tubing that directs gas flow both within the ventilator (the internal circuit) that directs gas flow from the source gas through the ventilator to the external or patient circuit. (**Ch 12**)

International Organization for Standardization (ISO)   Sets the design and performance standards for heat and moisture exchangers. (**Ch 6**)

intrinsic positive end-expiratory pressure (iPEEP)   The level of pressure in the airway as a result of pressure trapped in the lung at the end of exhalation. Also called *auto-PEEP*. (**Ch 13**)

invasive   Characterized by a tendency to spread or infiltrate. Also refers to the use of diagnostic or therapeutic methods that require access to the inside of the body. (**Ch 10**)

inverse ratio ventilation (IRV)   Ventilation in which inspiratory time exceeds expiratory time. See also *pressure-controlled inverse ratio ventilation*.

in vitro   Occurring in a laboratory apparatus (said of a biological reaction). (**Ch 10**)

in vivo   Occurring in a living organism (said of a biological reaction). (**Ch 10**)

iron lung   A negative-pressure ventilator. Also called a *tank ventilator, artificial lung,* or *Drinker respirator*. (**Ch 12**)

isolation procedures   Infection control measures that combine barrier-type precautions (e.g., hand washing and the use of gloves, masks, and gowns) with the physical separation of infected patients in specific disease categories to disrupt the transmission of pathogenic microorganisms. (**Ch 2**)

isolation techniques   See *isolation procedures*. (**Ch 2**)

isothermic saturation boundary (ISB)   The point at which gases reach body temperature and full saturation. (**Ch 6**)

isovolumetric contraction   The period of ventricular systole that occurs during the period between closure of the atrioventricular valves and opening of the semilunar valves. (**Ch 9**)

isovolumetric relaxation   The period of ventricular diastole that occurs during the period between closure of the semilunar valves and opening of the atrioventricular valves. (**Ch 9**)

J

jet   A device using a gas-entrainment mechanism to mix gases or add aerosols to a mainstream gas flow.

jet solenoid   Controls the driving pressure to the exhalation valve jet Venturi and is controlled by the microprocessor. It is active when the flow rate control is set at 5 L/min or greater with a PEEP of 0 cm H_2O to 5 cm H_2O or when PEEP is set at 0 and flow at any setting. (**Ch 14**)

joule   A unit of energy or work in the meter-kilogram-second system. It is equivalent to 10^7 ergs, or 1 W-second. (**Ch 1**)

Joule-Kelvin effect   A physical phenomenon in which the rapid expansion of a gas without the application of external work causes a cooling of the gas. Used in the liquefaction of air to produce oxygen and nitrogen. Also called the *Joule-Thompson effect*. (**Ch 3**)

Joule-Kelvin-Thompson method   See *fractional distillation of liquid air*.

Joule-Thompson effect   See *Joule-Kelvin effect*.

junctional escape rhythm   Rhythm that is characterized by the atrioventricular node becoming the pacemaker of the heart (i.e., intrinsic rate of 40 to 60 beats/min). This type of rhythm typically occurs in cases of sinus block or sinus arrest. (**Ch 9**)

K

Kelvin (K)   An absolute temperature scale calculated in centigrade units from the point at which molecular activity apparently ceases (−273.15°C). To convert Celsius degrees to Kelvin, add 273.15 to the Celsius temperature. (**Ch 1**)

kilowatt   Unit of measure of electrical power (1000 W). (**Ch 1**)

kinetic activity   Molecular motion uses energy and produces heat as a by-product.

kinetic energy   The energy a body possesses by virtue of its motion. (**Ch 1**)

kinetic theory   Theory that states that the atoms and molecules that make up matter are in constant motion. (**Ch 1**)

Korotkoff sounds   Sounds heard during the measuring of blood pressure when a sphygmomanometer and stethoscope are used. (**Ch 9**)

kymograph   A device for graphically recording lung volume changes during spirometry. (**Ch 8**)

L

large-volume jet nebulizer   The device most commonly used to generate bland aerosol. (**Ch 6**)

large-volume nebulizer (LVN)   Used to provide continuous nebulization. (**Ch 6**)

laryngeal mask airway (LMA)   A custom-formed soft mask with a hollow tube fitting into the pyriform sinuses directly above the larynx. Used to establish and maintain a patent upper airway. (**Ch 5**)

laryngoscope   An endoscope for examining the larynx. (**Ch 5**)

latent heat   The amount of heat needed for a substance to change its state of matter. (**Ch 1**)

leaf-type valve   See *leaf valve*.

leaf valve   A thin membrane that overlays an orifice and that, when closed, prevents fluid (gas or liquid) transmission through the opening. (**Ch 5**)

leak compensation   A special features on the V.I.P. Bird that introduces a small amount of flow into the ventilator circuit to stabilize baseline pressure, prevent asynchrony, and optimize sensitivity in the presence of leaks. (**Ch 14**)

Levy-Jennings charts   The most common method of recording quality control data. These charts allow the operator to detect trends and shifts in performance and thus can help prevent problems associated with reporting inaccurate data caused by analyzer malfunction. (**Ch 10**)

light-emitting diode (LED)   An electronic component that emits light when exposed to current flow. Used in instruments to display digital data. (**Ch 10**)

limit variable   An element of breath delivery, including flow, volume, pressure, or time, given a set maximum value by the operator that cannot be exceeded during the breath. (**Ch 12**)

linear-drive piston   A piston with movement governed by linear (straight line) movement of a shaft that is connected to the piston head. See also *direct-drive piston*. (**Ch 12**)

liquefaction   The conversion of a substance into its liquid form. (**Ch 3**)

Low-flow PV loop   A special feature on the EvitaXL that can be used to generate a pressure-volume loop to evaluate upper and lower inflection points. (**Ch 13**)

low-level disinfection   Killing of most vegetative bacteria, some fungi, and some viruses. Compare *high-level disinfection* and *intermediate-level disinfection*. (**Ch 2**)

Lukens sputum trap   Used to obtain sterile sputum samples. (**Ch 5**)

lung and chest wall compliance   Value that is used to indicate the dispensability or elasticity of the lungs and chest wall. Note that compliance is the inverse of elasticity or C = 1/E. (**Ch 8**)

M

Macintosh blade   A curved laryngoscope blade, as opposed to a straight Miller type of blade. (**Ch 5**)

macroshock   A shock from an electric current of 1 mA or greater that is applied externally to the skin. (**Ch 1**)

magnetic valve resistors   A type of threshold resistor containing a bar magnet that attracts a ferromagnetic disk seated on the expiratory port of a pressurized circuit. (**Ch 7**)

magnetism   The branch of physics dealing with magnets and magnetic phenomena; also called *magnetics*. (**Ch 1**)

mainstream capnograph   See *capnograph*. (**Ch 8**)

mandatory breath   A breath initiated and ended by the mechanical ventilator. Mandatory breath delivery is completely determined by the ventilator. (**Ch 12**)

mandatory minute ventilation (MMV)   A closed-loop (servo-controlled) mode of ventilation that guarantees delivery of a set minute volume by monitoring the patient's spontaneous minute volume and supplementing breaths as necessary to achieve the set minute volume. (**Chs 12, 13**)

mandatory minute volume   See *mandatory minute ventilation*.

mass median aerodynamic diameter (MMAD)   The diameter at which the mass of aerosol particles is equally divided; that is, 50% of the particles are lighter than the MMAD, and 50% are heavier. (**Ch 6**)

maximum voluntary ventilation (MVV)   The maximum volume of air that a person can breathe over a 1-minute period. (**Ch 8**)

measured variables   One or more of the four elements of a breath (pressure, flow, volume, and time) monitored during ventilation.

mechanical insufflation–exsufflation device   A device that stimulates a cough and assists in the removal of secretions. It works by gradually inflating the lungs (insufflation) and then abruptly changing to negative pressure at the end of inspiration, producing a rapid exhalation (exsufflation). (**Ch 7**)

mechanics   The branch of physics dealing with the motion of material bodies and the phenomena of the action of forces on them. (**Ch 1**)

melting point   The temperature at which solids begin to turn into liquids. (**Ch 1**)

message log   Electronic record keeping system on the Dräger Babylog 8000 that keeps track of advisory, warning, and alarm messages that are digitally displayed on a ventilator screen. The message log records the time of occurrence, displayed text, and information on the response. It is capable of storing the 100 most recent entries. (**Ch 14**)

metabolic carts   Uses a bias flow of gas to keep the turbine constantly turning, thereby reducing the inertia of the vane. These devices are good for measuring unidirectional flow, but they are inaccurate for measuring bidirectional flows. (**Ch 8**)

metabolic energy expenditure   The total amount of energy used by an individual to accomplish a given amount of work. It is expressed in kilocalories per minute. (**Ch 13**)

metered-dose inhaler   Compact, portable device that offers a convenient method of delivering inhalants at the recommended dose volume. (**Ch 6**)

microcuvette   A small transparent tube or container with specific optical properties. The chemical composition of the container dictates the vessel's use (e.g., Pyrex glass for examining materials in the visible spectrum or silica for those in the ultraviolet range). (**Ch 10**)

microprocessor   A small, compact computer designed to monitor and control specific functions.

microshock   A shock from a usually imperceptible electrical current (<1 mA) that is allowed to bypass the skin and follow a direct, low-resistance pathway into the body. (**Ch 1**)

Miller blade A straight laryngoscope blade, as opposed to a curved Macintosh blade. (**Ch 5**)

minimum minute volume See *mandatory minute ventilation.*

minute ventilation The total ventilation per minute. The product of tidal volume and respiratory rate, as measured by expired gas collection for 1 to 3 minutes. The normal value is 5 to 10 L/min. Also called *minute volume.* (**Ch 8**)

mixture A substance composed of ingredients that are not chemically combined and do not necessarily occur in a fixed proportion. (**Ch 1**)

molecular sieve A term used to describe components of a type of oxygen concentrator that filters air and chemically removes nitrogen and some trace gases from the air. (**Ch 3**)

molecule The smallest unit that exhibits the properties of an element or compound. A molecule is composed of two or more covalently bonded atoms. (**Ch 1**)

Monel screen A specially designed screen that is composed of nickel alloys, copper, iron, and other trace elements. The screen provides a fixed resistance used in the design of pneumotachometers. Monel is a trademark of Special Metals Corporation. (**Ch 8**)

monodisperse Aerosols consisting of particles of similar size have a geometric standard deviation (GSD) less than or equal to 1.4. (**Ch 6**)

monoplace hyperbaric chamber A hyperbaric unit rated for single occupancy. (**Ch 4**)

multiplace hyperbaric chamber A walk-in hyperbaric unit that provides enough space to treat two or more patients simultaneously. (**Ch 4**)

multistage reducing valve See *multistage regulator.*

multistage regulator A pressure-reducing valve that has more than one level of pressure reduction between system pressure and working pressure. (**Ch 4**)

murmur A gentle blowing, fluttering, or humming sound, such as a heart murmur. (**Ch 9**)

mustache cannula A type of reservoir nasal cannula that can reduce oxygen supply use from that of a continuous-flow nasal cannula. (**Ch 4**)

N

nasal trumpet A type of artificial airway. Also called a *nasal,* or *nasopharyngeal, airway.*

nasopharyngeal airway A type of artificial airway inserted through the nose with the distal tip in the posterior part of the oropharynx. Also called *nasal trumpet* or *nasal airway.* (**Ch 5**)

nasotracheal intubation The use of the nose as the entry point for placement of tubes or catheters in the trachea. (**Ch 5**)

nebulizer A type of aerosol production device that consists of an "atomizer," or jet, and a baffle or baffles. (**Ch 6**)

negative-pressure ventilator A machine that provides ventilation by generating less pressure than ambient (atmospheric) around the thorax while maintaining the upper airway

at ambient. The iron lung and chest cuirass are examples. (**Ch 12**)

NeoFlow A special mode of ventilation on the Dräger EvitaXL and Infinity series (N500) that allows for ventilation of neonates (0.5 to 6 kg). The Neoflow setting requires a proximal airway sensor that enables respiratory rates up to 150 breaths/min. (**Ch 13**)

Nernst equation An expression of the relationship between the electrical potential across a membrane and the concentration ratio between permeable ions on either side of the membrane. (**Ch 10**)

neurally adjusted ventilatory assist (NAVA) A mode of ventilation available as an option on the Maquet Servo^i ventilator. It relies on detection of the electrical activity of the diaphragm (EAdi[a]) to control ventilator function. (**Chs 12, 13**)

Newton A Système Internationale d'Unités (SI) unit of force that would impart an acceleration of 1 m/s to 1 kg of mass. (**Ch 1**)

non–pressure-compensated The needle valve is located before the indicator tube. Restriction or high-resistance devices attached to the outlet of a non–pressure-compensated Thorpe tube flowmeter create back pressure, which is transmitted back to the needle valve. Because the needle valve is located proximal to the Thorpe tube, the back pressure causes the float to fall to a level that indicates a flow lower than the actual flow. (**Ch 4**)

nonforced vital capacity The maximum amount of air that can be slowly exhaled after a maximum inspiration.

noninvasive Pertains to a diagnostic or therapeutic technique that does not require the skin to be broken or a cavity or organ of the body to be entered (e.g., obtaining a blood pressure reading by auscultation with a stethoscope and sphygmomanometer). (**Ch 10**)

nonrebreathing valve A valve that opens, allowing gas to flow to the patient, then closes, allowing exhaled air to exit by another route. Examples are spring-loaded and diaphragm valves. Diaphragm valves are further subdivided into duckbill (or fishmouth) valves and leaf-type valves. (**Ch 5**)

normal flora Microorganisms that live on or within a body, that compete with disease-producing microorganisms, and that provide a natural immunity against certain infections. (**Ch 2**)

normal sinus rhythm A cardiac rhythm characterized by the presence of P waves and an effective ventricular rate of 60 to 100 beats/min. (**Ch 9**)

nosocomial Pertaining to or originating in a hospital (e.g., a nosocomial infection). (**Ch 2**)

O

occlusion pressure ($P_{0.1}$) or airway occlusion pressure See *$P_{0.1}$.* (**Ch 13**)

---

[a]Medical literature uses the abbreviation *EAdi* for electrical activity of the diaphragm; Maquet, manufacturer of the Servo^i ventilator, uses *Edi* in its literature.

ohm A unit of measurement of electrical resistance. One ohm is the resistance of a conductor in which an electrical potential of 1 V produces a current of 1 A. (**Ch 1**)

Ohm's law $V = I \times R$. (**Ch 1**)

one-point calibration Adjusting the electronic output of an instrument to a single known standard to help ensure quality assurance. It should be performed before analyzing an unknown sample, unless the analyzer is programmed to automatically perform a one-point calibration at regular intervals (e.g., every 20 to 30 minutes). (**Ch 10**)

open-circuit method The volumes of inspired and expired gases are measured, as well as the fractional concentrations of oxygen in each. (**Ch 8**)

open-loop system A microprocessor-controlled system that provides clinical data or advice but defers to the user, who must then take the appropriate action. (**Ch 12**)

optical plethysmography A technique for measuring blood volume changes in a specific body part (e.g., a digit or earlobe). These blood-volume changes are then used to define systolic and diastolic time periods during the cardiac cycle. (**Ch 10**)

optical shunting Transmitted light never comes in contact with the vascular bed; therefore SpO_2 values can be erroneously high or low, depending on whether this light is pulsatile. (**Ch 10**)

optics A field of study that deals with the electromagnetic radiation of wavelengths that are shorter than radio waves but longer than x-rays. (**Ch 1**)

optimal targeting A mode of ventilation in which one target of the ventilator is automatically adjusted to optimize another target according to some model of system behavior whose output can be maximized or minimized dynamically. (**Ch 12**)

oropharyngeal airway An artificial airway that is inserted into the mouth until the distal tip is behind the base of the tongue, providing an open channel to the laryngopharynx. (**Ch 5**)

oscillator subsystem A piston assembly on the CareFusion 3100A High Frequency Oscillatory Ventilator. The oscillator subsystem incorporates an electronic control circuit, or square-wave driver, which powers a linear-drive motor. (**Ch 14**)

oscillometry A method of measuring blood pressure that is accomplished by placing a person's arm in a pressure cuff. The blood pressure is determined by noting cuff pressure fluctuations that are associated with the pulsation of arm blood vessels. (**Ch 9**)

oximeter A device that monitors the amount of oxygen in a (physiological) system.

oxygen adder Simplest example of an oxygen proportioner. System consists of two flowmeters, one attached to an oxygen supply and the other attached to an air supply. (**Ch 4**)

oxygen analyzer A device used to determine the concentration of oxygen in a gas mixture. (**Ch 4**)

oxygen blender A device that mixes oxygen with air or other gases to provide precise oxygen concentrations. **(Ch 4)**

oxygen concentrator A device that increases the oxygen content of inspired gas by enriching or concentrating the oxygen in air. **(Ch 3)**

oxygen content (O$_2$ct) A measure of the total amount of oxygen carried by the blood. It is equal to the sum of the oxygen associated with hemoglobin as well as that which is dissolved in plasma. It is typically expressed as mL oxygen per 100 mL of whole blood or volume %. **(Ch 10)**

oxygen controller/blender See *oxygen blender*.

P

P$_{0.1}$ The mouth pressure 100 milliseconds after the start of a patient's inspiratory effort that is measured in a closed (occluded) system; a measure of the output of the respiratory center. **(Chs 8, 13)**

PaCO$_2$ Partial pressure of arterial carbon dioxide. **(Ch 10)**

PaO$_2$ Partial pressure of arterial oxygen. **(Ch 10)**

palpebral conjunctiva Surrounds the eyeball. **(Ch 10)**

paramagnetic Of or pertaining to a characteristic that causes a substance to be attracted to magnetic fields. **(Ch 8)**

passover humidifier A humidification system in which the patient's gas supply flows over a water supply.

pasteurization The process of applying moist heat, usually to a liquid such as milk, for a specific time to kill or retard the development of pathogenic bacteria. **(Ch 2)**

pathogenic Capable of producing disease. **(Ch 2)**

patient circuit The portion of the pneumatic circuit consisting of tubing from a ventilator to a patient. Also called *external*, or *ventilator, circuit*. **(Ch 12)**

patient triggering When pressure, flow, or volume begins the breath; that is, the patient controls the beginning of inspiration. **(Ch 12)**

peak flowmeter A device that regulates the maximum flow a ventilator delivers. **(Ch 8)**

peak inspiratory pressure (PIP) A measurement of the maximum pressure in the patient circuit that occurs during the delivery of a mandatory breath from a ventilator. Also called *peak pressure (P$_{peak}$)*. **(Chs 8, 12)**

peak pressure See *peak inspiratory pressure*.

pedestal ventilator A term used in reference to a Covidien Puritan Bennett PR series respirator. **(Ch 7)**

PEEP See positive end-expiratory pressure.

pendant cannula A type of reservoir nasal cannula that can reduce oxygen supply use (compared with a continuous-flow nasal cannula). The reservoir is attached as connecting tubing that is a conduit to a pendant, which hangs below the chin. **(Ch 4)**

pendelluft German for "pendulum breath," this term describes the movement of gas, from "fast" to "slow," filling spaces during breathing. Alternatively, the ineffective movement of gas back and forth (accompanied by mediastinal shifting) from a healthy lung to one with a flail segment; caused by a crushing chest injury. **(Ch 12)**

PEP therapy Similar to that for the use of continuous positive airway pressure (CPAP) and expiratory positive airway pressure (EPAP), except that positive expiratory pressure (PEP) seems to be less cumbersome and more manageable for patients. **(Ch 7)**

percutaneous dilatory tracheostomy (PDT) A common means of providing direct tracheal access for long-term airway management. **(Ch 5)**

pH Abbreviation for potential hydrogen, a scale representing the relative acidity (or alkalinity) of a solution, in which a value of 7.0 is neutral, below 7.0 is acidic, and above 7.0 is alkaline. **(Ch 10)**

phase variables During breath delivery, the variables controlled by the ventilator that are responsible for each of the four parts of a breath, including triggering (begins inspiratory flow), cycling (ends inspiratory flow), and limiting (places a maximum on a control variable: pressure, volume, flow, and/or time). **(Ch 12)**

Phasitron A sliding Venturi mechanism incorporated into the Percussionaire Intrapulmonary Percussive Ventilator. The Phasitron functions to increase and decrease air pressures. **(Ch 7)**

phonocardiogram The third and fourth heart sounds are not typically heard with a stethoscope but can be amplified and recorded graphically as a phonocardiogram. **(Ch 9)**

photoplethysmography The use of light waves to detect changes in the volume of an organ or tissue. Pulse oximeters use this principle to measure the arterial pulse. **(Ch 10)**

physical separation Process of producing enriched oxygen mixtures from atmospheric air by using molecular sieves and semipermeable membranes to filter room air. See *oxygen concentrator*. **(Ch 3)**

piezoelectric ceramic transducer The ability of a substance to change shape in response to and at the frequency of an electrical current, thus changing electrical energy into mechanical energy. **(Ch 6)**

Pin Index Safety System (PISS) A standardized scheme to prevent accidental mismatching of reducing valves and pressurized gases in small-capacity cylinders (E or smaller). **(Ch 3)**

PISS See *Pin Index Safety System*.

piston assembly See *oscillator subsystem*. **(Ch 14)**

piston compressor A gas source in which a volume of gas is reduced in volume and pressurized by a piston. **(Ch 3)**

plateau pressure (P$_{plat}$) The pressure measured in the patient circuit of a ventilator during an inspiratory hold maneuver. Also the pressure needed to overcome the elastic component of the lungs (static compliance) during breath delivery. **(Chs 8, 12)**

plug-and-play modules Part of a computer-integrated circuitry that enables the discovery of new hardware components introduced without the need for a user intervention. **(Ch 13)**

pneumatic circuit A series of tubing that directs the gas flow in a ventilator and from a ventilator to a patient. **(Ch 12)**

pneumatic safety valve A safety feature incorporated into a ventilator that directs excessive pressure buildup within the ventilator system through the exhalation valve. **(Ch 14)**

pneumatically powered Energy supplied by high-pressure gas or air. **(Ch 12)**

pneumotachograph An instrument that incorporates a pneumotachometer to record variations in respiratory gas flow. **(Ch 8)**

point-of-care (POC) testing Testing that is done outside the main hospital laboratory. POC testing typically involves the use of portable devices that can be located at or near the point of patient care. **(Ch 10)**

point-of-care ultrasonography of the airway Refers to the use of portable ultrasonography at a patient's bedside for diagnostic and therapeutic purposes. **(Ch 5)**

polarity voltage Control function of the piston assembly mechanism in the oscillator subsystem of the CareFusion 3100A High Frequency Oscillatory Ventilator. The amount of polarity voltage applied to the electrical coil determines the distance that the piston will be driven toward or away from the patient airway. **(Ch 14)**

polarographic electrode A device that uses the flow of electric current between the negative (cathode) and positive (anode) electrodes to measure a physical phenomenon such as the partial pressure of oxygen in the blood. **(Ch 8)**

positive-pressure ventilator A device that applies positive pressure to the lungs to improve gas exchange. **(Ch 12)**

potential energy The energy a body possesses by virtue of its position. **(Ch 1)**

potentiometric Refers to measuring voltage. **(Ch 10)**

power A source of physical or mechanical force or energy. Force or energy that can be put to work (e.g., electrical power). **(Ch 1)**

precision/imprecision In measurement, precision is freedom from random errors; imprecision is inaccuracy caused by random error. **(Ch 8)**

premature ventricular beats A ventricular depolarization occurring earlier than expected. **(Ch 9)**

premature ventricular depolarizations See *premature ventricular beats*. **(Ch 9)**

preset reducing valve See *preset regulator*.

preset regulator A device that decreases the pressure from a gas supply system to a predetermined lower pressure. **(Ch 4)**

pressure-compensated The most commonly used flowmeters in respiratory care, they provide accurate estimates of flow regardless of the downstream pressure. **(Ch 4)**

pressure control The mechanism that determines the pressure level generated by the ventilator. **(Ch 12)**

pressure-controlled breath Mode of ventilatory support in which mandatory support breaths are delivered to the patient at a set inspiratory pressure. (**Ch 12**)

pressure-controlled inverse ratio ventilation (PC-IRV) Pressure-targeted, time-cycled ventilation in which the inspiratory time exceeds the expiratory time. (**Ch 12**)

pressure-controlled ventilation (PCV) A mode of ventilation in which the maximum preset pressure is delivered, regardless of the volume achieved. (**Ch 12**)

pressure-limited ventilation A mode of ventilation in which inspiration is stopped when a selected pressure value is reached. (**Ch 12**)

pressure-regulated volume control (PRVC) The name given to a mode of ventilation on the Servo-i ventilator that provides pressure-targeted, time-cycled ventilation that is volume guaranteed. (**Ch 12**)

pressure-relief valve A safety device that vents pressure in excess of a preset value; the pressure is vented to the atmosphere. (**Ch 15**)

pressure support See *pressure-support ventilation.*

pressure-support ventilation (PSV) A mode of ventilatory support designed to augment spontaneous breathing. Patient-triggered, pressure-targeted, flow-cycled ventilation. (**Ch 12**)

pressure swing adsorption (PSA) A technique used in some oxygen sieve concentrators to produce an enriched oxygen mixture. In this technique, room air is drawn through one or more filters by a compressor and eventually compressed to a pressure of 15 to 25 psig and then passed through an air-cooled heat exchanger before entering two or more sieve beds containing a porous material such as zeolite. The PSA method attempts to minimize the problems associated with the accumulation of moisture and other contaminants building up on the sieve bed and allows for the pressurization of one sieve bed while the other bed is purged at a rate of 1 to 5 times per minute. (**Ch 3**)

pressure triggering Inspiration begins when the ventilator senses a drop in circuit pressure. (**Ch 12**)

pressure ventilation Setting a desired pressure. Also called *pressure-limited ventilation, pressure-controlled ventilation,* and *pressure-targeted ventilation.*

pressurized metered-dose inhaler (pMDI) See *metered-dose inhaler.* (**Ch 6**)

principle of continuity The velocity of a fluid flowing through a tube at a constant rate varies inversely with the cross-sectional area of the tube. (**Ch 1**)

prokaryotic Of or pertaining to an organism that does not contain a true nucleus surrounded by a nuclear membrane. Characteristic of lower life forms, such as bacteria, viruses, and blue-green algae. Division of the organism occurs through simple fission. (**Ch 2**)

proportional assist ventilation plus (PAV+) A method of assisting spontaneous ventilation in which the practitioner adjusts the amount of work the ventilator will perform. (**Chs 12, 13**)

proportional solenoid valve A valve designed to modify gas flow. Typically, an electrical current flows through an electromagnet, creating a magnetic field that controls a plunger. The plunger governs the valve opening and gas delivery. (**Ch 12**)

proportioning valve A system in which two or more valves vary the amounts of the gases they control as these gases enter the gas-delivery system. This dictates the final composition of the gas mixture. (**Ch 14**)

PSV See *pressure-support ventilation.*

pulmonary vascular resistance The impedance to right ventricular blood flow offered by the pulmonary circulation. (**Ch 9**)

pulsation dampener A device on the CareFusion V.I.P. Bird infant/pediatric ventilator used to stabilize pressure and maintain driving pressure to the flow-control valve. It is located between the regulator and the flow-control valve. (**Ch 14**)

pulse-demand oxygen delivery system A system that delivers oxygen to the patient only during inspiration (i.e., on demand). (**Ch 4**)

purge valve A valve that maintains a moisture-free, pressure-monitoring line of the endotracheal tube by allowing pressurized gas from the ventilator to pass through the line. (**Ch 14**)

Q

quality assurance Any evaluation of services provided and the results achieved as compared with accepted standards. (**Ch 10**)

quality control A planned, systematic approach to designing, measuring, assessing, and improving performance. (**Ch 10**)

quenching A process of removing or reducing an energy source, such as heat or light. Also, stopping or diminishing a chemical or enzymatic reaction. (**Ch 8**)

quick-connect adapter A device that allows rapid connection and disconnection of compressed-gas appliances to high-pressure gas delivery systems. (**Ch 3**)

quick-connect outlet See *quick-connect adapter.*

R

Raman effect Occurs when light interacts with gas molecules to cause rotational or vibrational energy changes in the gas molecules. (**Ch 8**)

Rankine The fourth temperature scale, used in the engineering sciences. (**Ch 1**)

relative humidity The ratio of actual to potential water vapor in a volume of gas (i.e., how much is present as opposed to how much could be present). (**Chs 1, 6**)

relative refractory period The time period during phase 3 of a ventricular action potential in which a depressed response to a strong stimulus is possible. (**Ch 9**)

repeatability A measure of the closeness of agreement for a series of successive measurements of the same variable when they are recorded under identical conditions over a period of time. (**Ch 8**)

reproducibility Describes the closeness of agreement of successive measurements of a variable when the conditions have changed. (**Ch 8**)

residual volume (RV) The volume of gas remaining in the lungs after a complete exhalation. (**Chs 6, 8**)

resistors Passive electrical components that impede the movement of electrons through an electrical circuit. (**Ch 1**)

respirable mass Product of the inhaled mass multiplied by the fine-particle fraction. (**Ch 6**)

respiratory system compliance The distensibility of the lungs and chest wall, which is determined by dividing the V_T by the pressure. Normal compliance averages 0.05 to 0.1 L/cm H_2O. (**Ch 8**)

retrograde wire intubation Another means of placing an endotracheal tube with the added benefit of not requiring manipulation of the cervical spine. (**Ch 5**)

rhythmicity See *automaticity.* (**Ch 9**)

rotary compressor A kind of fan or compressor in which a fanlike device spins at high speeds to produce a pressurized gas flow. (**Ch 3**)

rupture disks A thin, metal disk that ruptures or buckles when the pressure inside the cylinder exceeds a certain predetermined limit. Also called a *frangible disk.* (**Ch 3**)

S

Sanz electrode The standard electrode that measures pH. Composed of two half-cells that are connected by a potassium chloride bridge. (**Ch 10**)

scalars Graphic displays of pressure, volume, and flow over time. (**Ch 12**)

semiconductors Materials with conductivity characteristics that are intermediate between conductors and insulators. (**Ch 1**)

sedimentation The deposition of insoluble materials at the bottom of a liquid or out of suspension in an aerosol. (**Ch 6**)

semipermeable membrane A biological or synthetic membrane that permits the passage of certain molecules (e.g., based on size or electrical charge). (**Ch 3**)

separation bubble A low-pressure vortex. (**Ch 12**)

servo-controlled A closed-loop system in which a microprocessor compares a set parameter with a measured parameter and alerts the operator or makes specific changes to the set value based on its findings. (**Chs 6, 10**)

servo targeting A ventilator targeting scheme in which the output of the ventilator automatically follows a varying input. (**Ch 12**)

sidestream A gas analyzer that extracts a small sample of gas from the main gas flow for analysis. A nebulizer in which the aerosol cloud is formed outside of the main gas flow. (**Ch 8**)

sidestream capnograph See *capnograph* (**Ch 8**)

Siggaard-Andersen alignment nomogram A graph for calculating actual and standard bicarbonate, buffer base, and base excess concentrations. (**Ch 10**)

SIMV See *synchronized intermittent mandatory ventilation.*

single-stage reducing valve See *single-stage regulator.*

single-stage regulator A pressure-reducing system that lowers primary equipment pressure to working pressure (approximately 50 psig) in one step. **(Ch 4)**

sinus arrhythmia Cardiac rhythm characterized by a waxing and waning of the heart rate. The rhythm appears to be related to the breathing cycle, with heart rate increasing during inspiration and decreasing during expiration. **(Ch 9)**

sinus bradycardia Cardiac rhythm characterized by the presence of P waves preceding each QRS complex with an effective ventricular rate of less than 60 beats/min. **(Ch 9)**

sinus tachycardia Cardiac rhythm characterized by the presence of P waves preceding each QRS complex with an effective ventricular rate greater than 100 beats/min. **(Ch 9)**

sinusoidal Of or pertaining to the shape of a sine wave. **(Ch 12)**

small-volume nebulizer (SVN) A pneumatic aerosol generator. It may be used with a gas-flow circuit used for intermittent positive-pressure breathing (IPPB) therapy or mechanical ventilation or as a handheld nebulizer powered by low-flow oxygen or compressed air. **(Ch 6)**

SmartCare/PS A closed-loop form of ventilation available on the Dräger Evita Infinity V500 and N500 and EvitaXL that is designed to shorten weaning time for intubated or tracheotomized patients who are ready for ventilator discontinuation. **(Ch 13)**

Smart Pulmonary View A feature on the Dräger Evita V500 that allows for real-time visualization of pulmonary function data. In addition to this information, the ventilator can show several extended displays of monitoring data. **(Ch 13)**

sniffing position Extension of the occiput with flexion of the lower cervical spine; the optimal position to establish and maintain a patent upper airway, as well as for oral intubation. Also called *extreme extension.* **(Ch 5)**

spacer An accessory to enhance aerosol delivery from a metered-dose inhaler (MDI). **(Ch 6)**

sphygmomanometer An instrument for indirect measurements of arterial blood pressure. It consists of an inflatable cuff that fits around the arm, a bulb for controlling air pressure within the cuff, and a mercury or aneroid manometer. **(Ch 9)**

spirochete A general term for any microorganism of the order Spirochaetales. **(Ch 2)**

SpiroDynamics A module on the GE Care-Station Ventilator that allows for the measurements of intrinsic PEEP using a tracheal catheter. **(Ch 13)**

spirogram A graphic representation of lung volumes and ventilatory flow rates. **(Ch 8)**

spontaneous breaths Breaths initiated and ended by the patient with no ventilatory support provided. The ventilatory muscles must assume all responsibility for breathing. **(Ch 12)**

spring-loaded device A device that functions based on its ability to overcome the tension imposed by a spring. **(Ch 3)**

spring-loaded resistors A type of threshold resistor that relies on a spring to hold a disk or diaphragm down over the expiratory port of a pressurized circuit. **(Ch 7)**

spring-loaded valve A valve that functions based on its ability to overcome the tension imposed by a spring. **(Ch 5)**

square-wave driver See *oscillator subsystem.* **(Ch 14)**

standard bicarbonate The plasma concentration of HCO_3^- in milliequivalents/liter that would exist if the PCO_2 were normal (40 mm Hg). **(Ch 10)**

standard precautions Guidelines recommended by the Centers for Disease Control and Prevention (CDC) to reduce the risk for transmission of blood-borne and other pathogens in hospitals. Standard precautions apply to blood, all body fluids (secretions and excretions [except sweat]), nonintact skin, and mucous membranes. **(Ch 2)**

Staphylococcus A genus of nonmotile, spherical Gram-positive bacteria. Some species are normally found on the skin. Certain species cause severe purulent infections or produce an enterotoxin, which may cause nausea, vomiting, and diarrhea. Life-threatening staphylococcal infections may arise in hospitals. **(Ch 2)**

static compliance A lung characteristic associated with the elastic properties of the lungs such that a delivered volume is associated with a specific delivered pressure under conditions of no gas flow. Mathematically expressed as the change in volume divided by the change in pressure. **(Ch 12)**

Stead-Wells spirometer A type of water-sealed device that uses a plastic instead of a metal bell to measure volume changes in the airway opening. **(Ch 8)**

sterilization The complete destruction of all microorganisms, usually by heat or chemical means. **(Ch 2)**

streptobacilli Chains of bacilli. **(Ch 2)**

Streptococcus A genus of nonmotile, Gram-positive cocci classified by serological type (Lancefield groups A through T), hemolytic action (α, β, γ), reaction to bacterial viruses (phage types 1 to 86), and growth on blood agar. The various species occur in pairs, short chains, and chains. Some are facultative aerobes; some are anaerobic. Some species are also hemolytic, but others are nonhemolytic. Many species cause disease in humans. **(Ch 2)**

sublimation The direct transition of a substance from solid to the gas or vapor state. **(Ch 1)**

sulfhemoglobin A form of hemoglobin containing an irreversibly bound sulfur molecule that prevents normal oxygen binding. **(Ch 10)**

supercooled liquid An amorphous solid (e.g., margarine). **(Ch 1)**

sustained maximum inspiration (SMI) A therapeutic breathing maneuver in which patients are coached to inspire from the resting expiratory level up to their inspiratory capacity (IC), with an end-inspiratory pause. **(Ch 7)**

synchronized intermittent mandatory ventilation (SIMV) A mode of ventilation in which the patient breathes spontaneously with mandatory breaths periodically imposed after an inspiratory effort.

synchronized minimum mandatory ventilation (SMMV) A ventilator mode available on the Smiths Medical Pneupac ventiPAC that allows the patient to breathe spontaneously without the risk for stacking mandatory breaths on top of spontaneous breaths. **(Ch 15)**

Système Internationale d'Unités (SI) An internationally accepted scientific system of expressing length, mass, and time in base units (IU) of meters, kilograms, and seconds, replacing the old centimeter-gram-second system (CGS). The SI system includes the ampere, Kelvin, candela, and mole as standard measurements. **(Ch 1)**

systemic vascular resistance The resistance to left ventricular blood flow offered by systemic circulation. **(Ch 9)**

T

termination sensitivity A parameter that when measured can allow the RT to adjust the flow termination point of the breath, preventing air trapping and an inverse I:E ratio, thus providing expiratory synchrony. **(Ch 14)**

therapeutic index Improved therapeutic action with fewer systemic side effects provides a higher therapeutic index. **(Ch 6)**

thermal flowmeter A device that measures gas flow by using a temperature-sensitive, temperature-resistive element. **(Ch 8)**

thermistor A metal oxide bead whose resistance changes according to its temperature. **(Ch 1)**

thermodynamics The science of the interconversion of heat and work. **(Ch 1)**

thermometer An instrument for measuring temperature. Usually consists of a sealed glass tube that is marked in degrees Celsius or Fahrenheit and contains a liquid such as mercury or alcohol. The liquid rises or falls as it expands or contracts according to changes in temperature. **(Ch 1)**

Thorpe tube See *Thorpe tube flowmeter.*

Thorpe tube flowmeter A type of flowmeter in which the gas stream suspends a steel ball in a tapered tube. As the ball obstructs a greater proportion of the cross-section of the tapered tube, flow is reduced. **(Chs 3, 4)**

Thorpe tube/reducing-valve regulator A combination of a pressure-reducing valve and a Thorpe tube–type of flowmeter that can regulate both pressure and flow.

three-point calibration Adjusting the electronic output of an instrument to two known standards, as in a two-point calibration, and then adding a third standard intermediate to the other two to ensure linearity of the response. It should be performed every 6 months or whenever an electrode is replaced. **(Ch 10)**

threshold resistance Usually the amount of pressure needed to overcome resistance to flow. **(Ch 12)**

time triggering The ventilator controls the beginning of inspiration based on the total cycle time (TCT), which, in turn, controls the set mandatory rate. (**Ch 12**)

total cycle time (TCT) The time required for both inspiration (T_I) and expiration (T_E). Also called *total respiratory cycle* and *ventilatory cycle time*. (**Ch 12**)

total hemoglobin (THb) The sum of all types of hemoglobin present in a sample of whole blood (e.g., HbA, carboxyhemoglobin, MetHb). (**Ch 10**)

total lung capacity (TLC) The total amount of gas in the lungs after a maximum inspiration. (**Ch 8**)

tracheostomy tube An artificial airway surgically inserted into the trachea through the neck. (**Ch 5**)

transmission-based precautions In hospitals, safeguards designed for patients documented or suspected to be infected with highly transmissible or epidemiologically important pathogens for which additional precautions (beyond standard precautions) are needed to interrupt transmission. There are three types of transmission-based precautions: airborne precautions, droplet precautions, and contact precautions, which may be combined for diseases with multiple transmission routes. Whether these types are used singularly or in combination, they are to be used in addition to standard precautions. (**Ch 2**)

trigger sensitivity The amount of patient effort needed to begin inspiratory gas flow from a ventilator. Usually determined by measured pressure or flow changes. (**Ch 12**)

trigger variable That which begins inspiration. A ventilator may be time triggered, pressure triggered, flow triggered, or volume triggered. (**Ch 12**)

Troop Elevation Pillow Positioning product, provides patients with the head elevated laryngoscopy position (HELP). It is most helpful in morbidly obese patients and establishes a position that maximizes alignment of the oropharyngeal axis. Additionally, it is helpful in the obese, awake patient because it allows the patient to breathe more comfortably and helps to unload the weight of a large chest from the lungs. (**Ch 5**)

tube compensation (TC) Mode of ventilation that attempts to maintain tracheal pressure equal to end-expiratory pressure during both inspiration and expiration. (**Chs 12, 13**)

tubing compliance factor A measure of the volume of air loss as a result of compression of the gas within the ventilator tubing during mechanical ventilation (i.e., tubing compressibility). It is equal to the number of milliliters of volume lost for every centimeter of water pressure generated during ventilation. (**Ch 12**)

tubing compressibility See *tubing compliance factor*. (**Ch 12**)

two-point calibration Adjusting the electronic output of an instrument to two known standards to ensure quality assurance. Usually performed at least three times daily, or approximately every 8 hours. (**Ch 10**)

U

ultrasonic nebulizer (USN) A device that uses high-intensity sound waves to break water into very fine particles. (**Ch 6**)

underwater seal resistor A type of threshold resistor in which tubing attached to the expiratory port of a pressurized circuit is submerged beneath a column of water. (**Ch 7**)

universal precautions An approach to infection control designed to prevent transmission of bloodborne diseases, such as human immunodeficiency virus and hepatitis B, in health care settings. Universal precautions were initially developed in 1987 by the CDC in the United States and in 1989 by the Bureau of Communicable Disease Epidemiology in Canada. The guidelines for universal precautions include specific recommendations for use of gloves, masks, and protective eyewear when contact with blood or body secretions containing blood is anticipated. (**Ch 2**)

user interface The control panel where the operator sets the controls. Also called the *front panel*. (**Ch 12**)

user interface module (UIM) Front panel of a ventilator device. (**Ch 13**)

V

Van der Waals forces Physical intermolecular forces that cause molecules to be attracted to each other. (**Ch 1**)

vapor A transition state between a liquid and a gas during which, through application of pressure/temperature changes, the transition may be reversed. (**Ch 1**)

vapor pressure The force exerted by vapors on a gas or a mixture of gases. (**Ch 1**)

vaporization The process whereby matter in its liquid form is changed into its vapor or gaseous form. (**Ch 1**)

variable-orifice (flow) pneumotachometer Bidirectional, flow-measuring devices that use a variable area, flexible obstruction for measuring flow as a function of the pressure differential generated by the obstruction. (**Chs 8, 13**)

variable-performance oxygen delivery system Oxygen therapy equipment that delivers oxygen at a flow that provides only part of the patient's inspired gas needs. Also called a *low-flow system*. (**Ch 4**)

vector An animal carrier, especially an insect, of infectious organisms. (**Ch 2**)

vegetative cells All cells of animal and plant origin except reproductive cells. (**Ch 2**)

vehicle Any substance, such as food or water, that can be a mode of transmission for infectious agents. (**Ch 2**)

ventricular asystole The cessation of ventricular contractions. (**Ch 9**)

ventricular diastole The period of the cardiac cycle that encompasses the filling period for cardiac ventricular muscle. (**Ch 9**)

ventricular fibrillation No effective ventricular contractions occur and, consequently, there is no cardiac output. (**Ch 9**)

ventricular systole The contraction period for cardiac ventricular muscle. (**Ch 9**)

ventricular tachycardia Cardiac rhythm that is characterized by at least three consecutive ventricular complexes with a rate of more than 100 beats/min. It usually originates in a focus distal to the branching part of the bundle of His. (**Ch 9**)

vibrating mesh (VM) Electromechanical devices that pump or push liquid through a mesh (aperture plate) to form droplets. Unlike with an SVN, aerosol is emitted at the intended particle size and does not require baffling, or recirculation. VM nebulizers rely on two different operating principles: passive and active. (**Ch 6**)

virucide Any agent that destroys or inactivates viruses. (**Ch 2**)

vital capacity (VC) The total amount of air that can be exhaled after a maximum inspiration. The sum of the inspiratory reserve volume, the tidal volume (V_T), and the expiratory reserve volume. (**Ch 8**)

volt (V) The unit of electrical potential. In an electric circuit, a volt is the force required to send 1 A of current through 1 ohm of resistance, or the difference in potential between two points on a conductor carrying a charge of 1 A when there is a dissipation of 1 W between them. (**Ch 1**)

voltmeter An instrument, such as a galvanometer, that measures (in volts) the differences in potential between different points of an electric circuit. (**Ch 1**)

volume conductor The heart is surrounded by tissues that contain ions that can conduct electrical impulses generated in the heart to the body surface where these electrical signals can be detected by electrodes placed on the skin. (**Ch 9**)

volume control plus (VC+) Enhanced mode of ventilation available on the Covidien PB 840 ventilator; it uses a clinician-set inspiratory time and clinician-set target tidal volume. The ventilator initially delivers a single standard volume test breath with a decelerating flow pattern and plateau to determine the relative lung compliance. If the delivered tidal volume is either greater or less than the preset value, the target pressures for subsequent breaths are adjusted to correct for any discrepancies. (**Ch 13**)

volume-controlled ventilation One of the primary breath-control variables. In volume-controlled ventilation the delivered volume remains constant, but pressure can vary. (**Ch 12**)

volume-displacement incentive spirometer A device that encourages a patient to take slow, deep breaths (as in sighing or yawning) to inspire a preset volume of air. The device measures and visually displays the volume of air that the patient inspires during a sustained maximum inspiration. (**Ch 7**)

volume limit A setting that determines the maximum deliverable volume on a ventilator. (**Ch 13**)

volume median diameter (VMD) For laser diffraction; the average particle size is expressed with a measure of central tendency. (**Ch 6**)

volume-pressure constant   Gas volume contained in a cylinder is directly related to the regulator's gauge pressure. (**Ch 3**).

W

watt   A unit of power, equivalent to work done at the rate of 1 J/s. (**Ch 1**)

weight density   Weight divided by its volume, or $d_w = $ Mass/Volume. (**Ch 1**)

weighted-ball resistors   A type of resistor in which a steel ball is placed over a calibrated orifice that is attached directly above the expiratory port of a pressurized circuit. (**Ch 7**)

Wheatstone bridge   A particular arrangement of multiple resistors in an electrical circuit. (**Chs 1, 8**)

wick humidifier   A type of humidification system in which the flow is exposed to a water-saturated cloth, paper, or polyethylene membrane. (**Ch 6**)

Wolff-Parkinson-White syndrome   Cardiac rhythm that is characterized as a preexcitation syndrome. In this arrhythmia, ventricular depolarizations are initiated when impulses initiated in the atria bypass the atrioventricular node and travel through an ancillary Kent bundle, resulting in the presence of characteristic delta waves. (**Ch 9**)

Wood's metal   A metal alloy commonly used in fusible plugs. (**Ch 3**)

work of breathing   The amount of force needed to move a given volume into the lung with a relaxed chest wall. It can be reduced when applied properly with mechanical ventilation. (**Ch 8**)

Page numbers followed by *f* indicate figures; *t*, tables; *b*, boxes.

ABBREVIATIONS

Δ — change in
μ — micro-
AARC — American Association for Respiratory Care
ABG(s) — arterial blood gas(es)
A/C — assist/control
ADH — antidiuretic hormone
a-et PCO$_2$ — arterial to end-tidal partial pressure of carbon dioxide
Ag/AgCl — silver–silver chloride
AIDS — acquired immunodeficiency syndrome
ALV — adaptive lung ventilation
ANP — atrial natriuretic peptide
APRV — airway pressure-release ventilation
ARDS — acute respiratory distress syndrome
ASV — adaptive support ventilation
ATC — automatic tube compensation
ATM — atmospheric pressure
AV — atrioventricular
AVP — arginine vasopressin
BE — base excess
bilevel PAP — bilevel positive airway pressure
BiPAP — registered trade name for a bilevel PAP device
BP — blood pressure
BPD — bronchopulmonary dysplasia
BSA — body surface area
BTPS — body temperature and pressure, saturated
BUN — blood urea nitrogen
°C — degrees Celsius
CaO$_2$ — oxygen content of arterial blood
C(a-v̄)O$_2$ — arterial-to-mixed venous oxygen content difference
cc — cubic centimeter
C$_D$ — dynamic characteristic or dynamic compliance
CDH — congenital diaphragmatic hernia
CHF — congestive heart failure
CI — cardiac index
C$_{LUNG}$ or C$_L$ — lung compliance
cm — centimeter(s)
cm H$_2$O — centimeters of water pressure
CMV — continuous mandatory ventilation
CNS — central nervous system
CO — cardiac output
CO$_2$ — carbon dioxide
COPD — chronic obstructive pulmonary disease
CPAP — continuous positive airway pressure
CPP — cerebral perfusion pressure
CPPB — continuous positive-pressure breathing
CPPV — continuous positive-pressure ventilation
CPR — cardiopulmonary resuscitation
CPU — central processing unit
CRT — cathode ray tube
C$_S$ — static compliance
CSF — cerebral spinal fluid
CSV — continuous spontaneous ventilation
CT — computed tomography
C$_T$ — tubing compliance (also C$_{tubing}$)
Cv̄O$_2$ — mixed venous oxygen content
CVP — central venous pressure
d — diameter
DIC — disseminated intravascular coagulation

DPAP — demand positive airway pressure
DPPC — dipalmitoyl phosphatidylcholine
e — elastance
EAdi — electrical activity of the diaphragm
ECCO$_2$R — extracorporeal carbon dioxide removal
ECG — electrocardiogram
ECMO — extracorporeal membrane oxygenation
EDV — end-diastolic volume
EDV — ventricular end-diastolic volume
EE — energy expenditure
EEP — end-expiratory pressure
EPAP — (end-)expiratory positive airway pressure
ERV — expiratory reserve volume
ET — endotracheal
ETCO$_2$ — end-tidal CO$_2$ (or etCO$_2$)
°F — degrees Fahrenheit
f — respiratory frequency; respiratory rate
FDA — US Food and Drug Administration
FEV$_1$ — forced expiratory volume in 1 second
F$_I$CO$_2$ — fractional inspired carbon dioxide
F$_I$O$_2$ — fractional inspired oxygen
FRC — functional residual capacity
ft — foot
f/V$_T$ — rapid shallow breathing index (frequency divided by tidal volume)
μg — microgram(s)
g/dL — gram(s) per deciliter
[H$^+$] — hydrogen ion
Hb — hemoglobin
HbCO — carboxyhemoglobin
HCH — hygroscopic condenser humidifier
HCO$_3^-$ — bicarbonate
H$_2$CO$_3$ — carbonic acid
He — helium
He:O$_2$ — helium-oxygen mixture, heliox
HFFI — high-frequency flow interrupter
HFJV — high-frequency jet ventilation
HFO — high-frequency oscillation
HFOV — high-frequency oscillatory ventilation
HFPPV — high-frequency positive pressure ventilation
HFV — high-frequency ventilation
HHb — reduced or deoxygenated hemoglobin
HME — heat and moisture exchanger
HR — heart rate
ht — height
IBW — ideal body weight
IC — inspiratory capacity
ICP — intracranial pressure
ICU — intensive care unit
ID — inner diameter
I:E — inspiratory-to-expiratory ratio
IMV — intermittent mandatory ventilation
IPAP — inspiratory positive airway pressure
IPPB — intermittent positive-pressure breathing
IPPV — intermittent positive-pressure ventilation
IR — infrared

IRDS — infant respiratory distress syndrome
IRV — inspiratory reserve volume
IRV — inverse ratio ventilation
ISO — International Organization for Standardization
IV — intravenous
IVC — inferior vena cava
IVH — intraventricular hemorrhage
IVOX — intravascular oxygenator
KBS — knowledge-based system
kcal — kilocalorie(s)
kg — kilogram(s)
kg-m — kilogram-meter
kPa — kilopascal
L — liter(s)
LAP — left atrial pressure
lb — pound(s)
LED — light-emitting diode
LFPPV-ECCO$_2$R — low-frequency positive-pressure ventilation with extracorporeal carbon dioxide removal
LV — left ventricle
LVEDP — left ventricular end-diastolic pressure
LVEDV — left ventricular end-diastolic volume
m^2 — meters squared
μm — micrometer(s)
MABP — mean arterial blood pressure
MalvP — mean alveolar pressure
MAP — mean arterial pressure
MAS — meconium aspiration syndrome
MDI — metered-dose inhaler
MEP — maximum expiratory pressure
mEq/L — milliequivalent(s)/liter
metHb — methemoglobin
mg — milligram(s)
mg% — milligram percent
mg/dL — milligrams per deciliter
MI-E — mechanical insufflation-exsufflation
MIF — maximum inspiratory force
min — minute
MIP — maximum inspiratory pressure
mL — milliliter(s)
MLT — minimum leak technique
mm — millimeter(s)
mm Hg — millimeters of mercury
mmol — millimole
MMV — mandatory minute ventilation
Mo — month
MOV — minimal occluding volume
ms — millisecond(s)
MVV — maximum voluntary ventilation
NaBr — sodium bromide
NaCl — sodium chloride
NAVA — neurally adjusted ventilatory assist
NEEP — negative end-expiratory pressure
NICU — neonatal intensive care unit
NIF — negative inspiratory force (also see MIP and MIF)
NIH — National Institutes of Health
NIV — noninvasive positive-pressure ventilation (also NIPPV)
nM — nanomole
nM/L — nanomole/liter
nm — nanometer(s)
NO — nitric oxide
N$_2$O — nitrous oxide
NP — nasopharyngeal
NPO — nothing by mouth